BERNADETTE F. RODAK, MS, CLSpH(NCA), MT(ASCP)SH

Assistant Professor
Medical Technology Program
Indiana University
Indianapolis, Indiana

DIAGNOSTIC HEMATOLOGY

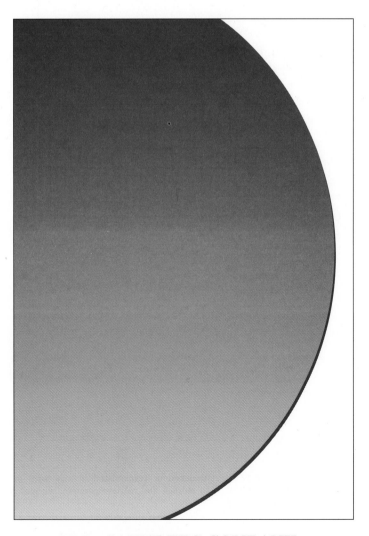

W.B. SAUNDERS COMPANY
A Division of Harcourt Brace & Company
Philadelphia London Toronto Montreal Sydney Tokyo

W.B. SAUNDERS COMPANY
A Division of Harcourt Brace & Company

The Curtis Center
Independence Square West
Philadelphia, Pennsylvania 19106

Library of Congress Cataloging-in-Publication Data

Diagnostic hematology / [edited by] Bernadette F. Rodak.
        p.   cm.
    ISBN 0-7216-4727-8
    1. Hematology.   2. Blood—Analysis.   I. Rodak, Bernadette F.
    [DNLM: 1. Hematologic Diseases—diagnosis. 2. Hematologic Tests—methods. 3. Hematopoiesis. 4. Blood Cells.
WH 100 D536 1995]
RB45.D49   1995   616.07′561—dc20
DNLM/DLC
                                                                          95-11097

Diagnostic Hematology

ISBN 0-7216-4727-8

MUST
IAHT 2819

Printed in the United States of America

Last digit is the print number: 9   8   7   6   5   4   3   2   1

To my mother
who inspired me to love learning,
nourished my quest for knowledge,
taught me an appreciation of the written word,
and, by her example,
motivated me to persevere in the face of adversity.

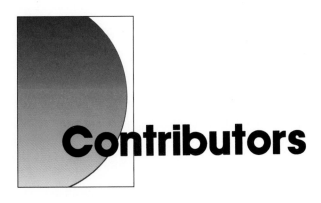

Contributors

JEFF BAILEY, BS, MT(ASCP)SH
Assistant Supervisor, Department of Pathology and Laboratory Medicine, Division of Hematopathology, Indiana University Medical Center, Indianapolis, Indiana
Cytochemistry and Immunohistochemistry

ANN BELL, MS, SH(ASCP), CLSpH(NCA)
Assistant Professor of Medicine and Professor of Clinical Laboratory Sciences, University of Tennessee, Memphis, Tennessee
Introduction to the Anemias: Approach to Diagnosis; Anemias Caused by Increased Destruction of Erythrocytes

JACQUELINE CARR, MS, MT(ASCP)SH
Administrative Supervisor, Department of Pathology and Laboratory Medicine, Division of Hematopathology, Indiana University Medical Center, Indianapolis, Indiana
Myelodysplastic Syndromes

KAREN CLARK, MT(ASCP)SH
Hematology Clinical Instructor, Shelby State Community College and The University of Tennessee Medical Center; Technical Specialist and Hematology Phlebotomy Instructor, Baptist Memorial Hospital East, Memphis, Tennessee
Miscellaneous Erythrocyte Disorders

JEANNE M. CLERC, EdD, MT(ASCP)SH
Dean of Instruction and Student Services, College of Health Sciences, Community Hospital of Roanoke Valley, Roanoke, Virginia
Platelet Anomalies and Hemorrhagic Diathesis; Coagulation Disorders

CRISTIN A. COATES, MS, MT(ASCP)
Medical Technologist, Department of Pathology, University of Pittsburgh Medical Center, Pittsburgh, Pennsylvania
Routine Testing in Hematology

MARY COLEMAN, MS, MT(ASCP), CLS, CLSpH, CLSpCG(NCA)
Instructor, Department of Pathology, University of North Dakota School of Medicine, Grand Forks, North Dakota
Hemoglobin and Iron Metabolism; Anemias Caused by Impaired Production of Erythrocytes

LEILANI COLLINS, BA, MT(ASCP)SH
Assistant Supervisor, Hematology, Baptist Memorial Hospital, Memphis, Tennessee
Cerebrospinal, Serous, and Synovial Fluids

v

CHRISTINE DANIELE, BS, MT(ASCP)

Senior Technologist, Coagulation Department, Lutheran General Hospital, Park Ridge, Illinois

Cell-Counting and Coagulation Instrumentation

GORDON E. ENS, BA, MT(ASCP)

Laboratory Director, Colorado Coagulation, Denver, Colorado

Normal Hemostasis

MARALIE G. EXTON, BA, MT(ASCP)SH

Associate in Medicine, Vanderbilt University School of Medicine; Director, Program of Medical Technology, Vanderbilt University Medical Center, Nashville, Tennessee

Cell-Counting and Coagulation Instrumentation

SHEILA A. FINCH, MS, MT(ASCP), CHMM

Director of Safety Operations, Sinai Hospital, Detroit, Michigan

Safety in the Hematology Laboratory

GEORGE A. FRITSMA, MS, MT(ASCP), CLS(NCA)

Associate Professor, Clinical Laboratory Sciences Division, The University of Alabama at Birmingham, Birmingham, Alabama

Laboratory Evaluation of Hemorrhage and Thrombosis

KIMBERLY GATZIMOS, MD

Department of Pathology, Indiana University Medical Center, Indianapolis, Indiana

Lymphoproliferative Disorders

JOHN GRIEP, MD

Clinical Professor of Pathology, Indiana University, Indianapolis; Medical Director, Pathology and Laboratory Service, Saint Catherine Hospital, East Chicago, Indiana

Metabolism of the Erythrocyte; Myeloproliferative Disorders

SALLY HAMBY, MS, MT(ASCP)

Assistant Professor, Clinical Laboratory Sciences, University of Tennessee, Memphis, Tennessee

Anemias Caused by Increased Destruction of Erythrocytes

TERESA G. HIPPEL, BS, MT(ASCP)SH

Hematology Clinical Instructor, University of Tennessee Medical Center; Laboratory Resource Management Consultant, Baptist Memorial Hospital East, Memphis, Tennessee

Miscellaneous Erythrocyte Disorders

ROBERT HROMAS, MD

Assistant Professor of Medicine and Biochemistry, Indiana University; Bone Marrow Transplant Specialist, Indiana University Medical Center, Indianapolis, Indiana

Origins of Leukocyte Neoplasia; Treatment of Leukocyte Neoplasia

KARLA JOHN, BS, MT(ASCP)

Supervisor, Immunohistology, Department of Pathology and Laboratory Medicine, Division of Hematopathology, Indiana University Medical Center, Indianapolis, Indiana

Cytochemistry and Immunohistochemistry

PATRICIA K. KOTYLO, MD

Assistant Professor of Pathology, Indiana University School of Medicine; Director, Clinical Flow Cytometry Faculty, Hematopathology Department, Indiana University Hospitals, Indianapolis, Indiana

Lymphoproliferative Disorders; Flow Cytometric Analysis in Diagnostic Hematology

JOHN KRAUSE, MD

Professor of Pathology, Tulane University Medical Center; Director of Laboratories, Tulane Medical Center Hospital and Clinic, New Orleans, Louisiana

Quality Control/Quality Assurance; Bone Marrow Overview; Lymphoproliferative Disorders

SUSAN J. LECLAIR, MS, CLS(NCA)

Professor, Department of Medical Laboratory Science, University of Massachusetts at Dartmouth, North Dartmouth, Massachusetts

Leukopoiesis; Benign Disorders of Leukocytes; Platelet Maturation and Function

LYNN B. MAEDEL, MS, MT(ASCP)SH

Education Coordinator, University of Colorado Health Sciences Center, Medical Laboratory Sciences Program, Denver, Colorado

Examination of the Peripheral Blood Smear

DORIS B. MCGHEE, MPA, MT(ASCP)

Assistant Professor, Clinical Laboratory Sciences, University of Tennessee, Memphis; Chief Supervisor, Hematology Laboratory, Regional Medical Center, Memphis, Tennessee

Hemoglobinopathies and Hemoglobin Defects; Appendix: Special Procedures

MARTHA K. MIERS, MS, MBA, MT(ASCP)

Senior Associate in Medicine, Vanderbilt University School of Medicine; Assistant Director, Hematology Laboratory, Vanderbilt University Medical Center, Nashville, Tennessee

Cell-Counting and Coagulation Instrumentation

ANN T. MORIARTY, MD

Clinical Pathologist and Hematopathologist, Methodist Hospital of Indiana, Indianapolis, Indiana

Acute and Chronic Leukemias

CAROLE MULLINS, MPA, CL Dir(NCA)

Associate Faculty, Indiana Vocational Tech College—Northcentral, South Bend; Consultant, ABP, Inc., Granger, Indiana

Specimen Collection

MARTHA PAYNE, MPA, MT(ASCP)SH

Associate Professor, Clinical Laboratory Sciences, University of Tennessee, Memphis, Tennessee

Anemias Caused by Impaired Production of Erythrocytes; Anemias Caused by Increased Destruction of Erythrocytes; Hemoglobinopathies and Hemoglobin Defects

KEILA B. POULSEN, BS, MT(ASCP)SH, CLSpH(NCA)

Adjunct Teacher, Brigham Young University, Provo, Utah; Hematology Supervisor, Eastern Idaho Regional Medical Center, Idaho Falls, Idaho

Morphology and Function of Cellular Components

DEAN PUTT, MBA, MT(ASCP)SH, DLM
Hematology/Oncology Laboratory Manager, University Hospital, Indiana University Medical Center, Indianapolis, Indiana
Origins of Leukocyte Neoplasia; Treatment of Leukocyte Neoplasia

BERNADETTE F. RODAK, MS, CLSpH(NCA), MT(ASCP)SH
Assistant Professor, Medical Technology Program, Indiana University, Indianapolis, Indiana
Overview of Hematology; Myelodysplastic Syndromes

DEBORAH ROPER, BS, MT(ASCP)SH
Hematology Instructor, Saint Francis Hospital School of Medical Technology; Laboratory Services Coordinator, AMI Saint Francis Hospital, Memphis, Tennessee
Anemias Caused by Impaired Production of Erythrocytes

SHERRI A. SCHEIRER-FOCHLER, MS, MT(ASCP)
Medical Technologist, Image Department, University of Pittsburgh Medical Center, Pittsburgh, Pennsylvania
Lipid Storage Disorders and Lupus Erythematosus

JOHN R. SNYDER, PhD, MT(ASCP)SH
Dean and Professor, Indiana University School of Allied Health Sciences, and Associate Dean, Indiana University School of Medicine, Indianapolis, Indiana
Management and Supervision in the Hematology Laboratory

DAN SOUTHERN, MS, CLSpH(NCA)
CLS Program Director/Associate Professor, Clinical Laboratory Sciences Program, Western Carolina University, Cullowhee, North Carolina
Platelet Maturation and Function; Normal Hemostasis

SUSAN STEIN, BS, MT(ASCP)SH
Supervisor of Hematology, AMI Saint Francis Hospital, Memphis, Tennessee
Anemias Caused by Impaired Production of Erythrocytes

MARCELLA STEVENS, MA, MS, CLS(NCA), MT(ASCP)
Assistant Professor of Life Sciences and Coordinator of the Center for Clinical Laboratory Science, Indiana State University, Terre Haute, Indiana
Pediatric and Geriatric Hematology

AMY TONTE, BS, MT(ASCP)
Senior Technologist, Department of Pathology and Laboratory Medicine, Division of Hematopathology, Indiana University Medical Center, Indianapolis, Indiana
Pediatric and Geriatric Hematology

GAIL H. VANCE, MD
Assistant Professor, Department of Medical and Molecular Genetics, Indiana University School of Medicine; Staff, University Hospitals, Indiana University School of Medicine, Indianapolis, Indiana
Cytogenetics

M. ANN WALLACE, MS, MT(ASCP), CLS(NCA)
Assistant Professor, Department of Clinical Laboratory Science, Wayne State University, Detroit, Michigan
Care and Use of the Microscope; Hematopoietic Theory; Erythrocyte Production and Destruction

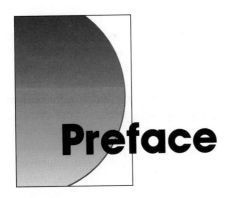

Preface

As the technology and information explosion influences clinical laboratory medicine, the quantity and difficulty of material that the clinical laboratory scientist must assimilate increase. There was a time when hematology consisted almost exclusively of cell counting, morphology differentiation and evaluation, and detection of bleeding disorders. Although those procedures are still the mainstays of hematology, several ancillary areas have increased the speed and precision of diagnosis and treatment.

The purpose of this text is to present a complete hematology course for Clinical Laboratory Science (CLS) students, as well as to provide a resource for clinical laboratory practitioners, medical students, and residents. It presents an in-depth study of cell counting, morphologic differentiation and evaluation, and related areas, such as flow cytometry, immunohistochemistry, and cytogenetics. A chapter on specific age groups covers the unique aspects of hematology in the pediatric and geriatric populations. A section on the etiology and treatment of leukocyte neoplasms has been included to provide some insight into the special considerations of oncologic disorders.

Diagnostic Hematology is organized in an easy-to-follow format for teaching and learning. Each chapter starts with an outline and learning objectives, in order to provide a quick overview of content that will be covered. Color figures are presented as close to the citation as possible to facilitate understanding of the discussion. Most chapters end with a summary. In many cases, review questions or case studies are included to assess or reinforce understanding of material.

One of the superior features of this text is the inclusion of four-color illustrations. In order to aid comprehension, the same diagram that illustrates general hematopoietic theory is broken down into component parts in the sections on erythropoiesis, granulopoiesis, lymphopoiesis, and so forth.

The introductory chapter presents an overview of hematology that should be beneficial to the beginning student. The specimen collection chapter, written by a CLS author with many years of experience in teaching phlebotomy, addresses not only the proper collection of specimens by venipuncture and microcollection but also the psychological and professional approach to the patient.

The next few chapters provide general information that is needed for working in a hematology laboratory: safety, microscope care and use, and quality control.

The section on hematopoiesis reviews the parts and functions of the cell to provide a reference for study of particular cell types. The chapter on general hematopoietic stem cell theory is followed by chapters on erythropoiesis, hemoglobin, erythrocyte metabolism, and leukopoiesis.

The section on routine laboratory evaluation of blood cells includes chapters on routine manual hematology testing and examination of the peripheral blood smear. The essentials of each procedure are provided, as are sources of error and comments. An overview of bone marrow examination follows, in preparation for the study of hematologic disorders.

The anemias and erythrocyte disorders are presented from a pathophysiologic approach, starting with an overview of general introduction to anemias and erythrocyte shapes before a description of the distinguishing features of these disorders and diseases.

The section on leukocyte disorders includes malignant and nonmalignant disorders and ancillary areas, such as cytochemistry, immunohistochemistry, cytogenetics, and flow cytometry. Principles and interpretation of cytochemical and immunohistochemical staining are included; definitive procedures, however, have not been included in this edition, because many are available as kits with accompanying instructions. As chromosome resolution techniques have improved, the ability to relate certain abnormalities to diagnosis and prognosis has increased, making an understanding of cytogenetics valuable. The chapter on cytogenetics, written by a medical geneticist, provides an introduction for the student and a more detailed presentation for the working technologist. Two chapters of this section discuss the etiology and treatment of leukocyte neoplasms. Although not essential for entry-level CLS, the information provided in these two chapters is valuable to practitioners whose interest has been piqued. The chapter on flow cytometry includes a discussion of the principle of flow cytometry and its use in the analysis of malignant disorders. A discussion of the more common lipidoses (Gaucher, Niemann-Pick, and Tay-Sachs diseases) is covered in the chapter on lipid storage disorders.

The hemostasis section covers the development and function of platelets, the newest theories of normal coagulation, and excellent discussions of platelet abnormalities and disorders of coagulation. A thorough discussion of laboratory evaluation of bleeding disorders is included. The chapter on pediatric and geriatric hematology was included because technology is enabling more preterm infants to survive and is expanding the life expectancy of the elderly. The hematologic and hemostatic values to expect in these two populations are discussed.

The instrumentation chapter describes coagulation instrumentation and then compares and contrasts four major instruments for cell counting and differentiation, including many examples of scatterplots and histograms.

The chapter on body fluids includes flow charts on how to determine dilutions for the most accurate cell counts and many color figures of morphology.

A chapter on supervision and management by a well-known author in the field of laboratory administration and supervision concludes the technical section. Not only is this knowledge necessary in view of legislation and regulations, but with the changing role of the CLS, supervisory skills are becoming increasingly desired.

The appendix describes the specialized procedures associated with hemoglobinopathies and hemolytic disorders.

Most of the contributors are clinical laboratory practitioners and educators. We have endeavored to satisfy as many needs as feasible in a text this size. Ideas for improvements and additions for the second edition began developing even before this edition was finished. We welcome yours also.

BERNADETTE F. RODAK

Acknowledgments

I want to express my appreciation to all the contributors who shared their time, talent, and expertise in order to make this text possible, especially those who accepted additional responsibilities with often very short deadlines.

I am grateful to the staff at the W.B. Saunders Company, who were able to guide me and *Diagnostic Hematology* through production in spite of many obstacles. Special thanks go to Melissa McGrath and Shirley Kuhn, Developmental Editors; Selma Ozmat, Senior Editor, Health-Related Professions; Anne Ostroff, Copy Editor; Cecilia Roberts, Illustration Specialist; Peter Faber and Carolyn Naylor, Production Managers; Susan Thomas, Indexer; Bill Donnelly, Designer; and Sandy Won, Editorial Assistant, Health-Related Professions.

I would also like to thank my fellow faculty members in the Clinical Laboratory Science program at Indiana University for their understanding and patience during this endeavor.

Contents

PART X
Management.. **649**

Introduction to Hematology

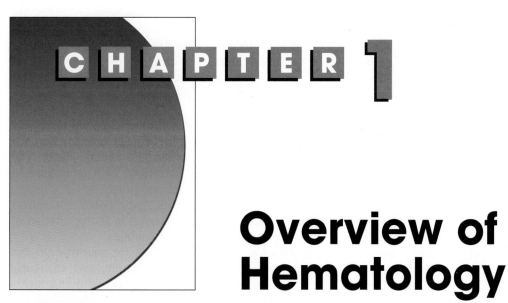

CHAPTER 1

Overview of Hematology

Bernadette F. Rodak

Outline

DEFINITION AND BRIEF HISTORY
QUANTITATION
DIFFERENTIATION
STUDIES ANCILLARY TO ROUTINE
  HEMATOLOGY
TREATMENT OF HEMATOLOGIC
  DISORDERS
BODY FLUIDS
HEMOSTASIS

Objectives

AFTER COMPLETION OF THIS CHAPTER, THE READER WILL BE ABLE TO

1. Present a brief overview of routine hematology and hemostasis.
2. List specialized areas that contribute to diagnosis of hematologic diseases.

DEFINITION AND BRIEF HISTORY

The term *hematology* is derived from Greek, meaning the study of blood. Basic hematology involves analysis of the concentration, structure, and functions of the formed elements (cells) of blood and their products. In the past, hematology was essentially limited to quantitation and differentiation of cells on a morphologic basis. Through advanced technology, it is now possible to supplement morphology with staining of specific elements in cells and detection of cellular antigens. Adjunct studies such as cytogenetics and flow cytometry have enabled more rapid and definitive diagnoses of hematologic disorders.

This brief chapter presents an overview of routine hematology and some specialized areas that contribute to knowledge of normal hematologic status and aid in the diagnosis of hematologic diseases. It is by no means meant to be comprehensive; rather, it serves as an introduction for the beginning student. Each area presented here is discussed in greater detail in subsequent chapters.

QUANTITATION

Basic or routine hematology, as discussed in this text, includes quantitation of hematologic parameters and differentiation of formed elements. For many years the mainstay of hematologic measurements included manual counting of cells and measurement of hemoglobin and hematocrit (Chapter 12). Cell counting was performed with the use of Thoma pipettes and a counting chamber. The pipettes enabled the mixing of small quantities of blood in appropriate proportions with fluids that would either retain all formed elements or destroy those not desired in the count. These pipettes were somewhat awkward to use and required special aspirating tubes or other apparatus for suction. They are still retained for occasional use but have been largely replaced by self-contained diluting devices, such as Unopettes.

The heart of the counting procedure was the hemocytometer, or counting chamber, which is still used for manual cell counts. It consists of two raised platforms, each containing a 3×3 mm square divided into smaller increments. Although there are standard dilutions and standard counting areas for erythrocytes, leukocytes, platelets, eosinophils, and body fluids, a thorough understanding of the hemocytometer enables the technologist to make adjustments as necessary to increase the accuracy of an abnormally high or low count.

Hemoglobin is synthesized in the bone marrow in developing erythrocytes. Measurement of hemo-globin concentration provides an estimate of the oxygen-carrying capacity of blood. The reference method is the cyanmethemoglobin reaction, in which hemoglobin is converted to cyanmethemoglobin and absorbance (or transmittance) is read in a spectrophotometer, with the use of a reagent blank.[1] This same principle or a variation thereof is used in most dedicated and multiparameter instruments.

The term *hematocrit* originally applied to the instrument used to pack blood cells, but it is now the term used for the packed cell volume itself. The manual procedure is performed as a micromethod with the use of a special centrifuge.

The erythrocyte count, hemoglobin concentration, and hematocrit are useful in the evaluation of the degree and etiology of anemias.

All of the manual methods for quantitation can be performed precisely, accurately, and efficiently by automated methods. The use of instruments currently available entails one or more of the following principles: electrical impedance, light scatter, hydrodynamic focusing, and cytochemistry. Many of the multiparameter instruments also provide a screening differential count of leukocytes (Chapter 37).

DIFFERENTIATION

Manual differentiation and evaluation of blood cells are achieved under a microscope with a Wright's stained blood smear (Chapter 13). The three main classes of cells observed are the thrombocytes, erythrocytes, and leukocytes. An example of a normal blood smear as it would appear under the microscope is shown in Figure 1–1.

Thrombocytes, or platelets, participate in the clotting function of blood. On the peripheral smear, they appear as small, blue to purple granular bodies, approximately 2–4 μm in diameter. In recent years, their granules and the substances secreted by them have been studied extensively.

Erythrocytes, or red blood cells, normally appear as biconcave discs, or doughnuts with the hole partially filled in. They turn a reddish-pink when stained and are approximately 7 μm in diameter. The size, shape, and color of the erythrocytes are evaluated as part of the routine blood smear examination. Some examples of abnormal erythrocytes that can be observed include macrocytes (larger than normal, found in specimens from patients with pernicious anemia and liver disease), microcytes (smaller than normal, found in specimens from patients with iron deficiency anemia and a genetic disorder called thalassemia), sickle cells (sickle-shaped, found in specimens from patients

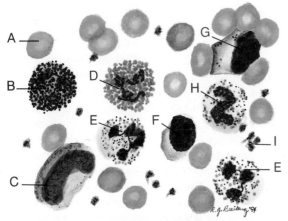

Figure 1–1 Cell types in peripheral blood as they would appear under the microscope with Wright's stain. The ratio of leukocytes to erythrocytes and thrombocytes is greater than would be observed under normal conditions. *Abbreviations:* A, erythrocyte; B, basophil; C, monocyte; D, eosinophil; E, polymorphonuclear neutrophil; F, lymphocyte; G, large lymphocyte; H, band neutrophil; I, thrombocyte.

with sickle cell anemia), and target cells (bull's-eye appearance, found in specimens from patients with liver disease, thalassemias, and some hemoglobin disorders). The causes of these various abnormalities, along with others, will be discussed in the chapters on erythrocytes (Chapters 15–19).

During examination of the blood smear, it is also possible to observe parasites, such as those that cause malaria.

A leukocyte, or white blood cell, differential count gives the percentage of the various leukocyte types, based on morphologic features. In general, leukocytes are larger than erythrocytes, have a definite nucleus, and turn purple when stained. The exception is the eosinophil, which has orange-pink granules in the cytoplasm. The leukocytes normally found on the blood film include polymorphonuclear neutrophils, band neutrophils, lymphocytes, monocytes, eosinophils, and basophils. The percentages of specific cells indicate a normal state or provide diagnostic clues. In adults, the most prevalent cell is the polymorphonuclear neutrophil; the lymphocyte is the second most common. A reverse of these proportions in adults may indicate a viral illness.

Abnormalities in leukocyte morphology may be malignant or nonmalignant. Some nonmalignant changes are toxic granulation (which may be seen in specimens from patients with severe infections) and the presence of atypical or reactive lymphocytes (seen in specimens from patients with viral illnesses, such as infectious mononucleosis). Malignant cells are usually larger than their normal counterparts and have immature nuclei. Some examples of malignancies are acute and chronic leukemias.

STUDIES ANCILLARY TO ROUTINE HEMATOLOGY

When leukocytes are mature, it is usually fairly easy to differentiate them by morphology alone. However, immature cells are more difficult to classify, and it may be necessary to perform additional studies. When immature cells are seen on the peripheral blood smear, it may be desirable to obtain specimens from the major site of blood production, the bone marrow. Specimens may be taken from either the sternum or the iliac crest. Morphology can be studied by routine Wright's stain or by cytochemical stains that stain specific substances, such as enzymes in early cells or glycogen.

Determination of antigens on white blood cells may also help to determine or confirm the cell type when morphology is uncertain. This may be done by immunohistochemistry or by flow cytometry. In immunohistochemistry, antibodies specific to a cell type are mixed with a cell suspension, and visualization of the antigen-antibody bond is achieved by tagging the antibody with an enzyme or fluorochrome, which can then be observed under the microscope. In flow cytometry, a laser light source is used to study surface antigenic characteristics and nuclear DNA content of neoplastic cells.

Cytogenetics is the study of chromosomes. Chromosome abnormalities are found in many hematologic disorders, and some patterns are diagnostic or suggestive of specific diseases. The number or type of abnormality may provide important diagnostic and/or prognostic information.

A combination of information from several or all of the adjunct areas (bone marrow morphology, cytochemistry, immunohistochemistry, flow cytometry, and cytogenetics), along with peripheral blood studies, provides more diagnostic clues than any single area individually, enabling more accurate classification of diseases, prediction of clinical outcome, and determination of optimal therapeutic protocols.

TREATMENT OF HEMATOLOGIC DISORDERS

Medications can affect the production of blood cells. Some medications, such as iron and vitamin B_{12}, are given to stimulate production of cells. Others cause interruption of cell cycles in order to cause decreased production or destruction of malignant cells. These medications also affect the normal cell lines. An overview of treatment protocols and their effects is presented in Chapter 28 in order to alert the laboratorian to some of the resultant hematologic changes.

BODY FLUIDS

In addition to blood, various body fluids such as cerebrospinal, pleural (lung), pericardial (heart), peritoneal (abdomen), and synovial (joint) fluids may be examined. The examination routinely includes cell counts and differential counts and may include other tests, as indicated.

HEMOSTASIS

Hemostasis (coagulation) is the study of the ability of blood to form clots and to dissolve clots spontaneously to prevent occlusion of vessels. The hemostatic mechanism is complex, and research in hemostasis has caused rapid growth in this field.

Routine testing usually includes screening procedures, such as the prothrombin and activated partial thromboplastin times. When results of these tests are abnormal, further testing is conducted to determine the nature of the abnormality. Disorders such as hemophilia and von Willebrand's disease are discovered and monitored by coagulation tests. To prevent formation of small clots, such as those responsible for coronary artery disease, the coagulation laboratory also provides monitoring of anticoagulant therapy for patients who are medicated.

Readers are encouraged to keep this overall picture of hematology in mind as they study the individual sections. Correlation and integration of the various units will make the study of hematology both more realistic and enjoyable.

Reference

1. National Committee for Clinical Laboratory Standards (NCCLS): Reference Procedure for the Quantitative Determination of Hemoglobin in Blood, vol 4, no. 3. Villanova, PA: NCCLS, 1984.

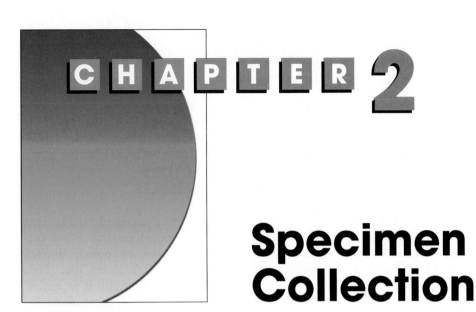

CHAPTER 2

Specimen Collection

Carole Mullins

Outline

Objectives

AFTER COMPLETION OF THIS CHAPTER, THE READER WILL BE ABLE TO

1. Follow universal precautions when collecting a blood specimen.
2. List collection equipment used for both venipuncture and
 skin puncture.
3. Correlate tube stopper color with additive, if any, and with
 its use in the laboratory.
4. Discuss selection of a vein for venipuncture.
5. Enumerate the steps recommended by the National Committee for Clinical Laboratory Standards (NCCLS) for venipuncture in adults.
6. Discuss complications encountered in blood collection and
 proper response of phlebotomist.
7. Explain appropriate use of skin puncture equipment and
 procedure to be followed.
8. Discuss essentials of quality assurance in specimen collection.
9. List reasons for specimen rejection.

SAFETY

Universal precautions must be followed in the collection of blood, and all specimens must be treated as potentially infectious. Regulations from the Occupational Health and Safety Administration (OSHA) that took effect on March 6, 1992, outlined in detail what must be done to protect health care workers from exposure to bloodborne pathogens, such as those that cause non-A, non-B hepatitis, hepatitis B, delta hepatitis, syphilis, and malaria, and the human immunodeficiency virus (HIV).[1]

Bloodborne pathogens may enter the body by way of an accidental injury by a sharp object such as a contaminated needle, a scalpel, broken glass, or anything else that can pierce the skin. Cuts, dermatitis abrasions, and even the mucous membranes of the mouth, eyes, and nose may provide a portal of entry. Indirect transmission can occur when a person touches a contaminated surface or object and then touches the mouth, eyes, nose, or open skin without washing the hands. Hepatitis B virus can survive on inanimate or dried surfaces at room temperature for at least a week.

Handwashing is the most important procedure to prevent the spread of infectious diseases. The clinician should wash hands with a nonabrasive soap and running water between patients and every time gloves are removed. If handwashing facilities are not available, an antiseptic hand cleanser or an antiseptic towelette may be used as a temporary measure. *Gloves* are essential protective equipment and must be worn when venipunctures are per-formed. When gloves are removed, it is important that no substances from the soiled gloves come in contact with the hands. Glove removal is covered in detail in Chapter 3.

Contaminated sharps and infectious wastes should be placed in designated puncture-resistant containers. The red or orange *biohazard* sign (Fig. 2–1) indicates that a container holds potentially infectious materials. Biohazard containers should be easily accessible and not be overfilled.

PHYSIOLOGIC FACTORS AFFECTING TEST RESULTS

Certain physiologic factors specific to the patient may affect results of laboratory testing. These factors include posture (supine or erect), diurnal rhythms (day or night), exercise, stress, diet (fasting or not), and smoking.[2] Therefore, it is important that the phlebotomist adhere to requests for specimens to be drawn at a specific time and to record the time of collection.

COLLECTION EQUIPMENT FOR VENIPUNCTURE

The most common means of collecting blood specimens is with the use of an evacuated tube system. The system includes a tube, which can be either plastic or glass; a needle; and an adapter, which is used to secure both the needle and the tube. The tubes contain a premeasured amount of an additive sealed in a vacuum. They are usually coated with silicone to help decrease the possibility of hemolysis and to prevent the clot from adhering to the sides of the tube. The tubes come in various sizes and contain a variety of additives. Although there are several manufacturers of evacuated tubes, all follow a universal color code in which the stopper color indicates the type of additive contained within the tube (Fig. 2–2).

Additives in Collection Tubes

Anti-glycolytic Agent. This substance inhibits the use of glucose by blood cells. Such inhibition may be necessary if testing for glucose level is delayed. Examples of anti-glycolytic agents are sodium fluoride, iodoacetate, and potassium oxalate.

Anti-coagulant. This substance prevents blood from clotting. The mechanism by which clotting is prevented varies with the anti-coagulant; for example, some remove calcium, whereas others inactivate thrombin and thromboplastin. Examples of anti-coagulants are ethylenediaminetetraacetic acid

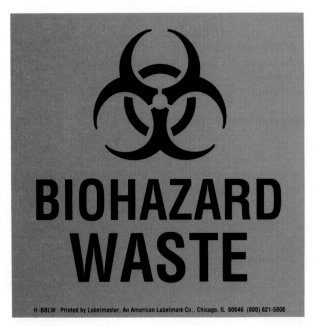

Figure 2–1 Biohazard symbol.

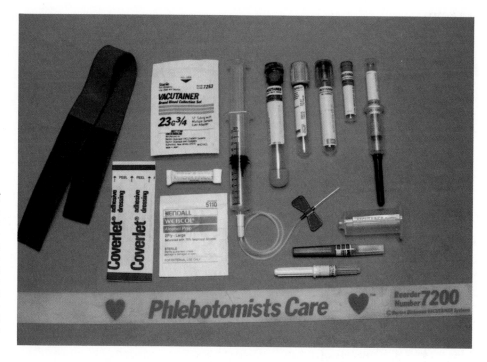

Figure 2–2 Examples of equipment used in venipuncture. *Top left to right:* Velcro tourniquet; winged infusion set (butterfly) packaging; syringe with butterfly attached; and evacuated tubes, one attached to tube holder and multiple-sample needle. *Middle left to right:* adhesive bandage, ammonia ampule, alcohol preparation, tube holder, and needles. *Bottom:* rubber tourniquet. (Photo by Steve Kasper.)

(EDTA), sodium citrate, and lithium heparin. Tubes must be inverted several times to ensure proper mixing after collection, according to the manufacturer's instructions.

Clot Activator. This substance helps initiate the clotting mechanism. It can be either an inert additive or a coating in the tube. Examples are silica gel and silicone coating.

Separator Gel. This inert material undergoes a temporary change in viscosity during the centrifugation process, enabling it to serve as a separation barrier between serum and cells or between plasma and cells. Because this gel may interfere with some testing, serum from these tubes cannot be used for blood bank procedures and with certain instruments. See Table 2–1 for a summary of collection tubes.

Needles

Sterile needles come in a variety of lengths and gauges (bore or opening size). Needles are made either to fit the vacuum tube holder by screwing in or to be attached to the tips of syringes. Most evacuated tube needles are considered "multiple-sample" because they have a rubber sleeve that prevents blood from dripping into the holders when tubes are changed. In syringes, "single-sample" needles are used. The end of the needle that is inserted into the vein has a point with a slanted side (bevel), which must be facing up when the needle is inserted. Needle tips should be examined for burrs or bends before a venipuncture is performed. Gauge numbers are related inversely to the bore size: the smaller the gauge number, the larger the bore. The most common size needle for adult venipuncture is 21-gauge with a length of 1 or 1½ inches. The advantage of using a 1-inch needle is that it provides better control.

Needle Holders

Needle holders are usually made to fit specific manufacturers' needles and tubes and, for best results, should not be interchanged. The holders are disposable and can be discarded after a single use, or they may be cleaned by soaking in a 10% bleach solution. Because needle sticks continue to be a safety concern, several new needle holders on the market have sheaths that lock into place after use. There is also one that projects the needle into a sharps container.[3]

Tourniquet

A tourniquet is used to provide a barrier against venous blood flow in order to help locate a vein. A tourniquet can be a disposable latex strap, a heavier Velcro strap, or a blood pressure cuff. The tourniquet should be applied 3–4 inches above the venipuncture site and left on for no longer than 1 minute before the venipuncture is performed.

Syringes

Syringes consist of a barrel that is graduated in milliliters and a plunger onto which the needle fits. Syringes come with different types of needle at-

Table 2-1. LIST OF COMMON STOPPERS, ADDITIVES, AND LABORATORY USES

Conventional Stopper Color*		Hemogard Closure†	Additive/Additive Function	Laboratory Use‡
Yellow		Yellow	Sodium polyanetholsulfonate (SPS): prevents blood from clotting and stabilizes bacterial growth	Blood or body fluid cultures
Red		Red	None	Serum testing: chemistry, blood bank, serology
Red/Gray (marbled)		Gold	None, but contains silica particles to enhance clot formation	Serum testing
Light Blue		Light Blue	Sodium citrate: removes calcium to prevent blood from clotting	Coagulation testing
Green		Green	Heparin (sodium/lithium/ammonium): inhibits thrombin formation to prevent clotting	Chemistry testing
Green/Gray (marbled)		Light Green	Lithium heparin and gel for plasma separation	Plasma determinations in chemistry
Yellow/Gray (marbled)		Orange	Thrombin	Stat serum demonstrations in chemistry
Lavender		Lavender	Ethylenediaminetetraacetic acid (EDTA): removes calcium to prevent blood from clotting	Hematology testing
Gray		Gray	Potassium oxalate/sodium fluoride: removes calcium to prevent blood from clotting; fluoride inhibits glycolysis	Chemistry testing, especially glucose/alcohol
Royal Blue		Royal Blue	Sodium heparin: inhibits thrombin formation to prevent clotting; also sodium EDTA	Chemistry trace elements

* Stopper colors based on Becton-Dickinson Vacutainer tubes.
† Hemogard closures provide protective plastic cover over the subber stopper as an additional safety feature.
‡ Sterile needles come in a variety of lengths and gauges (bore or opening size). Needles are also made to fit the evacuated tube holder by screwing in or to be attached to the tips of syringes. Most evacuated tube needles have a rubber sleeve to prevent blood from dripping into the holders when tubes are changed, and are called multi-sample needles. The open end of the needle containing the point has a slanted side (bevel), which must be facing up when the needle is inserted into the vein. Needle positioning is very important in drawing blood. The angle of entry should be 15 degrees. The most common size needle for adult venipuncture is 21-gauge.

tachments, as well as in different sizes. It is important to attach the needle securely to the syringe in order to prevent air from entering the system. Syringes may be useful in drawing blood from pediatric, geriatric, or other patients with tiny, fragile, or "rolling" veins that would not be able to withstand the vacuum pressure from the evacuated tubes. With a syringe, the amount of pressure exerted is controlled by the phlebotomist. Other suggestions for drawing blood from geriatric and pediatric patients are discussed in Chapter 36.

Winged Infusion Sets (Butterflies)

A butterfly is an intravenous device that consists of a short needle and a thin tube with attached plastic wings. The butterfly can be connected to Vacutainer holders, syringes, or blood culture bottles with the use of special adapters. Butterflies are very useful in collecting specimens from children or other patients from whom it is difficult to draw blood. Many butterflies now come with resheathing devices in order to minimize the risk of needle stick injury.

Solutions for Skin Preparation

The most common skin cleanser is 70% isopropyl alcohol. It can be applied by a commercially prepared alcohol pad or by a cotton ball or piece of gauze soaked in the alcohol. The site should be cleaned in a circular motion, beginning in the center and working outward. It is important to allow the area to dry before the venipuncture is performed, so that the patient does not experience a burning sensation and to prevent contamination of the specimen. When a sterile site is prepared for collection of blood cultures, povidone-iodine or 1–2% tincture of iodine is used, in addition to the isopropyl alcohol. To avoid contamination when legal blood alcohol level is measured, benzalkonium chloride (Zephiran chloride) is used.

SELECTING A VEIN FOR ROUTINE VENIPUNCTURE

The superficial veins of the anterior surface of the upper extremity are the most common sites for venipuncture. The three primary veins that are used are (1) the cephalic vein, located on the upper forearm and on the thumb side of the hand; (2) the basilic vein, located on the lower forearm and the little finger side of the hand; and (3) the median cubital vein, which connects the basilic and cephalic veins in the antecubital fossa (bend in elbow) and is the vein of choice (Fig. 2–3).

If the patient makes a fist after application of the tourniquet, the vein should become prominent. The patient should not do any vigorous pumping of the fist, as it may affect some of the test values. The clinician should palpate the vein with his or her index finger to be certain of its location and direction. If a vein cannot be located in either arm, it may be necessary to examine the veins in the wrist, hands, or feet. The policy in some institutions is to request that a second phlebotomist attempt to locate a vein in the arm before one of these three sites is used.

VENIPUNCTURE PROCEDURE IN ADULTS

The following steps are recommended by the National Committee for Clinical Laboratory Standards (NCCLS, Document H3, 1991):[2]

■ Prepare the accession order, if necessary.
■ Identify the patient.
■ Verify the patient's diet restrictions.
■ Assemble supplies and put on gloves.
■ Reassure the patient.
■ Position the patient.
■ Verify paperwork and tubes.
■ Ensure that the patient's hand is closed.
■ Select the venipuncture site.
■ Cleanse the venipuncture site.
■ Apply the tourniquet.
■ Inspect the needle and other equipment.
■ Perform the venipuncture.
■ Mix tubes with additives by gentle inversion after each tube is drawn.
■ Release and remove the tourniquet.
■ Ensure that the patient's hand is open.
■ Place gauze or cotton ball over the site.

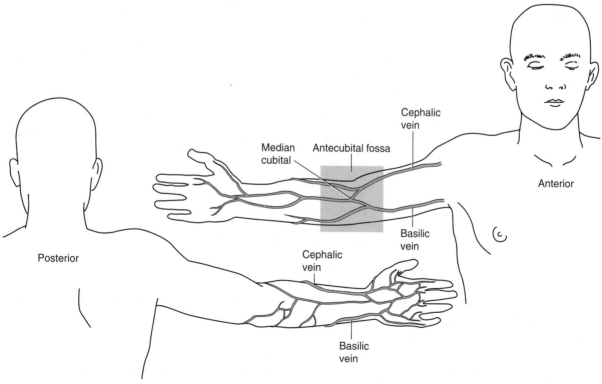

Figure 2–3 Veins of forearm; two views.

- Release last tube from the back of the needle.
- Remove the needle.
- Bandage the patient's arm.
- If a syringe has been used, fill the tubes.
- Dispose of the puncturing unit in the biohazard container.
- Chill the specimen, if procedure requires chilling.
- Eliminate diet restrictions.
- Time-stamp paperwork.
- Send properly labeled tubes to appropriate laboratories.

The most critical steps in the process are identification of the patient and specimen labeling. The patient must tell the phlebotomist his or her name, or someone must identify the patient for the phlebotomist. A hospitalized patient must also be identified by his or her identification bracelet.

The patient's name and identification number or Social Security number must match the information on the test requisition. If there are discrepancies, they must be resolved before the procedure can continue. Failure to confirm proper identification could result in a life-threatening situation for the patient and possible legal ramifications for the phlebotomist. Labeling should be performed or confirmed at the patient's bedside. The minimal amount of information that should be on each tube is

patient's full name
patient's identification number
date and time of collection
phlebotomist's initials or code

The recommended order of draw when the evacuated tube system is used is as follows:

blood culture tubes or bottles
nonadditive or plain red stopper tube
coagulation or light blue stopper tube
other additive or gel separator tube (e.g., lavender)

In order to prevent cross-contamination between different additives, the following order of draw is recommended:

light blue stopper (sodium citrate)
green stopper (heparin)
lavender stopper (EDTA)
gray stopper (oxalate/fluoride)

When tubes are filled from a syringe, the recommended order of filling is as follows:

blood culture
light blue stopper
other additive
nonadditive or red stopper/gel separator tubes

Tubes containing specimens drawn for coagulation testing (light blue stopper) require special handling. Collection and handling of these specimens are discussed in Chapter 35.

VENIPUNCTURE PROCEDURE IN CHILDREN AND INFANTS

Pediatric phlebotomy requires experience, special skills, and a tender touch. Excellent interpersonal skills are needed in order to deal with distraught parents, as well as with crying, screaming, and scared children. Ideally, only experienced phlebotomists should draw blood from children. Unfortunately, the only way to gain experience is through practice. Through experience, one learns what works in different situations. Frequently, smaller gauge (23 or 25) needles are used. Syringes or butterflies may be advantageous with some infants' veins. No matter what equipment is used, the real secret to a successful venipuncture is a good child holder! The child's arm should be immobilized as much as possible in order to successfully get the needle into the vein and be able to keep it there if the child tries to move. Use of special stickers or character bandages as rewards may serve as incentive for cooperation; however, protocol of the institution with regard to their distribution must be followed.

COMPLICATIONS ENCOUNTERED IN BLOOD COLLECTION

Ecchymosis (Bruise). This is the most common complication encountered in obtaining a blood specimen. It is caused by leakage of a small amount of fluid around the tissue.

Syncope (Fainting). Fainting is probably the second most common complication. Before drawing blood, the collector should always ask the patient whether he or she has had any prior episodes of fainting during or after blood collection. An ammonia inhalant should always be within reach of the collector. If the patient begins to faint, the clinician should immediately remove the needle, lower the patient's head, and apply cold compresses to the back of the patient's neck. The patient should take some deep breaths, and some cold water to drink should be offered.

Hematoma. Leakage of a large amount of fluid around the puncture site that causes the area to swell results in a hematoma. If swelling begins, the needle should be removed immediately and pressure applied to the site for at least 2 minutes. The most common causes of a hematoma are the needle's going through the vein, the bevel of the needle being only partially in the vein, and failure to apply enough pressure after venipuncture.

Failure to Draw Blood. One reason for failure to draw blood is that the vein is missed, often because of improper needle positioning. The needle should be inserted completely into the vein with the slanted side (bevel) up, at an angle of 15 degrees. Figure 2–4 demonstrates reasons for unsatisfactory flow of blood. It is sometimes possible to enter the vein with slight manipulation of the needle, but this should be attempted only by an experienced phlebotomist because such manipulation can cause discomfort to the patient.

Occasionally a vacuum tube has insufficient suction, and insertion of another tube will yield blood.

Petechiae. Petechiae are small red spots that indicate that small amounts of blood have escaped into the skin epithelium. Petechiae indicate a possible coagulation problem and should alert the phlebotomist to be aware of possible prolonged bleeding.

Edema. Swelling caused by an abnormal accumulation of fluid in the intercellular spaces of the tissues is termed *edema.* The most common cause is infiltration of the tissues by the solution running through an incorrectly positioned intravenous (IV) catheter. Edematous sites should be avoided for venipuncture because the veins are hard to find and the specimens may become contaminated with the tissue fluid.

Obesity. In obese patients, veins may be neither readily visible nor easy to palpate. Sometimes the use of a blood pressure cuff can aid in locating a vein. It is not advisable to probe blindly in the patient's arm.

Intravenous Therapy. Blood should not be drawn from an arm with an IV catheter. If there is no alternative, blood should be drawn *below* the catheter with the tourniquet placed *below* the catheter site. It is preferable to have the nurse stop the infusion for 2 minutes before the specimen is drawn. NCCLS recommends that 5 mL of blood be drawn for discard before samples that will be used for testing are obtained. It is important to note on the requisition that the specimen was obtained from an arm in which an IV solution was running.[2]

Hemoconcentration. Hemoconcentration is an increased concentration of larger molecules and analytes in the blood as a result of a shift in water balance. This can be caused by leaving the tourniquet on the patient's arm for too long or by probing or massaging the site. It is recommended that the tourniquet not remain on for more than 1 minute before venipuncture. If it is left on for a longer time because of difficulty in finding a vein, it should be removed for 2 to 3 minutes and then reapplied before the venipuncture is performed.[4]

Hemolysis. The rupture of red blood cells with the consequent escape of hemoglobin—a process termed hemolysis—can cause the plasma or serum to appear pink or red. Hemolysis can occur during a difficult draw if too small a needle was used; if the clinician pulls back too quickly on the plunger of a syringe, forces blood into a tube from a syringe, or shakes a tube too hard; or because of contamination by alcohol or water at the veni-

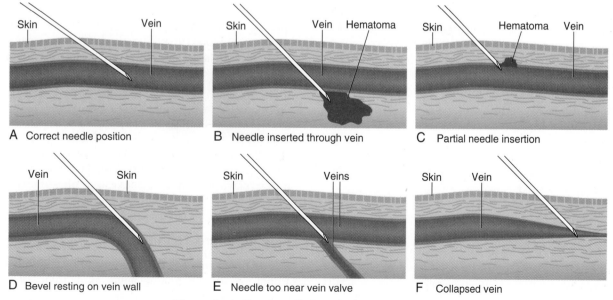

A Correct needle position

B Needle inserted through vein

C Partial needle insertion

D Bevel resting on vein wall

E Needle too near vein valve

F Collapsed vein

Figure 2–4 Proper needle insertion for venipuncture.

puncture site or in the tubes. Hemolysis can also occur physiologically as a result of hemolytic anemias or severe renal problems.

Burned, Damaged, Scarred, and Occluded Veins. All such veins should be avoided because they do not allow the blood to flow freely and may make it difficult to obtain an acceptable specimen.

Seizures, Tremors. Patients occasionally experience seizures, either because of a pre-existing condition or as a response to the needle stick. If a seizure occurs, the needle should be removed immediately. The patient's safety should be ensured by preventing injury from nearby objects.

Vomiting, Choking. Turn the patient's head so that he or she does not aspirate any vomit. Keep the patient from hitting his or her head.

Allergies. Some patients may be allergic to skin antiseptic substances other than alcohol. Adhesive bandages and tape may also cause an allergic reaction. Hypoallergenic tape should be used or pressure applied manually until the bleeding has completely stopped.

Inability to Obtain a Blood Specimen

Each institution should have a policy covering proper procedure when a blood specimen cannot be collected. Some of the most common are mentioned here. If two unsuccessful attempts at collection have been made, both the nurse in charge of that patient and the phlebotomy supervisor should be notified. Another person can make two attempts to obtain a specimen. If a second person is unsuccessful, the physician should be notified.

The patient has the right to refuse to give a blood specimen. If gentle urging does not persuade the patient to allow blood to be drawn, the clinician should alert the nurse, who will either talk to the patient or notify the physician. The clinician must not try to force an uncooperative patient to have blood drawn; it can be unsafe for the clinician and for the patient. If the patient is a child and the parents offer to help hold the child, it is normally all right to proceed. Any refusals or problems should be documented for legal reasons.

If the patient is not in his or her room, the absence should be reported to the nursing unit, so that the nurses will be aware that the specimen was not obtained.

SKIN PUNCTURES

Skin punctures are often performed in newborns; in pediatric patients under 2 years of age; in adults who are severely burned, who have thrombotic tendencies, and whose veins are being reserved for therapeutic purposes; and in geriatric patients with fragile veins. However, when peripheral circulation is poor, accurate results may not be obtained with specimens obtained by skin puncture.

Capillary blood is actually a mixture of venous, arterial, and capillary blood. When the puncture site is warmed, the specimen more closely resembles arterial blood. Because capillary specimens may generate slightly different test results, a notation should be made when the specimen is obtained by skin puncture.[5] White blood cell counts in specimens obtained by skin puncture may be 15–20% higher than those in venous specimens.[6] Clinically significant higher glucose values are found in specimens obtained by skin puncture than in specimens obtained by venipuncture. This is especially important to note when a glucose tolerance test is performed or when glucometer results are compared with findings from venous samples.

Collection Sites

In most patients, skin punctures may be performed on the heel, big toe, or finger. In infants the finger should not be punctured because the lancets could cause serious injury to the bones in the fingers. The site of choice in infants is the lateral (outside) or medial (inside) surface of the plantar side (bottom) of the heel, although there have been some problems with using the medial heel surface and puncturing the posterior tibial artery. The plantar surface of the big toe is also an acceptable site if the infant has large feet (Fig. 2–5A). In older children and adults, the palmar surface of the distal portion of the second, third, or fourth finger may be used; the third (middle) finger is the recommended site.[5] The puncture on the finger should be made perpendicular to the fingerprint lines (Fig. 2–5B). Warming can increase the blood flow sevenfold. The site can be warmed with a warm, moist wash cloth or a commercial heel warmer. A temperature no higher than 42°C for no longer than 3 minutes should be used, unless the collection is for capillary blood gases. The skin puncture site should be cleansed with 70% isopropyl alcohol and allowed to dry. Povidone-iodine should not be used because of possible blood contamination, which would produce falsely elevated levels of potassium, phosphorus, or uric acid.

Skin Puncture Technique

The finger or heel must be securely immobilized. Punctures should not be made more than 2.4 mm deep because of the risk of bone injury and possible infection (osteomyelitis). In premature infants,

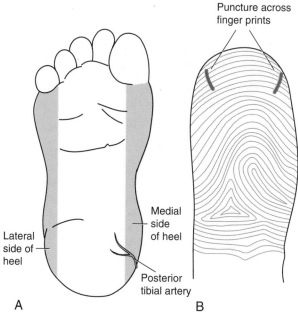

Figure 2–5 Areas for skin puncture—heel (*A*) and finger (*B*).

it is advisable to use a puncture device with even less depth. Most of the devices on the market for performing skin punctures come in varying depths.

Do not puncture an area that is swollen, is bruised, or has already been punctured. The first drop of blood should be wiped away to prevent contamination of the specimen with tissue fluid and to facilitate the free flow of blood.[5]

DEVICES FOR COLLECTING BLOOD FROM SKIN PUNCTURE[7]

Capillary tubes (Fig. 2–6) of various sizes are available with or without heparin added.

Microtainer tubes have virtually replaced Caraway/Natelson tubes, which are large-bore glass collecting tubes. Microtainers are available with or without additives, and the cap colors on the tubes correspond to the colors on the vacuum tubes. The order of drawing is different for Microtainer tubes. The EDTA Microtainer should be collected first to ensure adequate volume and accurate hematology results, especially for platelets, which tend to aggregate at the site of puncture. Other additive tubes should be collected next and followed by nonadditive tubes.

Unopettes, which are available in various dilutions and with varied diluents, come with their own calibrated micropipettes and are used in the preparation of specimens for cell counting.[4]

Labeling for capillary specimens should contain the same information as for vacuum tubes. This may be facilitated by placing the Microtainer in a labeled large tube.

PREPARATION OF BLOOD SMEARS

Blood smears can be made directly from capillary blood or from venous blood by either wedge or coverslip method. In either method, the clinician must remember to wipe the first drop of blood

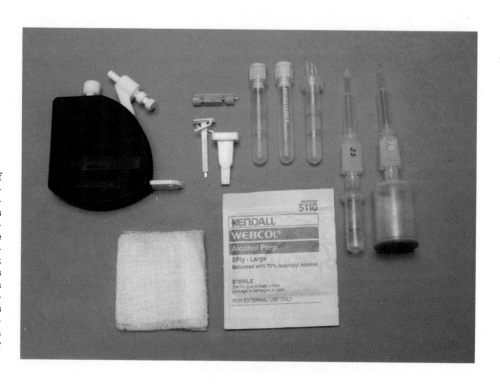

Figure 2–6 Examples of equipment used for skin puncture. *Left to right:* Autolet blood-drawing device; other examples of lancets, both opened to expose cutting edge, although the larger (yellow) one is self-contained and the blade will retract into the housing once it has been used; Microtainer (Becton Dickinson) tubes, one with collection top attached; Unopettes (Becton Dickinson). Also pictured are an alcohol preparation and a gauze square. (Photo by Steve Kasper.)

away and use the second drop to make the smear, if blood from a finger or heel stick is used. (See Chapter 13.)

QUALITY ASSURANCE IN SPECIMEN COLLECTION

In order to obtain a good-quality specimen, the laboratory is responsible for ensuring that the patient has been properly prepared before the specimen is collected. The phlebotomist must be adequately trained and have knowledge of the protocol needed to handle the specimen appropriately. Proper specimen handling includes selection of the appropriate tube, knowledge of the required amount of blood, and correct specimen transport and storage. Tubes must be checked for expiration dates and cracks. Tubes that contain additives must be completely mixed by gentle inversion at the time of collection.

Reasons for Specimen Rejection

A laboratory procedure is only as good as the specimen provided. At times a specimen does not yield accurate results and must therefore be rejected. Table 2–2 lists some reasons for specimen rejection.

Responsibility of Phlebotomist in Infection Control

Because phlebotomists interact with patients and staff throughout the day, they could potentially infect numerous people. A phlebotomist must maintain good personal health and hygiene, making sure to have clean clothes, clean hair, and clean fingernails. Universal precautions must be followed at all times, with special attention to the use of gloves and handwashing.

Table 2–2. REASONS FOR SPECIMEN REJECTION

The test order requisition and the tube identification do not match

The tube is unlabeled, or the labeling, including patient identification number, is incorrect

The specimen is hemolyzed

The specimen was collected at the wrong time

The specimen was collected in the wrong tube

The specimen was clotted, and the test requires whole blood

The specimen was contaminated with intravenous fluid

The specimen is lipemic*

* Lipemic specimens cannot be used for certain tests; however, the phlebotomist has no control over this aspect. Collection of a fasting specimen may be requested to try to reduce the potential for lipemia.

SUMMARY

Laboratory test results are only as good as the specimens tested. All of the newest equipment and innovative technology cannot compensate for an improperly collected or mishandled specimen. It is vital to the quality of care that everything possible be done to ensure the integrity of the patient's blood specimen.

To reduce the potential for errors, the phlebotomist or the person collecting the blood specimen must be properly trained in collection and specimen handling procedures. The phlebotomist should be provided with all the materials needed to perform a proper venipuncture and must be experienced in their proper use.

REVIEW QUESTIONS

1. The most important precaution in preventing infections is
   a. wearing a mask
   b. handwashing
   c. wearing a gown
   d. wearing gloves

2. The vein of choice for performing a venipuncture is the
   a. basilic
   b. cephalic
   c. median cubital
   d. femoral

3. One of the most common reasons for failure to obtain blood when a venipuncture is performed is
   a. Incorrect needle positioning.
   b. Movement of the patient.
   c. Inadequate vacuum in the tube.
   d. Collapsed vein.

4. What is the recommended order of drawing when the evacuated tube system is used?
   a. Gel separator, nonadditive, coagulation, and blood culture.
   b. Additive, nonadditive, gel separator, and blood culture.
   c. Nonadditive, blood culture, coagulation, and other additive.
   d. Blood culture, nonadditive, coagulation, and gel separator or other additive

5. Acceptable sites for skin puncture on infants are
   a. Middle of the heel and tip of the big toe.
   b. Lateral or medial surface of the bottom of the heel and plantar surface of the big toe.
   c. Inside of the heel, close to the arch of foot, and any of the toes, close to the tip.
   d. Middle of the bottom of the heel and middle of the big toe.

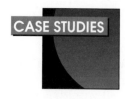
CASE STUDIES

1. A 2-year-old on the pediatric floor starts to scream as soon as the phlebotomist walks into the room. The mother is there and tells the child not to worry because "this won't hurt." What should the phlebotomist do?

2. As soon as the phlebotomist enters the room, the patient immediately tells the phlebotomist that it will be hard to draw blood and that the phlebotomist had better be good at it, because he or she will only get one chance. What should the phlebotomist do?

References

1. Rules and regulations: bloodborne pathogens. Federal Register 1991; 56(235):64175–64182.
2. National Committee for Clinical Laboratory Standards (NCCLS): Procedures for the Collection of Diagnostic Blood Specimens by Venipuncture, 3rd ed (NCCLS Document H3-A3). Villanova, PA: NCCLS, 1991.
3. Pendergraph GE: Handbook of Phlebotomy, 3rd ed. Philadelphia: Lea & Febiger, 1992.
4. Garza D, Becan-McBride K. Phlebotomy Handbook, 3rd ed. Norwalk, CT: Appleton & Lange, 1992.
5. NCCLS: Procedures for the Collection of Diagnostic Blood Specimens by Skin Puncture, 3rd ed (NCCLS Document H4-A3). Villanova, PA: NCCLS, 1991.
6. American Society of Clinical Pathologists (ASCP): Effect of Sample Collection on Laboratory Test Results (ASCP Spring 1992 Teleconference; Presenter: J. Geller, MT[ASCP]).
7. NCCLS: Devices for Collection of Skin Puncture Blood Specimens, 2nd ed (NCCLS Document H14-A2). Villanova, PA: NCCLS, 1990.

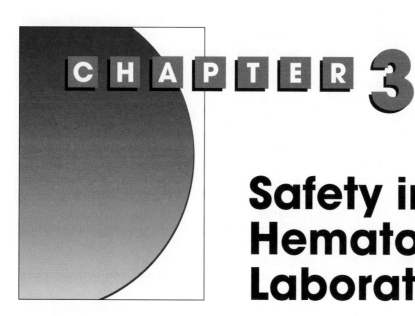

CHAPTER 3

Safety in the Hematology Laboratory

Sheila A. Finch

Outline

Objectives

AFTER COMPLETION OF THIS CHAPTER, THE READER WILL BE ABLE TO
1. Discuss the development of a safety management program.
2. Define universal precautions.
3. List infectious materials included in universal precautions.
4. Identify occupational hazards that exist in the hematology laboratory.
5. Describe the safe practices required in the "Occupational Exposure to Bloodborne Pathogens" standard.
6. Describe the principles of a fire prevention program.
7. Identify the requirements of the "Occupational Exposure to Hazardous Chemicals in Laboratories" standard.

Many conditions in the laboratory have the potential for causing injury to personnel and damage to the building or to the community. Patients' specimens, needles, chemicals, electrical equipment, reagents, and glassware can all be possible sources of accidents or injury. Management and employees must be knowledgeable about safe work practices and incorporate these practices into the operation of the hematology laboratory. The key to prevention of accidents and laboratory-acquired infections is a well-defined safety program.

Safety is a very broad subject and cannot be covered in one chapter. This chapter simply highlights some of the key safe practices that should be followed in the laboratory. Omission of a safe practice from this chapter does not imply that it is not important or that it should not be considered in the development of a safety curriculum or a safety program.

UNIVERSAL PRECAUTIONS

One of the biggest risks associated with the hematology laboratory is the exposure to blood and body fluids. Universal precautions, which require that most human blood and body fluids be treated as if they were infectious, must be adopted by the laboratory. Universal precautions apply to the following potentially infectious materials: blood, semen, vaginal secretions, cerebrospinal fluid, synovial fluid, pleural fluid, any body fluid with visible blood, any unidentified body fluid, and saliva from dental procedures. Past practice was to label specimens from patients known to have infectious diseases; however, experience has demonstrated that even patients without visible symptoms can have infectious diseases. Adopting universal precautions will protect workers from exposure and reduce the risk of becoming infected.

In December 1991, the Occupational Safety and Health Administration (OSHA) issued the *Occupational Exposure to Bloodborne Pathogens* standard, which specifies universal precautions in order to protect laboratory workers and other health care professionals. Bloodborne pathogens are pathogenic microorganisms that, when present in human blood, can cause disease. They include, but are not limited to, hepatitis B virus (HBV) and human immunodeficiency virus (HIV). This chapter does not cover the complete details of the standard; it covers only those sections that apply directly to the hematology laboratory.

Safe Practices

The following standards must be enforced:

1. *Handwashing* is one of the most important safety precautions. Hands must be washed with soap and water. Only if water is not available should antiseptic hand cleaners with paper towels be used. The proper technique for handwashing is as follows:
   a. Wet hands *and wrists* thoroughly under running water.
   b. Apply germicidal soap and rub hands vigorously for 10–15 seconds.
   c. Rinse hands thoroughly under running water.
   d. Dry hands with paper towel. Use the paper towel to turn off the faucet handles.

   Hands must be washed
   a. Whenever there is visible contamination with blood or body fluids.
   b. After completion of work.
   c. After gloves are removed and between glove changes.
   d. Before the worker leaves the laboratory.
   e. Before and after the worker eats, drinks, smokes, applies cosmetics or lip balm, changes contact lens, and uses the lavatory.
   f. Before and after all other activities that entail hand contact with mucous membranes, eyes, or breaks in skin.

2. *Eating, drinking, smoking, and applying cosmetics or lip balm must be prohibited* in the laboratory work area.

3. Hands, pens, and other fomites must be kept away from the worker's mouth and all mucous membranes.

4. *Food and drink* must not be kept in the same refrigerator as laboratory specimens or reagents or where potentially infectious materials are stored or tested.

5. *Mouth pipetting* is prohibited.

6. Needles and other sharp objects contaminated with blood and other potentially infectious materials should not be manipulated in any way. Such manipulation includes resheathing, bending, clipping, or removing the sharp object. If resheathing is unavoidable, an appropriate resheathing device or approved one-handed techniques can be used.

7. *Contaminated sharps* (include, but are not limited to, needles, blades, pipettes, syringes with needles, glass slides) must be placed in a puncture-resistant container that is appropriately labeled with the universal biohazard symbol (see Fig. 2–1) or a red container that adheres to the standard. The container must be leakproof (Fig. 3–1).

8. Procedures, such as removing caps when checking for clots, filling hemocytometer chambers, making slides, discarding specimens,

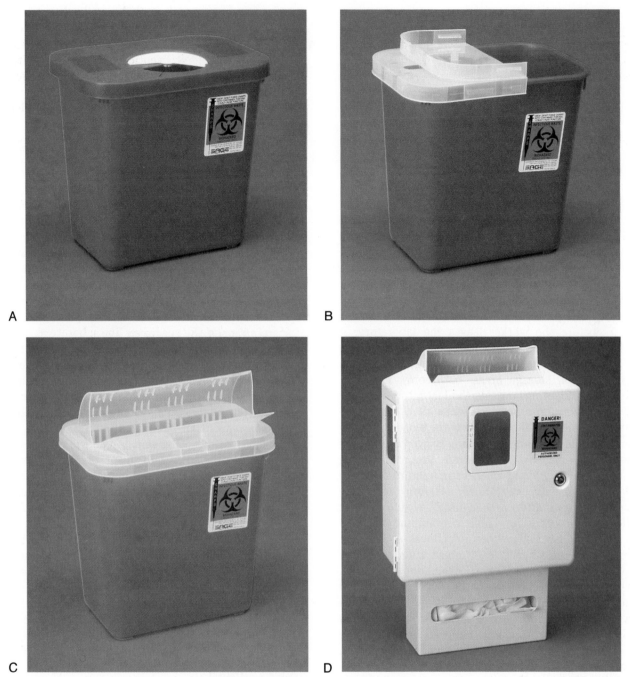

Figure 3–1 Examples of sharps disposal systems: *A*, rotor opening container; *B*, clear hinged lid for larger items; *C*, transparent red container with horizontal drop; *D*, wall unit with horizontal drop; glove dispenser attached. (Courtesy of Sage Products, Inc., Crystal Lake, IL.)

making dilutions, and pouring specimens or fluids must be performed so that they prevent splashing, spraying, or production of droplets of the specimen manipulated. These procedures may be performed behind a barrier, such as a plastic shield, or protective eyewear should be worn (Fig. 3–2).

9. *Personal protective clothing* and equipment must be provided to the worker. The most common forms of personal protective equipment are as follows:

a. *Outercoverings*—gowns, laboratory coats, and/or sleeve protectors—should be worn when there is a chance of splashing or spilling on work clothing. The outercovering must be made of fluid-resistant material, must be long-sleeved, and must remain buttoned at all times. If contamination or strike-through occurs, the protective clothing should be removed immediately and treated as infectious material.

When a phlebotomy is performed, cloth

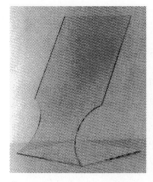
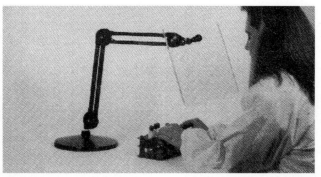

Figure 3–2 Examples of safety shields: *A,* tabletop; *B,* adjustable swing arm. (Courtesy of Peter E. Johnson & Associates.)

A   B

laboratory coats may be worn; the same guidelines for changing them apply. If cloth laboratory coats are worn, they must be laundered at the institution. This clothing must never be taken home to be washed or discarded.

All protective clothing should be removed before the worker leaves the laboratory; it should not be worn into public areas. These areas include, but are not limited to, break rooms, storage areas, bathrooms, cafeteria, and meetings outside the laboratory.

b. *Gloves* must be worn when there exists the potential for contact with blood or body fluids (including handling bagged biohazardous material and when decontaminating benchtops) and when venipuncture or finger sticks are performed. Gloves must be changed after each contact with a patient when there is visible contamination, or if physical damage occurs. Gloves should not be worn when "clean" areas, such as a copy machine or a "clean" telephone, are used. The gloves must not be reworn or washed and should be discarded into a biohazardous container. Once one glove is removed, the second glove can be removed by sliding the index finger of the ungloved hand between the glove and the hand and slipping the second glove off. This technique prevents contamination of the "clean" hand by the "dirty" second glove.[1]

c. *Eyewear*—face shields, or goggles, and masks—should be used when there is potential for aerosol mists, splashes, or sprays to the mouth, eyes, or nose. Removing caps from specimen tubes, working at the cell counter, and centrifuging specimens are examples of tasks that could result in aerosol mist.

10. *Phlebotomy trays* should be appropriately labeled to indicate potentially infectious materials. Specimens should be placed into a secondary container, such as a resealable bag.

11. If a *pneumatic tube system* is used to transport specimens, the specimens should be placed into a special leakproof bag, appropriately labeled with the biohazard symbol. If there is potential for leakage, a secondary container should be used. Requisition forms should be placed outside of the secondary container to prevent contamination if the specimen leaks.

When specimens are received in the laboratory, they should be handled by someone wearing gloves, a laboratory coat, and other protective clothing, in accordance with the type and condition of specimen. Contaminated containers or requisitions must be decontaminated or replaced before being sent to the work area.

12. When *equipment* used to process specimens becomes visibly contaminated or requires maintenance or service, it must be decontaminated, whether service is performed in-house or equipment is sent out. If it is difficult to decontaminate the equipment, it must be labeled with the biohazard symbol to indicate potentially infectious material. *Routine cleaning* should be performed on equipment that has the potential for splashes, sprays, and so forth, such as inside the lid of the microhematocrit centrifuge.

Housekeeping

Work surfaces should be cleaned at the completion of the procedures and whenever the bench area or floor becomes visibly contaminated. An appropriate disinfectant solution is household bleach, used in a 1:10 volume/volume dilution (2½ cups bleach per gallon of water), to accomplish the recommended concentration of chlorine of 5500 ppm. Because this solution is not stable, it must be made fresh *daily.* Bleach is not recommended for aluminum surfaces. Other solutions used to decontaminate include, but are not limited to, Amphyl and 70% ethanol. All paper towels used in the decontamination process should be disposed of as biohazardous.

Laundry

If nondisposable laboratory coats are used, they must be placed in appropriate containers for transport to the laundry at the facility and not taken to the employee's home.

HBV Vaccination

Laboratory workers should receive the HBV (hepatitis B) vaccination series before or within 10 days after beginning work in the laboratory at no cost. An employee must sign a release form if he or she refuses the series. If an exposure incident (needle puncture; exposure to skin, eye, face, mucous membrane) occurs, postexposure evaluation and follow-up, including prophylaxis and medical consultation, should be made available to the employee at no cost. Employees should be encouraged to report all exposure incidents, and such reporting should be enforced as standard policy.

Training and Documentation

Hematology personnel should be properly educated in epidemiology and symptoms of bloodborne diseases, modes of transmission of bloodborne diseases, use of protective equipment, work practices, ways to recognize tasks and other activities that may result in an exposure, and the location of the written exposure plan for the laboratory. Education should be documented and should occur at the time of initial assignment to the laboratory and at least annually thereafter.

Waste Management

The specimens from the laboratory are identified as regulated waste. State and local regulations for disposal of medical waste must be followed. In 1988, OSHA developed a Medical Waste Tracking Act that required generators (producers) of medical waste to be responsible for the handling and disposal of waste. This standard should be reviewed before any waste from the hematology laboratory is disposed of.

OCCUPATIONAL HAZARDS

Four important occupational hazards in the laboratory are discussed in this chapter: fire, chemical hazards, electrical hazards, and needle puncture. There are other hazards to be considered when a safety management program is developed, and the reader is referred to the Department of Labor reference for detailed regulations.[2]

Fire Hazard

Because of the number of flammable and combustible chemicals used in the laboratory, fire is a potential hazard. However, complying with standards established by the National Fire Protection Agency, OSHA, the Joint Commission on the Accreditation of Healthcare Organizations (JCAHO), the College of American Pathologists (CAP), and other organizations can minimize the dangers. A good fire safety/prevention plan is necessary and should consist of the following:

1. Enforcement of a no-smoking policy.
2. Installation of appropriate fire extinguishers. There are several types of extinguishers for use on specific types of fire, some of which are multipurpose.
3. Placement of fire extinguishers every 75 feet (22.9 m). A distinct system for marking the locations of fire extinguishers enables quick access when they are needed.
4. Placement of adequate fire detection systems (alarms, sprinklers), which should be tested every 3 months.
5. Placement of manual fire alarm boxes near the exit doors. Travel distance should not exceed 200 feet (61 m).
6. Written fire prevention and response procedures. All personnel in the laboratory should be knowledgeable about the procedures. Workers should be given assignments for specific responsibilities in case of fire, including responsibilities for patients' care, if applicable. Total count of employees in the laboratory should be known for any given day and a buddy system should be developed in case evacuation is necessary. Equipment shutdown procedures should be addressed in the plan, as should responsibility for implementation of those procedures.
7. Regular fire drills should be conducted so that response to a fire situation is routine and not a panic response. A summary of the laboratory's fire response plan can be copied on a quick reference card and attached to workers' identification badges, to be readily available in a fire situation.
8. Written storage requirements for any flammable or combustible chemicals stored in the laboratory. Chemicals should be arranged according to hazard class and not alphabetically.
9. A well-organized fire safety training program should be completed by all employees. Activities that require walking evacuation routes and locating fire extinguishers and pull boxes in the laboratory area should be scheduled. Types of fires likely to occur and use of the fire extinguisher should be discussed. Local fire depart-

ments work with facilities to conduct fire safety programs.

Chemical Hazards

Some of the chemicals used in the hematology laboratory are considered hazardous and thus are governed by the Occupational Exposure to Hazardous Chemicals in Laboratories standard, which requires laboratories to develop a chemical hygiene plan that outlines safe work practices to minimize exposures to hazardous chemicals. The full text of this standard can be found in the January 31, 1990, Federal Register.[2]

Some general principles should be followed in working with chemicals:

1. Properly label all chemicals. Do not use a chemical that is not properly labeled as to identity or content.
2. Follow all handling and storage requirements for the chemical.
3. Store alcohol and other flammable chemicals in approved safety cans or storage cabinets. Limit the quantity of flammable chemicals stored on the workbench to 2 working days' supply. Do not store chemicals in a hood, where they could react with other chemicals.
4. Use adequate ventilation when working with hazardous chemicals.
5. Use personal protective equipment and clothing, such as fume hoods, eye wash stations, rubber gloves, rubber aprons, and face shields. Safety showers should be available in the immediate area where the hazardous chemicals are used.
6. Use bottle carriers for bottles containing over 500 mL.
7. Alcohol-based solvents, rather than xylene or other potentially dangerous solutions, should be used to clean microscope objectives.
8. The wearing of contact lenses should not be permitted when an employee is working with xylene, acetone, alcohols, formaldehyde, and other solvents. They can make it difficult to wash the eyes in the event of a chemical splash in the eyes.
9. Spill response procedures should be included in the chemical safety procedures, and all employees must receive training in these procedures. Absorbent material should be available for spill response. Spill response kits and absorbent material should be stored in a room other than the area where they are likely to be needed. This prevents the necessity of walking through the spilled chemical to get the kit.
10. Material Safety Data Sheets (MSDSs) are written by the manufacturer of the chemicals

to provide information on the chemical. When an MSDS is received in the laboratory, it must be retained and reviewed with laboratory personnel. MSDSs give information on the identity of the chemical, hazardous ingredients, physical and chemical characteristics, data on fire and explosion hazard, reactivity and health hazard, precautions for safe handling and use, control measures, personal protective clothing, and equipment required for use with the chemical (Fig. 3–3).

Electrical Hazard

Electrical equipment and outlets are other sources of hazards. Faulty wiring may cause fires or serious injury. A few guidelines should be followed:

1. Equipment must be grounded or double-insulated. (Grounded equipment has a three-prong plug.)
2. Use of "cheater adapters" (adapters that allow three-pronged plugs to fit into a two-pronged outlet) should be prohibited.
3. Use of gang plugs (plugs that allow several cords to be plugged into one outlet) should be prohibited.
4. Use of extension cords should be avoided.
5. Equipment with loose plugs or frayed cords should not be used.
6. Stepping on cords, rolling heavy equipment over them, and other abuse of cords should be prohibited.
7. When cords are unplugged, the plug, not the cord, should be pulled.
8. Equipment that causes shock or a tingling sensation should be turned off, the instrument unplugged and identified as defective, and the problem reported.
9. Before repair or adjustment is attempted on electrical equipment, the following should be done:
   a. Unplug equipment.
   b. Make sure hands are dry.
   c. Remove jewelry.

Needle Puncture

Needle puncture is a serious occupational hazard for laboratory workers. Handling procedures should be written and followed, with special attention to phlebotomy procedures and disposal of contaminated needles. Sedimentation rate tubes, applicator sticks, capillary tubes, glass slides, and transfer pipettes are a few of the items that can cause a puncture similar to a needle puncture.

BECTON DICKINSON

Becton Dickinson and Company

Material Safety Data Sheet

SECTION 1 - IDENTITY

NAME
Becton Dickinson VACUTAINER Systems

ADDRESS
Stanley Street, E. Rutherford, NJ 07073

TELEPHONE NUMBER
(201) 460-2615

FOR ADDITIONAL INFORMATION CONTACT:
Fu-chung Lin, Ph.D.

DATE PREPARED
November 25, 1987

COMMON NAME (USED ON LABEL)
UNOPETTE Brand Test 5854, 5855

CHEMICAL FAMILY
Saline Diluent

CHEMICAL NAME
Does not apply

FORMULA
Does not apply

TRADE NAME & SYNONYMS
UNOPETTE, trademark of Becton Dickinson and Company

SECTION 2 - HAZARDOUS INGREDIENTS

HAZARDOUS COMPONENT	CAS #	% (wt)	TLV	PEL
Proprietary Mixture The ingredients of this mixture do not exist in concentrations greater than those described in 29 CFR 1910.1200(g)(2)(i)(c)(1)& (2) and listed in sources identified in 29 CFR 1910.1200(d)(3)&(4)				

PEL: Permissible Exposure Limit established by the Occupational Safety and Health Administration (OSHA).
TLV: Threshold Limit Value established by the American Conference of Governmental Industrial Hygienists, 1986-87.

SECTION 3 - PHYSICAL DATA

BOILING POINT
Not determined

SPECIFIC GRAVITY ($H_2O=1$)
Not determined

VAPOR PRESSURE (mm Hg)
Not determined

PERCENT VOLATILE BY VOLUME (%)
Not determined

VAPOR DENSITY (AIR=1)
Not determined

EVAPORATION RATE (_____ =1)
Not determined

SOLUBILITY IN WATER
Soluble

REACTIVITY IN WATER
Not reactive

APPEARANCE AND ODOR
Clear, colorless liquid; no characteristic odor, if any

SECTION 4 - FIRE AND EXPLOSION DATA

FLASH POINT
None

FLAMMABLE LIMITS IN AIR (% by VOLUME)
LOWER: Not applicable   UPPER: Not applicable

EXTINGUISHING MEDIA
Water, carbon dioxide, dry chemical

AUTO IGNITION TEMPERATURE
Not applicable

UNUSUAL FIRE AND EXPLOSION HAZARDS
May emit sulfur dioxide, mercury, oxides of phosphorus on decomposition by heat.

SPECIAL FIRE FIGHTING PROCEDURES
Wear full protective clothing including self-contained breathing apparatus.

BD/VS0003   *Continued on Reverse Side*

Figure 3–3 Material Safety Data Sheet (MSDS). (Courtesy of Becton Dickinson Vacutainer Systems, E. Rutherford, NJ.)

BD/VS0003

SECTION 5 - HEALTH INFORMATION

PRIMARY ROUTES OF EXPOSURE
Skin or eye contact, inhalation, ingestion

SIGNS AND SYMPTOMS OF EXPOSURE Some components are corrosive and may produce severe delayed chemical burns on contact
(1) ACUTE OVEREXPOSURE - with skin or mucous membranes.

(2) CHRONIC OVEREXPOSURE- Ammonium oxalate component is readily absorbed internally causing kidney damage.

MEDICAL CONDITIONS GENERALLY AGGRAVATED BY EXPOSURE
Kidney disfunction

CHEMICAL/COMPONENT LISTED AS CARCINOGEN OR POTENTIAL CARCINOGEN	**NTP**	**IARC**	**OSHA**
None	☐ Yes ☒ No	☐ Yes ☒ No	☐ Yes ☒ No

OTHER EXPOSURE LIMITS None

EMERGENCY & FIRST AID PROCEDURES
SKIN or EYES: wash with water for at least 15 minutes; get medical attention for persistent dermatitis. INGESTION and
INHALATION: get medical assistance.

SECTION 6 - REACTIVITY DATA

STABILITY | **CONDITIONS TO AVOID** Not determined
Unstable ☐ Stable ☒

INCOMPATIBILITY (MATERIALS TO AVOID)
Not determined

HAZARDOUS DECOMPOSITION PRODUCTS
Sulfur dioxide, mercury, oxides of phosphorus on decomposition by heat

HAZARDOUS POLYMERIZATION | **CONDITIONS TO AVOID**
May Occur ☐ Will Not Occur ☒ | Not determined

SECTION 7 - SPILL OR LEAK PROCEDURES

STEPS TO BE TAKEN IN CASE MATERIAL IS LEAKED OR SPILLED
Absorb, rinse, flush to sewer, avoid skin or eye contact

WASTE DISPOSAL METHOD
Dispose of wastes in accordance with local, state and Federal codes.

SECTION 8 - PERSONAL PROTECTION INFORMATION

RESPIRATORY PROTECTION Respiratory protection is not required under normal and intended uses

VENTILATION
General room ventilation is expected to be adequate

PROTECTIVE GLOVES | **EYE PROTECTION** Normally not required, except when
Not required, except during spill clean-up | chance of splashing exists.

OTHER PROTECTIVE CLOTHING OR EQUIPMENT
None

SECTION 9 - SPECIAL PRECAUTIONS

PRECAUTIONS TO BE TAKEN IN HANDLING & STORING

Store and handle according to packaged instructions

OTHER PRECAUTIONS
None

THE INFORMATION CONTAINED WITHIN WAS OBTAINED FROM AUTHORITATIVE SOURCES AND IS BELIEVED TO BE ACCURATE FOR
THE MANNER IN WHICH THE PRODUCT IS INTENDED TO BE USED. OTHER USES COULD RESULT IN CONSEQUENCES WHICH ARE NOT
CONSIDERED WITHIN THIS DOCUMENT.

Figure 3-3 *Continued*

Disposal procedures should be followed and enforced. The most frequent cause of a needle puncture or a puncture from other sharp objects is improper disposal. Failure to check sharps containers on a regular basis and to replace them when they are full encourages overstuffing them, which sometimes leads to injury. Portable bedside containers are available for workers when performing venipunctures or capillary punctures. Wall-mounted needle disposal containers are also available and make disposal very convenient.

As mentioned earlier, all needle punctures should be reported to the health services or proper authorities within the institution.

DEVELOPING A SAFETY MANAGEMENT PROGRAM

Every laboratory accredited by the CAP is required to have a safety management program. A safety management program is a program that identifies the guidelines necessary to provide a safe working environment that is free from recognizable hazards that can cause harm or injury. Many medical technologists assume positions as supervisors or laboratory safety officers. Responsibilities in these positions require knowledge of the safety principles and the development of a laboratory safety program.

This section provides an overview of the elements that should be considered in developing a safety program.

Beginning Stages: Research

Awareness of the standards and regulations that govern laboratories is a required step in the development of a safety program. Taking the time to become knowledgeable about the regulations and standards that relate to the procedures performed in the hematology laboratory is an essential first step. Some of the regulatory agencies that have standards, requirements, and guidelines are listed in Table 3-1.

Sorting through the regulatory maze can be frustrating, but the government agencies and voluntary organizations are quite willing to assist employers in complying with their standards.

Safety Program Elements

A proactive program should include the following ingredients:

Written Safety Plan—Written policies and procedures that explain the steps to be taken for all of the occupational hazards that exist in the lab.

Training Programs—Conducted annually for all employees. New employees should receive safety information on the first day that they are assigned to the hematology laboratory.

Job Safety Analysis—Can identify all of the tasks performed in hematology, the steps involved in performing the procedures, and the risk associated with the procedures.

Table 3-1. GOVERNMENT REGULATIONS

Department of Labor: 29 Code of Federal Regulations Parts 1900-1910

Hazard Communication Standard (right to know)	29 CFR 1910.1200
Occupational Exposure to Bloodborne Pathogens standard	29 CFR 1910.1030
Occupational Exposure to Hazardous Chemicals in Laboratories standard	29 CFR 1910.1450
Formaldehyde standard	29 CFR 1910.1048
Air contaminants: permissible exposure limits	29 CFR 1910.1000
Occupational Noise Level standard	29 CFR 1910.95
Hazardous Waste and Emergency Response standard	29 CFR 1910.126
Personal protective equipment	29 CFR 1910.132
Eye and face protection	29 CFR 1910.133
Respiratory protection	29 CFR 1910.134

Department of Interior: Environmental Protection Agency 40 Code of Federal Regulations Parts 200-399

Resource Conservation and Recovery Act (RCRA)
Medical Waste Tracking Act
Clean Air Act
Clean Water Act
Toxic Substances Control Act (TSCA)
Comprehensive Environmental Response, Compensation, and Liability Act (CERCLA)
Superfund Amendments and Reauthorization Act (SARA)
  SARA Title III: Community Right to Know Act

Voluntary Agencies/Accrediting Agencies
Joint Commission on the Accreditation of Healthcare Organizations (JCAHO)
College of American Pathologists (CAP)
State Public Health Departments
Centers for Disease Control and Prevention (CDC)

Abbreviation: CFR, Code of Federal Regulation.

Safety Awareness Program—Promotes a team concept and encourages employees to take an active part in the safety program.

Safety Audits and Follow-Up—A safety checklist should be developed for the hematology laboratory.

Reporting and Investigation of All Accidents, "Near Misses," or Unsafe Conditions—The causes of all incidents should be reviewed and corrective action taken, if necessary.

Emergency Drill and Evaluation—Periodic drills for all potential internal and external disasters. Drills should address the potential accident or disaster before it occurs and test the preparedness of the staff for an emergency situation. Planning for the accident and practicing the response to that accident reduces the panic that results when employees do not know the correct response to a situation.

Safety Committee/Department Safety Meetings—To communicate safety policies to the employees.

Review of Any Equipment Purchased for the Laboratory—For code compliance and safety features.

Annual Evaluation of the Safety Program—Review of the regulations for compliance in your laboratory.

SUMMARY

Working safely in the hematology laboratory is a performance issue. The day-to-day expectation of a medical technologist is to perform the analytic procedures accurately, precisely, and safely. Safety is included in that same error-free performance expectation. Safe practices must be incorporated into all the laboratory procedures and should be followed by every worker. Some common sense rules for safety are as follows:

- Be knowledgeable about the procedures that are being performed. If in doubt, ask for further instructions.
- Wear protective clothing and use protective equipment when required.
- Clean up all spills immediately.
- Keep work stations clean and corridors free from obstruction.
- Report injuries and unsafe conditions. Review accidents and incidents for the root cause of an accident. Take corrective action to prevent further injuries.
- Follow universal precautions in the laboratory at all times.

Safety is not a separate program; it is a part of the day-to-day activities in the laboratory, involving and requiring the cooperation of all staff members.

REVIEW QUESTIONS

1. What are the requirements of the Occupational Exposure to Bloodborne Pathogens standard?
2. Define universal precautions.
3. Describe the procedures for proper handwashing.
4. What is the proper disposal of sharps?

References

1. Garza D, Becan-McBride K: Phlebotomy Handbook, 3rd ed. Norwalk, CT: Appleton & Lange, 1993.
2. Department of Labor: 29 Code of Federal Regulations Parts 1900–1910. Federal Register, January 3, 1990.

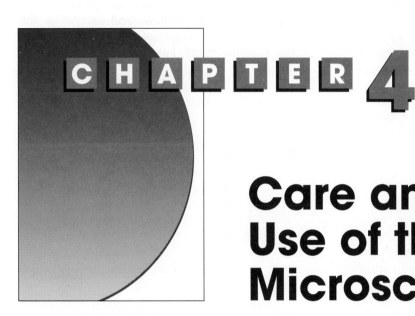

CHAPTER 4

Care and Use of the Microscope

M. Ann Wallace

Outline

Objectives

AFTER COMPLETION OF THIS CHAPTER, THE READER WILL BE ABLE TO

1. Identify the component parts of the microscope and explain the function of each.
2. Properly adjust a microscope by use of Koehler illumination.
3. Using correct technique, focus a stained blood film, with both dry and oil immersion objectives.
4. Demonstrate proper care and cleaning of the microscope.
5. Describe types of microscopy used in the clinical laboratory and their uses.

Microscopes available today reflect improvement in every aspect since the first microscope of Anton van Leeuwenhoek (1632–1723).[1] Advanced technology as applied to microscopy has resulted in computer-designed lens systems, sturdier stands, perfected condensers, and built-in illumination systems. Continued care and proper cleaning ensures the use of a powerful diagnostic instrument. The references listed at the end of the chapter deal with the physical laws of light and illumination as applied to microscopy.

PRINCIPLE OF MICROSCOPY

By the use of the compound microscope, an intermediate image of the illuminated specimen is formed by the objective lens in the optical tube. This image is then magnified and viewed through the eyepieces (Fig. 4–1).

An example of a *simple microscope* is a magnifying lens that enlarges objects that are difficult to view with the unaided eye. The 35-mm slide projector incorporates this system efficiently.

The *compound microscope* employs two separate lens systems, the product of which produces the final magnification. In standard microscopes, the brightfield illumination system, which passes light directly through the transparent specimen, is used.

COMPONENT PARTS AND FUNCTION OF EACH PART
(Fig. 4–2)

1. The *eyepieces,* or *oculars,* are usually equipped with 10× lenses (degree of magnification is 10 times). The lenses magnify the intermediate image formed by the objective lens in the optical tube; they also limit the area of visibility. Most microscopes have one fixed and one adjustable ocular. Both should be used correctly for optimal focus (see section on operating procedures). Eyepieces should not be interchanged with those of other models of microscopes. The eyepieces in a pair are optically matched.

2. The *interpupillary control* is used to adjust the lateral separation of the eyepieces for each individual. When properly adjusted, the user should be able to comfortably focus both eyes on the specimen and visualize *one* clear image.

3. The *optical tube* connects the eyepieces with the objective lens. The intermediate image is formed in this component. The standard length is 160 mm, which, functionally, is the distance from the real image plane (eyepieces) to the objective lenses.

4. The *neck,* or *arm,* provides a structural site of attachment for the revolving nosepiece.

5. The *stand* is the main vertical support of the microscope. The stage assembly, together with the condenser and base, is supported by the stand.

6. The *revolving nosepiece* holds the objectives and allows for easy rotation from one objective

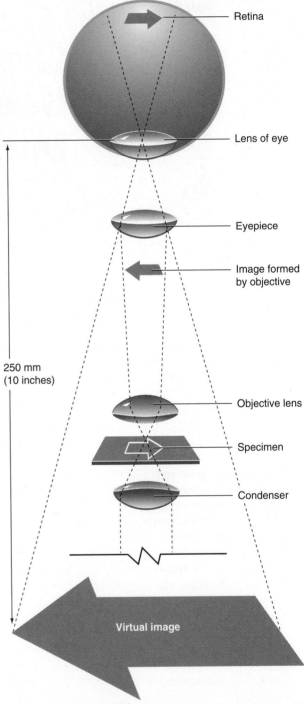

Figure 4–1 Compound microscope. (From Abramowitz M: The Microscope and Beyond, Vol. 1. Lake Success, NY: Olympus Corp., 1985:2. Reprinted courtesy of Eastman Kodak Company, Rochester, NY.)

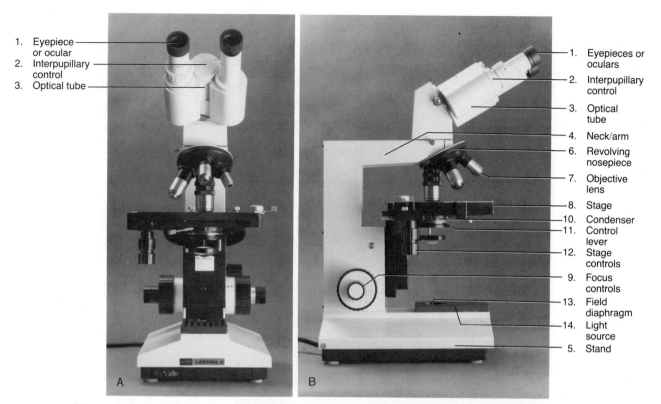

Figure 4–2 Components of a microscope. (Courtesy of Commercial Imaging & Design, Inc., Brighton, MI.)

lens to another. The working distance between the objectives and the slide varies with the make and model of the microscope.

7. There are usually three or four *objective lenses* (Fig. 4–3), each with a specific power of magnification. Engraved on the barrel of each objective lens is the power of magnification and numerical aperture (n.a.). The n.a. is related to the angle of light collected by the objective; in essence, it indicates the light-gathering ability of the objective lens. Functionally, the larger the n.a., the greater the *resolution* or the ability to distinguish between fine details of two closely situated objects.

Three standard powers of magnification/n.a. used in the hematology laboratory are 10×/ 0.25 (low power), 40×/0.65 (high power, dry), and 100×/1.25 (immersion oil). The smaller the magnification, the larger the viewing field; the larger the magnification, the smaller the viewing field. Total magnification is calculated by multiplying the magnification of the eyepiece by the magnification of the objective lens; for example, 10× (eyepiece) multiplied by 100× (oil immersion) is 1000 times total magnification.

Microscopes employed in the clinical laboratory are used with achromatic or planachromatic objective lenses, whose function is to correct for chromatic and spheric aberrations. *Chromatic aberrations* are caused by the spheric surface of the lens, which acts as a prism. As the various wavelengths pass through the lens, each focuses at a different point, causing concentric rings of color near the periphery of the lens. *Spheric aberrations* result as light waves travel through the varying thicknesses of the lens, blurring the image. The *achromatic objective lens* brings light of two colors into focus, partially correcting for the aberrations. When achromatic objective lenses are used, the center of the field is in focus, whereas the periphery is not. A *planachromatic lens,* which is more expensive, also corrects for curvature of the field, which results in a flat field with uniform focus.[23] Hence planachromatic lenses are sometimes referred to as "flat field" lenses. For critical microscopy, a *planapochromatic lens,* which brings light of three colors into focus and thereby almost completely corrects for chromatic aberration, may be used. This objective lens is extremely expensive and rarely needed for routine laboratory use.

A set of lenses with corresponding focal points all in the same plane is said to be *parfocal.* As the nosepiece is rotated from one magnification to another, the specimen remains in

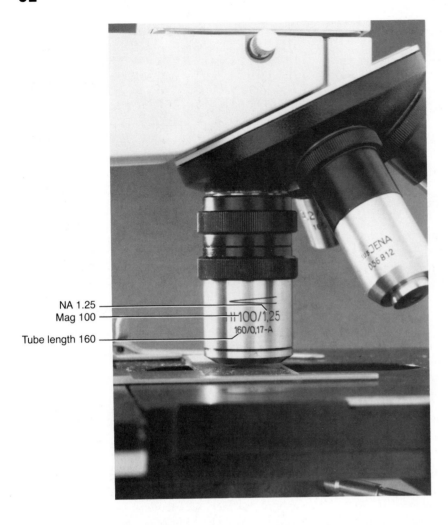

NA 1.25
Mag 100
Tube length 160

Figure 4–3 Microscope objective lens. (Courtesy of Commercial Imaging & Design, Inc., Brighton, MI.)

focus, and only minimal fine adjustment is necessary.

8. The *stage* supports the prepared microscopic slide to be reviewed. A spring assembly secures the slide to the stage.

9. The *focus controls* (or adjustments) can be incorporated into one knob or can be two separate controls. When one knob is used, it is moved in only one direction, engaging the coarse control; reversal of the knob activates the fine control. One gradation interval of turning is equivalent to 2 μm. Many microscopes are equipped with two separate adjustments: the coarse and the fine. The order of usage is the same: engage the coarse adjustment first and then fine-tune with the fine adjustment.

10. The *condenser,* consisting of several lenses in a unit, may be permanently mounted or vertically adjustable with a rack-and-pinion mechanism. It gathers, organizes, and directs the light through the specimen. Attached to and at the bottom of the condenser is the *aperture diaphragm,* an adjustable iris containing a number of leaves that control the angle and amount of the light sent through the specimen. The angle, also expressed as an n.a., regulates the balance between *contrast* (ability to enhance parts within a cell) and *resolution* (ability to differentiate fine details of two closely situated objects). The best resolution is achieved when this iris is used fully open, but there is some sacrifice in image contrast. In practice, this iris is closed only enough to create a slight increase in image contrast. Closing it beyond that point will lead to a loss of resolution and to the introduction of false detail.

Some microscopes are equipped with a swing-out lens immediately above or below the main condenser lens. This lens is used to permit a wider field of illumination when the n.a. of the objective lens is less than 0.25 (e.g., the 4×/0.12 objective lens).[4] If the swing-out lens is *above* the main condenser, it should be *out* for use with the 4× objective lens and *in* for lenses of magnification 10× and above. If it is *below* the condenser, it should be *in* for use with the 4X objective lens and *out* for lenses of magnification 10X and higher.

Stage and condenser (Fig. 4–4) consist of (a) a control lever for swing-out lens, (b) an aperture diaphragm stop lever, (c) a vertical adjustment of condenser, and (d) a condenser diaphragm.

11. The *control lever* swings the condenser top lens out of position.

12. The *stage controls* located under the stage move it in an x or a y axis.

13. The *field diaphragm* is located below the condenser within the base. When it is open, it allows a maximal-size circle of light to illuminate the slide. An almost closed diaphragm, when low power is used, assists in centralizing the condenser apparatus by the use of two centering screws. Some microscopes have permanently centralized condensers, whereas in others these screws are used for this function. The glass on top of the field diaphragm protects the diaphragm from dust and mechanical damage.

is imaged at the specimen, resulting in in-

14. Microscopes are dependent on electricity as the primary source for illumination power. There are two types of *brightfield illumination:* (1) critical illumination, in which the light source creased but uneven brightness, and (2) the Koehler (or Köhler) system, in which the light source is imaged at the condenser aperture diaphragm. The end result of Koehler illumination is a field of evenly distributed brightness across the specimen. Tungsten-halogen light bulbs are most frequently used as the illumination source. They consist of a tungsten filament enclosed in a very small quartz bulb that is filled with a halogen gas. Tungsten possesses a very high melting point and gives off very bright but yellowish light. A blue filter should be used to eliminate the yellow color emitted by tungsten. The light control knob turns on the light and should be the *only* control used to regulate the intensity of the light needed to visualize the specimen.

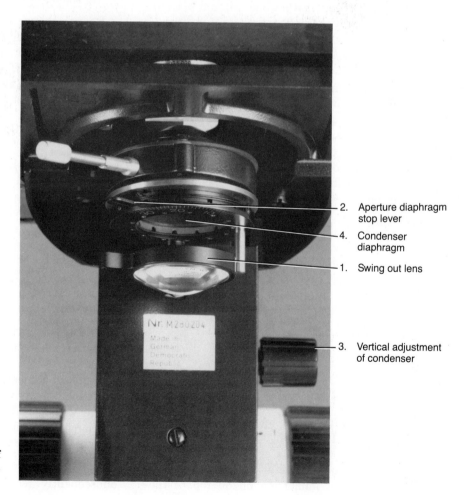

2. Aperture diaphragm stop lever

4. Condenser diaphragm

1. Swing out lens

3. Vertical adjustment of condenser

Figure 4–4 Condenser. (Courtesy of Commercial Imaging & Design, Inc., Brighton, MI.)

OPERATING PROCEDURE WITH KOEHLER ILLUMINATION

This applies to microscopes with a nonfixed condenser.

1. Connect the microscope to the power supply.
2. Turn on the light source.
3. Open all diaphragms.
4. Revolve the nosepiece until the 10× objective lens is directly above the stage.
5. Adjust the interpupillary control so that looking through both oculars yields one clear image.
6. Place a stained blood film on the stage and focus on it, using the fixed ocular, while covering the other eye. (Do not simply close the other eye, because this will necessitate adjustment of the pupil when you focus with the other ocular.)
7. Using the adjustable ocular and covering the opposite eye, focus on the specimen. Start with the eyepiece all the way out, and adjust inward.
8. Raise the condenser to its upper limit.
9. Focus the field so that the cells become sharp and clear. Concentrate on one cell and place it in the center of the field.
10. Close the field (lower) diaphragm. Look through the eyepieces. A small circle of light should be seen. If the light is not in the center of the field, center it by using the two centering screws located on the condenser. This step is essential as an off-center condenser will result in uneven distribution of light. Adjust the vertical height of the condenser so that you see a sharp image of the field diaphragm, ringed by a magenta halo. If the substage condenser is raised too much, the halo will be orange; if it is lowered too far, the halo will be blue.
11. Reopen the field diaphragm until the image is nearly at the edge of the field, and fine-tune the centering process.
12. Open the diaphragm slightly until the image just disappears.
13. Remove one ocular and, while looking through the microscope (without the ocular), close the condenser diaphragm completely. Reopen the condenser diaphragm until the leaves just disappear from view. Replace the ocular.
14. Rotate the nosepiece until the 40× objective lens is above the slide. Adjust the focus (which should be minimal) and find the cell that you had centered. If it is slightly off center, centralize it again with the stage x-y control. Note the greater amount of detail that you can see.
15. Place a drop of immersion oil on top of the slide. Rotate the nosepiece until the 100× objective lens is directly above the slide. Adjust the focus (which should be minimal) and observe the detail of the cell: the nucleus, its chromatin pattern, the cytoplasm, its color, and its texture. The objective lens should dip into the oil slightly.

Considerations

1. When revolving the nosepiece from one power to another, rotate it in such a direction that the 10× and 40× objective lenses never come into contact with the oil on a slide.
2. *Parcentric* is a term referring to the ability to center a cell in question in the microscopic field, rotating from one magnification power to another while retaining the cell close to the center of the viewing field. Re-centralizing the cell at each step is minimal. Most laboratory microscopes have this feature.
3. In general, when the 10× or 40× objective, lenses are used, the light intensity should be low. When the 100× objective lens is used, increase the intensity of light by using *only* the light control knob or neutral density filters.

Do not change the position of the condenser or the aperture lever to regulate light intensity. The condenser should always be in its upward position. The aperture lever is used only to achieve contrast of the features of the specimen being viewed.

IMMERSION OIL AND TYPES

Immersion oil is required when the 100× objective lens is used to increase the *refractive index.* The refractive index is the speed at which light travels in air, divided by the speed at which light travels through a substance. This oil, which has the same properties as glass, allows the objective lens to collect light from a very wide n.a., thus providing very high resolution of detail.

Three types of immersion oil differing in viscosity are employed in the clinical laboratory:

Type A—Very low viscosity, used in fluorescence and darkfield studies.
Type B—High viscosity, used in brightfield and standard clinical microscopy. In hematology, this oil is routinely used.
Type C—Very high viscosity, used with inclined microscopes with long-focus objective lenses and wide condenser gaps.

Bubbles in the oil tend to act as prisms and subsequently reduce resolution. Bubbles may be created when oil is applied to the slide. More often they are caused by lowering of the objective immediately into the oil. Sweeping the objective from right to left in the oil will eliminate bubbles.[2]

CARE OF THE MICROSCOPE

1. When not in use, the microscope should always be covered.
2. Before use, inspect the component parts. If dust is found, use an air syringe, a camel hair brush, or a soft nonlint cloth to remove it. Lens paper used directly on a dirty lens without removal of the dust first may scratch the lens.
3. Avoid placing your fingers on the lens surface. Fingerprints affect the contrast and resolution of the image.
4. Use solvent sparingly. The use of Xylol is discouraged because it contains a carcinogen component (benzene). Xylol is also a poor cleaning agent, leaving an oily film on the lens. Windex (or a similar solution) or 70% isopropyl alcohol used sparingly on a cotton applicator stick can be used to clean the objective lenses. Alcohol should be kept away from the periphery of the lenses, because alcohol can dissolve the cement and seep into the back side of the lens.
5. When fresh oil is added to residual oil on the 100× objective lens, there may be loss of contrast. First, clean off all residual oil.
6. Do not use water to clean lenses. Your condensed breath on the lens surface may be useful in cleaning slightly soiled lenses.
7. When transporting the microscope, place one hand under the base as support and one hand firmly around the arm.

BASIC TROUBLESHOOTING

The majority of common problems are related to inability to focus. Questions to be considered when the clinician is unable to focus a slide include the following:

1. Are you trying to obtain a "flat field" with an objective lens that is not planachromatic?
2. Is the slide right side up on the stage?
3. Are the oculars clean?
4. Are the oculars securely assembled?
5. Is the objective lens screwed in tightly?
6. Are the dry objective lenses and condenser free of oil?
7. Is the condenser adjusted to the proper height?
8. Is the coverslip on the right side of the smear? Are there two coverslips on the slide?
9. Is mounting media on the top of the coverslip?

THE MICROMETER RETICLE: ITS CALIBRATION AND USE

Size is one criterion used in the identification of blood cells. It is also one of the most important criteria in identifying parasites. The micrometer reticle, which is an ocular disc with an arbitrary scale etched on its surface, can be used to make measurements through the microscope. It must be calibrated in order to ascribe a specific measurement value to each ocular unit. The micrometer disc is inserted into one of the 10× eyepieces; a hemacytometer (see Chapter 12) is placed on the stage. The red blood cell (RBC) counting area of the hemacytometer is used. The entire square measures 1 mm² and is subdivided several times. The first subdivision is into 25 squares, each measuring 0.04 mm². Each of these 25 squares is further subdivided into 16 squares, each measuring 0.0025 mm², or 0.05 mm per side in length. This final measurement is used to convert ocular units to measurement in millimeters. (Fig. 4-5).

Procedure for Converting Ocular Units to Millimeters

1. With both the ocular disc and the hemacytometer in place, line up the "0" line of the ocular unit scale on the left with the inner line of the tri-line boundary of the hemacytometer.
2. Without moving the hemacytometer, find the first point to the right of the line where two lines are exactly superimposed. The distance will vary with the objective and the microscope. Proceed to the right and find the next point where two lines are exactly superimposed. Count the number of ocular units and the smallest red cell squares between these two points. In the example in Figure 4-4, the number of ocular points is 5, and the number of the smallest squares is 3.
3. Knowing that the linear measurement of each of the smallest divisions equals 0.05 mm, determine the total distance in millimeters between the two points of superimposition.

Calculation

1. The number of RBC small squares × 0.05 = distance in millimeters, so 3 × 0.05 = 0.15.
2. 1 ocular unit = $\dfrac{\text{total distance in mm}}{\text{total number of ocular units}}$

   $\dfrac{0.15}{5} = 0.03$ mm
3. To convert millimeters to microns, multiply by 1000: 0.03 × 1000 = 30 μ.

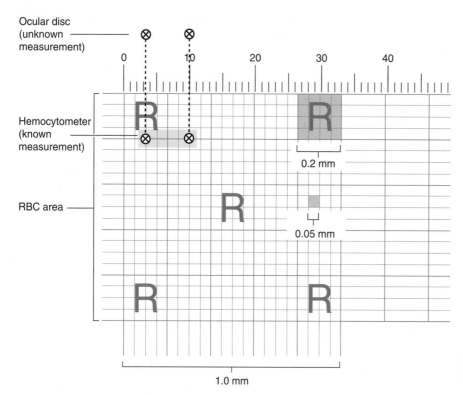

Ocular disc (unknown measurement)

Hemocytometer (known measurement)

RBC area

0.2 mm

0.05 mm

1.0 mm

Figure 4–5 Alignment of ocular disk with red blood cell area of hemacytometer.

THE MICROLOCATOR SLIDE

The microlocator slide is a commercially manufactured standard glass slide with an etched consecutive alphabet-number sequence running along the x and y axes (A1–A50; A1–Y1) (Fig. 4–6).

1. When a microscopist locates a cell of interest on a prepared slide, the cell should be centered under high dry or oil and then under the 10× objective lens. *Note whether the feathered edge of the blood film faces right or left.*
2. The slide should be carefully removed from the spring assembly, and the microlocator slide should be placed onto the stage.

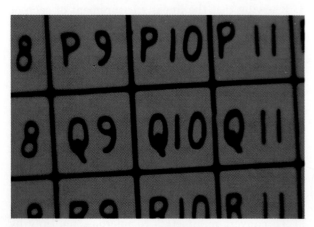

Figure 4–6 Microlocator slide.

3. The microlocator should be viewed through the eyepiece, and the letter/number combination should be recorded.
4. To relocate the cell, place the microlocator onto the stage and place the recorded letter/number combination in the center of the stage.
5. Remove the locator slide carefully and replace it with the initial blood smear. The cell of interest should be in the field.

OTHER MICROSCOPES USED IN THE CLINICAL LABORATORY

Phase Contrast Microscopy

In brightfield microscopy, a stained specimen may be viewed because of its ability to absorb the light passing through it. With unstained specimens, the degree of light absorption may be so light as to render the specimen mostly invisible. In phase contrast, special equipment is employed to enable these unstained specimens to be clearly seen. The phase contrast equipment accomplishes this by converting the phase wave shift of light passing through the specimen into an amplitude shift (absorption) that can be seen. Phase contrast is used to perform manual platelet counts, urinalysis, histologic studies, and cytologic studies.

Polarized Light Microscopy

Polarized light microscopy is another contrasting technique used to identify certain crystalline chemicals. Crystals affect the plane of polarization of light passing through it. The wave energy of light is normally transmitted in all planes perpendicular to the direction of propagation. A polarizing filter transmits light vibrating in only one of these planes, creating polarized light. If two filters (polarizers) were used with their transmission axes oriented at right angles, no light would pass through the pair. Certain crystals rotate a plane of polarized light passing through them. When the crystal is viewed between a pair of crossed filters (one in the condenser side of the microscope and the other in the ocular side), the crystal is seen magnified against a black background because the rotated plane of light emerging from the crystal is no longer perpendicular to the second filter. The effect may be highly dependent on the orientation of the crystal (as with birefringent crystals). The effect that these crystals have on polarized light yields clues to their specific chemical composition. Polarized microscopy is used to identify crystals in synovial fluid (see Chapter 38) and in chemistry studies and in urinalysis.

Darkfield Microscopy

Darkfield microscopy is a contrasting technique that employs a special condenser. The condenser sends light up toward the specimen in a hollow cone. Because of the high angle of this cone, none of the illuminating rays enter the objective lens. Without the specimen in place, the field would appear black because of the absence of light. However, where fine detail exists in the specimen, light is diffracted in all directions. This diffracted light is picked up by the objective lens and appears as bright detail on a black background. Darkfield is used in microbiology in the identification of the causative agent of syphilis. When combined with the use of fluorochrome dyes, darkfield fluorescence microscopy can be used to identify lymphocyte subsets.

SUMMARY

Standard microscopes employing Koehler illumination are used in routine studies in the clinical laboratory. Various methods of modifying the illumination system have resulted in phase contrast, polarized light, darkfield, fluorescence, and electron microscopy. These systems have provided increased visibility of specimen features not visualized with brightfield illumination. With continued care, the microscope will provide a valuable diagnostic tool to the user.

REVIEW QUESTIONS

1. Use of which of the following objective lenses causes the center of the microscope field to be in focus, while the periphery is blurred?
   a. planachromatic
   b. achromatic
   c. planapochromatic
   d. flat field

2. Which of the following gathers, organizes, and directs light through the specimen?
   a. ocular
   b. objective lens
   c. condenser
   d. optical tube

3. After focusing a specimen by using the 40× objective, the technologist switches to a 10× objective. The specimen remains in focus. This characteristic is referred to as
   a. parfocality
   b. parcentrality
   c. compensation
   d. Koehler magnification

4. The objective with the greatest degree of color correction is the
   a. achromatic
   b. planapochromatic
   c. bichromatic
   d. planachromatic

5. The total magnification obtained when a 10× ocular and a 10× objective lens is used is
   a. 1×
   b. 10×
   c. 100×
   d. 1000×

6. Once a microscope has been adjusted for Koehler illumination, light intensity should *never* be regulated by using the
   a. transformer
   b. neutral density filter
   c. Koehler magnifier
   d. condenser

7. The recommended cleaner for removing oil from objectives is
   a. 70% alcohol or Windex
   b. xylol
   c. water
   d. benzene

References

1. Asimov I. Understanding Physics: Light, Magnetism, and Electricity. London: George Allen & Unwin, 1966.
2. Oldham AD. Care and use of the microscope. *In* Wentworth BB (ed): Diagnostic Procedures for Mycotic and Parasitic Infections, 7th ed. Washington, DC: American Public Health Association, 1988:567–597.
3. Benford JR: The Theory of the Microscope, 4th ed. Rochester, New York: Bausch & Lomb, 1965.
4. Leitz E: Leitz Teaching and Routine Microscope—Operating Instructions. Wetzlar, Germany: E. Leitz, undated.

Suggested Readings

Eggert AA: Electronics and Instrumentation for the Clinical Laboratory. New York: Wiley Medical, 1983.

Brown BA: Hematology: Principles and Procedures, 6th ed. Philadelphia: Lea & Febiger, 1993.

CHAPTER 5

Quality Control/Quality Assurance

John Krause

Outline

Objectives

AFTER COMPLETION OF THIS CHAPTER, THE READER WILL BE ABLE TO

1. Define terms commonly used in quality control.
2. Discuss statistics involved in describing populations.
3. Distinguish between types of errors in test systems or methods.
4. Differentiate between internal and external quality control.
5. Discuss several methods used to monitor internal quality control.
6. List organizations offering external quality control programs.
7. Discuss the role of continuing education in maintaining a quality laboratory.
8. Briefly discuss the role that quality control plays in a total quality assurance program.

There is much emphasis today in the health care arena for the implementation of quality assurance procedures to monitor the delivery of health care in the presence of rapidly rising health care costs. The Joint Commission on Accreditation of Healthcare Organizations (JCAHO) is focusing extensively and intensively on quality assurance procedures to evaluate the outcome of the quality of medical care delivered by all providers. This chapter is limited to quality control and quality assurance procedures in the clinical laboratory and, in particular, the clinical hematology laboratory.

The terms *quality control* and *quality assurance* are used to refer to the control of the testing process to ensure that the test results meet their quality requirements. The terms have overlapping definitions and are frequently used interchangeably. *Quality assurance* is the coordinated effort to organize all the various activities in the laboratory in order to provide the best possible service to the patient and to the physician. It is not a single activity; rather, it includes controlling and monitoring the competence of personnel, quality of materials, method, reagents, instruments, and the reporting of test results, as well as patient/physician satisfaction and the financial costs attributable to the laboratory. *Quality control* involves the process of monitoring the characteristics of the testing system. This is done by studying control samples along with the patient's sample and analyzing the results with appropriate statistical methods to establish accuracy and precision, which are benchmarks for determining conformance and, hence, acceptability of results. It also involves taking any necessary corrective actions to bring the results into conformance. Quality control is an important part of the quality assurance program. Quality assurance, however, is more expansive and entails monitoring of numerous parameters.

DEFINITIONS

The following definitions are used in the monitoring of quality control in the clinical laboratory.

Accuracy—The *exactness* of a measurement in comparison with the true value. This true value is normally not known in the laboratory unless the specimen is a *reference material.*

Precision—The extent to which replicate analyses of a sample agree with each other. In the laboratory this is known as *reproducibility.* Precision provides an indication of the random error of the measurement; the more precise a measurement is, the less random error and the better the repeatability. Precision is often expressed as

the coefficient of variation. A method may yield precise results but not accurate results. Results that are both accurate and precise are desirable. See Figure 5–1.

Delta Checks—Involves comparing the result from the analysis of a sample with the result from the previous sample for the same analyte. A difference greater than the expected run-to-run precision, day-to-day precision, or a clinically defined significant value established for that method must be considered an analytic error (exceeds delta check) until it is proved to be otherwise by inquiry into the patient's condition or review of the patient's chart. This way of evaluating the precision or accuracy of a method is much easier if a laboratory computer is available to search each patient's file of laboratory results.

Reference (Normal) Range—The term *normal range* is frequently used in reference to the range of values for an analyte in healthy persons. There is always some uncertainty about what "normal" or healthy is, and the term *reference interval* or *reference range* has been suggested as more appropriate. A reference population, therefore, is a group of persons from whom the data was obtained to establish the reference interval. Each laboratory must define its own reference intervals for the instruments that it uses and for the population that it serves. Reference intervals should be established for adults (male and female), as well as for children. Within the pediatric group, "normal" values may change dramatically over short age intervals, and it is appropriate to establish reference intervals for newborns, infants, and the various pediatric age groups (see Chapter 36). The number of people needed for determining a reference interval is dependent on the method of calculating the reference interval. With carefully selected groups, the sample size may be as small as 25. With less carefully chosen groups, data from 500 or more persons may be necessary to establish an appropriate distribution of values.

Reliability—Refers to the extent to which a method is able to maintain both accuracy and precision over a period of time. The methods in use in the clinical laboratory should have a high degree of reliability. All aspects of a testing system (instrument, reagent, and ancillary quality control materials) must be monitored to ensure continued reliability.

Primary Standard—A reference material that is of fixed and known composition and capable of being prepared in essentially pure form; also, any certified reference material that is generally accepted or officially recognized as the unique

Poor precision and poor accuracy   Good precision and poor accuracy   Good precision and good accuracy

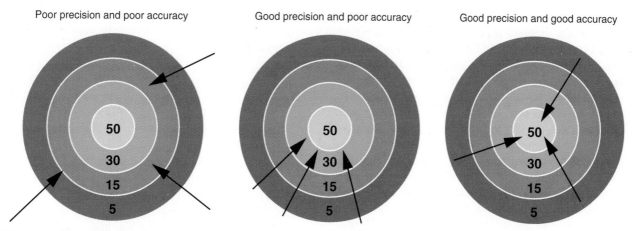

Figure 5–1 Examples of precision and accuracy.

standard for the assay, regardless of its level of purity.

Secondary Standard—A reference material in which the analyte concentration has been ascertained by reference to a primary standard.

STATISTICAL DESCRIPTION OF POPULATIONS

A laboratory measurement is inexact. If a single specimen is repeatedly analyzed under identical conditions, a series of nonidentical results is obtained. These nonidentical values arise from the random variation that is present in all measured parameters. When numerous results are obtained from the repeated analysis, their frequency distribution will approximate a *normal,* or *gaussian,* distribution (Fig. 5–2). Distribution of many medical measurements in populations approximates the gaussian curve. The value at the center of a gaus-

sian distribution is the *mean* $(\overline{x})$. The mean is a measure of central tendency and is calculated by dividing the sum of all results by the number of results. The distribution of gaussian data about this mean is expressed as the *standard deviation (s),* which is a statistical measurement of the imprecision among observations of analytic results. According to Figure 5–2, 68.26% of the results are located within the interval bounded by the $\overline{x} \pm 1.0s$ line, 95.46% are within the $\overline{x} \pm 2.0s$ lines, and 99.73% are within the $\overline{x} \pm 3.0s$ lines. These intervals represent specific *confidence intervals.* The $\overline{x} \pm 2s$ interval is the 95.5% confidence interval, which means that there is a 95.5% probability that any given results will fall within the $\overline{x} \pm 2.0s$ line. If a population has a gaussian distribution, only the mean and standard deviation are necessary to describe the population. Virtually all quality control procedures in the clinical laboratory assume a gaussian distribution. Causes of deviation include outliers, shifts, nonrandom variation, and instabil-

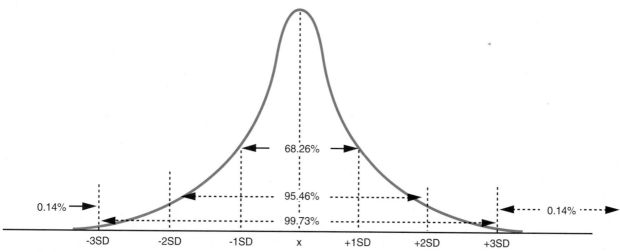

Figure 5–2 Gaussian distribution.

ity of the analytic method. The *coefficient of variation (CV)* is a unitless number that is calculated as $100s/\bar{x}$; the smaller the CV value, the more precise is the analytic method. Examples of the calculations for the terms just described are included in Table 5–1.[1]

Other parameters that are used to describe test results are sensitivity and specificity. The diagnostic *sensitivity* is the proportion of patients with the disease who have a positive test result. It is defined by the ratio ($a/a + b \times 100$), where a is the number of true positive results and b is the number of false negative results. The diagnostic *specificity* is the proportion of patients who are correctly identified by the test as not having the disease. It is defined by the ratio ($c/c + d \times 100$), where c is the number of false positive results and d is the number of true negative results. The diagnostic sensitivity and specificity of a test also influence how the test should be used when there is a clinical suspicion of a disease. A very sensitive test should be used when normal serves to rule out a suspected disease, whereas a very specific test should be used when abnormal serves to confirm the presence of a disease.

TYPES OF ERRORS

SYSTEMATIC

Systematic errors are errors within the test system or method. These may be caused by incorrect calibration procedures, malfunctioning components, or failure of some part of the testing process to perform accurately or precisely. Systematic errors are further subdivided into proportional and constant systematic errors.

Constant Systematic. These are errors in the test system in which the magnitude of an error remains constant throughout the range of the test measurement; this situation is also known as a constant bias.

Proportional Systematic. These are errors in the test system in which the magnitude of an error increases with the concentration of the substance being measured.

RANDOM

Random errors are mistakes that occur without prediction or regularity.

INTERNAL QUALITY CONTROL

Internal quality control involves the analysis of control samples along with patients' specimens and evaluation of the results statistically to determine the acceptability of the analytic run. In internal quality control, a test method's precision and analytic bias are monitored. A control sample is a special specimen inserted into the testing process and treated as if it were a patient's sample. It should have appropriate concentrations at medically significant levels that the physician uses to make decisions concerning treatment. A distinction must be made between controls and calibrators or standards. Calibrators and standards are used to adjust instrumentation or to define a standard curve for analysis. In addition to having an accurately assigned value that has been assayed by a reference method, the calibrator should have the same characteristics as the control method. *Calibration and control materials are not interchangeable.* The control must be completely independent of the calibration process so that systematic errors caused by deterioration of the calibrator or a change in the analytic process are detected.

The attributes of the ideal hematology control material have been described by Bachner[2] and are listed in Table 5–2.

Although control materials for clinical chemistry perform reasonably well, most of the commercially available hematology control products unfortunately fall short of this ideal performance. Even

Table 5–1. SELECTED CALCULATIONS USED IN QUALITY CONTROL		
Hemoglobin Value (g/dL)	$x - \bar{x}$	$(x - \bar{x})^2$
12.2	0.1	0.01
12.3	0.0	0
12.5	0.2	0.04
12.5	0.2	0.04
11.9	0.4	0.16
12.5	0.2	0.04
12.8	0.5	0.25
12.3	0.0	0
11.8	0.5	0.25
12.2	0.1	0.01
12.7	0.4	0.16
12.4	0.1	0.01
11.9	0.4	0.16
12.2	0.1	0.01

CONFIDENCE INTERVALS

     1 *s* (65% of values) = 12.0–12.6
     2 *s* (95% of values) = 11.7–12.9
     3 *s* (99% of values) = 11.4–13.2

Sum (Σ) = 172.2. Mean $\bar{x} = \dfrac{\Sigma x}{n}$, where n = number of values;

$\bar{x} = \dfrac{172.2}{14} = 12.3$.

Standard deviation (s) = $\sqrt{\dfrac{+\Sigma(x - \bar{x})^2}{n - 1}}$; $s = \sqrt{\dfrac{1.14}{13}} = 0.3$. (Use n if number of observations is ≥30, $n - 1$ if <30.)

Coefficient of variation (CV) = $\dfrac{100(s)}{\bar{x}}$; CV = $100\left(\dfrac{0.3}{12.3}\right) = 2.4\%$.

Table 5-2. AN IDEAL HEMATOLOGY CONTROL SUBSTANCE
Inexpensive
Prolonged stability
Sampled directly
Suspends easily and does not agglutinate
Flow characteristics similar to those of blood
Optical and electrical proportions similar to blood
Particle size and shape similar to blood
Assayable by independent methods

Modified from Bachner P: Quality assurance in hematology. *In* Howanitz JF, Howanitz JH (eds): Laboratory Quality Assurance, New York: McGraw-Hill, 1987:214–243.

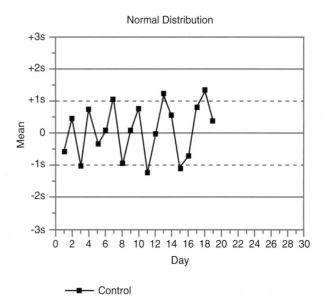

Figure 5-3 Normal Levey-Jennings control plot.

though current hematology controls are not ideal, they do have several advantages over retained patients' specimens. Because they are assayed materials, they can be used to verify calibration after maintenance procedures and daily start-up. They are also convenient and are more stable than retained patients' specimens.

Quantitative Procedures

Levey-Jennings Control Charts. In 1950, Levey and Jennings suggested the use of control charts in the clinical laboratory.[3] This suggestion was based on the observation that in a stable test environment, the distribution of the results of the same sample analyzed a number of times has a gaussian distribution. The Levey-Jennings control chart indicates the mean and the one-, two-, and three-standard deviation ranges on both sides of the mean. Deviation from this distribution indicates the occurrence of an analytic systematic error. In a random distribution, therefore, approximately 65% of the values will be between the ±1s (standard deviation) ranges and will be evenly distributed on either side of the mean. In a properly operating system, 95% of the values should fall between the ±2s ranges, and 99%, between the ±3s limits. This means that one data point in 20 should be located between either of the 2s and 3s limits, and one data point will occur outside of the 3s limits once in every 100 analyses. More than one point outside of the 3s limits per 100 analyses signifies that some form of error has occurred and that investigation is necessary. The ±2s limits are considered warning limits. Values that exceed the 2s and 3s limits indicate that the analysis should be repeated. The ±3s limits are rejection limits. When a point exceeds the limits expected, the analysis should stop, the patients' results held, and the system investigated. An example of a normal Levey-Jennings control plot is illustrated in Figure 5-3.

The pattern of the data points plotted over time is important for spotting shifts and trends in the calibration of the test method. A *shift* is a drift of values from one level of the control chart to another (Fig. 5-4). The shift may be sudden or gradual; in the latter case, it is referred to as a *trend*. A trend is the continuous movement of values in one direction over six or more consecutive values (Fig. 5-5). In hematology, trends may be caused by deterioration of reagents or problems with pump tubing or light sources.

The occurrence of shifts or trends is the result of either proportional or constant systematic analytic error. Random error is evidenced by an increased

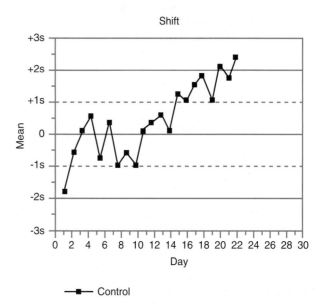

Figure 5-4 Shift.

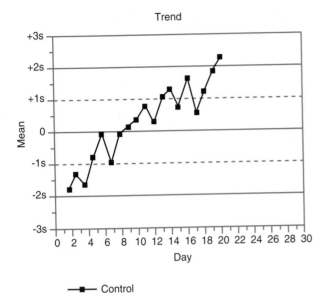

Figure 5–5 Trend.

number of values beyond the ±2s limits. More than one in 20 values beyond this limit is indicative of increased random error.

Multi-Rule (Westgard) Analysis

Although a single level of control at a decision level enables monitoring of the test process at that particular concentration, two levels of control at different concentrations will be more effective for statistically evaluating and monitoring the method. One control should have a low concentration and the other a high concentration at medically significant levels or at the ends of the test methods linearity range. Westgard and associates have formulated a series of multi-rules to help evaluate paired control runs.[4] Running and evaluating the results of two controls simultaneously allows shifts and trends to be detected earlier. These multi-rules are as follows:

1_{2s} **Rule**—A control value is outside a 2s limit. This is a warning of a possible error of the instrument or method malfunction.

1_{3s} **Rule**—One value is outside a 3s limit. This may be the result of a random error and should be investigated.

2_{2s} **Rule**—Two consecutive values are outside the same 2s limits. This may be within the same control run involving both levels of control exceeding the same +2 or −2 limit or two consecutive analyses of the same control material exceeding the same 2s limit. Investigate as out of control.

R_{4s} **Rule**—Two consecutive values are more than 4s apart involving both control materials. One

control is beyond the +2 limit and the other beyond the −2 limit. Investigate as out of control. See Figure 5–6 as an example of this violation.

4_{1s} **Rule**—Four consecutive values have been plotted on the same side of the 1s range. This may be within or across control materials. Violation of this rule indicates a shift or trend in the analytic process.

10_x **Rule**—Violation occurs when 10 consecutive values fall on the same side of the mean either within the same control or across both controls. This indicates a shift in the analytic process.

These rules can be adapted to a control chart similar to the Levey-Jennings chart: violation of the rules indicates the type of error that occurs. Rejection by the 1_{3s} and R_{4s} rules suggests random error. Rejection by the 2_{2s}, 4_{1s}, and 10_x rules either by themselves or in combination with others suggests that systematic errors have occurred in the system.

Moving Averages of the Red Blood Cell Indices

In 1974, Bull and colleagues[5] proposed a method of using patients' red blood cell indices to monitor the performance of hematology analyzers. Their formula for calculation of the moving average is beyond the scope of this text; however, several of the manufacturers of multichannel analyzers have incorporated this formula and calculation into the computerization of their data analysis. The red blood cell indices, MCV, MCH, and MCHC, are

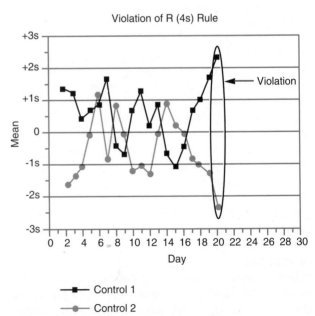

Figure 5–6 Violation of R_{4s} rule.

relatively constant throughout a population and change little. By calculating a moving average on the patients' values, an indication of the method's precision and accuracy can be determined. Values from groups of 20 patients are collected. Bull and colleagues' algorithm smoothes and trims data so as to control the effect of outliers. This calculation is also referred to as an $\overline{X}b$. As long as the majority of the patients are from the same population, any trend or shift of the moving averages when plotted on a control chart strongly suggests an instrument error.

To set up an individual hematologic analysis for using this moving average method, the instrument must be calibrated and the precision determined to be acceptable. The indices of 500 consecutive patients are analyzed and averaged to determine the mean values for the MCV, MCH, and MCHC, respectively. Control ranges are calculated to be ±3% of the mean. Action is then taken when points fall on or are outside the control limits. Use of computerization to calculate the $\overline{X}b$ values on each group of 20 patients makes life much easier.

This method is not sensitive to random errors and is less sensitive than commercial controls to small systematic shifts. The method is sensitive to the patient population; a number of oncology patients, for example, could affect the calculation in the absence of instrument malfunction. Finally, this method does not directly monitor the white blood cell and platelet counts.

Automated Differential Counting

The imprecision and inaccuracy of the routine manual differential count has been well documented.[6] This imprecision is attributable to nonrandom cell distribution, cell identification errors, and statistical sampling errors caused by the small numbers of cell counted (usually 100–200).[7] The automated screening differential instruments count thousands of cells, thus greatly reducing the statistical sampling error and allowing for a high degree of precision. However, quality control of the automated screening differential poses a new challenge. Manufacturers offer fixed cells or particles as controls for differential counts. These controls are not without problems. The imprecision of manual counts, with the limited number of cells examined, clearly limits their usefulness as a dependable control for the automated differential. Each laboratory must also establish its own criteria for when the automated differential should be reviewed. These criteria will vary in accordance with the type of instrument being used and the population served.

EXTERNAL QUALITY CONTROL

In internal quality control programs in which control materials analyzed at specific intervals are used, the precision of a test method, but not its accuracy, is monitored. The accuracy of a test procedure can be evaluated by comparing the performance of the analysis with an external quality control program, such as proficiency surveys, and/or with required control programs, such as state surveys. The external control programs provide a means whereby the performance of each laboratory or participant on an identical specimen can be evaluated and compared against the performance of laboratories with the same or similar methods. The group mean or consensus result of the group is considered to be the "true," or accurate, value. A laboratory performance is evaluated by how close its results compare with those of the mean opinion of the group. External quality control programs exist for both quantitative and qualitative methods. The College of American Pathologists (CAP) Survey Program is probably the best known and is representative of most proficiency surveys. Participation in such an external program is necessary for meeting the requirements of regulatory and accrediting agencies such as the JCAHO, as well as of the Clinical Laboratory Improvement Act (CLIA) 88.

CONTINUING EDUCATION

An active continuing education program will help maintain technical performance at a continued high level. Programs and workshops on peripheral blood cell identification are a means of improving and maintaining a good level of intralaboratory precision. Lectures and seminars correlating the cytograms and histograms obtained from the automated differential instruments with peripheral blood findings maintain a high level of awareness on the part of the technologist for abnormalities that may be present on the peripheral blood smear. This helps to detect spurious, specimen-related variables that can produce a variety of inaccurate results in automated hematology, such as spurious macrocytosis due to cold agglutinins, particulate interference that may be produced by cryoglobulins, and pseudoleukocytosis and pseudothrombocytopenia in ethylenediaminetetraacetic acid (EDTA) collected blood. As Stewart and Koepke pointed out, "The best prevention of errors and mistakes is a well-trained and conscientious technologist."[1]

QUALITY ASSURANCE

This chapter has emphasized quality control, which is only one portion of the total quality assurance program. Space restrictions limit the discussion of quality assurance. The JCAHO defined a 10-step program for the monitoring and evaluation process; this program is divided into preanalytic, analytic, and postanalytic phases.[8] In the laboratory, the measurement step has received the most attention, although the other phases are now being included.

In 1988, Q probes, a subscription program under the auspices of the CAP, was developed.[9] The aim of this program was to provide a formatted program for institutions that have not been able to develop programs themselves. Experts in quality assurance were assembled to develop a consensus of appropriate indicators of quality for pathology and laboratory medicine. The aim was also to provide a program that would document practice patterns, provide scientific evidence on which improvement could occur, and improve the care of the patients served. This program has been very successful.

Each institution should develop activities that generally follow the 10-step monitoring and evaluation process of the JCAHO. Each laboratory, after studying the scope of services they provide, should develop and implement a set of *indicators* unique for their own setting. Furthermore, for each indicator, a threshold that the laboratory should attempt to meet should be defined and set. Some of these indicators might include the appropriateness of the test ordered, the turnaround time, proper identification of the patient at the time of phlebotomy, complications of phlebotomy, specimen adequacy, correct specimen drawn, number of tests per patient per day, number of stat tests, reporting errors in tests, and customer satisfaction (both patient and physician.) Obviously there are many other indicators that might be included in a laboratory quality assurance program. The ability of the laboratory and the personnel to meet the thresholds of these indicators should be discussed at monthly quality assurance laboratory meetings, and the minutes should be recorded. Results and/or suggestions from the laboratory quality assurance team should be presented and discussed at the Hospital Quality Assurance meeting, at which representatives from other areas and divisions of the hospital are included. The ability to improve laboratory services and care of patients can often be implemented at this level as the important indicators and findings are discussed. Quality assurance is becoming increasingly more important, and it is necessary for all levels of laboratory personnel to participate in and help define the best and proper indicators that will ensure the optimal and most effective health care.

SUMMARY

Quality assurance is the coordinated effort of personnel to enhance care of patients through the monitoring, evaluation, and improvement of all aspects of laboratory service. A set of indicators, such as turnaround time, reporting errors in tests, and customer satisfaction should be determined for each laboratory on the basis of the scope of services provided. Quality control is the component of quality assurance that involves the process of monitoring the characteristics of the testing system, primarily statistical. Quality control includes internal and external components, as well as continuing education to maintain technical performance.

Because quality assurance is desirable not only within an institution but within the entire health care system, the JCAHO closely monitors the outcome of the quality of health care delivered by all providers. Several commercial programs are available, or an institution may wish to develop its own program.

REVIEW QUESTIONS

1. The reference range for hemoglobin on a control sample is 13.0 ± 0.4 g/dL. A hemoglobin determination is performed five times in succession. The results are (in grams per deciliter) 12.0, 12.3, 12.0, 12.2, and 12.1. These results are
   a. precise, but not accurate
   b. both accurate and precise
   c. accurate, but not precise
   d. neither accurate nor precise

2. A mean value of 6.0×10^9/L is determined for a leukocyte count. One standard deviation (s) is 0.3×10^9/L. The 95.5% confidence limits would be (as 10^9 per liter)
   a. 3.0–9.0
   b. 5.4–6.6
   c. 5.5–6.5
   d. 5.7–6.3

3. On a run of 20 hemoglobin samples, 95% are 0.4 g/dL above known values. This type of error is known as
   a. random
   b. proportional systematic
   c. constant systematic
   d. coefficient of variation

4. The following data for leukocyte counts is extracted from the last 10 control specimens run on an automated instrument (in 10^9 per liter): 7.2, 7.6, 6.8, 7.2, 6.9, 6.8, 7.4, 7.5, 6.9, 7.2. These data
   a. represent a normal distribution
   b. represent a trend
   c. represent a shift
   d. are impossible to interpret

5. The control value for an erythrocyte count is $4.00 \pm 0.4 \times 10^{12}/L$ (2s). On two successive days, the technologist obtains a value of $4.65 \times 10^{12}/L$. According to Levey-Jennings control charts, this value is
   a. a warning limit
   b. acceptable, because it could be repeated
   c. a rejection limit
   d. within normal random error

6. Given the following values for hemoglobin, calculate the mean. (All values in grams per deciliters.) 7.3, 7.7, 7.3, 7.2, 7.5, 7.4, 7.5, 7.3, 7.6, 7.2

7. For the example in Question 6, calculate the standard deviation.

References

1. Stewart CE, Koepke, JA: Basic quality assurance practices for clinical laboratories. Philadelphia: JB Lippincott, 1987:216.
2. Bachner P: Quality assurance in hematology. In Howanitz JF, Howanitz JH (eds): Laboratory Quality Assurance. New York: McGraw-Hill, 1987:214–243.
3. Levey S, Jennings ER: The use of control charts in the clinical laboratory. Am J Clin Pathol 1950; 20:1059–1066.
4. Westgard JO, Barry PL, Hunt MR, Groth T: A multi-rule Shewhart chart for quality control in clinical chemistry. Clin Chem 1981; 27:493–501.
5. Bull BS, Elashoff RM, Heilbron DC, et al: A study of various estimators for the derivation of quality control procedures from patient erythrocyte indices. Am J Clin Pathol 1974; 61:473–481.
6. Koepke JA, Dotson MA, Shifman MA: A critical evaluation of the manual/visual differential leukocyte counting method. Blood Cells 1985; 11:173–186.
7. Pierre RV: Differential counting. In Koepke JA (ed): Laboratory Hematology. New York: Churchill Livingstone, 1984: 973–997.
8. Fromberg R: Monitoring and Evaluation. Chicago: Pathology and Medical Laboratory Services, Joint Commission on Accreditation of Health Care Organizations, 1987.
9. Howanitz PJ, Schifman RB, Steindel SJ, et al: A nationwide quality assurance program can describe standards for the practice of pathology and laboratory medicine. Qual Assur Health Care 1992; 3:245–256.

Hematopoiesis

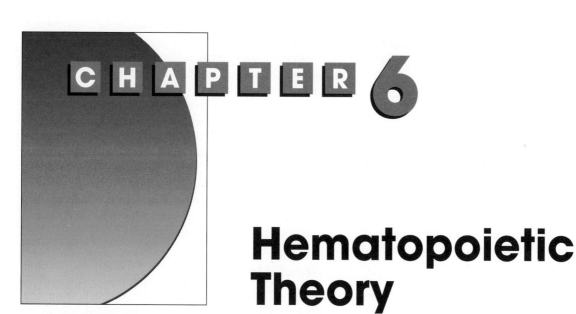

CHAPTER 6

Hematopoietic Theory

M. Ann Wallace

Outline

Objectives

AFTER COMPLETION OF THIS CHAPTER, THE READER WILL BE ABLE TO

1. Define hematopoiesis.
2. Discuss the evolutionary (embryonic, fetal, and adult) formation of blood cells.
3. Relate architecture of hematopoietic tissue to role in cellular formation.
4. Identify the blood cells in hierarchical order of elaboration.
5. Identify the various growth factors, their modes of action, and their target cells.
6. Discuss the general hematopoietic stem cell theories.

HEMATOPOIETIC DEVELOPMENT

Hematopoiesis encompasses the formation, development, and specialization of all formed elements into functional blood cells. Hematopoiesis progresses in three phases: mesoblastic, hepatic, and medullary.

Mesoblastic Phase

Shortly after fertilization (2–3 weeks), the blastocyst differentiates into three distinct layers: the ectoderm, the mesoderm, and the endoderm. The mesoderm gives rise to basophilic cells collectively known as "blood islands."[1] The peripheral cells of these islands flatten while their nuclei elongate as they develop into a continuous system of tubular blood vessels.[2] By day 28, a circulation is established between the embryo, the yolk sac, and the chorionic vesicle. Blood of the embryo then circulates through the newly formed vascular system.[3]

Simultaneously, the central cells of the island become detached and enter the primitive plasma. A number of yolk sac stem cells further differentiate into primitive erythroblasts. These cells are the earliest recognizable hemoglobin-synthesizing cells. Morphologically, they appear megaloblastic (large and asynchronous; see Chapter 16), exhibiting a nucleus with coarse clumped chromatin and very basophilic cytoplasm.[4] Unlike pronormoblasts of adult bone marrow, the primitive erythroblasts do not give rise to mature anucleated erythrocytes.

These primitive pluripotential cells, which ex-hibit ameboid movement in the embryo, represent the precursors of all blood cell lines.[5] There is, however, evidence that these cells have a shortened life span.

Because mesoderm is so widespread in the developing tissues, blood cells are formed in many areas. Eventually, with tissue specialization, blood cell production is restricted to specific limited sites. The yolk sac proper evaginates and differentiates into tissue, giving rise to the digestive organs and the liver.[3] By the sixth week, yolk sac hematopoiesis is undetectable. Measurable hematopoietic products at this time include Portland, Gower-1 and Gower-2 hemoglobins (see Chapter 9), primitive erythroblasts, granulocytes, and non-platelet producing megakaryocytes.

Hepatic Phase

These primitive erythroblasts migrate from the yolk sac to the liver, and by the third month of embryonic development, the liver reaches its peak in both erythropoiesis and granulopoiesis (Fig. 6–1). During this stage of intrauterine life, red blood cells in all forms of maturity are seen, giving evidence to *definitive* erythropoiesis. Erythrocytes arise from endothelial cells lining the sinusoids and from the erythroblasts closely associated with them. By the end of the fourth month, the primitive cells have disappeared entirely.[6]

Shortly thereafter, megakaryocytic development, together with splenic activity involving erythropoiesis, granulopoiesis, and lymphopoiesis, is ob-

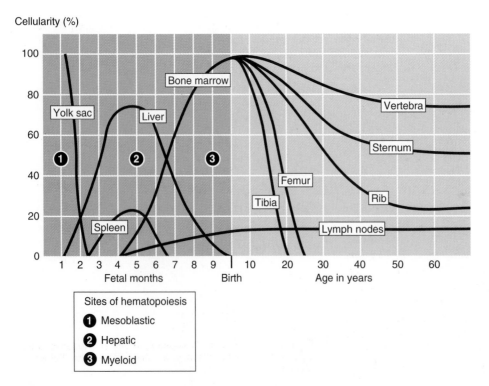

Figure 6–1 Sites of hematopoiesis.

served. To a lesser degree, hematopoietic activity has begun in the lymph nodes and the thymus. Splenic activity gradually decreases, terminating granulopoiesis.

The thymus is the first organ of the lymphatic system to develop fully in the fetus. It continues to grow and enlarge until late childhood, involving itself solely with lymphocytic specialization. Medullary (myeloid) production begins with ossification and development of marrow within its core. The clavicle is the first bone to demonstrate marrow hematopoietic activity.[7] This is followed by rapid ossification of the entire skeleton with subsequent development of active marrow.

Red blood cell production continues in the liver but decreases a few days after birth. Measurable products at this time include primitive erythroblasts, definitive erythroblasts, granulocytes, monocytes, lymphocytes, megakaryocytes, and hemoglobins F, A, and A_2.[6]

Medullary (Myeloid) Phase

About the fifth month of fetal development, the scattered islands of mesenchymal cells begin to differentiate into blood cells of all types. The bone marrow activity increases, resulting in extremely hyperplastic red marrow. By the sixth month, the marrow has become the primary site of hematopoiesis and the exclusive site of all cellular production. Measurable products at this time include representatives of the various stages of maturation of all the cell lines, erythropoietin, fetal hemoglobin, and adult hemoglobins.

ADULT HEMATOPOIETIC TISSUE

The Bone Marrow

Early in bone formation, a space is left at the center by the resorption first of cartilage and then of endosteal bone. This space is invaded by the mesenchyme, which develops into an organ entity. The mesenchyme differentiates into three types of cells that give rise to reticular tissue, adipose tissue, and hematopoietic tissue. Some of the reticular cells in the bone marrow are positioned on the outside surface of the venous sinuses, their long narrow branches extending into the perivascular space, thus providing a support for the developing hematopoietic cells, macrophages, and mast cells.[8] During early childhood, the marrow remains exclusively red. By ages 5–7 years, fat appears in the long bones in the areas previously occupied by red marrow. Retrogression occurs, and thus active red marrow is restricted to the flat bones, the sternum,

vertebrae, pelvis, ribs, skull, and the proximal portion of the long bones. Hematopoietic cells gradually disappear from specific areas, leaving only reticular tissue and fat cells, which constitute the yellow marrow (Fig. 6–2). *Yellow marrow proper* is an admixture of fat cells and undifferentiated mesenchymal cells, scattered throughout the red marrow. The yellow marrow serves as a storage organ (fat) and as a reserve of hematopoietic tissue. In times of excessive loss of blood or destruction of red marrow by chemicals or irradiation, the mesenchymal cells, having retained the potential to transform and revert to red marrow, engage in hematopoiesis.[7]

RED MARROW

The arrangement of the red marrow (Figs. 6–3, 6–4) consists of extravascular cords composed of all developing blood cell lines, stem cells, adventitial cells, and macrophages. This area is separated

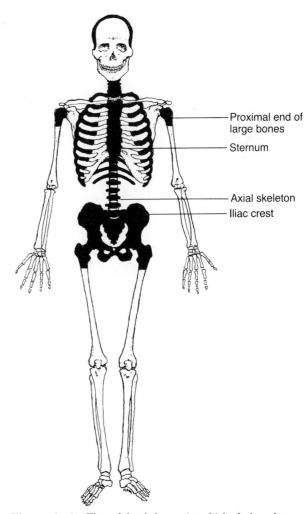

Proximal end of large bones

Sternum

Axial skeleton

Iliac crest

Figure 6–2 The adult skeleton, in which darkened areas depict active red marrow hematopoiesis. (Drawn by Robert A. Mitchell.)

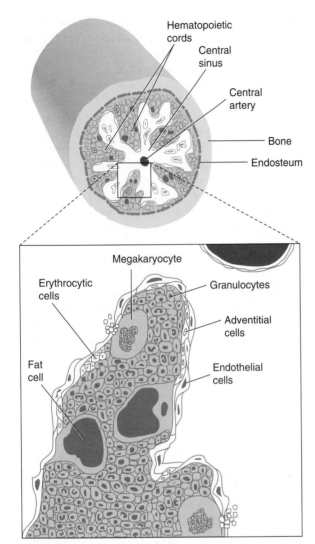

Figure 6–3 Graphic illustration of the arrangement of the extravascular area in hematopoietic tissue.

MARROW CIRCULATION

There are numerous blood vessels that supply necessary nutrients and gases to the red and yellow marrow. Close to the middle of the shaft of long bones is a foramen (opening) that provides the entrance for the medullary, or nutrient, canal that passes through the bone and into the marrow cavity. The nutrient artery passes through this canal, giving off branches to the canal on the way. In the marrow cavity, it divides into ascending and descending branches, both of which supply the nutritional substances to the marrow.[8] Bone matrix is impervious to some radiation but pervious to x-rays, gamma rays, and neutrons. These types of radiation are capable of completely disrupting DNA synthesis of developing blood cells, which results in aplastic marrow. Chemicals or drugs that cause suppressant activity and that are administered intravenously enter the marrow cavity via this route, also causing hypoplasia of the red marrow.

from the lumen of the sinusoids by endothelium and adventitial cells. Developing cell lines appear to be territorial in their locale of development. The erythrocytes are localized in small clusters against the outer surfaces of the vascular sinuses (Fig. 6–5); some are characteristically found surrounding iron-laden macrophages (Fig. 6–6). The megakaryocytes are directly outside the vascular walls of the sinusoids; this location facilitates release of their platelets into the lumen of the sinusoids. The granulocytic cells are situated deeper in the cords until the maturation of the metamyelocyte, at which time they move closer to the vascular sinuses.[7]

All cells leaving the marrow penetrate the sinusoidal wall by passing between adventitial cells and egressing through spaces in the endothelial lining.

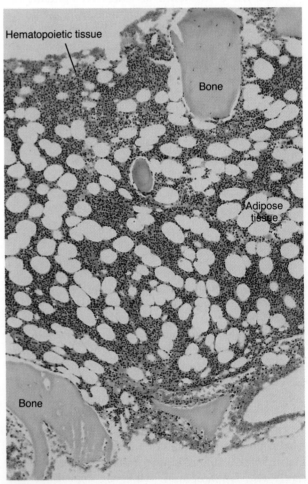

Figure 6–4 Fixed and stained bone marrow tissue (hematoxylin and eosin, 100×). The extravascular tissue consists of blood cell precursors and various tissue cells with scattered fat tissue. A normal bone marrow displays 50% tissue, 50% fat.

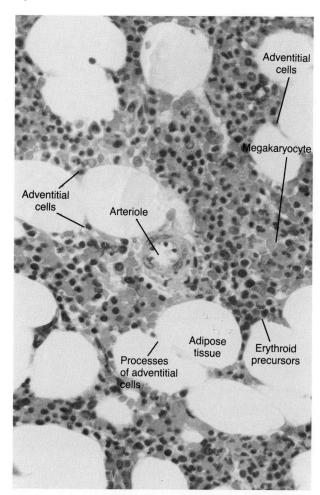

Figure 6–5 Fixed and stained bone marrow tissue (hematoxylin and eosin, 400X). Hematopoietic tissue reveals areas of granulopoiesis (lighter staining cells), erythropoiesis (darker staining nuclei). One megakaryocyte can be seen. Adventitial cells and their processes give support to the hematopoietic cells; they also guard apertures of the basement membrane.

NEEDS OF DEVELOPING CELLS

Microenvironmental needs of developing cells in the extravascular cords consist of (1) a predominantly CO_2 environment, (2) a wet sticky surface on which to anchor (provided by the layering of endothelial cells, macrophages, fibroblasts, and T lymphocytes), and (3) a "normal" population of red marrow cells necessary for cellular interaction and for provision of growth stimulating factors.

The Liver

Although the main function of the liver is not related to hematopoiesis, its dysfunction or partial absence seriously affects homeostasis. Its involvement with hematopoiesis begins in the second trimester, when it constitutes the principal site of all cell production. In adults, the liver has many cellular production functions: synthesizing and pro-

viding transport proteins, storing essential minerals and vitamins that are utilized in both DNA and RNA synthesis, conjugating bilirubin from hemoglobin degradation, and transporting the bilirubin to the small intestine for eventual excretion.

The liver consists of two lobes situated beneath the diaphragm in the abdominal cavity. The position of the liver with regard to the circulatory system is optimal for gathering, transferring, and eliminating substances via the bile.[9] Anatomically, the liver cells are arranged in radiating hepatic lobules emanating from a central vein (Fig. 6–7). Adjacent to the longitudinal lobes of the liver and separated only by a small space are sinusoids, which are lined by two types of cells: Kupffer cells and epithelial cells. The Kupffer cells function as macrophages, removing cellular and foreign debris from the blood that circulates through the liver;[10] they are also responsible for protein synthesis. The epithelial cells are arranged in the lining so as to be separated from one another by a noncellular area; this arrangement allows plasma direct access

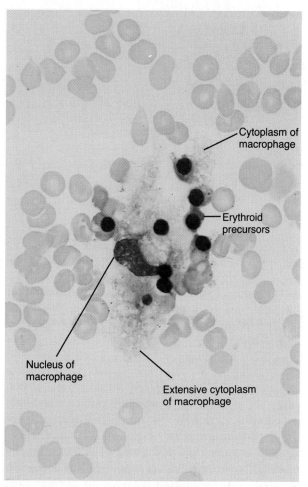

Figure 6–6 Bone marrow smear (Wright-Giemsa, 1000X). Macrophage with extensive iron-laden cytoplasm, surrounded by developing erythroid precursors.

Fat-
storing
cells   Sinusoid   Central   Liver   Sinusoid
                     vein   plates   endothelial
                                         cell

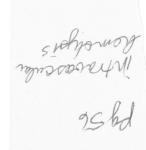

Distibuting   Hepatic   Portal   Bile   Kupffer
vein   artery   vein   duct   cells

        Inlet   Bile
        venule   canaliculi

Figure 6–7 Three-dimensional schematic of the normal liver.

---

to the hepatocytes. This unusual organization of the liver and its location in the body enables it to be involved in many and varied functions.

PATHOPHYSIOLOGY

The liver is often involved in blood-related diseases. In porphyrias, the liver exhibits enzymatic deficiencies, which result in the accumulation of the various intermediary porphyrins. In severe hemolytic anemias and red blood cell dysplasia, the conjugation of bilirubin is increased, as is storage of iron. The liver sequesters membrane-damaged red blood cells, thus impeding intravascular hemolysis. The liver is capable of extramedullary pro-

duction in cases of marrow shutdown. It is directly affected by storage diseases of the monocyte/macrophage (Kupffer) cells as a result of enzymatic deficiencies that cause hepatomegaly with ultimate dysfunction of the liver (Gaucher, Niemann Pick, and Tay Sachs diseases; see Chapter 30).

The Spleen

The spleen is the largest lymphoid organ in the body. It is vital but not essential for life. It is directly below the diaphragm and behind the fundus of the stomach. It is ovoid, and its shape can vary considerably from one individual to another and even within the same individual at different times. In a healthy person, the spleen contains approximately 100–150 mL of blood.[8]

The splenic structure relates closely to its manner of functioning. The spleen is covered outwardly by peritoneum and inwardly by a connective tissue capsule that sends extensions (trabeculae) that inwardly divide the interior of the spleen. The spaces between the trabeculae contain three types of splenic tissue: (1) the *white pulp,* which consists of scattered follicles with germinal centers, loose reticular connective tissue packed with lymphocytes, and free macrophages; (2) the *marginal zone,* a reticular meshwork with narrow interstices, blood vessels, and few cells, which separates the red and white pulp ~~and is a reticular meshwork with narrow interstices, blood vessels, and few cells;~~ and (3) *the red pulp,* composed primarily of vascular sinusoids and sinuses separated by cords of tissue, the *cords of Billroth,* which contain sensitive macrophages. Increasing numbers of circulating red blood cells pass slowly through the cords, thus depleting the glucose supply. Blood flow that is stag-

nant as a result of the increased concentration of cells, together with an almost glucose-free environment, stresses damaged or senescent cells beyond their ability to maintain their integrity. These cells are then *culled* (phagocytosed with subsequent degradation of cell parts). Other cells, having limited membrane injury or small inclusions, are *pitted,* a "pinching" process by which the macrophages remove the inclusion or the damaged membrane area. Other functions include immunoglobulin M (IgM) synthesis that takes place in the germinal centers. The spleen also serves as a storage site for platelets. In a healthy person, 20–30% of the total platelet count is sequestered in the spleen.

The central splenic artery enters the spleen at the hilum and branches outwardly through a dense accumulation of lymphocytes in the white pulp. It branches further, forming arterioles and eventually capillaries, which supply the red pulp. Venous sinuses, which are located in the red pulp, unite and leave the spleen as splenic veins[11] (Figs. 6–8, 6–9).

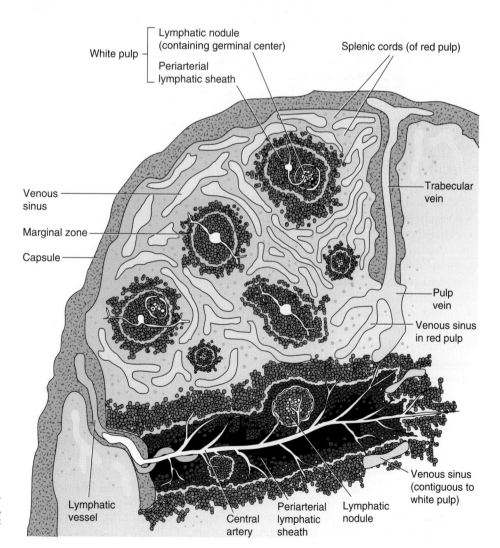

Figure 6–8 Schematic of normal spleen. (From Weiss L, Greep RO: Histology. New York: McGraw-Hill, 1977.)

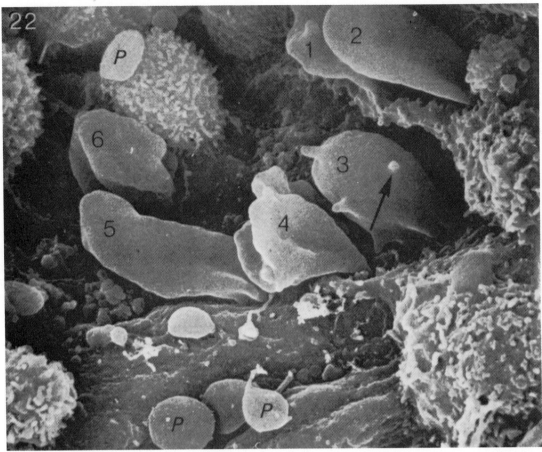

Figure 6–9 Scanning electron micrograph of spleen, demonstrating erythrocytes (numbered 1–6) squeezing through the fenestrated wall in transit from the splenic cord to the sinus. The view shows the endothelial lining of the sinus wall, to which platelets (P) adhere, along with "hairy" white cells, probably macrophages. The arrow shows a protrusion on a red blood cell (×5000). (From Weiss L: A scanning electron microscopic study of the spleen. Blood 1974, 43:665.)

PATHOPHYSIOLOGY

In splenomegaly, the spleen is large and palpable as a result of a variety of both red and white blood cell conditions, such as chronic leukemias, genetically defective red blood cells, hemoglobins S and C, Hodgkin's disease, thalassemia intermedia, malaria, and the myeloproliferative disorders.

Splenectomy is advised in cases of excessive red blood cell destruction, severe hereditary spherocytosis, and autoimmune hemolytic anemias when treatment with corticosteroids does not effectively suppress hemolysis.[1] It may also be indicated in severe cases of agnogenic myeloid metaplasia that is associated with splenomegaly, severe refractory hemolytic anemia, thrombocytopenia, or qualitative platelet defect syndromes. Platelet counts eventually reach normal levels within 10 days after splenectomy.[12] Repeated splenic infarcts caused by drepanocytes (sickle cells) trapped in the small circulation of the spleen cause tissue damage and necrosis, often resulting in *autosplenectomy*.

Hypersplenism is an enlargement of the spleen with some degree of pancytopenia despite the presence of very hyperactive bone marrow. The most common cause is congestive splenomegaly secondary to cirrhosis of the liver and portal hypertension. Other causes include thrombosis, vascular stenosis, other vascular deformities such as aneurysm of the splenic artery, and cysts. In such cases, "It is better out than in."

The Lymph Nodes (Figure 6–10)

Lymph nodes are members of the lymphatic system located along the lymphatic capillaries that parallel, but are not part of, the circulatory system. The afferent lymphatic vessels carry lymph (a fluid similar to blood but characterized by a low protein concentration and the absence of red blood cells) to the nodes. Lymph circulates throughout the node and leaves via the efferent lymphatic vessels located at the hilus of the lymph node.

The lymph nodes are bean-shaped bodies (1–5 mm in diameter), occurring mostly in chains at intervals along the lymphatic vessels. They are superficial (inguinal, axillary, cervical, supratrochlear) or deep (mesenteric, retroperitoneal).

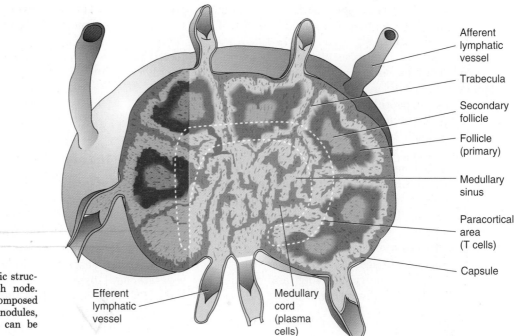

Figure 6–10 Histologic structure of a normal lymph node. The cortical layer is composed mainly of lymphatic nodules, whose germinal centers can be clearly seen.

Afferent lymphatic vessel

Trabecula

Secondary follicle

Follicle (primary)

Medullary sinus

Paracortical area (T cells)

Capsule

Efferent lymphatic vessel

Medullary cord (plasma cells)

Similar in structure to the spleen, the lymph nodes consist of an outer capsule that forms trabeculae and provides a support for macrophages, and the predominant population of lymphocytes. The trabeculae divide the interior of the lymph nodes into specific areas. Between the trabeculae lie *cortical* nodules. Within these nodules are follicles, most of which have a focus of B cell proliferation called a germinal center.[7] These nodules are arranged in circles along the outer layer of the lymph node. The paracortex contains mostly T cells. The medullary cords lie toward the interior of the lymph node and surround the efferent lymphatic vessels. They consist of cords of plasma cells and B lymphocytes.

Lymph nodes are involved in three main functions: (1) the formation of new lymphocytes from the germinal centers, (2) the processing of specific immunoglobulins, and (3) the filtration of particulate matter, debris, and bacteria entering the lymph node via the lymph.

PATHOPHYSIOLOGY

Lymph nodes, by their nature, are vulnerable to the very organisms that circulate through the tissue. Sometimes, increased numbers of microorganisms enter the nodes, overwhelming the macrophages and causing adenitis (infection of the lymph node). More serious is the frequent entry of malignant cells that have broken loose from malignant tumors. They establish new growths, which in

turn metastasize to other lymph nodes in the same group.

The Thymus

To understand the role of the thymus in the adult, certain formative intrauterine processes that affect function must be considered: (1) the thymus tissue originates from endodermal as well as mesenchyme tissue, and (2) the thymus is populated initially by lymphocytes from both the yolk sac and the liver. This increased lymphoid population physically pushes the epithelial cells apart, and yet their long processes remain attached to each other by *desmosomes.*

At birth, the thymus is an efficient, well-developed organ in the upper part of the anterior mediastinum at about the level of the great vessels of the heart.[7] It is small, consisting of two lobules each 0.5–2 mm in diameter. It resembles other lymphoid tissue in that the lobules are subdivided into two areas: the cortex (a peripheral zone) and the medulla (a central zone). Both areas are populated with the same cellular components—lymphocytes, mesenchymal cells, reticular cells, and many macrophages—although in different proportions. The *cortex* is characterized by a blood supply system that is unique in that it consists only of capillaries. Its function appears to be of a waiting zone, densely populated with lymphocytes that originated in the bone marrow. These cells have no identifiable surface markers. Those that receive surface antigens move toward the medulla and eventually leave to populate specific regions of other lymphoid tissue (Fig. 6–11). It is theorized that the cytoplasmic processes of the epithelial reticular cells contain the secretory products, thymic hormones, thymic factor, and thymic humoral hormones (protein/peptides extracted from the thymus), which promote differentiation of pre–T (nonmarked) from mature T lymphocytes. The cells that are not marked die in the cortex and are phagocytosed by macrophages before release. The *medulla* contains only 5% mature T lymphocytes and appears to be a holding zone for conditioned cells until those cells are needed by the peripheral lymphoid tissues.[12]

According to gross examination, the size of the thymus is related to age. At birth, the thymus weighs 12–15 g; at puberty, 30–40 g; and at later ages, 10–15 g. It is hardly recognizable at old age, having atrophied (Fig. 6–12).

Pathophysiology

Nondevelopment of the thymus during gestation results in the lack of formation of T lymphocytes. Related manifestations involve failure to thrive, uncontrollable infections, and death in infancy. Adults with any thymic disturbance are not affected because they have maintained a pool of T lymphocytes for life.

STEM CELLS

Stem Cell Theory

The exact structure and interrelationships of hematopoietic stem cell compartment fully understood. Morphologic observations indicate that all blood cells are derived from a single stem cell; this thinking represents the *monophyletic theory*. Other observers postulate that there is a separate and distinct stem cell compartment for each of the blood cells; this thinking best describes the *polyphyletic theory*. Still others propose an intermediate between these two theories. Current evidence suggests that both theories are correct.[1]

According to current information obtained from culture studies, the hierarchical lineage of cells is based on activity rather than morphology. It is

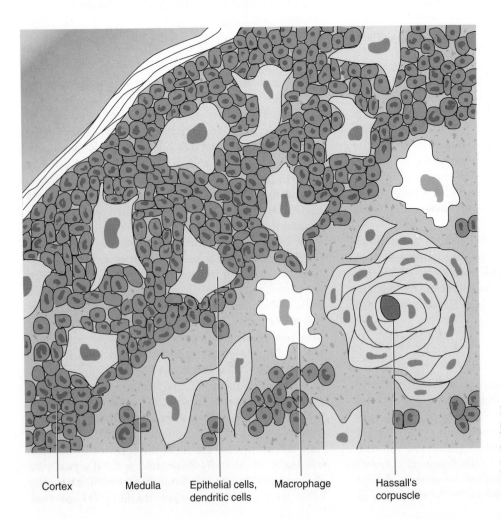

Cortex   Medulla   Epithelial cells, dendritic cells   Macrophage   Hassall's corpuscle

Figure 6–11 Schematic diagram of the edge of a lobule of the thymus, showing cells of the cortex and medulla. (From Abbas AK, Lichtman AH, Pober JS: Cellular and Molecular Immunology. WB Saunders, Philadelphia, 1991.)

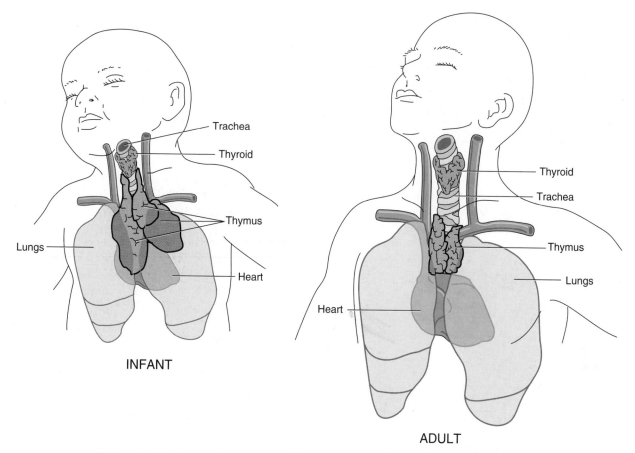

Figure 6–12 Diagram demonstrating difference in size of thymus of the infant and the adult.

interesting to note how closely the recent findings substantiate the two proposed theories (Fig. 6–13).

Stem Cell Cycle Kinetics: The Generative Cycle

It has been estimated that the bone marrow is capable of producing approximately 3 billion red blood cells, 2.5 billion platelets, and 1.5 billion granulocytes per kilogram of body weight daily. The determining factor controlling the rate of production is basic body need. Included in the marrow is a hierarchical realm of cells characterized by the ability to self-replicate and differentiate. These stem cells exist in a ratio of 1:1000. These hematopoietic cells are capable of two mitotic divisions when stimulated by specific growth factors. Information generated from activity demonstrated in culture in response to colony stimulating factors (CSF) is depicted in a schematic to describe the state of activity in which each cell is involved (Fig. 6–14).

From this data, a *mitotic index (MI)* is calculated to establish the percentage of cells in mitosis in relation to the total number of cells. Factors affecting the MI are duration of mitosis and length of resting state, G_0. Normally, the MI is approximately 1–2%. An increased MI implies increased proliferation. (One exception to this rule is in the case of megaloblastic anemia, when mitosis is prolonged.[12]) Understanding the mechanism of the generative cycle aids in understanding the mode of action of specific drugs used in the treatment and maintenance of the proliferative disorders.

Stimulating Growth Factors

THE ERYTHROCYTIC CELL LINE

Erythropoietin is an erythropoietic stimulating factor composed of erythropoietin (produced in the kidney) and an alpha globulin (produced in the liver). It is a glycoprotein consisting of sialic acid, hexosamine, and hexoses. Upon removal of sialic acid, the erythropoietic activity is lost in vivo but retained in vitro. It is involved primarily with the processes of differentiation, mitosis, and maturation.

In 1961, Till and McCullock irradiated spleens and bone marrow of mice and intravenously injected marrow cells. Seven to eight days later, discrete macroscopic colonies were observed growing

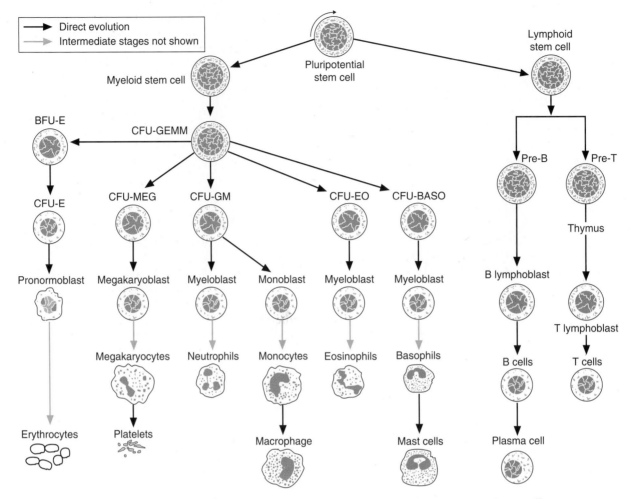

Figure 6–13 Hematopoiesis demonstrating derivation of cells from the pluripotential stem cell.

on the spleens. The stem cell progenitors of these colonies were termed *colony-forming unit–spleen (CFU-S.)*[13]

A second study involving plasma clots in culture media with added marrow cells generated colonies of cells numbering 8–64 cells. The term *colony-forming unit–erythrocytic* (CFU-E) was used to describe the unit growth. A second group of colonies giving rise to 1000 or more cells was later observed. These were termed *burst-forming units–erythrocytic* (BFU-E) because all the cells in the colony were committed to erythropoiesis. BFU-E has been identified as the most primitive erythrocyte precursor. CFU-E is dependent on BFU-E for differentiation[1] (see Fig. 8–2). Studies identifying and measuring BFU-E units have generated sufficient data in order to establish normal values. In a study involving fetal blood of over 3400 fetuses, the number of BFU-E was increased threefold at mid-gestation. The erythropoietin levels were found to be stable.[14]

Also identified by the use of the culture model are interleukin 3 (IL-3), which is an erythrocytic

growth stimulating factor, and more recently a new system labeled KL.[15]

MEGAKARYOCYTIC CELL LINE

Thrombopoietin, the stimulating hormonal factor, controls the production and release of platelets. It has never been identified or assayed but has been convincingly demonstrated in the plasma from a thrombocytopenic animal and some thrombocytopenic humans.[10]

IL-3 stimulates both megakaryoblasts and promegakaryocytes, whereas IL-1α stimulates only the promegakaryocyte. Stem cell factor, with its receptor, *c-kit*, has been shown to promote increases in erythrocytes and platelets.[15]

LEUKOCYTES

Leukopoietin was for many years regarded as the sole stimulating factor inducing white blood cell proliferation. It also has potential for limiting mitosis and maturation of later white cell precursors.

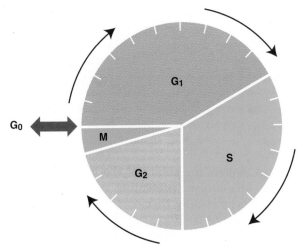

Figure 6-14 Cell cycle schematic. G_0, resting stage; G_1, RNA and protein synthesis; S, DNA synthesis; G_2, premitotic phase; M, mitosis.

Culture studies have identified an interleukin and a KL system that affect the early progenitors of the white blood cell lines.

INTERLEUKINS

The discovery and naming of all secreted regulatory proteins of the immune system (i.e., cytokines, monokines, lymphokines, interleukins) are subject for approval by a subcommittee of the International Union of Immunological Studies (IUIS). Figure 6-15 illustrates the hematopoietic system and the sites of action of colony forming units (CFUs) and growth stimulating factors. These factors are discussed in detail in the appropriate chapters.

Interleukins are growth factors that were discovered during investigation of liquid culture systems devised to study B and T cell proliferation and differentiation. Interleukins stimulate proliferation and differentiation in specific cell lines, or work synergistically and in conjunction with CSFs. Characteristics shared by the interleukins include the following:

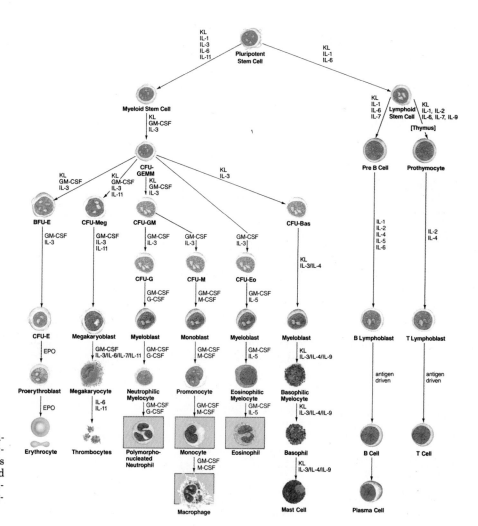

Figure 6-15 Derivation of hematopoietic cells, illustrating sites of activity of colony stimulating factors (CSFs) and interleukins. (Reprinted by permission of Sandoz Pharmaceuticals Corporation and Schering-Plough, 1991.)

1. Proteins that exhibit multiple biologic activity.
2. Synergistic action.
3. Ability to affect targets directly and indirectly.
4. Interacting systems with amplification potential.
5. Effectiveness in low concentrations.

Interleukin-1 (IL-1) is a soluble factor released by monocytes,[11,16] macrophages, and the active T helper cell. It is also referred to as lymphocyte activating factor. Targets include pluripotential cells, pre–B lymphoblasts, and pre–T lymphoblasts. IL-1 regulates expression of GM-CSF and G-CSF in vivo. It is produced by the stromal cells in the bone marrow. In older age, the stroma appears to be less sensitive to IL-1.[17]

IL-2 is a major stimulating factor for T lymphoid stem cells and for the pre–T and pre–B lymphocytes.[18] It is secreted by CD4+ cells[19] (see Chapter 29).

IL-3 is the earliest discovered interleukin. It is regarded as a multilineage CSF and competes with GM-CSF for binding to receptors. Human recombinant granulocyte-macrophage CSF and IL-3 have overlapping but distinct hematopoietic activities.[20] IL-3 also stimulates early eosinophilic precursors.[21]

IL-4, when used with polyclonal activation, causes a percentage of resting splenic B lymphocytes to increase proliferation by about 40%.[22] IL-4 was seen to enhance the proliferation of normal peripheral blood BFU-E.[23] It is able to regulate the induction of lymphokine-activated killer activity in both T cell–replete and T cell–depleted bone marrow and may play a role in modulating the effector cells with potential antileukemic reactivity in vivo.[24] It also stimulates early eosinophil precursors[25] and interacts with IL-2 in activating macrophages.[26] IL-4 with IL-2 exhibits reciprocal interrelationships in human thymocyte cultures.[27]

IL-5 is a B lymphocyte growth factor and exhibits control over the maturation of terminal eosinophils.[21] IL-5 induces responsiveness in small splenic B lymphocytes when stimulated by IL-4, anti-IgM + LPS (lipopolysaccharide), and TI-2 (thymus independent antigen type 2) analog.[22]

IL-6 synergizes with CSF-M in stimulating monocyte/macrophage colony formation. It is also involved in B lymphocyte proliferation.[28]

IL-7 is derived from stromal cells and targets T and B lymphoid stem cells that induce differentiation.[29]

IL-8 is a member of a family of pro-inflammatory cytokines.[30] IL-1 and tumor necrosis factor are potent inducers of IL-8 chemotactic attraction of neutrophils. IL-8 is significantly increased in synovial fluid in many cases of rheumatoid arthritis.[31] IL-8 induces histamine and leukotriene release in human basophils exposed to IL-3. Pretreatment low concentration of IL-8 inhibits the response.[32,33] IL-8 activates polymorphonuclear neutrophils and elicits selective diapedesis of these neutrophils into the extracellular space.[34] IL-8 recruits both neutrophils and lymphocytes in vitro and in vivo.[35]

The loci for IL-9 is on chromosome 5.[36] It supports the growth of helper T cell clones, mast cells, and megakaryoblastic leukemia cells. IL-1 plus a T cell receptor–mediated signal increases IL-9 secretion.[37]

IL-10 inhibits the ability of the macrophage, but not B cell, antigen presenting cells to stimulate cytokine synthesis by thymocyte 1 cell clones. The potent action of IL-10 on the macrophage, particularly at the level of monokine production, supports an important role for this cytokine in regulation of not only T cell responses but also acute inflammatory responses.[38–41]

IL-11 has been derived from culture studies. It targets pluripotential stem cells and the megakaryocytic cell line.[42,43]

IL-12 has a multiple regulatory effect on blood lymphocytes, natural killer cells, and T cell subsets. It is derived from B cells and monocytes. Its activity includes induction of lymphokine production, mitogenesis, and enhancement of spontaneous activity.[44]

IL-13 is secreted by activated T cells and shares certain characteristics and functions with IL-4.[45]

CULTURE-DERIVED COLONY-FORMING UNITS

CFUs are dependent on CSFs and colony stimulating activity (CSA). In its purified state, CSA has been shown to be a sialic acid–containing protein with a molecular weight of 45,000.[46] CSA is produced in human tissue; it has also been derived from human urine. See Table 6–1 for a listing of CFUs.

Table 6-1. CULTURE-DERIVED COLONY-FORMING UNITS

Abbreviation	Cell Line
CFU-GEMM	Granulocytic, erythrocytic, megakaryocytic, monocytic
CFU-E	Erythrocytic
CFU-M	Megakaryocytic
CFU-GM	Granulocytic, monocytic
CFU-BASO	Myeloid to basophil
CFU-EO	Myeloid to eosinophil
CFU-G	Myeloid to neutrophil
CFU-LT	T lymphocyte
CFU-LB	B lymphocyte

ANALYTIC AND THERAPEUTIC APPLICATION

The use of the growth factors has contributed options in the treatment of malignancies involving the bone marrow, leukemias, and aplastic anemia.

Applications of the interleukins found in the literature include the following:

IL-1—Used in cases of inflammation, such as fever, and as a defense mechanism during infection.[47]

IL-2—Enhances migration of cells with anti-tumor activity into tissues; induces release of IL-6, TNF, and interferon, which may have anti-tumor effect.[48]

IL-3—Used in treatment of refractory anemia with or without ringed sideroblasts; also used to stimulate megakaryopoiesis.

IL-4—Used to potentiate anti-tumor activity, especially in cases of gastric carcinoma.[50]

IL-6—Used in treatment of acute myeloid leukemia; has been found to initiate both increases and suppression of blast cells.[51]

IL-7—Enhances allocytolytic activity of lymphokine-activated killer cells.[52]

IL-8—Acts as principal mediator of inflammation, which can be acted upon by IL-4.[53]

IL-10—Is being investigated for use in immune suppression as a consequence of transplantation, tolerance, cancer therapy, and infectious disease.[54]

IL-11—Has demonstrated activity in pre-clinical studies in association with myelosuppression, cancer therapy, neutropenia, and thrombocytopenia.[55]

IL-12—Used in stimulating proliferation of peripheral blood mononuclear cells and tumor-infiltrating lymphocytes in melanoma patients.[44]

CSA and GM-CFU were assayed in 17 patients with chronic drug-induced neutropenia. Leukocyte-derived CSA and monocyte-macrophage–derived CSA were found to be significantly decreased in comparison with the levels in the control group.[56] In cases of an adult with immune thrombocytopenic purpura, levels of IL-6 were found to be within normal range, but an increased number of megakaryocyte progenitors were present. This was possibly caused by an increase in megakaryocyte CSA.[57] In many studies, patients who had received the pretransplant chemotherapeutic regimen were given GM-CSF, and hematopoietic reconstitution was successful.[58-64] Patients with aplastic anemia were found to have markedly decreased production of IL-1.[65]

SUMMARY

The evolution of the hematopoietic system begins shortly after conception through the specialization of the mesoderm. Characteristic abilities and functions of lymphoid tissue are determined during the second and third trimesters. In the adult, the red marrow, the sole site for blood cell development, is confined to the axial skeleton and the epiphysis of the long bones. The discovery and identification of the various cytokines that control the development of blood cells has resulted in innovative therapeutic applications in the treatment of patients affected with malignant and myeloproliferative disorders.

REVIEW QUESTIONS

1. What is the significance of the presence of mesenchymal cells in the bone marrow?
2. Differentiate between primitive and definitive erythroblasts.
3. Describe the thymus of an 83-year-old man.
4. What purpose does yellow marrow serve in the body?
5. Where does hematopoiesis take place in the adult?
6. What type of agents can destroy red marrow?
7. Describe the cords of Billroth.
8. When is a splenectomy advised?
9. Of what use is the mitotic index?
10. Of what significance is the study of Till and McCullock?
11. The multi-CSF among the interleukins is
    a. IL-1
    b. IL-2
    c. IL-3
    d. IL-4
12. Illustrate the application of CSF in the practice of medicine.

References

1. Beck W: Hematology, 4th ed. Cambridge, MA: MIT Press, 1985.
2. Mengle CE: Hematology: Principles and Practice. Chicago: Year Book Medical, 1990.
3. Potter EL: Pathology of the Fetus and Newborn. Chicago: Year Book, 1953.
4. Simmons A: Hematology: A Combined Theoretical and Technical Approach. Philadelphia: WB Saunders, 1989.

5. Smith CH: Blood Disease—Infancy and Childhood. St. Louis: CV Mosby, 1960.
6. Gallichio VS: Hematopoiesis and review of genetics. *In* Lotspeich-Steininger CA, Stein-Martin EA, Koepke JA: Clinical Hematology: Principles, Procedures, Correlations. Philadelphia: JB Lippincott, 1992.
7. Junqueira LC, Carneior J, Long JA: Basic Histology, 6th ed. Los Altos, CA: Lange Medical, 1989.
8. Bevelander G: Essentials of Histology, 6th ed. St. Louis: CV Mosby, 1970.
9. Anthony CP: Textbook of Anatomy and Physiology, 7th ed. St. Louis: CV Mosby, 1967.
10. Williams JW, Beutler E, Erslev AJ, Lichtman MA: Hematology, 4th ed. New York: McGraw-Hill, 1990.
11. Seeley RR, Stephens TD, Tate PDA: Anatomy and Physiology. St. Louis: Times Mirror/Mosby College, 1989.
12. Lee GR, Bethell TC, Foerster J, et al (eds): Wintrobe's Clinical Hematology, 9th ed. Philadelphia: Lea & Febiger, 1993.
13. Till TE, McCullock EA: A direct measurement of the radiation sensitivity of normal mouse bone marrow cells. Radiat Res 1961; 14:213.
14. Forestier F, Daffos F, Catherine N, et al: Developmental hematopoiesis in normal human fetal blood. Blood 1991; 77(11):2360–2363.
15. Zsebo KM, Williams DA, Geissler EN, et al: Stem cell factor is encoded at the SI locus of the mouse and is the ligand for the *c-kit* tyrosine kinase receptor. Cell 1990; 63:213–224.
16. Rapaport SI: Introduction to Hematology, 2nd ed. Philadelphia: JB Lippincott, 1987.
17. Lee MA, Segal GM, Bagby GC: The hematopoietic microenvironment in the elderly: defects in IL-1 induced CSF expression in vitro. Exp Hematol 1989; 17(9):952–956.
18. Mostyn G, Burgess AW: Hematopoietic growth factors: a review. Cancer Res 1988; 48:5624.
19. Bass H, Adkins B, Strober S: Thymic irradiation inhibits the rapid recovery of Th1 but not Th2-like functions of CD4+ T cells after total lymphoid irradiation of cell. Immunol 1991; 137(2)316–328.
20. Emerson SG, Yang YC, Clark SC, Long MW: Human recombinant granulocyte-macrophage colony stimulating factor and interleukin have overlapping but distinct hematopoietic activities. J Clin Invest 1988; 82(4):1282–1287.
21. Sonoda Y, Arai N, Ogawa M: Humoral regulation of eosinophilopoiesis in vitro: analysis of the targets of interleukin-3, granulocyte/macrophage colony-stimulating factor (GM-CSF), and interleukin-5. Leukemia 1989; 3(1):14–18.
22. Wetzel GD: Induction of interleukin-5 responsiveness in resting B cells by engagement of the antigen receptor and perception of a second polyclonal activation signal. Cell Immunol 1991; 137(2):358–366.
23. Dewolf JT, Hendriks DW, Beentjes JA, et al: Erythroid progenitors in polycythemia vera demonstrate a different response pattern to IL-4 compared to normal BFU-E from peripheral blood. Exp Hematol 1991; 19(9):888–892.
24. Drobyski WR, LeFever AV, Truitt RL: Regulation of lymphokine-activated killer activity in T-replete and T-cell–depleted human bone marrow by interleukin 4. Exp Hematol 1991; 19(9):950–957.
25. King CL, Nutman TB: Regulation of the immune response in lymphatic filariasis and onchocerciasis. Immunol Today 1991; 12(3):A54–A58.
26. Nacy CA, Meltzer MS: T-cell mediated activation of macrophages. Curr Opin Immunol 1991; 3(3):330–335.
27. Barcena A, Torribio ML, Gutierrez-Ramos JC, et al: Interplay of IL-2 and IL-4 in human thymocytic differentiation. Int Immunol 1991; 3(5):419–425.
28. Bot FJ, van Eijk L, Broeders L, et al: Interleukin-6 synergizes with M-CSF in the formation of macrophage colonies from purified human marrow progenitor cells. Blood 1989; 73(2):358–366.
29. Billips LG, Pettite D, Dorshkind K, et al: Differential roles of stromal cells, interleukin-7 and *kit*-ligand in the regulation of B lymphopoiesis. Blood 1992; 79(5):1185–1192.
30. Murphy PM, Tiffany HL: Cloning of complementary DNA

31. encoding a functional human interleukin-8. Science 1991; 253(5025):1280–1283.
31. Peichi P, Ceska M, Effenberger F, et al: Presence of NAP-1/IL-8 in synovial fluids indicates a possible pathogenic role in rheumatoid arthritis. Scand J Immunol 1991; 34(3):333–339.
32. Bischoff SC, Baggiolini M, deWeck AL, Dahinden CA: Interleukin 8-inhibitor and inducer of histamine and leukotriene release in human basophils. Biochem Biophys Res Commun 1991; 179(11):628–633.
33. Kuna P, Reddigari SR, Kornfeld D, Kaplan AP: IL-8 inhibits histamine release from human basophils induced by histamine-releasing factors, connective tissue activating peptide III, and IL-3. J Immunol 1991; 147(6):1920–1924.
34. Kusner DJ, Luebbers EL, Nowinski RJ; et al: Cytokine- and LPS-induced synthesis of interleukin-8 from human mesangial cells. Kidney Int 1991; 39(6):1240–1248.
35. Holmes WE, Lee J, Kuang WJ, et al: Structure and functional expression of a human interleukin-8-receptor. Science 1991; 253(5025):1278–1280.
36. Modi WS, Pollack DD, Mock BA, et al: Regional localization of the human glutaminase (GLS) and interleukin-9 (IL-9) genes by in situ hybridization. Cytogenet Cell Genet 1991; 57(2–3):114–116.
37. Schmitt E, Beuscher HV, Huels C, et al: IL-1 serves as a signal for IL-9 expression. J Immunol 1991; 147(11):3848–3854.
38. Fiorentino DF, Zlotnik A, Mosmann TR, et al: IL-10 inhibits cytokine production by activated macrophages. J Immunol 1991; 147(11):3815–3822.
39. Mosmann TR: Regulation of immune responses by T cells with different cytokine secretion phenotypes: role of a new cytokine, cytokine synthesis inhibitory factor IL-10. Int Arch Allergy Appl Immunol 1991; 94:110–115.
40. deWaal MR, Abrams J, Bennet B, et al: Interleukin 10 (IL-10) inhibits cytokine synthesis by human monocytes: an autoregulatory role of IL-10 produced by monocytes. J Exp Med 1991; 174(5):1209–1220.
41. deWaal MR, Haanen J, Spits H, et al: Interleukin 10 (IL-10) and viral IL-10 strongly reduce antigen-specific human T cell proliferation by diminishing the antigen-presenting capacity of monocytes via down-regulation of class II major histocompatibility complex expression. J Exp Med 1991; 174(4):915–924.
42. Paul SR, Bennett F, Calvetti JA, et al: Molecular cloning of a cDNA encoding interleukin II, a stromal cell-derived lymphopoietic and hematopoietic cytokine. Genetics 1990; 87:7512–7516.
43. Bruno E, Briddel RA, Cooper RJ, Hoffman R: Effects of recombinant interleukin II on human megakaryocyte progenitor cells. Exp Hematol 1991; 19:378–381.
44. Zeh HJ, Hurd S, Strojus WJ, Lotze MT: Interleukin-12 promotes the proliferation and cytolytic maturation of immune effectors: implications for the immunotherapy of cancer. J Immunother 1993; 14:155–161.
45. Zurawks S, Vega F, Huygle B: Receptors for interleukin-13 and interleukin-4 are complex and share a novel component and function in signal transduction. EMBO J 1993; 12:2663–2670.
46. Spivak JL: Fundamentals of Clinical Hematology. Philadelphia: Harper & Row, 1984.
47. Scales WE, Kunkel SL: Regulatory interactions between interleukin-1, tumor necrosis factor and other inflammatory mediators. *In* Bomford R, Henderson B (eds): Interleukin-1 Inflammation and Disease. New York: Elsevier, 1989.
48. Rosenberg SA, Lotze MT, Muul LM, et al: A progress report of the treatment of 157 patients with advanced cancer using lymphokine-activated killer cells and IL-2 on high dose or high dose IL-2 alone. New Engl J Med 1987; 316:889–897.
49. Vrhovac R, Kusee R, Jaksic B: Myeloid hematopoietic growth factor. Int J Clin Pharm 1993; 31:241–252.
50. Morisake T, Yuzuki D, Lin R, et al: Interleukin-4. Receptor expression and growth inhibition of gastric carcinoma cells by IL-4. Cancer Res 1992; 52(21):6059–6065.
51. Suzuki T, Morio T, Tohda S, et al: Effects of interleukin-6

and granulocytic colony-stimulating factor on the proliferation of leukemic blast progenitor from acute myeloblastic leukemia patients. Jpn J Cancer Res 1990; 81:979–986.

52. Lotze MT: T-cell growth factors and the treatment of patients with cancer. Clin Immun Immunopathol 1992; 62:2663–2670.

53. Schroder JM: Peptides and cytokines. Arch Dermatol Res 1992; 284:22–26.

54. Spits H, Malefy R: Functional characterization of human IL-10. J Int Arch Allergy Immunol 1992; 1:8–15.

55. Neber S, Terner K: The biology of interleukin-11. Stem Cell 1993; 11:156–162.

56. Eliopoulos G, Meletis J, Fessas P, Anagnou NP: Defective CSA-dependent granulopoiesis in patients with chronic drug-induced neutropenia. Haematologia 1990; 23(2):101–109.

57. Bellucci S, Han ZC, Caen JP: Studies of in vitro megakaryocytopoiesis in adult immune thrombocytopenic purpura (ITP). Eur J Haematol 1991; 47(2):86–90.

58. Vadhan-Raj S, Hittleman WN, Broxmeyer HE, et al: In vivo biologic activities of recombinant human granulocyte-macrophage colony-stimulating factor. Ann NY Acad Sci 1989; 554:231–240.

59. Vadhan-Raj S, Buescher S, LeMaistre A, et al: Stimulation of hematopoeisis in patients with bone marrow failure and in patients with malignancy by recombinant human granulocyte-macrophage colony-stimulating factor. Blood 1988; 72(1):134–141.

60. Laporte JP, Fouillard L, Douay L, et al: GM-CSF instead of autologous bone-marrow transplantation after the BEAM. Lancet 1991; 338(8767):601–602

61. Brandwein JM, Nayar R, Baker MA, et al: GM-CSF therapy for delayed engraftment after autologous bone marrow transplantation. Exp Hematol 1991; 19(3):191–195.

62. Bettelheim P, Valent P, Andreeff M, et al: Recombinant human granulocyte-macrophage colony-stimulating factor in combination with standard induction chemotherapy in de novo acute myeloid leukemia. Blood 1991; 77(4):700–711.

63. Gianni AM, Siena S, Bregni M, et al: Granulocyte-macrophage colony-stimulating factor to harvest circulating hemopoietic stem cells for autotransplantation. Lancet 1989; 2(8663):580–585.

64. Visani G, Tosi P, Gamberi B, et al: Accelerated hemopoietic recovery after chemotherapy and autologous bone marrow transplantation in hematological malignancies using recombinant GM-CSF, preliminary results obtained in 14 cases. Haematologica 1990; 75(6):551–554.

65. Gascon P, Scala G: Decreased interleukin-1 in aplastic anemia. Am J Med 1988, 85(5):668–674.

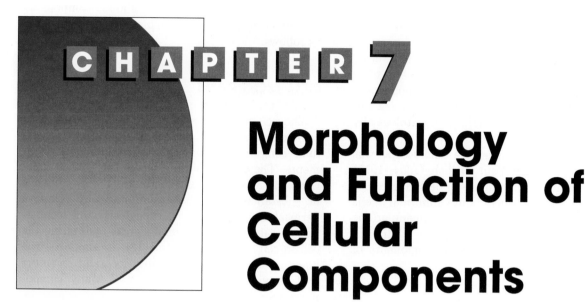

CHAPTER 7

Morphology and Function of Cellular Components

Keila B. Poulsen

Outline

Objectives

AFTER COMPLETION OF THIS CHAPTER, THE READER WILL BE ABLE TO

1. Describe the general function and chemical composition of cellular membranes.
2. Describe the features of the cytoplasm.
3. Name the cytoplasmic organelles found in the cell.
4. Describe the features of the nucleus.
5. Correlate the nuclear structures to the activities of the cell.
6. Correlate the cytoplasmic structures to the activities of the cell.

The study of hematology has been revolutionized with the numerous multichannel instruments that have become available for the clinical diagnostic process. The technologies of light scatter, electrical impedance, and conductivity have added parameters and scatterplots whose significance are yet to be fully realized and clinically applied, but morphologic examination of the peripheral blood smear with light microscopy still remains of hallmark importance for clinical evaluation of hematologically abnormal patients.

The study of cells under the microscope was greatly enhanced when Paul Ehrlich (1854–1915) developed staining techniques to better differentiate the various normal and abnormal cells present in human blood. The development of the electron microscope revolutionized the ability to study and understand the internal components of the cell.[1]

CELL ORGANIZATION (Figure 7–1)

Cells are structural units that constitute living organisms. Many cells have specialized functions and contain the components necessary to perform and perpetuate these functions. Regardless of shape, size, or function, most cells have three basic parts: unit membranes, the cytoplasm, and the nu-

cleus. Each of these basic parts has components or subdivisions that assist in their varied functions. Table 7–1 summarizes the cellular components and functions, which are explained in more detail as follows.

CELL MEMBRANE

The cell membrane (see Fig. 8–11) serves as a semipermeable outer boundary separating the cellular components from their surrounding environments. The cell membrane serves three basic functions: (1) it restricts and facilitates the interchange of substances with the environment by selective permeability, endocytosis, exocytosis, and locomotion; (2) it detects hormonal signals facilitating the cell-to-cell recognition; and (3) it supports the blood groups, histocompatibility loci, and receptors that provide for cellular identity.[2] Many components found within the cell (e.g., the mitochondria, nucleus, and endoplasmic reticulum) have similarly constructed membrane systems. The red blood cell membrane has been widely studied and serves as an example of a cell membrane.

To accomplish its many requirements, this cell membrane must be resilient and elastic; it achieves these qualities by being a fluid structure of globular proteins floating in lipids. The lipids are made

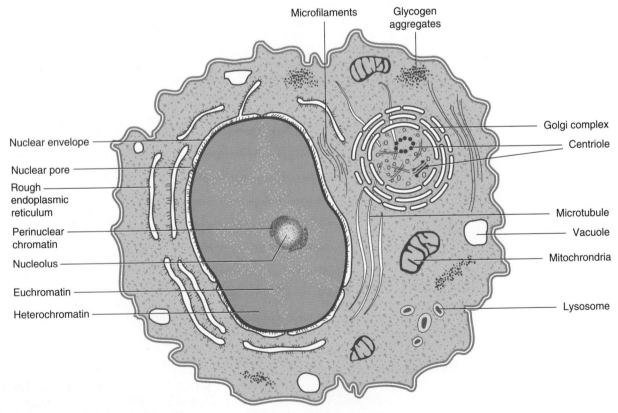

Figure 7–1 Cell organization.

Table 7-1. SUMMARY OF CELLULAR COMPONENTS AND FUNCTIONS

Organelle	Location	Appearance and Size	Function	Comments
Membranes: plasma, nuclear, mitochondrial, endoplasmic reticulum	Outer boundary of cell, nucleus, endoplasmic reticulum, mitochondria and other organelles	Usually a lipid bilayer consisting of proteins, cholesterol, phospholipids, and polysaccharides; membrane thickness varies with the cell or organelle	Separates the various cellular components; facilitates and restricts cellular exchange of substances	Membrane must be resilient and flexible
Nucleus	Within cell	Usually round or oval but varies depending on cell; varies in size; composed of DNA	The control center of the cell and contains the genetic blueprint	Governs the cellular activity and transmits information for cellular control
Nucleolus	Within nucleus	Usually round or irregular in shape; 2–4 μm in size; composed of RNA; there may be 1–4 within nucleus	Site of synthesis and processing of various ribosomal RNA	Appearance will vary with activity of the cells; larger when cell is actively involved in protein synthesis
Golgi body	Between nucleus and luminal surface of the cell	System of stacked membrane-bound flattened sacs; horseshoe shaped; varies in size	Involved in modifying and packaging macromolecules for secretion	Well developed in cells with large secretion responsibilities
Endoplasmic reticulum	Randomly throughout cytoplasm	Membrane-lined tubules that branch and connect to nucleus and plasma membrane	Stores and transports fluids and chemicals	Two types: smooth with no ribosomes; rough with ribosomes on the surface
Ribosomes	Free in cytoplasm. Outer surface of rough endoplasmic reticulum	Small granule, 100–300 Å; composed of protein and nucleic acid	Protein production, such as enzymes and blood proteins	Large proteins are synthesized from polyribosomes (chains of ribosomes)
Mitochondria	Randomly in cytoplasm	Round or oval structures; 3–14 nm in length, 2–10 nm in width; membrane has 2 layers; inner layer has folds called cristae	Cell's "powerhouse"; makes ATP, the energy source for the cell	Active cells have more present than do inactive ones
Lysosomes	Randomly in cytoplasm	Membrane bound sacs; size varies	Contain hydrolytic enzymes for cellular digestive system	If the membrane breaks, the hydrolytic enzymes can destroy the cell
Microfilaments	Near nuclear envelope and within proximity of mitotic process	Small, solid structure approximately 5 nm in diameter	Support of cytoskeleton and motility	Consist of actin and myosin (contractile proteins)
Microtubules	Cytoskeleton, near nuclear envelope and component part of centriole near Golgi body	Hollow cylinder with protofilaments surrounding the outside tube; 20–25 nm in diameter, variable length	Maintenance of cell shape, motility and the mitotic process	Produced from tubulin polymerization; make up mitotic spindles and part of the structure of centriole.
Centriole	In centrosome near nucleus	Cylinders; 150 nm in diameter, 300–500 nm in length	Serve as insertion points for mitotic spindle fibers	Nine sets of triplet microtubles

up of phospholipids and cholesterol arranged in two layers. The phosphate end of the phospholipid and the hydroxyl radical of cholesterol are polar-charged hydrophilic (water-soluble) lipids oriented toward the inner and outer surfaces of the cell membrane. The fatty acid portion of the phospholipid and the steroid nucleus of cholesterol are non–polar-charged hydrophobic (water-insoluble) lipids directed toward each other in the center of the cell membrane. Other lipids such as lipoproteins and lipopolysaccharides contribute to the membrane structure.

Membrane Proteins

Most of the proteins found in the cell membrane are called glycoproteins and are found floating in the lipid bilayers. Two types of proteins, integral and peripheral, have been described in the cell membrane. *Integral proteins* may traverse the whole lipid bilayers and penetrate the outside of the membrane or only the cytoplasmic side of the membrane. These transmembrane proteins are thought to serve as a communication and transport system between the cell's interior and the external environment. *Peripheral proteins* are only found on the inner cytoplasmic side of the membrane and form the cell's cytoskeleton. Peripheral proteins are also attached to the cytoplasmic ends of integral proteins to form a reticular network for maintaining structural integrity and holding the integral proteins in a fixed position.

Membrane Carbohydrates

Membrane carbohydrates occur in combination with proteins (glycoproteins) and lipids (glycolipids). The carbohydrate portion almost always extends beyond the outer cell surface, giving the cell a carbohydrate coat often referred to as the glycocalyx. These carbohydrate moieties function in cell-to-cell recognition and provide a negative surface charge, surface receptor sites, and cell adhesion capabilities.[3] The function of the red blood cell membrane is discussed in detail in Chapter 8.

NUCLEUS

The nucleus is made up of three components: the chromatin, nuclear envelope, and the nucleoli. It is the control center of the cell and the largest organelle within the cell. The nucleus is made up largely of DNA and is the site of DNA replication and transcription. It is responsible for the chemical reactions within the cell and the cell's reproductive process. The nucleus has an affinity to the basic dyes because of the nucleic acids contained within it.

Chromatin

The *chromatin* consists of nucleic acids and proteins. Two types are present: the histones, which are negatively charged, and the nonhistones, which are positively charged. Chromatin has been divided into two types: (1) the heterochromatin, which is represented by the more darkly stained condensed clumping pattern and is the genetically inactive area of the nucleus, and (2) the euchromatin, which has diffuse, uncondensed chromatin and is the genetically active portion of the nucleus in that RNA transcription is able to occur in it. This genetic material is loosely coiled and when stained turns a pale blue.

Nuclear Envelope

Surrounding the nucleus is a *nuclear envelope* consisting of an inner and an outer membrane. The outer membrane is continuous with an extension of the endoplasmic reticulum. Between the two membranes is a diaphragm of approximately 50 nm in thickness that is continuous with the lumen of endoplasmic reticulum. Nuclear pores penetrate the nuclear envelope, allowing communication between the nucleus and the cytoplasm. The number of these pores decreases as the cell matures.

Nucleoli

The nucleus contains one to four *nucleoli*. These organelles contain a large amount of RNA and other proteins in a loose fibrillar form. The nucleolus is the site for the synthesis of various forms of RNA, which is transported through the nuclear pores for ribosomal assembly and protein synthesis.

CYTOPLASM

Cytoplasmic matrix is a homogeneous continuous aqueous solution called cytosol. It is the environment in which the organelles join and function. These organelles are discussed individually.

Golgi Complex

The *Golgi complex* is a system of stacked, membrane-bound, flattened sacs referred to as cisternae involved in modifying, sorting, and packaging macromolecules for secretion or delivery to other organelles. The number of stacked cisternae ranges from 6 to 30 per cell, depending on the cell type. The Golgi complex is normally located between the nucleus and luminal surface of the cell. The Golgi complex is horseshoe-shaped and usually arranged around the centriole pair. The concave aspect has numerous enzymes for synthetic activities. The convex side is the "maturing surface" and is where the various products are packaged.[3]

Membrane-bound vesicles are closely associated with the stacks of cisternae. Some of the vesicles are coated and bud off for transport to other areas of the cell. The Golgi complex seems to direct traffic in the cell. The exact mechanisms of macromolecule modification and sorting is still being defined, though it is clearly a responsibility of the Golgi complex.

Endoplasmic Reticulum

The endoplasmic reticulum (ER) (Fig. 7–2) is a lace-like network found throughout the cytoplasm of cells and appears as flattened sheets, sacs, and tubes of membrane. The ER subdivides the cytoplasm into various compartments. The outer membrane of the nuclear envelope is in continuity with the ER membrane and specializes in making and transporting lipid and membrane proteins.

Rough endoplasmic reticulum (RER) has a studded look on its outer surface caused by the presence of ribosomes engaged in synthesis of proteins. The amount of ER found within a cell is proportional with the protein production required by the cell. More ER is necessary for increased protein synthesis. Smooth ER does not contain ribosomes and may serve as storage sites for the newly synthesized protein. Also, it has been suggested as a site for steroid hormone production and synthesis of lipid substances.

Ribosomes

Ribosomes are small particles composed of near-equal amounts of protein and RNA. Ribosomes are found free in the cytoplasm, on the surface of RER, and in the nucleus and nucleoli of a cell. These bodies may exist singly (monoribosome) or form chains (polyribosomes). The more ribosomes present within the cell, the more basophilia observed with Wright's stain.

Ribosomes serve as the site of protein synthesis. This is accomplished with the assistance of transfer RNA, for amino acid transport to the ribosome, and messenger RNA, which provides the necessary information for the sequencing order of the amino acids for each protein.[4]

Mitochondria

The awareness of *mitochondria* (Fig. 7–3) within the cell has existed since the 19th century, but their function has only recently been clearly defined. Structurally, the mitochondria has a continuous outer membrane. Running parallel to it is an inner membrane that invaginates at various intervals, giving the interior a shelf appearance, referred to as cristae mitochondriales, where oxidative enzymes are attached. The two membranes differ chemically: the inner membrane has a higher protein content and a lower lipid content. The convoluted inner membrane increases the surface area to enhance the respiratory capability of the cell. The interior of the mitochondria consists of a homogenous material called the mitochondrial matrix that contains many enzymes for the extraction of energy from nutrients.

The mitochondria are responsible for the metabolic processes of energy-producing reactions and electron transfer-oxidative reactions. The oxidative systems described within the mitochondria are the Krebs cycle, the fatty acid cycle, and the respiratory chain.[5] Also present in the mitochondria are proteins, phosphorylase, ribosomes, and DNA.[6]

The mitochondria are capable of self-replication. It has recently been documented that this organelle has its own DNA and RNA for the mitochondrial division cycle. There may be fewer than 100 to thousands of mitochondria per cell. The number is directly related to the amount of energy required by the cell.

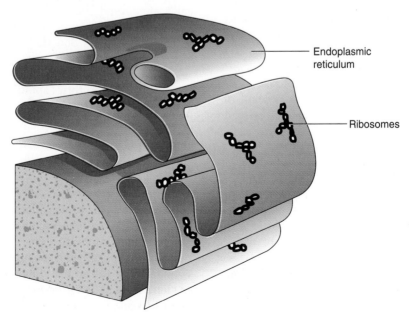

Endoplasmic reticulum

Ribosomes

Figure 7–2 Endoplasmic reticulum.

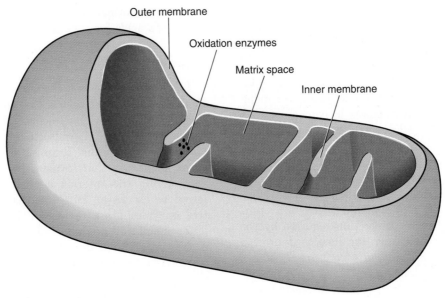

Outer membrane

Oxidation enzymes

Matrix space

Inner membrane

Figure 7–3   Mitochondria.

Mitochondria do not turn color with Wright's stain but instead give a negative image or clear impression against the stained cytoplasm. At times these organelles become so swollen that they appear as short white rods against a blue cytoplasmic background.

Lysosomes

Lysosomes contain hydrolytic enzymes bound within a membrane and are involved in the cell's intracellular digestive process. The membrane prevents the enzymes from attacking the protein, nucleic acids, mucopolysaccharides, lipids, and glycogen within the cell.[7] The enzymes become active when lysosomes bind to the phagocytic vacuole and the membrane ruptures, allowing the escape of the hydrolytic enzymes into the phagosome.

With Wright's stain, these lysosomes are visualized as granules. When stained, many of the granules appear azurophilic unless they are too small to be visualized under the light microscope. Special staining techniques are required in order to indicate the presence of the smaller granules.

Microfilaments

Microfilaments are solid structures approximately 5 nm in diameter and consist of actin and myosin proteins. These fibrils or groups of fibrils are located near the nuclear envelope or in the proximity of the nucleus and assist in cell division. They are also present near the membrane for cytoskeletal support and motility.

Microtubules

Microtubules are approximately 25 nm in diameter and vary in length. These organelles are organized from tubulin through self-assembly. The tubulin polypeptides form protofilaments. Usually 13 protofilaments are lined up in parallel rows of hollow spheres.[8] This arrangement gives the microtubules structural strength. A variety of conditions cause microtubules to become disorganized and disappear, especially after mitosis. Tubulin can then polymerize and reform the microtubule as needed.

Microtubules have several functions. Their contribution to the cytoskeleton helps maintain the cell's shape and the movement of some intracellular organelles. The microtubule makes up the mitotic spindle fibers and the centrioles during mitosis.[9] In the peripheral smear, the microtubules and microfilaments are not directly seen, but in special conditions the mitotic spindles may cluster and form Cabot rings.[6]

Centrioles

Centrioles are paired structures consisting of nine bundles of three microtubules within each bundle. They are shaped like cylinders and serve as insertion points for the mitotic spindle fibers during metaphase and anaphase of mitosis. The cylinders are 150 nm in diameter and 300–500 nm in length. The long axes are typically at right angles to one another.

SUMMARY

Cells are the building blocks of the living organism. Through numerous complex mechanisms, the cell provides the basis for all life processes. The nucleus serves as the control center by directing, educating, and maintaining the cell. Many organelles found within the cell serve as functional units, each providing a different activity in maintaining the cell's integrity or purpose. Many of these organelles are located in the cytoplasm. The cell is protected from its environment by a cell membrane. It is also able to regulate and communicate with its environment through the membrane barrier system.

The ultrastructure and function of the cell have been areas of intense research for years. The findings have greatly increased knowledge of the cell, and yet the ability to alter or direct a cell that has lost its regulatory or functional control is still lacking.

REVIEW QUESTIONS

1. Organelle(s) involved in synthesis of granules is (are)
   a. the nucleus
   b. the Golgi complex
   c. the mitochondria
   d. membrane-bound ribosomes
2. The most common protein found in the cell membrane is
   a. lipoprotein
   b. mucoprotein
   c. glycoprotein
   d. nucleoprotein
3. The "control center" of the cell is
   a. the nucleus
   b. the cytoplasm
   c. the membrane
   d. the microtubules
4. The nucleus is made largely of
   a. RNA
   d. DNA
   c. ribosomes
   d. glycoproteins
5. Protein synthesis occurs in
   a. the nucleus
   b. the mitochondria
   c. the Golgi complex
   d. ribosomes
6. The shape of a cell is maintained by which of the following? (1) microtubules, (2) microfilaments, (3) spindle fibers, (4) ribosomes.
   a. 1 and 2
   b. 1 and 3
   c. 2 and 4
   d. only 4
7. Functions of the cell membrane include
   a. interchange of substances
   b. cell-cell recognition
   c. receptors for cellular identity
   d. all of the above
8. The energy source for cells is
   a. the Golgi complex
   b. the endoplasmic reticulum
   c. the nucleolus
   d. the mitochondria

References

1. Wintrobe MM: Blood, Pure and Eloquent. New York: McGraw-Hill, 1980.
2. Bennington JL: Dictionary and Encyclopedia of Laboratory Medicine and Technology. Philadelphia: WB Saunders, 1984.
3. Guyton AC: Textbook of Medical Physiology, 8th ed. Philadelphia: WB Saunders, 1991.
4. Koss LB: Diagnostic Cytology and Its Histopathologic Bases, 3rd ed, vol 1. Philadelphia: JB Lippincott, 1979.
5. Prebble JN: Mitochondria, Chloroplasts and Bacterial Membranes. New York: Longman, 1981.
6. Bessis M: Blood Smears Reinterpreted. Berlin: Springer International, 1977.
7. Deduve C, Wattiaux R: Functions of lysosomes. Ann Rev Physiol 1966; 28:435.
8. Alberts B, Bray D, Lewis J, et al: Molecular Biology of the Cell. New York: Garland, 1983.
9. Stephens RE, Edds KT: Microtubules: structure, chemistry and function. Physiol Rev 1976; 56:709.

Suggested Reading

Avers CJ: Molecular Cell Biology. Menlo Park, CA: Benjamin Cummings, 1986.

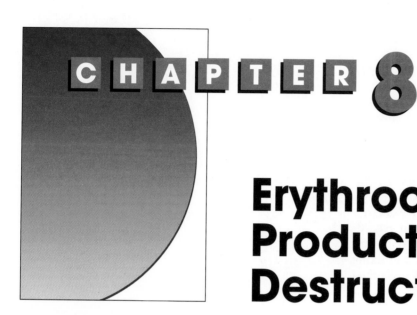

CHAPTER 8

Erythrocyte Production and Destruction

M. Ann Wallace

Objectives

AFTER COMPLETION OF THIS CHAPTER, THE READER WILL BE ABLE TO

1. Identify the features of the bone marrow that contribute to establishing the microenvironment necessary for the proliferation of cells.
2. Describe the chemical composition of erythropoietin and the functional attributes of each component.
3. Discuss the various mechanisms by which erythropoietin effects erythropoiesis.
4. List the erythroid precursors in order of maturity, including the morphologic characteristics, cellular activity, and functional capabilities of each.
5. Explain the formation and development of each stage of normoblastic maturation.
6. Identify the component substances of the erythrocyte membrane, together with their individual and collective function.
7. Identify the cellular organelles and describe their specific function.
8. Discuss the characteristics of the erythrocyte that mark it for destruction.
9. Discuss and identify the pathways used for erythrocyte destruction and subsequent degradation, including the recycling mechanism.

The erythrocyte was one of the first elements observed through the newly developed microscope in the year 1723. The oxygen-carrying capacity of the cell was discovered by Hoppe-Seyler in 1865. However, until the late 19th century, erythrocytes were believed to originate and develop specifically in the lymph nodes and/or the liver and spleen. In 1886, Neuman and Bizzazero independently observed nucleated blood cells in material squeezed from the ribs of human cadavers, and they proposed that the bone marrow was the major source of blood cell production. Soon after, the physiologist Claude Bernard pinpointed capillaries of medullary tissue as the site of erythropoiesis.[1]

During the next decade, postmortem examinations of bone marrow yielded information regarding the morphology of immature cells. With improved methods of obtaining, sectioning, and fixing bone marrow tissue, the identification of individual cells began.

Since the early 1950s, the revolutionary development of technologic instruments and methods, including the use of fluid and semisolid culture techniques, has contributed valuable information regarding the process of erythropoiesis as stimulated by erythropoietin. The various mechanisms by which erythropoietin can stimulate erythrocyte proliferation have been observed and documented.

With the maturation of molecular biology, the use of DNA-based clinical procedures will soon become part of routine laboratory testing. The information generated from this field will more accurately define and describe the relationship in erythrocytes between morphology and physiology.

THE ERYTHRON

By definition, the erythron encompasses all stages of erythrocytes in designated areas of the body: the developing normoblasts in the bone marrow, the circulating mature erythrocytes in the peripheral blood, and the vascular spaces within specific organs. When the term *erythron* is used, the concept of a unified functional tissue is implied.

Erythropoietin

In 1878, Paul Bert proposed the existence of a feedback loop (Fig. 8–1) between the erythroid marrow and the body tissues. Early in the 20th century, Carnot and DeFlandre postulated the existence of a humoral agent that adjusted erythropoiesis in response to tissue hypoxia. The agent was referred to as erythropoiesis stimulating factor,

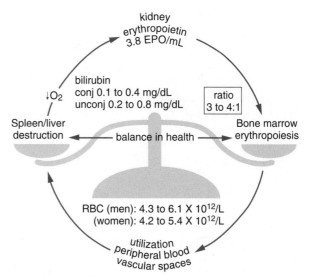

Figure 8–1 Feedback loop.

or erythropoietin. This factor was demonstrated by Erslev in 1953 in work with anemic rats. He concluded that stimulating dormant marrow cells with a very small dose of erythropoietin elicited production of erythroblasts. He further discovered evidence of receptor sites for transferrin and erythropoietin on the membrane of developing erythroid precursors. He observed that when these erythroid precursors possessed sufficient receptor sites on their membranes, they transformed into colony-forming units–erythroid (CFU-E).[1]

Biochemically, erythropoietin is a thermostable, nondialyzable, glycoprotein hormone with a molecular weight of between 20,000 and 30,000. It consists of a carbohydrate unit (34%), which is believed to convey specificity in recognizing target cell receptor sites, and a terminal sialic acid unit (10–15%), which is necessary for biologic activity in vivo. Upon desialation, this activity ceases totally.

A peritubular interstitial cell located in the kidney has been identified as the probable site for synthesis of erythropoietin.[1] Erythropoietin, when stimulated by tissue hypoxia, is capable of increasing the red cell mass through many mechanisms. By binding to the membrane surface receptors of erythroid precursors, erythropoietin stimulates the synthesis of RNA and perhaps cyclic adenosine monophosphate (cAMP). Once erythropoietin binds to specific membrane receptors,[2] it can stimulate CFU-E and control the production of erythrocytes by

1. Regulating the three division-reduction stages of normoblastic production.
2. Controlling the rate of production by shortening

the time element of either the division or the maturation process, or of both.[3]

3. Increasing the rate of the pentose-phosphate shunt.

4. Assisting in the egression of mature erythrocytes through small gaps of the endothelium into the sinusoids by working on the walls of the bone marrow sinuses.

5. Stimulating the early release of shift reticulocytes.

6. Increasing the rate of hemoglobin synthesis by transferring iron from transferrin to developing erythroid precursors.

In addition to tissue hypoxia, other factors that may have an influence on stimulating the production of erythropoietin have been identified. It is well documented that testosterone stimulates erythropoiesis, which partially explains the difference in hemoglobin concentration norms associated with sex and age categories. Also, through patients identified with pituitary, thyroid, and adrenal malfunction, evidence of the activity or absence of their specific hormones has been associated with either an increase or a decrease in the production of erythropoietin.[4] Excessive amounts of erythropoietin may be produced by cysts and tumors, causing polycythemia. Erythroblasts (pronormoblasts) have been shown to respond to erythropoietin with an increase of intracellular free calcium concentration. It is believed that the bone marrow cannot differentiate between physiologic and pathologic stimuli.[5]

Quantitative measurements of erythropoietin are performed on urine and plasma samples. Although normal levels of erythropoietin in urine are low (1–4 U/μL), urine is the preferred source for isolation of erythropoietin because urine is usually available in large quantities.[6] Increased amounts of erythropoietin are found in the urine of patients with anemias, except for those with anemia caused by renal disease.[7] Plasma values of 3–18 mU/mL of plasma reflect the amount of erythropoietin necessary to maintain a steady state of erythropoiesis. However, 2000–5000 mU/mL are necessary to compensate for severe hemolytic anemia or acute blood loss.[8]

In red blood cell aplasia, there is no response to stimulus by erythropoietin, which indicates the existence of a possible inhibitor. Antisera to human urine erythropoietin show highly specific biologic activity. Two types of anti-erythropoietin antibodies have been demonstrated: Type I causes the neutralization of the biologic activity of erythropoietin, and Type II causes hemagglutination. Some antisera contain both types.[9]

Microenvironment of the Bone Marrow

CARBON DIOXIDE CONTENT

Within the bone marrow exists a microenvironment that is conducive to elaboration of blood cells. The marrow can be described as a tissue with nonanastomosing arterial vessels emptying into a rich plexus of venous sinusoids. The sluggish circulation results in blood stasis, which contributes to a relatively high level of carbon dioxide. This promotes the elaboration of hemoglobin and the formation of primordial blood cells.[10] (Refer to O_2 dissociation curve in Chapter 9.)

WETTED STICKY SUBSTANCE

The formation of the stromal environment created by a multilayering of cells provides a sticky surface suitable for anchoring. Adherence of cells is essential to hematopoietic proliferation. The development of such a surface follows a very systematic programming. When monocytes attach to this wettable surface, a fertile bed that supports stem cell growth is produced. Here the monocytes transform into large activated macrophages. Once the macrophages establish connections through the extrusion of reticulum, these connections are stabilized by fibroblasts. Within 10 days, these structural elements coalesce, and endothelial cells overgrow the initial layer. Epithelial cells become flat, and macrophages become affixed to them.[11] This cellular bed appears to be essential in controlling differentiation and development of various cell lines.

LOCALE

Hematopoiesis takes place in marrow cords formed by the extravascular areas. Erythropoiesis localizes in the central sinus beds. Within these beds are iron-laden macrophages, often surrounded by erythroid precursors in various stages of development. These macrophages provide easily accessible iron to be used by the cells in the synthesis of hemoglobin. The extravascular area is separated from the intravascular area by a single layer of epithelial cells and processes of adventitial cells.

NORMOBLASTIC MATURATION

Normoblastic proliferation is a continuous process of replication and maturation. In the steady state, this process is controlled, reflecting the mechanism of the feedback loop. The pluripotential stem cells supply recognizable blasts commit-

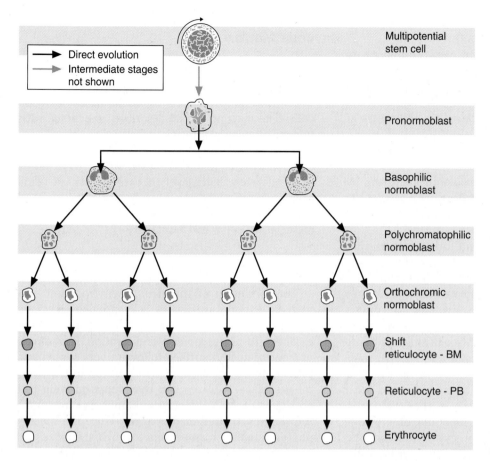

Figure 8–2 Maximum production of erythrocytes from one pronormoblast.

ted to erythropoiesis. This cell line undergoes three divisions with simultaneous nuclear and cytoplasmic maturation. As the cells mature, the development of hemoglobin progressively increases, with resultant decrease of RNA. Each division or maturation stage results in smaller cells, reflecting condensation of nuclear chromatin. Severe anemias involving increased cell loss can realize the *maximal potential* of mitotic divisions (two during the polychromatic normoblast stage), resulting in 16 mature erythrocytes from one pronormoblast (Figure 8–2).

Terminology

Three nomenclatures are used in identifying the erythroid precursors. The proerythroblast terminology is used primarily in Europe (Table 8–1).

Criteria Used in the Identification of the Erythroid Precursors

Identification of blood cells is dependent on a good working stain. In hematology, a modified Romanowsky stain, such as Wright's or Wright-Giemsa, is commonly used. Table 8–2 summarizes criteria for the identification of erythroid precursors with Wright's stain.

When the stage of maturation of any blood cell is determined, both the nucleus and the cytoplasm must be carefully examined. In the nucleus, the investigator should carefully observe the chromatin pattern (texture, density, homogeneity), size, nucleus-to-cytoplasm ratio, presence or absence of nucleoli, placement of nucleus in cell (central or eccentric), shape, color, and whether it is mononuclear, lobulated, or segmented.

Table 8-1. NOMENCLATURE FOR ERYTHROID PRECURSORS		
Normoblastic	**Rubriblastic**	**Erythroblastic**
Pronormoblast	Rubriblast	Proerythroblast
Basophilic normoblast	Prorubricyte	Basophilic erythroblast
Polychromatic normoblast (polychromatophilic)	Rubricyte	Polychromic erythroblast
Orthochromic normoblast	Metarubricyte	Orthochromic erythroblast
Reticulocyte	Reticulocyte	Reticulocyte
Erythrocyte	Erythrocyte	Erythrocyte

Table 8–2. NORMOBLASTIC SERIES: COMPARATIVE FACTUAL INFORMATION

Cell	Size (μm)	Nucleus-to-Cytoplasm Ratio	Nucleoli	% In Bone Marrow	Transit Time (hours In Bone Marrow)
Pronormoblast	12–20	8:1	1–2	1	12
Basophilic normoblast	10–15	6:1	0–1	1–4	20
Polychromatic normoblast	10–12	4:1	0	10–20	30
Orthochromic normoblast	8–10	1:2	0	5–10	48
Reticulocyte, shift	8–10	—	0	1	48–72
Reticulocyte	8–8.5	—	0	—	24–48 (PB)

The cytoplasm should be examined for amount of basophilia, which reflects the amount of RNA. Organelles (mitochondria, rough endoplasmic reticulum, polyribosomes, and ribosomes) react with the basic component of the stain to generate this blue color. Increased numbers of organelles generate a deeper blue color.

Maturation Sequence

PRONORMOBLAST (Fig. 8–3)

Nucleus. The nucleus is round to oval, containing one or two nucleoli. The chromatin contains fine clumps.

Cytoplasm. The cytoplasm, when stained, becomes intensely blue. The Golgi complex may be visible next to the nucleus. The color helps differentiate the pronormoblast from the myeloblast. When there is an abundance of red blood cell (RBC) precursors in the bone marrow, the color is striking.

Evidence of iron uptake and hemoglobin synthesis within the pronormoblast has been documented. The large content of RNA masks any hemoglobin color development. Blasts characteristically demonstrate small tufts of irregular cytoplasm along the periphery of the membrane. The pronormoblast undergoes mitosis and gives rise to two daughter pronormoblasts. These mature into basophilic normoblasts.

BASOPHILIC NORMOBLAST (Fig. 8–4)

Nucleus. The chromatin has begun to condense, thus revealing clumps along the periphery of the nuclear membrane and a few in the interior. As the chromatin condenses, the parachromatin areas become larger and sharper. The staining reaction is one of a deep purple-red.

Cytoplasm. When stained, the cytoplasm is a deeper, richer blue than the blast. Increased hemoglobin synthesis takes place, but the increased amounts of RNA completely mask the hemoglobin pigmentation. The basophilic normoblast undergoes mitosis, giving rise to two daughter cells that mature into two polychromatic normoblasts.

POLYCHROMATIC NORMOBLAST (Fig. 8–5)

Nucleus. The appearance of the chromatin pattern is quite variable at this stage of development. The condensation of chromatin has reduced the size of the cell considerably. Further condensation

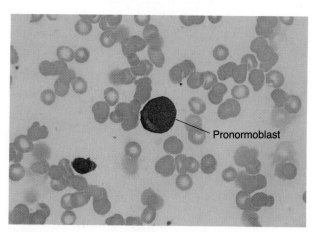

Figure 8–3 Pronormoblast (rubriblast), bone marrow; 1000×, Wright's stain.

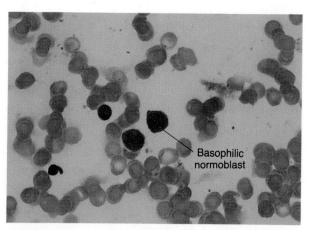

Figure 8–4 Basophilic normoblast (prorubricyte), bone marrow; 1000×, Wright's stain.

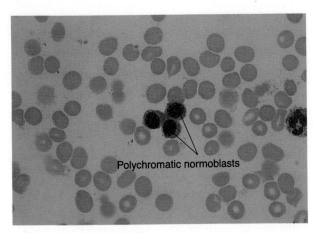

Figure 8–5 Polychromatic normoblasts, (rubricyte), bone marrow; 1000X, Wright's stain.

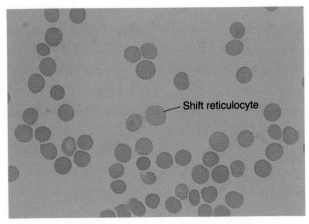

Figure 8–7 Shift reticulocyte, bone marrow; 1000X, Wright's stain.

can reveal the appearance of chromatin, which ranges from a spoke-wheel–like pattern to no pattern at all.

Cytoplasm. The color staining reaction of this cell demonstrates the greatest variety, reflecting the inverse relationship of increasing production of hemoglobin pigmentation and decreasing amounts of RNA. The color produced is a murky gray-blue.

The polychromatic normoblast goes through mitosis, producing two daughter cells that mature and develop into orthochromic normoblasts. In severe anemias, two divisions may take place at this stage. This is the last stage in which the cell is capable of undergoing mitosis.

ORTHOCHROMIC NORMOBLAST (Fig. 8–6)

Nucleus. The nucleus is almost or completely pyknotic. It is incapable of DNA synthesis and is usually ejected from the cell at this stage.

Cytoplasm. The cytoplasm reflects the full complement of hemoglobin production and, when stained, turns pink-orange. The residual organelles, mitochondria, rough endoplasmic reticulum, and polyribosomes react with the basic component of the stain and contribute a slightly bluish hue to the cell.

RETICULOCYTE

The cytoplasm can be easily compared with that of the orthochromic normoblast in that the predominant pigment is that of hemoglobin. Residual RNA, in varying amounts, continues to cast a bluish hue to the cell until eventual absorption of the organelles. This *shift reticulocyte* (Fig. 8–7) egresses through the wall of the sinusoids and enters the vascular system. When reticulocytes in the peripheral blood are observed with the use of a modified Romanowsky stain, a slightly larger cell is seen to demonstrate either residual RNA by dif-

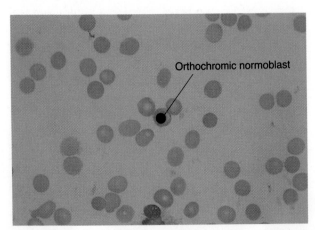

Figure 8–6 Orthochromic normoblast, (metarubricyte), bone marrow; 1000X, Wright's stain.

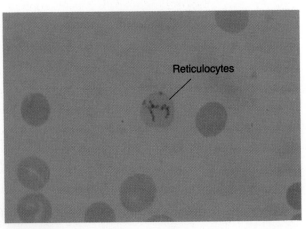

Figure 8–8 Reticulocytes, peripheral blood; 1000X, new methylene blue.

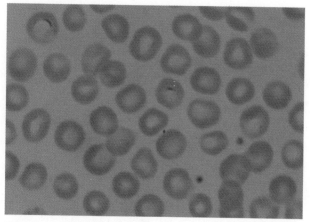

Figure 8–9 Mature erythrocytes, peripheral blood; 1000×, Wright's stain.

fuse *polychromatophilia* or aggregated RNA visualized as *basophilic stippling*. The reticulocyte (Fig. 8–8) can be examined with a supravital stain, such as new methylene blue, which precipitates the reticulum and results in clearly visible blue knotty strands. The reticulocyte count is an excellent index of bone marrow activity (discussed further in Chapter 12).

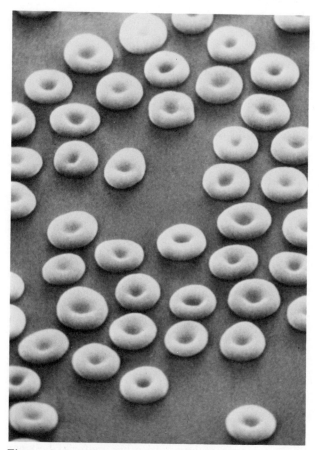

Figure 8–10 Scanning electron micrograph of red blood cells.

ERYTHROCYTE (Figs. 8–9, 8–10)

The mature circulating erythrocyte is a biconcave disc measuring 7–8 μm in diameter with a thickness of about 1.5–2.5 μm. It has a surface-to-volume ratio that enables optimal gaseous exchange to occur. The cell's main function of oxygen delivery throughout the body requires a membrane whose component parts interact, thus imparting to the cell the capabilities of selective permeability and deformability. It has been estimated that in the 120-day lifetime of the erythrocyte, it has traversed over 300 miles, constantly subjected to changes in pH, glucose concentration, osmotic pressure, surfaces, gases, and so forth. The interior of the erythrocyte contains 90% hemoglobin and 10% water.

THE ERYTHROCYTE MEMBRANE

Functions

The ability of the circulating erythrocyte to perform the function of gaseous exchange relies almost exclusively on the integral composition and functional capabilities of the membrane components (Fig. 8–11) and sufficient generated adenosine triphosphate (ATP). The RBC membrane (after a hemolyzing process resulting in ghost cells with intact membranes), when viewed through transmission electron microscopy, is shown to be a trilaminar structure that consists of approximately 40% lipid, 52% protein, and 8% carbohydrate.[12] Its arrangement is a double matrix of phospholipids in which specific proteins and phospholipids are located, some of which are strategically placed. The interplay of these components contributes to the structure and fluidity of the membrane. Any variability in this composition may alter the functional capabilities of the membrane and ultimately results in early cell death. The main physiologic functions of the RBC membrane are (1) to maintain cell shape deformability for osmotic balance between plasma and the cell cytoplasm, (2) to act as a supporting skeletal system for surface antigens, and (3) to help in the transportation of essential cellular ions and gases. This involves *passive transportation,* which occurs by simple diffusion through cell pores (gases, glucose), and *active transportation,* which involves the movement of substances against an electrochemical gradient (Na$^+$, K$^+$).[3]

Osmotic Balance and Permeability

The selectively permeable membrane allows water and anions (HCO$_3^-$, Cl$^-$) to freely enter the

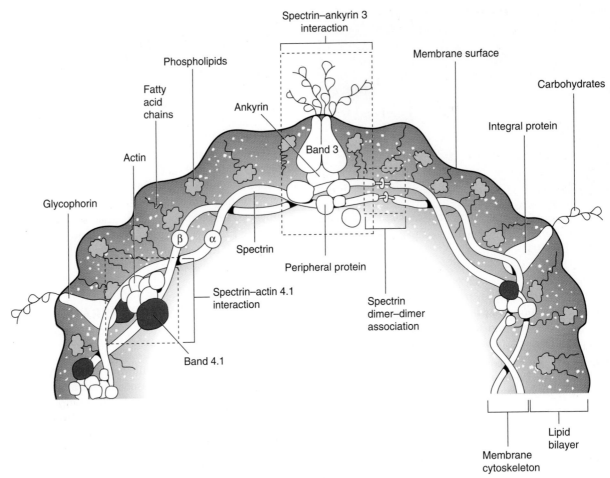

Figure 8-11 Schematic of erythrocyte membrane.

cell. These substances enter through pores or channels possibly formed by integral proteins. Their positive surface charges impart a unidirectional valve action. The active cation pump regulates the balance of intracellular and extracellular Na^+ and K^+, maintaining ratios of 1:12 and 25:1, respectively. This mechanism enables the erythrocyte to maintain a normal structure. Any slight deviation in the membrane selective permeability causes an influx of Na^+, resulting in a defective membrane. The cell assumes a spheroid shape with subsequent loss of hemoglobin.

Calcium, another cation, has been identified as also being necessary for maintenance of cell integrity. It is associated with the ATPase activity of spectrin and has an enzymatic control over the intracellular content of calcium ions. Intracellular levels of 5-10 $\mu M/L$ RBCs are maintained by the energy-dependent calcium ATPase cationic pump.[13] Calmodulin, a cytoplasmic Ca^+-binding protein, is believed to control the pumps.[14] With failure of active cation transport, altered membrane permeability incurs a process known as *colloid osmotic hemolysis,* in which intracellular equilibrium is lost

by the increase of water and ions, resulting in complete cell hemolysis. One example of increased cation permeability is sickle cell disease; in the process of deoxygenation in the sickle cell, there is measurably increased cation permeability of Na^+, K^+, and Ca^+.[15]

Composition

THE LIPID LAYER

The RBC membrane consists of two interrelated parts: the outer bilayer of lipids with integral proteins embedded in it and the underlying protein membrane skeleton[16,17] (see Fig. 8-11). The insoluble lipid portion of the membrane serves as a barrier to separate the vastly different ion and metabolite concentrations of the interior of the RBC from its external environment, the blood plasma.[16] The protein portion of the membrane is responsible for the shape, structure, and deformability of the RBC. It also contains the pumps and channels for movement of ions and other material between the RBC's interior and the blood plasma. Various proteins in the membrane act as receptors, RBC antigens, and enzymes. The outer lipid bilayer (by weight, 50% of the RBC membrane) consists of almost equimolar quantities of phospholipids and non-esterified cholesterol and smaller amounts of glycolipids.[18]

Several phospholipids compose a lipid bilayer (a bimolecular leaflet): phosphatidylcholine and sphingomyelin are located in the outer layer, and phosphatidylethanolamine and phosphatidylserine are in the inner layer. In this leaflet the polar heads of each lipid layer face away from the center of the membrane and toward the aqueous hydrophilic environment of the plasma. The long acyl tails of these lipids form a hydrophobic core of the membrane.[19] The cholesterol is embedded in this leaflet lipid bilayer and apparently stabilizes it. Glycolipids are also embedded here and located entirely in the external half of the bilayer; their carbohydrate moieties extend into the aqueous phase. They carry several important RBC antigens, including A, B, H, and P.[18, 20] Studies performed on several Rh genotypes demonstrated that $Rh_0(D)$, C/c, and E/e antigen-containing polypeptides span the lipid bilayer, having cytoplasmic domains susceptible to the action of proteases.[21] It appears that these antigens are necessary for normal membrane integrity. Therefore, the absence of these antigens on the RBC membrane elicits hemolysis[22] (Chapter 17).

MEMBRANE PROTEINS

The lipid membrane bilayer is coupled to a protein membrane skeleton that contains 10–12 major proteins and many minor proteins.[23] These proteins can be extracted from RBC membranes in sodium dodecyl sulfate, separated on polyacrylamide gel electrophoresis (SDS-PAGE) according to

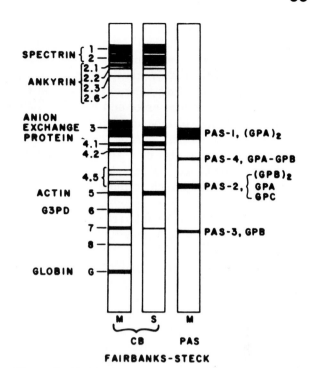

Figure 8–12 Bands of protein in red blood cell membrane.

their size, and then stained with Coomassie blue for membrane and skeletal proteins and with periodic acid Schiff (PAS) for the sialoglycoproteins, also known as glycophorins[18, 24, 25] (Fig. 8–12). The bands are numbered 1–8, beginning at the top of the gel. Table 8–3 lists these bands, their names, and their characteristics.

The membrane proteins are classified as integral or peripheral. The integral proteins penetrate or go across the lipid bilayer and can interact with the hydrophobic lipid area. Integral proteins include the glycophorins (A, B, C, and D), which are rich in carbohydrates, give the RBC its negative charge through membrane sialic acid, and carry membrane

Table 8–3. MAJOR MEMBRANE POLYPEPTIDES

Electrophoretic Designation	Molecular Weight	Percent of Protein	Name	Relation to Membrane
1	240.000	15 ⎫	Spectrin ⎧ α	Peripheral
2	225.000	15 ⎭	⎩ β	
2.1	206.000			
2.2	190.000	⎬ 5	Ankyrin	Peripheral
3	90–105.000	24	Anion channel	Integral
4.1	78.000	4.2		
4.2	72.000	5.0	Protein kinase	
4.5	45–75.000	5.0	Glucose transporter	Integral
5	43.000	4.5	Actin	Peripheral
6	35.000	5.5	G-3PD	Peripheral
7	29.000	3.4		
PAS-1 ⎱ PAS-2 ⎰	39.000	6.7	Glycophorin A	Integral

Modified from Steck TL: The organization of proteins in the human red blood cell membrane. J Cell Biol 1974, 62:1.

receptors and RBC antigens.[26] These are the proteins in the PAS 1, 2, and 3 bands. Protein 3 (band 3 on membrane proteins) is also an integral protein and functions as a transport or anion exchange protein that forms an anion channel in the membrane. Chloride ions enter and leave the RBC as the intracellular bicarbonate ion concentration varies with the carbon dioxide content of the blood.[27] Band 3 may also be a key site of attachment of the RBC membrane cytoskeleton to the lipid layer and may attach membrane hemoglobin and certain enzymes.

The peripheral proteins interact with protein or lipids at the membrane surface but do not penetrate the bilayer area. They line the inner membrane surface and interact to form a "membrane skeleton," or cytoskeleton. These fibrous proteins include the five major proteins: (1) spectrin (bands 1 and 2), (2) actin (band 5), (3) protein (band 4.1), (4) ankyrin (bands 2.2, 2.3, and 2.6 being isoforms), and (5) glyceraldehyde-3-phosphate dehydrogenase (GPD) (band 6).[18] Current research is defining the function of these proteins and the role they play as the cytoskeleton, which modulates cell shape and deformability. However, several abnormalities in these proteins have been shown to be related to morphologic disorders, such as spherocytosis and elliptocytosis, that clinically result in hemolytic processes.

Electron micrographs show a hexagonal lattice with long filaments of spectrin tetramers and higher oligomers joining complexes of actin and band 4.1[18, 28] (Fig. 8–13). Ankyrin appears as small globular areas when it is bound near the head groups of spectrin dimers. As seen in Figure 8–11, the membrane cytoskeleton is attached to the bilayer by at least one, and probably two, integral membrane proteins (band 3 and glycophorin C.)[18]

The strength of the skeleton appears to be derived from spectrin, a long fiber-like molecule composed of twisted flexible polymers of heterodimers (α and β) that join at their head ends to form heterotetramers (αβ)₂ and high-order oligomers, in which each molecule joins to two others in a radial arrangement.[29] This structure produces a strong but flexible scaffolding for the weak bilayer.

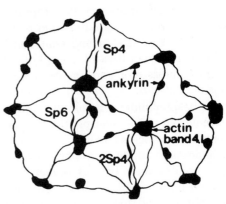

Figure 8–13 Hexagonal lattice of red blood cell membrane. (From Nathan DG, Oski FA [eds]: Hematology of Infancy and Childhood, 5th ed. Philadelphia: WB Saunders, 1993:543.)

Spectrin composes 50–70% of the skeletal mass and consists of two large polypeptide subunits that are structurally related but functionally distinct. These are the alpha chain, which is 267,000 D in length, and the beta chain, which is 246,000 D in length. The chains of this long, slender and twisted molecule line up side by side to form heterodimers.[30] The two chains are weakly associated except at the ends, which makes the molecule very flexible and therefore contributes to RBC membrane pliancy.[31]

Sequencing of the amino acids of the protein shows that each chain is composed of 106 amino acid triple helical segments or subunits (12,000 D) that have been duplicated many times. These subunits are linked to each other by short nonhelical regions (Fig. 8–14). The spectrin chains can be divided into a series of structural domains linked by trypsin-sensitive regions. (When the molecule is treated with trypsin, it cleaves in these areas, and the fragments or domains are obtained.) These domains are useful for detecting structural abnormalities because the molecule is so large that single amino acid substitutions are difficult to see. The domains are numbered from the head end of the molecule which contains the spectrin self-association site. There are five unique alpha chain domains, numbered from alpha I to alpha V, and four beta chain domains, numbered from beta I to beta IV. The alpha I domain attaches to a complemen-

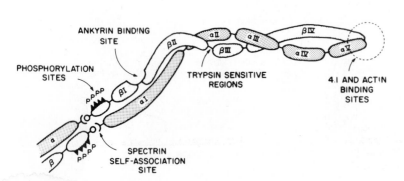

Figure 8–14 Schematic of spectrin structure.

tary site on a small phosphorylated region of the beta chain.[18] These tetramers of spectrin are bound by interactions with band 4.1 and actin-tropomyosin[18, 32] (see Fig. 8–11). Branching occurs at this interaction and leads to a two-dimensional skeletal network. This network is attached to the lipid bilayer by ankyrin, a large pyramid-shaped protein, which binds to the spectrin beta chain linking it to protein 3.[32] The protein network provides the physical integrity and morphologic shape of the normal RBC. Disorders associated with defective membranes are discussed in Chapter 17.

ERYTHROCYTE DESTRUCTION

The erythrocyte, having engaged in oxygen dissociation during its circulative life, begins to undergo senescence. A sequence of activities is initiated by decreased generation of ATP by the nonoxidative glycolytic pathway. Decreased amounts of cholesterol and phospholipids cause loss of selective permeability, resulting in increased Na^+ and loss of K^+, which in turn result in eventual decreased surface-to-volume ratio. Morphologically, the erythrocyte disc becomes spheroidal. The membrane accumulates IgG on its surface, which further impedes function. Internally, methemoglobin reductase ceases activity, which results in an accumulation of methemoglobin, a nonfunctional form of iron. All metabolic activities gradually shut down.

EXTRAVASCULAR HEMOLYSIS

As the erythrocyte circulates through the spleen, the glucose-free environment further stresses the erythrocyte, rendering it vulnerable to the sensitive macrophages located in the architectural maze of the splenic tissue. Phagocytosis occurs, and the RBC is degraded by strong digestive enzymatic activity of the macrophage. As the hemoglobin molecules are disassembled, iron is bound to transferrin and is transported to the hepatocytes to be stored.

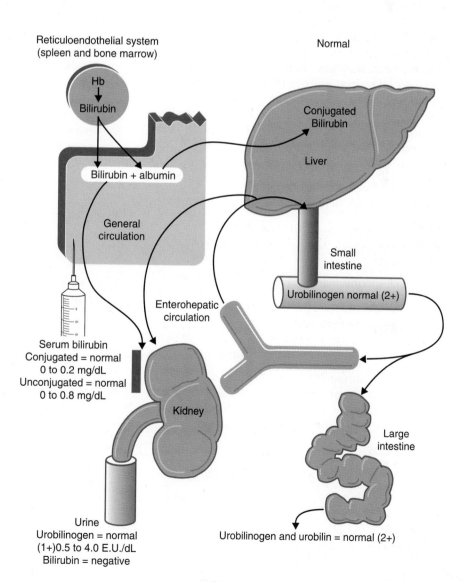

Figure 8–15 Schematic of erythrocyte extravascular destruction pathway. (From Tietz NW: *Fundamentals of Clinical Chemistry,* 3rd ed. Philadelphia: WB Saunders, 1987.)

Amino acids are transferred to body amino acid pools. The components of protoporphyrin are chemically separated, the alpha carbon is exhaled as CO_2, and the open tetrapyrrole ring is converted to biliverdin, which when conveyed to the liver is further conjugated into bilirubin glucuronide. This enters the intestine via the bile, where it is excreted as urobilinogen. This routine destruction of senescent erythrocytes takes place in lymphoid tissue and accounts for 90% of RBC degradation. This process of *extravascular hemolysis* balances RBC number with production and use (Fig. 8–15).

INTRAVASCULAR HEMOLYSIS

Ten percent of RBC hemolysis occurs *intravascularly* (within the lumen of the blood vessels). Conditions that cause increased hemolysis by this route include microangiopathic hemolytic anemias, septicemias, prostheses (e.g., an artificial heart valve), malarial parasites, and occasionally trauma and thermal burns. When continual hemolysis takes place intravascularly, the RBC components enter the circulating plasma. Hemoglobin chains dissociate into free dimers, are bound to plasma haptoglobin, and are transported to the liver for storage. Iron is bound to transferrin and is conveyed to body iron stores. The breakdown of protoporphyrin is identical to the procedure in extravascular pathway. Excessive continual hemolysis is consistent with the following measurable substances:

increased indirect bilirubin
depleted haptoglobin and hemopexin
increased lactate dehydrogenase (LD), isoenzymes 1 and 2
increased reticulocyte count
measurable methemalbumin
increased iron stores
hyperplastic bone marrow.

SUMMARY

The bone marrow provides a microenvironment essential for normoblastic production and maturation. The resultant normoblast consists of a trilaminar membrane that facilitates the delivery of oxygen from the red blood cell to the tissues and exercises selective permeability. An integral membrane is essential for normal function. Two distinct processes exist within the body for eventual red blood cell destruction.

REVIEW QUESTIONS

1. What is meant by the "feedback mechanism"?
2. What conditions can alter this balance?
3. Discuss several pathways erythropoietin can be employed in stimulating erythropoiesis.
4. Match the following erythroid precursors with their identifying characteristics.

Red Blood Cell Precursor	Characteristics
A. pronormoblast	a. released into the vascular system; capable of 35% hemoglobin production
B. basophilic normoblast	b. incapable of mitosis; nucleus is characteristically ejected at this stage
C. polychromatic normoblast	c. homogenous nucleus; 8:1 nucleus-to-cytoplasm ratio; observable iron uptake with minimal hemoglobin production
D. orthochromic normoblast	d. demonstrates variable morphologic changes involving inverse amounts of RNA/hemoglobin production
E. reticulocyte	e. chromatin has condensed, resulting in clumps along periphery of the nuclear membrane

5. Illustrate how several components of the RBC membrane complex ensure membrane integrity.
6. Give several characteristics of the RBC that contribute to senescence.
7. Contrast extravascular and intravascular hemolysis.
8. List several red blood cell conditions and specify the defect of the membrane component.

References

1. Beck WS: Hematology, 5th ed. Cambridge, MA: MIT Press, 1991.
2. Atkins HL, Broudy VC, Papayannopoulow T: Characterization of the structure of the erythropoietin receptor by ligand blotting. Blood 1991, 77(12):2577–2582.
3. Simmons A: Hematology: A Combined Theoretical and Technical Approach. Philadelphia: WB Saunders, 1989.
4. McKenzie SB: Textbook of Hematology. Philadelphia: Lea & Febiger, 1988.
5. Miller BA, Foster K, Robishaw JD, et al: Role of pertussis toxin–sensitive guanosine triphosphate binding proteins in the response of erythroblasts to erythropoietin. Blood 1991, 77(3):486–492.
6. Erslev AJ: Production of erythrocytes. *In* Williams WJ,

Beutler E, Erslev A, Lichtman MA (eds): Hematology, 4th ed. New York: McGraw-Hill, 1990:389–407.

7. Floyd PB, Gallagher PG, Valentino LA, et al: Heterogeneity of the molecular basis of hereditary pyropoikilocytosis and hereditary elliptocytosis associated with increased levels of the spectrin alpha 1/74-kilodalton tryptic peptide. Blood 1991, 78(5):1364–1372.

8. Erslev AJ, Kansu E, Caro J: The biogenesis and metabolism of erythropoietin. *In* Golde DW, Cline MJ, Metcalf D, Fox CF (eds): Hematopoietic Differentiation. New York: Academic Press, 1978:1–14.

9. Lange RD, McDonald TP, Jordan T: Antisera to erythropoietin: partial characterization of two different antibodies. J Lab Clin Med 1969, 73:78–90.

10. Smith BH. Blood Diseases—Infancy and Childhood. St. Louis: CV Mosby, 1960.

11. Dexter TM, Spooner E, Schofield R, et al: Hematopoietic stem cell and the problem of self-renewal. Blood Cells 1984, 10:315.

12. Steck TL: The organization of proteins in the human red blood cell membrane. J Cell Biol 1974; 62:1–19.

13. James PH, Pruschy M, Vorhers TE, et al: Primary structure of the cAMP-dependent phosphorylation site of the plasma membrane calcium pump. Biochemistry 1989; 28(10):4253.

14. Takakuwa Y, Mohandas N: Modulation of erythrocyte membrane material properties by Ca^{2+} and calmodulin. Implication for their role of skeletal proteins and interaction. J Clin Invest 1988, 82(1):394.

15. Rhoda MD, Apovo N, Beuzard Y, Giraud F: Ca^{++} permeability in deoxygenated sickle cells. Blood 1990, 75(12):2453–2458.

16. Stephen, BS, Beutler E: The red cell membrane. *In* Williams WJ, Beutler E, Erslev A, Lichtman MA (eds): Hematology, 4th ed. New York: McGraw-Hill, 1990:369–371.

17. Singer SJ, Nicholson GL: The fluid mosaic model of the structure of cell membranes. Science 1972, 175:720.

18. Becher PS, Lux SE: Disorders of the red cell membrane. *In* Nathan DG, Oski FA (eds): Hematology of Infancy and Childhood, 4th ed. Philadelphia: WB Saunders, 1993:529–556.

19. Sweeley CC, Dawson G: Lipids of the erythrocyte. *In* Jamison GA, Greenwalt TJ (eds): Red Cell Membrane Structure and Function. Philadelphia: JB Lippincott, 1969:121.

20. Watkins WM: Blood group substances: their nature and genetics. *In* Surgenor DM (ed): The Red Blood Cell, 2nd ed, vol 1. New York: Academic Press, 1974:293–360.

21. Suyama K, Goldstein J: Enzymatic evidence for differences in the placement of Rh antigens within the red cell membrane. Blood 1991; 75(1):255–260.

22. Agre P, Cartron JP: Molecular biology of the Rh antigens. Blood 1991, 78(3):551–563.

23. Bennett V: The membrane skeleton of human erythrocytes and its implications for more complex cells. Annu Rev Biochem 1985, 54:273.

24. Fairbanks G, Steck TL, Wallach DF: Electrophoretic analysis of the major polypeptides of the human erythrocyte membrane. Biochemistry 1971, 10:2606.

25. Lux SE: Disorders of the red cell membrane skeleton: Hereditary spherocytosis and hereditary elliptocytosis. *In* Stanbury JB, Wyngaarden DS, Goldstein JL, Brown MS (eds): The Metabolic Basis of Inherited Disease, 5th ed. New York: McGraw-Hill, 1983:1573–1605.

26. Furthmayr H: Glycophorins A, B, and C: A family of sialoglycoproteins, isolation and preliminary characterization of trypsin derived peptides. *In* Lux SE, Marchesi VT, Fox CJ (eds): Normal and Abnormal Red Cell Membranes. New York: AR Liss, 1979:195–211.

27. Jennings ML: Topical review: Oligometric structure and the anion transport function of human erythrocyte band 3 protein. J Membr Biol 1984, 80:150.

28. Lui SC, Derick LH, Palek KJ: Visualization of the hexagonal lattice in the erythrocyte membrane skeleton. J Cell Biol 1987, 104:527.

29. Lux SE: Dissection of the red cell membrane skeleton. Nature 1979, 281:426.

30. Shotton DM, Burke BE, et al: The molecular structure of human erythrocyte spectrin: biophysical and electron microscope studies. J Mol Biol 1979, 131:313.

31. Speicher DW, Marchesi VT: Erythrocyte spectrin is composed of many homologous triple helical segments. Nature 1984, 311:177.

32. Lux SE: Spectrin-actin membrane skeleton of normal and abnormal red blood cells. Semin Hematol 1979, 16:21.

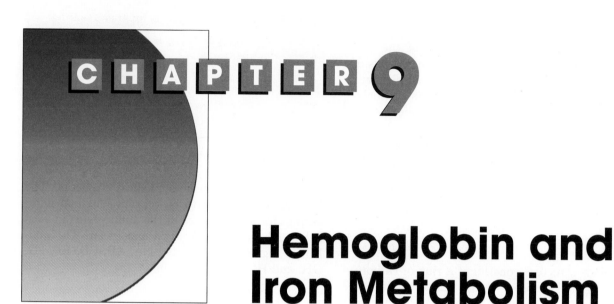

CHAPTER 9

Hemoglobin and Iron Metabolism

Mary Coleman

Outline

Objectives

AFTER COMPLETION OF THIS CHAPTER, THE READER WILL BE ABLE TO

1. Identify the structure of hemoglobin.
2. Describe the biosynthesis of heme and globin.
3. Describe the regulatory effects of hemoglobin metabolism.
4. Identify the important role that hemoglobin plays in maintaining body functions.
5. Describe the mechanism by which hemoglobin carries oxygen to the tissue.
6. Describe the Bohr effect.
7. Identify the three types of normal hemoglobin in adults and their normal values.
8. Discuss the ontogeny of hemoglobin.
9. Discuss the absorption, regulation, transport, and storage of iron in the body.

HEMOGLOBIN METABOLISM

Structure

Hemoglobin is the main component of the red blood cells; its concentration within the red blood cells is approximately 34 g/dL. It is a red pigment with a molecular weight of 64.5 kD and is a vehicle for the transport of oxygen and carbon dioxide in the body.

The hemoglobin molecule is a conjugated protein. It was the first protein whose structure was described by x-ray chromatography.[1-4] Each molecule consists of four heme groups and a protein portion called globin.

HEME

The heme structure consists of a ring of carbon, hydrogen, and nitrogen atoms called protoporphyrin IX with an atom of ferrous (Fe^{+2}) iron attached (ferroprotoporphyrin) (Fig. 9–1). Each heme group is positioned in a pocket of the polypeptide chain near the surface of the hemoglobin molecule. The heme component can combine reversibly with one molecule of oxygen or carbon dioxide. The heme component also renders blood red.

GLOBIN

The globin in the hemoglobin molecule consists of two pairs of polypeptide chains. These chains are made up of 141–146 amino acids each. Variations in the amino acid sequences give rise to different types of globin chains (Table 9–1).[5]

Each of the polypeptide chains is divided into

Table 9–1. GLOBIN CHAINS		
Symbol	Name	No. of Amino Acids
α	Alpha	141
β	Beta	146
γ_A	Gamma A	146 (position 136: alanine)
γ_G	Gamma G	146 (position 136: glycine)
δ	Delta	146
ϵ	Epsilon	Unknown
ζ	Zeta	141
θ	Theta	Unknown

eight helices and seven nonhelical segments. The helices, designated A to H, contain subgroup numberings for the sequence of the amino acids in each helix and are relatively rigid and linear. The nonhelical segments, designated NA, AB, CD, EF, FG, GH, and HC are more flexible.

COMPLETE MOLECULE

The globin chains are looped to form a cleft pocket for heme. Heme is suspended between the E and F helices of the polypeptide chain (Fig. 9–2). Amino acids in the cleft are hydrophobic, and each chain contains a heme group with iron positioned between two histidine radicals. Amino acids on the outside are hydrophilic, rendering the molecule water-soluble. The arrangement also helps iron stay in the ferrous form.

A complete hemoglobin molecule is spherical, has four heme groups attached to four polypeptide chains, and may carry up to four molecules of oxygen.

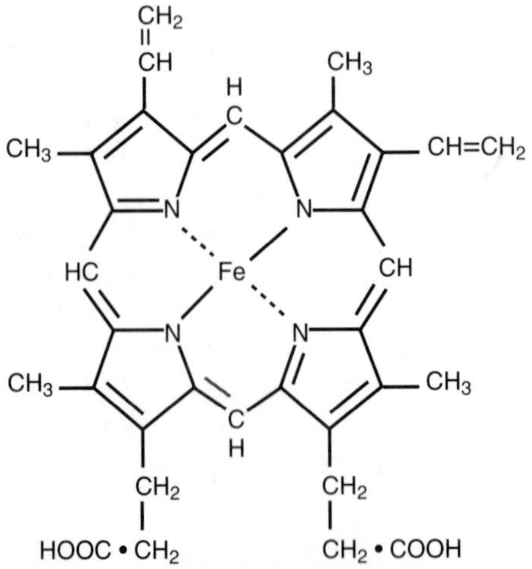

Figure 9–1 Pathophysiology of heme synthesis. (From Bottomley SS, Muller-Eberhard UM: Pathophysiology of heme synthesis. Semin Hematol 1988; 25:282–302.)

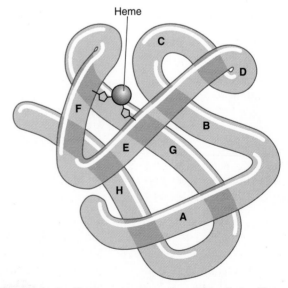

Figure 9–2 Tertiary structure of a globin chain. Heme is suspended between the E and F helices of the polypeptide chain.

Biosynthesis

HEME

Biosynthesis of heme takes place in the mitochondria and cytoplasm of the erythrocyte precursors from the pronormoblast to the reticulocyte in the bone marrow. Mature erythrocytes cannot make hemoglobin because they lose their mitochondria and the capability of using the tricarboxylic cycle necessary for hemoglobin synthesis.

Heme biosynthesis begins with the condensation of glycine and succinyl coenzyme A (CoA), catalyzed by δ-aminolevulinic acid (δ-ALA) synthase to form ALA. δ-ALA synthase requires pyridoxal 5'-phosphate as a cofactor. This pathway continues until, in the final step of production of heme, Fe^{+2} combines with protoporphyrin IX in the presence of ferrochelatase to make heme (Fig. 9–3).[6]

Transferrin, a plasma protein, carries iron in the ferric (Fe^{+3}) form to developing red blood cells. Iron goes through the red blood cell membrane to the mitochondria and is united with protoporphyrin IX to make heme. Heme leaves the mitochondria and is joined to the globin chains in the cytoplasm.

GLOBIN

Six structural genes control the synthesis of the six globin chains. Alpha and zeta genes are on chromosome 16; gamma, beta, delta, and epsilon genes are linked on chromosome 11.

The protein synthetic pathway is followed in the translation of the genetic code to the final globin polypeptide chain. Each set of single chains is synthesized in equal amounts, and the chains are released from the ribosomes in the cytoplasm. An alpha chain and a non-alpha chain combine to form dimers, and two dimers spontaneously combine to form tetramers. These chains are immediately incorporated into the heme moiety and complete the molecule.[7]

The combination of alpha and beta chains is most common, followed by combinations of alpha with gamma and alpha with delta globin chains.[1]

Progression of Hemoglobin Production: Ontogeny Through Adult Forms of Hemoglobin

The hemoglobin composition in the erythrocyte differs, depending on gestational or postnatal age of the person. This change is due to changes in the activation and inactivation or switching of the globin genes, progressing from the zeta to the alpha gene on chromosome 16 and from the epsilon to the gamma, delta, or beta genes on chromosome

11. The zeta and epsilon genes normally appear only during the first 3 months of embryonic development. These two chains in addition to the alpha and gamma chains are constituents of embryonic hemoglobins (Fig. 9–4). Another globin gene on chromsome 16 has been identified as a theta gene.[5]

A normal adult has primarily hemoglobin A ($\alpha_2\beta_2$) with small amounts of hemoglobins A_2 ($\alpha_2\delta_2$) and F ($\alpha_2\gamma_2$) (Table 9–2).

Hemoglobin A also has minor amounts of hemoglobin that have been modified after translation. Usually a component has been added to the N-terminus of the beta chain. The most common one is hemoglobin A_1C, in which glucose has been added. Normally, about 4% of hemoglobin A is in the A_1C form. In uncontrolled diabetes mellitus, the amount of A_1C is increased.[5]

Regulation

HEME

Regulation of heme production takes place in the heme production pathway. The key rate-limiting step in heme synthesis is thought to be the initial reaction of glycine and succinyl-CoA to form 5-aminolevulinic acid (δ-ALA). ALA synthase is inhibited by heme, which leads to a decrease in heme production (a negative feedback mechanism). Other enzymes in the heme pathway inhibited by heme are ALA dehydratase and porphobilinogen deaminase. An increased demand for heme would induce an increased synthesis in ALA synthase.[6]

Some research suggests that ferrochelatase (heme synthase) also plays a regulatory role in heme biosynthesis. A negative feedback mechanism by protoporphyrin IX and heme inhibits the enzyme.[8]

GLOBIN

Globin production is regulated by the rate at which the DNA code is transcribed to messenger RNA (mRNA). The amount of the specific globins synthesized is proportional in general to the content of their individual globin mRNAs.

Heme (in the form of hemin) is important in controlling the rate of globin synthesis in intact reticulocytes and various cell-free extracts, and in its absence, globin production decreases. The end result is that normal mature red blood cells contain only complete hemoglobin molecules. Pools of free heme or globin chains are minute.[9, 10]

Function

The main function of hemoglobin is transport of oxygen from lungs to the tissues and carbon diox-

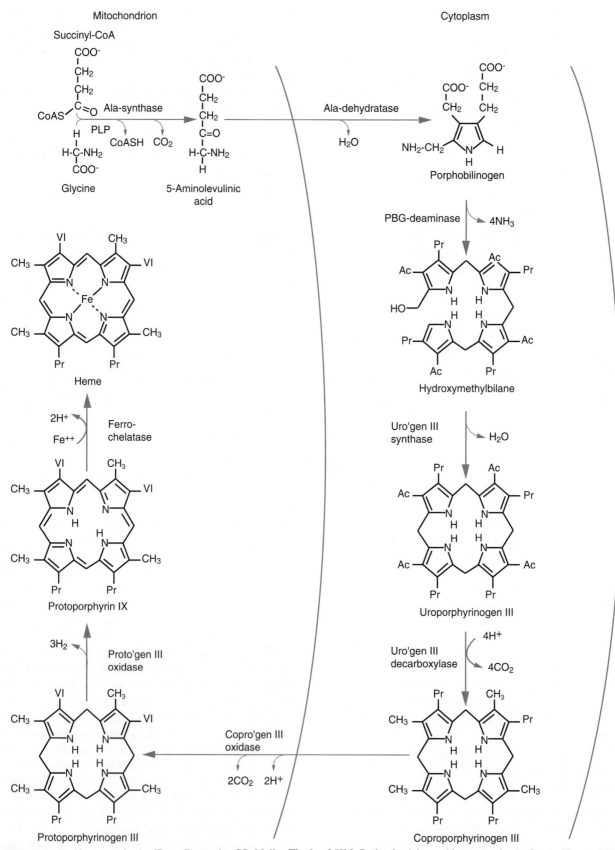

Figure 9–3 Heme synthesis. (From Bottomley SS, Muller-Eberhard UM: Pathophysiology of heme synthesis. Semin Hematol 1988; 25:282–302.)

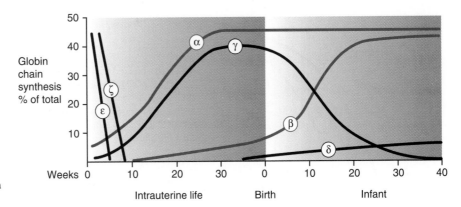

Figure 9–4 Globin chain production from intrauterine life to adulthood.

ide back to the lungs. Hemoglobin also plays a role in electron transport, oxygen reduction, and transfer of oxygen for hydroxylation reactions.

Myoglobin, which is present in cardiac and skeletal muscle, is an oxygen-binding heme protein. It exists in a monomer form and binds oxygen with greater affinity than does hemoglobin. Its oxygen dissociation curve is hyperbolic (Fig. 9–5).[11,12] It is not effective in delivering oxygen to the tissues.

Hemoglobin is an allosteric molecule; that is, its function and structure are influenced by other molecules. A major controller of hemoglobin-oxygen affinity in human erythrocytes is 2,3-diphosphoglycerate (2,3-DPG). As 2,3-DPG increases in concentration in the hemoglobin solution, the oxygen affinity progressively decreases. As oxygen is unloaded by hemoglobin, there is a widening of the space between beta chains and the binding of 2,3-DPG. Anionic salt bridges form between the beta chains. The deoxyhemoglobin molecule is known as the tense form and has lower affinity for oxygen. The oxyhemoglobin molecule, when loaded with oxygen, is known as the relaxed form of hemoglobin. In the relaxed form, the salt bridges have been broken and beta chains are pulled to-

gether, expelling 2,3-DPG. The relaxed form has a higher affinity for oxygen[12, 13] (Fig. 9–6).

Each of the four heme components in the hemoglobin molecule can reversibly bind one oxygen molecule, thus resulting in oxygenation of hemoglobin (not oxidation). The amount of oxygen picked up and released by the red blood cells is dependent on the partial pressure of oxygen (pO_2) present.

The relationship between the oxygen saturation of hemoglobin (%) and pO_2 is described by the oxygen dissociation curve of hemoglobin. This curve is distinctly sigmoidal (see Fig. 9–5). The affinity of hemoglobin for oxygen is often defined in terms of the amount of O_2 needed to saturate 50% of the hemoglobin (P_{50}). Normally a pO_2 of 27 mm Hg results in 50% O_2 saturation. The sigmoidal curve shifts to the left or right if there are changes in pH of blood (this phenomenon is known as the Bohr effect), in body temperature, in 2,3-DPG concentration, in the type of globin structure in the heme molecule, and in the overall stability of the heme molecule.[4]

If there is a shift to the left in the curve, as seen with a decreased H^+ concentration (increased pH), decreased 2,3-DPG concentration, or decreased body temperature, a pO_2 of less than 27 mm Hg is required for 50% hemoglobin saturation. A patient with a normal arterial pO_2 concentration (90–150 mm Hg) would have a higher percentage of oxygen saturation of hemoglobin and an increased oxygen affinity. The patient would pick up more oxygen in the lungs and give up less oxygen in the tissues. Conditions causing a shift to the left include multiple transfusions of stored blood with depleted 2,3-DPG, rapid correction of metabolic acidosis, presence of hemoglobin F, and the presence of methemoglobin, carboxyhemoglobin, and some other hemoglobin variants. These conditions are further explained later.

If there is a shift to the right in the curve, as seen with an increased H^+ concentration (decreased pH), increased 2,3-DPG concentration, or

Table 9-2. NORMAL HEMOGLOBINS		
Time	**Globin Chain**	**Hemoglobin**
INTRAUTERINE		
Early embryogenesis	$\zeta + \epsilon$	Gower-1
(product of the yolk	$\alpha + \epsilon$	Gower-2
sac erythroblasts)	$\delta + \gamma$	Portland
Begins in early embryo-	$\alpha + \gamma$	F
genesis; peaks during		
midgestation and		
begins rapid decline		
just before birth		
BIRTH	$\alpha + \gamma$	F, 60–90%
	$\alpha + \beta$	A, 10–40%
ADULTHOOD	$\alpha + \gamma$	F, <1–2%
	$\alpha + \delta$	A_2, <3.5%
	$\alpha + \beta$	A, >95%

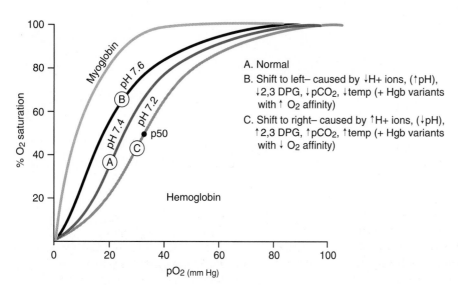

Figure 9-5 Oxygen dissociation curve.

increased body temperature, a pO_2 of more than 27 mm Hg is required for 50% hemoglobin saturation. A patient with a normal pO_2 would have a lower percentage of oxygen saturation and decreased oxygen affinity. The patient would thus pick up less oxygen in the lungs and give up more oxygen in the tissues. A shift to the right occurs in conditions causing hypoxia, such as high altitude, pulmonary insufficiency, congestive heart failure, severe anemia, and cardiac right-to-left shunt.[14]

Hemoglobin F (fetal hemoglobin) has poor binding capacity with 2,3-DPG, resulting in a shift to the left in the dissociation curve. Cord blood made up primarily of hemoglobin F has a P_{50} of 19-21 mm Hg. This results in increased oxygen saturation of hemoglobin and increased oxygen affinity. Thus the fetus has the physiologic ability to extract oxygen from the maternal blood supply via hemoglobin F. After birth, hemoglobin F is less functional because oxygen unloading is constrained.

Methemoglobin is a form of hemoglobin that contains iron in the ferric state (Fe^{+3}). A small amount is normally present in the blood. Methemoglobin is continuously being formed within erythrocytes because of spontaneous oxidation of hemoglobin, but it is prevented from accumulation within the red blood cells by the reduction of oxidized heme by a number of enzyme systems that restrict the normal concentration of methemoglobin to <1% of total hemoglobin.

If methemoglobin is increased in blood, there is a shift to the left in the oxygen dissociation curve, and oxygen affinity is increased. This results in delivery of less oxygen to the tissues, and patients present with cyanosis.[5]

Elevated levels of methemoglobin are seen when there is excess production of methemoglobin as a result of presence of oxidants (e.g., nitrites) or if there is decreased activity of methemoglobin reductase (usually a genetic deficiency). It is also seen in patients who inherit a hemoglobin M dis-

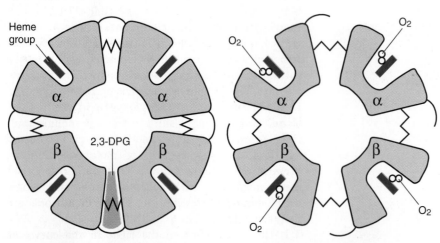

Deoxyhemoglobin tense (T) structure   Oxyhemoglobin relaxed (R) structure

Figure 9-6 Hemoglobin molecular changes.

ease, which is caused by an abnormality in the structure of the globin portion of the hemoglobin molecule.

Methemoglobin levels can be detected by spectrum absorption instruments. Methemoglobin peaks in the range of 620–640 nm. Treatment is administration of ascorbic acid or methylene blue.

Sulfhemoglobin is a chemically altered hemoglobin formed by the irreversible oxidation of hemoglobin by certain drugs and chemicals. Ingestion of drugs such as sulfonamides and acetanilid have been associated with the disorder. In vitro it is formed by the addition of hydrogen sulfide to hemoglobin. It is ineffective for oxygen transport (100 times less affinity for oxygen), and patients with elevated levels (>3–4%) present with cyanosis. Sulfhemoglobin cannot be converted to hemoglobin; thus it persists for the life of the cell. Treatment consists of avoidance of the offending agent.[15]

Sulfhemoglobin, like methemoglobin, peaks at 620 nm on a spectrum instrument. Air-equilibrated and carbon monoxide–equilibrated samples can be used to distinguish methemoglobin from sulfhemoglobin. Sulfhemoglobin can then be confirmed by isoelectric focusing.[16]

Carboxyhemoglobin results from the binding of carbon monoxide to heme iron. Hemoglobin has about 200 times more affinity for carbon monoxide than for oxygen.

Some carboxyhemoglobin is produced endogenously. Normal values range from 0.2% to 0.8%. Exogenous carbon monoxide is derived from the exhaust of automobiles and from industrial pollutants such as coal, gas, charcoal burning, and tobacco smoke. In smokers, levels may vary from 4% to 20%. Toxic effects such as headaches and dizziness may be present at levels of 10–15%. Levels of more than 50% may cause coma and convulsions. Carboxyhemoglobin may be detected by spectrum absorption instruments. In severe carbon monoxide poisoning, hyperbaric oxygen treatments may be used.[17]

IRON METABOLISM

Iron is essential for human life. Most functional iron is in the form of hemoglobin and myoglobin, but a small, significant portion of iron is used to bind with cofactors essential to basic metabolic oxidative and reduction reactions (Table 9–3). The regulation of body iron is complex and exquisitely done so as to preserve iron needed but not to allow highly toxic excesses.[18]

Table 9–3. IRON COMPARTMENTS IN NORMAL HUMANS

Compartment	Total Body Iron
Hemoglobin iron	Approximately 70%
Storage iron (hemosiderin ferritin)	Approximately 25%
Myoglobin iron	Approximately 5%
Other sources	<1%
In peroxidase, catalase	
In cytochromes	
In riboflavin enzymes	

Dietary Iron

Iron is absorbed most efficiently in the duodenum of the gastrointestinal tract. It is absorbed in two forms: heme and nonheme iron. Heme iron is well absorbed. It is present in forms of hemoglobin, myoglobin, and heme enzymes in meat sources. Approximately 20–30% of heme iron is absorbed.

Nonheme iron, found in nonmeat sources such as legumes and leafy vegetables, accounts for approximately 90% of dietary iron, but only about 10% of it is absorbed. An average American diet may contain 10–20 mg of iron per day, but of that, only 1–2 mg is absorbed.

The amount of iron absorbed is dependent on the composition of the meal. Caffeine, fiber, phylates, tannates, and phosphates hamper iron absorption. Ascorbic acid enhances iron absorption. Cooking in iron pots and pans increases the amount of iron found in food. Iron absorption is also influenced by gastrointestinal factors such as gastric secretion, intestinal motility, and consequences of surgery or bowel disease.[19]

Absorption

Upon entering the gastrointestinal tract, iron is most effectively absorbed in the duodenum, and less so in the lower gastrointestinal tract. Iron is absorbed in both the heme and nonheme forms and must traverse the mucosal epithelium and pass into the submucosal capillary network. Heme iron is absorbed intact and processed within the mucosal cell. It is degraded to free iron and a tetrapyrrole by a heme-splitting enzyme, heme oxygenase.

Nonheme iron either may be absorbed bound to transferrin or may pass the mucosa by diffusion. Upon entering the mucosal cells, both heme and nonheme iron enters a common pool. Some of the absorbed iron is held by ferritin, a storage form of iron, until the cell is exfoliated. Some iron is only temporarily stored as ferritin to be released and absorbed over a period of a few hours.[20, 21]

Iron enters the circulation bound to transferrin, nonspecifically bound to albumin, or perhaps in the form of low–molecular-weight iron chelates. Iron may also be taken up by macrophages to be carried back into the intestinal lumen.

Regulation

Humans are unique in their lack of any effective means to excrete excess iron. Therefore they regulate iron by controlling absorption. The amount of iron absorbed is inversely related to the amount of iron stores and the rate of erythropoiesis. Both in vivo and in vitro animal studies, as well as studies of human duodenal mucosal obtained by biopsy, show this to be true. Some evidence suggests that this is achieved, at least in part, by altering the number of specific iron receptors on the mucosal surface.[18] Normal absorption of iron is 1–2 mg/day. With decreased iron stores, iron absorption may be 3–4 mg/day. In iron overload, only 0.5 mg/day is absorbed.

Humans conserve iron very efficiently. There is a 35- to 40-mg/day turnover of iron, and a normal male may lose 1 mg/day, mostly through normal shedding of the epithelial cells from the intestine. A menstruating female will lose, on the average, 2 mg/day. Patients with iron overload may lose up to 4 mg/day.[21]

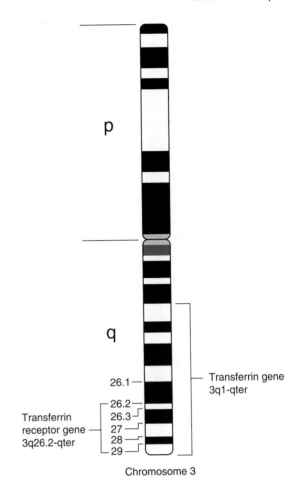

Chromosome 3

Cycle and Transport

Iron cycles through the body moving from absorption in the gastrointestinal tract via the circulation to the bone marrow, where it is incorporated with protoporphyrin IX in the mitochondria of the erythroid precursors to make heme. Iron circulates in red blood cells in the ferrous form in the hemoglobin molecule. The iron in senescent red blood cells is turned over to macrophages and reused. A glycoprotein, transferrin, has a key role in the iron cycling process.

The transferrin molecule contains two terminal lobes, an N and a C, each of which can bind independently to a ferric (Fe^{+3}) ion. A bicarbonate ion locks the iron in place within the molecule by serving as a bridging ligand between the proteins and iron. The transferrin molecule can exist as apoferritin, as a single chain glycoprotein with no iron attached, or in a monoferric or diferric form.[18, 20]

The transferrin gene is located on the long arm of chromosome 3, 3q21-qter (Fig. 9–7). Most transferrin is produced by hepatocytes.[19] The transferrin receptor is a glycoprotein dimer located on virtually all cells and present in large numbers in erythroid precursors, the placenta, and the liver. The transferrin receptor can bind two molecules of transferrin. Transferrin receptor's affinity for transferrin depends on both the iron content and the physiologic pH. At a pH of 7.4 and with sufficient amounts of iron-bearing transferrin, the transferrin receptor has highest affinity for diferric transferrin, as opposed to monoferric transferrin or apotransferrin.[19] The transferrin receptor gene is located near the transferrin gene at chromosome 3q26.2-qter (see Fig. 9–7).[19]

Cellular uptake of iron is mediated largely by interaction of the transferrin receptor and the transferrin molecule. The ferric-transferrin-receptor complex is endocytosed, iron is released into the cell, and the receptor-transferrin complex is returned to the cell surface, whereupon transferrin is released for reuse.[20]

Iron enters a "chelatable" soluble pool, where it is used either for synthesis of essential cellular constituents or for deposition as ferritin, an apparently nontoxic storage form of iron.

Storage

Iron may be stored in an accessible reserve form as ferritin or as partially degraded or precipitated ferritin called hemosiderin.

Apoferritin, the ferritin molecule without iron, is a spherical protein shell about 12 nm in diameter and 1 nm in width and is composed of mixtures of light and heavy subunits. The liver and spleen, which function as major iron storage deposits, have a large amount of light subunits. Tissues such as heart tissue that do not act normally as iron storage sites have a higher proportion of heavy subunits.

Genes for the heavy and light chains belong to multigene families with members of several chromosomes. The gene for two types of light chains is on chromosome 19; the gene for heavy chains is on chromosome 11. Intracellular ferritin is synthesized by smooth endoplasmic reticulum to be used in the cell. Small amounts are secreted into the plasma. It is believed that plasma ferritin is synthesized by rough endoplasmic reticulum and glycosylated by the Golgi apparatus.[19] Within the apoferritin shell, ferric ions, hydroxyl ions, and oxygen are distributed in a lattice-like relationship.

Hemosiderin is thought to be a degradation product of ferritin produced by the partial digestion of protein and release of iron micelles, which then form insoluble aggregates. Normally, most of the stored iron is in the ferritin form, but as iron stores increase, so does the proportion of hemosiderin in relation to ferritin.

Ferritin and hemosiderin stores are found in liver, bone marrow, and spleen. The majority are found in the liver. When iron is required from iron stores, it is returned to transferrin to be used by the cells that need the iron for metabolism.

SUMMARY

Hemoglobin is a vital component of the red blood cell. Its structure, synthesis, and regulation have been studied extensively. From M. F. Perutz's elegant studies to current research, it has been a fascinating molecule to study. Hemoglobin's ability to change its structure and function when influenced by other molecules provides the body with an efficient molecule capable of adjusting to the demands of tissue for oxygen.

Iron plays an important role in the production of hemoglobin and oxygen transport to the tissue. To clarify the process of absorption and regulation of iron by the body, however, further research is needed; the material discussed in this chapter should provide a basis for studying the various types of anemia and their underlying causes.

REVIEW QUESTIONS

1. A hemoglobin molecule is composed of
   a. one heme and four globin chains
   b. ferrous iron, protoporphyrin IX, and a globin chain
   c. red blood cells, globulin, and iron
   d. four heme and four globin chains

2. Normal adult hemoglobin A contains the following polypeptide chains:
   a. alpha and beta
   b. alpha and delta
   c. alpha and gamma
   d. alpha and epsilon

3. A key rate-limiting step in heme synthesis is
   a. suppression of δ-amino levulinic acid synthase
   b. suppression of transferrin
   c. suppression of iron
   d. suppression of protoporphyrin IX

4. Which of the following forms of hemoglobin molecule has the *lowest* affinity for oxygen?
   a. tense form
   b. relaxed form
   c. arterial form
   d. venous form

5. How does an increase in hydrogen ions affect the hemoglobin-oxygen dissociation curve?
   a. a shift to the right in the curve, a decreased oxygen affinity, and an increase in oxygen release to the tissues
   b. a shift to the right in the curve, an increased oxygen affinity, and a decrease in oxygen release to the tissues
   c. a shift to the left in the curve, a decreased oxygen affinity, and an increase in oxygen release to the tissues
   d. a shift to the left in the curve, an increased oxygen affinity, and a decrease in oxygen release to the tissues

6. The predominant hemoglobin found in a normal newborn is
   a. Gower 1
   b. Gower 2
   c. A
   d. F

7. What is the composition of normal adult hemoglobin?
   a. 80–90% Hb A, 5–10% Hb A_2, 1–5% Hb F
   b. 80–90% Hb A_2, 5–10% Hb A, 1–5% Hb F

   c. >95% Hb A, <3.5% Hb A_2, <1–2% Hb F

   d. >90% Hb A, 5% Hb F, 1% Hb A_2

8. Approximately 70% of body iron is found in the form of

   a. transferrin

   b. hemosiderin

   c. free ferric ion

   d. hemoglobin

9. Iron is incorporated into the heme molecule in which of the following forms?

   a. ferro

   b. ferrous

   c. ferric

   d. apoferritin

10. The transport protein for iron is

   a. transferrin

   b. hemosiderin

   c. apoferritin

   d. ferritin

11. Iron is stored in the body in the forms of

   a. hemosiderin and ferritin

   b. apoferritin and transferrin

   c. macrophages and hemoglobin

   d. hemosiderin and transferrin

References

1. Perutz MF: Molecular anatomy, physiology, and pathology of hemoglobin. *In* Stamatoyannopoulos G, Nienhuis AW, Leder P (eds): Molecular Basis of Blood Diseases. Philadelphia: WB Saunders, 1987: 127–173.
2. Perutz MF, Rossman MG, Cullis AF, et al: Structure of hemoglobin. A three dimensional fourier synthesis at 5.5A resolution obtained by x-ray analysis. Nature 1960; 185:416–422.
3. Perutz MF, Kendrew JC, Watson HC: Structure and function of hemoglobin II. Some relations between polypeptide chain configuration and amino acid sequence. J Mol Biol 1965; 13:699–673.
4. Perutz MF, Muirhead H, Cox JM, Goaman LCG: Three dimensional fourier synthesis of horse oxyhaemoglobin at 2.8A resolution: the atomic model. Nature 1968; 219:131–139.
5. Ranney HM, Sharma V: Structure and function of hemoglobin. *In* Williams WJ, Beutler E, Erslev AJ, Lichtman MA (eds): Hematology, 4th ed. New York: McGraw-Hill, 1990:377–387.
6. Bottomley SS, Muller-Eberhard UM: Pathophysiology of heme synthesis. Semin Hematol 1988; 25:282–302.
7. Jandl JH: Blood: Textbook of Hematology. Boston: Little, Brown, 1987:49–109.
8. Jones MS, Jones OTG: Permeability properties of mitochondrial membranes and the regulation of heme biosynthesis. Biochem Biophys Res Commun 1970; 41:1072–1079.
9. Benz EJ Jr, Forget BG: The biosynthesis of hemoglobin. Semin Hematol 1974; 11:463–523.
10. Dessypris EW: Erythropoiesis. *In* Lee GR, Bithell TC, Foerster J, et al (eds): Wintrobe's Clinical Haematology, 9th ed. Philadelphia: Lea & Febiger, 1993: 134–157.
11. Telen M: The mature erythrocyte. *In* Lee GR, Bithell TC, Foerster J, et al (eds): Wintrobe's Clinical Haematology, 9th ed. Philadelphia: Lea & Febiger, 1993: 101–133.
12. Steinberg MH, Benz EJ: Hemoglobin: Synthesis, structure and function. *In* Hoffman R, Benz EJ, Shattil SJ, et al. (eds): Hematology: Basic Principles and Practice. New York: Churchill Livingstone, 1991:291–302.
13. Bunn HF, Forget BG: Oxygen and carbon dioxide transport in health and disease. *In* Hemoglobin: Molecular, Genetic and Clinical Aspects. Philadelphia: WB Saunders, 1986:91–125.
14. Bunn HF: Hemoglobin I. Structure and function. *In* Beck WS (ed): Hematology, 5th ed. Cambridge, MA: MIT Press, 1991:173–186.
15. Lukens JN: Methemoglobinemia and other disorders accompanied by cyanosis. *In* Lee GR, Bithell TC, Foerster J, et al (eds): Wintrobe's Clinical Haematology, 9th ed. Philadelphia: Lea & Febiger, 1993:1262–1271.
16. Park CM, Nagel RL: Sulfhemoglobinemia. N Engl J Med 1984; 310:1579–1583.
17. Bauer JD: Hemoglobin, porphyria and iron metabolism. *In* Kaplan LA, Pesce AJ (eds): Clinical Chemistry: Theory, Analysis and Correlation, 2nd ed. St. Louis: CV Mosby, 1989:611–655.
18. Woods S, DeMarco T, Friedland M: Iron metabolism. Am J Gastroenterol 1990; 85:1–8.
19. Bittenham GM: Disorders of iron metabolism: iron deficiency and overload. *In* Hoffman R, Benz EJ, Shattil SJ, (eds): Hematology: Basic Principles and Practice. New York: Churchill Livingstone, 1991:327–349.
20. Seligman PA, Klausner RD, Hubers HA: Molecular mechanisms of iron metabolism. *In* Stamatoyannopoulos G, Nienhuis AW, Leder P (eds): Molecular Basis of Blood Diseases. Philadelphia: WB Saunders, 1987:219–244.
21. Fairbanks WF, Beutler E: Iron metabolism. *In* Williams WJ, Beutler E, Erslv AJ, Lichtman MA (eds): Hematology, 4th ed. New York: McGraw-Hill, 1990:329–338.

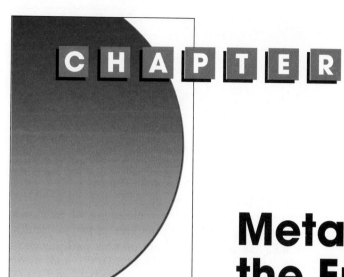

CHAPTER 10

Metabolism of the Erythrocyte

John Griep

Outline

Objectives

AFTER COMPLETION OF THIS CHAPTER, THE READER WILL BE ABLE TO

1. List the red blood cell processes that require energy.
2. Discuss the Embden-Meyerhof anaerobic glycolytic pathway in the erythrocyte to include ATP generation and consumption.
3. Identify the enzyme deficiency in the EMP responsible for the most cases of hereditary nonspherocytic hemolytic anemia.
4. Identify the glycolytic enzyme involved in NADH-linked methemoglobin reductase.
5. Describe the role of 2,3-diphosphoglycerate (2,3-DPG) in erythrocyte metabolism.
6. Explain the main function of the hexose monophosphate (HMP) shunt.
7. Identify the enzyme deficiency in the HMP that causes erythrocytes to be vulnerable to oxidative damage.
8. Discuss methods used to determine erythrocyte survival.
9. Distinguish between an erythrocyte survival curve that reflects senescent loss and another that reflects random loss.

After its release from the bone marrow as a reticulocyte, the erythrocyte survives about 120 days. The most important function of the erythrocyte is to deliver oxygen to body tissues and organs. This function, which involves oxygen and carbon dioxide transport and exchange, does not require consumption of energy.[1] Metabolic processes in the erythrocyte that do require energy are listed in Table 10–1. The mature erythrocyte, lacking a nucleus, mitochondria, and other organelles, is unable to synthesize proteins and lipids or to perform oxidative phosphorylation. If energy is not available for these common metabolic needs, the erythrocyte will be destroyed prematurely. Necessary elements for sustenance of the erythrocyte include an intact erythrocyte membrane, a functioning glycolytic pathway, and nucleotide metabolism. The erythrocyte membrane is discussed in detail in Chapter 8. Glycolytic pathways and nucleotide metabolism are discussed in this chapter.

Membrane exchange pathways allow maintenance of an intracellular cationic composition of high levels of potassium and low levels of sodium and calcium against extracellular gradients of low levels of potassium and high levels of sodium and calcium. These pump mechanisms prevent adverse accumulations of intracellular sodium and calcium. They consume approximately 15% of erythrocyte ATP production. When deprived of this energy, the erythrocyte swells and is destroyed.

Energy is stored and available as adenosine triphosphate (ATP), adenosine diphosphate (ADP), and adenosine monophosphate (AMP). Glycolysis serves to generate ATP from ADP. ATP, a high-energy phosphate, represents the greatest reservoir of energy.

Plasma glucose enters the erythrocyte glucose catabolic process through a facilitated membrane transport system.[2] It is metabolized both anaerobically and aerobically. Anaerobic glycolysis, responsible for approximately 90–95% of the erythrocyte's glucose consumption, occurs in the Embden-Meyerhof pathway (EMP). By means of this pathway, glucose is metabolized to lactic acid,

Table 10-2. GLUCOSE CATABOLISM: FIRST PHASE		
Substrates	**Enzyme**	**Products**
Glucose, ATP	Hexokinase	G6P, ADP
G6P	Glucose phosphate isomerase	F6P
F6P, ATP	Phosphofructokinase	F-1,6-P, ADP
F-1,6-P	Fructodiphosphate adolase	DHAP, G3P

Abbreviations: G6P, glucose-6-phosphate; F6P, fructose-6-phosphate; F-1,6-P, fructose 1,6 diphosphate; DHAP, dihydroxyacetone phosphate; G3P, glyceraldehyde-3-phosphate.

utilizing two molecules of ATP per molecule of glucose and providing four molecules of ATP per molecule of glucose, for a net gain of two molecules of ATP. In addition, shunts off this pathway provide 2,3-diphosphoglycerate (2,3-DPG) and nicotinamide-adenine dinucleotide (NADH). 2,3-DPG regulates oxygen delivery to tissues; NADH is a cofactor in the methemoglobin reductase reaction, which maintains hemoglobin in its functionally reduced state. In aerobic glycolysis, which is responsible for 5–10% of glucose consumption, glucose is diverted into the hexose monophosphate pathway, which provides a pool of reduced glutathione to combat potential oxidant injury to the erythrocyte.

ANAEROBIC GLYCOLYSIS

The first phase of glucose catabolism involves glucose phosphorylation, isomerization, and diphosphorylation to yield fructose-1,6-diphosphate (F-1,6-P). This then serves as the substrate for aldolase cleavage for the final product of phase 1 glycolysis: glyceraldehyde-3-phosphate (G3P) (Fig. 10–1; Table 10–2).

Hexokinase (HK) has the lowest activity of all the glycolytic enzymes. It requires magnesium and exhibits increase in activity with increase in pH. Phosphofructokinase (PFK) requires magnesium and is sensitive to pH, inorganic phosphates, and ADP. HK and PFK are rate limiting in steady-state anaerobic glycolysis. Deficiency of HK is inherited as an autosomal recessive trait and is a rare cause of hereditary non-spherocytic hemolytic anemia (HNSHA).[3] Phosphofructokinase, inherited as an autosomal recessive trait, may be associated with severe muscle dysfunction (type VII glycogen storage disease). It may cause mild HNSHA.[4]

The second phase of glucose catabolism converts G3P to 3-phosphoglycerate. The substrates, enzymes, and products for this phase of glycolytic metabolism are summarized in Table 10–3. During the first reaction step, G3P is phosphorylated with

Table 10-1. ERYTHROCYTE METABOLIC PROCESSES REQUIRING ENERGY
Maintenance of intracellular cationic electrochemical gradients
Maintenance of membrane phospholipid
Maintenance of skeletal protein plasticity
Maintenance of functional ferrous hemoglobin
Protection of cell proteins from oxidative denaturation
Initiation and maintenance of glycolysis
Synthesis of glutathione
Mediation of nucleotide salvage reactions

**Embden-Meyerhof Pathway
(Anaerobic Pathway of Glucose Metabolism)**

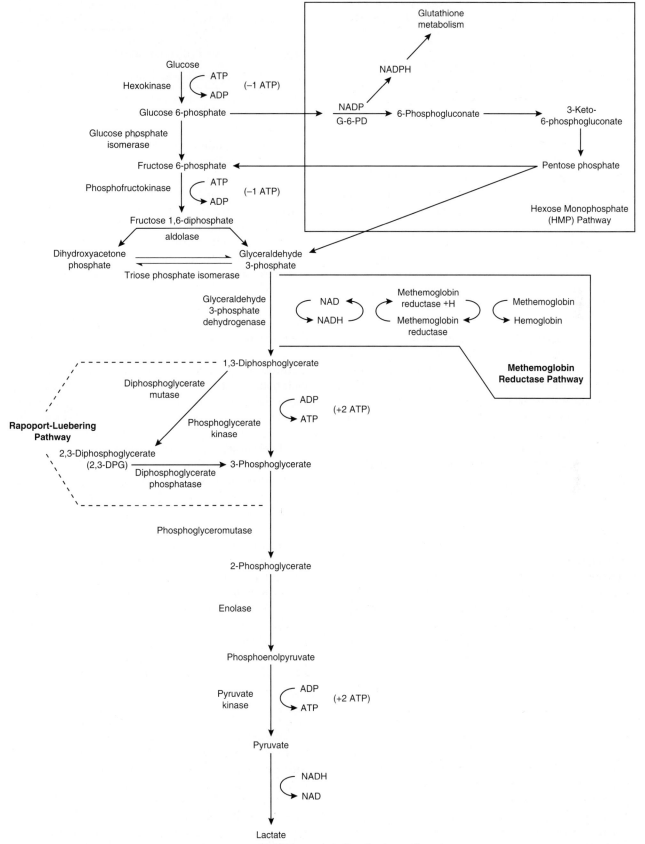

Figure 10–1 Glucose metabolism in the erythrocyte.

Table 10-3. GLUCOSE CATABOLISM: SECOND PHASE		
Substrates	**Enzyme**	**Product**
G3P	Glyceraldehyde-phosphate dehydrogenase	1,3 DPG
1,3-DPG, ADP	Phosphoglycerate kinase	3PG, ATP
1,3-DPG	Diphosphoglyceromutase	2,3-DPG
2,3-DPG	Diphosphoglycerate phosphatase	3-PG

Abbreviations: G3P, glyceraldehyde-3-phosphate; DPG, diphosphoglycerate (1,3/2,3); 3PG, 3-phosphoglycerate.

Table 10-4. GLUCOSE CATABOLISM: THIRD PHASE		
Substrates	**Enzyme**	**Product**
3-PG	Monophosphoglyceromutase	2-PG
2-PG	Phosphopyruvate hydratase (enolase)	PEP
PEP, ADP	Pyruvate kinase	Pyruvate, ATP

Abbreviations: 3-PG, 3-phosphoglycerate; 2-PG, 2-phosphoglycerate; PEP, phosphoenolpyruvate.

a high-energy phosphate and oxidized to 1,3-diphosphoglycerate (1,3-DPG), through the action of glyceraldehyde phosphate dehydrogenase (GAPD). This reaction is coupled to NAD^+ reduction to NADH, which is available as an essential cofactor for the reduction of methemoglobin to hemoglobin by methemoglobin reductase (methemoglobin reductase pathway).[5] 1,3-DPG may be dephosphorylated by phosphoglycerate kinase (PGK), thus generating ATP, or it may be shunted into the Luebering-Rapaport pathway, where it is isomerized to 2,3-DPG by diphosphoglyceromutase. 2,3-DPG essentially competes with oxygen for hemoglobin, effectively enhancing release of oxygen from hemoglobin (see Chapter 9). 2,3-DPG, the most concentrated organophosphate in the erythrocyte, forms 3-phosphoglycerate (3-PG) by the action of diphosphoglycerate phosphatase. Diphosphoglyceromutase and diphosphoglycerate phosphatase are the same protein molecule.[6] The concentration of 2,3-DPG varies inversely with the hydrogen ion concentration (pH), which is inhibitory to catalytic action of DPG mutase. Deficiency of PGK is X-linked and may be associated with neurologic disturbances and HNSHA.[7]

There is a delicate balance between the need to generate ATP to support energy requirements for cell metabolism and the need to maintain appropriate oxygenation/deoxygenation status of hemoglobin. This balance is maintained by dephosphorylation of 1,3-DPG to 3-PG with the generation of ATP or by mutation of 1,3-DPG to 2,3-DPG, which enhances the deoxygenation of hemoglobin. Low (acidic) pH inhibits the activity of diphosphoglyceromutase and activates diphosphoglycerate phosphatase, which favors generation of ATP.

The third phase of anaerobic glucose catabolism involves conversion of 3-PG to pyruvate with the generation of ATP. Substrates, enzymes, and products are listed in Table 10-4.

2,3-DPG is a cofactor in the monophosphoglyceromutase reaction. Pyruvate kinase (PK) activity is allosterically modulated by increased concentrations of fructose-1,6-phosphate (F-1,6-P), which

increases the affinity of PK for phosphoenolpyruvate (PEP).[8] Pyruvic acid may diffuse from the erythrocyte or may become a substrate for lactic dehydrogenase (LD) with regeneration of NAD^+. The ratio of NAD^+ to NADH may modify the activity of this enzyme.

PK deficiency is inherited as an autosomal recessive trait and is the most common cause of HNSHA. This deficiency is discussed in Chapter 17.

AEROBIC GLYCOLYSIS

Aerobic or oxidative glycolysis diverts glucose metabolism into the hexose monophosphate pathway (HMS; also known as the pentose phosphate shunt) for the purpose of maintaining reduced glutathione (GSH) and reduced NADP.[8] During steady-state erythropoiesis, approximately 5–10% of glucose-6-phosphate (G6P) is diverted into the HMS. After oxidative challenge, activity of the HMS may be increased 20- to 30-fold.[8] This pathway catabolizes G6P to ribulose-5-phosphate and CO_2 by oxidizing G6P at carbon 1. Ribulose-5-phosphate may be utilized during nucleotide metabolism or re-enter anaerobic glycolysis pathways as fructose-6-phosphate (F6P) or G3P under enzymatic activity of pentose epimerase, isomerase, transketolase, and transaldolase. The substrates, enzymes, and products for the HMS are listed in Table 10-5.

During the conversion of glucose to pentose, NADPH is generated, which reduces oxidized glu-

Table 10-5. GLUCOSE CATABOLISM: HEXOSE MONOPHOSPHATE SHUNT		
Substrates	**Enzyme**	**Product**
G6P	Glucose-6-phosphate dehydrogenase	6PG
6PG	Phosphogluconolactonase Phosphogluconate dehydrogenase	R5P

Abbreviations: G6P, glucose-6-phosphate; 6PG, 6-phosphogluconate; R5P, ribulose-5-phosphate.

tathione via glutathione reductase and, in the presence of glutathione peroxidase, can convert hydrogen peroxide to water. Hydrogen peroxide, regularly produced in small amounts, may be generated in large amounts by oxidant drugs.

The enzyme glucose-6-phosphate dehydrogenase (G6PD) functions to reduce NADP while oxidizing G6P. It governs the rate of reduction of NADP, which restores GSH through H^+ transfer by glutathione reductase.[9] G6PD provides the only means of generating NADPH, and in its absence of erythrocytes are particularly vulnerable to oxidative damage.[10] Erythrocytes with normal G6PD activity are able to detoxify the oxidative compounds and safeguard the hemoglobin SH–containing enzymes and membrane thiols (sulfhydrals), allowing normally functioning red blood cells to carry enormous quantities of O_2 safely.[8]

NUCLEOTIDE METABOLISM

Nucleotides, present in mature erythrocytes, cannot be synthesized de novo and must be maintained to preserve the energy requirements of the cell. The adenine nucleotide pool is the largest pool and is composed of approximately 88% ATP, 10% ADP, and 2% AMP. This relative proportion of nucleotides is maintained by the action of adenylate kinase and by the generation of ATP from ADP during glycolytic metabolism. AMP may be deaminated to inosine-5′-monophosphate (IMP) or dephosphorylated to adenosine, which is diffusible across the erythrocyte membrane.

Nucleotide salvage may be possible through the relative activities of adenosine kinase and adenosine deaminase. Deficient activity of adenosine deaminase leads to accumulations of deoxyadenine nucleotides, whereas increased activity of adenosine deaminase leads to depletions of deoxyadenine nucleotides. A second potential salvage pathway is related to the activity of adenosine phosphoribosyl transferase which converts adenine to AMP. This activity is likely limited by the availability of adenine.

ERYTHROCYTE KINETICS

The term *erythrocyte kinetics* refers to an attempt to quantify the processes of red blood cell production and destruction, which may occur directly or prematurely in loss of red blood cells from the body. The presumption underlying erythrocyte kinetic studies is that the rate of erythrocyte production equals the rate of loss, thus providing a steady-state pattern. This maintains circulating

erythrocytes at the normal parameters for erythrocytes, hemoglobin, and packed cell volume. Alterations in plasma volume may have a slight bearing on measurements taken to assess erythrocyte kinetics. The measurement of the rate of erythrocyte production is generally estimated from the reticulocyte count (see Chapter 12).

ERYTHROCYTE SURVIVAL

The measurement of erythrocyte survival may be undertaken by either random or cohort label method. Cohort studies require approximately 3 to 4 months to complete, involve labeling of erythrocytes by pre-administration of the labeled substance, and necessitate a stable label within the erythrocyte for this period. The dynamics of the cohort survival curve are relatively complex and generally divided into three phases: an uptake phase, a phase reflecting the relatively long range of survival, and a phase in which erythrocytes are lost relatively rapidly from circulation. The interpretations of the patterns may be complicated by the metabolism of the label or by the re-utilization of the label within the red blood cell pool. Cohort studies are rarely performed in clinical medicine.

The most common measurement for erythrocyte survival is the random label method, which involves the removal of erythrocytes from circulation, the labeling with an appropriate label (commonly a radioactive substance), and the introduction of the labeled cells into circulation. This type of study takes approximately one month.

For a valid study, certain assumptions must be present:

1. There is no significant change in circulating erythrocyte mass.
2. All erythrocytes of all ages are properly labeled.
3. All erythrocytes die of senescence or other age-related causes.
4. No free label is available after initial exposure of the erythrocytes.
5. Appropriate corrections can be made for any radioactive decay.

Chromium 51 is commonly used to label the globin chain of the hemoglobin molecule. Approximately 0.7–1.3% of this label leaks from the erythrocytes per day and a small portion of the label may not be fixed and thus may be deleted during the first 24 hours. The study is measured by calculating the rate of loss of one half of the label after correcting for radioactive decay. In normal persons the range is approximately 25 to 35 days. Chromium 51 survival times of less than 25 days are considered to reflect an increased rate of erythrocyte loss. A half-life of 15 days indicates an average length of survival, which is one half of the expected observation. Shortened survival time of the erythrocyte indicates hemolytic anemia and/or early blood loss.

SUMMARY

The mature erythrocyte, lacking a nucleus and other organelles, must derive energy from other sources to survive its 120-day life span. The greatest reservoir of energy is ATP, which is generated by glycolysis. Glucose enters the erythrocyte by facilitated membrane transport. Glycolysis occurs both aerobically and anaerobically. Through anaerobic glycolysis in the EMP glucose is metabolized to lactic acid, utilizing two molecules of ATP per molecule of glucose, and providing four molecules of ATP per molecule of glucose, for a net gain of two molecules. By means of the Luebering-Rapaport pathway (a shunt off the EMP), 2,3-DPG necessary for facilitation of oxygen delivery to the tissues is generated. The methemoglobin reductase pathway (also a bypass from the EMP), is responsible for maintaining iron in its reduced state.

Aerobic glycolysis occurs in the hexose monophosphate shunt, which converts glucose into pentose with the generation of NADPH. NADPH reduces glutathione, which protects the cell from oxidative injury.

The steady state of the erythrocyte refers to equal production and destruction. Erythrocyte production can be approximated by the reticulocyte count. When destruction exceeds production, the possibility of a hemolytic anemia exists.

Erythrocyte survival can be measured through the use of random labeling with radioactive substances. The range of survival is normally 25 to 35 days.

References

1. Beutler E: Energy metabolism and maintenance of erythrocytes. *In* Williams WJ, Beutler E, Erslev AJ, Lichtman MA (eds): Hematology. New York: McGraw-Hill, 1990:355–368.
2. Kondo T, Beutler E: Developmental changes in glucose transport of guinea pig erythrocytes. J Clin Invest 1980; 65:1–4.
3. Netzloff WL: Clinical consequences of enzyme deficiencies in the erythrocyte. Ann Clin Lab Sci 1980; 10:414–424.
4. Vora S: Isoenzymes of human phosphofructokinase: biochemical and genetic aspects. *In* Rattazz MC, Scandalios JG, Whitt GS (eds): Isozymes: Current Topics in Biological and Medical Research, 2nd ed. New York: AR Liss, 1983:119–167.
5. Schwartz JM, Reiss AL, Jaffe ER: Hereditary methemoglobinemia with deficiency of NADH cytochrome b₅ reductase. *In* Stanbury JB, Wyngaarden JB, Fredrickson DS, et al (eds): The Metabolic Basis of Inherited Disease. New York: McGraw-Hill, 1983:1654–1665.
6. Rosa R, Gaillardon J, Rosa J: Diphosphoglycerate mutase and 2,3 diphosphoglycerate phosphatase activities of red cells. Comparative electrophorectic studies. Biochem Biophys Res Comm 1973; 51:536–542.
7. Beutler E: Hemolytic anemia in disorders of red cell metabolism. New York: Plenum, 1978.
8. Paglia DE: Biochemistry of the red cell. *In* Hoffman R, Benz EJ, Shattil SJ, et al (eds): Hematology: Basic Principles and Practice. New York: Churchill Livingstone, 1991:269–273.
9. Beutler E: Glucose-6-phosphate dehydrogenase deficiency. N Engl J Med 1991; 324:169–174.
10. Beutler E: The genetics of glucose-6-phosphate dehydrogenase deficiency. Semin Hemat 1990; 27:137–167.

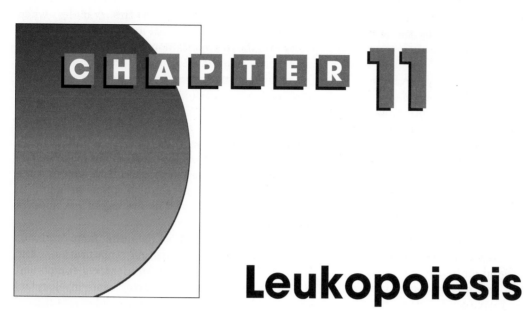

CHAPTER 11

Leukopoiesis

Susan J. Leclair

Outline

LEUKOCYTES
 Granulocytes
 Monocyte/Macrophage
 Lymphocytes
PERIPHERAL BLOOD
 CONSIDERATIONS
 Quantity
 Alterations in Granulocyte
  Number and Maturity
 Alterations in Eosinophil
  Number
 Alterations in Basophil Number
 Alterations in Monocyte/
  Macrophage Number
 Alterations in Lymphocyte
  Number

Objectives

AFTER COMPLETION OF THIS CHAPTER, THE READER WILL BE ABLE TO

1. Discuss the role of the interleukins in the development of white blood cells, including their origin, sites of activity, function, and interrelationships.
2. Explain the differentiation sequence required for producing neutrophilic granulocytes.
3. Explain the differentiation sequence required for producing monocytes/macrophages.
4. Explain the differentiation sequence required for producing lymphocytes.
5. List the important compounds synthesized or stored in the various leukocytes.
6. Correlate neutrophilic function to morphology and maturation.
7. Correlate peripheral blood cell numbers and cell types with possible causes.
8. Compare and contrast the morphology of the peripheral blood lymphocyte against the various stages of immunologic activity.

Leukopoiesis, or the development of white blood cells (WBCs), occurs in the same locations as erythrocytes, with the exception of lymphocytes.[1]

Although the term *erythron* defines the sum of erythrocytic development, there is no such term for leukocyte development and function. The lack of a term is influenced by the complexity of the WBC populations and the different compartments that they occupy during their lives. In addition, control mechanisms that influence cellular behavior are more complex in leukocytes than those seen in the erythrocyte. Thus there are many ways to evaluate the needs and functions of these cells throughout their lives. This chapter relates developmental needs and consequences to environmental constraints and controls.

At birth, all available marrow space is taken up by hematopoiesis. By the end of adolescence, active marrow is typically found only in the proximal ends of the long bones and in flat bones, such as the skull and sternum. Inactive, or "fatty," marrow can be converted to active marrow if the demands for a blood cell line become excessive.

LEUKOCYTES

Human blood leukocytes can be divided into various categories on the basis of their specific function, site of origin, or their morphology. In essence, all leukocytes exist to defend the organism against non-self agents. This is accomplished through intricate cooperation among cells. Independently of lymphocyte control, phagocytes attack and destroy a wide variety of matter. However, it is through lymphokines (biologic response mediators released by both B and T lymphocytes and by macrophages) that lymphocytes direct and amplify phagocytic action. For this discussion, leukocytes are divided into granulocytes and lymphocytes by virtue of the differentiation apparent at the primitive stem cell level (Fig. 11–1). Lymphocytes are produced in both bone marrow and lymphoid tissue. They are under the control of environmental and hormonal stimuli very different from those that control granulocytes and monocytes. Granulocytes such as the neutrophils function primarily as destroyers of pyogenic bacteria, whereas monocyte/macrophages are less discriminating in their phagocytic activities.

Granulocytes are cells containing visible granules and develop solely in the bone marrow. Subdivided according to morphology, granulocytes can be categorized as those containing large and easily visualized granules and those containing minute or barely visible granules. By convention, cells containing large visible granules are usually called granulocytes; these are further subdivided according to the type of reaction (neutrophilic, eosinophilic, basophilic) found in the granules when stained differentially with a Romanowsky-based stain. Monocytes contain minute granules, which, as a result of the resolution limitation of most bright-light microscopes, have a grainy appearance.

Granulocytes

As a group, these cells can be found in high concentrations in four locations: bone marrow, circulating freely in the peripheral blood, marginating up against the endothelium of blood vessels, and in the tissues. These locations are called granulocyte pools.

The bone marrow pool is quite large and has three functions: proliferation, maturation, and storage. Cells found in the proliferating component (i.e., myeloblasts, promyelocytes, and myelocytes) are capable of mitotic divisions. The maturation portion consists of metamyelocytes and bands—that is, cells that are no longer capable of mitosis but are not yet fully functional. The storage component of the bone marrow, which consists of bands and polymorphonuclear leukocytes, contains approximately 25 times as many cells as are in the circulation. Once a cell has fully matured and has been stimulated by chemotactic factors, it leaves the marrow and enters the peripheral blood, in which it can become part of either the marginating pool or the circulating pool. The marginating pool consists of approximately 50% of total peripheral blood granulocyte levels. These cells have adhered to the vessel endothelium or are engaged in diapedesis (egressing through vessel walls) into the tissue. The circulating pool contains the remaining 50% of total peripheral blood granulocyte levels; these are the cells counted in a WBC count. A freedom of movement between pools is seen most often between cells of the marginating and circulating pools. Marginating cells can "drop off" into the circulating pool for a variety of reasons; likewise, circulating cells may become marginating.

MATURATION

Stem Cell to Myeloblast. The earliest leukopoietic precursor was identified from mouse spleen cells and is referred to as either the colony forming unit–spleen (CFU-S) or the pluripotential stem cell (PSC).[2] Its identification with traditional Romanowsky-based stains is not possible. This cell apparently can move among various activity sites and may look like a large, nongranular lymphocyte. It responds to circumstances as yet undefined and commits its progeny to cells of either lymphoid or

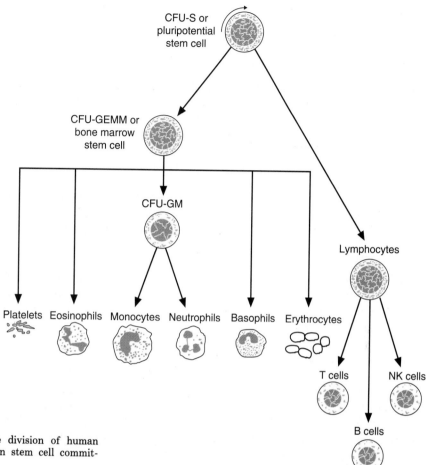

Figure 11–1 A representation of the division of human blood cells into major categories based on stem cell commitment.

bone marrow (myeloid) origin.[3] For granulopoiesis, the PSC undergoes stimulation, mitosis, and maturation into a stem cell that is specific for bone marrow–derived or myeloid cells. This colony forming unit–granulocyte–erythrocyte–monocyte/ macrophage–megakaryocyte (CFU-GEMM) matures into yet another stem cell called the colony forming unit–granulocyte–monocyte/macrophage (CFU-GM). This in turn finally matures into the earliest recognizable cell of the neutrophilic series, the myeloblast. The stability of cell numbers and functionality is controlled by a complex interaction of humoral factors such as interleukins (ILs) and various colony stimulating factors (CSFs)[4] (Fig. 11–2A). CSFs are categorized by the type of cell stimulated. So, for example, GM-CSF stimulates cells to form both granulocytes and monocyte/macrophages, whereas G-CSF stimulates only granulocyte development. Specificity for CSFs is mediated by receptor sites on precursors as well as mature cells.

Cells in the bone marrow proliferation pool usually take approximately 24–48 hours for a single cell cycle. Less than 1% of the normal bone marrow compartment is composed of myeloblasts.

They are variable in size but usually large (15– 20 μm). The nucleus is delicate, with prominent nucleoli. The meager cytoplasm contains rough endoplasmic reticulum, a developing Golgi apparatus, and, as it matures through its life cycle, an increasing number of azurophilic granules that, when stained, color positively for the enzyme myeloperoxidase. Myeloperoxidase is required for intracellular kill, which means that the killing function is the first to be operational. Unfortunately, the cell is incapable of motility, adhesion, and phagocytosis, so it is, in essence, a nonfunctional cell (Fig. 11–2B).

Promyelocyte (Progranulocyte). After several days in the blast stage, the cell progresses to the promyelocyte stage. This cell is almost as rare as the myeloblast (1–5%), and its size is variable, often exceeding 20 μm, which is occasionally larger than the size of its precursor cell. The nuclear chromatin pattern may be as delicate as that of a myeloblast or may show slight clumping. Nucleoli begin to fade. Granules are present throughout the larger cytoplasm and on top of the nucleus (Fig. 11–2C).

Myeloperoxidase can be found throughout the

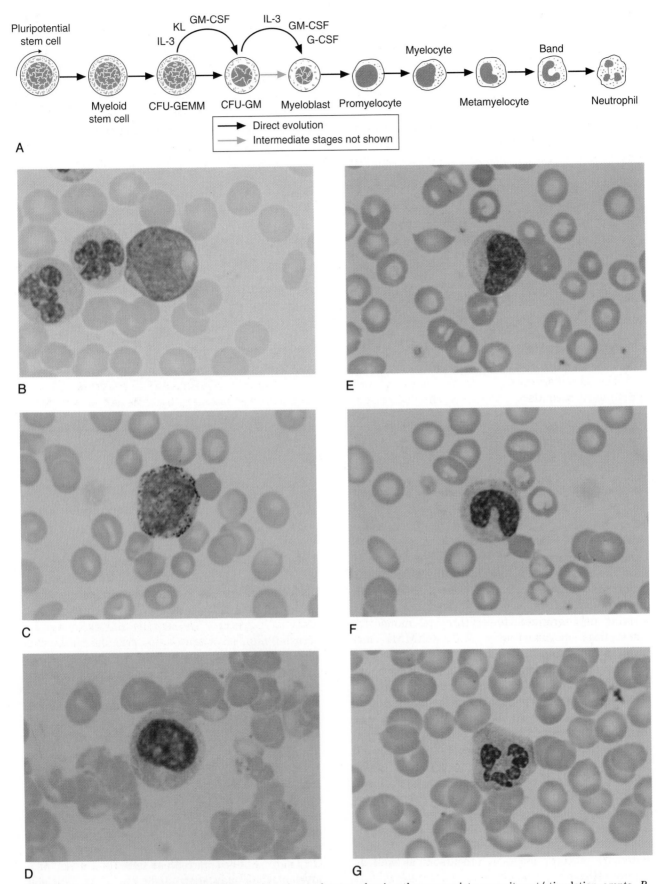

Figure 11-2 *A*, Schematic for the differentiation of granulocytes, showing the appropriate commitment/stimulation agents. *B*, Myeloblast showing delicate chromatin, multiple nucleoli and nongranular cytoplasm. *C*, Promyelocyte showing the concentration of primary granules throughout the cytoplasm and on top of the nucleus. *D*, Neutrophilic myelocyte, so named because of the presence of secondary granules that when stained appear neutrophilic. Notice the absence of nucleoli and the beginning condensation of chromatin in the nucleus. *E*, Metamyelocyte with the classic kidney bean–shaped nucleus. *F*, Band form with a nucleus whose indentation is greater than 50% the width of the nucleus. Notice that the remaining primary granules are less apparent and, when stained, turn a lighter blue. *G*, A polymorphonuclear cell with a typically twisted and segmented nucleus.

cell and, together with the other enzymes necessary for the peroxidase/superoxide burst, this cell has the capability of intracellular kill. Intracellular kill is initiated by a complex system of signals that link the cell membrane receptors to the production of a respiratory burst oxidase, reduced nicotinamide-adenine dinucleotide phosphate (NADPH)-dependent oxidase, which generates oxygen containing compounds such as superoxide, hydroxyl radicals, and hydrogen peroxide. This reaction requires cytochrome B, flavoprotein, and a functional electron transport system within the mitochondria. In the presence of halide ions, peroxide reacts with superoxide to produce bactericidal hydroxyl radicals or aldehydes. Remaining peroxidase is neutralized by catalase or reduced glutathione. All portions of this system must be functional if the entire process is to provide complete intracellular kill.

Neutrophilic Myelocyte. When the cell ceases to produce primary azurophilic granules, it begins to make secondary or neutrophilic granules. Accumulation of secondary granules is characteristic of the myelocyte, the last cell of the bone marrow compartment capable of mitosis. The myelocyte demonstrates a good deal of morphologic variability, for this stage of development is the longest, and the development of the granules over a period of 4–5 days causes considerable alteration in the staining reaction of the cell.[5] This cell is usually smaller than the promyelocyte and constitutes less than 10% of the total marrow cell population. The nucleus may be round to oval with a flattened side near the well-developed Golgi apparatus. The nuclear chromatin shows clumping, and nucleoli are usually no longer visible. The secondary granules alter the staining reaction within the cytoplasm. They cause a "dawn of neutrophilia," or faint blush of pink first seen near the Golgi apparatus within the cytoplasm. Some of the important compounds contained within secondary granules are alkaline phosphatase, lactoferrin, lysozyme, and plasminogen activators. As the cell matures, secondary granule formation overshadows the primary granules. Alteration in the granule membrane causes the remaining primary granules to color less intensely with staining; they are light bluish and less noticeable. The cell also acquires some motility (Fig. 11–2D).

Neutrophilic Metamyelocyte. After the cessation of all active DNA synthesis, the myelocyte becomes a metamyelocyte. The traditional discriminator between myelocyte and metamyelocyte is the shape of the nucleus; that of the metamyelocyte becomes indented. However, it is far better to assess the relative maturity (nonclumped vs. clumped chromatin pattern) of the nucleus, because microcinematography has shown that the

shape of the myelocyte nucleus varies from round to deeply indented.[6] By this stage, the cytoplasm has a complete collection of primary and secondary granules with which to kill and degrade toxic, infectious, or non-self agents. However, the cell is still incapable of responding to chemotactic factors and initiating phagocytosis. Metamyelocytes, which are not seen in the typical peripheral blood smear, constitute approximately 5–15% of the normal marrow differential.[7] Because this cell is still not fully functional, it is considered part of the maturation component of the marrow (Fig. 11–2E).

Neutrophilic Band (Nonsegmented Form). After a time, the metamyelocyte assumes a transitional form, because it is in both the peripheral blood and the bone marrow and is considered to be part of both the maturation and storage pools. Within the marrow, it constitutes one of the most common leukocytes, its numbers averaging as high as 40% of the WBCs therein. The definition and name of this intermediate form have been debated extensively. In one classification system, its discrimination is based on the presence or absence of nuclear segments made up of dense heterochromatin. The terms *segmented* and *nonsegmented* are used in this definition of these cells.[8] Another classification requires that the outer shape of the nucleus have uniform or parallel width (C or S shape) as its basis and identifies a cell whose nucleus is so described as a "band" and cells with all other nuclear forms as "polymorphonuclear neutrophils." Finally, a third classification system defines a band as a cell whose nuclear indentation is less than half the width of the nucleus and a polymorphonuclear neutrophil as a cell whose nuclear indentation is more than half the width of the nucleus.[9] This third system reflects an appreciation of the role of change and maturity within the cell, for chromatin maturity is also used as a criterion. Regardless of which classification is used, the band form is thought to represent the almost mature cell. It has been shown to possess full motility, active adhesion properties, and some phagocytic ability. Membrane maturity is characterized by changes in the cytoskeleton, changes in surface charge, and the presence of receptors for complement (CR), specifically for CR_1 and CR_3.[10] Adhesion capabilities are associated with the presence of certain secondary granules.[11] Once out in the peripheral blood, bands usually account for less than 6% of the WBCs. In the peripheral blood, they can be found in both marginating and circulating pools (Fig. 11–2F).

Polymorphonuclear Neutrophil (Segmented Neutrophil). The cell's nucleus continues its indentation until thin strands of membrane and heterochromatin form into segments and create a lobated nucleus. This nucleus is easily deformable because of the active motility of the cell. The name *polymorphonuclear* means "many-shaped nucleus" and accurately describes the nuclear shapes. Most nuclei have visible segments, although some appear grossly twisted or folded. According to the traditional Arneth count, nuclei should have between two and four lobes.[12] A lesser amount indicates either immaturity or genetic anomaly; a greater amount suggests difficulty in maturation. Regardless of the number of nuclear segments, this cell is completely functional. These cells spend time both in bone marrow (as part of the storage pool) and in the marginating and circulating pools of the peripheral blood, in which they constitute between 40% and 50% of the total (Fig. 11–2*G*).

The functioning neutrophil spends its life performing phagocytosis and pinocytosis. These are essentially the same event at two sizes; phagocytosis usually involves larger material and can be seen at the light microscope level, whereas pinocytosis involves small material and can be seen adequately only with an electron microscope. These activities can be performed in the blood stream, as in transient bacteremia, or in the tissues (Table 11–1). Neutrophils are attracted to particles by several mechanisms. Chemotactic factors, antibodies, or complement fixation causes the polymorphonuclear cell to migrate to the source. Chemotactic recognition ability, mobility, and adhesion are all required for phagocytosis to occur. Cells deficient in any of these characteristics defend poorly against infections.[13] Normal cells adhere to particles whose presence has initiated the attraction. Pseudopods extend around the particle, engulfing it and forming a phagosome. Cytoplasmic granules surround the material and, by fusing their granules, dump their contents into the phagosome. Combined primary granule release of peroxide, myeloperoxidase, superoxide, and anions contribute to the oxidative killing of live organisms. Secondary granules contain complement activators that increase both complement fixation of the foreign material and the chemotactic response by the neutrophil. In addition, the concentration of collagenase, lysozyme, and proteases from the secondary granules cause degradation and detoxification of material. The release of many of these agents is deleterious to the neutrophil itself, and cell content leakage or cell disruption can cause the release of endogenous pyrogens into the blood; such leakage is partially responsible for the sign of fever.

EOSINOPHIL DEVELOPMENT

A close relative of the neutrophilic granulocyte is the eosinophil, whose prominent secondary granules are stained heavily with the eosin or acidophilic dye used in conventional Romanowsky-based stains. The cell develops from the CFU-GEMM into a stem cell specific for eosinophils (CFU-Eo), then into a myeloblast stage similar to that seen in the neutrophils. The promyelocyte stage produces the same type of primary granules and is indistinguishable from other promyelocytes. In the myelocyte stage, the eosinophil is distinguished from the neutrophil by the presence of numerous, large, round granules containing a crystalloid compound made up of major basic protein (MBP). MBP may be responsible for the staining qualities of the granules.[14] Eosinophil granules contain various proteolytic enzymes (Table 11–2) but do not contain lysozyme or alkaline phosphatase.

Eosinophils spend less than 1 week in the peripheral blood, but there is a large storage capacity in the marrow that allows for rapid mobilization on demand.[14] Upon stimulation, eosinophils leave the marrow and pass quickly through the peripheral blood into the tissues. They are actively motile and use the same migration as neutrophils. Because of the short time that eosinophils spend in transit in the peripheral blood, day-to-day variation in eosinophil numbers is quite high. In the absence of an allergic response, eosinophils should not number more than 4%.

Table 11–1. PHAGOCYTOSIS/PINOCYTOSIS

Recognition-Attachment Phase
Requires mediation by immunoglobulin C or unknown factors
Stimulation of actin, myosin, and binding proteins

Ingestion Phase (Phagocytosis)
Pseudopod extension
Microfilament rearrangement
Engulfment

Intracellular Kill: Oxidative Mechanism
Respiratory burst via superoxide (30% hydrogen peroxide) generation

Digestion Phase: Degradation
Secondary lysosomal formation
Usually proteinases, hydrolases and arylsulfatases, phosphatases, etc.

Exocytosis
Removal of indigestible elements
Reverse of phagocytosis

Table 11–2. EOSINOPHILIC GRANULE CONTENTS

Acid phosphatase
Arylsulfatase
β-Glucuronidase
Cathepsin
Peroxidase
Phospholipase

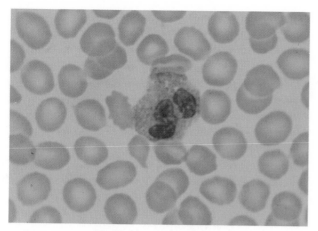

Figure 11-3 Eosinophil.

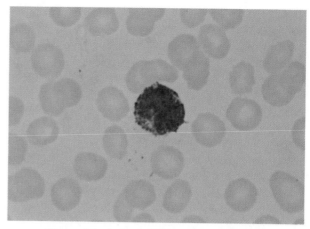

Figure 11-4 Basophil with obscured nucleus.

The adult eosinophil typically contains a nucleus that is in band form or bilobed. Nuclei with higher lobe counts are seen rarely. The cell is slightly larger than the average neutrophil and may have an irregular border as a result of motility[7] (Fig. 11-3).

BASOPHIL DEVELOPMENT

Like their eosinophilic counterparts, basophils are characterized by the presence of large, heavily staining granules. These granules differ from those of the eosinophil in that they are irregularly shaped, unevenly distributed throughout the cell, and turn a deep purple to black with Romanowsky stains. The process of maturation of the basophil from the stem cell is not as well known as for the other peripheral blood cells. It may parallel the development of eosinophils. Basophils can be differentiated into myelocytes, metamyelocytes, bands, and polymorphonuclear cells on the basis of nuclear development, although mature nuclei with more than 2 lobes are extremely rare. The granules contain heparin, chondroitin sulfate, proteoglycans, histamine, and other inflammatory mediators.[15] These granules are water-soluble, may be partially or completely washed out in cells that are poorly fixed, and may appear as empty areas within the cytoplasm. When the slides are fixed correctly, it is possible for granules to overshadow the nucleus,

making it difficult to discern any nuclear detail. Basophils are the least common cell in the peripheral blood; on average, they represent less than 2%. Human basophil membranes have specific high affinity receptors for the Fc region of immunoglobulin E (IgE). When IgE antibodies bound to the plasma membrane are connected to specific antigens, degranulation occurs[16] (Fig. 11-4).

Maturation

MONOCYTE/MACROPHAGE

Stem Cell to Monoblast. Current theory holds that monocyte/macrophage cells are divided into monoblasts, promonocytes, blood monocytes, and free and fixed macrophages.[17] As stated in the section on granulocyte development, the commitment from PSC to CFU-GEMM is little understood. By the action of IL-3, GM-CSF, and M-CSF, the monoblast is generated from the CFU-GEMM and is found primarily in the bone marrow although possible secondary sites include the spleen and other reticuloendothelial sites (RES) (Fig. 11-5). Monoblasts are found in low numbers in the bone marrow, and their only function is in mitosis. They are large cells with an eccentrically placed nucleus containing one or two noticeable nucleoli. Their cytoplasm is nongranular and when stained may appear weakly positive for peroxidase (Fig. 11-6).

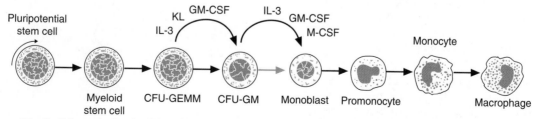

Figure 11-5 Schematic for the differentiation of monocytes, showing the appropriate commitment/stimulation agents.

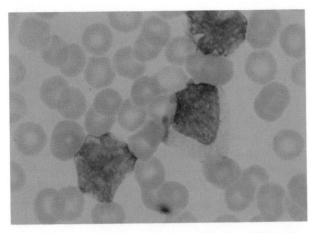

Figure 11–6 Although usually quite difficult to differentiate from a myeloblast, monoblasts can be identified by the presence of a single large nucleolus, an irregularly shaped nucleus, and delicate chromatin.

Monoblast to Promonocyte. After mitosis and maturation, the blast becomes a promonocyte. Promonocytes are similar in size to the blast but have some granulation. They begin to assume a more monocytoid appearance with folded, twisted, or indented nuclei and irregularly shaped cytoplasm. They can be motile and participate in phagocytosis.[17] Of major interest are the nonmorphologic changes present at this and subsequent stages.

Promonocyte to Monocyte. Granular content and number vary considerably as the cell gets older. More than 50 secretory compounds such as transport proteins, nonspecific inflammatory agents, storage materials, and humoral acting agents have been identified[18] (Table 11–3). Peripheral blood monocytes have great morphologic variability. Because of their aggressive motility and adherence, cells may be distorted as they cling to both the push and smear slides. The monocyte nucleus is usually indented or curved with chromatin that is lacy with small clumps, and it is typically described as the largest cell in the peripheral blood. The monocyte's abundant cytoplasm is filled with swirls of minute granules that produce a cloudy or turbid appearance. The cytoplasmic membrane may be quite irregular. Pseudopods and phagocytic vacuoles are common (Fig. 11–7).

This cell may also be thought of as a transitional cell because it leaves the bone marrow to enter circulation and then leaves the circulation as it enters tissues in response to chemotactic factors. Monocytes account for less than 15% of the peripheral blood WBC differential. They are highly motile, tend to marginate along vessel walls, and have a strong tendency to adhere to surfaces. With appropriate stimuli, they undergo diapedesis through vessel walls and differentiate into larger

Table 11–3. MONOCYTE-ASSOCIATED COMPOUNDS
Transport Proteins
Transferrin
Transcobalamin
Nonspecific Inflammatory Agents
Lysozyme
Endogenous pyrogens (interleukin-1)
Tissue Activators
Coagulation factors V, VII, IX, and X and tissue thromboplastin
Plasminogen activator
Complement (1 to 5)
Properdin
Specific/Humoral Agents
Colony stimulating factors for CFU-GEM, T and B cells, epithelial cells
Erythropoietin
Storage
Iron
Vitamin B$_{12}$
Self-/Non-Self-Recognition/Defense Agents
Interferon
Tumor inhibitory factors such as tissue necrosis factor

free macrophages, which have greater phagocytic activity and a higher concentration of hydrolytic enzymes.

Monocyte to Macrophage. The function of the monocyte/macrophage is phagocytosis, and the material ingested is more variable than the material ingested by the neutrophil. The process is similar to neutrophil phagocytosis but much quicker. Monocytes require less opsonization (sensitization to phagocytosis) or complement and can be initiated by simple contact. Pinocytosis occurs with items less than 2 μm large and requires receptor mediation and some degree of protein synthesis. Both activities require the same multistep process found in neutrophils and include recognition/at-

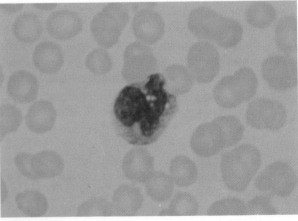

Figure 11–7 Typical monocyte showing vacuolated cytoplasm and cerebriform nucleus.

tachment, ingestion (phagocytosis), intracellular kill, digestion/degradation, and exocytosis. Monocytes kill any recognizable non-self agent: dead or dying cells, bacteria, fungi, and viruses.[19] They play a role in processing specific antigens for lymphocyte recognition and stimulation of lymphocyte transformation. They may function as an antitumor agent by phagocytic action of non-self cells through the elaboration of tumor necrosis factor and stimulation of lymphocyte activity.[20]

Macrophages can be divided into two categories: free and fixed. Free macrophages are found in varying concentrations in all sites of inflammation and repair, alveolar spaces, and peritoneal and synovial fluids, whereas fixed (tissue) macrophages are found in specific concentrations and in such specific sites as the nervous system (microglial cells) and hepatic (Kupffer cells), splenic, bone marrow, and lymph nodes. They are large cells with ample cytoplasm filled with granules and frequently have multiple vacuoles. The nucleus is typically round to reniform and may contain one or two nucleoli (Fig. 11–8).

Lymphocytes

Lymphocytes are the human blood leukocytes whose site of development is not solely the bone marrow. The cells circulate throughout the body in both peripheral blood and lymph, and these carrier streams bring them to sites of activity. Migrating lymphocytes travel from the thoracic duct through vessel endothelium to lymph nodes into the blood stream and back again. The hand mirror shape of peripheral blood lymphocytes is a result of their characteristic form of locomotion. As with other cell lines that have subpopulations, lymphocytes can be categorized in a variety of ways: they may be short-lived or long-lived cells;[21] they may pro-

Table 11-4. SOME IMPORTANT LYMPHOKINES*	
B cell growth factor B cell differentiation B cell stimulatory factor	As a group, these three control proliferation, growth rate, maturation, and stimulation of B cells
Colony stimulating factors	Hematopoietic factors regulating proliferation and differentiation of myeloid cells
Macrophage inhibitory factor	Inhibits macrophages from migration
Histamine-producing cell-stimulating factor	Induces histamine synthesis by basophils and mast cells
T cell–activating factor	Influences the cytotoxic T cells and natural killer cells to become cytolytic

* Lymphokines are biologically active molecules elaborated by lymphocytes in response to specific needs. Listed is a selection of the more important lymphokines. The range of the activity can be appreciated by the variety of cell types influenced by these agents.

duce antibodies or lymphokines (Table 11–4); and they have different surface charges, densities, and antigen receptors.[22]

DEVELOPMENT (Fig. 11–9)

Probably the result of specific hormone stimuli, the earliest maturation of the PSC results in a stem cell for the lymphoid cell (CFU-L), which matures in several environments.[23] The primary lymphatic tissues are the thymus and bone marrow. They give rise to lymphocytes, foster differentiation, and are independent of antigenic stimulation. These environments determine to a great extent the functionality of the cell. Cells that develop under the influence of the thymus are called T cells and have a specific, unique set of receptors and responses. B cells are derived from the bone marrow and have a different set of functions and capabilities. Once the environmental effects have been achieved, lymphocytes migrate to secondary lymphatic tissues such as the spleen and tonsils, the main repositories of already differentiated lymphocytes. These cells are now responsive to specific antigens. Regardless of the environment, the cells can, when seen through traditional staining methods, be divided into three basic morphologic stages: lymphoblast, prolymphocyte, and mature lymphocyte.

Lymphocyte percentages in the peripheral blood vary, depending on the age of the person. Children under the age of 4 years have a much higher proportion of lymphocytes in the peripheral blood than do adults, although, in adults, lymphocytes

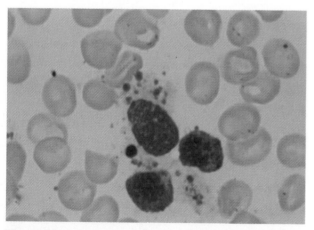

Figure 11–8 A bone marrow macrophage with an eccentrically placed nucleus and granulated cytoplasm.

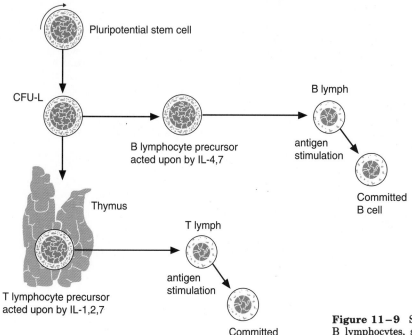

Figure 11–9 Schematic for the differentiation of both T and B lymphocytes, showing the appropriate commitment/stimulation agents.

are the second most common cell of the peripheral blood differential, accounting for 20–55% of WBCs. Further differentiation into subpopulations reveals that approximately 20–35% of total circulating lymphocytes are B cells.

Lymphoblast to Prolymphocyte (Fig. 11–10). The lymphoblast is a small to medium-size cell (10–18 µm) with a round to oval nucleus containing loose chromatin and one or more active nucleoli. The cytoplasm is scanty and has basophilia in proportion to the amount of RNA present. The next stage may be difficult to distinguish from the blast stage, as the prolymphocyte differs from the blast by subtle changes such as slightly more clumped chromatin, a lessening of nucleolar prominence, and a change in the thickness of the nuclear membrane.

Prolymphocyte to Lymphocyte (Fig. 11–11). The morphology of the lymphocyte, when seen with the aid of Wright's stain, varies mostly by size. The size discrepancy may be due to the activity of the cell or the location in the smear in which it is found. Cells in thick areas of the smear tend to be rounded up and to appear smaller and thicker than they actually are. The most common form is the small lymphocyte, which is approximately 9 µm in diameter with skimpy cytoplasm and a few azurophilic granules. The nucleus is round to oval, and its chromatin pattern is a block type. This cell has been described as nondividing or resting.

The medium-sized lymphocyte is approximately 11–14 µm in diameter. Its cytoplasm usually contains azurophilic granules that are more clearly

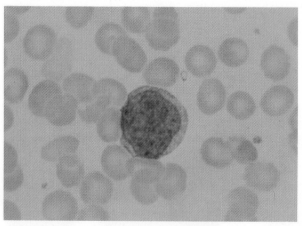

Figure 11–10 Lymphoblast.

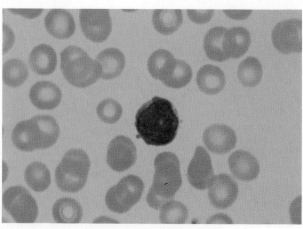

Figure 11–11 Lymphocyte.

discerned, probably as a result of the larger amount of cytoplasm in which they are found. Although these cells are larger than the small lymphocytes, their nucleus-to-cytoplasm ratios are essentially the same. Like the small lymphocytes, these cells are considered nondividing.

The rarest of the peripheral blood lymphocytes are the large lymphocytes. It is approximately 15 μm or more in diameter, and its more generous cytoplasm usually turns a deeper shade of blue when stained. The usual block-type DNA is spread a little more loosely. The cell may be considered to be in transformation in association with active cell proliferation. According to examination by immunologic techniques, this cell, if it contains adequate granulation, may be part of a subpopulation of thymus dependent cells called natural killer cells. Morphologic variants of lymphocytes are summarized in Table 11-5.

IMMUNOLOGIC DIFFERENTIATION

Lymphocytes may be categorized by their immunologic function, and some connections to morphology may be made. The earliest cells show only the marker of a nuclear enzyme, terminal deoxynucleotidyl transferase (TdT) and may be the CFU-L.[24] Later stages show nonspecific immunoglobulin gene structures and TdT (morphologically, these may be what are called blasts).

B Cells. As they mature into pre-B cells, or prolymphocytes, the cells begin immunoglobulin gene rearrangements and cytoplasmic immunoglob-

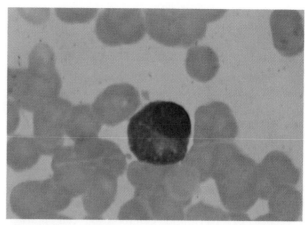

Figure 11-12 Plasma cell showing the typical abundant cytoplasm and perinuclear halo usually ascribed to the presence of the high lipid content of the Golgi apparatus. Notice the dense packing of the heterochromatin in the nucleus.

ulin concentrations of mostly IgD and IgM. Some membrane receptors are apparent. Mature B cells that are committed to specific antibody production have a full complement of IgM and IgD on their membranes and a full amount of cytoplasmic immunoglobulins.[25] All receptors are functional. The fully committed B lymphocyte is the plasma cell (Fig. 11-12). At the end stage of cell development, there is a specificity of surface immunoglobulins and other receptors with copious amounts of cytoplasmic immunoglobulins. Other surface immunologic markers include receptors for the crystallizable fragment of IgG, complement, Epstein-Barr virus, Class I and Class II antigens (HLA-A;

Table 11-5. MORPHOLOGIC VARIATIONS OF LYMPHOCYTES

| | Nucleus | | | | Cytoplasm | | |
CELL	SHAPE	COLOR	CHROMATIN	NUCLEOLI	AMOUNT	COLOR	GRANULATION
Small lymphocyte	Round, oval; indented; stretched	Medium purple	Clumped, smudged, or streaked; not distinct	Not usually	Scanty to moderate	Colorless through shades of blue; clear	If present, few large azurophilic
Large lymphocyte	Round, oval; indented; stretched; usually not folded	Light to medium purple	Variable; clumped, smudged, or reticular	Variable	Moderate to abundant	Colorless through shades of azurophilic blue; clear	If present, few large Tend to localize
Basophilic lymphocyte	Round	Dense; medium to deep purple	Clumped	If present, indistinct; not in late stages	Moderate	Royal blue to deep purple	None or in blocks
Plasma cell	Round; eccentrically placed	Dense; medium to deep purple	Very coarse; clumping; sharp definition of parachromatin	None	Moderate to abundant	Deep blue; may have perinuclear halo	None

HLA-B; HLA-C and HLA-D; HLA-DR), and pokeweed mitogens.

T Cells. T cells are somewhat harder to characterize because the receptors and markers appear, disappear, and reappear throughout the development of the cell, which indicates that these markers may serve some developmental or proliferative function.[26] These markers have been given an alphanumerical code CD__; CD stands for clusters of differentiation. The primitive T cell is the CFU-L, which travels to the thymus for maturation and commitment. The earliest cell within the thymus is the pre-T cell and demonstrates the presence of TdT and common T cell marker (CD2), whereas the prothymocyte possesses TdT but loses CD2 and acquires a transferrin receptor that is apparently not specific to differentiation, but to cell proliferation. The common cortical thymocyte is characterized by the presence of TdT, CD1, CD2, and either CD4 (helper/inducer subset marker) or CD8 (cytotoxic/suppressor subset marker). Mature T cells lose all precursor markers and have an active helper or suppressor function. T cells are further differentiated through the presence or absence of HLA-D class antigens. T cells also possess sheep erythrocyte rosetting receptor and receptors for phytohemagglutinin, concanavalin A, and class I antigens (HLA-A, HLA-B, HLA-C). (A further discussion of cell markers is in Chapter 29.)

Lymphocyte Activity: Regulation of Cellular Response. The main function of the lymphocyte is the regulation of immune function. If foreign material (exogenous antigenic matter; altered endogenous material such as dead, dying, or malignant cells) is completely engulfed, degraded, and disposed of by phagocytes, no immune response occurs. But if complete engulfment does not occur, antigenic fragments are fixed to the exterior surface of the macrophage. The macrophage releases interleukin-1; T cells release factors that increase activation of antigen-specific CD8+ T cells and the development of clones of antigen-specific B lymphs and cytotoxic T cells begins by the action of cytotoxic lymphocyte differentiation factor. Cytotoxic cells require prior activation and major histocompatibility complex class I antigens. T cells release a number of soluble factors that activate effector cells. Suppressor cells then complete the feedback loop by damping the specific response, not immune responsiveness in general, and quench the activated T cells.

If a B cell meets up with a polysaccharide antigen, it does not need T cell stimulation. Induction of a specific helper factor in turn stimulates IgM secretion, and activated B cells expose surface receptors for the lymphokine B cell growth factor (BCGF), which with IL-1 stimulates cell division. A second lymphokine, B cell differentiation factor (BCDF), promotes differentiation into plasma cells. Meanwhile, cytotoxic T cells have CD8+-like suppressors and lyse cells by surface-to-surface contact independent of antibody.

MORPHOLOGY OF ACTIVATION

The activity that accompanies clonal expansion necessary for successful removal of antigen can be seen to a certain degree in the morphology of the cells called *reactive,* or *transformed,* lymphocytes. An older term, *atypical,* although inaccurate, is occasionally still used. Cells must recognize the appropriate antigen (at times modified and presented by the macrophage), commit to producing the correct antibody or lymphokines necessary for the type of antigen attack, undergo clonal expansion to increase numbers of committed cells, and attempt to neutralize or eliminate the antigen in question. Doing all this requires both frequent and significant amounts of morphologic change. These cells should not be confused with distinctly abnormal lymphocytes seen in such conditions as lymphoma (see Chapter 25).

Causes of an increase in reactive lymphocytes are many. In essence, anything that is antigenic or material that is incompletely eliminated by phagocytes results in the presence of reactive lymphocytes (Table 11–6).

As a result of antigen stimulation, lymphocytes may become quite large, sometimes more than $30 \mu m$ in diameter. The cells are highly pleomorphic. In comparison with the nucleus of a common lymphocyte, the nucleus of the reactive lymphocyte is less clumped; faintly stained multiple nucleoli are more likely to be seen. Chromatin patterns are generally less striking in the reactive lymphocyte; some patterns appear quite similar to those of a blast. The shape of the common lymphocyte nucleus is round to oval; that of the reactive cell nucleus ranges from elliptic to cleft to folded. The cytoplasm has greater variability in morphology than does the nucleus. The cytoplasm may range from large, deeply basophilic, and abundant to un-

Table 11–6. CAUSES OF REACTIVE LYMPHOCYTOSIS
β-Streptococcus
Cytomegalovirus
Drugs
Epstein-Barr virus (infectious mononucleosis)
Syphilis
Toxoplasmosis
Vaccination
Viral hepatitis

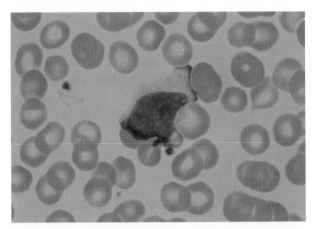

Figure 11–13 The typical reactive lymphocyte seen in most antigenic responses; this cell has a large flared cytoplasm with a loose chromatin structure to its nucleus.

evenly stained and granular. A Golgi apparatus is commonly seen. A variant of reactive lymphocyte is the plasmacytoid lymphocyte whose appearance is somewhere in between those of the lymphocyte and plasma cell (Figs. 11–13, 11–14).

The reporting protocol for reactive lymphocytes is dependent on individual facilities. Some institutions term all cells that are not small lymphocytes as reactive; others have more lenient criteria. However it is done, every clinical laboratory scientist within a given facility must use the same protocol in order to achieve reliability within the institution.

PERIPHERAL BLOOD CONSIDERATIONS

The number, population type, and significance of leukocytes found in the peripheral blood vary with

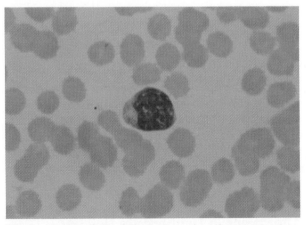

Figure 11–14 Quite different from the other reactive lymphocyte (Fig. 11–13), this cell has a plasmacytoid appearance with a deeply basophilic cytoplasm, easily visualized Golgi apparatus, and dense nucleus.

the individual patient. Certain assumptions about these topics, however, should be kept in mind when peripheral blood smears are evaluated. Although normal values must be established for each population group, some ballpark figures can be used. The calculation of absolute values is necessary to determine whether a patient has a significant increase or decrease in a particular cell type. Instruments that perform a differential reveal both relative values (percentage of cell type) and absolute values (total number per 10^9/L). The absolute value may be manually determined by multiplying the total leukocyte count by the relative value; for example, 10.0×10^9/L (WBC) $\times$ 0.40 (percentage of neutrophils) = 4.0×10^9/L neutrophils.

Quantity

The number of circulating (and countable) WBCs is dependent on three factors. The first factor is the age of the patient. In comparison with the accepted norms, the WBC counts of neonates are elevated; they begin to drop within days after birth (see Chapter 36). Although the high end of the accepted range for children is higher than that for an adult, the range gradually narrows until the teenage years, at which time a relatively steady-state WBC count is maintained. Elderly patients may have lower WBC counts. Spuriously elevated counts may be seen when the granulocytic marginating pool is decreased. Spuriously decreased counts may be seen when a larger-than-expected number of granulocytes are in the marginating or storage pool, thus lessening the circulating pool.

Overall granulocyte kinetics are influenced by (1) input from bone marrow pools, (2) changes in proportion of marginating to circulating pools, and (3) changes caused by disease. The causes of both leukocytosis and leukopenia are many, and in view of the dynamic interactions that are required for WBC number and quality, it is not surprising that many of the causes of leukocytosis are also the causes of leukopenia.

Alterations in Granulocyte Number and Maturity

Neutrophilia is defined as an absolute count of neutrohils that is higher than 8.0×10^9/L with granulocytic hyperplasia of bone marrow and a lack of eosinophils, basophils, and nucleated red blood cells in the peripheral blood, or when the combined percentage of polymorphonuclear cells and bands is greater than 80%. Benign elevations in neutrophils occurs most often in such conditions as stress, tachycardia, fever, strenuous exercise, and ingestion of certain medications such as epinephrine and cortisone. Benign transient neutropenia can be seen after exposure to certain medications such as tranquilizers, sedatives, or antimicrobial agents and procedures such as hemodialysis.[27] If input from the bone marrow functional storage pool exceeds the demand in the tissues, an elevated number of matured cells is found in the peripheral blood. Causes of neutrophilia include inflammatory states, intoxication, acute hemorrhage or hemolysis, and malignancy (in which the condition is termed *leukoerythroblastic picture* because of the presence of nucleated red blood cells). The most dramatic example of neutrophilia is termed a *leukemoid reaction*. This is defined as a WBC count higher than 50.0×10^9/L and may be considered a "hysterical reaction" to a not-so-significant cause when the patient's total picture is assessed. Differential evaluation of leukemoid reaction and leukemia includes the leukocyte alkaline phosphatase (LAP) stain, which is discussed in greater detail in Chapter 21.

Leukopenia is defined as less than 2.5×10^9/L WBC. It is necessary to refer to absolute cell counts to decide whether the situation is caused by neutropenia or lymphopenia. If input from the bone marrow functional storage pool fails to satisfy tissue demand, fewer cells will be found in the peripheral blood, and these cells may be less mature as the depletion of storage pool forces cells from the maturation pool to enter the blood stream. Causes of neutropenia with fully mature granulocytes include diminishing of bone marrow mitotic pool as a result of vitamin B_{12}/folate deficiency, ingestion of medications, and "lazy leukocyte" syndrome[28] (Table 11–7). In rare cases, cells are trapped in the spleen or portal circulation or have shortened lives.[29] Autoinfection becomes a possibility if the WBC count is below 1.0×10^9/L and is an almost certainty below 0.5×10^9/L. Because of the many recognizable stages in neutro-

philic maturation, evaluation of the total number of cells without consideration of their maturity is of limited value. One general conclusion is that an elevated count is preferable to a decreased one, because elevation implies adequate storage and sufficient time to allow for cell maturation. Another interpretation is that an elevated WBC count with an increase in mature neutrophils is probably a better prognostic sign than an elevated WBC count with immature forms, because the latter situation implies a diminution of storage pools and a stress on the maturation pool. In a third evaluation, the quality of the cells in the peripheral blood is considered. Although cytoplasmic abnormalities such as Döhle bodies, toxic granulation, degranulated areas, and vacuoles are considered in greater detail in Chapter 20, it is important to list them here as qualitative changes that have significance for the patient's peripheral blood differential. In this case, the fewer abnormalities seen, the better the prognosis.

Alterations in Eosinophil Number

Eosinophilia is seen commonly in a wide spectrum of allergic responses, medication usage, many skin diseases such as dermatitis, parasitic infestations, some autoimmune disorders, and malignancy. Numbers of eosinophils may be reduced in response to adrenocorticotropic hormone and emotional stress.

Alterations in Basophil Number

Basophilia is seen in patients with hypoactive thyroid conditions, ulcerative colitis, and some types of nephrosis, as well as in certain malignancies. Increases in tissue basophils are seen in patients with contact dermatitis and in instances of delayed hypersensitivity reactions. Basophil concentration is low in patients with hyperthyroidism and stress.

Alterations in Monocyte/Macrophage Number

Monocytosis is seen whenever there is increased amount of cell damage; conditions causing this increase include active tuberculosis, subacute bacterial endocarditis and syphilis, parasitic and rickettsial infections, certain autoimmune diseases, and trauma.

Alterations in Lymphocyte Number

Reference values for peripheral blood lymphocytes average approximately 34% of WBCs in adult

Table 11–7. CAUSES OF NEUTROPHILIA AND NEUTROPENIA	
Neutrophilia	**Neutropenia**
Acute infections	Acute infections
Hemorrhage or hemolysis	Hemodialysis
Inflammatory changes	Overwhelming inflammation/infection
Intoxications (drugs, metabolic, poisons)	Medications
Medications	Physical agents (x-rays)
Myeloproliferative disorders	Secondary to autoimmune disorders
Malignancy (leukoerythroblastic picture)	Aplastic/hypoplastic states
Physiologic response to stress	

blood, or $0.6-5.5 \times 10^9/L$. This value is higher in children and ranges up to 70%, or $2.0-7.0 \times 10^9/L$. Lymphocytosis is considered to be present in an adult when the absolute lymphocyte count is higher than $5.5 \times 10^9/L$.

Relative lymphocytosis can sometimes be seen in patients with exanthems (skin rashes) from certain viral diseases such as measles and mumps; in patients with thyrotoxicosis; and in patients convalescencing from certain acute infections.

Lymphocytosis is rare in children with bacterial infection. The exception, *Bordetella pertussis* infection, causes a significant elevation in the presence of small lymphocytes. More common in viral infections, lymphocytosis is seen with hepatitis A, infectious mononucleosis, and infectious lymphocytosis. It is also seen in cases of congenital and secondary-stage syphilis and brucellosis. An important benign case of lymphocytosis occurs as a result of absolute neutropenia. Relative lymphopenia is seen in patients with heart failure, uremia, lupus erythematosus, and malaria, to name but a few.[27]

Absolute lymphopenia or a peripheral blood lymphocyte count less than $0.6 \times 10^9/L$ can be seen in patients with infectious hepatitis, is secondary to various malignancies, is seen in patients with certain types of Hodgkin's lymphoma, and is a result of drug exposure. Relative lymphopenia is associated with any event of benign or malignant neutrophilia that manifests with a leukoerythroblastic picture and, in the elderly, with bone marrow depletion.

SUMMARY

Leukocytes are a primary defense of the body. They are directed to eliminate all non-self agents, which include bacteria, fungi, viruses, and dead and dying cells from the body. In addition, they are sensitive to alterations in homeostasis caused by internal stressors, such as hormonal (e.g., epinephrine), physical (e.g., temperature), and biochemical (e.g., blood urea nitrogen) stressors, or external stressors, such as radiation (e.g., high energy particles), position (e.g., recumbent), and chemical agents (e.g., drugs). Their reflective variability is important evidence in the development of a diagnosis, choice of appropriate therapy, and prognosis.

Their development is complex, requiring delicate control and maturation for proper cellular function. As limited as knowledge is of how these cells perform their tasks, the relationship among the cells themselves is only now being explored with any depth. Communication, control, and cellular "decision making" are not yet understood. Future investigations concerning the action of colony stimulating factors and cytokine elaboration may reveal additional functions for leukocytes.

REVIEW QUESTIONS

1. The stem cell committed to the production of granulocytes is the
   a. PSC
   b. CFU-S
   c. CFU-E
   d. CFU-G

2. The presence of major basic protein in the cytoplasm confirms that the cell is
   a. basophilic
   b. eosinophilic
   c. neutrophilic
   d. monocytic

3. IL-3 causes increased production of
   a. granulocytes only
   b. monocytes only
   c. granulocytes, monocytes, and platelets
   d. all blood cells except lymphocytes

4. The choice of therapy for a patient with absolute neutropenia would be to provide
   a. erythropoietin
   b. IL-3
   c. G-CSF
   d. M-CSF

5. A patient's complete blood cell (CBC) count reveals a $4.0 \times 10^9/L$ total WBC count with a differential of 25% polymorphonuclear cells, 70% lymphocytes, and 5% monocytes. One interpretation of this data is that
   a. the patient has an absolute neutrophilia caused by a bacterial infection
   b. the patient has an absolute lymphopenia caused by a viral infection
   c. the patient may be a healthy 1-year-old
   d. the patient is elderly and has a relative neutropenia as a result of age related marrow hypoplasia

6. The expected CBC results for women in active labor would include
   a. low total WBC count, many lymphocytes
   b. low total WBC count, many polymorphonuclear cells
   c. high total WBC count, many lymphocytes
   d. high total WBC count, many polymorphonuclear cells

7. The presence of small numbers of reactive lymphocytes in a peripheral blood differential would support the inference that
   a. the patient may be healthy
   b. the patient has infectious mononucleosis

c. the patient has toxoplasmosis

d. this finding could be caused by the presence of an intoxicant such as ethanol

8. A patient's record shows the following laboratory data:

	Day 1	Day 4
WBC	8×10^9/L	2×10^9/L
polymorphonuclear cells	70%	20%
bands	4%	30%
lymphocytes	20%	30%
monocytes	4%	12%
eosinophils	2%	6%
metamyelocytes	0	2%

One conclusion might be that

a. the patient is getting sicker

b. the patient is getting better

c. the data are insufficient for establishing a conclusion

d. there is essentially no change in the patient's status

9. Examination of a peripheral blood smear reveals the presence of a large number of pleomorphic lymphocytes with round to oval and eccentrically placed nuclei, abundant cytoplasm, and mild to marked basophilia, with a clear area adjacent to the nucleus. One possible explanation might be that

a. the patient is responding to a bacterial infection such as *Staphylococcus aureus*

b. the patient has a viral infection, probably mumps

c. the patient is producing a large number of committed b cells

d. the patient is having a generalized response to stress

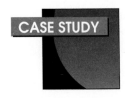

CASE STUDY

A patient with the diagnosis of colon cancer has an admitting CBC count that includes a WBC count of 25.0×10^9/L and a differential of 70% polymorphonuclear cells, 10% bands, 5% metamyelocytes, 10% lymphocytes and 5% monocytes. Two nucleated red blood cells are seen in the 100-cell differential. Appropriate oncologic therapy is instituted, and 48 hours later, the WBC count is 2.1×10^9/L with 35% polymorphonuclear cells, 55% lymphocytes and 10% monocytes. Forty-eight hours later, the WBC count had dropped to 0.9×10^9/L with a similar differential. Infusion of G-CSF was started. On the fifth day after the infusion of G-CSF, the WBC count was up to 3.4×10^9/L with a differential of 45% polymorphonuclear cells, 5% bands, 42% lymphocytes, and 8% monocytes.

1. What was the interpretation of the first CBC count?

2. When the WBC count dropped below 1×10^9/L, what possible outcome became a serious concern?

3. Why was G-CSF used?

References

1. Jandl JH: Blood: Textbook of Hematology. Boston: Little, Brown, 1987.
2. Blackburn AJ, Pratt HM: Increased survival of haemopoietic pluripotent stem cells in vivo induced by a marrow fibroblast factor. Br J Haemotol 1977; 37:337.
3. Platzer E: Human hemopoietic growth factors. Eur J Hematol 1989; 42:1.
4. Metcalf D: The Hemopoietic Colony Stimulating Factors. Amsterdam: Elsevier, 1984.
5. Bell A. Hematopoiesis: morphology of human blood and marrow cells. *In* Harmening DM (ed): Clinical Hematology and Fundamentals of Hemostasis, 2nd ed. Philadelphia: FA Davis, 1991:21–41.
6. Bull I, Kuhn A: Granulocytopoiesis in human bone marrow culture studies by means of kinematography. Blood 1965; 26:449.
7. Diggs LW, Sturm D, Bell A: The Morphology of Human Blood Cells, 5th ed. Abbott Park, IL: Abbott Laboratories, 1985.
8. Ponder E, Mineola LI: The polycyte. J Lab Clin Med 1942; 27:866.
9. Edwin E: The segmentation of polymorphonuclear neutrophils. Acta Med Scand 1967; 182:401.
10. Wallace PJ, Packman CH, Lichtman MA: Maturation-associated changes in the peripheral cytoplasm of human neutrophil: a review. Exp Hematol 1987; 15:34.
11. Bainton DF, Miller LJ, Kishimoto TK, Springer TA: Leukocyte adhesion receptors are stored in peroxidase-negative granules of human neutrophils. J Exp Med 1987; 166:1641.
12. Arneth J: Die neutrophilen wiessen blutkoorperchen bei infectious-krankheiten. Jena, Germany: Fischer, 1904.
13. Strauss RG, Bove KI, Jones JF, et al: An anomaly of neutrophil morphology with impaired function. N Engl J Med 1974; 290:478.
14. Williams WJ, Beutler E, Erslev AJ, Lichtman MA (eds): Hematology, 3rd ed. New York: McGraw-Hill, 1989.
15. Galli SJ, Dvorak AM, Dvorak HF: Basophils and mast cells: morphologic insights into their biology, secretory patterns, and functions. Prog Allergy 1984; 34:1.
16. Galli SJ, Lichtenstein LM: Biology of basophils and mast cells. *In* Middleton E Jr, Reed CE, Ellis EF, Adkinson NF

Jr (eds): Allergy: Principles and Practice, 3rd ed. St. Louis: CV Mosby, 1988:1.

17. van Furth E (ed): Mononuclear Phagocytes: Characteristics, Physiology and Function. Dordrecht, The Netherlands: Martinus Mijhoff, 1985.

18. Nathan CF, Murray HW, Cohen ZA: The macrophage as an effector cell. N Engl J Med 1980; 303:622.

19. Biano C, Griffin FM Jr, Silverstein SC: Studies on the macrophage complement receptor. Alteration of receptor function upon macrophage activation. J Exp Med 1975; 141:1278.

20. Fink MA (ed): The Macrophage in Neoplasia. New York: Academic Press, 1976.

21. Ford WL, Gowans JL: The traffic of lymphocytes. Semin Hematol 1969; 6:67.

22. Miller RG: Physical separation of lymphocytes in the lymphocyte structure and function. *In* Marchalonis JJ (ed): Immunology Series, vol 5. New York: Marcel Dekker, 1977:227.

23. Gupta S, Good RA: Markers of human lymphocyte subpopulations in primary immunodeficiency and lymphoproliferative disorders. Semin Hematol 1980; 17:1.

24. Janossy G: Differentiation of human bone marrow cells and thymocytes. *In* Knapp W (ed): Leukemic Markers. London: Academic Press, 1981:45.

25. Vogler LB, Grossi CE, Cooper MD: Human lymphocyte subpopulations. *In* Brown EB, Moore CV (eds): Progress in Hematology XI. New York: Grune & Stratton, 1979:1.

26. Reinherz EL, Kung PC, Goldstein G et al: Discrete stages of human intrathymic differentiation: analysis of normal thymocytes and leukemic lymphoblasts of T-cell lineage. Proc Natl Acad Sci USA 1980; 77:1588.

27. Wintrobe MM, Lee GR, Boggs DR, et al (eds). Variations of leukocytes in disease. *In* Clinical Hematology, 8th ed. Philadelphia: Lea & Febiger, 1981:1284–1312.

28. Miller ME, Oski FA, Harris MB: Lazy-leucocyte syndrome. A new disorder of neutrophil function. Lancet 1971; 1:665.

29. Wiseman BK, Doan CA: A newly recognized granulopenic syndrome caused by excessive splenic leukolysis and successfully treated by splenectomy. J Clin Invest 1939; 18:473.

PART III

Routine Laboratory Evaluation of Blood Cells and Bone Marrow

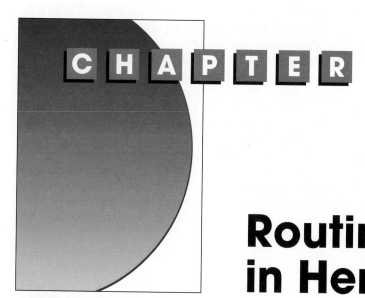

CHAPTER 12

Routine Testing in Hematology

Cristin A. Coates

Objectives

AFTER COMPLETION OF THIS CHAPTER, THE READER WILL BE ABLE TO

1. Perform manual cell counts for leukocytes, erythrocytes, platelets, and eosinophils.
2. Perform manual hemoglobin determinations, including construction of a standard curve.
3. Determine a microhematocrit.
4. Identify sources of error in routine manual procedures.
5. Calculate mean corpuscular volume, hemoglobin, and hemoglobin concentration (erythrocyte indices).
6. Classify erythrocytes according to size and hemoglobin content, using results of red blood cell indices.
7. Perform a reticulocyte count and calculate the relative, absolute, and corrected values.
8. Calculate and interpret the reticulocyte production index.
9. State the diagnostic value of erythrocyte sedimentation rates and identify the differences between the Westergren and Wintrobe erythrocyte sedimentation rates.

Although most routine testing procedures in the hematology laboratory are automated, manual methods may need to be used for counts that exceed the linearity of an instrument or when an instrument is nonfunctional and there is no backup.

MANUAL CELL COUNTS

Manual cell counts are performed with the use of a hemacytometer, or counting chamber, and manual dilutions, made either in Thoma pipettes or with self-contained diluting devices, such as Unopettes (Becton-Dickinson, Rutherford, NJ). The principle for performance of cell counts is essentially the same for leukocytes, erythrocytes, platelets, and eosinophils; only the dilution, diluting fluid, and area counted are varied. In fact, any particle (e.g., sperm) can be counted through the use of this system.

Equipment

THE HEMACYTOMETER

The "heart" of the manual cell count is the hemacytometer, or counting chamber. The most common one is the Levy chamber with improved Neubauer ruling. It is composed of two raised areas, each in the shape of a 3×3 mm square (total area, 9 mm^2). As shown in Figure 12–1, this large square is made up of nine 1×1 mm squares. The center square is subdivided into 25 squares, and each of these is further divided into 16 squares. A coverslip is placed on top of the counting areas. The distance between each counting area and the coverslip is 0.1 mm; thus the total volume is 9 mm^3. Hemacytometers must meet specifications of the National Bureau of Standards, as indicated by the initials NBS on the chamber.

Once the dimensions of the hemacytometer are thoroughly understood, it is possible to count any convenient and significant area and insert that number into the calculation, as discussed later in this chapter.

SUCTION DEVICES

A suction apparatus available from Clay Adams (Parsippany, NJ) is used to make the dilutions in Thoma pipettes. The tip of the pipette closest to the bulb is placed into the black rubber holder. The knob on the end of the device is then carefully turned to aspirate first the blood and then the diluting fluid. Placing a finger over the end of the pipette when it is removed from the device prevents loss of fluid from the pipette (Fig. 12–2).

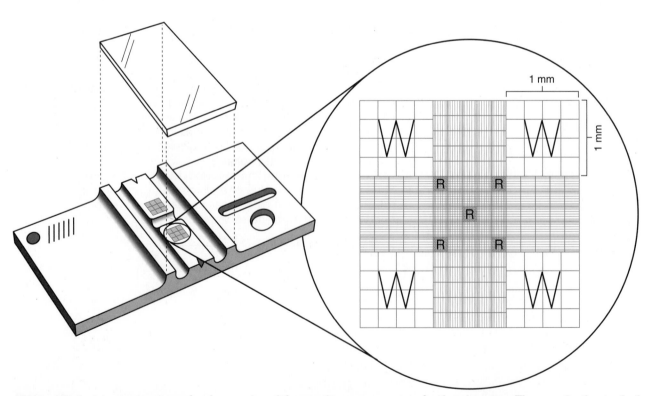

Figure 12–1 A hemacytometer and a close-up view of the counting areas as seen under the microscope. The areas for the standard WBC are labeled by W, and those for RBC, by R.

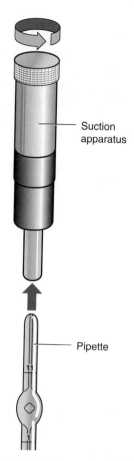

Figure 12-2 Suction device used to facilitate pipetting.

THOMA PIPETTES

Thoma pipettes were standard diluting devices for cell counting until Unopettes were developed in the late 1950s. They are still used in some places, especially when a nonstandard dilution is required. Traditionally, red blood cell (RBC) pipettes have a red mixing bead in the bulb, and white blood cell (WBC) pipettes have a white mixing bead (Fig. 12-3). However, the pipettes can be used to count whatever cells require the possible dilutions; for example, a 1:100 dilution might be made in an RBC pipette in order to determine a very high WBC count more accurately.

The WBC pipette has markings of 0.5, 1, and 11. These markings simply signify parts, and no unit is associated with them. A dilution is made by drawing blood to the 0.5 mark; care must be taken not to introduce bubbles into the pipette. Blood is wiped from the outside of the pipette with a tissue or gauze square, which is not allowed to touch the tip of the pipette and pull liquid out. Diluting fluid is drawn to the 11 mark with steady suction, and no bubbles are allowed in. The dilution itself is made in the bulb; the diluting fluid remaining in the stem does not participate in the dilution. Therefore, the dilution in this example would be

0.5:10, or 1:20. The same pipette can be used to make a 1:10 dilution by drawing blood to the 1 mark and diluting fluid to the 11 mark.

The RBC pipette has markings of 0.5, 1, and 101. A dilution made by drawing blood to the 0.5 mark, and diluting fluid to the 101 mark would be a 1:200 dilution (0.5:100). The same pipette can be used to make a 1:100 dilution by drawing blood to the 1 mark and drawing diluting fluid to the 101 mark.

THE UNOPETTE SYSTEM

The Unopette is a commercially available self-contained diluting device available from Becton-Dickinson (Rutherford, NJ). Unopettes have eliminated many of the pipetting errors and make the manual methods easier and more accurate. Unopettes are available for WBC, RBC, platelet, and eosinophil counts; for hemoglobin (Hb) determinations; and for reticulocyte counts. Kits are also available for more specialized testing (e.g., osmotic fragility).

The reservoir of the Unopette (Fig. 12-4) contains the appropriate diluting fluid and is covered at the top by a thin plastic diaphragm. The pipette

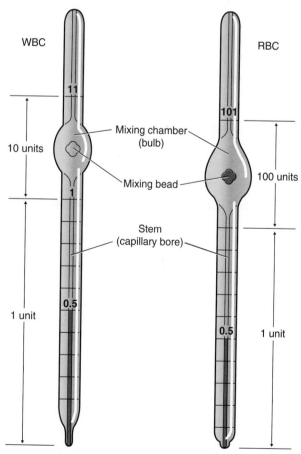

Figure 12-3 Thoma pipettes for manual cell counting.

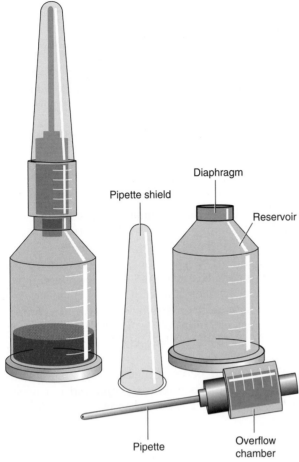

Pipette shield

Diaphragm

Reservoir

Pipette

Overflow chamber

Figure 12–4 Unopette.

varies in volume, depending on the dilution required. An overflow chamber is located at the end of the pipette tip. The pipette shield is used to protect the pipette and to puncture the reservoir diaphragm.

PROCEDURE

1. To open the reservoir, puncture the diaphragm, using the pointed end of the pipette shield. The hole should be large enough to easily insert the pipette into the reservoir.
2. Remove the pipette from the shield with a twisting motion.
3. Fill the pipette by capillary action from EDTA anti-coagulated blood or capillary puncture. Wipe excess blood from outside of pipette.
4. Place an index finger over the top of the overflow chamber. With the other hand, squeeze the reservoir enough to expel air without allowing liquid out.
5. Seat the pipette into the reservoir and release the finger from the top of pipette, while releasing pressure on the reservoir. The sample will thus be drawn into the diluting fluid.

6. Squeeze and release the reservoir several times to rinse pipette, allowing fluid to enter the overflow chamber without overflowing it.
7. With a finger covering the overflow chamber, invert the unit several times to mix.
8. After the incubation period (if required for procedure), convert the unit to a dropper assembly. Mix well, invert, and expel a few drops onto a tissue.
9. Maintaining steady pressure on the unit to prevent air bubbles, charge the hemocytometer, and proceed with the count, as specified in procedure.

Calculations

The general formula for manual cell counts is as follows:

$$\text{Total count} = \frac{\substack{\text{number of cells counted} \\ \times \text{ dilution factor}}}{\text{area counted (mm}^2\text{)} \times \text{depth (0.1)}}$$

$$= \frac{\substack{\text{number of cells counted} \\ \times \text{ dilution factor} \times 10}}{\text{area (mm}^2\text{)}}$$

WHITE BLOOD CELL COUNT

The leukocyte, or WBC, count represents the number of WBCs in a liter of whole blood. Whole blood from a capillary puncture or anti-coagulated with ethylenediaminetetraacetic acid (EDTA) is mixed with a diluting fluid that contains a weak acid (hydrochloric acid, acetic acid) to lyse the nonnucleated erythrocytes. In general, a 1:20 dilution is made. A hemacytometer is charged (filled) with the dilution and placed under a microscope in order to count the number of cells.

PROCEDURE

1. A 1:20 dilution is made in a Unopette containing 3% glacial acetic acid, or in a Thoma Pipette. When a Thoma pipette is used, the following guidelines should be followed:
   a. Attach suction device to pipette.
   b. Draw blood to the desired mark (for WBC, 0.5).
   c. Wipe outside of pipette, being careful not to touch the bore, and remove liquid portion of blood.
   d. Aspirate diluting fluid, with steady suction to the desired mark (for WBC, 11), allowing no bubbles.
   e. Clean the outside of the pipette carefully.

f. Detach the device from the pipette carefully, ensuring no fluid loss. Placing an index finger on the open end of the pipette may prevent this from happening.

g. Mix the contents of the pipette for 3 minutes to facilitate hemolysis of the erythrocytes. Mixing can be done on a mechanical shaker, or by placing the pipette between two fingers and rotating it in a figure eight pattern.

h. Before filling the hemacytometer, discard the first four to five drops of the mixture on a piece of gauze to expel the diluent from the stem.

2. Charge both sides of the hemacytometer by holding the pipette at a 45 degree angle, and touch the tip of the pipette to the coverslip edge where it meets the chamber floor. Often there is a V-shaped indentation. The hemacytometer fills by capillary action. The chamber should be filled with a steady flow of fluid and be completely filled without overflowing.

3. After charging the counting chamber, place it in a moist chamber for 1–2 minutes before counting the cells, to give them time to settle. Care should be taken not to disturb the coverslip. A moist chamber may be made by placing a piece of damp filter paper in the bottom of a Petri dish. An applicator stick broken in half can serve as a support for the chamber.

4. While keeping the hemacytometer in a horizontal position, place it on the microscope stage.

5. Lower the condenser on the microscope and focus by using the low-power (10×) objective lens. The cells should be evenly distributed in all of the squares.

6. For WBCs, count all of the cells in the four large corner squares, starting with the square in the left hand corner (see Fig. 12–1). The variation in the counts from each square should not differ by more than 10 cells. Cells that touch the top and left lines should be counted; those that touch the bottom and right lines should be ignored (Fig. 12–5).

7. Repeat the count on the other side of the counting chamber. The counts in the eight squares should not differ from one another by more than 15 cells.

8. Calculate the WBC count:

$$\frac{\text{cells counted} \times \text{depth factor (10)} \times \text{dilution factor (20)}}{\text{area counted (mm}^2)}$$

Example: If 200 cells were counted in the four large squares,

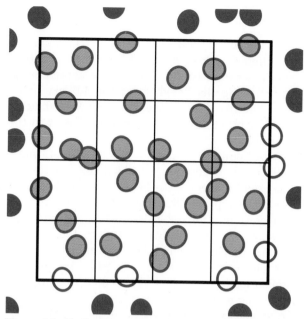

Figure 12–5 One square of hemacytometer indicating which cells to count. Cells touching the right and bottom lines (solid circles) are counted. Cells touching bottom and right (open circles) are not counted.

$$\text{WBC count} = \frac{200 \times 10 \times 20}{4}$$
$$= 40,000/4$$
$$= 10,000/\text{mm}^3$$
$$= 10.0 \times 10^9/\text{L}$$

9. After calculating the WBC count for each side of the chamber, average the numbers together and report the average.

REFERENCE VALUES*

Age	Male and Female ($\times 10^9$/L)
1 day	9.0–38.0
2 months	5.5–18.0
12 years	4.5–13.5
Adult	4.5–11.0

Values may vary slightly according to the population tested and should be established for each institution.

SOURCES OF ERROR AND COMMENTS

1. The hemacytometer and coverslip should be properly cleaned before they are used. Dust and fingerprints may cause difficulty in distinguishing the cells and, therefore, errors.

2. Pipettes must also be cleaned properly. If the pipette is damaged at the tip, the dilution will not be accurate.

_____

* From the University of Pittsburgh Medical Center.

3. The diluting fluid should be free of contaminants.
4. If the count is less than 3.0×10^9/L, a smaller dilution of blood should be used to ensure a more accurate count. This can be accomplished by drawing the blood up to the 1.0 mark and the diluting fluid to the 11 mark. The dilution will then be 1:10, and the dilution factor in the calculation will be 10.
5. If the count is greater than 30.0×10^9/L, more dilution is needed. A red blood cell pipette can be used by drawing the blood up to the 1.0 mark and the diluting fluid to the 101 mark. This yields a dilution of 1:100, which changes the dilution factor in the calculation to 100.
6. After the chamber is filled, 1–2 minutes' pause should be allowed to let cells settle, but a pause much longer than that allows fluid to start evaporating and causes inaccuracies in the count.
7. Any nucleated erythrocytes present in the sample are not lysed by the diluting fluid. The nucleated erythrocytes are counted as WBCs because they are undistinguishable when seen on the hemocytometer. If five or more nucleated RBCs (nRBCs) per 100 WBCs on the differential are discovered, the WBC count must be corrected for these cells. This is accomplished by using the following formula:

$$\frac{\text{uncorrected WBC count} \times 100}{\text{number of nRBCs/100 WBCs} + 100}$$

Report the result as the "corrected" WBC count.
8. The accuracy of the manual WBC count can be assessed by performing a WBC estimate on the peripheral blood smear (see Chapter 13).
9. The error in the manual WBC count with Thoma pipettes is approximately 16%.[1] With Unopettes, it is 5.6% (Becton-Dickinson product information).

PLATELET COUNT

A phase-contrast microscope is used in the reference method for performing a manual platelet count. Platelets are very adhesive to foreign objects and to each other, which makes it very difficult to count them. They are also small and could be easily confused with dirt. In this procedure, whole blood, with EDTA as the anti-coagulant, is diluted with 1% ammonium oxalate, which lyses the nonnucleated erythrocytes. The platelets can then be counted with the use of a phase-contrast microscope as described by Brecher and Cronkite.[2]

Procedure

1. Make a 1:100 dilution in a red blood cell pipette, using ammonium oxalate. Repeat with a second pipette. Alternatively, a Unopette containing ammonium oxalate may be used.
2. Mix both Thoma pipettes for 10–15 minutes on a mechanical shaker.
3. Place the charged hemacytometer in this moist environment for 15 minutes to allow platelets to settle.
4. Platelets are counted with the use of the 40× objective lens. The platelets have a diameter of 2–4 μm and appear round or oval, displaying a light purple sheen when phase-contrast microscopy is used. The shape and color help distinguish the platelets from dirt and debris, which are very refractile. "Ghost" red blood cells are often seen in the background.
5. Count the 25 small squares in the center square of the grid. The area of this center square is 1 mm². Each side of the hemacytometer should be counted, and the counts should not differ by more than 10%.
6. Calculate the number of platelets per liter by using the following formula:

$$\frac{\text{cells counted} \times \text{depth factor (10)} \times \text{dilution factor}}{\text{area counted (mm}^2)}$$

Example: If 200 platelets were counted in the entire center square,

$$\frac{200 \times 10 \times 100}{1} = 200,000/\text{mm}^3$$

$$= 200 \times 10^9/\text{L}$$

7. Platelet counts should be verified by performing an estimate on the Wright's stained peripheral blood smear, as described in Chapter 13.

Reference Value

Male and female: $150–450 \times 10^9$/L.

Sources of Error and Comments

1. Inadequate mixing and poor collection of the sample can cause the platelets to clump on the hemacytometer. If the problem persists after rediluting, a new sample is needed. A fingerstick sample is less desirable because of the adhesive quality of the platelets.
2. Dirt in the pipette, hemacytometer, or diluting fluid may cause the counts to be inaccurate.
3. If fewer than 50 platelets are counted on each side, the procedure should be repeated with the use of a WBC pipette and by diluting the blood

to 1:20 as outlined in the procedure for a manual WBC count. If there are more than 500 platelets counted on each side, a 1:200 dilution should be made in an RBC pipette. The appropriate dilution factor should be used in calculating the results.

4. The error in performing a manual platelet count with Thoma Pipettes is ±10–22%.[1,3]

EOSINOPHIL COUNT

The diluting fluid for eosinophil counts contains propylene glycol to lyse the erythrocytes, sodium carbonate and water to lyse all WBCs except eosinophils, and phloxine to stain the eosinophils a bright pink.

Procedure

1. Make a 1:10 dilution in a WBC pipette, using the appropriate diluting fluid. Repeat with a second pipette. The Unopette for eosinophil counts is used with a 1:32 dilution.
2. Mix the contents of each pipette for 2 minutes.
3. Expel the first four drops from the tip of the pipette and fill the hemacytometer, using one pipette per side.
4. Place the charged hemacytometer in a moist environment. Allow the contents to settle for approximately 15 minutes.
5. Count eosinophils in the entire ruled area on both sides of the pipette under the 10× objective lens.
6. Calculate the number of eosinophils per liter, using the following formula:

$$\frac{\text{cells counted}}{\text{area counted (mm}^2)} \times \text{depth factor (10)} \times \text{dilution factor}$$

Example with the use of Thoma pipettes and Neubauer chamber: The number of cells in all 18 squares is 55.

$$\frac{55 \times 10 \times 10}{18} = 305/\text{mm}^3$$
$$= 0.3 \times 10^9/\text{L}$$

Example with the use of a Unopette with 1:32 dilution:

$$\frac{55 \times 10 \times 32}{18} = 978/\text{mm}^3$$
$$= 1.0 \times 10^9/\text{L}$$

7. Results should approximate those obtained by performing an indirect absolute count from the peripheral blood smear differential. The indirect eosinophil count is calculated by multiplying the total WBC count by the percentage of eosinophils in the differential. Example:
a. WBC = $10.0 \times 10^9/\text{L}$
b. eosinophils = 3%
c. $10.0 \times 0.03 = 0.3 \times 10^9/\text{L}$

Reference Value

The reference range is $0–450/\text{mm}^3$, or $0–0.45 \times 10^9/\text{L}$, although each laboratory should determine the range for its particular population.[3]

Sources of Error and Comments

1. EDTA is the preferred anti-coagulant. If oxalate is used as the anti-coagulant, the blood must be tested within 4 hours after collection.
2. The error in the chamber count when a Neubauer hemacytometer and Thoma pipettes are used is approximately ±30%.
3. The indirect count of eosinophils is not as accurate as the direct chamber count. Instruments that provide a five-part differential have decreased the necessity of manual eosinophil counts, because absolute counts obtained from the instrument are based on many thousands of cells.

RED BLOOD CELL COUNT

Whole blood is diluted with an isotonic fluid. Manual erythrocyte counts are rarely performed, because of both the inaccuracy of the count and questionable necessity, when other more accurate manual RBC parameters, such as microhematocrit and Hb, are available.

A summary of manual cell counts is given in Table 12–1.

HEMOGLOBIN DETERMINATION

The primary function of Hb within the erythrocyte is the carrying of oxygen and carbon dioxide to and from the tissues. The cyanmethemoglobin method for Hb determination is the reference method.

PRINCIPLE

In the cyanmethemoglobin method, blood is diluted in a solution of potassium ferricyanide and potassium cyanide. The Hb is oxidized to methemoglobin by the potassium ferricyanide. The potassium cyanide then converts the methemoglobin

Table 12-1. SUMMARY OF MANUAL CELL COUNTS*

Cell Counted	Diluting Fluid	Dilution	Objective	Area Counted	Adult Reference Range†
leukocyte	weak acid	1:20	10×	4 mm²	4.5-11.0 × 10⁹/L
erythrocyte	isotonic saline	1:200	40×	0.2 mm² (5 small squares of center mm²)	4.35-5.87 × 10¹²/L (male) 3.79-5.23 × 10¹²/L (female)
eosinophil	propylene glycol, phloxine and sodium carbonate	1:10	10×	18 mm²	0-450/mm3 (0-0.45 × 10⁹/L)
platelet	ammonium oxalate	1:100	40× (phase)	1 mm²	150-450 × 10⁹/L

* General formula: # cells counted × depth factor (10) × dilution factor/area (mm²).
† University of Pittsburgh Medical Center, Department of Hematology, 1993.

to cyanmethemoglobin (Fig. 12–6). The absorbance of the cyanmethemoglobin at 540 nm is directly proportional to the Hb concentration. Sulfhemoglobin is not converted to cyanmethemoglobin; therefore, it cannot be measured by this method.

PROCEDURE: CYANMETHEMOGLOBIN METHOD

Cyanmethemoglobin Reagent (Drabkin's reagent, commercially available)

	Amount
Sodium bicarbonate	1.00 g
Potassium cyanide	0.05 g
Potassium ferricyanide	0.02 g
Distilled water	1000 mL

1. Create a standard curve, using a commercially available cyanmethemoglobin standard.
   a. When a standard containing 80 mg/dL of Hb is used, the following dilutions should be made:

Hb Concentration (g/dL)	Blank	5	10	15	20
Cyanmethemoglobin standard	0.0	1.5	3.0	4.5	6.0
Cyanmethemoglobin reagent	6.0	4.5	3.0	1.5	0.0

   b. Transfer the dilutions to cuvettes. Starting with the blank, measure the absorbance on a spectrophotometer (Fig. 12–7) at 540 nm.
   c. Using semilogarithmic paper, plot percentage

transmittance on the y-axis and the Hb concentration on the x-axis. The Hb concentrations of the controls' and patients' samples can be read from this standard curve, as shown in Figure 12–8.
   d. A standard curve should be set up with each new lot of reagents. It should also be checked when alterations (e.g., bulb change) are made to the instrument.
2. Controls should be run with each batch of specimens. Commercial controls are available.
3. Using the patient's whole blood anti-coagulated with EDTA or heparin or from a capillary puncture, make a 1:251 dilution by adding 0.02 mL (20 μL) of blood to 5.0 mL of cyanmethemoglobin reagent. The pipette should be thoroughly rinsed with the reagent to ensure that no blood remains. Follow the same procedure for the control samples.
4. Cover and mix well by inversion or using a vortex mixer. Let stand for 10 minutes at room temperature to allow full conversion of hemoglobin to cyanmethemoglobin.

$$Hb(Fe^{++}) \xrightarrow{K_3Fe(CN)_6} Methemoglobin (Fe^{+++}) \xrightarrow{KCN} cyanmethemoglobin$$

Figure 12–6 The reaction that takes place during the hemoglobin determination.

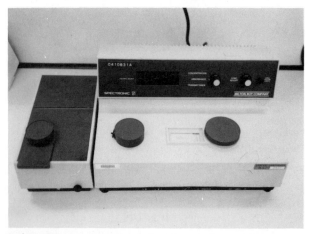

Figure 12–7 A spectrophotometer, used to measure transmittance or absorbance.

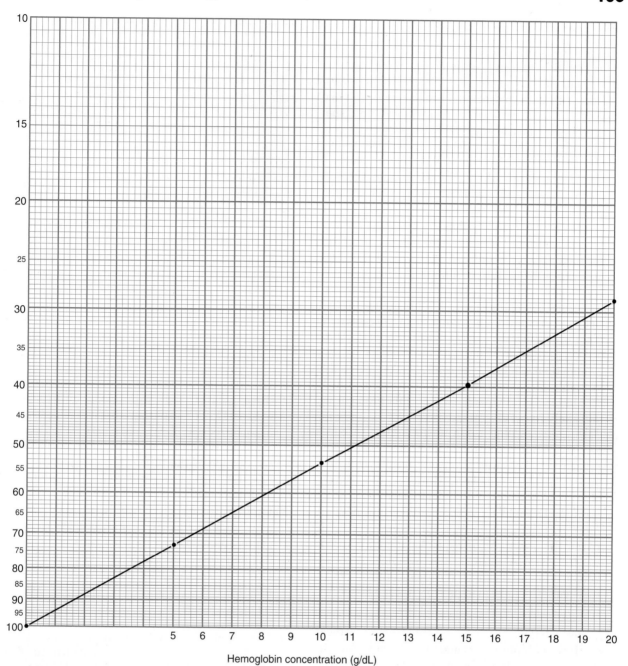

Figure 12–8 A standard curve obtained when a cyanmethemoglobin standard of 80 mg/dL is used. A blank (100% transmittance) and four dilutions were made: 5 g/dL (72.9% transmittance); 10 g/dL (53.2% transmittance); 15 g/dL (39.1% transmittance); 20 g/dL (28.7% transmittance).

5. Transfer all of the solutions to cuvettes. Set the spectrophotometer to 100% transmittance at the wavelength of 540 nm, using cyanmethemoglobin reagent as a blank.

6. Using a matched cuvette, continue reading the patients' samples and record the percentage transmittance.

7. Determine the Hb values of the control samples and the patients' samples from the standard curve.

REFERENCE RANGES*

Age	Male (g/dL)	Female (g/dL)
1 day	15.0–24.6	15.0–24.6
6 months	10.5–12.9	10.5–12.9
10 years	10.8–15.6	10.8–15.6
Adult	13.3–17.7	11.7–15.7

* From the University of Pittsburgh Medical Center.

SOURCES OF ERROR AND COMMENTS

1. Drabkin's reagent is sensitive to light. It should be stored in a brown bottle or in a dark place.
2. A high leukocyte count ($>30.0 \times 10^9/L$) can cause turbidity and a falsely high result. In this case the solution can be centrifuged and the supernatant measured.
3. Lipemia can also interfere, and a false result can be corrected by adding 0.02 mL of the patient's plasma to 5.0 mL of the cyanmethemoglobin reagent, this solution being used as the reagent blank.
4. Hemoglobins S and C may be resistant to hemolysis, causing turbidity. This can be corrected by making a 1:1 dilution with distilled water and multiplying the results from the spectrophotometer by 2.
5. Abnormal globulins, such as those found in patients with multiple myeloma or Waldenström's macroglobulinemia, may precipitate. If this occurs, add 0.1 g of potassium carbonate to the cyanmethemoglobin reagent. Commercially available Drabkin's reagent has been modified to contain KH_2PO_4 salt, and so this problem is not likely to occur.
6. Carboxyhemoglobin takes up to 1 hour to convert to cyanmethemoglobin and, therefore, theoretically could cause erroneous results in samples from heavy smokers. However, the degree of error is probably not clinically significant.
7. Because Drabkin's reagent contains cyanide, it must be used cautiously; a minimum of 4 L of reagent is lethal. Acid-free sinks should be used for disposal of reagent and samples, because acidification of cyanide releases hydrogen cyanide gas. Copious amounts of water should be used to flush the sink after disposal.

A method that has been accepted among office practitioners involves conversion of hemoglobin to azide methemoglobin, which is read photometrically at two wavelengths. This method avoids the necessity of sample dilution and interference from turbidity.[4]

Another more recent method that has been used in automated instruments involves the use of sodium lauryl sulfate (SLS) to convert hemoglobin to SLS-methemoglobin. This method does not generate toxic wastes.[5-8]

MICROHEMATOCRIT[9]

The hematocrit (Hct) is the volume of packed RBCs that occupies a given volume of whole blood, stated as a percentage.

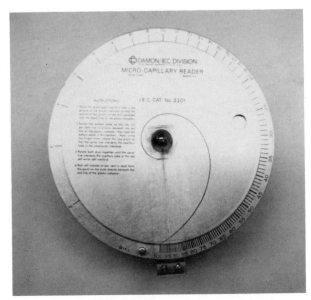

Figure 12–9 Microhematocrit reader.

PROCEDURE

1. Fill two plain capillary tubes approximately three quarters full with blood anti-coagulated with EDTA or heparin. Alternatively, blood for heparinized capillary tubes may be collected by capillary puncture. Wipe any excess blood from the outside of the tube.
2. Seal the end of the tube with the colored ring with nonabsorbent clay.
3. Balance the tubes in the centrifuge with the clay ends facing the outside away from the center, touching the rubber gasket.
4. Tighten the head cover on the centrifuge and close the top. Activate the centrifuge for 5 minutes between 10,000 and 15,000 rpm (see comments). Do not use the brake to stop the centrifuge.
5. Determine the Hct by using a microhematocrit reading device such as that shown in Figure 12–9. Read the level of RBC packing; do not include the buffy coat (leukocytes and platelets) when reading (Fig. 12–10).
6. The values of the two Hcts should agree within 2% (0.02).

REFERENCE RANGES*

Age	Male (L/L)	(%)	Female (L/L)	(%)
1 day	0.44–0.72	(44–72)	0.44–0.72	(44–72)
6 months	0.32–0.40	(32–40)	0.32–0.40	(32–40)
10 years	0.33–0.45	(33–45)	0.33–0.45	(33–45)
Adult	0.40–0.52	(40–52)	0.35–0.47	(35–47)

* From the University of Pittsburgh Medical Center.

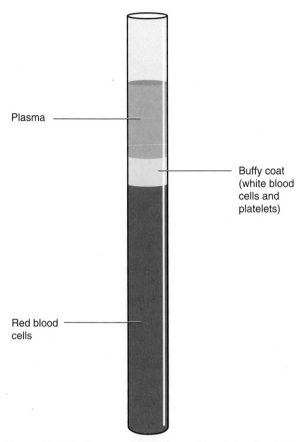

Figure 12–10 Representation of a capillary tube after it has been spun. Notice the layers containing plasma, the buffy coat (leukocytes and platelets), and the erythrocytes.

Plasma

Buffy coat (white blood cells and platelets)

Red blood cells

SOURCES OF ERROR AND COMMENTS

1. Improper sealing of the capillary tube causes a decreased Hct reading as a result of loss of blood during centrifugation. A higher number of erythrocytes are lost in relation to the plasma.
2. An increased amount of anti-coagulant decreases the Hct reading as a result of erythrocyte shrinkage.
3. A decreased or increased result may occur if the specimen was not properly mixed.
4. The time and speed of the centrifugation and the time when the results are read are very important. Insufficient centrifugation or a delay in reading results after centrifugation cause Hct readings to increase. Time for complete packing should be determined for each centrifuge and rechecked at regular intervals.[9]
5. The buffy coat of the specimen should not be included in the Hct reading, because its inclusion falsely elevates the result.
6. A decrease or increase in the readings may be seen if the microhematocrit reader is not used properly.
7. A number of disorders such as sickle cell ane-

mia, macrocytic anemias, hypochromic anemias, spherocytosis, and thalassemia may cause plasma to be trapped in the erythrocytes even if the procedure was performed properly. The trapping of the plasma causes the microhematocrit to be 1–3% (0.01–0.03 L/L) higher than that obtained on automated instruments, which calculate the Hct and are unaffected by the trapped plasma.

8. A temporarily low Hct reading may result immediately after a blood loss, because plasma is replaced faster than are erythrocytes.
9. The fluid loss of dehydration causes a decrease in plasma volume and falsely increases the Hct reading.
10. Proper specimen collection is an important consideration. The introduction of interstitial fluid from a skin puncture or the improper flushing of a catheter causes decreased Hct readings.

THE RULE OF THREE

When specimens are analyzed, by either automated or manual methods, a quick visual check of the results of the erythrocyte count, Hb, and Hct can be done by applying the "rule of three." This rule applies only to specimens that have normal erythrocytes. The value of the Hb should be three times the RBC count, and the Hct should be three times the value of the Hb plus or minus 3. Numerically, this would appear as RBC × 3 = Hb; Hb × 3 = Hct ± 0.03. It should become habit for the analyst to multiply the Hb by 3 mentally for every specimen; a discrepancy in this rule is often the first indication of error.

Example: The following results are obtained from a patient:

RBC = 4.0 × 10¹²/L	RBC (4.0) × 3 = 12; Hb = 12.0 g/dL
Hb = 12.0 g/dL	Hb (12) × 3 = 36; Hct = 0.36 L/L
Hct = 0.36 L/L	Acceptable range for the Hct would be 0.33–0.39 L/L

These values conform to the rule of three. Those in the following example do not:

RBC = 4.5 × 10¹²/L	RBC (4.5) × 3 = 13.5; but Hb = 9.0 g/dL
Hb = 9.0 g/dL	Hb (9.0) × 3 = 27.0; but Hct = 0.32 L/L
Hct = 0.32 L/L	Acceptable range for Hct would be 0.24–0.30 L/L

If values do not agree, the blood smear should be examined for abnormal erythrocytes. In the second example, the blood smear reveals erythrocytes that are abnormal in size and in Hb content. If erythrocytes do appear normal, the problem should be investigated. When a discrepancy is found, the samples before and after the sample in question should be checked for whether they conform to the rule. If they do not conform, further investigation should be done to find the problem. A control sample should be run when a discrepancy is found. If the instrument is in control, random error may have occurred (see Chapter 5).

RED BLOOD CELL INDICES

The mean corpuscular volume (MCV), mean corpuscular Hb (MCH), and the mean corpuscular Hb concentration (MCHC) are RBC indices. These are calculated to determine the size and Hb content of the average RBC. In addition to serving as a quality control check, the indices may be used to differentiate anemias (see Chapter 15).

MEAN CORPUSCULAR VOLUME

The MCV is the average volume of the RBC in femtoliters (fL), or 10^{-15} L:

$$MCV = \frac{Hct\ (\%) \times 10}{RBC\ count\ (10^{12}/L)}$$

Example: Hct = 45%, RBC count = 5.0×10^{12}/L; therefore,

$$MCV = \frac{45.0 \times 10}{5.0} = 90\ fL$$

Note: For the purpose of calculating only indices, units may be disregarded to facilitate calculations.

RBCs are *normocytic* if the MCV is 80–100 fL, *microcytic* if the MCV is less than 80 fL, and *macrocytic* if the MCV is greater than 100 fL. In general, microcytic cells are found in patients with iron deficiency anemia, thalassemia, or other conditions of defective iron utilization. Macrocytic cells are found (1) in patients with liver disease or hypothyroidism; (2) in situations in which there is a large increase in young erythrocytes (reticulocytes), such as chronic hemolytic anemias; (3) when there is asynchrony in RBC maturation (termed megaloblastic anemias), such as folate and vitamin B_{12} deficiencies; and (4) in patients undergoing treatment with drugs that interfere with RBC maturation, such as some chemotherapeutic agents and zidovudine.

MEAN CORPUSCULAR HEMOGLOBIN (MCH)

The MCH is the average weight of Hb in an RBC, expressed in the units of picograms (pg), or 10^{-12} g:

$$MCH = \frac{Hb\ (g/dL) \times 10}{RBC\ count\ (10^{12}/L)}$$

Example: Hb = 16.0 g/dL, RBC count = 5.0×10^{12}/L;

$$MCH = \frac{16.0 \times 10}{5.0} = 32.0\ pg$$

The reference range for adults is 28–32 pg. The MCH is not generally considered in the classification of anemias.

MEAN CORPUSCULAR HEMOGLOBIN CONCENTRATION (MCHC)

The MCHC is the average concentration of Hb in each individual erythrocyte. The units used are grams per deciliter (formerly referred to as a percentage).

$$MCHC = \frac{Hb\ (g/dL) \times 100}{Hct\ (\%)}$$

Example: Hb = 16 g/dL, Hct = 48%;

$$MCHC = \frac{16 \times 100}{48} = 33.3\ g/dL$$

Values of normochromic cells range from 32 to 37 g/dL, those of hypochromic cells are less than 32 g/dL, and those of hyperchromic cells are greater than 37 g/dL. Hypochromic erythrocytes occur in thalassemias and iron deficiency. The term *hyperchromic* is actually a misnomer: a cell does not really contain more than 37 g/dL of Hb, but its shape may have become spherocytic, making the cell appear full. An MCHC >37 g/dL should be scrutinized carefully for an error in Hb value (see sources of error in the section on Hb determination).

RETICULOCYTE COUNT

The reticulocyte is the last immature erythrocyte stage. Normally, a reticulocyte spends 2 days in the bone marrow and 1 day in the peripheral blood before developing into a mature erythrocyte. The reticulocyte contains remnant cytoplasmic RNA and organelles such as the mitochondria and ribosomes. The reticulocyte count is used to assess erythropoietic activity of the bone marrow.

PRINCIPLE

Whole blood, anti-coagulated with EDTA, is stained with a supravital stain such as new methylene blue. Any nonnucleated erythrocyte that contains two or more particles of blue-stained, granulofilamentous material after new methylene blue staining is defined as a reticulocyte (Fig. 12–11).

PROCEDURE

1. Equal amounts of blood and new methylene blue stain (two to three drops, or 50 μL each) are mixed and allowed to incubate at room temperature for 10 minutes.
2. Two wedge smears are prepared (see Chapter 13).
3. In an area in which cells are close together but not touching, 1000 RBCs are counted under the oil immersion objective lens. Reticulocytes are included in the total RBC count (i.e., a reticulocyte counts as both an RBC and a reticulocyte).
4. To ensure accuracy, another technologist counts the other smear; values should agree within 20%.
5. Calculate the reticulocyte count:

$$\frac{\text{number of reticulocytes}}{1000 \text{ (RBCs observed)}} \times 100$$

Example: If 15 reticulocytes are counted,

$$\text{reticulocyte (\%)} = \frac{15}{1000} \times 100 = 1.5\%$$

It is easy to see from this formula that the number of reticulocytes counted can be multiplied by 0.1 (100/1000) to obtain the result.

MILLER DISC METHOD OF COUNTING

1. The Miller disc (Fig. 12–12) may be placed in one of the ocular lenses to aid in the counting of the reticulocytes. The disc has two squares; square B is one ninth of square A.
2. Five hundred RBCs are counted in square B in consecutive fields, while reticulocytes are counted in squares A and B. If a reticulocyte is seen during counting in square B, it is counted both as an RBC and as a reticulocyte. When the counting is finished, the number of reticulocytes

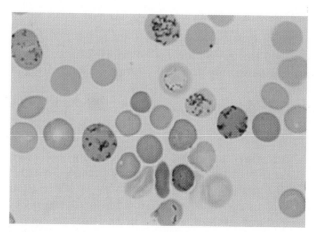

Figure 12–11 Reticulocytes under an oil immersion lens.

in 4500 erythrocytes has theoretically been counted.
3. Calculate the reticulocyte count:

Reticulocyte (%)

$$= \frac{\text{total reticulocytes in square A} \times 100}{\text{total RBCs in square B} \times 9}$$

Example: 100 reticulocytes were seen in square A, 500 red blood cells were counted in square B;

$$\text{reticulocyte (\%)} = \frac{100 \times 100}{500 \times 9} = 2.2\%$$

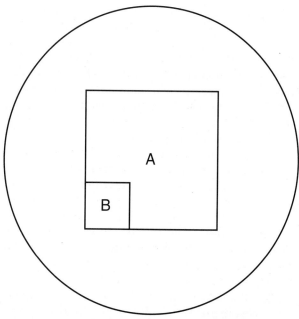

Figure 12–12 Miller counting disc for reticulocytes. Five hundred erythrocytes are counted in square B; reticulocytes are counted in squares A and B. Another format has square B in the center of square A.

REFERENCE RANGE

The reference range for adults is 0.5–2.0%. Although the range for newborns is 2.0–6.0%, the values move into the adult range usually within a few weeks.

SOURCES OF ERROR

1. An error may occur if the blood and stain are not mixed before the smears are made. The specific gravity of the reticulocytes is lower than that of the mature erythrocytes, and thus reticulocytes settle at the top of the mixture during incubation.
2. Moisture in the air and/or poor drying of the slide may cause areas of the slide to appear refractile and could be confused for reticulocytes. The RNA remnants in a reticulocyte are not refractile.
3. Other RBC inclusions that stain supravitally include Heinz, Howell-Jolly, and Pappenheimer bodies. Heinz bodies represent precipitated Hb, usually appear round or oval, and tend to cling to the cell membrane. Howell-Jolly bodies are round nuclear fragments and are usually singular. Pappenheimer bodies are iron fragments in the mitochondria whose presence can be confirmed with an iron stain such as Prussian blue.

FLOW CYTOMETRY

Reticulocyte counts may be performed by flow cytometry on such instruments as the Coulter and the Baxter R1000. Both the percentage and the absolute count are provided. These results are statistically more valid because of the large number of cells counted.[11]

The 1993 laboratory inspection checklist of the College of American Pathologists (CAP) requires that reticulocytes be counted either by automated methods or by the use of a restricted field ocular, such as the Miller disc.

ABSOLUTE RETICULOCYTE COUNT (ARC)

Principle

The absolute reticulocyte count is the actual number of reticulocytes in 1 L of whole blood.

Calculation

absolute reticulocyte count

$$= \frac{\text{reticulocytes}(\%) \times \text{RBC count} (\times 10^{12}) \times 1000}{100}$$

Example: If a patient's reticulocyte count is 2%

and the RBC count is 2.20×10^{12}/L, the ARC would be calculated as follows:

$$\text{ARC} = \frac{2 \times (2.20 \times 10^{12}/\text{L}) \times 1000}{100}$$

$$= 44.0 \times 10^{9}/\text{L}$$

Reference Range

Values between 25 and 75×10^{9}/L are within the reference range.[10]

CORRECTED RETICULOCYTE COUNT

Principle

In specimens with a low Hct, the percentage of reticulocytes may be falsely elevated because whole blood contains fewer RBCs. A correction factor is used, considering the average normal Hct to be 0.45 L/L.

Calculation

corrected reticulocyte count

$$= \text{reticulocytes}(\%) \times \frac{\text{Hct (L/L)}}{0.45 \text{ L/L}}$$

Reference Range

Patients with an Hct of 0.35 L/L are expected to have a corrected reticulocyte count of 2–3%. In patients with an Hct below 0.25 L/L, the count should increase to 3–5%. The corrected reticulocyte count is dependent on the degree of anemia.

RETICULOCYTE PRODUCTION INDEX

Principle

Reticulocytes that are released from the marrow prematurely are called shift reticulocytes. These reticulocytes are "shifted" from the bone marrow to the peripheral blood in order to compensate for anemia. Instead of losing their reticulum in 1 day like normal reticulocytes, these cells take up to 2.5 days to lose their reticulum. When erythropoiesis is evaluated, a correction should be made for the presence of shift reticulocytes, because the amount of reticulocytes in the peripheral blood may be increased without an increase in bone marrow erythropoiesis.

Calculation: Patient's Hematocrit

reticulocyte production index (RPI)

$$= \frac{\text{reticulocyte}(\%) \times 0.45 \text{ (L/L)}}{2 \text{ days (maturation time)}}$$

or

$$\text{RPI} = \frac{\text{corrected reticulocyte count}}{2 \text{ (maturation time)}}$$

Reference Range

An adequate bone marrow response is usually indicated by an RPI that is greater than 3. An inadequate response is seen when the RPI is less than 2.[10]

RETICULOCYTE CONTROL

A commercial control is now available for the use of monitoring both the manual and automated reticulocyte counts. The Retic-Chex (Streck Laboratories, Omaha, NE) is a tri-level whole blood reticulocyte control manufactured from human erythrocytes. The three levels available include vials for 1%, 3%, and 5%. The control samples are treated in the same manner as the clinical specimens. The control can be used to verify the technologist's accuracy and precision when manual counts are performed.

ERYTHROCYTE SEDIMENTATION RATE

The erythrocyte sedimentation rate (ESR) is useful for monitoring the course of an existing inflammatory disease or for differentiating between similar diseases. The erythrocyte sedimentation rate is normal in patients with osteoarthritis but is elevated in patients with rheumatic fever, rheumatoid arthritis, or pyogenic arthritis. The ESR is elevated in the early stage of acute pelvic inflammatory disease or a ruptured ectopic pregnancy but normal in the first 24 hours of acute appendicitis. The ESR may be used to indicate the activity of pulmonary tuberculosis.

PRINCIPLE

When anti-coagulated blood is allowed to stand at room temperature undisturbed for a period of time, the RBCs settle to the bottom of the tube. The ESR is the rate in millimeters at which the RBCs fall in 1 hr. The ESR is affected by erythrocytes, plasma, and mechanical and technical factors.

Normal erythrocytes have a relatively small mass and settle slowly. Certain diseases can cause rouleaux formation, in which the plasma fibrinogen and globulins are altered. This alteration changes the erythrocyte surface, leading to aggregation of the RBCs, increased RBC mass, and a more rapid ESR. The ESR is directly proportional to the RBC mass and inversely proportional to plasma viscosity.

WESTERGREN ERYTHROCYTE SEDIMENTATION RATE

Procedure

1. Using blood collected in 3.8% sodium citrate, fill the Westergren pipette to the zero mark. No air bubbles should be in the pipette. Alternatively, 2.0 mL of blood anti-coagulated with EDTA may be diluted with 0.5 mL of 0.85% sodium chloride or 3.8% sodium citrate.
2. Place the pipette into the rack (Fig. 12–13) and allow to stand undisturbed for 60 minutes.
3. Record the number of millimeters the RBCs have fallen. The buffy coat should not be included in the reading. The ESR is reported as 1 hour = _____ mm.

Reference Range

Age	mm/hour
Children[12]	0–10
Male	
<50 years	0–15
>50 years	0–20
Female[13]	
<50 years	0–20
>50 years	0–30

WINTROBE ERYTHROCYTE SEDIMENTATION RATE

Procedure

1. Fill the Wintrobe tube to the zero mark with approximately 1 mL of EDTA–anti-coagulated blood, avoiding air bubbles.

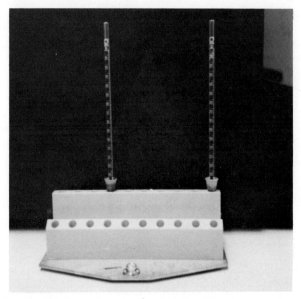

Figure 12–13 Westergren system for determining erythrocyte sedimentation rate.

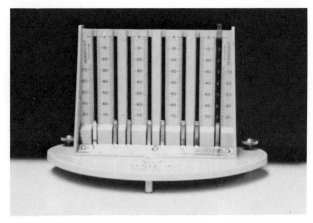

Figure 12–14 Wintrobe system for determining erythrocyte sedimentation rate.

2. Allow to stand undisturbed in Wintrobe rack at room temperature for 1 hour.
3. Afterwards, read the level of erythrocytes. This result is the ESR and is reported as 1 hour = _____ mm (Fig. 12–14).

Reference Range[14]

Population	mm/hour
Children	0–13
Men	0–9
Women	0–20

Sources of Error

1. If the concentration of anti-coagulant is increased, the ESR will be falsely low.
2. The anti-coagulants sodium or potassium oxalate and heparin cause the RBCs to shrink and falsely elevate the ESR.
3. A significant change in the temperature of the room alters the ESR.
4. Even a slight tilt of the pipette causes the ESR to increase.
5. If the specimen is allowed to sit at room temperature for more than 2 hours before being tested, the erythrocytes start to become spherical and may inhibit the formation of rouleaux.
6. Bubbles in the column of blood invalidate the test results.
7. The blood must be properly set to the zero mark at the beginning of the test.
8. A clotted specimen cannot be used.
9. Hematologic disorders that prevent the formation of rouleaux (e.g., sickle cells and spherocytes) decrease the ESR.
10. The ESR of patients with severe anemia is of little diagnostic value.

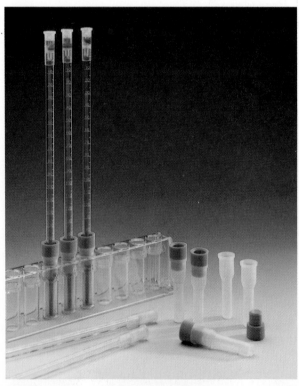

Figure 12–15 Sediplast (Polymedco) disposable sedimentation rate system. (Courtesy of Polymedco, Cortlandt Manor, NY.)

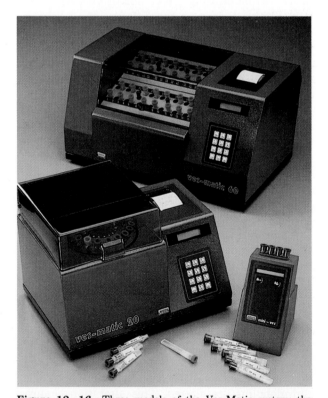

Figure 12–16 Three models of the Ves-Matic system: the Mini-Ves (for up to four samples) and the Ves-Matic 20 and Ves-Matic 60 (which analyze up to 20 and 60 samples simultaneously, respectively). Some Vacu-Tec primary sample collection tubes (black tops) and a quality control tube (orange top) are in the foreground. (Photograph courtesy of HiChem, Lincoln, RI.)

DISPOSABLE ERYTHROCYTE SEDIMENTATION RATE

Commercial kits are now available for a disposable ESR test. Several kits include safety caps for the pipettes that allow the blood to precisely fill to the zero mark. This makes the pipette a closed system and eliminates the error involved with manually setting the blood at the zero mark. One example is shown in Figure 12–15.

AUTOMATED ERYTHROCYTE SEDIMENTATION RATE

The Ves-Matic system is a benchtop analyzer designed to determine ESR by use of an optoelectronic sensor, which measures the change in opacity of a column of blood as sedimentation of blood progresses. Blood is collected in special Ves-Tec or Vacu-Tec tubes, which contain anti-coagulant and are compatible with the Vacutainer system. These tubes are used directly in the instrument. Acceleration of sedimentation is achieved by positioning the tubes at an 18 degree angle in relation to the vertical axis. Results comparable with Westergren 1-hour values are obtained in 20 minutes[15] (Fig. 12–16).

SUMMARY

Although most laboratories are highly automated, the manual tests discussed in this chapter, such as the cyanmethemoglobin method of Hb determination and the microhematocrit, are used as a part of many laboratories' quality control and backup methods of analysis.

The hemacytometer enables performance of counts of any type of cell or particle (e.g., WBCs, platelets, and eosinophils). The Unopette is a self-contained diluting system that simplifies dilutions for manual counts. Hb determination is based on the absorbance of cyanmethemoglobin at 540 nm. A standard curve is used to obtain the results. The microhematocrit is a measure of packed RBC volume. RBC indices—the MCV, MCH, and MCHC—are calculated to determine the size and Hb content of erythrocytes. The indices give an indication of the etiology of a patient's anemia. The reticulocyte count, which is used to assess the erythropoietic activity of the bone marrow, is accomplished through the use of supravital stains (such as new methylene blue) or by flow cytometric methods. The ESR, a measure of the settling of erythrocytes in a 1-hour period, is dependent on the erythrocytes' ability to form rouleaux. It is an indication of inflammation and may be used to differentiate various diseases or to monitor therapy for certain disorders.

REVIEW QUESTIONS

1. A 1:20 dilution is made in a Unopette, with glacial acetic acid as the diluent. One hundred WBCs are counted in the four corner squares. What is the total WBC count?

2. The total WBC count is 20.0×10^9/L. Twenty-five nRBCs are seen on the peripheral blood smear. What is the corrected WBC count?

3. List the reagents used in the cyanmethemoglobin method for Hb determination.

4. List three physiologic conditions that may interfere with Hb determination by the cyanmethemoglobin method and describe correction techniques.

5. A patient has an Hb of 8.0 g/dL. According to the rule of three, in what range would the Hct be expected?

6. Calculate the MCV and MCHC for the following values:
   A. RBC = 5.00×10^9/L
   B. Hb = 9.0 g/dL
   C. Hct = 0.30 L/L

7. On the basis of the indices calculated from the values in question 6, suggest potential diagnoses.

8. What information can be obtained from a reticulocyte count?

9. Given the following values, calculate and interpret the RPI:
   A. Observed reticulocyte count = 6.0%
   B. Hct = 0.30 L/L

10. State the diagnostic value of an erythrocyte sedimentation rate.

References

1. Cartwright GE: Diagnostic Laboratory Hematology, 4th ed. New York: Grune & Stratton, 1968.
2. Brecher G, Cronkite EP: Morphology and enumeration of human blood platelets. J Appl Physiol 1950; 3:365.
3. Seiverd CED: Hematology for Medical Technologists, 5th ed. Philadelphia: Lea & Febiger, 1983.
4. von Schenck H, Falkensson M, Lundberg B: Evaluation of "HemoCue", a new device for determining hemoglobin. Clin Chem 1986; 32:526–529.
5. MacLaren IA, Conn DM, Wadsworth LD: Comparison of two automated hemoglobin methods using Sysmex SULFOLYSER™ and STROMATOLYSER™. Sysmex J Int 1991; 1(1):59–61.
6. Oshiro I, Takenaka T, Maeda J: New method for hemoglo-

bin determination by using sodium lauryl sulfate (SLS). Clin Biochem 1982; 15:83–88.

7. Matsubara T, Mimura T: Reaction mechanism of SLS-Hb Method. Sysmex J (Japan) 1990; 13:206–211.

8. Fujiwara C, Hamaguchi Y, Toda S, Hayashi M: The reagent SULFOLYSER^R for hemoglobin measurement by hematology analyzers. Sysmex J (Japan) 1990; 13:212–219.

9. National Committee for Clinical Laboratory Standards (NCCLS), H7-A2: Procedure for Determining Packed Cell Volume by the Microhematocrit Method, 2nd ed, vol 13(9). Villanova, PA: NCCLS, 1993.

10. Koepke JF, Koepke JA: Reticulocytes. Clin Lab Haematol 1986; 8:169.

11. Burton S, O'Connell J, Mercolino T: A rapid, vital staining procedure for flow cytometric analysis of human reticulocytes. Cytometry 1983; 4:222–227.

12. Westergren A: Die Senkungsreaction. Ergeb Inn Med Inderheild 1924; 26:577.

13. Böttiger LE, Svedberg CA: Normal erythrocyte sedimentation rate and age. Br Med J 1967; 2:85.

14. Wintrobe MM, Landsberg JW: A standardized technique for blood sedimentation test. Am J Med Sci 1935; 189:102.

15. MINI-VES Erythrocyte Sedimentation Rate [manual]. Lincoln, RI: Diesse-Vega Biomedical, April 1991:4–8.

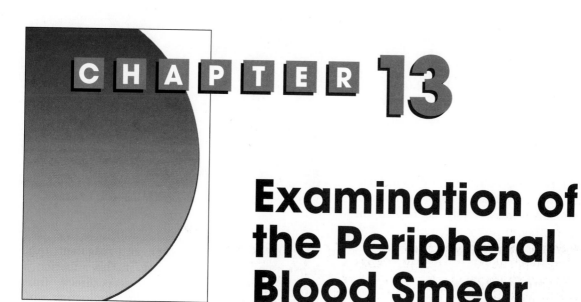

CHAPTER 13

Examination of the Peripheral Blood Smear

Lynn B. Maedel

Objectives

AFTER COMPLETION OF THIS CHAPTER, THE READER WILL BE ABLE TO

1. List the specimen sources and collection processes that are acceptable for blood smear preparation.
2. Describe the techniques for making peripheral blood smears.
3. Describe the qualities of a well-prepared peripheral blood smear and troubleshoot problems with poorly prepared smears.
4. Explain the principle, purpose, and basic method of Wright's staining blood smears.
5. Identify and troubleshoot problems that cause poorly stained blood smears.
6. Properly examine a peripheral blood smear, including selection of ''correct'' area, sequence of examination, and observations to be made at each magnification.

A well-made, well-stained, and carefully examined peripheral blood smear can provide some of the most valuable information possible regarding a patient's health. In fact, more can be learned from this test than from many of the other routinely performed hematologic tests. White blood cell (WBC) and platelet estimates can be achieved, relative proportions of the different types of WBCs may be obtained, and the morphology of all three cell lines can be evaluated for any abnormalities. Even though much of the routine work can now be handled by sophisticated automation found in most hematology laboratories, skilled and talented technologists are still essential. Proper peripheral smear evaluation will most likely be needed for some time.

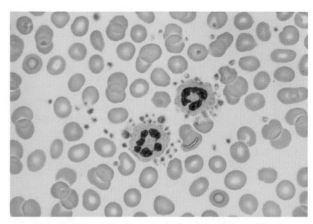

Figure 13–1 Photomicrograph of platelet satellitosis.

SPECIMEN COLLECTION AND PERIPHERAL SMEAR PREPARATION

Sources of Specimens

Today, most specimens received in the hematology laboratory for routine testing are in lavender-top tubes, which contain disodium or tripotassium ethylenediamine tetraacetic acid (EDTA). EDTA anticoagulates the blood by chelating the calcium, which is essential for coagulation. Liquid K_3EDTA is often preferred because it is easy to mix with blood. High-quality blood smears can be made from the EDTA tube as long as they are made within 2 to 3 hours of the blood's being drawn.[1] Smears made from EDTA tubes that sit at room temperature for more than 5 hours often have unacceptable artifact of the blood cells (echinocytic red blood cells, spherocytes, and necrobiotic leukocytes). Vacuolization of monocytes generally occurs with EDTA but causes no evaluation problems.

One of the main advantages of making smears from the EDTA blood is that multiple slides can be made if necessary; this task is not always performed easily with the Vacutainer or the syringe needle at the patient's side. In addition, EDTA prevents platelets from clumping on the slide, making it easier to more accurately estimate platelets. There are purists, however, who believe that anti-coagulant-free blood is still the most acceptable for evaluation of blood cell morphology.[2]

In certain conditions, however, a different anti-coagulant or no anti-coagulant at all may be helpful. The blood from some patients that is anti-coagulated with EDTA undergoes a phenomenon called *platelet satellitosis*,[3] in which the platelets surround or adhere to the neutrophils, potentially causing pseudothrombocytopenia by automated methods[4] (Fig. 13–1). To eliminate this problem in affected specimens, another anti-coagulant (e.g., heparin) can be used. In fact, in this situation it may be desirable to make the smears directly from the syringe or Vacutainer needle, eliminating anti-coagulant altogether.

Another source of blood for smears is finger and heel punctures. In general, the smears are made immediately at the patient's side. There are a couple of limitations to this procedure: first, there will be platelet clumping if smears are made directly from a drop of finger or heel blood; second, only a very limited number of slides can be made before the puncture site stops bleeding. If slides are made correctly, however, cell distribution and morphology should be adequate.

Types of Smears

MANUAL WEDGE TECHNIQUE

The wedge smear is probably the easiest to master. It is the most convenient and commonly used technique for making peripheral blood smears. This technique requires at least two 3 × 1 inch (75 × 25 mm) clean glass slides. High-quality, beveled-edge microscopic (bevel-edged) slides with chamfered corners for good lateral borders are recommended. It is a good idea to keep a few more slides handy in case a good-quality smear is not made immediately. One slide serves as the smear slide and the other is the pusher or spreader slide. They can then be reversed. It is also possible to make good wedge smears by using a hemacytometer coverslip attached to a handle (pinch clip or tongue depressor) as the spreader. A drop of blood (about 3 mm in diameter) from a finger, heel, or microhematocrit tube (nonheparinized for EDTA blood or heparinized for capillary blood) is placed at one end of the slide. The size of the drop of blood is important: too large a drop creates a very long or thick smear, and too small a drop often makes a short or thin blood smear. The pusher slide, held securely in the hand at about a 30 to 45-degree angle, backs into the drop of blood, allowing it to spread across the width of the slide. It is then quickly and smoothly pushed forward to the end of the slide, creating a wedge smear (Fig. 13–2). It is important that the whole drop is picked up and spread. Moving the pusher slide forward too slowly accentuates poor leukocyte distribution by pushing larger cells, such as monocytes and granulocytes, to the very end and sides of the smear. Maintaining an even, gentle pressure on the slide is essential. It is also critical to keep the same angle all the way to the end of the smear. For higher-than-normal hematocrits, as in patients with polycythemia or in newborns, the angle should be lowered so the smear is not too short and thick. For extremely low hematocrits, the angle may need to be raised. If two or three smears are made, the best one is chosen for staining and the others are disposed of properly. Some laboratories make two good smears and save one unstained in case another slide is desired.

Features of a Well-Made Wedge Peripheral Blood Smear (Fig. 13–3)

1. About two thirds to three fourths of the length of the slide.

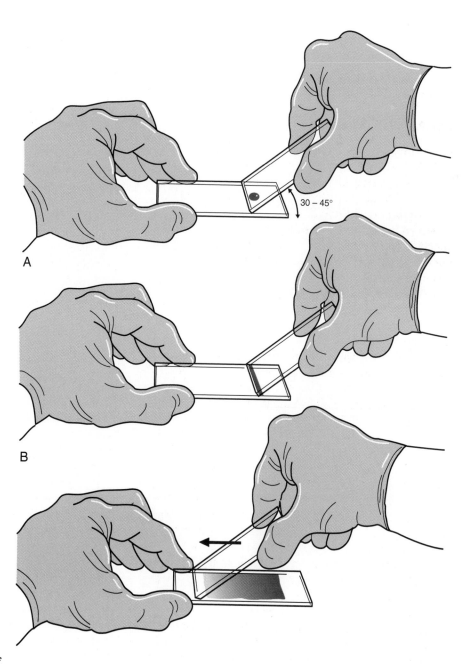

Figure 13–2 Wedge technique of making a peripheral blood smear.

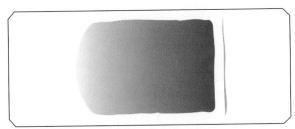

Figure 13-3 Well-made peripheral blood smear.

2. Finger-shaped, very slightly rounded at feather edge; not bullet-shaped.
3. Lateral edges of smear should be visible.
4. Smooth without irregularities, holes, or streaks.
5. When slide is held up to light, the thin portion (feather edge) of the smear should have a "rainbow" appearance.
6. Whole drop is picked up and spread.

Figure 13-4 demonstrates unacceptable smears.

COVERSLIP TECHNIQUE

The coverslip method of smear preparation is an older technique that is now only rarely used for peripheral blood smears. The only advantage of this preparation is its excellent leukocyte distribution, which in turn lends itself to more accurate differentials. For routine morphologic evaluation, this technique is neither convenient nor practical. Impeccably clean glass coverslips must be used.[5] The labeling, transporting, staining, and storage of these small breakable smears present many problems; however, coverslip preparations are sometimes used for making smears from bone marrow.

A small drop of blood or bone marrow is placed on one clean coverslip (22 × 22 mm), and another coverslip is placed on top, allowing the blood to spread across the two coverslips. Then one is pulled across the other to create two thin smears, one smear on each coverslip (Fig. 13-5). The two

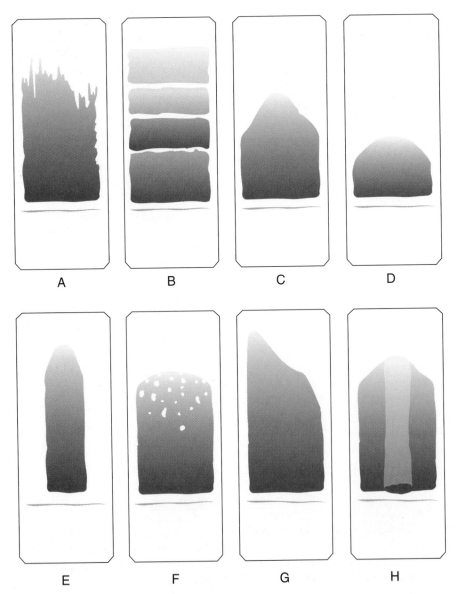

A   B   C   D

E   F   G   H

Figure 13-4 Unacceptable peripheral blood smears.

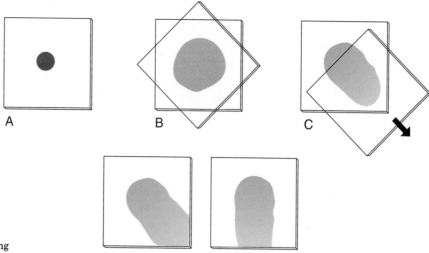

Figure 13–5 Coverslip method of making a peripheral blood smear.

smears can then be stained and mounted on a 1 × 3 inch glass slide. When bone marrow smears are made by this technique, very slight pressure is applied to the coverslips between the index finger and thumb (hence sometimes called a crush prep) to help spread the bone marrow spicule before the two smears are pulled apart. Refining the skills required to make high-quality crush prep bone marrow smears takes practice. Too much pressure on the coverslips causes cell rupture, making morphologic evaluation impossible, and inadequate pressure prevents the spicule from adequately spreading to a satisfactory monolayer. In a bone marrow crush prep similar to this, regular glass slides are used instead of coverslips, and the smears are of equal quality.

SEMI-AUTOMATED SPUN TECHNIQUE

The third technique for making a peripheral blood smear is the semi-automated spun prep, (spinner slide). The Hemaspinner is manufactured by Geometric Data Corporation. In some image-processing automated leukocyte differential systems, a monolayer spun smear is used. Manual microscopic smear evaluations can also be performed from these spun preps. To make a spun blood smear, a plain, nonfrosted or frosted glass slide is secured on the platen, and a large drop of blood (about 5 mm in diameter) in placed in the middle of the slide. The lid is closed, and centrifugal force spins the cells out into a monolayer smear. A light source under the slide shines up through it to a sensor. The instrument automatically stops spinning when the correct monolayer is reached. Too small a drop creates a smear that does not cover the entire slide and looks more like a centrifugally painted picture made at a fair or carnival. This is not satisfactory for evaluation. In addition, maintaining a clean instrument at all times is essential for high-quality smears. Even then, artifactual cellular changes, such as target cells, spherocytes, and rouleaux, can occur. Only anticoagulated blood can be used; therefore, smears must be made in the laboratory. Overall, the quality of the smear is good, WBC distribution is excellent, and the technique is easy.

SEMI-AUTOMATED WEDGE TECHNIQUE: MINIPREP

The Miniprep slide maker (Geometric Data Corp) is a lightweight and portable device that makes a wedge smear of adequate quality. A slide is secured in place on the apparatus, and a drop of blood is placed at one end of the slide. A lever is depressed, and a small pusher blade is drawn back into the blood and then released, making a wedge smear. The pusher blade must be kept clean to prevent carryover from slide to slide. This instrument provides consistency of blood smear preparation and is ideal for high-volume laboratories (Fig. 13–6). The designer of the Miniprep is currently designing a newer, automated version of the slide-making device, to be marketed by Alpha Scientific Corporation (personal communication, Dan Levine, Product Design Supervisor, Alpha Scientific Corp.).

Regardless of smear preparation method, all blood smears should be dried as quickly as possible to avoid slow drying artifact. In some laboratories, a small fan is used to facilitate drying. Blowing on a slide is counterproductive, because the moisture in breath causes red blood cells to look echinocytic and moth-eaten with punched-out centers. It is difficult to avoid drying artifact on extremely anemic patients' smears because of the very high ratio of plasma to red blood cells.

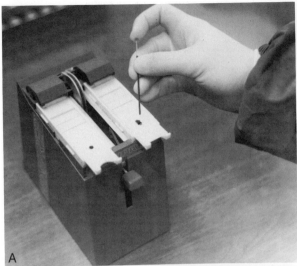

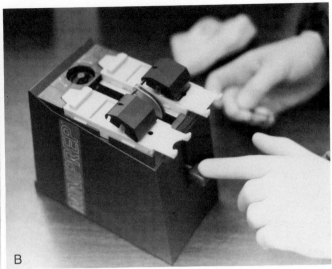

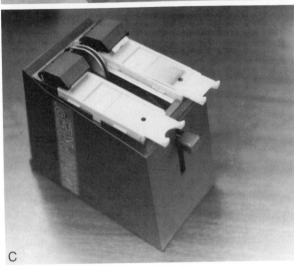

Figure 13–6 Miniprep apparatus.

STAINING OF PERIPHERAL BLOOD SMEARS

Pure Wright's stain or a Wright-Giemsa stain (Romanowsky stain)[6] is used for staining peripheral blood smears and bone marrow smears. These are considered polychrome stains because they contain both eosin and methylene blue. Giemsa stains additionally contain methylene blue azure. Obviously, the purpose of staining blood smears is simply to see the cells and evaluate their morphology.

Methanol in the stain fixes the cells to the slide. Actual staining of cells or cellular components does not occur until the buffer is added. The oxidized methylene blue and eosin form a thiazine-eosinate complex, staining neutral components. The buffer that is added to the stain should be 0.05-mol sodium phosphate (pH 6.4) or aged distilled water (distilled water placed in a glass bottle for at least 24 hours, pH 6.4–6.8). Staining reactions are pH dependent. Free methylene blue is basic and stains

acidic (or basophilic) cellular components such as RNA. Free eosin is acidic and stains basic (or eosinophilic) components such as hemoglobin or eosinophilic granules. Neutrophils are so names because they have cytoplasmic granules that have a neutral pH and pick up some staining characteristics from both stains. The slides must be completely dry before staining or the thick part of the blood smear may come off of the slide in the staining process.

Water artifact has been a long-lived nuisance to hematology laboratories. Multiple reasons contribute to this problem. Humidity in the air as the slide dries may add to the punched-out, moth-eaten, or echinocytic appearance of the red blood cells. Drying the slide as quickly as possible helps, and keeping stopper tightly on the stain bottle keeps moisture out. In some laboratories, 3 gm of Sephadex (Sigma) powder is added to 1 liter of Wright's stain to absorb any water that may have gotten into the hygroscopic methanol stain as it aged.[7] In other laboratories, slides are fixed in pure, anhydrous methanol before staining, to help alleviate water artifact.

Wright's Staining Methods

MANUAL TECHNIQUE

Traditionally, Wright's staining has been performed over a sink or pan with a staining rack. Slides are placed on the rack, smear side up. The Wright's stain may be filtered before use or may be poured directly from the bottle through a filter onto the slide (Fig. 13–7). It is important to completely flood the slide. The stain should remain on the slide at least 1–3 minutes to fix the cells to the glass. Then an approximately equal amount of buffer is added to the slide. Surface tension allows very little of the buffer to run off. Gently blow on the slide to mix the aqueous buffer and the alcohol stain. A metallic sheen (or green "scum") should appear on the slide if mixing is correct. Add more buffer if necessary. Allow the mixture to remain on the slide for 3 minutes or more (bone marrow smears take longer to stain than peripheral blood smears). The timing may be adjusted to acquire the best staining characteristics. When staining is complete, rinse the slide with a steady but gentle stream of neutral-pH water, wipe the back of the slide to remove any stain residue, and air dry in a vertical position. Coverslip blood smears must be stained by the manual method. These smears are placed on evacuated test tube rubber stoppers over the staining rack or sink (Fig. 13–8).

The manual Wright's staining technique is desirable for staining peripheral blood smears containing very high white blood cell counts, as in the smears from leukemic patients. As with bone marrow smears, the time can easily be lengthened to enhance the staining required by the increased numbers of cells. Understaining is not uncommon

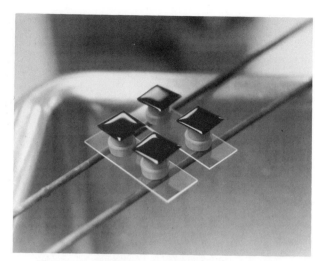

Figure 13–8 Manual Wright staining of coverslips.

when a leukemia slide is placed on an automated slide stainer. The main disadvantages of the manual technique are the increased risk of spilling the stain and the slower, more time-consuming procedure. This technique is best suited for low-volume laboratories.

AUTOMATED SLIDE STAINERS

There are numerous manufacturers of slide stainers on the market. For high-volume laboratories, these instruments are essential. Once set up and loaded with slides, they have walk-away capabilities. In general, it takes about 5–10 minutes to stain a batch of slides, depending on their number. The processes of fixing/staining and buffering are actually very similar in practice to those of the manual method. The slides may be automatically dipped in stain and then in buffer and a series of rinses (Midas II [Fig. 13–9] and Hemastainer [Fig. 13–10]) or propelled along a platen surface by two conveyor spirals (Hema-Tek [Fig. 13–11]). In the Hema-Tek, stain, buffer, and rinse are pumped through holes in the platen surface, flooding the slide at the appropriate time. Smear quality and color consistency is usually very good with any of these instruments. Some commercially prepared stain, buffer, and rinse packages do vary from lot to lot or manufacturer to manufacturer, and so testing is recommended. A couple of disadvantages of the batch, dip-type stainers are that (1) once the staining process has begun, stat slides cannot be added to the batch and (2) working or aqueous solutions of stain are stable only 3–6 hours and thus need to be made often. These instruments, however, require less maintenance on the whole. Stats can be added any time to the Hema-Tek stainer, and stain packages are stable for about 6

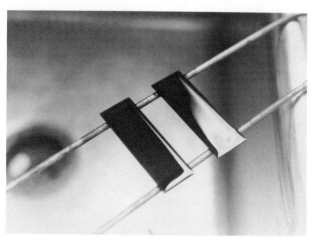

Figure 13–7 Manual Wright staining of slides.

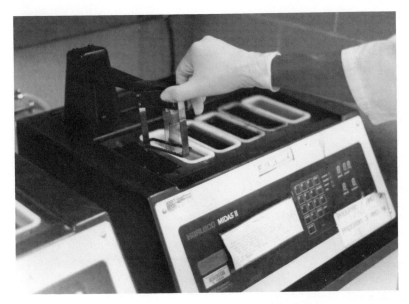

Figure 13-9 Harleco Midas II slide stainer.

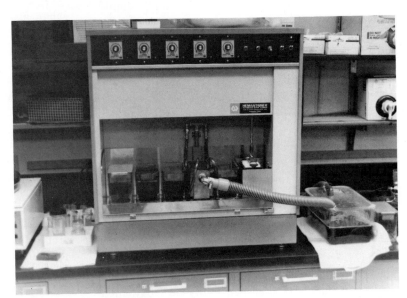

Figure 13-10 Geometric Data Hemastainer slide stainer.

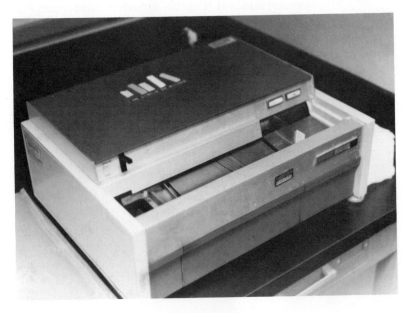

Figure 13-11 Ames Hema-Tek slide stainer.

months. This instrument, however, requires more daily and monthly maintenance.

QUICK STAINS

These stains, as the name implies, are fast and easy. The whole process takes about 1 minute. The stain is purchased in a bottle as a modified Wright's or Wright-Giemsa stain. The needed quantity can then be filtered into a Coplin jar or a staining dish, depending on the quantity of slides to be stained. Aged distilled water is used as the buffer. Stained slides are finally rinsed under a gentle stream of tap water and allowed to air dry. It is helpful to wipe off the back of the slide with alcohol to remove any excess stain. Quick stains are convenient and cost effective for low-volume laboratories, such as clinics and physicians' office laboratories, or whenever rapid turnaround time is essential. One complaint about the quick stains has concerned quality. However, with a little time and patience for adjusting the staining and buffering times, color quality can be acceptable.

The proper staining of a peripheral blood smear is of equal importance to making a good smear. Macroscopically, a well-stained blood smear should be pink to purple. Microscopically, the red blood cells should appear orange to salmon pink; WBC nuclei should be purple to blue. The cytoplasm of neutrophils should be a pink to tan with violet or lilac granules. Eosinophils should have bright orange refractile granules. Faulty staining can be very troublesome for reading the smears, from causing minor shifts in color to causing the inability to identify cells and morphology. Trying to interpret a poorly prepared or poorly stained blood smear is extremely frustrating. If at all possible, a newly stained smear should be studied. Hints for

troubleshooting poorly stained blood smears are in Table 13–1.

The best staining results are obtained on fresh slides because the blood itself acts as a buffer in the staining process. Slides stained after a week or more turn out too blue. In addition, specimens that have increased proteins (i.e., globulins) produce bluer staining blood smears.

PERIPHERAL SMEAR EXAMINATION

Macroscopic Examination

Examining the smear before placing it on the microscope stage can sometimes give the evaluator an indication of abnormalities or tests that need rechecking. For instance, a smear that is, overall, bluer than normal may indicate, as mentioned before, that the patient has increased blood proteins, as in multiple myeloma, and that rouleaux may be seen on the smear. A grainy appearance to the smear may indicate red blood cell agglutination, as found in cold hemagglutinin diseases. In addition, holes all over the smear could mean the patient has increased lipids, and some of the automated complete blood cell count parameters should be rechecked for interferences from lipemia. Markedly increased WBC counts and platelet counts can be detected from the blue specks out at the feather edge. Therefore, added information might be helpful even before the evaluator looks through the microscope.

Microscopic Examination

The microscope should be adjusted correctly for blood smear evaluation. The light from the illuminator should be properly centered; the condenser should be almost all the way up and adjusted correctly for the magnification used; and the iris diaphragm should be opened to allow a comfortable amount of light to the eye. Many people prefer to use a neutral-density filter over the illuminator to create a whiter light from a tungsten light source. If the microscope has been adjusted for Koehler illumination, all these conditions should have been met.

10X EXAMINATION

Blood smear evaluation begins with the 10X or low-power objective lens. Not much time needs to be spent at this magnification. It is, however, a common error to omit this step altogether and go directly to the higher power oil immersion lens. At the low-power magnification, overall smear quality,

---

Table 13–1. TROUBLESHOOTING POORLY STAINED BLOOD SMEARS

First Scenario

PROBLEMS
Red blood cells appear gray
White blood cells are too dark
Eosinophil granules are gray, not orange

CAUSES
Stain or buffer too alkaline (most common)
Inadequate rinsing
Prolonged staining

Second Scenario

PROBLEMS
Red blood cells too pale or red color
White blood cells barely visible

CAUSES
Stain or buffer too acidic (most common)
Underbuffering (too short)
Overrinsing

color, and distribution of cells can be assessed. The feather edge and lateral edges can be quickly checked for WBC distribution. A disproportionately number of larger cells, such as monocytes, seen at any of the edges may indicate that the smear was poorly made (i.e., a "snow plow" effect), and the smear should be remade. Under 10× magnification, it is possible to check for the presence of fibrin strands; if they are present, the sample should be rejected and another one collected. Red blood cell distribution can be noted as well. Rouleau formation or red blood cell agglutination is easy to recognize at this power. Finally, the smear can be quickly scanned for any large abnormal cells such as blasts, reactive lymphocytes, or even unexpected parasites.

40× EXAMINATION

The next step is using the 40× high dry objective lens. At this magnification, it is easy to select the correct area of the smear in which to begin the differential and to evaluate cellular morphology. The WBC estimate can also be performed at this power. To perform a WBC estimate, the evaluator selects an area in which two or three red blood cells overlap, but most red blood cells are lying out by themselves. The average number of WBCs per high-power field is multiplied by 2000 to get an adequate approximation of the WBC count. For example, after 8–10 fields were scanned, it was determined that there are four to five WBCs per field. This would be a WBC estimate of 8000–10,000/mm³ (8.0–10.0 × 10⁹/L). This technique can be very helpful for internal quality control. If a discrepancy exists between the estimate and the instrument WBC, a smear made on the wrong patient's blood sample or a mislabeled smear could be more easily discovered. In many laboratories, WBC estimates are performed on a routine basis; in others, these estimates are performed only as needed.

100× OBJECTIVE OIL IMMERSION EXAMINATION

This is the highest magnification for most standard binocular microscopes (10× eyepiece × 100× objective lens = 1000× magnification). The WBC differential is generally performed under 100× oil. The differential normally includes counting and classifying 100 WBCs and reporting the WBC percentages. The red blood cell, WBC, and platelet morphology evaluation and the platelet estimate are also performed under the 100× oil immersion objective lens. At this magnification, segmented neutrophils can easily be differentiated from

bands. Red blood cell inclusions, like Howell-Jolly bodies and WBC inclusions, like Döhle bodies can easily be seen if present. Reactive or abnormal cells are enumerated under the 100× lens as well. If present, nucleated red blood cells (NRBCs) are counted and reported as NRBCs/100 WBCs (see Chapter 12).

The tasks just described need to be performed in the best possible area of the peripheral blood smear. That occurs between the thick area, or "heel," where the drop of blood was initially placed and spread, and the very thin feather edge. Microscopically, the red blood cells are uniformly and singly distributed, with few touching or overlapping, and have their normal biconcave appearance (central pallor) (Fig. 13–12). An area that is too thin, in which there are holes in the smear and the red blood cells look flat, large, and distorted, is not acceptable. An area too thick also distorts the red blood cells by piling them on top of one another like rouleaux (Fig. 13–13). WBCs are similarly distorted, making morphologic evaluation more difficult and classification potentially incorrect. When viewing the correct area of a specimen from a patient with a normal red blood cell count, there are generally about 200–250 red blood cells per oil immersion field (OIF).

Although mentioned in the microscopy chapter, a common "problem" encountered with the oil immersion objective lens is worth mentioning again here. If the blood smear was in focus under 10× and 40×, but is impossible to bring into focus under 100×, the slide is probably upside down. The oil must be completely removed before the smear is put on the stage right side up.

PERFORMANCE OF THE DIFFERENTIAL

The differential should be performed in a systematic manner. Once the correct area has been selected, a back-and-forth serpentine, or "battle-

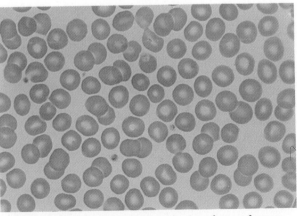

Figure 13–12 Photomicrograph of good area of smear.

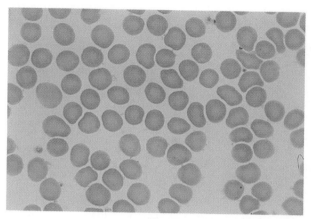
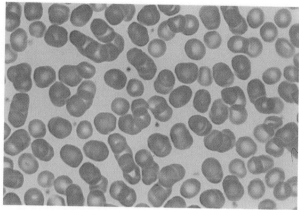

A   B

Figure 13–13 Photomicrograph of areas too thin and too thick to read.

ment," track is preferred for minimizing distributional errors[8] (Fig. 13–14). One hundred WBCs are counted and classified through the use of push-down button counters (Fig. 13–15) or newer computer-interfaced touch pads (Fig. 13–16). To increase the accuracy, it is advisable to count at least 200 cells when the WBC count is greater than 40.0×10^9/L. The results are reported as percentages: for example, 54% segmented neutrophils, 6% bands, 28% lymphocytes, 9% monocytes, 3% eosinophils. The evaluator should always check to be sure the percentages do indeed total 100%.

Performing 100 cell differentials on extremely low WBC counts can become tedious and time consuming. In some laboratories, the WBCs are concentrated and buffy coat smears are made. In others, evaluators perform a 25- or 50-cell differential, multiply the results by 4 or 2, respectively, to get a percentage, and document that this was done. The accuracy of this practice is questionable and should be avoided if possible.

It is important to include the side margins of the blood smear, so that the larger cells such as monocytes, reactive lymphocytes, and immature cells are not excluded. If present, WBC abnormalities, such as toxic granulation, Döhle bodies, reactive lymphocytes, and Auer rods (see Chapter 20), are also evaluated and reported. The exact method in which these are reported varies from laboratory to laboratory. For example, reactive lymphocytes may be reported in percentages or semiquantitatively (occasional to many). Toxic granulation is generally reported either as present or semiquantitatively (slight to marked, or 1+ to 3+).

Because the differential alone provides only partial information, the absolute cell counts are calculated for each cell type (see Chapter 11) in some laboratories. Automated differentials already include this step.

RED BLOOD CELL MORPHOLOGY

Red blood cell morphology is an important part of the blood smear evaluation (see Chapter 15). Some laboratories have specific terminology for reporting abnormal morphology, such as slight, moderate, or marked, or on a 1+-to-3+ scale. Other laboratories have instituted a summary statement regarding the overall red blood cell morphology that is consistent with the red blood cell indices.

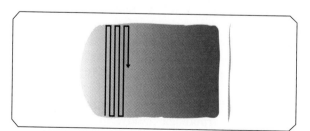

Figure 13–14 "Battlement" or "meander" pattern for performing a differential.

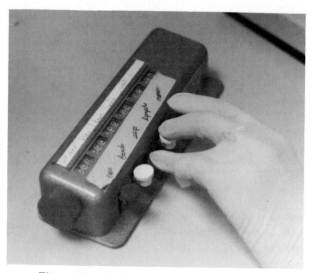

Figure 13–15 Clay Adams Laboratory Counter.

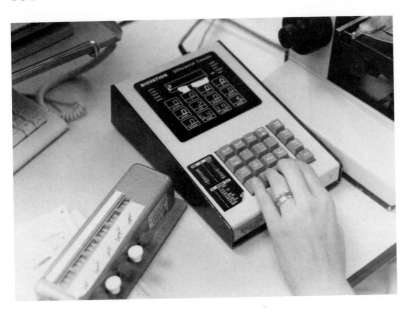

Figure 13–16 Biovation Differential Counter.

The latter method is becoming more popular with the increased computer interfacing in most laboratories. Regardless of the reporting method, the microscopic red blood cell morphology should be congruent with the information given by the automated parameters. If not, further investigation is needed.

PLATELET ESTIMATE

As previously mentioned, the platelet estimate is performed under the 100× oil immersion objective lens. In an area of the smear where the red blood cells barely touch, the number of platelets in 10 OIFs is counted. The average number of platelets per OIF ×20,000 approximates the platelet count. For example, 12–16 platelets per OIF would equal about 280,000 platelets/mm³ and would be considered adequate. A rougher estimate states that if there are 7–25 platelets per OIF, the platelet count is adequate, provided that there are approximately 200 red blood cells per OIF. In situations in which the patient is anemic or has erythrocytosis, the relative proportions of platelets to red blood cells is altered. In these instances, a more involved formula for estimates may be used:

$$\frac{\text{Average no. of platelets} \times \text{red blood cell count}}{200}$$
$$= \text{platelet estimate}$$

(200 is the average number of red blood cells per OIF in a patient with a normal red blood cell count).

Regardless of whether an "official" estimate is done, verification of the instrument platelet count should be included in the overall examination.

In many laboratories, microscopes are being upgraded with 40× to 50× oil immersion objective lenses. These lenses are of top quality and have very good resolution, enabling differentials to be performed more quickly than under the 100× objective lens. If this is the practice, any abnormal findings should be inspected under the 100× objective lens.

As mentioned in the microscopy chapter, immersion oils with different viscosities do not mix well. If slides are taken to another microscope for review, oil should be wiped off first.

SUMMARY

Much information can be obtained from a properly prepared, stained, and examined peripheral blood smear. In most laboratories, a wedge technique smear made from EDTA blood and a Wright's or Wright-Giemsa stain are used, generally with an automated stainer. Observing the blood smear macroscopically before placing it on the microscope stage can help predict what might be seen microscopically. It may also support the need to recheck other complete blood cell count parameters for accuracy. Peripheral blood smears should always be evaluated in a systematic manner, beginning with the 10× objective lens and finishing with the 100× oil immersion objective lens. Leukocyte differential and morphologic study, erythrocyte morphologic study, and platelet estimate and morphologic study are included in the evaluation.

REVIEW QUESTIONS

1. A laboratory science student consistently makes wedge technique blood smears that are too long and thin. Which of the following changes in technique would improve the smears?
   a. increasing the downward pressure on the pusher slide
   b. decreasing the acute angle of the pusher slide
   c. decreasing the size of the drop of blood used
   d. increasing the acute angle of the pusher slide

2. When a blood smear is viewed through the microscope, the red blood cells appear redder than normal, the neutrophils are barely visible, and the eosinophils are bright orange. What is the most likely cause?
   a. The slide is overstained.
   b. The stain is too alkaline.
   c. The buffer is too acidic.
   d. Inadequate rinsing.

3. A stained blood smear is held up to the light and observed to be bluer than normal. What microscopic abnormality might be expected on this smear?
   a. rouleaux
   b. spherocytosis
   c. reactive lymphocytosis
   d. toxic granulation

4. A technologist using the 40X objective lens sees the following numbers of white blood cells in 10 fields: 8, 4, 7, 5, 4, 7, 8, 6, 4, 6. Which of the following WBC counts most closely correlates with the estimate?
   a. 1.5×10^9/L
   b. 5.9×10^9/L
   c. 11.8×10^9/L
   d. 24.0×10^9/L

5. A very anemic patient with a red blood cell count of 1.25×10^{12}/L, has an average of 7 platelets per OIF. Which of the following amounts most closely correlates with the estimate per cubic millimeter?
   a. 14,000
   b. 44,000
   c. 140,000
   d. 280,000

6. A patient with a normal red blood cell count has an average of 10 platelets per OIF. Which of the following amounts best correlates with the estimate per cubic millimeter?
   a. 20,000
   b. 100,000
   c. 200,000
   d. 400,000

References

1. Kennedy JB, Machara KT, Baker AM: Cell and platelet stability in disodium and tripotassium EDTA. Am J Med Technol 1981; 47:89.
2. Dacie JV, Lewis SM: Practical Hematology, 4th ed. London: Churchill, 1984.
3. Bauer HM: In vitro platelet-neutrophil adherence. Am J Clin Pathol 1975; 63:824.
4. Shreiner DP, Bell WR: Pseudothrombocytopenia: manifestation of a new type of platelet agglutinin. Blood 1973; 42:541.
5. Kjeldsberg CR: Principles of hematologic examination. In Lee GR, Bithell TC, Foerster J, et al (eds): Wintrobe's Clinical Hematology, 9th ed. Philadelphia: Lea & Febiger, 1993:7–37.
6. Power KT: The Romanowsky stains. A review. Am J Med Technol 1982; 48(6):519.
7. Jurivich Z: Personal communication. Rush–Presbyterian–St. Luke's Medical Center bone marrow laboratory, Chicago, IL, 1994.
8. MacGregor RG, Scott RW, Loh GL: The differential leukocyte count. J Pathol Bact 1940; 51:337.

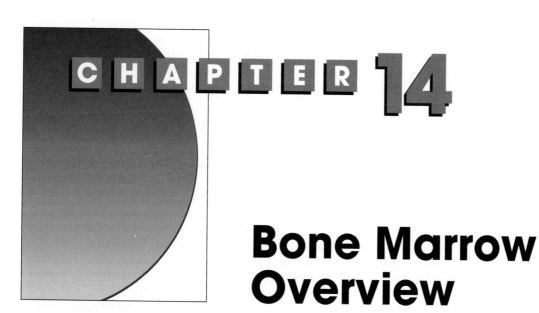

CHAPTER 14

Bone Marrow Overview

John Krause

Objectives

AFTER COMPLETION OF THIS CHAPTER, THE READER WILL BE ABLE TO

1. Compare the location of red marrow at various age intervals.
2. Specify sites for bone marrow aspirate and/or biopsy in the child and adult.
3. Discuss indications for bone marrow sampling.
4. Discuss advantages of bone marrow aspirate plus biopsy.
5. Review procedure for bone marrow aspirate and biopsy.
6. Summarize examination of bone marrow under low-power and oil immersion microscopy.
7. Describe cytologic features of hematopoietic cells found in the aspirate and core biopsy specimen.
8. Describe features of osteoblasts and osteoclasts.
9. Characterize features of tumor cells.
10. List the three components of a bone marrow evaluation.
11. Discuss the importance of a systematic approach to bone marrow review in total patient assessment.

In adults, bone marrow approximates 3.4–5.9% of total body weight, which translates into roughly 1600–3700 g.[1] At birth nearly all the bones in the body contain hematopoietic (red) marrow. In the fifth to seventh year, fat cells (yellow marrow) begin to replace the red marrow in the long bones of the extremities, and so by adulthood the hematopoietic tissue becomes limited to the axial skeleton and the proximal portions of the extremities.[2] The site chosen for bone marrow sampling therefore depends somewhat on the age of the patient. Most aspirates and biopsy samples of marrow are now obtained from the iliac crest (posterior-superior iliac spine) (Fig. 14–1). In adults, the anterior iliac crest can also be used and occasionally the ribs or vertebrae can be sampled, particularly if a suspicious lesion is seen on a roentgenogram. A good cellular aspirate can be obtained from the sternum at the second intercostal space, but obtaining a biopsy sample from this structure is not recommended because of the underlying heart and great vessels. In children younger than 1 year old, the anteromedial (front and middle) surface of the tibia is sometimes used.

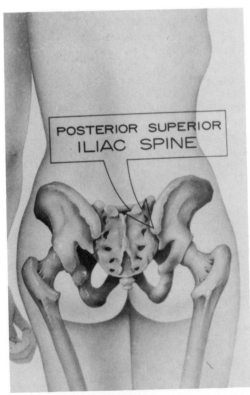

Figure 14–1 Bone marrow biopsy site. The posterior superior iliac spine is a good site for obtaining the aspirate smear and core biopsy. (From Ellis LD, Jensen WJ, Westerman MP: Needle biopsy of bone and marrow. Arch Intern Med 1964; 114:213. Copyright 1964, American Medical Association.)

BONE MARROW ASPIRATION AND BIOPSY

Marrow fills the spaces between the trabeculae of bone in the marrow cavity and is soft and semifluid. It is, therefore, amenable to sampling. A bone marrow sample usually consists of two parts: the aspirate and the core biopsy specimen. Aspiration provides a specimen that is useful for determining the cytologic types and proportions of hematopoietic cells in the marrow. The core biopsy provides another dimension and is extremely useful for determining cellularity and the anatomic relation of cells to fat and connective tissue stroma. The core biopsy is particularly important for evaluating diseases that characteristically produce focal lesions rather than diffuse involvement of the marrow, such as Hodgkin's disease, non-Hodgkin's lymphoma, multiple myeloma, metastatic tumor, amyloid and granulomas. It also allows evaluation of bone spicules, which may reveal changes in hyperparathyroidism or Paget's disease.[3] A core biopsy is mandatory for the so-called dry tap on aspiration (no cells obtained), which may be the result of true hypocellularity (aplastic anemia), fibrosis, or the marrow cavity's being too "tightly packed" with cells (leukemia) to yield a specimen.

The most common and familiar needles used for marrow sampling include the Jamshidi (Kormed, Minneapolis, MN) and the Westerman-Jensen (Becton Dickinson, Rutherford, NJ). The use of these needles makes it possible to obtain a core of bone and its enclosed marrow. Then, by means of an attached syringe, the bone marrow aspirate can be obtained. The procedure using the Westerman-Jensen needle is illustrated in Fig. 14–2.

For the biopsy procedure, the patient is placed in the right or left lateral decubitus position (lying on right or left side). Universal precautions are observed throughout the procedure. The skin area that will be penetrated is cleansed with a disinfectant and draped. The skin, dermis, and subcutaneous tissue are infiltrated with a local anesthetic solution such as 1% or 2% lidocaine or procaine through a 25-gauge needle, producing a 5-mm to 1-cm papule (bubble). The 25-gauge needle is then replaced with a 21-gauge needle, which is inserted through the papule to the periosteum. With the point of the needle on the periosteum, approximately 2 mL of anesthetic is injected over a dime-sized area as the needle is rotated, after which the anesthesia needle is withdrawn. Next, a 3-mm skin incision is made over the biopsy site with a No. 11 scalpel blade to facilitate insertion of the biopsy needle. Following this, the biopsy needle with the obturator locked in place is inserted through the

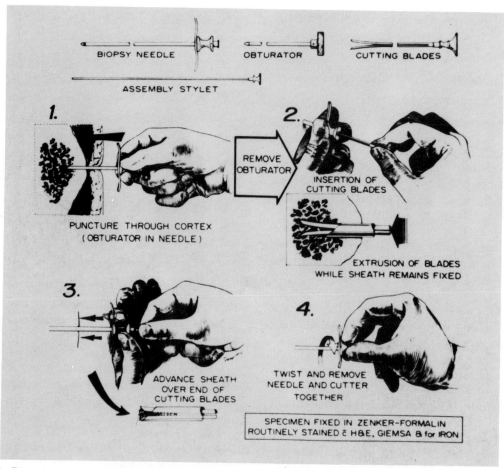

BIOPSY NEEDLE   OBTURATOR   CUTTING BLADES

ASSEMBLY STYLET

1.
PUNCTURE THROUGH CORTEX
(OBTURATOR IN NEEDLE)

2.
REMOVE OBTURATOR
INSERTION OF CUTTING BLADES
EXTRUSION OF BLADES WHILE SHEATH REMAINS FIXED

3.
ADVANCE SHEATH OVER END OF CUTTING BLADES

4.
TWIST AND REMOVE NEEDLE AND CUTTER TOGETHER

SPECIMEN FIXED IN ZENKER-FORMALIN
ROUTINELY STAINED c̄ H&E, GIEMSA & for IRON

Figure 14–2 Biopsy technique with the use of the Westerman-Jensen needle. (From Ellis LD, Jensen WJ, Westerman MP. Needle biopsy of bone and marrow. Arch Intern Med 1964; 114:213. Copyright 1964, American Medical Association.)

skin and bone cortex. A rotating movement eases the anterior advancement of the needle.

A subtle decrease in resistance is felt as the medullary cavity of the bone is entered; the stylet is then removed. A 10- to 20-mL syringe is attached, and 1–2 cm³ of marrow is aspirated. Aspirated particles are expelled from the syringe onto glass coverslips that have been previously washed in 70% ethanol. Each coverslip is quickly tilted, or the excess blood is removed with a small capillary tube, leaving pale grey-white marrow fragments and a small amount of blood. A second coverslip is then placed on top of the first, and a smear is made by pulling the coverslips apart in a sliding motion. Some practitioners prefer to use two alcohol-cleansed microscope slides in a manner similar to that described for coverslips (see Chapter 13). Additional specimens may be taken at this time for flow cytometric analysis, cytogenetics, or other studies as deemed necessary. Marrow aspirates are stained with a polychrome dye, usually Wright's or Wright-Giemsa stain.

Once the aspirate has been taken, the cutting blades of the biopsy device are inserted into the outer cannula and are advanced until the medullary cavity is entered. The cutting blades are then pressed into the medullary bone, with the outer cannula held firmly in a stationary position. After this, the outer cannula is advanced over the cutting blades with entrapment of the tissue and the entire unit is withdrawn. The marrow core inside the needle is removed by inserting the probe through the cutting tip and extruding the specimen through the hub of the needle. Touch preparations may be made from the marrow core before the latter is fixed in Zenker's 5% glacial acetic acid solution, B5, or buffered neutral formalin.

Fixation in Zenker's glacial acetic acid solution provides optimal specimens for morphologic interpretations. In each case at least three sections are cut and routinely stained with hematoxylin and eosin (H&E), Giemsa, and Prussian blue stain for iron.

After biopsy the care of the patient ordinarily consists of applying pressure over the posterior ilium for about 60 minutes, which is accomplished with a pressure dressing and having the patient remain recumbent. Patients with bleeding disorders or other complications are carefully observed for longer periods.

CHARACTERISTICS OF NORMAL BONE MARROW

Aspirate

The preparation is examined under low power to detect the presence of bone spicules, which stain dark blue or purple (Fig. 14–3). The cellularity may be estimated by observing the proportion of cells to empty fat vacuoles in the vicinity of the bone spicules. The smear is either cellular or relatively acellular. A better estimate of true cellularity must be obtained from the core biopsy sample.

After the low-power microscopic examination, the preparation should be examined with the oil immersion lens to determine the various types of hematopoietic cells present. Under normal situations, a large number of cell types are usually present. Because the distribution pattern may be irregular, it is preferable to count 300–500 nucleated cells to obtain a reliable differential count and to determine the myeloid/erythroid (M:E) ratio, both of which are useful parameters in evaluating marrow function. For adults, the normal M:E range is 1.5–3.3.[4] Other normal values are found in the bone marrow report form (see Fig. 14–20).

Cytologic Features

The majority of cells in the normal bone marrow consist of the myeloid and erythroid series. The myeloid (or granulocytic) series is represented by the neutrophilic, eosinophilic, and basophilic lineages (Figs. 14–4 to 14–7) (see Chapters 8 and 11

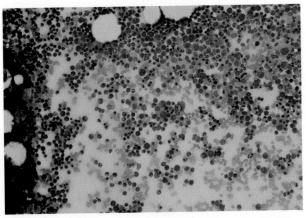

Figure 14–3 Bone marrow aspirate specimen. Cellular area that would provide a good site for cytological evaluation and cell counting. Wright's stain, 100X.

for description of morphology). Although some laboratories differentiate erythrocyte precursors, others simply report nucleated erythroid cells. Others distinguish pronormoblasts and group all other erythroid precursors together. The majority of normoblasts in the normal marrow are at the polychromatophilic or the orthochromic stage (Fig. 14–8).

The largest cells in the normal marrow are megakaryocytes (Fig. 14–9). They may be pleomorphic in both nuclear morphology and size. Megakaryoblasts have a single nucleus with blue cytoplasm. They undergo a process called endomitosis (nuclear division without cytoplasmic division) one or two times, yielding a larger cell with two to four nuclei called a promegakaryocyte. As the maturation process continues with cycles of endomitosis, large cells with polylobulated nuclei containing ploidy of 8, 16, and 32 may be found. In the developing megakaryocytes red granules first appear about the

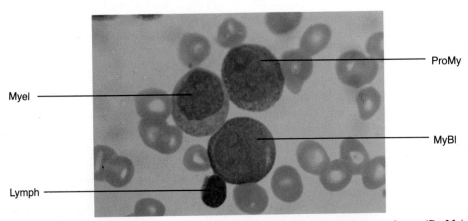

Figure 14–4 Bone marrow aspirate specimen. Cells present include a myeloblast (MyBl), promyelocyte (ProMy), myelocyte (Myel) and lymphocyte (Lymph). Wright's stain, 1000X.

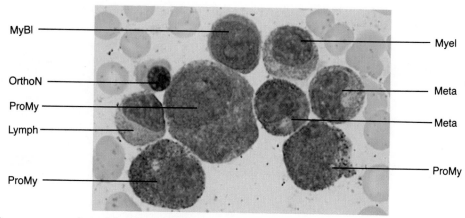

Figure 14–5 Bone marrow aspirate. Myeloblast (MyBl), promyelocyte (ProMy), myelocyte (Myel), metamyelocyte (Meta), orthochromic normoblast (OrthoN) and lymphocyte (Lymph). Wright's stain, 1000×.

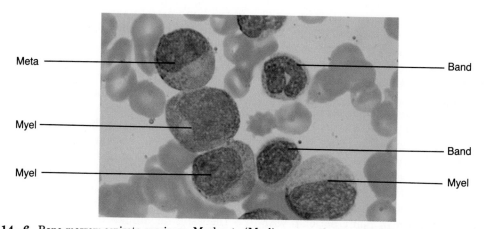

Figure 14–6 Bone marrow aspirate specimen. Myelocyte (Myel), metamyelocyte (Meta), band. Wright's stain, 1000×.

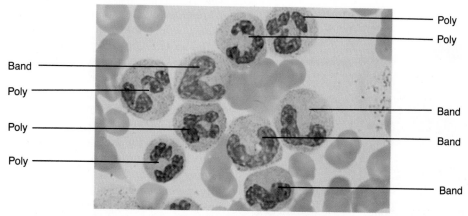

Figure 14–7 Bone marrow aspirate specimen. Bands and polymorphonuclear (Polys) granulocytes. Wright's stain, 1000×.

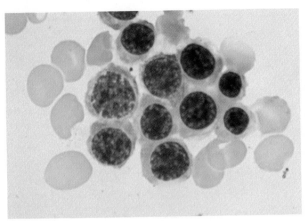

Figure 14–8 Bone marrow aspirate specimen. A nest of nucleated red blood cell precursors with polychromatophilic and orthochromic normoblasts. Wright's stain, 1000×.

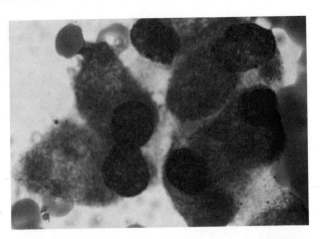

Figure 14–10 Bone marrow aspirate specimen. Cluster of osteoblasts that superficially resemble plasma cells. Osteoblasts have round to oval eccentric nuclei and mottled blue cytoplasm that is devoid of secretory granules. They may have a clear area within the cytoplasm but lack the well-defined "hof" of the plasma cell. Wright's stain, 1000×.

periphery of the cells (platelets). The most mature megakaryocytes have abundant pink cytoplasm that is diffusely filled with red granules. There is little evidence that platelets are formed from cytoplasmic buds often seen in the megakaryocyte. The terms *stage I, II,* and *III* are sometimes used in reference to the degree of maturity and correspond to the designations of megakaryoblast, promegakaryocyte, and granular megakaryocyte, respectively. Megakaryocyte stages are not usually differentiated in the normal marrow.

Abnormal megakaryocytes with small mononuclear, binuclear, or bilobed nuclei and abundant hypogranular cytoplasm are often seen in the bone marrow of individuals with myelodysplastic syndromes and myeloproliferative disorders. Morphologic abnormalities are seen in many patients with idiopathic thrombocytopenic purpura. Megakaryocytes with multiple nonconnected nuclei (multinucleated cells) are sometimes found in individuals with megaloblastic anemias.

Osteoblasts and osteoclasts, occasionally seen in

the bone marrow, are important to note because of their similarity to other cells. Osteoblasts are the cells responsible for the formation and remodeling of bone. They are thought to be descendants of fibroblasts. When dislodged from bone they look very much like plasma cells (Fig. 14–10). Osteoblasts have eccentric round to oval nuclei and abundant blue, somewhat mottled cytoplasm. They may also have a clear area within the cytoplasm but not a well-defined "hof" like the plasma cell. Osteoblasts also lack secretory granules. Osteoblasts are usually found in a single cluster, and it would be unusual to find large numbers of these in the aspirate, unlike plasma cells, which would be diffusely present in the marrow. Osteoclasts are large cells with multiple, evenly spaced nuclei, which should distinguish them from polylobulated megakaryocytes and from the Langerhans giant cells of chronic inflammation, which have palisaded nuclei. Osteoclasts are giant cells formed by the fusion of monocytes/macrophages. They are physiologically responsible for the resorption of bone. Osteoclasts are most easily seen and recognized in the core biopsy specimen, being multinucleated giant cells close to the endosteal surface of the bone spicule (see Fig. 14–19).

While scanning under the low-power objective one should be alert for abnormal clusters of cells, such as metastatic tumor or lymphoid aggregates. In scanning for tumor cells, the observer should look for the presence of clusters of molded cells (syncytia) (Fig. 14–11). Tumor cell nuclei are usually darkly stained (hyperchromatic), and vacuoles are frequently seen in the cytoplasm. Tumor cell clusters are often found at or near the edge of the coverslip or glass slide.

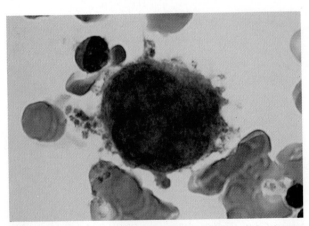

Figure 14–9 Bone marrow aspirate specimen. Megakaryocyte with platelet budding. Wright's stain, 1000×.

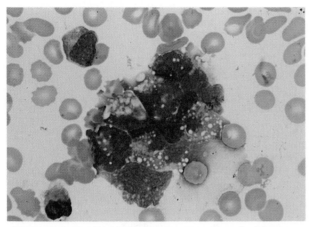

Figure 14–11 Bone marrow aspirate specimen. Cluster or syncytia of tumor cells. Nuclei are irregular and hyperchromatic, and vacuoles are found within the cytoplasm of many cells. Cytoplasmic margins are not well delineated. Wright's stain, 400×.

Core Biopsy Specimen

The core biopsy specimen provides an intact portion of the bone marrow for examination. A typical specimen is approximately 3/4 inch in length by 1/16–1/18 inch in diameter and weighs about 150 mg; thus, it represents only a minute fraction of the total body marrow (Fig. 14–12A). However, in most instances the specimen is a representative sample of the total marrow picture as pertains to cellularity, the proportion of myeloid and erythroid cells present, and iron stores. Examples of hypocellular and hypercellular core biopsy specimens are illustrated for comparison with normocellular marrow in Figure 14–12B and C, respectively.

As described previously in the illustrations, the marrow is fixed in Zenker's solution and sections are cut and stained with H&E, Giemsa, and Prussian blue stain, for iron. The value of the Giemsa stain lies in its ability to differentially stain cells of the myeloid, lymphoid, and plasma cell series.[3]

Neutrophilic myelocytes and metamyelocytes are recognized in Giemsa-stained marrow by the light pink appearance of their cytoplasm. Mature neutrophils and bands are recognized by their smaller size and darkly stained C-shaped nuclei (bands) or multiple nuclear lobes (polys); the cytoplasm of these mature cells may be a very light pink or may not seem to stain at all (Fig. 14–13). Myeloblasts and promyelocytes have oval or round nuclei with cytoplasm that stains blue (Fig. 14–14). It may be difficult to differentiate these cells from pronormoblasts other than through the tendency of the latter to cluster with more mature normoblasts. The cytoplasm of eosinophils has a more intense red staining, and these cells are easily recognized as the most brightly stained cells of the marrow

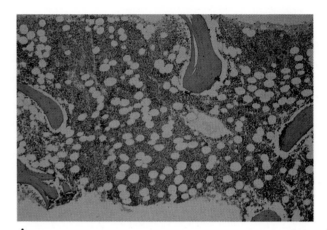

A

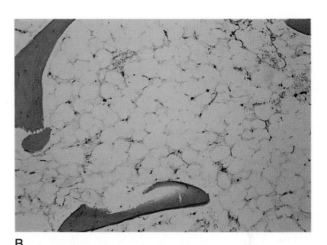

B

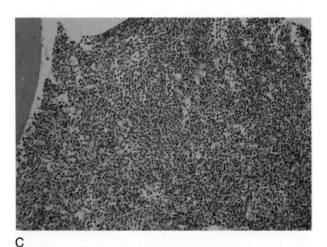

C

Figure 14–12 *A,* Representative sample of core biopsy that may be obtained with biopsy needle. Cellularity is better estimated from the core biopsy, which in this case is approximately 50% fat and 50% cellularity. H&E, 40×. *B,* Hypocellular bone marrow core biopsy specimen from individual with aplastic anemia. Only fat and connective tissue cells are found. H&E, 100×. *C,* Hypercellular bone marrow specimen from individual with chronic myelogenous leukemia. There is virtually 100% cellularity with no marrow fat visible. H&E, 100×.

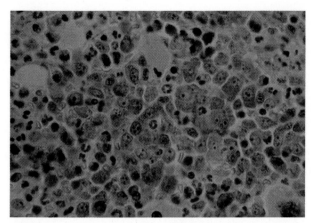

Figure 14–13 Bone marrow core biopsy specimen. Granulocytic area with myelocytes, metamyelocytes, bands, polymorphonuclear granulocytes, and eosinophils (dark red). Giemsa, 400×.

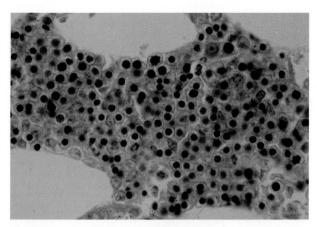

Figure 14–15 Erythroid island in bone marrow core biopsy specimen. Late-stage normoblasts often have a fried-egg appearance. Giemsa, 400×.

(Fig. 14–13). Basophils cannot be recognized on marrow specimens fixed with Zenker's solution.

The more mature or older normoblasts have centrally placed, round nuclei that stain very intensely, being so dark that light does not penetrate the nucleus to any extent (Fig. 14–15). The cytoplasm of these cells is not appreciably stained, but the plasma membrane margin is often clearly discerned, giving the cells a "fried egg" appearance. Normoblasts have a tendency to cluster in small groups and are often easily recognized at lower power.

Lymphocytes are among the most difficult cells to recognize, other than when they occur in clusters. In the latter situation, the small, round, mature lymphocytes have a speckled nuclear chromatin in a small, round nucleus, along with a scant amount of blue cytoplasm (Fig. 14–16). More immature lymphocytes will have larger round or lo-

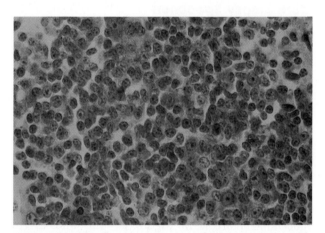

Figure 14–16 Bone marrow core biopsy specimen with lymphoid collection. Most lymphocytes are small and mature. A few lymphocytes are immature with a larger nucleus that contains a single prominent nucleolus. Giemsa, 400×.

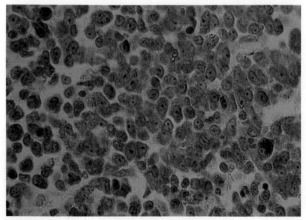

Figure 14–14 Core biopsy specimen showing infiltration with blasts (blue cytoplasm) and a few myelocytes (pink cytoplasm). Giemsa, 400×.

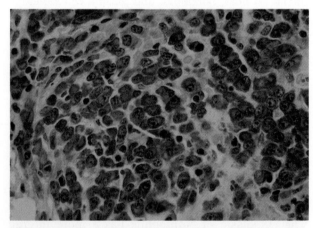

Figure 14–17 Collection of plasma cells in core biopsy specimen. Nuclei are eccentric, and a cytoplasmic clearing, or "hof," can be seen. Giemsa, 400×.

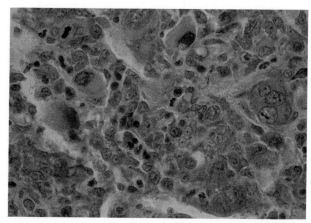

Figure 14–18 Bone marrow core biopsy specimen containing many large polylobated megakaryocytes and increased blasts. Giemsa, 400×.

bulated nuclei but still only a small rim of blue cytoplasm.

Plasma cells can be difficult to distinguish from myelocytes in H&E-stained sections but are **recognized** with Giemsa staining as cells with eccentric dark nuclei and blue cytoplasm with a pale, perinuclear Golgi zone located next to the nucleus (Fig. 14–17). Plasma cells are characteristically located around blood vessels.

Megakaryocytes are easily recognized as the largest cells of the marrow and have a characteristic polylobulated nucleus. The nucleus of older megakaryocytes becomes smaller and more darkly stained on H&E staining. The cytoplasm varies from a light pink in younger cells to a dark pink in older cells (Fig. 14–18).

BONE MARROW REPORTS

A bone marrow evaluation should include examination of the peripheral blood smear, the bone marrow aspirate, and the bone marrow core biopsy specimen. Each of these is important in the total assessment of the patient, and they complement one another. A systematic approach is recommended in evaluating each patient. This is especially useful in the training of clinical laboratory scientists, interns, residents, and fellows, since it emphasizes the need to examine all facets of the bone marrow and not just to focus on a single abnormality, thereby missing any associated or incidental findings.

The peripheral blood is examined first. The examination includes red cell morphology (e.g., size, shape, inclusions), white blood cell numbers and morphology, and platelets (estimate and morphology). Examination of the peripheral blood will

often help considerably in interpreting bone marrow findings. The bone marrow aspirate or smear is examined next. A differential count is done on each smear for teaching purposes, with recognition of the variability that may occur if only a small area of the aspirate is counted. After the careful examination of each smear, a 300-cell (or more) differential count is done in a cellular area close to a bone spicule. The results of the differential count are then related to the impression of the smear as a whole and then to the core biopsy specimen. Finally, the core biopsy specimen is examined. Because of the sample size obtained with the procedure discussed, the cellularity and M:E ratio of biopsy samples tend to be more representative than the aspirate smear, as well as providing numerous other advantages that have been mentioned previously.[3] The systematic approach that the author uses in examining the marrow smear or core biopsy includes evaluation of

Cellularity
M:E ratio
Maturation of myeloid series
Maturation of erythroid series (normoblastic/megaloblastic)
Eosinophils/basophils, including mast cells
Megakaryocytes
Presence of other cells: lymphocytes, plasma cells, histiocytes, osteoclasts, fibroblasts (Fig. 14–19)
Stromal abnormalities (e.g., granulomas, fibrosis, necrosis, serous atrophy of fat)
Hemosiderin content
Vessel abnormalities (e.g., amyloid deposits)
Bone changes (e.g., Paget's disease, osteodystrophy)

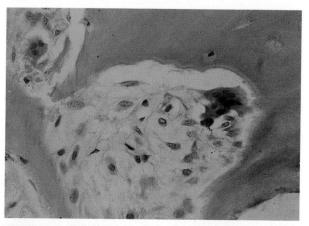

Figure 14–19 Bone marrow core biopsy specimen. Note presence of large multinucleated cell near endosteal surface of bone. This is an osteoclast, which is a cell involved in resorption of bone. The spindle-shaped cells are fibroblasts. This specimen is from an individual with hyperparathyroidism. H&E, 400×.

A PORT ASSOCIATES (412) 422 2079   10/79/9

UNIVERSITY HEALTH CENTER OF PITTSBURGH
CENTRAL HEMATOLOGY LABORATORY
BONE MARROW REPORT

ASP. NO. _H-92-000_

NAME _SMITH, WALTER_   LOCATION _11300-00_   BX. NO. _S-92-000_

UNIT NO. _100-00-000_   PHYSICIAN _Dr. Watson_   DATE _02/01/92_

CLIN. HX. _82 year old male with anemia._

MARROW DIFFERENTIAL: %

NEUTROPHIL SERIES:	MEAN	± 2 S.D.	PATIENT	ERYTHROID SERIES:	MEAN	± 2 S.D.	PATIENT
Blast	1	0-2	1	Total NRBC	26	15-37	24
Promyelocyte	3	2-5	2	Pronormoblast	1	0-2	29
Myelocyte	13	9-17	8				
Metamyelocyte	16	7-25	12	LYMPHOCYTE	16	8-24	1
Band	12	9-15	7	PLASMA CELL	1	0-4	1
PMN	7	3-11	9	MONOCYTE	1	0-2	1
				OTHER CELLS		1	
EOSINOPHIL SERIES:							
Myelocyte	1)	0-2)	1				
Band	1) 3	0-2) 1-7	1	M: E RATIO	2.3:1	1.5-3.3:1	0.8:1
Eosinophil	1)	0-3)	3				

PATIENT HEMATOLOGIC VALUES

HGB: 5.8 **gms; HCT** 15.8 **%; MCV:** 114.2µ³ **: MCH** 34.2 µµg; **WBC:** 3,160 /mm³;

Plts: 87,000 /mm³

IMPRESSION

PB: The RBC's are normochromic with prominent anisocytosis. Many macrocytes, microcytes, are present including oval forms. The WBC differential is: polys 66% (2086), bands 1% (32), lymphs 25% (790), monos 5% (158), eos 3% (95). Several multilobed (6 and 7 lobes) polys are seen. The platelets are reduced in number.

BMA: Cellular spicules are present. The M:E ratio is 0.8:1. Myeloid maturation is megaloblastic with giant bands and metamyelocytes present. Erythroid maturation is megaloblastic with numerous promegaloblasts. Megakaryocytes are present.

BMBX: The trabeculae are nomal. The cell to fat ratio is 40-60%. The M:E ratio is approximately 1:1. There is a preponderance of large round to polygonal cells (promegaloblasts) containing vesicular nuclei, 1-3 basophilic nucleoli and a small to moderate amount of amphophilic cytoplasm. Megakaryocytes are seen 0-1 per hpf. Iron stores are markedly increased.

DX: 1. Peripheral blood with macrocytic anemia, thrombocytopenia and mild leukopenia.
2. Bone marrow aspirate and bone marrow biopsy with erythroid predominance and marked megaloblastic changes.
3. Bone marrow biopsy with increased iron stores.

NOTE: There are striking megaloblastic features in this case. B12 and folate levels will be necessary to determine the type of megaloblastic anemia.

RESIDENT   PATHOLOGIST

FORM NO. ■■ ■■ ■ ■

Figure 14-20 Sample of bone marrow report, including normal values. HGB, hemoglobin; HCT, hematocrit; MCV, mean corpuscular volume; MCH, mean corpuscular hemoglobin; WBC, white blood cell count; Plts, platelet count; PB, peripheral blood; BMA, bone marrow aspirate; BMBX, bone marrow biopsy; Dx, diagnosis.

The final step is correlation of all results into a diagnosis, using morphologic features as well as supplementary laboratory and clinical material as available (Fig. 14-20). After the diagnosis, comments or notes may be added, especially if a differential diagnosis is involved or a definite diagnosis cannot be established. Finally, recommendations are offered for additional studies.

SUMMARY

The bone marrow evaluation is a valuable adjunct to peripheral smear examination when hematologic diseases are suspected. Obtaining a core biopsy sample also allows evaluation of bony spicules and a search for focal lesions.

REVIEW QUESTIONS

1. The preferred site for bone marrow biopsy in an adult is the
   a. sternum
   b. vertebrae
   c. anterior or posterior iliac crest
   d. femur

2. The aspirate should be examined under low power to assess
   a. number of megakaryocytes
   b. cellularity
   c. presence of tumor cells
   d. all of the above

3. The normal M:E ratio range in adults is approximately
   a. 1.5 to 3.5
   b. 5.1 to 6.2
   c. 8.6 to 10.2
   d. 10 to 12

4. The majority of normoblasts in the normal marrow are
   a. pronomoblasts
   b. pronomoblasts and basophilic normoblasts
   c. basophilic and polychromatophilic normoblasts
   d. polychromatophilic and orthochromic normoblasts

5. Cells occasionally seen in the bone marrow that are responsible for formation of bone are
   a. plasma cells
   b. osteoblasts
   c. osteoclasts
   d. macrophages

6. List characteristics of tumor cells in a bone marrow aspirate or biopsy specimen.

7. Give indications for a bone marrow examination.

8. Discuss the importance of a systematic approach to bone marrow evaluation in total patient assessment.

References

1. Mechanik N: Untersuchungen uber das Gewicht des Knochenmarkes des Menschen. Z Gesamte Anat 1926; 79:58.
2. Kent DL, Larson EB: Magnetic resonance imaging of the brain and spine: Is clinical efficacy established after the first decade? Ann Intern Med 1988; 108:402–424.
3. Krause JR: Bone Marrow Biopsy. New York: Churchill Livingstone, 1981.
4. Rothstein G: Origin and development of the blood and blood-forming tissues. In Lee GR, Bithell TC, Foerster J, et al (eds): Wintrobe's Clinical Hematology, 9th ed. Philadelphia: Lea & Febiger, 1993:41–78.

PART IV

Hemato-pathology: Erythrocyte Disorders

CHAPTER 15

Introduction to the Anemias: Approach to Diagnosis

Ann Bell

Outline

Objectives

AFTER COMPLETION OF THIS CHAPTER, THE READER WILL BE ABLE TO

1. Define anemia in "ideal" terms and discuss problems with the definition.
2. Discuss the importance of the history and the physical examination in the diagnosis of anemia.
3. Describe clinical symptoms of anemia.
4. List procedures that are commonly performed for the detection and diagnosis of anemia.
5. Distinguish between effective and ineffective erythropoiesis.
6. Explain the two general classifications (morphologic and pathophysiologic) of anemic states.
7. Characterize the three morphologic groups of anemias that are based on the mean cell volume and give one example of each.
8. Describe the use of the red blood cell distribution width in the classification of anemias.
9. Define the two major categories of anemia on the basis of pathophysiology.
10. Briefly explain how the body adapts to anemia over time.

Erythrocytes serve mainly as transport mechanisms for hemoglobin to deliver oxygen to the tissues for proper metabolic function.[1] A decrease in the ability of the blood to deliver sufficient oxygen to the tissues results in hypoxia. Anemia is the consequence of the oxygen-carrying capacity of the blood and is related to the tissue hypoxia. Anemia is not a disease or a diagnosis in itself but a manifestation of an underlying disease.[2, 3] Anemia is the most common manifestation of disease worldwide. This chapter provides an overview of the diagnosis, mechanism, and classification of anemia. In the following chapters, each anemia is discussed in detail.

DEFINITION OF ANEMIA

Anemia is defined ideally as a reduction of more than 10% from the normal value for the total number of red blood cells (RBCs), amount of circulating hemoglobin, and RBC mass for a particular patient. However, this definition is not applicable because patients' usual normal values are often not known. A more conventional definition is a decrease in RBCs, hemoglobin (Hb), and hematocrit (Hct) below the previously established normal values for healthy persons of the same age, gender, and race and under similar environmental conditions.[1-6]

Problems with this conventional definition may occur for several reasons. The blood values of nonanemic persons may fall just below the "normal" level. Those of mildly anemic persons may fall within the low normal range. This latter group usually is not recognized unless the blood smear is evaluated or the RBC indices and RBC distribution width (RDW) are appreciated.

Hematologic reference values for adults are listed in Chapter 12. The values may vary in different areas according to age, gender, race, and environment but are given for the purpose of discussion in the approach to anemias. Table 15–1 gives reference ranges for hemoglobin at different ages.[1] Each laboratory should determine its reference ranges in accordance with the patient population. Geographic elevation influences hemoglobin levels, as do other factors. A patient whose values fall below those listed in these tables is considered most likely to be anemic.

CLINICAL FINDINGS

The clinical diagnosis of anemia is made from the history, physical examination, signs, symptoms,

Table 15-1. REFERENCE RANGES FOR HEMOGLOBIN AT DIFFERENT AGES

Age Group	Hemoglobin (Range in g/dL)
Newborn (<1 week old)	14–22
6 months old	11–14
Children (1–15 years old)	11–15
Adults	
Men	14–16
Women	12–16

* From Glassman AB: Anemia: diagnosis and clinical considerations. *In* Harmening DM (ed): Clinical Hematology and Fundamentals of Hemostasis, 2nd ed. Philadelphia: FA Davis, 1992.

hematologic values, and other procedures and findings.

History and Physical Examination

The approach to the patient with anemia begins with a complete history and physical examination.[1-6] The history and physical findings can yield information that may prove valuable in identifying and narrowing the possible cause or causes of anemia and in lessening the need for ordering expensive special tests.

Obtaining a good history requires questioning of the patient, particularly in regard to diet, drug ingestion, exposure to chemicals, occupation, hobbies, travel, bleeding history, ethnic group, family history of disease, neurologic symptoms, previous medication, jaundice, and various underlying diseases that produce anemia.[2, 3, 6] (Note: This is only a partial list of questions to be asked.)

In the physical examination, certain features should be evaluated closely, such as skin (e.g., pallor, jaundice, petechiae), eyes (hemorrhage), mouth (mucosal bleeding), sternal tenderness, lymphadenopathy, cardiac murmurs, splenomegaly, and hepatomegaly.[2, 3] (Note: This is by no means a complete list.) Many anemias have common manifestations.

Moderate anemias (Hb 7–10 g/dL) may not produce clinical signs or symptoms if the onset of anemia is slow.[1] Depending on the patient's age and cardiovascular state, however, moderate anemias may be associated with pallor of conjunctivae and of nail beds, dyspnea, vertigo, headache, muscle weakness, lethargy, and other symptoms.[2, 3] Severe anemias (Hb <7 g/dL) usually produce tachycardia, hypotension, and other symptoms and volume loss, in addition to symptoms listed earlier. The severity of the anemia is gauged by the degree of reduction in blood volume, cardiopulmonary adaptation, and the rapidity of progression of the anemia.[1]

The history and physical examination are essential for establishing the clinical diagnosis of anemia.

LABORATORY PROCEDURES

Complete Blood Cell Count with Cell Indices

To detect the presence of anemia, the medical technologist performs a complete blood count on a hematology cell analyzer to determine the RBC count, hemoglobin, hematocrit, RBC indices, white blood cell (WBC) count, and platelet count. Normal reference ranges for these determinations are listed in Chapter 12. Some electronic counters also provide for an RBC histogram (to be described) and/or a calculated value for the RDW (to be described). A relative and absolute reticulocyte count (to be described) should be performed for every patient when anemia is suspected or observed. Several automated analyzers are available for performance of reticulocyte counts and increase the accuracy of the count.

Modern automated counters generate an RBC histogram (RBC size frequency distribution curve) with relative number of cells plotted on the ordinate and RBC volume in femtoliters on the abscissa. The curve is approximately gaussian for normal RBCs. Abnormalities include a shift to left in the curve (microcytosis) or to the right (macrocytosis), a widening caused by a greater variation about the mean, and two populations of cells. The histogram complements the blood smear in identifying variant RBC populations.[2, 6] (Histograms are further discussed with examples in Chapter 37.)

RDW is the mathematical expression of variation in size of RBCs (or anisocytosis), which is calculated by cell counters. The RDW is the coefficient of variation of the normally gaussian curve-shaped RBC volume distribution histogram. The RDW is determined by dividing the standard deviation of the mean corpuscular volume (MCV) by the MCV and multiplying by 100 to convert to a percentage value. Thus the RDW is a quantitative measure of the size variation of circulating RBCs. The normal value for RDW is 12–15%.[1, 2, 6]

Reticulocyte Count

A reticulocyte count permits effective assessment of RBC production by the bone marrow. Reticulocytes are young RBCs that have just left the marrow but still contain residual RNA; they remain for only 1–1.5 days in the blood; the normal range is 0.5–2%.[1, 3] In addition to the percentage of reticulocytes present, an absolute reticulocyte count should be determined. The low normal absolute reticulocyte count is 25×10^9/L; the upper range has been given as $75-90 \times 10^9$/L.[1, 7] A patient with a severe anemia may appear to be producing increased numbers of reticulocytes if only the percentage is considered. For example, a patient with 1.5×10^{12}/L RBCs and 3.0% reticulocytes has an absolute reticulocyte count of 45×10^9/L, which is in the normal range, but for the degree of anemia the count should be much higher.[3] In other words, production of reticulocytes at a normal rate does not compensate for an RBC count that is approximately one third of normal.

The reticulocyte count may be corrected for anemia if the absolute count is not performed. The corrected reticulocyte count (CRC) is determined by multiplying the reticulocyte percentage by the patient's hematocrit and dividing the result by the normal hematocrit. If the reticulocytes are released prematurely from the bone marrow and remain in the circulation 2–3 days (instead of 1–1.5 days), the CRC must be divided by 2 in order to find a better indication of the rate of RBC production.[3] Reticulocytes and related calculations are further discussed in Chapter 12.

Blood Smear Examination

The most important evaluation in the workup of an anemia is to examine the peripheral blood smear, giving particular attention to the RBCs as to variation in size, shape, color content, and inclusions. Normal RBCs on a Wright's stained blood film are nearly uniform in size, being 7.0–7.9 μm in diameter. Small or microcytic cells are less than 6 μm in diameter, and large or macrocytic RBCs are more than 9 μm in diameter. Certain abnormalities of diagnostic value, such as sickle-shaped RBCs or malarial parasites, can be detected only by studying the RBCs on a peripheral blood smear carefully. Some examples of abnormal shapes are seen in Figure 15–1.

The types of WBCs should be differentiated, and any WBC abnormalities should be noted. The number of platelets per oil immersion field (oif) must be determined by counting 10 consecutive oifs in an area of the smear in which the RBCs are separated or gently touch one another. If the platelets are decreased, then 50–100 oifs should be counted in order to obtain an estimate of the number of platelets per oifs. (See Chapter 13 for a complete discussion of the peripheral blood film.)

Additional information from the blood smear examination always complements the helpful analytic information from the cell counter.

Hematologic values that may be observed in patients with anemia are given in Table 15–2.

Erythrocyte shapes

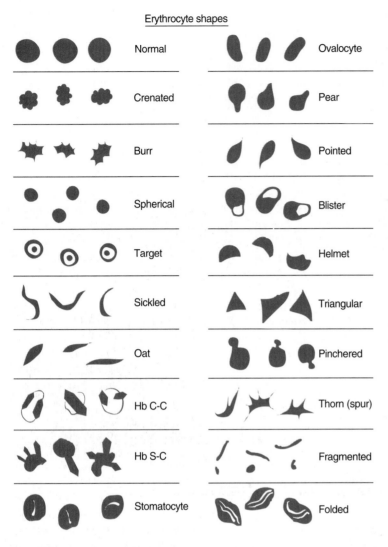

Figure 15-1 Artist's rendition of normal and abnormal erythrocyte shapes (poikilocytes). Examples of some poikilocytes and the disorders with which they are associated are described as follows and, along with other erythrocyte abnormalities, are discussed in detail in Chapters 16-19. *Crenated and burr cells (echinocytes):* seen in renal disease. *Spherical cells (spherocytes):* seen in hereditary spherocytosis, hemolytic processes, severe burns, transfused blood. *Target cells (codocytes):* seen in hemoglobinopathies (e.g., CC, SS, DD, EE, S-thalassemia), thalassemia, iron deficiency, post-splenectomy, obstructive liver disease. *Sickled and oat cells (drepanocytes):* common in Hb SS disease; fewer in Hb SC disease, HbS-β thalassemia, HbC-Harlem disease, Hb S-Memphis disease. *Hb CC:* crystals are hexagonal and may be difficult to find. *Stomatocytes:* have a mouth-shaped central pallor; a few may be seen on normal blood smears; increased numbers in hereditary stomatocytosis, obstructive liver disease, cirrhosis, alcoholism, Rh null disease. *Hb SC:* often described as "catcher's mitt" or "finger in glove"; found with Hb SC. *Pear shaped and pointed (dacryocytes):* seen in myelofibrosis with myeloid metaplasia, beta thalassemia, tuberculosis, metastatic cancer, other causes of extramedullary hematopoiesis. *Blister, helmet, triangle, pinchered, fragmented (shizocytes or schistocytes):* cells that have been damaged by trying to pass through fibrin strands, such as those in microangiopathic hemolytic anemia, thrombotic thrombocytopenia, disseminated intravascular coagulation, hemolytic uremic syndrome, severe burns. *Thorn cells (acanthocytes):* fewer and blunter points than echinocytes; seen in abetalipoproteinemia, in alcoholic cirrhosis with hemolytic anemia, after splenectomy, in malabsorption, in pyruvate kinase deficiency, in hypothyroidism, in vitamin E deficiency. *Folded:* seen with Hb CC; a few may be seen on normal smears. Increased numbers are seen in iron deficiency, megaloblastic anemia, myelofibrosis, and sickle cell anemia. There is also a hereditary form. (Redrawn from Miller SE, Weller JM: Textbook of Clinical Pathology. Baltimore: Williams & Wilkins, 1971:59. Original drawing courtesy of L.W. Diggs, M.D.)

Bone Marrow Examination

In the determination of the type of anemia, a marrow aspiration and biopsy are important procedures for inclusion in the workup studies.[1, 2] A bone marrow examination reveals the morphologic patterns of RBCs and WBCs, the presence of megakaryocytes, the myeloid-to-erythroid (M:E) ratio, results of stains for iron and from other stains that may be needed, and the presence of granuloma and tumor cells in hematoxylin and eosin-stained marrow sections. (Chapter 14 discusses the bone marrow procedure and examination in detail.)

Table 15-2. HEMATOLOGIC VALUES IN ADULTS WITH ANEMIA			
Test	**Men**	**Women**	**Both Sexes**
Red blood cell count ($\times 10^{12}$/L)	<4.6	<4.2	
Hemoglobin (g/dL)	<14.0	<12.0	
Hematocrit (L/L)	<0.42	<0.37	
Mean corpuscular volume (fL)			<80->100
Mean corpuscular hemoglobin (pg)			<27->32
Mean corpuscular hemoglobin concentration (g/dL or %)			<32-36
Red blood cell distribution width			>15%
Platelets ($\times 10^9$/L)			150-350
Reticulocytes			
Relative			<0.5->2.0%
Absolute			<25->90 $\times 10^9$/L

Other needed laboratory tests are a complete urinalysis, including microscopic examination, and a fecal analysis with occult blood test and microscopic examination for parasites.

After the hematologic laboratory studies are completed, the anemia may be classified morphologically (to be discussed). Particular special tests may be indicated on the basis of the morphologic type of anemia present, such as serum iron, iron-binding capacity, and serum ferritin if microcytic hypochromic anemia is present. The physician eventually determines the pathophysiologic cause of the anemia and makes the final diagnosis after the results from all the procedures are available. The cause of the anemia must be determined before replacement therapy (such as iron for iron deficiency anemia) or supportive therapy (such as transfusion) is begun.[1]

MECHANISMS OF ANEMIA

The lifespan of the RBC in the circulation is about 120 days. In a healthy person with no anemia, approximately 1% of the senescent circulating RBCs are lost daily, and the bone marrow normally continues to produce RBCs to replace those lost. Hematopoietic stem cells must function satisfactorily by maturing the erythroid precursor cells and releasing mature RBCs into the peripheral blood. Adequate RBC production requires several nutritional factors, such as iron, vitamin B_{12}, and folic acid. Hemoglobin synthesis must also function normally. The maintenance of a stable hematocrit requires the production of an amount of blood equaling the amount normally lost.[1-3]

Erythropoiesis

Several terms are used in referring to marrow erythroid proliferative activity, or erythropoiesis. *Erythropoiesis* is the formation of red blood cells in the bone marrow (Chapter 8). Total erythropoiesis represents total erythroid proliferative activity in marrow. Total erythropoiesis is composed of two main divisions: effective and ineffective.[1, 2, 3, 6]

Effective erythropoiesis results in the production of 90% mature differentiated RBCs in the circulation. In ineffective erythropoiesis, 10% or more of the progenitor cells are destroyed in the marrow before they reach the mature stage or immediately after release from the marrow.[1, 2, 3, 6]

Two general mechanisms are involved in anemic states:[1, 2, 3] (1) increased destruction or loss of blood from bleeding or hemolysis results in anemia although there is total and effective erythropoiesis, such as that seen in patients with hereditary spherocytosis, and (2) decreased production of RBCs leads to decreased total and effective erythropoiesis such as that found in patients with aplastic anemia, or increased ineffective erythropoiesis, such as that observed in patients with vitamin B_{12} deficiency.[1-3]

Note that effective erythropoiesis does not necessarily imply that an anemia is compensated; it means only that the erythrocytes produced actually reach the circulation and are not destroyed immediately.

CLASSIFICATION OF ANEMIAS

The two common methods of classification of anemia are morphologic and pathophysiologic. In the morphologic classification, anemia is subdivided into three large groups according to blood counts, cell indices, particularly MCV, reticulocyte count, and examination of RBC on a blood smear: normocytic, normochromic anemia; microcytic, hypochromic anemia; and macrocytic anemia. In Figure 15–2, anemias are classified into the three morphologic groups on the basis of the MCV. Anemias may also be classified by RDW.

The pathophysiologic classification of anemia relates the disease process to the current concept of the two mechanisms or causes of anemia: (1) anemia caused by decreased RBC production and (2) anemia caused by increased RBC destruction or loss.

Morphologic Classification[1-3, 5, 8-11]

Normocytic, normochromic anemia has an MCV in the range of 80–100 fL and a mean corpuscular hemoglobin concentration (MCHC) of 32–36%. (The RBCs on the smear must be examined in order to rule out a bimodal population of microcytes and macrocytes, which would yield a normal mean range.) The number of reticulocytes may be increased, normal, or decreased. Normocytic anemias are usually caused by hemolysis, acute bleeding, malignancy (leukemia, lymphoma, carcinoma), splenomegaly (RBCs are trapped and destroyed in spleen), agents that produce toxicity (radiation, cytotoxic drugs), chronic disease states, infections, rheumatoid arthritis, and renal and liver diseases. Chronic disease, malignancy, splenomegaly, and exposure to toxic agents may also produce a microcytic (normochromic) anemia.

Microcytic, hypochromic anemia is revealed by an MCV of less than 80 fL and an MCHC of less than 32% with small cells that have increased central pallor on the smear. Microcytic anemias are generally caused by an abnormality of hemoglobin

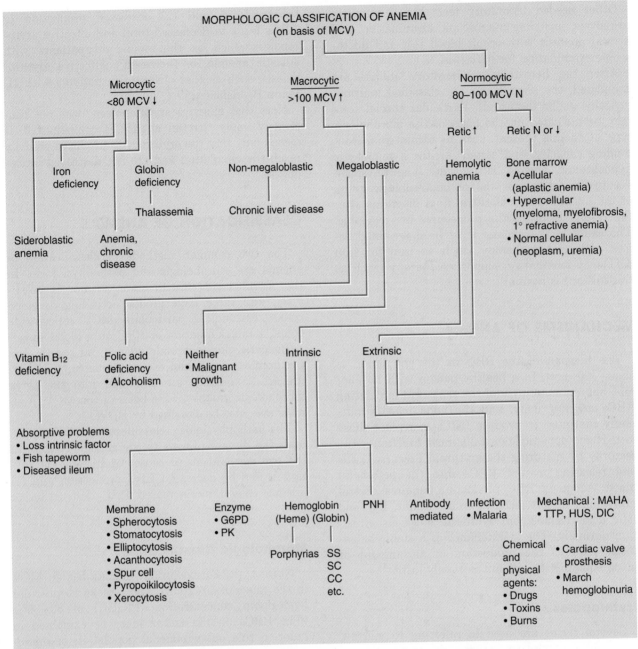

Figure 15–2 Morphologic classification of anemia on the basis of mean corpuscular volume.

synthesis: iron deficiency, deficiency of heme synthesis (sideroblastic anemia), deficiency of globin synthesis (thalassemia), and chronic disease states. Microcytic anemia results from an iron level insufficient for maintaining normal erythropoiesis and is characterized by abnormal results of iron studies. Early development of a microcytic anemia may reveal reduced iron stores, but an obvious anemia has not developed. The causes of iron deficiency vary in infants, children, adolescents, and adults, and it is necessary to find the cause before treatment begins.

Macrocytic, normochromic anemias are revealed when the MCV is higher than 100 fL, the MCHC is higher than 32%, and RBCs appear macrocytic. Macrocytic anemias may be megaloblastic or non-megaloblastic.

Megaloblastic anemias are commonly caused by vitamin B_{12} deficiency or folate deficiency. Pernicious anemia is one result of vitamin B_{12} deficiency. Alcoholism is one cause of folate deficiency but it also is a cause of nutritional deficiency. A megaloblastic anemia is characterized by oval macrocytes and teardrop-shaped cells in blood and by megaloblasts or large nucleated RBC precursors in marrow. Nuclear maturation lags behind cytoplasmic development as a result of lack of vitamin B_{12} or folate. All cells of the body are affected by the deficiency in the production of DNA (see Chapter 16).

Nonmegaloblastic anemia is also characterized by large RBCs that are mostly round, but the marrow nucleated RBCs do not display megaloblastic maturation changes. Macrocytic anemias are seen in patients with chronic liver disease, chronic hemolytic anemia with a high reticulocyte count, myelodysplastic refractory anemia, and other types of anemias.

Classification by Red Blood Cell Distribution Width

Each of the three morphologic categories mentioned earlier can also be subclassified by the automated RDW as homogeneous (normal RDW) or heterogeneous (increased or high RDW), according to Bessman and associates.[12, 13] A few examples are given:

Normocytic Anemias (MCV = 80–100 fL)

RDW normal: Hemolytic anemia without high reticulocyte count
RDW high: Early deficiency of iron, vitamin B_{12}, or folate

Microcytic Anemia (MCV < 80 fL)

RDW normal: Heterozygous thalassemia
RDW high: Iron deficiency anemia

Macrocytic Anemia (MCV > 100 fL)

RDW normal: Aplastic anemia
RDW high: Vitamin B_{12} or folate deficiency; hemolytic anemia with high reticulocyte count

Pathophysiologic Classification[10]

A pathophysiologic classification of anemias relates disease processes to associated causes and currently described mechanisms. It is based on concepts that may later be changed, but at present they serve as an aid to physicians in the clinical investigation of anemia. In the pathophysiologic classification, the anemias caused by decreased RBC production (such as disorders of DNA synthesis) are distinguished from the anemias caused by increased RBC destruction or loss (intracorpuscular or extracorpuscular abnormalities of RBCs). Table 15–3 presents the pathophysiologic classification of anemia, lists the causes of the abnormal-

---

Table 15–3. PATHOPHYSIOLOGIC CLASSIFICATION OF ANEMIAS

Anemia Caused by Decreased Production of Red Blood Cells

Disorder of hematopoietic stem cell proliferation and differentiation: aplastic anemia
Disorder of DNA synthesis: megaloblastic anemia
Disorder of hemoglobin synthesis: iron deficiency anemia, thalassemia
Disorder of proliferation and differentiation of precursor erythroid cells: anemia of chronic renal failure, anemia of endocrine disorders
Unknown mechanisms: anemia of chronic disease, anemia associated with marrow infiltration, sideroblastic anemia

Anemia Caused by Increased Destruction or Loss

INTRACORPUSCULAR ABNORMALITY

Membrane defect: hereditary spherocytosis, hereditary elliptocytosis
Enzyme deficiency: glucose-6-phosphate dehydrogenase, pyruvate kinase
Globin abnormality: hemoglobinopathies (e.g., Hb SS)
Paroxysmal nocturnal hemoglobinuria

EXTRACORPUSCULAR ABNORMALITY

Mechanical: microangiopathic hemolytic anemia (thrombotic thrombocytopenic purpura, hemolytic uremic syndrome)
Infection: hemolytic anemia due to infection with malaria, babesia, bartonella
Chemical and physical agents: drugs, toxins, burns
Antibody-mediated: acquired hemolytic anemia
Blood loss: acute blood loss anemia

Modified from Erslev AJ: Clinical manifestations and classification of erythrocyte disorders. *In* Williams WF, Beutler E, Erslev AJ, Lichtman MA (eds): Hematology, 4th ed. New York: McGraw-Hill, 1990

---

ity, and gives one or more examples of a type of anemia.

PHYSIOLOGIC ADAPTATIONS

In anemia that develops slowly with few symptoms, the body adapts to anemia over a period of time. Reduced delivery of oxygen to tissue secondary to reduced hemoglobin causes increased erythropoietin secretion by the kidneys. With persistent anemia, physiologic adaptations consist of mechanisms that increase the oxygen-carrying capacity of a reduced amount of hemoglobin. There is more rapid delivery of blood with reduced oxygen content. Heart rate and respiratory rate are increased. Cardiac output is increased. With tissue hypoxia, there is an increase in RBC 2,3-diphosphoglycerate (2,3-DPG), which shifts the oxygen dissociation curve to the right (decreased oxygen affinity of hemoglobin) and results in increased delivery of oxygen to tissues[8] (see Chapter 9). This is a highly significant mechanism in chronic anemias, in such a way that a patient with anemia may be relatively asymptomatic at very low levels of hemoglobin.

SUMMARY

An approach to the diagnosis of anemia is through obtaining a careful history and thorough physical examination, and accurately performing a complete blood count with cell indices on a cell counter, a reticulocyte count, blood smear examination, bone marrow examination, urinalysis, fecal analysis, and additional studies as ordered. Modern sophisticated counters provide much useful diagnostic information but merely complement the precise examination of the blood smear, which remains the most important study in the workup of a patient with anemia. Two general mechanisms of anemia that lead to effective or ineffective erythropoiesis are increased destruction or loss of RBCs and decreased production of RBCs. The morphologic classifications of anemia are normocytic, microcytic, and macrocytic. Physiologic adaptations to anemia are briefly mentioned.

REVIEW QUESTIONS

1. Is anemia a disease? Explain.
2. Give a conventional definition of anemia.
3. What are the two essential clinical features that are performed by the physician in an approach to the diagnosis of anemia?
4. Identify essential hematology tests needed in the workup of a patient with anemia.
5. Name the three morphologic classifications of anemia.
6. Give the MCV in the three morphologic types of anemia.
7. Name the two pathophysiologic causes or mechanisms of anemia.
8. Name one anemia that is caused by a disorder of hemoglobin synthesis.
9. What laboratory procedure is the most important in the workup of a patient with anemia?

References

1. Glassman AB: Anemia: diagnosis and clinical considerations. *In* Harmening DM (ed): Clinical Hematology and Fundamentals of Hemostasis, 2nd ed. Philadelphia: FA Davis, 1992:54–64.
2. Kjeldsberg C., Beutler E, Bell C, et al: Practical Diagnosis of Hematologic Disorders. Chicago: ASCP Press, 1989.
3. Schumacher HR, Gavin DF, Triplett DA: Introduction to Laboratory Hematology and Hematopathology. New York: AR Liss, 1984.
4. Van Assenfeldt ON: Anemia and polycythemia: Interpretation of laboratory tests and differential diagnosis. *In* Koepke JA (ed): Laboratory Hematology. New York: Churchill Livingstone, 1984:865–902.
5. Jandl JH: Blood: Pathophysiology. Boston: Blackwell Scientific, 1991.
6. Rapaport SI: Introduction to Hematology, 2nd ed. Philadelphia: JB Lippincott, 1987.
7. Koepke JF, Koepke JA: Reticulocytes. Clin Lab Haematol 1986; 8:169.
8. Beck WS (ed): Hematology, 5th ed. Cambridge, MA: MIT Press, 1991.
9. Powers LW: Diagnostic Hematology: Clinical and Technical Principles. St. Louis: CV Mosby, 1989.
10. Erslev AJ: Clinical manifestations and classification of erythrocyte disorders. *In* Williams WF, Beutler E, Erslev AJ, Lichtman MA (eds): Hematology, 4th ed. New York: McGraw-Hill, 1990:423–429.
11. Wintrobe MM, Lukens JN, Lee GR: Approach to the patient with anemia. *In* Lee GR, Bithell TC, Foerster J, et al (eds): Wintrobe's Clinical Hematology, 9th ed. Malvern, PA: Lea & Febiger, 1993:715–744.
12. Bessman JD, Gilmer PR, Gardner FH: Improved classification of anemia by MCV and RDW. Am J Clin Pathol 1983; 80:322–326.
13. Bessman JD, Gilmer PR, Gardner FH: Education program of American Society of Hematology, 25th Annual Meeting, Dec 3–6, 1983, pp 54–56.

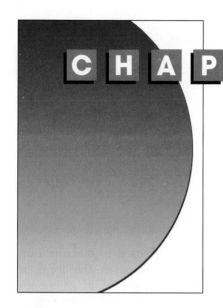

CHAPTER 16

Anemias Caused by Impaired Production of Erythrocytes

Deborah Roper, Susan Stein,
Martha Payne, and Mary Coleman

Outline

Objectives

AFTER COMPLETION OF THIS CHAPTER, THE READER WILL BE ABLE TO

1. Describe peripheral blood and bone marrow morphology characteristic of iron deficiency anemia.
2. Describe iron absorption and metabolism.
3. Describe causes for iron deficiency.
4. Utilize morphology and iron values to distinguish among (a) iron deficiency anemia, (b) sideroblastic anemia and lead poisoning, (c) thalassemia, and (d) anemia of chronic disease.
5. Discuss treatment of iron deficiency anemia.
6. Describe peripheral blood and bone marrow morphology characteristic of megaloblastic anemias.
7. Describe vitamin B_{12} and folate metabolism, including sites and mechanisms of absorption, and carrier proteins.
8. Describe the roles of vitamin B_{12} and folate in nuclear maturation.
9. Describe causes for vitamin B_{12} and/or folate deficiencies.
10. Explain the laboratory testing sequence, including rationale, for the megaloblastic anemias.
11. Discuss treatment of the megaloblastic anemias.
12. Describe the defect in sideroblastic anemias.
13. Summarize the peripheral blood and bone marrow morphology in sideroblastic anemias.
14. Explain the relationship between lead poisoning and sideroblastic anemia.
15. Define aplastic anemia.
16. Compare and contrast aplastic anemia with other types of pancytopenia.
17. List the criteria for diagnosis of severe aplastic anemia.

18. Discuss the etiology and pathogenesis of aplastic anemia.

19. List at least three drug or chemical agents associated with the development of severe aplastic anemia.

20. List at least three biological agents associated with the development of severe aplastic anemia.

21. Describe Fanconi's anemia.

22. Discuss the clinical and laboratory findings in aplastic anemia including clinical signs, peripheral blood and bone marrow findings.

23. Compare and contrast the treatment regimens and prognosis in aplastic anemia: bone marrow transplants, antiviral drugs, immunosuppressive therapy, red cell transfusions, and androgen therapy.

24. Describe the morphologic features of congenital dyserythropoietic anemias (CDA).

25. List characteristics of CDA types I, II, and III.

Among the most common hematologic disorders is iron deficiency anemia (IDA). It is widespread throughout the world and is among the most common human disorders, affecting approximately 30% of the world's population.[1] Iron deficiency anemia is defined as the state in which the body's iron stores are inadequate for normal homeostasis.[2] The most common causes of iron deficiency are lack of dietary iron, insufficient iron absorption, chronic bleeding, and rapid growth in children.[3, 4]

Patients exhibit a variety of signs and symptoms, depending on the degree of anemia, including pallor (skin, mucous membranes, and conjunctivae), lack of energy, and spoon nails (koilonychia). Because iron is a necessary component in the erythrocyte's ability to carry oxygen to the tissue, shortness of breath becomes a major patient complaint as hemoglobin levels decrease. Extreme cases of iron deficiency may result in leakage of electrolytes from the intestines ("leaky-gut" syndrome) and may lead to heart failure and death. Because iron deficiency is so common and so easily treated, the clinical laboratory scientist must be attuned to the sometimes subtle hematologic changes that assist in a rapid diagnosis.

IRON METABOLISM

Iron is absorbed from foodstuffs in the duodenum and jejunum. The amount of absorption depends on several factors, including the amount of stored body iron, the amount and type of iron in ingested food, the status of gastrointestinal mucosa, and the body's need for replacement erythrocytes.

Iron is stored by the liver in one of two forms: ferritin or hemosiderin, with ferritin predominating. The amount of ferritin circulating in the blood stream is in equilibrium with stored ferritin; thus serum ferritin assays can be used to measure iron stores. Biochemically, ferritin is in the form of apoferritin. Apoferritin is composed of 24 monomers of ferritin arranged to form a spherical shell. Hemosiderin is very similar to ferritin except that it is water insoluble and portions of the apoferritin shell are missing. Hemosiderin increases when a rapid turnover of erythrocytes occurs, as in hemolytic anemias, or when a defect in iron metabolism exists, such as in sideroblastic anemias or iron overload states.

Most dietary iron is in the ferric form. Some foods contain more available iron for absorption; for example, meat contains heme iron from both myoglobin and hemoglobin. The body can absorb 20–30% of heme iron. Non–heme iron sources generally are foods of plant origin. Even though most diets contain more non–heme iron sources, absorption is inefficient; only 1–5% of non–heme iron is absorbed. Optimal absorption of non–heme iron occurs when the gastric mucosa pH is less than 4.0 and reducing substances such as ascorbic acid are present. Common foods that inhibit non–heme iron absorption include tea, coffee, whole grain phytates, bran, corn, and the oxalates found in chocolate and spinach.

Another major factor that influences iron absorption is the amount of stored iron. A healthy adult absorbs approximately 5–10% of dietary iron, whereas an iron-deficient individual absorbs 10–20%. Minimum daily requirements (MDR) of iron vary depending on age, sex, weight, and state of health. The recommended dietary allowance (RDA) for adult males is 10 mg/day; for adult females, 15 mg/day; and for pregnant females 30 mg/day.[3] More important than the amount of iron ingested is the amount of iron absorbed. A more complete discussion of iron requirements is discussed later in this chapter.

Iron is absorbed quickly in the ferrous state.

Once in the blood stream, ferrous iron is converted back to the ferric state so that the iron may be bound to transferrin, a beta-globulin that carries iron to the bone marrow for subsequent use in red cell production. Each transferrin molecule can transport up to two atoms of iron, although normally only one third of serum transferrin is saturated. Liver cells (and other iron-storing tissues) have many specific binding sites for the iron-transferrin complexes. These binding sites increase as the need for iron increases and decrease when the liver cells are adequately filled with iron. Some absorbed iron is used by cells as an enzyme cofactor and also in oxidative phosphorylation. The largest amount of iron is transported to the bone marrow to become incorporated into hemoglobin.

The body conserves iron tenaciously. The iron released when senescent erythrocytes are destroyed by the monocyte/macrophage system is retained and recycled into more developing erythroblasts. Iron is normally lost from the body through sweating, skin desquamation, and menstruation in females.

IRON DEFICIENCY

Definition

Iron deficiency is progressive; three stages have been described as leading up to the most severe form, that of iron deficiency anemia. According to the laboratory definition of anemia, a patient's hemoglobin must be below 95% of the reference range for age.[3, 4] Patients' signs and symptoms are also progressive, relating to the presence and degree of anemia.

Stages

In stage 1 (iron depletion), stores of iron in the bone marrow and liver decrease. The patient has no symptoms, and the hemoglobin level is in the normal range. Serum ferritin and bone marrow stainable iron are decreased and are sensitive tests for this stage. The major physiologic consequence is increased absorption of non–heme iron, indicating a greater vulnerability or potential for developing iron deficiency.[3, 4] This stage is relatively common among healthy children.[3]

Stage 2 (iron deficient erythropoiesis) is sometimes referred to as iron deficiency without anemia. Erythropoiesis slows because of lack of iron available for insertion into the heme portion of the hemoglobin molecule.[3, 4] The patient's hemoglobin level begins to decrease, and the raw material for hemoglobin synthesis, free erythrocyte protoporphrin, increases (see Fig. 9–1). This stage is also characterized by an absent or decreased storage iron, low serum iron, elevated total iron binding capacity, and low transferrin saturation. The hematocrit remains near normal. If anemia is present, it is normochromic and normocytic.

Stage 3 (iron deficiency anemia) is the most advanced. Ferritin levels and percentage transferrin saturation levels are very low. Other laboratory indications are absent iron stores, low serum iron, elevated total iron-binding capacity (TIBC), elevated free erythrocyte protoporphyrin, and low hemoglobin levels.[3] In an effort to maintain the correct hemoglobin concentration, more mitotic divisions occur. The result is a microcytic erythrocyte with a normal mean corpuscular hemoglobin concentration (MCHC).[1, 3] Hypochromia finally occurs when the red cells can no longer divide. The hypochromic microcytic red cells then demonstrate the anisopoikilocytosis characteristic of full blown iron deficiency anemia. Figure 16–1 shows that microcytosis occurs before hypochromia. Table 16–1 summarizes the progressive stages of IDA.

Etiology

Iron deficiency affects all ages and both sexes and is seen worldwide. Iron deficiency in infants most often results from milk diets unsupplemented by iron.[5, 6] A typical newborn has stores of approximately 300 mg of iron (80 mg/kg of body weight), all of which was supplied in utero from the mother.[7] The infant requires approximately 160 mg iron during the first year for use in erythropoiesis.[8] Approximately 50 mg are recycled from the destruction of red blood cells during the first week of life; the rest must come from diet. Premature infants will develop iron deficiency without supplements because iron stores are incomplete in utero.[9]

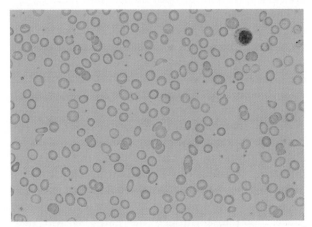

Figure 16–1 Hypochromic, microcytic anemia with increased red blood cell distribution width. Note lymphocyte at upper right.

Table 16-1. DEVELOPMENT OF IRON DEFICIENCY ANEMIA

Stage I: Iron Depletion	Stage II: Iron Deficient Erythropoiesis	Stage III: Iron Deficiency Anemia
Serum ferritin ↓ Bone marrow Iron ↓	Serum ferritin ↓ Bone marrow Iron ↓ Serum iron ↓ TIBC ↑	Serum ferritin ↓ Bone marrow iron ↓ Serum iron ↓ TIBC ↑ Hemoglobin ↓ Hematocrit ↓ MCV ↓ RDW ↑

Abbreviations: TIBC, total iron-binding capacity; MCV, mean corpuscular volume; RDW, red blood cell distribution width. ↑, increased; ↓, decreased.

Another group at risk for iron deficiency is the elderly. They may lack sufficient iron in their diets because they cannot or will not cook adequate meals. Many aged people fall into the habit of quick and easy meals, such as tea and toast. In other age groups, iron deficiency may also be caused by fad or binge diets.

Iron requirements increase with normal growth spurts around 2 years of age and during adolescent years, which begin at age 11 for girls and 14 for boys. Males have twice the lean body mass as females; therefore, the minimum requirement is greater, approximately 3.5 mg/kg. In females, the adolescent spurt is usually coupled with the onset of menstrual periods, and the daily requirement for menstruating females is 2.1 mg/kg.[3] Adolescent females are also at high risk for eating disorders and may fail to supplement their diets with iron.[10] This age group, therefore, is at risk for iron deficiency.

Increased iron requirements also exist in pregnant and lactating females. The developing fetus in the second trimester takes 3–4 mg iron/day from the maternal stores and 6 mg/day in the last trimester.[9] Once nursing, the mother's iron stores are again challenged by the baby. Frequent pregnancies without supplemental iron can result in iron deficiency anemia for both mother and child.

The second most common cause of iron deficiency is chronic blood loss. Adult males do not require as much iron as other age groups or any female group. They are rarely iron deficient due to diet alone. In addition to blood loss with menstruation, however, females may develop chronic bleeding from uterine fibroid tumors or neoplasms.[11] In males and post menopausal females, the most common cause of iron deficiency is occult bleeding from the gastrointestinal tract. Gastrointestinal bleeding can be caused by peptic ulcer, hiatal hernia, gastritis, hemorrhoids, and vascular anomalies.[2] Chronic aspirin ingestion can also cause blood loss through the gut,[12] as will neoplasms and growths such as rectal polyps. Gastritis due to alcohol ingestion may also cause significant blood loss.[2] Other less common causes of blood loss are through hemoglobinuria due to intravascular hemolysis,[13] or recurrent hemoptysis (bleeding in the respiratory tract) resulting from vascular anomalies, infections, neoplasms, idiopathic pulmonary hemosiderosis, or Goodpasture syndrome.[2]

Outside the United States, hookworm infestations are a common source of iron deficiency.[14, 15] The worm, *Ancylostoma duodenale* or *Necator americanus,* attaches itself to the gut wall and sucks blood from submucosal vessels. The amount of bleeding is generally proportional to the number of worms.[16] Excessive blood donation is another recognized cause of iron deficiency.[2]

"Runner's anemia" was first reported in 1981 in a group of Danish runners.[17] It was found that 56% of a group of obviously healthy, top-trained runners were iron deficient with no anemia. The runners were treated with oral iron supplements, and their iron deficiency was corrected. In fact, three male runners broke their personal records. It is especially important that athletes meet their required daily allowances for iron.[18]

Differential Diagnosis

Iron deficiency states must be differentiated from other anemias that appear microcytic and hypochromic. These include sideroblastic anemia, anemias of chronic disorders (see Chapter 19) and thalassemias (see Chapter 18). Table 16–2 summarizes laboratory values in microcytic, hypochromic anemias.

Laboratory Diagnosis

Early stages of iron deficiency pose the greatest diagnostic problems for the clinician. The typical patient does not present with symptoms of anemia or anemia demonstrable through hematologic investigation. Depleted iron stores may be an incidental finding. Owing to lack of non-erythroid iron compound assays in the past, many physicians

Table 16-2. DIFFERENTIATION OF THE MICROCYTIC, HYPOCHROMIC ANEMIAS

	Iron Deficiency	Thalassemia Minor	Anemia of Chronic Disease	Sideroblastic Anemia	Lead Poisoning
Serum ferritin	↓	↑/N	↑/N	↑	N
Serum iron	↓/N	↑/N	↓	↑	Variable
TIBC	↑	N	↓	↓/N	N
Transferrin saturation	↓	↑/N	↓	↑	↑
FEP/ZPP	↑	N	↑	↑	↑ (marked)
BM iron (Prussian Blue reaction)	No stainable iron	↑/N	↑/N	↑	N
Sideroblasts in BM	None	N	None/very few	↑ (ringed)	N (ringed)
Other special tests		↑ Hb A$_2$ (β-thalassemia minor)	Specific tests for inflammatory disorders, rheumatoid arthritis or cancer		↑ ALA in urine ↑ whole blood lead levels

Abbreviations: N, normal; ↑, increased; ↓, decreased; TIBC, total iron-binding capacity; FEP/ZPP, free erythrocyte protoporphyrin or zinc protoporphyrin; BM, bone marrow; ALA, δ-aminolevulinic acid.

continue to choose to treat symptoms of iron deficiency without laboratory investigation. Some physicians also choose to treat high-risk patients with iron supplements to avoid iron deficiency.

In the modern laboratory, several tests are available to assist the physician in assessing iron status. The most sensitive test for iron stores (other than the demonstration of stainable iron in the bone marrow) is the serum ferritin. The presence of a chronic disease, such as rheumatoid arthritis, malignancies, or hepatitis, may result in a normal value and must be interpreted with care. Other sensitive indicators of iron deficiency include increased red blood cell distribution width (RDW), low serum iron (less than 50 μg/dL), increased total iron binding capacity, and low percentage transferrin saturation (less than 15%).

In patients with *classic iron deficiency anemia* (IDA), stage 3, hemoglobin is less than 10.0 g/dL, erythrocyte morphology is consistent with an increased RDW, and certain indices (e.g., mean corpuscular volume) decrease. Red blood cell counts may be greater than 5.50×10^{12}/L in infants and children. The peripheral smear shows striking poikilocytosis, including ovalocytes, elliptocytes, and bizarre forms. Erythrocytes are microcytic and hypochromic. The reticulocyte count is usually normal or decreased, but occasional counts up to 2.0 or 3.0% may be encountered. Leukocyte and platelet counts may be elevated, particularly after a recent blood loss.

Bone marrow examination is usually not indicated in simple IDA due to lack of dietary iron. If the patient is evaluated for apparent chronic blood loss, however, a bone marrow examination may be performed to demonstrate adequate megakaryocytes or absence of tumor in cases where bleeding is due to neoplasms. Typically, stainable iron is

absent in both developing erythroblasts and macrophages. The polychromatophilic normoblast (rubricyte) shows the most striking morphologic changes. This cell is smaller than normal and there is nuclear:cytoplasmic asynchrony with the cytoplasm lagging behind the nucleus. The cytoplasm has been described as "shaggy" and appears basophilic due to poor hemoglobinization. Erythroid hyperplasia is present with a decreased myeloid:erythroid (M:E) ratio most common (Fig. 16-2).

Treatment

Clinical manifestations of IDA were known in ancient times. Iron therapy was used as a "cure" for chlorosis, or "green sickness," in 17th century France.[2,19] Thomas Sydenham, recognized as the father of English medicine, recommended iron or

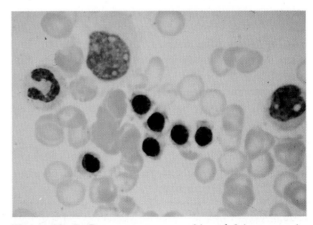

Figure 16-2 Bone marrow smear of iron-deficiency anemia. The late nucleated red blood cells show the characteristic "shaggy blue" cytoplasm due to asynchronism in maturation. (Courtesy of Ann Bell, University of Tennessee, Memphis.)

steel filings, steeped in cold Rhine wine.[20] Pierre Blaud in 1832 described his now famous pills.[21] The pills contained 0.3 g of ferrous sulfate and 0.1 g of potassium carbonate and provided 64 mg of iron per pill. It was only in the 20th century that the cause of chlorosis was directly linked to iron deficiency.

Modern treatment of IDA is very similar to Blaud's pills. Oral iron supplements are usually given as ferrous sulfate.[2,3,4] Side effects of oral iron include epigastric pain, nausea, diarrhea, and constipation.[2] Parenteral iron (iron dextrans) is rarely given, but may be indicated in cases of malabsorption, intolerance to oral iron, or lack of patient cooperation. Nutritional counseling is essential in dietary IDA. In cases of chronic bleeding, correction of the underlying disorder is most desirable. Blood transfusions are rarely warranted because of their hazards, and in most circumstances, there is time to wait for normal mechanisms of erythropoiesis with iron therapy. This allows for the gradual adjustment of the cardiovascular system for the re-expansion of the total circulating erythrocyte volume.[2]

Response to Therapy

The first hematologic response to iron therapy is the appearance of reticulocytes, which reach a maximum (5–10%) on the fifth to tenth day[22] of therapy and gradually return to normal as the hemoglobin increases. The hemoglobin level is the most accurate monitor of anemia in iron deficiency, because red blood cells may temporarily increase during therapy. Red blood cell indices may remain low for up to 3–4 months, as the normal red cell population gradually replaces the microcytic, hypochromic cells of IDA. Treatment must continue for 3–6 months after the anemia is relieved.[22] If treatment is terminated too early, iron stores will not be repleted and relapse may occur.

The rate of change of hemoglobin levels depends on the degree of anemia, with the hemoglobin increasing more rapidly in more severe anemias. Approximately two months are usually required to regain normal values. Other nonhematologic symptoms will generally return to normal within 3–6 months of start of treatment.

If the patient is unresponsive to iron therapy as determined by lack of reticulocytes and lack of hemoglobin improvement, the failure must be evaluated. The following explanations, in order of importance, must be evaluated to explain and correct a treatment failure: (1) incorrect diagnosis; (2) complicating illness; (3) failure of patient to take prescribed dose; (4) inadequate dose or incorrect form; (5) continuing iron loss in excess of intake; and (6) malabsorption of iron.[22]

MEGALOBLASTIC ANEMIA

Before the 1920s, megaloblastic anemia was dreaded as much as leukemia.[23] It is caused by a deficiency of either vitamin B_{12} or folic acid, which are critical nutrients for DNA production and subsequent cell division.[24] Megaloblastic anemias are characterized by abnormally large erythrocytes and precursors and by striking nuclear/cytoplasmic asynchrony.[25] It is thought that the cells are large because of a prolonged intermitotic resting phase or a skipped cell division.[26] All rapidly proliferating cells of the body are affected, but changes are most easily demonstrated in the developing red blood cell precursors.

Morphology

All megaloblastic anemias are hematologically similar, which makes the technologist's job easier. The clinician has the harder task, because there are many reasons for a deficiency of vitamin B_{12} and/or folic acid. These are discussed later in this chapter.

PERIPHERAL BLOOD MORPHOLOGY

The first clues to a megaloblastic anemia lie in peripheral blood studies. Characteristically, there are oval macrocytes and pancytopenia. A few dacryocytes, microspherocytes, and fragments may be present,[27] resulting in an elevated RDW.[28] There is moderate to marked anemia, with hematocrits usually in the low 20s. The mean corpuscular hemoglobin concentration (MCHC) is usually normal. The macrocytosis is reflected by an elevated mean corpuscular volume (MCV), which can range from 100 to 150 fL or more. In uncomplicated megaloblastic anemia, increase in MCV is usually proportional to the anemia; however, coexisting blood disorders such as iron deficiency, thalassemia (alpha or beta), or anemia of chronic disease may prevent the macrocytosis.[29-31] Other red blood cell changes include nucleated red blood cells, basophilic stippling, Howell-Jolly bodies, and Cabot rings.[25] The reticulocyte count is usually low (Fig. 16–3).[25]

The typical white blood cell change seen is hypersegmentation of the neutrophil nuclei.[27] Megaloblastic hypersegmentation is indicated by any neutrophils with six or more lobes or five neutrophils/100 with five or more lobes, with the majority of neutrophils having four lobes (Fig. 16–4).[24,27] Giant bands or metamyelocytes may also be present. When the megaloblastic anemia is complicated by a microcytic anemia, these neutrophil changes will often provide the morphologic clues to the coexistent process.[24]

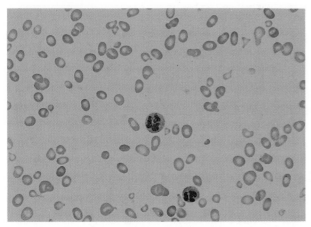

Figure 16–3 Oval macrocytes, other red blood cell abnormalities, and hypersegmented neutrophil in peripheral blood (×50).

BONE MARROW MORPHOLOGY

Megaloblastic anemias show characteristic bone marrow changes. As megaloblastic anemia develops, the first cells to show morphologic changes are the megakaryocytes.[32] They tend to be abnormally large, have decreased granulation, and have a bizarre nuclear appearance.[25,32] Chromatin appears stringy and exploded.

Granulocyte precursors are affected next. Many of these precursor cells become extremely large and have the same chromosomal abnormalities as the red cell precursors. The metamyelocyte is a giant cell, with a sausage-shaped nucleus. Chromatin is irregular and cytoplasm is basophilic with few granules. The segmented neutrophil is hyperlobulated or hypersegmented with greater than five lobes. Normally eosinophils have two to three lobes, but in megaloblastic anemias, it is not uncommon to see more than five lobes.

Red blood cell precursors are affected last as a result of the longer maturation and survival time of the red blood cells in general. All precursors are large, but the nuclear aberrations are cumulative with each division, because DNA replication is involved. Pronormoblasts and basophilic normoblasts (BNB) have particulate open chromatin patterns, described sometimes as "clock-face" or "exploded rice." The cytoplasm is deeply basophilic with a larger perinuclear halo. The nuclear/cytoplasmic asynchrony is most striking in the polychromatophilic normoblast (PNB) and orthochromic normoblast (ONB). The PNB nucleus resembles a BNB and the cytoplasm color is normal for the PNB. The ONB nucleus is not dense and pyknotic as in the normal ONB; instead, it has many spaces. The cytoplasm is greyish-green (Fig. 16–5).

Numerous mitotic figures are seen in the bone marrow, which suggests prolonged times for mitotic divisions. It is not unusual to see PNB and ONB with multiple Howell-Jolly bodies, again suggesting abnormalities in cell division.[25,27] A hypercellular bone marrow is often seen, and an M:E ratio of 1:1 is common because the red blood cell precursors are detained due to nuclear maturation arrest. Red blood cell death in the marrow, because of the abnormal nuclear division causing such delay that the cell disintegrates within the marrow sinuses, results in ineffective erythropoiesis and causes the anemia seen in the peripheral blood.[27] Red blood cell survival is decreased to 27–35 days. The red blood cell death causes a mild hemolytic anemia, as is evidenced by increased serum bilirubin and LDH.[25,33]

Clinical Presentation

Megaloblastic anemias have common symptoms, including those attributed to anemia, granulocytopenia, and thrombocytopenia, as well as gastrointestinal symptoms. In vitamin B_{12} deficiency, neurologic signs and symptoms also occur. Symptoms attributed to the anemia are weakness, palpitation, shortness of breath, easy fatigability, light-headed-

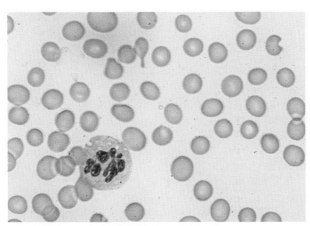

Figure 16–4 Hypersegmented neutrophil in peripheral blood (×100).

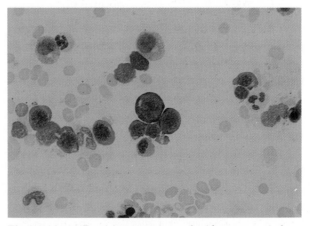

Figure 16–5 Pernicious anemia: erythroid precursors in bone marrow (×50).

ness, and pallor; congestive heart failure may supervene.[33] The granulocytopenia may lead to infection. Purpura due to thrombocytopenia may be present. Patients appear jaundiced as a result of increased bilirubin. Glossitis, or sore tongue, and stomatitis are common. Nausea, usually without vomiting, and constipation or diarrhea may be experienced. These symptoms are due to epithelial cell abnormalities.[34] This disorder and anemia develop slowly and may produce few symptoms until the hematocrit reaches a low level[33] (Table 16–3).

It is critical to correctly diagnose megaloblastic anemia due to vitamin B_{12} deficiency because of the neurologic damage that occurs if it is treated improperly. Megaloblastic anemias due to vitamin B_{12} deficiency, such as pernicious anemia, produce neurologic symptoms, such as tingling of the extremities (pins and needles), numbness, and weakness. Personality changes that may be seen in these patients have been termed "megaloblastic madness."[35] Although the anemia of vitamin B_{12} deficiency responds somewhat to large doses of folate, the neurologic defects are not corrected.

Vitamin B_{12} Metabolism

Vitamin B_{12} is synthesized by bacteria and fungi and is an essential vitamin in animals. As it is not required in plants, plants do not store the vitamin and so are poor dietary sources for man. The best sources are animal products, such as milk, eggs, and liver.[24]

Vitamin B_{12} is the largest vitamin and structurally resembles the porphyrins of hemoglobin and chlorophyll (see Fig. 16–6). Cobalt is the central

Table 16–3. SEQUENCE OF DEVELOPMENT OF MEGALOBLASTIC ANEMIAS

1. Vitamin levels decrease.
2. Hypersegmentation of neutrophils.
3. Macroovalocytosis of PB, megaloblastoid BM.
4. Definite megaloblastic BM.
5. Anemia.

Abbreviations: PB, peripheral blood; BM, bone marrow.
Note: Hypersegmentation of neutrophils is the first sign to manifest in the PB and is the last sign to disappear.[25]

atom and the basis for laboratory measurement of the vitamin in serum. Several forms exist with different side chains. Vitamin B_{12} (also known as cobalamin) is a coenzyme for two reactions in the body: the synthesis of methionine from homocystiene and 5-methyltetrahydrofolate[24,33,36] and the conversion of methylmalonyl coenzyme A to succinyl coenzyme A.[24,33,37,38] The first mechanism may account for impairment of DNA synthesis by trapping of folate in the nonfunctional state of N^5-methyltetrahydrofolate (Fig. 16–7). This impairs thymidylate synthesis and depresses DNA synthesis, causing accumulation of UTP which causes gradual misincorporation into DNA.[33] The mechanism underlying the neurologic damage is not clearly understood but may be related to impairment of methylmalonyl coenzyme A.[33] Both homocysteine and methylmalonic acid are potentially toxic to the body, and vitamin B_{12} assists with detoxification. In vitamin B_{12} deficiencies, both methylmalonic acid and homocysteine accumulate in the plasma and are subsequently excreted in the urine.

Dietary absorption of vitamin B_{12} (cobalamin) in

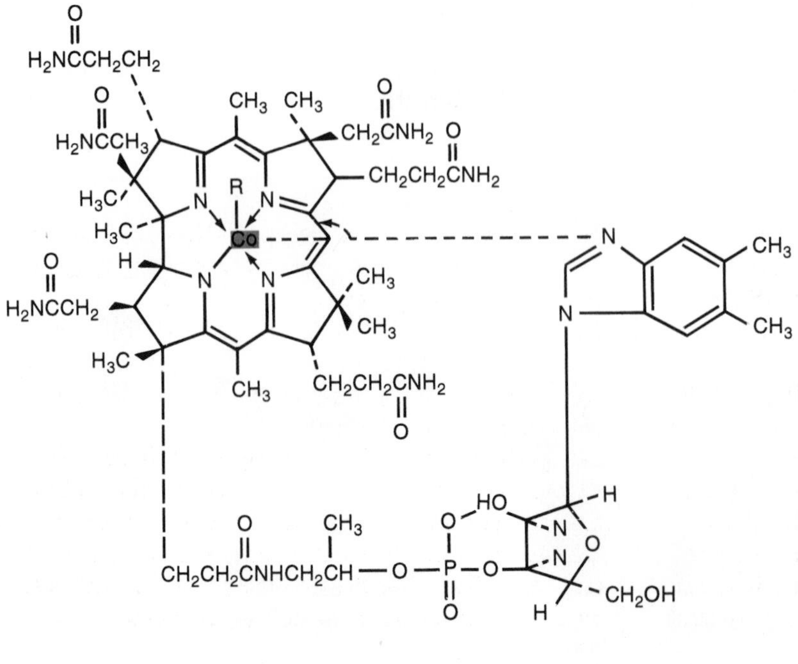

Figure 16–6 Structure of vitamin B_{12}.

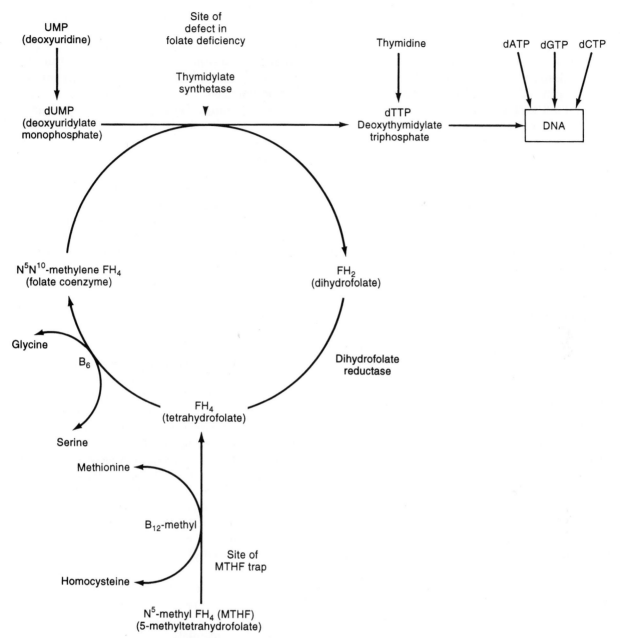

Figure 16-7 Diagram of DNA synthesis, showing folate trap.

the intestine occurs in stages. First, vitamin B_{12} is bound to the protein intrinsic factor (IF). IF is produced by the gastric parietal cells.[39] Patients with achlorhydria due to carcinoma or pernicious anemia produce no stomach acid and no IF. IF acts as a permease so that vitamin B_{12} can be transported across the mucosal cells of the ileum.[24] Pancreatic enzymes are a necessary cofactor for the process.[25] The cobalamin-IF complex binds to receptor sites of the ileal cells. When the cobalamin enters the plasma, it is immediately attached to another binding protein called transcobalamin (TC). IF remains attached to the ileal cells and

never enters the blood stream. TC, as is common with other plasma proteins, has a slightly different structure depending on the site in which it is produced. TCI and TCIII are produced by granulocytes, hence the increase in serum vitamin B_{12} levels in the myeloproliferative diseases. The most biologically active form is the II isomer, a 38,000-mol plasma α-globulin synthesized by hepatocytes. Its only known function is delivery of cobalamin to specific receptors in endothelial cells.[40] In order to deliver the vitamin to the cells, the TCII-cobalamin complex attaches to receptors on the cell membrane and enters the cell by endocytosis.[41]

CAUSES OF VITAMIN B_{12} DEFICIENCY

Dietary Insufficiency. Body stores of vitamin B_{12} are approximately 2–5 mg and the minimum daily requirement recommended by the World Health Organization (WHO) is about 1 μg for adults and 1.3 to 1.4 μg in lactating and pregnant women.[42] A decrease in dietary amounts or increase in need results in anemia in about 15 months. At risk are strict vegetarians (vegans), who consume no meat products, and infants of vegans. Infants who are born deficient and who do not receive supplements may have permanent neurologic damage.[24]

In India, where strict vegetarianism is common, however, few people show neurologic damage. It is thought that bacterial and fungal contamination of food through handling is the source of vitamin B_{12} in Asian countries.[43]

Pernicious Anemia. Pernicious anemia is defined as a lack of vitamin B_{12} absorption due to lack of functional IF.[24] Rare cases of pernicious anemia are caused by a genetically dysfunctional or absent IF. Most cases are caused by antibodies directed to the gastric parietal cells.[24,44] These antibodies can be readily demonstrated in the laboratory. Atrophy of the gastric mucosa reduces parietal cell numbers to the point where too little IF is secreted to handle daily cobalamin requirements.[25] The true pernicious anemia cases are usually seen in patients 50 years and older; however, it may be seen in persons as young as the early 20s. A pregnant woman with circulating IF antibodies can transfer these antibodies to the developing fetus. Most surveys indicate equal incidence among men and women. Although more predominant in whites, it is not absent in blacks, in whom it may appear at an earlier age.[24,37] Among whites, it is more common among those of northern European origin.[24,25]

Biologic Competition. Biologic competition is common in certain geographic areas, such as near the Baltic Sea and in Canada and Alaska, where it is due to infestation with the fish tapeworm, *Diphyllobothrium latum*.[25] Man is infected by eating undercooked or raw fish. The worm is carried in the ileum and can separate the vitamin B_{12}–IF complex and block absorption of B_{12}. Not all carriers of the worm become B_{12} deficient. Those with marginal IF levels become deficient, whereas those with normal gastric secretion do not.[24]

Blind loop syndrome is another recognized cause of vitamin B_{12} deficiency. These patients exhibit B_{12} malabsorption caused by stenotic areas in the small intestine due to anatomic lesions from striction diverticula or surgical blind loops or impaired mobility and subsequent accumulation of bacteria.[25] Bacterial overgrowth is normally prevented by gastric acidity and peristalsis. The bacteria take up ingested vitamin B_{12} before it can be absorbed from the intestine. In these patients, serum folate is often increased because of folate generation by the accumulated intestinal bacteria.

Gastrectomy. Both partial and total gastrectomy cause vitamin B_{12} deficiency because of lack of gastric acid and production of IF.[25]

There are other less common causes for B_{12} deficiency. Immerslund syndrome is select familial B_{12} malabsorption that responds to conventional B_{12} therapy.[24] Patients with chronic pancreatic disease lack pancreatic proteases that help in absorption of vitamin B_{12}. Zollinger-Ellison disease produces too acid an environment for optimal B_{12} absorption.[25] Other causes are congenital lack of TCII[23] and acquired nutritional disorders such as kwashiorkor and marasmus.

Folic Acid Metabolism

Folic acid is present in several forms in nature and in the body. Collectively, the forms found in various parts of the body are known as the "folate pool." Folic acid is present in green, leafy vegetables, liver, meats, and in some fruits, especially oranges and their juice.[24] Folic acid is known to be heat labile, thus, overcooking vegetables and infant formula destroys the folic acid. The main dietary form of folate is pteroylglutamate folate. When ingested, dietary folate undergoes three chemical reactions, including deconjugation, reduction and methylation. The resulting N-5 methyl tetrahydrofolate (N-5-methyl THF) is then absorbed by the mucosal cells of the duodenum and jejunum.[27,45] Once absorbed, the N-5-methyl THF is attached to carrier proteins for transport to the liver and the tissues. Liver stores are very small; consequently lack of folate in the diet rapidly produces a deficient state and subsequent megaloblastic anemia.

As vitamin B_{12} is crucial for DNA synthesis and proper nuclear maturation, folic acid is critical as a coenzyme in several metabolic systems.[33] The reaction that produces the majority of folate deficiency manifestations is the methylation of deoxyuridylate to thymidylate which is an essential preliminary step in the synthesis of DNA (Fig. 16–7). Limitation of thymidylate synthesis impairs DNA synthesis resulting in megaloblastic transformation.[33]

CAUSES OF FOLATE DEFICIENCY

Dietary. Minimum daily requirement is approximately 150–200 μg.[42] Folate requirements are greater in newborn infants, young children and pregnant women, in whom folate is shunted to the developing fetus.[24] For pregnant or lactating women, WHO suggests a 300–100 μg/day supplementation of folate.[24,42]

Deficiency of folate is common in persons with a poor diet, including the elderly, alcoholics, and persons who chronically overcook vegetables. Because body folate reserves are relatively small, folic acid deficiency develops rapidly in individuals with an inadequate diet.[33] It is believed that folate is excreted through the bile and is reabsorbed to the tissues. In alcoholics, however, this excretion is blocked and the folate remains in the liver and unavailable for use.[46]

Increased Need. There are several periods in life during which demand can outstrip supply. The need for folate is especially great in young infants, and in pregnant and nursing mothers.[47,48] Boiled infant formula is a poor source of folic acid. In pregnancy and in the perinatal period, women are advised to take folic acid supplements, both for themselves and their babies.[42] Folate deficiency in the first trimester of pregnancy has been linked to neural tube defects in babies.[24,49] The supplements have been credited with fewer such occurrences.

Chronic Hemolysis. Sickle cell anemia, thalassemia, hereditary spherocytosis, and other chronic hemolytic conditions stress the bone marrow with increased demand for red blood cells.[25] Because folic acid stores are small, after a series of hemolytic crises, the patient may experience a "megaloblastic crisis." Folate supplementation is a necessary tool in management of these patients.

Malabsorption Syndromes. The most common of the malabsorption syndromes causing folate deficiency is sprue. Two types are recognized: tropical and nontropical.[25,33] Tropical sprue is characterized as a wasting disorder with accompanying diarrhea, steatorrhea, and glossitis as seen in the tropics. The cause is unknown; however, some patients do respond to antibiotics. Nontropical sprue is associated with a gluten-induced enteropathy or adult celiac disease. Surgical resection of the intestine and Crohn's disease may also interfere with absorption or cause malabsorption of folic acid.

Folate Antagonists. Some drugs have been implicated in folate deficiency because of their mode of action in the body.[24] Folate antagonists are so named because they inhibit pyrimidine synthesis or they bind folic acid and make it unavailable for use. Examples include methotrexate (a chemotherapy drug), Dilantin (an anti-convulsant), isoniazid (INH) (given for tuberculosis), and pyrimethamine (an antimalarial drug). Oral contraceptives also have been implicated.

Hemodialysis. Patients undergoing hemodialysis for renal failure are susceptible to folate deficiency because folate is lost with the dialysate. Supplemental folic acid is given to these patients.

Testing Sequence for Megaloblastic Anemias

In the laboratory workup for megaloblastic anemias, the following should be considered:

1. MCV: in megaloblastic anemias, the MCV should be greater than 100 fL. A value closer to 125 fL is more common.
2. Peripheral blood smear: characteristic findings are pancytopenia, macro-ovalocytes and hypersegmented neutrophils.
3. Lactate dehydrogenase (LDH): LDH is elevated from rapid cell turnover caused by the premature death of megaloblastic red cell precursors in the bone marrow. Serum bilirubin is usually increased because of this cell destruction.

After the preliminary diagnosis of megaloblastic anemia is established from these three conditions, testing for megaloblastic anemia should continue with analysis of serum vitamin levels, concurrent bone marrow examination, gastric analysis, and the Schilling test.

Vitamin B_{12} levels below 150 pg/mL and/or folate levels below 3 ng/L constitute a deficiency. Formerly, bacterial bioassay with various species of *Lactobacillus* and *Euglena gracilis* were used to determine serum levels of vitamin B_{12} and folate and took several days to perform. Now testing is most commonly performed through radioimmunoassay methods. Vitamin B_{12} and folate can be determined simultaneously with the use of a Co57 isotope.

Most physicians opt to perform bone marrow examinations to demonstrate the characteristic nuclear changes seen in megaloblastic anemias and also to rule out malignancies. Gastric analysis, once routinely performed, now is sometimes still used to demonstrate the characteristic achlorhydria seen in pernicious anemia and/or gastric carcinoma.

The Schilling test consists of two doses of vitamin B_{12}. First, the test dose is given orally. It contains vitamin B_{12} labeled with Co57. One to two hours later, the flushing dose of 1000 mg of unlabeled vitamin B_{12} is given intramuscularly. Urine is collected for 24 hours and radioactivity is determined. The flushing dose saturates the liver binding sites for vitamin B_{12}, thus any radioactivity detected in the urine is indicative of the patient's ability to absorb vitamin B_{12} in the gut. In the patient with pernicious anemia, less than 7% radioactivity is detected in the urine, indicating that vitamin B_{12} is not being absorbed. The test can be repeated administering HCl to provide acidity in the patient's gut so that vitamin B_{12} can be absorbed if IF is present or functional. The test may also be performed with human or hog IF.[24]

The Schilling test should be performed last. The flushing dose of vitamin B_{12} corrects the vitamin deficiency, causes serum vitamin B_{12} levels to rise, and alters the bone marrow picture. A starved marrow will show alteration with normal cell morphology within 6 hours and may show complete remission after 72 hours.

Treatment of Megaloblastic Anemias

Because the metabolism of vitamin B_{12} and folate are closely related, specific therapy is the key to successful treatment of megaloblastic anemias. In a vitamin B_{12} deficiency, it is common for the serum folate to be elevated. Also, pharmacologic doses of vitamin B_{12} will correct a folic acid deficiency and vice versa. If there is a vitamin B_{12} deficiency, treatment with folic acid improves the patient's anemia, but the neurologic manifestations worsen. Pharmacologic doses of vitamin B_{12} are generally given intramuscularly, whereas physiologic doses are given orally. The intramuscular route bypasses the need for intrinsic factor and is essential in the patient with absent or impaired IF, such as those with pernicious anemia, and must be maintained throughout life. A maximal reticulocyte response should be observed by 6–8 days, and a normal hemoglobin by 20 days. Folic acid is given orally for 7–14 days; improvement is evident after 1–2 days.

SIDEROBLASTIC ANEMIA

Etiology and Pathophysiology

The sideroblastic anemias are a heterogeneous group of disorders characterized by ineffective erythropoiesis, elevated body iron stores, and microcytic, hypochromic red blood cells (Table 16–4), but all involve a defective function of the hematopoietic stem cell.[50] A low reticulocyte count and accumulation of iron in the mitochondria of the erythroid precursors (ringed sideroblasts) caused by defective heme synthesis characterizes the sideroblastic anemias.

It is clear that no single defect in heme synthesis accounts for the sideroblast formation in this heterogeneous group of disorders. The defect may be in intramitochondrial heme synthesis, and possibly in pyridoxine metabolism. The role of pyridoxine has been established, because even though sidero-

Table 16-4. DISORDERS INCLUDED IN SIDEROBLASTIC ANEMIAS
Hereditary
X-linked
Autosomal
Acquired
PRIMARY SIDEROBLASTIC ANEMIA (REFRACTORY)
SECONDARY SIDEROBLASTIC ANEMIAS
Drugs and bone marrow toxins
Antitubercular
Chloramphenicol
Alcohol
Lead
Chemotherapeutic agents

blastic anemias are not caused solely by pyridoxine deficiency, some do respond to pharmacologic doses of this vitamin.[50-52] Pyridoxine is a coenzyme in the initial step of protoporphyrin and heme synthesis, the condensation of glycine and succinyl coenzyme A to form aminolevulinic acid (ALA). (See section on heme synthesis in Chapter 9.)

Hereditary Sideroblastic Anemia

Hereditary sideroblastic anemia is a rare X-linked recessive disorder, therefore occurring primarily in males.[53] However, autosome-linked hereditary sideroblastic anemia has also been described.[54] The anemia usually manifests after age 7 or 8 years but may develop within a few months of birth. The anemia is progressive with hematocrit levels in the 20% range. Transfusions may be necessary to maintain an acceptable hematocrit. The stem cell dysfunction may also lead to significant thrombocytopenia and neutropenia.[50] The platelets may exhibit abnormal aggregation patterns and a prolonged bleeding time, which may be clinically manifested by hemorrhage. Neutrophil dysfunction may increase the risk of infection.

LABORATORY FINDINGS

Typically there are low hemoglobin and a low hematocrit. The red blood cell morphology demonstrates a dimorphic population with both normocytic, normochromic and microcytic, hypochromic red blood cells. In the microcytic, hypochromic population, there is a degree of poikilocytosis with target cells and basophilic stippling.[50-52] There may also be a mild to moderate indication of hemolysis.

Bone marrow examination reveals erythroid hyperplasia, but because of ineffective erythropoiesis, anemia is present. Slight megaloblastic changes occur because of the asynchronism between nuclear and cytoplasmic development in the erythroblasts.[50] A main diagnostic feature of sideroblastic anemia is the ringed sideroblast demonstrated by Perls' Prussian blue reaction on bone marrow preparations. This characteristic cell is a nucleated erythrocyte precursor with aggregates of iron surrounding the nucleus (blue staining)[55] (Fig. 16–8). On electron microscopy, these blue inclusions (siderotic granules) are shown to be mitochondria containing deposits of inorganic iron. In normal individuals, 30–50% of marrow erythroblasts contain an occasional siderotic granule which is not within the mitochondria or any organelle.[56] In hereditary sideroblastic anemia, 10–40% of the late erythroid precursors are ringed sideroblasts, whereas in acquired sideroblastic anemia, the ringed sideroblasts are early precursors. The iron stain reveals a marked increase in storage iron, as well. Both myeloid and megakaryocytic precursors may show morphologic abnormalities owing to the clonal nature of the disorder.[50]

Chromosome studies on bone marrow cells frequently show abnormalities such as 5q– and 7q– hypoploidy.[57] Many times the karyotype analysis reveals random loss or breakage in chromosomes. The hypoploid karyotype carries a poor prognosis.

Blood chemistries reveal an elevated serum iron, transferrin saturation, and serum ferritin, with a normal total iron-binding capacity.[50-52] Free erythrocyte protoporphyrin (FEP) levels are elevated in about 30% of patients with sideroblastic anemia.[58]

TREATMENT AND PROGNOSIS

Most patients with hereditary sideroblastic anemias do respond to some degree to pyridoxine in doses of 50–200 mg/day.[59,60] This response may increase the patients' hemoglobin level and decrease the transfusion requirement. In most patients, however, the correction does not totally eliminate the transfusion requirements. Iron over-

loading usually occurs in this disorder and can cause death. Desferrioxamine therapy is used to help chelate excess iron. For those who do not respond well to pyridoxine therapy, removing excess iron by phlebotomy has also been helpful.[61]

Acquired Sideroblastic Anemia

Most sideroblastic anemias are acquired in adulthood and may be considered a part of the myelodysoplastic syndromes (see the discussion of refractory anemia with ringed sideroblasts in Chapter 26); some may be secondary to marrow toxins such as drugs, alcohol, and lead poisoning. Acquired sideroblastic anemia shares with the hereditary form a derangement of heme synthesis, a dimorphic peripheral red blood cell morphology, and ringed sideroblasts in the bone marrow. The ringed sideroblasts are usually more numerous and prominent and appear in early erythroblasts.

ACQUIRED SIDEROBLASTIC ANEMIAS SECONDARY TO DRUGS AND BONE MARROW TOXINS

A reversible sideroblastic anemia may develop after the administration of certain drugs or the ingestion of alcohol. The syndrome includes a dimorphic red blood cell picture with microcytic, hypochromic red blood cells, hyperferremia, and numerous ringed sideroblasts. Some of the drugs that may occasionally cause this side effect are long-term use of the antituberculosis agent isoniazide (INH), especially in combination with other antituberculosis drugs, such as pyrazinamide, cycloserine, and ethionamide.[62] The mechanism involved in the cause of sideroblastic anemia by these drugs is interference with pyridoxine metabolism. Sideroblastic anemia is promptly reversed by administration of pyridoxine or withdrawal of the offending drugs. Other drugs implicated in sideroblastic anemia are chloramphenicol and various chemotherapeutic agents.[63]

Alcohol has a multiple suppressive effect on the bone marrow. Included in the various morphologic abnormalities that may be seen in alcoholism are ringed sideroblasts, associated with hyperferremia and elevated FEP.[64] These changes usually disappear within 2 weeks after the withdrawal of alcohol. Although alcohol does interfere with the conversion of pyridoxine to the coenzyme form of pyridoxyl-5-phosphate necessary for ALA synthetase and although alcoholics may suffer from many nutritional deficiencies, the exact mechanism for the development of sideroblastic anemia in alcoholics is unknown.

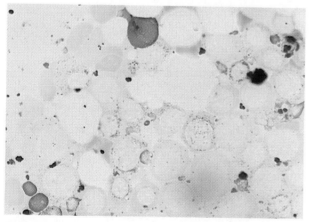

Figure 16–8 Ringed sideroblasts, shown with Prussian blue stain.

LEAD POISONING AND SIDEROBLASTIC
ANEMIA

Lead poisoning interferes with two enzymes in the sequence of heme synthesis, ALA dehydrase and ferrochelatase (heme synthetase).[65] This results in increased ALA and a marked accumulation of FEP in the cytoplasm of the red cell. Biochemically, a patient's profile reveals an elevated FEP, increased ALA excretion in the urine, and normal porphobilinogen. The last distinguishes lead poisoning from acute intermittent porphyria in which porphobilinogen is excreted in the urine.

Anemia does not evolve in chronic lead poisoning until later, unless the exposure is extremely high. In children, the clinical effects of excessive exposure to lead are apparent primarily in the central nervous system. In adults, peripheral neuropathy, abdominal colic, and anemia are the most common manifestations.[65] The anemia is microcytic, hypochromic with more pronounced decreases in hematocrit and hemoglobin in children than in adults. The reticulocyte count is usually elevated to the 10–15% range. Prominent basophilic stippling may occur in lead poisoning as the result of ribosomal DNA and mitochondrial fragments.[66] The bone marrow shows erythroid hyperplasia with increased marrow iron and ringed sideroblasts. Hyperferremia is also present.

APLASTIC ANEMIA

In 1888 Paul Ehrlich described what is believed to be the first reported case of aplastic anemia. The patient had severe anemia, neutropenia, and, on post mortem exam was found to have a yellow hypocellular marrow. The disease was subsequently given the name aplastic anemia by the French physician, A.M.E. Chauffard, in 1904. Aplastic anemia is a hematologic disorder characterized by a deficiency of hematopoietic cells resulting in severe hypoplasia of the bone marrow and pancytopenia in the peripheral blood. There is no evidence of any primary disease infiltrating or replacing active hematopoietic bone marrow tissue. Criteria for the diagnosis of severe aplastic anemia are listed in Table 16–5.

Incidence

The incidence of aplastic anemia in the United States is 2–5 cases per one million population per year. The male to female ratio is 1:1. The risk is 4 to 5 times higher in Japan and Korea.[67] Aplastic anemia can occur in any age group.

Table 16-5. CRITERIA FOR GRADING OF SEVERITY OF APLASTIC ANEMIA

Type	Criteria
Severe aplastic anemia	Peripheral blood: two out of three values decreased Granulocytes $<0.5 \times 10^9/L$ Platelets $<20 \times 10^9/L$ Reticulocytes $<1\%$ (corrected for the anemia) Bone marrow biopsy Markedly hypocellular, $<25\%$ cellularity Moderately hypocellular, 25–50% Normal cellularity with $<30\%$ of remaining cells hematopoietic
Very severe aplastic anemia	Above *plus* granulocytes $<0.2 \times 10^9/L$; infection present.

Differential Diagnosis

A differential diagnosis must be made between aplastic anemia and other pancytopenias which include nutritional depletions, hypersplenism, some infections, consumptive coagulopathies, and marrow infiltrative processes including leukemia, myelofibrosis, and lymphomas (Table 16–6). Aplastic anemia must also be differentiated from other hypoplastic conditions (Table 16–7).

Etiologic Classification

IDIOPATHIC

Acquired aplastic anemia is designated as idiopathic in about 50–75% of cases. In fewer than 25%, a prior exposure to drugs and chemicals, radiation, or a biologic agent can be found. Inherited forms of aplastic anemia also exist[68] and are dis-

Table 16-6. CAUSES OF PANCYTOPENIA

Aplastic Anemia
Marrow infiltrative processes
Acute leukemia
Hodgkin disease, malignant lymphoma
Lipid storage disease
Metastatic carcinoma
Myelodysplastic syndromes
Myelofibrosis, myelosclerosis
Multiple myeloma
Paroxysmal nocturnal hemoglobinuria
Hypersplenism
Infection
Disseminated tuberculosis
Disseminated fungal disease
Nutritional depletions
Vitamin B_{12} deficiency
Folate deficiency
Consumptive coagulopathy

Table 16-7. CAUSES OF HYPOPROLIFERATIVE ANEMIAS

Aplastic Anemia
Pure Red Blood Cell Aplasia
Acquired pure red cell aplasia
Diamond-Blackfan syndrome
Transitory infections
Other Hypoproliferative Anemias
Anemia associated with endocrine abnormalities
Anemia of chronic renal disease

cussed later in this chapter. The etiologic classification of aplastic anemias is listed in Table 16–8.

SECONDARY CAUSES

Two agents traditionally associated with aplastic anemia are chloramphenicol and benzene. California studies from the 1960s indicate chloramphenicol was linked to almost 50% of all drug-associated aplastic anemias. Traditionally two types of chloramphenicol drug-associated aplastic anemia have been described: a reversible dose-dependent type and an irreversible idiosyncratic type. The latter type can appear weeks or months after use of the drug and has a 25% fatality rate. It is believed that chloramphenicol renders the stem cells permanently incapable of differentiating by changing the genetic structure of the cells. The drug, because of its side effects, is not used much any more. It is believed that benzene, found in petroleum products, causes aplastic anemia by suppressing DNA

synthesis in differentiated precursor cells and inhibiting proliferation of progenitor cells.[69]

Two newer drugs that are associated with aplastic anemia are phenylbutazone and hydantoin. Table 16–9 lists drugs associated with aplastic anemia. Some researchers believe that a clear causal relationship between a drug and aplastic anemia has been established in very few instances.[69]

Hepatitis C has been associated with a very severe aplastic anemia. It may be caused by the virus itself or an immunologic mechanism such as production of lymphokines that depress the bone marrow. Other viruses that have been associated with aplastic anemia include the Epstein-Barr virus, cytomegalovirus, and the parvovirus. Parvovirus B19 and its interaction with hematopoietic cells and the immune system has been examined.[69]

Pregnancy and thymoma are other rare causes of acquired aplastic anemia. Aplasia in pregnancy may be related to estrogen inhibition of stem cell proliferation.[68]

In about 20% of paroxysmal nocturnal hemoglobinuria (PNH) patients, the diagnosis is preceded by a frank aplastic anemia. In other patients aplastic anemia develops as the terminal phase of PNH.[70]

Radiation has been associated with aplastic anemia. The mechanism is uncertain, but it is believed that peroxides, ions, and free radicals which damage large molecules generate electrons from the damaged molecules and cause the most damage to marrow and intestinal tissues. Among survivors of the Hiroshima and Nagasaki atomic bombings, however, only a few developed delayed aplastic anemia.[68, 69]

Table 16-8. ETIOLOGY OF ACQUIRED APLASTIC ANEMIA

Idiopathic
Secondary
DRUGS AND CHEMICALS
Cytotoxic agents
Benzene
Chloramphenicol
Nonsteroidal anti-inflammatory drugs
Anti-inflammatory drugs
Antiepileptics
Gold
Other drugs and chemicals
IMMUNOLOGIC
Humoral
Cellular
INFECTIONS
Hepatitis, Epstein-Barr
Bacterial: miliary tuberculosis
METABOLIC
Pancreatitis
Pregnancy
PAROXYSMAL NOCTURNAL HEMOGLOBINURIA
RADIATION

Table 16-9. DRUGS ASSOCIATED WITH APLASTIC ANEMIA

Acetazolamide	Oxyphenbutazone
Acetophenetidin	Penicillamine
Acetylsalicylic acid	Phenytoin
Carbamazepine	Phenylbutazone
Cephalosporins	Phenothiazine
Chloramphenicol	Potassium perchlorate
Chlordiazepoxide HCl	Primidone
Chlorothiazide	Prochlorperazine
Chlorpheniramine	Pyrimethamine
Chlorpromazine HCl	Quinacrine HCl
Chlorpropamide	Salicylamide
Colchicine	Streptomycin
Diphenylhydantoin sodium	Sulfadimethoxine
Epinephrine	Sulfamethoxypyridazine
Gold compounds	Sulfisoxazole
Indomethacin	Sulfonamides
Mezepine	Tolbutamide
Methazolamide	Trimethadione

Hereditary Causes

Hereditary forms of aplastic anemia usually become apparent in the first decade of life. The anemia first described in 1927 by Fanconi, and given his name, is an autosomal recessive form of aplastic anemia. Clinically the patients have brown pigmentation of the skin, microcephaly, short stature, mental and sexual retardation, absence or hypoplasia of the thumb, and hypoplasia of the spleen and kidney. The laboratory results are the same as in acquired aplastic anemia. The bone marrow cells have the i antigen and increased hemoglobin F. Chromosomal studies show increased instability, indicating a defect in rejoining of breaks in DNA chains.

The addition of a mutagenic agent such as diepoxybutane (DEB) to a sample of Fanconi anemia marrow cells causes chromosomal breaks and is usually considered a diagnostic test for the disease.[71]

Estren-Dameshek syndrome has the same hematologic features as Fanconi's but without physical abnormalities. Fanconi and Estren-Dameshek syndromes probably represent the same genetic abnormality.[68, 72]

Congenital erythroid hypoplasia of Diamond-Blackfan manifests in early infancy with chronic anemia, reticulocytopenia, and absent erythroblasts in the marrow.[73] Leukocytes, megakaryocytes, and platelets are normal. Hepatomegaly and splenomegaly may occur and may partially be related to congestive heart failure. The anemia is usually normocytic, normochromic and there may be persistence of the i antigen. Serum and urine erythropoietin levels are increased. Patients may experience growth retardation, failure of sexual maturation, osteoporosis, and portal hypertension. The course of the disease varies and there may be spontaneous remissions in some patients. For patients with insidious and progressive disease unresponsive to other forms of treatment, bone marrow transplantation may be successful.[74]

Other familial forms include Diamond-Blackfan and Shwachman-Diamond syndromes, familial aplastic anemia, and aplastic anemia associated with dyskeratosis congenita or amegakaryocytic thrombocytopenia.[75, 76]

Pathophysiology

Some possible causes of aplastic anemia are abnormal or damaged hematopoietic stem cells, failure of hematopoietic stroma or growth factors, and immunosuppression of hematopoiesis. Experiments have shown that some drugs such as busulfan can damage the stem cell of DNA. Stromal function may be affected or damaged by chemical toxins or viral pathogens, but this probably is not the primary defect in aplastic anemia.

Experimental studies and clinical treatment regimens have provided evidence for immune suppression as the cause of aplastic anemia. In vitro evidence has shown that normal marrow will fail to grow in the presence of an aplastic anemia patient's T suppressor cells. The suppressor cells may promote marrow inhibitor substances such as tumor necrosing factor and γ interferon. Treatment with immunosuppressive drugs has helped in some patients, possibly by suppressing the T suppressor cells themselves. Treatment with high doses of cyclophosphamide has worked successfully in some patients, possibly eliminating an abnormal population of autoreactive cells.[68]

Anti-γ interferon added to culture cells abolishes the T cell suppressor cell effect on the growth factor CFU-GM. Natural killer cells, deficient in aplastic anemia patients, return to normal in over half of the patients treated with antithymocyte globulin. This suggests a possible immune mediation, and further studies are needed. There may also be a viral pathogenesis to aplastic anemia in that is has been demonstrated that chronic parvovirus infection can exist in the bone marrow cells and has been associated with bone marrow aplasia.[67]

Clinical and Laboratory Findings

Aplastic anemia develops insidiously with symptoms relating to the cytopenias. The patient, because of anemia, may have fatigue, irritability, and pallor. Because of thrombocytopenia, bleeding gums, nose bleeds, retinal or other body hemorrhages, or petechiae may appear. Leukopenia may lead to infections and fever. Hepatomegaly and splenomegaly are rarely seen.

Laboratory findings include leukopenia from 0.5 to 3.5×10^9/L. Relative lymphocytosis with an absolute lymphopenia is frequently seen. Deficient or atypical granules may be seen in the neutrophils. There may also be a monocytopenia. Red blood cells are normochromic and may be moderately macrocytic resulting from earlier release of the red cells. The presence of nucleated red blood cells in the blood film is unusual and suggests marrow dysfunction rather than hypoplasia. The reticulocyte count corrected for the anemia is low. Platelet counts range from 25 to 75×10^9/L. Large bizarre forms may be seen. The serum iron is increased, total iron-binding capacity is decreased, and iron saturation is 100%. There may be increased ferritin, especially after transfusions. Erythropoietin levels are moderately to markedly elevated. Vitamin B_{12} and folate levels are normal or slightly elevated. Hemoglobin F may be elevated in children. Because of decreased platelet counts, the bleeding time and clot retraction time are prolonged.

The bone marrow is moderately or severely hypocellular. Less than 30% of the remaining cells are hematopoietic, although there may be some focal areas of normal or hypercellularity. The majority of nucleated cells will be lymphocytes, with small numbers of reticulum cells, fibroblasts, histiocytes, plasma cells, and mast cells. Increased iron stores are present (Figs. 16–9a and 16–9b).

Treatment and Prognosis

Initially the patient's history is reviewed to detect potential etiologic factors which should be avoided or discontinued. Hematologic recovery may occur after an offending drug or toxin is removed. Usually an etiologic factor is identified in less than 25% of the cases, and most patients do not recover despite removing the etiologic agent.

Supportive measures are given to maintain the hemoglobin and platelet levels, and to treat infections. Myelostimulatory therapy, androgen therapy, and hematopoietic growth factor treatment have all been used.

Marrow transplants should be considered if the patient's aplastic condition persists. Bone marrow from human leukocyte antigen (HLA)–identical siblings is used, with an 80% survival rate in patients less than 45–50 years old.[75] Graft versus host disease occurs in 10–15% of cases.

Immunosuppressive therapy has been used successfully in patients. Antithymocyte globulin and antilymphocyte globulin have allowed transfusion independence in 40–80% of patients.[75]

CONGENITAL DYSERYTHROPOIETIC ANEMIA

Patients with congenital dyserythropoietic anemia (CDA) exhibit refractory anemia, ineffective erythropoiesis and abnormalities of bone marrow–nucleated erythrocytes, including giantism, multinuclearity and karyorrhexis. These familial disorders are grouped into type I, II, or III, although some patients exhibit features that may overlap more than one type.

Type I CDA has been observed in both sexes and in siblings, and may become clinically apparent at any time in life. Erythrocytes are slightly macrocytic, anisocytic, and poikilocytic and may exhibit basophilic stippling and Cabot rings. Such characteristics of erythroblasts such as binucleation, multinucleation, megaloblastosis, incomplete nuclear segments, internuclear chromatin bridges, and spongy, unevenly dense nuclear chromatin are necessary for classification as Type I[77].

Type II CDA occurs in families and presents with moderate to severe anemia. Erythrocytes are normocytic, anisocytic, poikilocytic, and may exhibit basophilic stippling. The bone marrow manifests erythroid hyperplasia, and multinucleated erythrocytes are commonly identified.[78] The mature erythrocytes are susceptible to acid hemolysis[79] because a unique hereditary erythroblast multinuclearity with positive acidified serum (HEMPAS) antigen on cell surfaces reacts with an IgM antibody to cause activation of the classic complement pathway and a slight risk for in vivo hemolysis.

Type III CDA may manifest with anemia that is normocytic or macrocytic with up to 30% giant multinucleated erythroblasts in the bone marrow.[80] Erythrocytes from these patients are more readily

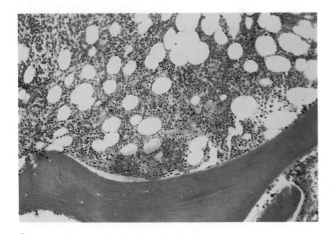

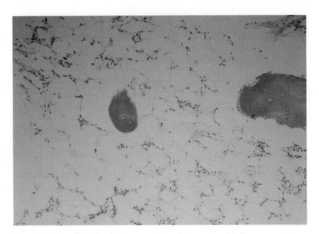

A   B

Figure 16–9 *A*, Normal bone marrow tissue section stained with hematoxylin and eosin (H&E). *B*, Hypoplastic bone marrow tissue section stained with H&E. The patient has aplastic anemia. (*A* and *B*, courtesy of Ann Bell, University of Tennessee, Memphis.)

agglutinated by anti-i antibodies than normal erythrocytes. An abnormal hemoglobin has been detected in one family.

SUMMARY

Production of erythrocytes may be impaired by delay in RNA maturation (hemoglobin development), DNA maturation (nuclear development), or aplasia of hemopoietic cells.

One of the most common disorders seen in the hematology laboratory is iron deficiency anemia (IDA). Iron from dietary sources is stored as both ferritin and hemosiderin with ferritin being the primary storage form. Iron is absorbed in the ferrous state and is converted to the ferric state in the blood stream. There iron is bound to transferrin, a beta globulin transport protein, which carries iron to the bone marrow for erythrocyte production.

Iron deficiency progresses through three stages: iron depletion, iron deficient erythropoiesis, and iron deficiency anemia. In iron depletion there is no anemia, but serum ferritin and bone marrow iron are decreased. In iron deficient erythropoiesis, hemoglobin levels begin to decrease, but not to the frankly anemic level. The ferritin is decreased, serum iron level is low, and total iron-binding capacity is elevated.

In iron deficiency anemia, true anemia exists and is characterized by microcytic, hypochromic RBCs on the peripheral blood smear, in addition to the values found in stages 1 and 2.

Iron deficiency affects all age groups and all populations. Poor diet is the primary cause of iron deficiency worldwide. Particularly at risk are infants and children, menstruating and pregnant females, and the elderly.

The second most common cause of IDA is chronic blood loss. In some countries, hookworm infestations, which suck blood from the gut, are an additional cause.

IDA is usually easily treated with oral supplements. Once hemoglobin has been restored to normal, treatment must continue until iron stores have been replenished.

IDA must be differentiated from other microcytic, hypochromic anemias, including thalassemias and anemia of chronic disease.

Megaloblastic anemias involve delayed nuclear maturation resulting primarily from vitamin B_{12} and folate deficiencies. Cells are abnormally large, and there is often asynchrony between the nucleus and cytoplasm.

In the peripheral blood, there is often pancytopenia with oval macrocytes and hypersegmented neutrophils. The bone marrow exhibits erythrocyte precursors in which hemoglobinization proceeds normally, but nuclear maturation lags behind, giving basophilic normoblasts a "clock face" appearance. Ineffective erythropoiesis results from cell disintegration in the bone marrow sinusoids caused by this delay In addition to symptoms attributable to anemia, neurologic symptoms in vitamin B_{12} deficiency may occur, such as tingling of the extremities and loss of position sense.

Vitamin B_{12} (cobalamin) is bound to intrinsic factor (IF), which is produced by parietal cells of the gastric mucosa. This cobalamin-IF complex is transported to the blood stream by transcobalamin. In the absence of normally functioning parietal cells or IF (e.g., in pernicious anemia), vitamin B_{12} cannot be bound for transport, and synthesis of DNA is impaired. If megaloblastic anemia is a result of impaired IF, parenteral treatment with vitamin B_{12} must be maintained throughout life.

Folic acid is critical in the methylation of deoxyuridylate to thymidilate which is essential in the synthesis of DNA. Folate deficiency is usually dietarily induced and can be replenished with oral folic acid.

When a megaloblastic anemia is suspected from the elevated MCV, characteristic peripheral blood morphology and elevated LDH, testing should proceed through serum vitamin levels, bone marrow exam, and lastly, the Schilling test.

Sideroblastic anemias are characterized by ineffective erythropoiesis, elevated iron stores, and microcytic, hypochromic erythrocytes. One diagnostic finding is the presence of ringed sideroblasts in the bone marrow. Sideroblastic anemia may be hereditary or acquired. Lead poisoning also produces ringed sideroblasts. In addition, there are basophilic stippling, elevated FEP, increased ALA, and a normal porphobilinogen.

Aplastic anemia is characterized by a deficiency of hematopoietic cells, resulting in a hypoplastic bone marrow and pancytopenia in the peripheral blood. The cause may be idiopathic or secondary to drugs, viruses, PNH, or radiation. There are also rare hereditary forms, such as Fanconi anemia.

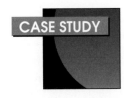
CASE STUDY

Case 1

An 80-year old female was admitted to the hospital with a 6-week history of progressive weakness, shortness of breath, and dyspnea upon exertion. The patient had a history of coronary artery disease with angina. She had been on nonsteroidal anti-inflammatory drugs. Antral gastritis and ulcer were noted on gastroscopic examination.

Admission laboratory values were as follows:

White blood cells (WBC): 8.1×10^9/L
Red blood cells (RBC): 2.90×10^{12}/L
Hemoglobin (Hgb): 5.0 g/dL
Hematocrit (HCT): 0.173 L/L
MCV: 60 fL
Mean corpuscular hemoglobin (MCH): 17.2 pg
MCHC: 29%
Platelets (Plt): 361.0×10^9/L
RDW: 19.9

Serum iron	11 μg/dL	(N: 50–150)
Total iron-binding capacity	404 μg/dL	(N: 250–400)
Percentage saturation	2.7%	(N: 20–40)
Ferritin	3 μg/L	(N: 10–186)

Differential:
Polymorphonuclear neutrophils, 77%
Lymphocytes, 18%
Monocytes, 3%
Eosinophils, 1%
Basophils, 1%

Nucleated red blood cells, 1/100 WBC
Reticulocytes, 3.1%

1. Which of the patient's results are abnormal?

2. What is the likely cause of her anemia?

3. Discuss the relationship between this anemia and the patient's medication.

4. What is the recommended treatment for this patient?

Case 2

A 75-year old male was admitted to the hospital with the differential diagnosis of pernicious anemia or liver disease or tumor.

Admission laboratory values were as follows:

WBC: 2.5×10^9/L
RBC: 1.68×10^{12}/L
Hgb: 7.3 g/dL
Hct: 0.207 L/L
MCV: 123fL
MCH: 45.4 pg
MCHC: 35.2%
Plt: 52.0×10^9/L

Differential:
Polymorphonuclear neutrophils, 27%
Lymphocytes, 65%
Monocytes, 2%
Eosinophils, 6%

Abnormal chemistry values included the following:

LDH: 2130 μ/L (N = 100–190)
Aspartate aminotransferase (AST): 53 μ/L (7–40)
Iron: 68μg/dL (50–150)
Total iron-binding capacity: 196 μg/dL (25–400)
Percentage saturation: 34.7%
Vitamin B_{12}: 150 pg/mL (N = 200–900)
Folic acid: 6 ng/mL (N > 2.5 ng/mL)

1. Which results are abnormal?

2. On the basis of laboratory values, what WBC changes would you expect on the peripheral blood smear?

3. Describe RBC morphologic changes expected in the bone marrow.

4. How can the clinician rule out or establish the preliminary diagnosis of pernicious anemia?

5. Why is it necessary to perform tests to measure vitamin B_{12} levels and do a bone marrow examination before the Schilling text?

REVIEW QUESTIONS

1. The main *diagnostic* feature of sideroblastic anemia is
   a. ringed sideroblasts
   b. oval macrocytes
   c. erythroid hyperplasia
   d. hypersegmented neutrophils

2. A prominent morphologic clue to lead poisoning is the presence of
   a. macrocytic, normochromic anemia
   b. dacryocytes
   c. basophilic stippling
   d. codocytes

3. The biochemical test which differentiates between lead poisoning and acute intermittent porphyria is
   a. free erythrocyte protoporphyrin (FEP)
   b. porphobilinogen in urine (PBG)
   c. aminolevulinic acid (ALA)
   d. ferritin

4. The diagnosis for severe aplastic anemia is associated with all of the following *except*
   a. granulocytes < 0.5 × 10^9/L
   b. platelets < 20 × 10^9/L
   c. reticulocytes <1% corrected
   d. lymphocytes <0.5 × 10^9/L

5. Etiologic factors of aplastic anemia include all of the following *except*
   a. myelofibrosis, myelophthisic anemia
   b. paroxysmal nocturnal hemoglobinuria
   c. hydantoin, phenylbutazone
   d. viral infections

6. The most consistent finding in aplastic anemia is
   a. neutropenia, anemia
   b. hypocellularity, lymphocyte proliferation
   c. anemia, nucleated red cells, splenomegaly
   d. reticulocytosis, pancytopenia

References

1. DeMayer E, Adiels-Tegman M: The prevalence of anemia in the world. World Health Stat Quart 1985; 38:302.
2. Fairbanks VF, Beutler E: Iron deficiency. *In* Williams WJ, Beutler E, Erslev AJ, Lichtman MA (eds): Hematology, 4th ed. New York: McGraw-Hill, 1990:482–505.
3. Dallman PR, Yip R, Oski FA: Iron deficiency and related nutritional anemias. *In* Nathan DG, Oski FA (eds): Hematology of Infancy and Childhood, 4th ed. Philadelphia: WB Saunders, 1993: 413–450.
4. Bothwell TH, Charlton RW, Cook JD, Finch CA: Iron Metabolism in Man. Boston: Blackwell, 1979.
5. Stekwl A, Olivares M, et al: Absorption of fortification iron from milk formulas in infants. Am J Clin Nutr 1986; 43:917.
6. Tunnessen WW, Oski FA: Consequences of starting whole cow milk at six months of age. J Pediatr 1987; 111:813.
7. Rios E, Lipschitz DA, Cook JD, Smith NJ: Relationship of maternal and infant iron stores as assessed by determination of plasma ferritin. Pediatrics 1975; 55:694.
8. Sculman I: Iron requirements in infancy. JAMA 1961; 175:118.
9. Lukens JN: Iron metabolism and iron deficiency. *In* Miller DR, Baehner RL (eds): Blood Diseases of Infancy and Childhood, 6th ed. St. Louis: CV Mosby, 1990.
10. Ten States Nutrition Survey (publication No. 72–8131). Washington, D.C.: U.S. Department of Health, Education, and Welfare, 1972.
11. Jacobs A, Butler EB: Menstrual blood loss in iron deficiency anemia. Lancet 1965; 2:407.
12. Roth WA, Waldes-Dapena A, Pieses P, Buchman E: Topical action of salicylates in gastrointestinal erosion and hemorrhage. Gastroenterology 1963; 44:146.

13. Sears DA, Anderson PR, Foy AL, et al: Urinary iron excretion and renal metabolism of hemoglobin in hemolytic diseases. Blood 1966; 28:708.
14. Farid A, Patwardham VN, Darby WJ: Parasitism and anemia. Am J Clin Nutr 1969; 22:498.
15. Bryan CP: The Papyrus Ebers. New York: Appleton-Century-Crofts, 1931.
16. Layrisse M, Roche M: The relationship between anemia and hookworm infection. Am J Hyg 1964; 79:279.
17. Hunding A, Jordal R, Paulev PE: Runner's anemia and iron deficiency. Acta Med Scand 1981; 209:315.
18. Weaver CM, Rajaram S: Exercise and iron status. J Nutr (US) 1992; 122:782.
19. London IM: Iron and heme: crucial carriers and catalysts. *In* Wintrobe MM (ed): Blood, Pure and Eloquent, 1st ed. New York: McGraw-Hill, 1980.
20. Latham RG: The Works of Thomas Sydenham, M.D., vol 11. London: C. and S. Allard, 1850.
21. Blaud P: Sur les maladies chlorotiques, et sur un mode de traitement spécifique dans ces affections. Rev Med Franc Étrang 1832; 45:341–367.
22. Lee GR: Iron deficiency and iron-deficiency anemia. *In* Lee GR, Bithell TC, Foerster J, et al (eds): Wintrobe's Clinical Hematology, 9th ed. Philadelphia: Lea & Febiger, 1993.
23. Wintrobe MM: Hematology, The Blossoming of a Science: A Story of Inspiration and Effort. Philadelphia: Lea & Febiger, 1985.
24. Cooper BA, Rosenblatt DS, Whitehead VM: Megaloblastic anemias. *In* Nathan DG, Oski FA (eds): Hematology of Infancy and Childhood, 4th ed. Philadelphia: WB Saunders, 1993: 354–390.
25. Babior BM: Erythrocyte disorders. Anemia related to disturbance of DNA synthesis (megaloblastic anemias). *In* Williams WJ, Beutler E, Erslev AJ, Lichtman MA (eds): Hematology, 4th ed. New York: McGraw-Hill, 1990: 453–481.
26. Steinberg SE, Fonda S, Campbell CL, Hillman RS: Cellular abnormalities of folate deficiency. Br. J. Haematol 1983; 54:605.
27. Jandl JH: Blood: Textbook of Hematology, 1st ed. Boston: Little, Brown, 1987.
28. Bessman JD, Gilmer PR, Jr, et al: Improved classification of anemias by MCV and RDW. Am J Clin Pathol 1983; 80:322.
29. Herbert V: Biology of disease. Megaloblastic anemias. Lab Invest 1985; 52:3.
30. Spivak JL: Masked megaloblastic anemias. Arch Intern Med 1982; 142:2111.
31. Green R, Kuhl W, Jacobsen R, et al: Masking of macrocytosis by alpha-beta chain deletions in blacks with pernicious anemia. N Engl J Med 1982; 307:1322.
32. Epstein RD: Cells of the megakaryocyte series in pernicious anemia. Am J Med 1958; 25:198.
33. Beck WS: Megaloblastic anemias I. *In* Hematology, 5th ed. Cambridge, MA: MIT, 1991.
34. Hoffbrand AV, Pettit JE: Essential Haematology, 3rd ed. Blackwell, London, 1993.
35. Smith ADM: Megaloblastic madness. Br Med J 1960; 281:1036.
36. Taylor RT: B_{12}-dependent methionine biosynthesis. *In* Dolphin D (ed): B_{12}: Biochemistry and Medicine, vol. 2. New York: Wiley, 1982.
37. Chananin I: The Megaloblastic Anaemias. London: Blackwell, 1979.
38. Retey J: Methylmalonyl-CoA mutase. *In* Dolphin D (ed): B_{12}: Biochemistry and Medicine, vol. 2. New York: Wiley, 1982.
39. Hardistry RM, Weatherall DJ: Blood and Its Disorders. London: Blackwell, 1982.
40. Hom BL, Ahlowalia BK: The vitamin B_{12} binding capacity of transcobalamin I and II of normal human serum. Scand J Haematol 1986; 5:64.
41. Suda R, et al: Receptor distribution and the endothelial uptake of transcobalamin II in liver cell suspensions. Blood 1985; 65:795.

42. Beaton, G: Requirements of Vitamin A, Iron, Folate, and Vitamin B_{12}: Report of a Joint FAO/WHO Expert Consultation. Rome: Food and Agriculture Organization of the United Nations, 1988.
43. Herbert V: Vitamin B_{12}: Plant sources, requirements, and assay. Am J Clin Nutr 1988; 48:852.
44. DeAzpurua HJ, Cosgrove LH, Ungar B, Toh BH: Autoantibodies cytotoxic to gastric parietal cells in serum of patients with pernicious anemia. N Engl J Med 1983; 309:625.
45. Rosenberg IH, Godwin HA: The digestion and absorption of dietary folate. Gastroenterology 1971; 60:445.
46. Hillman RS, McGuffin R, Campbell C: Alcohol interference with folate enterohepatic cycle. Trans Assoc Am Phys 1978; 91:145.
47. Shojania M: Folic acid and vitamin B_{12} deficiency in pregnancy and in the neonatal period. Clin Perinatol 1984; 11:2.
48. Ball EW, Giles C: Folic acid and vitamin B_{12} levels in pregnancy and their relation to megaloblastic anemia. J Clin Pathol 1964; 17:165.
49. Mulinare J, Cordero JF, et al: Periconception use of multivitamins and the occurrence of neural tube defects. JAMA 1988; 260:3141.
50. Bridges KR. Iron metabolism and sideroblastic anemia. *In* Nathan DG, Oski FA (eds): Hematology of Infancy and Childhood, 4th ed. Philadelphia: WB Saunders, 1993.
51. Bottomley SS. Sideroblastic anemia. Clin Haematol 1982; 11:389.
52. Beutler E. Hereditary and secondary acquired sideroblastic anemias. *In* Williams WJ, Beutler E, Allan JE, Lichtman MA (eds): Hematology, 4th ed. New York: McGraw-Hill, 1990:554–557.
53. Polino G, Ramella S, et al: Iron loading in congenital dyserythropoietic anemias and congenital sideroblastic anemias. Br J Haematol 1983; 54:649.
54. Kasturi J, Basha HM, et al: Hereditary sideroblastic anemia in four siblings of a Libyan family: autosomal inheritance. Acta Haematol 1982; 68:326.
55. Cartwright GE, Deiss A: Sideroblasts, siderocytes, and sideroblastic anemia. N Engl J Med 1975; 292:185.
56. Hansen HA, Weinfeld A. Hemosiderin estimation and sideroblast counts in the differential diagnosis of iron deficiency and other anemias. Acta Med Scand 1959; 165:333.
57. Neinhuis AW, Bunn A, et al: Expression of the human c-fms proto-oncogene in hematopoietic cells and its deletion in the 5q- syndrome. Cell 1985; 42:421.
58. Romslo I, Brun A, et al: Sideroblastic anemia with markedly increased free erythrocyte protoporphyrin without dermal photosensitivity. Blood 1982; 59:628.
59. Horrigan DL, Harris JW: Pyridoxine responsive anemia. Analysis of 62 cases. Adv Intern Med 1964; 12:103.
60. Mason DY, Emerson PM: Primary acquired sideroblastic anemias: response to treatment with pyridoxyl-5-phosphate. Br Med J 1973; 1:389.
61. Hines JD: Effect of pyridoxine plus chronic phlebotomy on the function and morphology of bone marrow and liver in pyridoxine-responsive sideroblastic anemia. Semin Hematol 1976; 13:133.
62. Verwilghen R, et al: Antituberculosis drugs and sideroblastic anemia. Br J Haematol 1965; 11:92.
63. Jandl JH: The hypochromic anemias and other disorders of iron metabolism. *In* Jandl JH (ed): Blood: Textbook of Hematology, 1st ed. Boston: Little, Brown, 1987.
64. Conrad ME, Barton C: Anemia and iron kinetics in alcoholism. Semin Hematol 1980; 17:149.
65. Piomelli S: Lead poisoning. *In* Nathan DG, Oski FA (eds): Hematology of Infancy and Childhood, 4th ed. Philadelphia: WB Saunders, 1993.
66. Paglia DE, Valentine WN, et al: Effects of low level lead exposure on pyrimidine-50 nucleotidase and other erythrocyte enzymes. Possible role of pyrimidine-5′ nucleotidase in the pathogenesis of lead-induced anemia. J Clin Invest 1975; 56:1164.
67. Bjorkholm M: Aplastic anemia: pathogenetic mechanisms and treatment with special reference to immunomodulation. J Intern Med 1992; 231:575–582.

68. Adamson JW, Erslev AJ: Aplastic anemia. *In* Williams WJ, Beutler E, Erslev AJ, Lichtman MA (eds): Hematology, 4th ed. New York: McGraw Hill, 1990:158–174.

69. Young NS: The pathogenesis and pathophysiology of aplastic anemia. *In* Hoffman R, Benz Jr EJ, Shattil SJ, et al (eds): Hematology. Basic Principles and Practice. New York: Churchill Livingstone, 1991:122–160.

70. Bick RL: Paroxysmal nocturnal hemoglobinuria. Laboratory Med 1994; 25:148–151.

71. Stewart FM: Hypoplastic/aplastic anemia. Med Clin North Am 1992; 76:683–697.

72. Gordon-Smith EC, Rutherford TR: Fanconi anemia: constitutional aplastic anemia. Semin Hematol 1991; 28:104–112.

73. Diamond LK. Congenital (erythroid) hypoplastic anemia. Adv Pediatr 1976; 122:349–378.

74. Iriondo A, Garijo J, Baro J, et al: Complete recovery of hemopoiesis following bone marrow transplant in a patient with unresponsive congenital hypoplastic anemia (Blackfan-Diamond syndrome). Blood 1984; 64:348–351.

75. Champlin RE: Aplastic anemia. *In* Bick RL (ed): Hematology. St. Louis, Mosby, 1993:471–481.

76. Alter BP, Young NS: The bone marrow failure syndromes. *In* Nathan DG, Oski FA (eds): Hematology of Infancy and Childhood, 4th ed. Philadelphia: WB Saunders, 1993:216–316.

77. Heimpel H, Forteza-Vila J, Queisser W, Spiertz E: Electron and light microscopic study of the erythroblasts of patients with congenital dyserythropoietic anemia. Blood 1971; 37:299–310.

78. DeLozzio CB, Valencia JI, Acame E: Chromosomal studies in erythroblastic endoploidy. Lancet 1962: 11:1004–5.

79. Crookston JH, Crookston MC, Burnie KL, et al: Hereditary erythroblastic multinuclearity associated with a positive acidified-serum test: a type of congenital dyserythropoietic anaemia. Br J Haematol 1969; 17:11–26.

80. Wolff JA, VonHofe FH: Familial erythroid multinuclearity. Blood 1951; 6:1274–1283.

CHAPTER 17

Anemias Caused by Increased Destruction of Erythrocytes

Martha Payne, Ann Bell, and
Sally Hamby

Outline

Objectives

AFTER COMPLETION OF THIS CHAPTER, THE READER WILL BE ABLE TO

1. Describe the membrane defects and membrane skeletal abnormalities associated with hereditary spherocytosis (HS).
2. Describe the hematologic and chemical laboratory results associated with the hemolytic process in HS.
3. Describe the peripheral blood and bone marrow morphology that is characteristic of HS.
4. Explain the clinical findings, therapy, and prognosis of HS.
5. Describe the osmotic fragility results in HS.
6. Describe the membrane defects and skeletal protein abnormalities associated with hereditary elliptocytosis (HE) and hereditary pyropoikilocytosis (HPP).
7. List laboratory results that are associated with HE.
8. List hematologic and chemical laboratory results that are associated with the hemolytic process of HPP.
9. Describe the morphology of red blood cells in the peripheral blood in the different types of HE.
10. Describe the peripheral blood and bone marrow morphology characteristic of HPP.
11. Explain the thermal sensitivity of red blood cells in HPP and the testing procedure.
12. List and explain the inherited disorders of red blood cell cation permeability and volume.
13. Explain the genetic inheritance pattern and the pathophysiology of glucose-6-phosphate dehydrogenase (G-6-PD) deficiency.
14. List the clinical and laboratory findings that would identify an individual with G-6-PD deficiency.
15. List the causes of hemolytic episodes in G-6-PD deficiency.

16. Define Heinz bodies and explain their relevance to G-6-PD deficiency.
17. State the principle of the screening test for G-6-PD deficiency.
18. Name the most common enzyme deficiency in the glycolytic pathway.
19. List the clinical findings of an individual with pyruvate kinase deficiency.
20. Give the principle of the screening test for pyruvate kinase deficiency.
21. Define porphyrias and explain the basic mechanism for the hereditary diseases.
22. Explain the main defect in paroxysmal hemoglobinuria (PNH).
23. Classify the subpopulation of PNH erythrocytes according to their susceptibility to complement-mediated lysis.
24. Describe the hemolytic anemia and the nocturnal hemoglobinuria that may be associated with PNH.
25. Give the principle of the sugar water test and the Ham test and the results expected for PNH.
26. List the five characteristics of thrombotic thrombocytopenic purpura.
27. Describe red blood cell morphology in thrombotic thrombocytopenic purpura.
28. State the triad of characteristics of hemolytic uremic syndrome.
29. Name the most common cause of hemolytic anemia worldwide.
30. Give the life cycle of the malarial parasite.
31. List at least four characteristics that distinguish *Plasmodium vivax*.
32. List three characteristics of *Plasmodium malariae*.
33. List three characteristics of *Plasmodium falciparum*.
34. Distinguish *Babesia microti* from *Plasmodium falciparum*.
35. Describe morphologic red cell changes in patients with third-degree burns involving more than 20% of the body.
36. Explain traumatic cardiac hemolytic anemia occurring after corrective cardiac surgery with aortic valve replacement.

INTRACORPUSCULAR ABNORMALITIES OF ERYTHROCYTES

Hereditary Defects of the Red Blood Cell Membrane

BIOCHEMISTRY AND STRUCTURE OF THE NORMAL RED BLOOD CELL MEMBRANE

The red blood cell (RBC) membrane has been studied in great detail. It consists of two interrelated parts: the outer bilayer of lipids with integral proteins embedded in it and the underlying protein membrane skeleton (see Fig. 8–11).[1, 2] The insoluble lipid portion of the membrane serves as a barrier to separate the vastly different ion and metabolite concentrations of the interior of the RBC from its external environment, the blood plasma.[1] The protein portion of the membrane is responsible for the shape, structure, and deformability of the RBC. It also contains the pumps and channels for the movement of ions and other material between the RBC's interior and the blood plasma. Various proteins in the membrane also act as receptors, RBC antigens, and enzymes. A more detailed discussion of the RBC membrane is included in Chapter 8; the reader is encouraged to review that chapter when studying defects in the membrane.

CLASSIFICATION OF HEREDITARY DEFECTS OF THE RED BLOOD CELL MEMBRANE

Hereditary defects of RBC membranes have historically been classified by morphologic features. The two major disorders are hereditary spherocytosis (HS), characterized by microspherocytes, and hereditary elliptocytosis (HE), characterized by a large number of elliptical RBCs (Fig. 17–1). Other rare membrane disorders include hereditary stomatocytosis (hydrocytosis), characterized by water-logged RBCs, and hereditary xerocytosis (desiccocytosis), characterized by dehydrated, shrunken red cells. Hereditary pyropoikilocytosis (HPP), now thought to be a variant of HE, involves bizarrely shaped, shrunken, and dehydrated cells that hemolyze when heated to temperatures 2–3 °C below that required for normal RBCs to hemolyze (49 °C).

Research has increased our knowledge of specific defects in the membrane skeleton that are associated with these morphologic abnormalities and clinical syndromes.

Hereditary Spherocytosis

History and Mode of Inheritance

HS is a hemolytic anemia characterized by numerous microspherocytes on the peripheral blood smear. It was first described in 1871 by Belgian physicians Vanlair and Masius.[3] In 1890, Wilson first identified the spleen as the cause of the anemia,[4] and at the turn of the century, Minkowski and Cauffard defined osmotic fragility and reticulocytosis as the hallmarks of the disease.[5] Its incidence is worldwide but is highest in Northern Europeans, in whom rates of 1 in 5000 persons have been reported. Among whites, it is the most commonly inherited anemia, with an incidence in the United States of approximately 220 per million. In 75% of families, it is inherited as an autosomal dominant trait expressed in heterozygotes who have one parent who is also affected. No homozygotes for this form of HS have been identified, suggesting possible incompatibility with life. In approximately 25% of cases, neither parent has this abnormality; thus, a recessive form of the disease apparently exists. A decreased penetrance of a dominant gene or a new mutation has also been suggested for some of these 25%.[6-8]

Pathophysiology (Table 17–1)

Almost all patients who have HS have some degree of spectrin deficiency of the membrane skele-

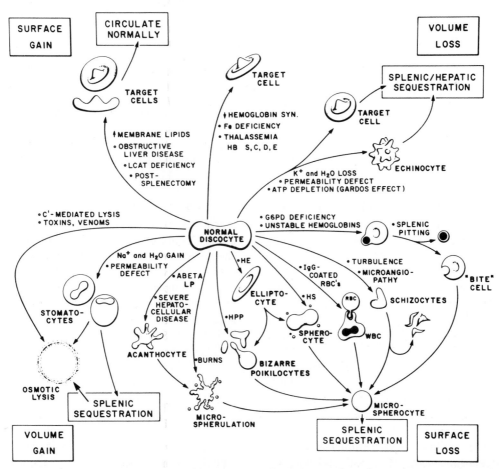

Figure 17–1 Schematic overview of major abnormalities of red blood cell shape and membranes in terms of their relative effects on red blood cell volume and surface area. (From Nathan DG, Oski FA: Hematology of Infancy and Childhood, 4th ed. Philadelphia: WB Saunders, 1993:557. Adapted from Lux SE, Glader BE: Hemolytic Anemias III. Membrane and Metabolic Disorders. *In* Beck WS (ed): Hematology. Cambridge, MA: MIT Press, 1977:269–298.)

Table 17-1. HEREDITARY DEFECTS OF RED BLOOD CELL SKELETAL PROTEINS IN SPHEROCYTES

Protein Deficit	Hereditary Characteristics
AUTOSOMAL DOMINANT SPHEROCYTOSIS	

Mild-to-moderate
   spectrin deficiency
      (spectrin = 60–90% of normal)
	Common (~75% of patients with HS have it)
	Usually comparable degree of ankyrin deficiency
	Severity proportional to spectrin/ankyrin deficiency

Primary ankyrin deficiency
   (ankyrin = 50–90%)
	Common and usually a similar degree of spectrin
	   deficiency

Ankyrin Prague	Small ankyrin content due to deletion of midpoint of regulatory domain

Primary protein 3 deficiency
   (protein 3 = 65–85%)
	Mild HS
	Probably 10–15% of dominant HS
	Normal or near-normal
	   spectrin content
	Not proved that primary defect is protein 3

AUTOSOMAL RECESSIVE HEREDITARY SPHEROCYTOSIS
Moderate-to-severe
   spectrin deficiency
      (spectrin = 30–75%)
	Less common (25%)
	Parents are silent carrier
	Expressed in homozygous state

PROTEIN 4.2 DEFICIENCY
   Heterozygous
      (protein 4.2 = 50%)
   Homozygous
      (protein 4.2 = 0%)
	Silent carrier
	Normal morphology
	May be common in Japanese
	Spherocytic or ovalostomatocytes
	Normal RBC spectrin
	Mild-to-moderate hemolytic anemias

HS, hereditary spherocytosis; RBC, red blood cells.

ton. The degree of deficiency correlates with the severity of the disease and with the degree of spherocytosis measured by the osmotic fragility test. As the molecular basis of more families with the disease is determined, it becomes apparent that the disorder is a heterogeneous group of spectrin and other membrane protein defects. Dominant HS has been linked to the ankyrin gene on chromosome 8 and is associated with defects in beta-chain spectrin.[6, 9, 10] Recent studies have shown that a combined spectrin and ankyrin deficiency is common in patients with HS.[11] Most autosomal dominant HS patients are deficient in both proteins to a similar degree. Other families with autosomal dominant HS have been linked to a protein 3 decrease.[12] Recessive HS is usually associated with defects in alpha-chain spectrin[13] or protein 4.2.[14] These membrane skeletal protein abnormalities cause the RBC to progressively lose membrane and therefore acquire a decreased surface-to-volume ratio and a spheroidal shape on the blood smear. These cells are rigid and are not as deformable as normal bioconcave disc RBCs, and their survival in the spleen is decreased.[15] The spleen selectively sequesters spherocytes from HS as they squeeze through spaces in the endothelial cells of the venous sinuses. As these spherocytes move more slowly through the narrow, elliptical fenestrations of the splenic sinusoids, which are smaller

than RBCs, they are especially susceptible to even further membrane loss and become so damaged that they are selectively removed by the macrophages of the red pulp of the spleen.[6]

The mechanism of this splenic conditioning and HS RBC destruction is uncertain. Various suggestions have been proposed to explain this phenomenon (Fig. 17-2). The longest-held theory is that because of the low glucose level in the spleen, less adenosine triphosphate is produced for these already leaky, membrane-defective cells. The cation pumps cannot maintain their electrolyte balance; therefore, the cells take on water and lyse. However, research has proved that this phenomenon could occur only if the cells were repeatedly metabolically deprived as they went through the spleen several times.[16] Other theories have suggested that HS RBCs have increased susceptibility to the acidic, oxidant-rich environment of the spleen because of their membrane abnormalities.[6] Other evidence points to another possible critical factor in splenic conditioning: splenic macrophage processing of the HS cells that results from their abnormal membranes.[6, 17] Whatever the mechanism, the life span of these HS RBCs is decreased, and a hemolytic process is present. Splenectomy, although it does not correct the basic defect of the cell, does increase the life span of these RBCs and corrects the hemolysis or anemia if present.[6]

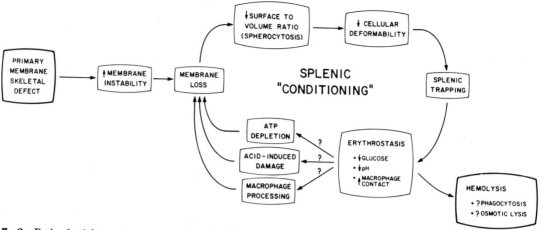

Figure 17–2 Pathophysiology of splenic conditioning and destruction of hereditary spherocytes. (From Nathan DG, Oski FA: Hematology of Infancy and Childhood, 4th ed. Philadelphia: WB Saunders, 1993:569.)

Clinical and Laboratory Findings

The three key clinical manifestations with which HS patients usually present are anemia, jaundice, and splenomegaly.[6, 18] Mild cases may not show all three of these signs. HS may manifest itself in early childhood, young adulthood, or even in old age. Children may be only minimally anemic most of the time because the bone marrow production of erythrocytes can increase to compensate for the increased hemolysis. Patients may be subject to various crises, classified as hemolytic, aplastic, and megaloblastic.[6] The hemolytic crises occur most frequently but are usually not severe. They are often associated with viral syndromes, and children may develop transient jaundice. During viral infections, often caused by parvovirus B19 (commonly called the fifth disease of childhood), which invades hematopoietic stem cells and inhibits their growth, the bone marrow function may decrease (aplastic crises) and the young patient may become rapidly and severely anemic.[19] These crises usually are observed in the first 6 years of life. Many HS patients may also have a folic acid deficiency resulting from the increased needs for this vitamin during chronic increased cell production in the bone marrow. This phenomenon is termed *megaloblastic crisis* and is particularly acute during pregnancy and during recovery from an aplastic crisis.[6] All HS patients with hemolytic anemia should routinely receive folic acid supplements. Quite often, however, the bone marrow compensates for the increased destruction well enough; therefore, HS is detected in adult life only when splenic enlargement increases with increased hemolysis and less efficient bone marrow compensation occurs, resulting in jaundice or anemia. Adults may present with the sudden onset of more severe jaundice, caused by pigment (bilirubinate) gallstones, a manifestation of a chronic hemolytic pro-

cess. These stones tend to occlude the common bile duct. Finally, some patients may present in old age, when bone marrow function normally becomes more sluggish. Compensation of the destruction lessens, and the anemia becomes more severe. Chronic ulceration of ankle skin may occur in 10–15% of adult patients.[17]

Blood Smear Morphology. The hallmark of HS is spherocytes on the blood smear.[6, 18] When present in patients with childhood hemolytic anemia and a family history of similar abnormalities, the spherocytes are highly suggestive of HS. Viewed under the microscope, these cells present a picture of increased numbers of uniformly round cells. Some of these are microspherocytes—small, round, dense RBCs—that are well filled with hemoglobin and lack a central pallor (Fig. 17–3). When examined in wet preparation or by electron microscopy, many of the HS RBCs may appear more as stomatocytes or spherostomatocytes.[6, 18] Normal-appearing RBCs, along with diffusely basophilic (polychromatophilic) RBCs and varying degrees of anisocytosis and poikilocytosis, are present.

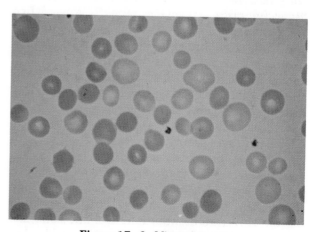

Figure 17–3 Microspherocytes.

Complete Blood Count. The most outstanding abnormality noted in the complete blood count is the increased mean cell hemoglobin concentration (>36%) in about 50% of patients. It may be as high as 40% greater in some patients.[20] This abnormality probably results from cellular dehydration of cells that have gone through the spleen and have low levels of water and potassium. The increased destruction in HS is usually compensated for, and the anemia, if present, is mild. The hemoglobin, hematocrit, and RBC counts reflect this balance of hemolysis and compensation. The hemoglobin usually ranges from 12 to 18 g/dL but varies among individuals. The mean corpuscular volume and mean corpuscular hemoglobin usually are normal but can also vary. Reticulocytes are usually between 5% and 20% but may be higher, especially during recovery from aplastic crisis.[20] The RBC distribution width is usually normal but may be increased, with high degrees of reticulocytosis. During the aplastic crisis, the hemoglobin, hematocrit, reticulocyte values, and RBC count decrease dramatically.

Other Laboratory Values. The bone marrow in HS shows erythrocyte hyperplasia resulting from the increased demand to compensate for the decreased life span of the circulating HS RBCs. The RBC precursors are morphologically normal because the morphologic defect is acquired in the circulation.[21]

Values of the chemistry profile reflect extravascular hemolysis. The unconjugated (indirect) bilirubin level is elevated from slight to moderate, fecal urobilinogen level is elevated, and haptoglobin levels are decreased.[6, 15, 18] The values associated with intravascular hemolysis, that is, hemoglobinemia, hemoglobinuria, and hemosiderinuria, are *not* features of HS.

Special Tests

Osmotic Fragility. The results of the osmotic fragility test are abnormal in blood samples that have decreased surface-to-volume ratios.[21] When RBCs are put in hypotonic solutions, water enters the cells until equilibrium is achieved. As this phenomenon occurs, the cells swell until the internal volume is too great, causing them to burst or lyse. Because spherocytes already have a decreased surface area–to-volume ratio, they lyse in less hypotonic solutions than normal-shaped, biconcave RBCs and therefore have increased osmotic fragility. The osmotic fragility is the most useful confirmatory test for HS; however, in about 25% of HS patients, the results of the initial osmotic fragility test are normal when fresh blood is used.[6] Increasing the difference between a normal and abnormal result is usually possible by incubating the blood at 37 °C for 24 hours before performing the test.

During this incubation period, HS cells become metabolically deprived and tend to lose membrane surface because of their relative membrane instability. Patients who have increased osmotic fragility only when their blood is incubated tend to be mildly affected and may have fewer than 1–2% spherocytes in the total RBC population; therefore, this disease is difficult to diagnose on morphologic grounds. If a patient has normal results on the incubated osmotic fragility test, it is highly unlikely that the patient has HS. In the unincubated osmotic fragility test, a distinct subpopulation of the most fragile cells, those most conditioned by the spleen, is reflected by a "tail" of the osmotic fragility curve (Fig. 17–4).[17, 18] After splenectomy is performed, the osmotic fragility improves, and this subpopulation of conditioned cells disappears.

Increased osmotic fragility simply indicates the presence of spherocytes and does not differentiate between hereditary spherocytosis and spherocytosis caused by other conditions, such as burns, immune hemolytic anemias, and other acquired conditions.

Autohemolysis. The autohemolysis test is relatively sensitive to HS but is not routinely used in many laboratories, because results are variable and false-positive results may be seen in normal populations.[6, 18] When normal RBCs are incubated in their own plasma, hemolysis gradually takes place. In HS, because of the loss of membrane and the inability to maintain the cation gradient, the hemolysis is much greater. Normal samples generally have less than 3.5% hemolysis at the end of the 48-hour incubation, and they have less than 0.6% if a source of glucose is added.[6] The glucose provides energy to drive the cation pumps to help maintain the cells. In HS, the hemolysis is be-

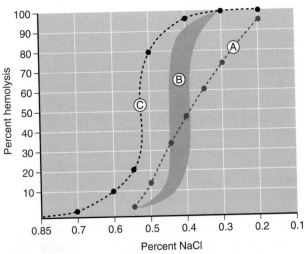

Figure 17–4 Erythrocyte osmotic fragility curve. *A,* Thalassemia demonstrating two cell populations: one with increased fragility *(lower left)* and one with decreased fragility *(upper right). B,* Normal curve. *C,* Increased fragility, as in hereditary spherocytosis.

tween 10 and 50%, which corrects considerably, but not necessarily to the normal range, when glucose is added. An HS patient with a large number of conditioned (in vivo by the spleen) microspherocytes may not correct the hemolysis with glucose.

Therapy and Prognosis

Splenectomy prevents clinically significant hemolysis, and patients with uncomplicated diseases always respond to this treatment.[6] In addition to curing the anemia, splenectomy prevents symptomatic gallbladder disease from occurring. This fact is important because of the risks associated with gallbladder surgery, especially in the elderly.

The major risk of splenectomy is sepsis, which may be life threatening.[22] Because children under 6 years of age have increased susceptibility after splenectomy to overwhelming bacterial infection, especially pneumococcal septicemia,[23] the surgery is usually postponed unless the anemia is very severe and life threatening. In older patients, the risk of surgery to prevent persisting hemolysis and pigment gallstones may outweigh the benefits; therefore, splenectomy is recommended by some investigators for all HS patients with anemia, significant hemolysis (indicated by repeated reticulocyte counts over 5%), or a strong family history of gallbladder disease.[6]

After a splenectomy is performed, spherocytes are still evident on the blood smear, but conditioned microspherocytes, as evidenced by the change in osmotic fragility, disappear. All of the typical changes in RBC morphology seen after splenectomy also exist, including Howell-Jolly bodies, target cells, siderocytes, and acanthocytes (Fig. 17–5).

Occasionally, an accidental autotransplantation of splenic tissue may occur during splenectomy. The hemolysis may resume again years later. The resumption of splenic function can be ascertained by the disappearance of the Howell-Jolly bodies from the peripheral blood smear and the increase in pitted RBCs.[6, 24]

Differential Diagnosis

Hereditary spherocytosis must be distinguished from hemolytic anemia with spherocytes that is associated with immune disorders. Family history and evaluation of family members, including both parents, siblings, and children of the patient, help differentiate the hereditary origin from the acquired disorder. The immune disorders with spherocytes are usually characterized by a positive result on the direct antiglobulin test, whereas the results are negative in HS.[6, 15, 17] The osmotic fragility test is not diagnostic of HS, because the cells in acquired hemolytic anemia with spherocytes also show increased osmotic fragility.

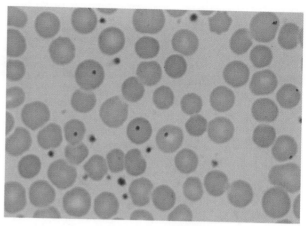

Figure 17–5 Hereditary spherocytosis after splenectomy, showing Howell-Jolly bodies and spherocytes.

Hereditary Elliptocytosis

History and Mode of Inheritance

HE was first reported in 1904 by Dresbach, who discovered elliptocytes on a student's blood smear in a histology class at Ohio State University.[25] HE is a very heterogeneous disorder clinically, genetically, and biochemically. HE reportedly exists in all of its forms in 250–500 per million people in the United States.[6] All racial and ethnic groups are represented, but certain types exist in certain racial and ethnic groups. Different types of HE have been linked with various blood group antigens, including Rh locus[26] and Duffy blood group locus.[27] Most of the variants are inherited in an autosomal dominant fashion.

Pathophysiology

HE is characterized by oval or elliptical RBCs on the peripheral smear. Recent studies have indicated the heterogeneity of this disorder and have also indicated several molecular defects in the RBC membrane skeleton that lead to this morphologic abnormality.[6, 7, 15, 17, 18] The type of structural change in the membrane protein spectrin appears to be associated with the clinical manifestations. These defects affect the RBCs' deformability and reflect the failure of RBCs to return to their normal disc shape after being deformed by the shear forces in the microcirculation.

Thirty percent of patients with common HE have abnormalities of the spectrin heterodimer head region, which cause an inability to associate the dimer form to tetramers and high-order oligomers. These abnormalities commonly involve the N-terminal peptide of the alpha-chain spectrin, the alpha I domain with a molecular mass of 80,000 D (αI^{80}) (Table 17–2). Six defects have been identified by using trypsin to cleave the molecule and using isoelectric focusing to identify the abnormal polypeptides. These polypeptides are smaller and

Table 17–2. HEREDITARY DEFECTS OF RED BLOOD CELL SKELETAL PROTEINS IN ELLIPTOCYTOSIS

Protein Deficit	Hereditary Characteristics
DEFECTS IN ALPHA-CHAIN SPECTRIN THAT IMPAIR SPECTRIN SELF-ASSOCIATION	
Spectrin alpha I/78	Silent carrier to moderately severe HE Heterogeneous defects seen in North African populations
Spectrin alpha I/74	Silent carrier to moderately severe HE Associated with HE with HPP and HE with infantile poikilocytosis Relatively common
Spectrin alpha I/65	Silent carrier to mild HE (heterozygous) Mild to moderately severe HE (homozygous) Common in blacks Homogeneous defect (extra amino acid (leucine) in alpha spectrin)
OTHER RARE DEFECTS REPORTED (Sometimes severe cases) Spectrin alpha I/50, Spectrin alpha I/43, Spectrin alpha II/31, Spectrin alpha II/21, Spectrin alpha II/20 Shortened alpha-chain spectrin Decreased amounts of alpha-chain spectrin	Mild-to-moderate HE Some cases associated in homozygous and heterozygous states with HPP
DEFECTS IN BETA-CHAIN SPECTRIN THAT IMPAIR SPECTRIN SELF-ASSOCIATION Shortened beta chain	Heterogeneous mutation that shortens and alters C-terminal sequences and phosphorylation of beta-chain spectrin

HE, hereditary elliptocytosis; HPP, hereditary pyropoikilocytosis.

are named by their size: αI^{78}, αI^{74}, αI^{65}, αI^{50}, and αI^{43}.[6, 17] Specific mutations have been identified that are responsible for three of these alpha-chain variants. A shortened alpha chain has also been discovered. One beta-chain abnormality has been found that involves a truncated chain. In HPP, both this alpha spectrin mutation that leads to defective spectrin heterodimers and a partial deficiency of spectrin exist. Rare defects in 4.1 protein and glycophorin C have been reported in HE.

HE patients all show decreased RBC thermal stability in varying degrees. Patients whose cells show marked thermal sensitivity with fragmentation are classified as having HPP.[17] This fragile self-association of spectrin to spectrin weakens the membrane skeleton of these HE cells and diminishes their resistance to shear stress. Several clinical syndromes are associated with these alpha-chain defects. Individuals who have only one abnormal allele are silent carriers or have mild common HE or common HE with infantile poikilocytosis.

Clinical and Laboratory Findings

HE has been subdivided into three types that have different clinical and morphologic syndromes: common HE, spherocytic HE, and Southeast Asian ovalocytosis.[6, 17] The most common form is common HE, which is composed of several subgroups, including the silent carrier, mild common HE, common HE with chronic hemolysis, and common

HE with infantile poikilocytosis. A rare subgroup of common HE that has an associated ineffective erythropoiesis and dyserythropoiesis has been described in Italian families. The patients affected are usually heterozygotes and have one abnormal gene.

The *silent carrier state* of HE has recently been identified as the result of studies of asymptomatic members of families with HE or HPP. Individuals with this condition have normal RBC morphology and no evidence of hemolysis, but detailed biochemical studies have revealed subtle defects in the RBC membranes. In *mild common HE*, many elliptocytes with rod forms are found on the blood smear (Fig. 17–6). The number of these cells always exceeds 30% and may be as many as 100%.[6, 17] The patients, however, have no anemia or splenomegaly. A mild compensated hemolysis may exist, as evidenced by a slight increase in the reticulocyte count and a decrease in haptoglobin.[6] No budding fragmentation of these cells occurs, and no spherocytes are present. Patients with mild HE may develop transient, uncompensated hemolytic anemia due to various conditions and infections, including infectious mononucleosis, malaria, cirrhosis, pregnancy, vitamin B_{12} deficiency, disseminated intravascular coagulation (DIC), and thrombotic thrombocytopenic purpura (TTP).[6] In some families with mild HE, a person will have more severe hemolysis and anemia, or *common HE with chronic hemolysis*. It has been suggested that

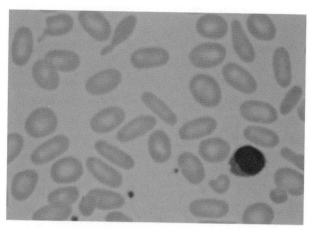

Figure 17–6 Hereditary elliptocytosis.

these individuals may have also inherited a modifier gene that causes the membrane defect to be worse, but this theory has not been proved.[28] In other cases, HE with chronic hemolysis is seen in most family members. These families usually have different molecular defects than those typically found in mild HE.[28] Fragmentation and poikilocytosis may be more prevalent in this group. These patients seem to respond to splenectomy.

Common HE with infantile poikilocytosis has budding, fragments, and bizarre poikilocytes and presents with moderate hemolysis at birth; however, the condition gradually (from 6 months to 2 years of age) converts to a morphologic and clinical picture resembling mild HE.[29] All of these common HEs have a normal osmotic fragility, and all respond well to splenectomy. Common HE RBCs are mildly heat sensitive. They become echinocytic and fragment at 47–48 °C, whereas normal RBCs are stable in temperatures up to 49 °C.

Rarely, parents with mild HE may have offspring who are homozygous for the abnormal gene (homozygous common HE) and present with a moderate to very severe hemolytic state. Some even have transfusion-dependent hemolytic anemia with gross fragmentation, poikilocytosis, and spherocytosis, along with elliptocytosis.[17, 30]

Hereditary Pyropoikilocytosis. In HPP, both this alpha spectrin mutation that leads to defective spectrin heterodimers and a partial deficiency of spectrin exist. *HPP* has traditionally been described as a separate disease, but many authors believe that there exists convincing evidence that it is a subtype of HE.[17] It appears to be transmitted as a recessive disease but is morphologically similar to homozygous HE. In one third of the reported cases of HPP, one of the parents or siblings has typical mild HE.[6, 17] In other families, the parents appear normal, but further investigation reveals that at least one of the parents is a silent

carrier; it has been suggested that the other parent may carry a gene that magnifies the defect in the biochemical nature of the RBC membrane.[6, 17, 28] Thus, the HPP phenotype may result from homozygosity for the silent carrier state, homozygosity for one of the mild HE genes, or double heterozygosity for any combination of these abnormal genes. In homozygous HE and HPP, osmotic fragility and autohemolysis are markedly increased. The RBCs show marked thermal sensitivity. After 10–15 minutes of heating at 45–46 °C, RBCs in HPP fragment, but normal cells do not fragment until 49 °C. RBCs in HPP even fragment at 37 °C when heated longer than 6 hours.[17]

Most patients who have HPP are black. They have a severe hemolytic anemia with facial bone abnormalities (resulting from expanding bone marrow mass), gallbladder disease (resulting from excessive RBC breakdown), and growth retardation. The RBC morphology of these patients shows marked poikilocytosis, including elliptocytes, RBC fragments, budding RBCs, spherocytes, and triangular and other bizarrely shaped cells (Figs. 17–7 and 17–8).[17] The mean cell volume is very low (50–70 fL) because of the RBC fragments. Patients with HPP partially respond to splenectomy, but some hemolysis still remains, probably as a result of the cells fragmenting even at body temperature.[6]

Spherocytic Hereditary Elliptocytosis. The second type of HE is a hybrid disorder that combines features of mild HE and mild HS. This disorder is seen in people of northern European origin and possibly the Japanese. Rounded elliptocytes and spherocytes are seen on the blood smear. The RBC morphology varies with different proportions of these abnormal cells, even in the same family. The incidence of this type HE is unknown but is judged to be about 5% of HE cases.[6] Most patients have evidence of a compensated mild hemolysis.[17] Gallbladder disease is common in these patients, and

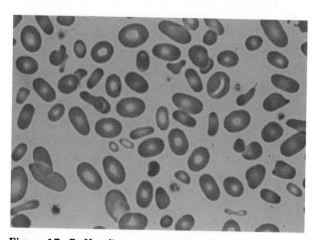

Figure 17–7 Hereditary pyropoikilocytosis before incubation.

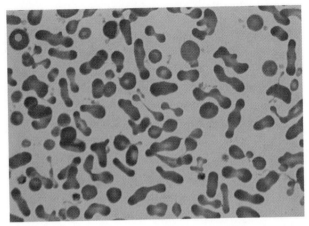

Figure 17–8 Hereditary pyropoikilocytosis after 1 hour at 45 °C.

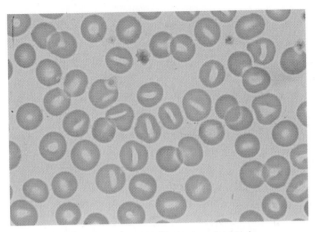

Figure 17–9 Hereditary stomatocytosis.

aplastic crises are a risk. The patients show a slightly increased osmotic fragility and an increased glucose-responsive autohemolysis test result. These patients' hemolysis responds well to splenectomy.

Stomatocytic Hereditary Elliptocytosis. The third major type of HE is *stomatocytic HE* and is common only in the Melanesian and Malaysian populations.[6, 17] The elliptocytes are rounded, and some have transverse bars so that they appear like double stomatocytes.[6] The osmotic fragility is usually normal. These cells are resistant to invasion of all forms of malaria.[6] The membrane appears more rigid than a normal RBC membrane, and hemolysis is mild or absent. Many of the blood group antigens are poorly expressed on these cells.[6] The RBCs in this disorder are unusually heat resistant, maintaining their shape up to 51–52 °C (normal, 49 °C). It has been suggested that the defect in these cells affects protein 3, the anion transport protein of the RBC membrane.[6]

Inherited Disorders of Red Blood Cell Cation Permeability and Volume

RBC hydration is determined by the intracellular concentration of the monovalent cations Na^+ and K^+. If the total cation content is increased, water enters the cell and forms a hydrocyte, or stomatocyte; if the total cation content is decreased, water leaves the cell and produces a dehydrated red cell, or xerocyte. Many congenital anemias have been described over the past 20 years that are clinically, morphologically, genetically, and biochemically diverse.[31]

HEREDITARY STOMATOCYTOSIS (HYDROCYTOSIS) (Fig. 17–9)

Hereditary stomatocytosis is a complex mixture of diseases in which hemolysis is mild to severe. It

is rare and is usually inherited in an autosomal dominant pattern.[31]

Pathophysiology

Hereditary stomatocytosis is characterized morphologically by stomatocytes and biochemically by the failure of the Na^+ and K^+ pumps and an increase in intracellular water.[6, 31] The influx of Na^+ exceeds the loss of K^+, and the cells swell, becoming less dense and more stomatocytic. In some patients, a deficiency of a membrane protein located in the band 7 region occurs.[6] This protein has been called "stomatin." It is presumed to regulate membrane sodium permeability. Studies of Japanese patients with this disorder, however, have shown some not to be deficient in stomatin.

Clinical and Laboratory Findings

The disease can cause mild, moderate, or severe hemolysis. The diagnostic features include stomatocytosis on the peripheral blood smear, macrocytosis, reduced K^+ concentration, elevated Na^+ concentration, and increased monovalent cation content in the erythrocytes. The red cells have an increased osmotic fragility and are moderately deficient in 2,3-diphosphoglycerate (2,3-DPG).[6] Patients who have severe hemolysis benefit from splenectomy.

ACQUIRED STOMATOCYTOSIS

Stomatocytosis occurs frequently as a drying artifact on Wright-stained peripheral blood smears; therefore, a laboratorian should examine many areas on several smears before categorizing the result as stomatocytosis. In normal people, up to 3% of RBCs may be stomatocytes.[6] Wet preparation with RBCs diluted in their own plasma and examined under phase microscopy shows stomatocytes to be bowl shaped or uniconcave rather than the normal biconcave shape. This technique can eliminate some of the artifactual stomatocytosis, but target cells may also appear bowl shaped in solution.

Some situations that have been associated with acquired stomatocytosis are acute alcoholism and drug therapy. Occasionally, the disorder has been seen transiently in marathon runners after a race.[6]

STOMATOCYTOSIS IN RH$_{null}$ DISEASE

In 1961, a rare condition was discovered in which patients lacked all of the Rh antigens on their RBC membranes.[6] They also had decreased expression of Ss and U antigens. These patients present clinically with a moderately severe hemolytic anemia, characterized morphologically by stomatocytes and spherocytes. Osmotic fragility is mildly increased. It has been suggested that the Rh antigens are associated with the membrane skeleton and that their loss affects the skeletal stability. Recently, a case of Rh$_{mod}$ in which the Rh antigens were suppressed but not absent was discovered. Stomatocytosis also occurs in this disorder, and clinically it manifests as a hemolytic anemia.

HEREDITARY XEROCYTOSIS

In the rare autosomal dominant hemolytic anemia, hereditary xerocytosis, the RBCs are dehydrated, as evidenced by the elevated mean cell hemoglobin concentration and a very decreased osmotic fragility.[6, 31] These cells lose K$^+$ because of an RBC membrane permeability defect; the specific defect has not been discovered. The RBC morphology includes stomatocytes, target cells, spiculated red blood cells, and macrocytes. RBCs in which the hemoglobin appears to be puddled in discrete areas on the cell periphery are characteristic. The 2,3-DPG concentration in RBCs is moderately decreased. Removal of the spleen in these patients does not totally correct the hemolysis.

Various other RBC permeability syndromes have been reported that have shared features of both hydrocytosis and xerocytosis; these have been termed the *intermediate syndromes*.[31]

ACANTHOCYTOSIS

Acanthocytes (spur cells) are RBCs with a few irregular projections that vary in width, length, and surface distribution. These are distinct from echinocytes (burr cells), which typically have small, uniform projections evenly spread on the cell circumference.[6] The differentiation is easier to make on scanning electron micrographs and on wet preparation than on dried smears. Echinocytes appear crenated on a stained smear, whereas acanthocytes appear as denser, more contracted, and irregular. Echinocytes have been associated with uremia, defects in glycolytic metabolism, and microangiopathic hemolytic anemias.[6] Acanthocytes have been associated with severe liver disease, abetalipoproteinemia, infantile pyknocytosis, anorexia nervosa, and the McLeod and *In(Lu)* blood groups.[6]

Abetalipoproteinemia is a rare autosomal recessive disorder manifested in the first month of life by steatorrhea. Also associated with the disorder is a progressive neurologic disease: retinitis pigmentosa, which often results in blindness. Low-density lipoproteins are absent.[32] The disease usually progresses to death in the second or third decade of life. Usually, 50–90% of the RBCs are acanthocytes.[32] Affected persons have a mild hemolytic anemia and normal RBC indices.

Pathophysiology

The RBCs in this disorder have a normal membrane protein composition, but the membrane lipids are abnormal. An increase in membrane sphingomyelin and a decrease in phosphatidylcholine are present in the membrane of acanthocytes.[32] These changes reflect abnormalities in the distribution of plasma phospholipids that decrease the lipid fluidity of the RBC membrane, resulting in the shape change. The shape defect is not present in developing nucleated RBCs or reticulocytes but progresses as RBCs age.[32]

Patients with other related disorders such as hypobetalipoproteinemia, normotriglyceridemic abetalipoproteinemia, and chylomicron retention disease, may also have acanthocytosis and neurologic disease, depending on the severity of the lipoprotein defect.[32]

Other Causes of Acanthocytosis

The McLeod blood group phenotype is an X-linked anomaly of the Kell blood group system that causes a lack of Kx, a membrane precursor of the Kell antigens.[33] Males who lack Kx on their RBCs have a variable acanthocytosis (8–85%) and a mild compensated anemia.[34] The acanthocytes are better appreciated on a wet preparation than on dried smears. Female heterozygote carriers may have an occasional acanthocyte as a result of the X chromosome inactivation. Patients with an *In(Lu)* gene, which is a dominantly acting inhibitor of Lutheran blood group antigens (Lu^a and Lu^b), have abnormally shaped RBCs but no hemolysis.[34] The morphology varies from normal to mild poikilocytosis to marked acanthocytosis. Patients who have malnutrition as a result of such causes as anorexia nervosa and cystic fibrosis may have acanthocytes on their blood smear that resolve after a normal nutritional state is obtained.[6]

Patients with vitamin E deficiency may have a variable number of acanthocytes.[6] A syndrome of neonatal jaundice and hemolysis in which a variable number of cells resembling acanthocytes is present has been described in neonates.[6] The abnormal cells peak at 3 to 4 weeks of age and then decline spontaneously. (See Chapter 19 for a discussion of the acanthocytes of spur cell anemia associated with liver disease.)

Red Blood Cell Enzymopathies

GLUCOSE-6-PHOSPHATE DEHYDROGENASE DEFICIENCY

Hemolysis due to glucose-6-phosphate dehydrogenase (G-6-PD) deficiency was recognized very early, with Pythagoras, the Greek philosopher and mathematician, warning his followers against the dangers of eating fava beans.[35] Physicians in Southern Italy wrote of the clinical picture of this disorder around the turn of this century.[36] The hemolytic effect of the antimalarial drug primaquine was recognized in the early 1950s. Carson and colleagues discovered that primaquine-sensitive people had low levels of G-6-PD activity in their RBCs.[37]

The gene for G-6-PD is located on the X chromosome and shows a characteristic X-linked pattern.[38] Males can be either a normal hemizygote (have the normal allele) or a deficient hemizygote (have a variant allele). Females can be a normal homozygote (both alleles normal), a deficient homozygote (both alleles abnormal), or a heterozygote (one normal allele and one abnormal allele).[39] The heterozygous woman's level of enzyme lies between normal and deficient. This disorder has been called X-linked recessive, but because heterozygous females have a decreased amount of the enzyme, it is biochemically codominant.[39] Some heterozygous females may even have hemolytic attacks, depending on the amount of RBC G-6-PD activity. Female heterozygotes have two populations of G-6-PD–producing cells because of the X chromosome inactivation (the Lyon hypothesis). This means that statistically half of the cells are G-6-PD normal and the other half are G-6-PD deficient. In reality, the activation is apparently statistically random; therefore, in female heterozygotes, the RBCs may be deficient in G-6-PD or they may have normal levels of G-6-PD.[38, 39] The G-6-PD locus has the greatest apparent extent of variability of any human genome.[40] All studies suggest that the abnormality is structural (point mutations) rather than resulting from a decrease in the number of normal molecules (deletions).[38] These changes in the primary structure (substitution of individual amino acids) cause G-6-PD deficiency either by decreasing its in vivo stability or by affecting its enzymatic functions, or possibly both, depending on the particular variant. Figure 17–10 shows the human G-6-PD gene, with a map of structural mutations of those variants for which a molecular basis has been elucidated.[39] The different genetic expressions of G-6-PD have been divided into classes by the World Health Organization, based on clinical symptoms and amount of enzyme activity.[39, 41] Class I has severe clinical symptoms (chronic, nonspherocytic hemolytic anemia) and less than 20% G-6-PD activity. Class II has mild clinical expression and less than 10% activity. Class III has mild clinical expression and 10–60% activity. Class IV has no clinical expression and 100% activity. Class V has no clinical expression and over 100% activity. Within these groups, different genetic mutations and enzymes exist that have different electrophoretic patterns.[39] The shaded areas on Figure 17–10 represent class I variants.

Normal G-6-PD has generally been designated G-6-PD-B. Some G-6-PD variants are not associated with significant reduced enzyme activity in the RBCs. A common mutant that is clinically normal, has no enzyme deficiency, and is present most often in those of African descent is G-6-PD-A. This common mutant has Asn→Asp at the 126-amino-acid position and moves faster on electrophoresis than does G-6-PD-B.[39] Twenty to forty percent of the X chromosomes of Africans have the gene for G-6-PD-A.[38] Three clinically deficient mutations are mutations of G-6-PD-A and are called G-6-PD-A⁻. These variants have the G-6-PD mutation plus an additional amino acid substitution. Those with a G-6-PD-A⁻ are a prototype for class III because of their clinical symptoms and the amount of enzyme activity in their RBCs.[38] Most (>90%) cases of G-6-PD-A⁻ result from the 68 Val→Met mutation. Eleven percent of African American males in the United States carry a gene that codes for G-6-PD-A⁻.[42] All other variants are designated by geographic names.[38] G-6-PD Mediterranean (G-6-PD Med) is the most common variant enzyme among whites.[39] In this variant, enzyme activity is barely detectable because the G-6-PD is synthesized in subnormal amounts and is unstable. Patients with this variant are a prototype for class II.[38] Its incidence among Kurdish Jews ranges from 3 to 50%.[38] The Mahidol variant has a high incidence in the population of Thailand and Vietnam, and the Canton variant is commonly found in the Chinese and in people of Southeast Asia. More than 400 variants of G-6-PD have been reported.[38]

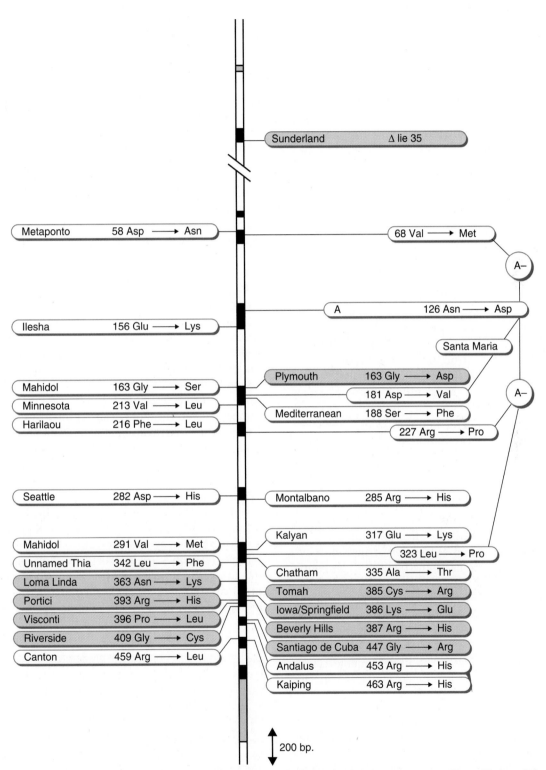

Figure 17–10 Map of structural mutations in human glucose-6-phosphate dehydrogenase gene. (From Nathan DG, Oski FA: Hematology of Infancy and Childhood, 4th ed. Philadelphia: WB Saunders, 1993:678.)

Pathophysiology

The enzyme G-6-PD reduces nicotinamide-adenine dinucleotide phosphate (NADP) while oxidizing glucose-6-phosphate. It governs the rate of reduction of NADP, which restores GSH-reduced glutathione through H^+ transfer by glutathione reductase in the hexose monophosphate shunt[43] (see Fig. 10–1). G-6-PD provides the only means of generating reduced nicotinamide-adenine dinucleotide phosphate, reduced form (NADPH), and in its absence, the erythrocyte is particularly vulnerable to oxidative damage.[38] Most oxidant drugs enable interaction between molecular oxygen and components of the RBC. RBCs with normal G-6-PD activity are able to detoxify the oxidative compounds and safeguard the hemoglobin, SH-containing enzymes, and membrane thiols (sulfhydryls), allowing normal-functioning RBCs to carry enormous quantities of oxygen safely.[43]

In patients with deficient G-6-PD activity, the exposure of RBCs to oxidative agents causes oxidation of membrane thiols, which produces several consequences, the most conspicuous being the appearance of Heinz bodies (irreversible intracellular precipitates of denatured hemoglobin) along with membrane skeletal structural abnormalities, causing K^+ and Na^+ leak rates to increase.[44] The mechanism of Heinz body formation is complex and poorly understood but most likely occurs when the NADPH-dependent counteroxidant defenses are overwhelmed and reduced glutathione (GSH) is oxidized to oxidized glutathione (GSSG). Conformational changes take place in the hemoglobin molecule, which exposes the interior thiols also to oxidation. With sustained intracellular production of oxygen free radicals, the three-dimensional structure of hemoglobin is affected sufficiently to lower its solubility, and aggregates of insoluble hemochromes aggregate as Heinz bodies.[44] The Heinz bodies adhere to the RBC membrane by hydrophobic bonds, a phenomenon that deforms the membrane. These hemoglobin precipitants are removed by the macrophages of the spleen, causing "bite" deformities in some of the RBCs.[39] Other RBCs are less pliable because of the undeformable Heinz body aggregates and are trapped and lysed in the spleen.[39]

Hemolytic Process

The following clinical syndromes associated with G-6-PD are recognized: acute hemolytic anemia (AHA), resulting from drug exposure or infection; favism; neonatal jaundice; and chronic, nonspherocytic hemolytic anemia.[40] Hemolysis has also been reported in association with diabetic ketoacidosis and hypoglycemia, but other factors, such as coexistent infection or an oxidant drug exposure, can not always be ruled out as a cause of the hemolysis.[40]

Acute hemolytic anemia due to drug exposure is the classic manifestation of G-6-PD deficiency. The actual discovery of G-6-PD deficiency was a direct consequence of investigations into the development of hemolysis after the ingestion of the antimalarial agent primaquine in some individuals (usually black males). Table 17–3 lists drugs that have a definite association with hemolytic episodes in persons with G-6-PD deficiency.[43] Other agents have a less direct association. With some of these drugs, hemolysis occurs in some populations and not in others, and different doses give rise to different degrees of hemolysis, depending on other circumstances, such as a coexisting infection or concomitant use of other drugs.[43] Also, because the oldest RBCs have the lowest amount of enzyme, the number of reticulocytes affects the hemolysis rate.

People with G-6-PD deficiency are clinically and hematologically normal until the offending drug is given. The acute hemolytic episode is caused by a genetic factor (the lack of functional G-6-PD) and an exogenous factor (the drug).[39] Clinical hemolysis and jaundice typically begin 2–3 days after the drug is started. Hemoglobinuria is a chief sign and indicates that the hemolysis is intravascular, even though some extravascular hemolysis probably also takes place.[39] The anemia worsens until the seventh to eighth day. Heinz bodies can be demonstrated by incubating the blood in a supravital stain. The reticulocyte count generally increases by the eighth to the tenth day, and the hemoglobin level begins to rise.[39] With some variants, the hemolytic episode is self-limiting because the newly formed reticulocytes have a degree of higher G-6-PD activity. However, with other variants that are more severely deficient, the hemolytic episode may be longer. The level of the drug dosage also plays a

Table 17–3. SUBSTANCES THAT CAN INDUCE HEMOLYSIS IN PATIENTS WITH GLUCOSE-6-PHOSPHATE DEHYDROGENASE DEFICIENCY
Acetanilid
Doxorubicin
Furazolidone
Methylene blue
Nalidixic acid
Niridazole
Nitrofurantoin
Phenazopyridine
Primaquine
Sulfamethoxazole

role in the severity and the length of the hemolytic episode.[39]

Infection is probably the most common cause of hemolysis in individuals with G-6-PD deficiency in areas where favism is not prevalent.[38-40] The clinical picture of hemolysis caused by infection is influenced by several factors, including the concomitant administration of oxidant drugs and the hemoglobin level, the liver function, and the age of the patient.[39] The mechanism of hemolysis induced by acute and subacute infection is poorly understood, but the generation of hydrogen peroxide by phagocytizing leukocytes may play a role,[39] or the RBC-containing G-6-PD variants may be unable to withstand the hyperthermia of infections.[42] Diminished liver function may further aggravate the oxidant stress on the RBCs by allowing the accumulation of metabolites capable of oxidizing RBC −SH groups.[42] Some of the infections associated with hemolysis in G-6-PD–deficient individuals are salmonellae, coliforms, beta-hemolytic streptococci, rickettsiae, influenza, and viral hepatitis.[45] In addition to hemolysis, viral hepatitis can cause acute renal failure and hyperbilirubinemia in G-6-PD–deficient patients.[40, 42]

Favism results when a small percentage of G-6-PD–deficient individuals are exposed to the fava bean (*Vicia fava* or broad bean, commonly grown in the Mediterranean area), either by ingesting the bean or inhaling the plant's pollen. Substances capable of oxidizing RBC reduced glutathione (GSH), and therefore capable of causing hemolysis, have been isolated from fava beans. Favism clinically manifests with a sudden onset of acute intravascular hemolysis within 24–48 hours of exposure. Hemoglobinuria is one of the first signs of the disorder. Only a small percentage of G-6-PD–deficient individuals are affected, and most of these have the G-6-PD Mediterranean variant; therefore, favism is seen primarily in the Mediterranean area. Rarely, a G-6-PD–deficient black patient may be susceptible.[39]

Neonatal jaundice due to G-6-PD deficiency occurs particularly in Greece, Sardinia, the Far East, and Africa and has been reported in the United States.[39] Jaundice usually appears by 1 to 4 days after birth, which is slightly earlier than physiologic jaundice but later than in blood group alloimmunization.[39] Genetic factors, which include the particular variant of G-6-PD, and environmental factors, such as drugs given to the mother or baby, infection, and gestational age, probably play an important role in this occurrence because a wide variation exists in the frequency and severity in different populations with G-6-PD deficiency.

Most G-6-PD patients are clinically normal and have only a slightly reduced RBC life span that is evidenced only by RBC survival studies unless they are challenged, as was discussed earlier. A very small group of G-6-PD–deficient patients have chronic, clinically detectable anemia evidenced by chronic hyperbilirubinemia, decreased haptoglobin level, and increased lactate dehydrogenase level. Most of these patients are diagnosed at birth as having neonatal jaundice, and the hemolysis continues into adulthood. They usually do not have hemoglobinuria, suggesting that the chronic hemolysis is extravascular, as opposed to the intravascular hemolysis associated with the AHA of G-6-PD deficiency.[39] There is evidence that normal oxidative stress causes the sulfhydryl groups of the membrane proteins (especially spectrin) to be oxidized and conformational changes to take place so that the RBCs are removed by the spleen, probably by the same mechanism as in hereditary spherocytosis. The RBC morphology is unremarkable and is referred to as "nonspherocytic."[39] These patients are also vulnerable to acute oxidative stress from the same agents as in other G-6-PD patients and may have acute attacks of hemoglobinuria. The severity associated with chronic, nonspherocytic hemolytic anemia is extremely variable, probably because almost every case that has been evaluated has resulted from a different mutation of the enzyme.[39]

An association between the distribution of G-6-PD deficiency and the incidence of *Plasmodium falciparum* has been suggested.[38] Many epidemiologic studies have supported the hypothesis that malaria selects for G-6-PD deficiency, which may also explain the genetic heterogeneity of the G-6-PD alleles and the frequency of the abnormal allele in particular geographic regions. The protection is apparently for G-6-PD–deficient heterozygous females and not for G-6-PD–deficient hemizygous males.[46] The *P. falciparum* parasite invades the G-6-PD–deficient cell normally, but intracellular development is impaired. This impairment is overcome by repeated schizogonic cycles of the parasite in G-6-PD–deficient RBCs.[47] This could explain why heterozygous females, who are genetic mosaics and have some G-6-PD–deficient RBCs and some G-6-PD–normal RBCs due to the X chromosome inactivation, are relatively protected, and hemizygous males, whose RBCs are all G-6-PD deficient, are not.

Clinical and Laboratory Findings

Most individuals with G-6-PD deficiency are usually asymptomatic and may never discover their genetic abnormality. Their only clinical manifestation may be acute hemolysis during oxidative stress resulting from drugs or other causes; this hemolysis may go undetected because the bone marrow rapidly compensates for the increased RBC destruction.[38-40] G-6-PD deficiency can cause clinically recognizable hemolysis, as is discussed later.

The anemia occurring during a hemolytic crisis may range from moderate to extremely severe and is usually normocytic, normochromic. The morphology of G-6-PD–deficient RBCs is normal except during a hemolytic episode. The change in morphology during a hemolytic episode can vary, depending on the amount of hemolysis. In some patients, such as G-6-PD-A⁻ individuals, the change is not striking,[42] but in individuals with other variants, marked anisocytosis and poikilocytosis may occur, with distorted RBCs and "bite cells" in which the cell's margin appears dented.[39] When an offending drug is administered, Heinz bodies (denatured hemoglobin) develop in the RBCs.[45] These are not able to be detected on Wright's stain, but when exposed to certain basic dyes or supravital stains, such as crystal violet, they assume a purple color and appear at the margin of the RBC. When they are removed by the spleen, "bite cells" are formed.[45] The reticulocyte count is increased and may reach up to 30%.[39] Haptoglobin level is severely decreased. In some cases, free hemoglobin may be detected in the plasma. The white blood cell count is usually moderately elevated,[39] and the platelet count is variable. The unconjugated (indirect) bilirubin level is elevated. The darkly colored urine tests strongly positive for blood. Few intact RBCs appear in the sediment because the color and blood reaction result from hemoglobinuria and not hematuria.[39]

Quantitative assays of the G-6-PD enzyme activity can be performed to enable the differential diagnosis in G-6-PD deficiency to be made, but screening tests are usually adequate.[42] The principle of both tests is based on the reduction of an oxidized pyridine nucleotide (NADP→NADPH) during the reaction shown in Figure 17–11.[48] In the quantitative assay, the hemolysate of the patient's blood is added to a mixture of reagents that has been constituted in such a way that the amount of enzyme represents the limiting step; the activity is read at 340 nm with the cuvette thermostat at 37 °C. The principle of the screening test is the same except that rather than measuring

the absorption of light by the reduced pyridine nucleotide (NADPH), the fluorescence of reduced nucleotide, when activated with long-wave ultraviolet light, is used to visually evaluate whether pyridine nucleotide (NADP) has been reduced.[48] This is done by mixing the reagents together, placing them on a filter paper, and observing the filter paper under fluorescent light. Because reticulocytes have higher G-6-PD levels than mature RBCs, assays or screening tests should not be prepared with samples collected after an individual has suffered a severe hemolytic crisis, because the G-6-PD levels may be falsely elevated. The testing should be performed after mature RBC levels have returned to normal. A normal and not an increased G-6-PD assay along with a high reticulocyte count should be a clue that the patient may be G-6-PD deficient.[40] Other tests that can be used to screen for G-6-PD deficiency are the methemoglobin reduction test,[49] (a sensitive test in which the erythrocytes that are G-6-PD deficient fail to reduce methemoglobin in the presence of methylene blue), and the ascorbate-cyanide test,[50] which measures peroxidative denaturation of hemoglobin. This last test is not specific for G-6-PD deficiency and gives positive results with pyruvate kinase (PK) deficiency, as well as with certain unstable hemoglobins.

Therapy and Prognosis

Therapy in G-6-PD patients involves preventing the common manifestation of AHA and neonatal jaundice. Most hemolytic episodes, especially in G-6-PD-A⁻ individuals, are self-limited. In more severe types, such as G-6-PD-Med, this is not always the case. Screening is important in populations that have a high incidence of this deficiency.[39] Because neonatal jaundice cannot be prevented, it must be looked for in the populations that are high risk and must be treated immediately. Neonatal jaundice is not a major problem in most populations in the United States. The prevention of AHA is more difficult because multiple causes exist; however, some cases of AHA are easily preventable, such as avoiding eating fava beans in families in which this sensitivity exists.

Favism is a relatively dangerous disease, and fatalities were common before transfusion services

Glucose-6-phosphate + NADP $\xrightarrow{\text{G-6-PD}}$ 6-Phosphogluconate + NADPH
(no fluorescence)   (fluorescence)

Figure 17–11 Principle of glucose-6-phosphate dehydrogenase–deficiency test. In the screening test, the nicotinamide-adenine dinucleotide phosphate, reduced form (NADPH), will fluoresce, whereas the nicotinamide-adenine dinucleotide phosphate, oxidized form (NADP), will not. If glucose-6-phosphate (G6P) is oxidized to 6-phosphogluconate (6PG), the coenzyme NADP is reduced to NADPH with a corresponding increase in fluorescence. G6PD, glucose-6-phosphate dehydrogenase.

were available.[39] Prevention of drug-induced AHA is possible by choosing alternate drugs when possible.[43] In cases in which the offending drugs must be used, especially in cases of G-6-PD-A⁻, the dosage can be lowered, and therefore the amount of hemolysis can be decreased to a manageable level.[43] Prevention of infection-induced hemolysis is more difficult but can be detected early in the course of the episode and treated if necessary. Most episodes of AHA resolve without treatment but may at times be severe enough to warrant a blood transfusion. Hemoglobin levels between 7 and 9 g/dL with evidence of continuing hemolysis have been recommended as criteria for a transfusion. In patients with hemoglobin levels above 9 g/dL with persistent hemoglobinuria, close monitoring is important.[39] Infants with neonatal jaundice due to G-6-PD deficiency may require exchange transfusion.

Differential Diagnosis

The drug-induced hemolysis of classes II and III G-6-PD must be differentiated from other drug-induced hemolytic anemias. This differentiation can be performed by the screening test or by quantitative assay for G-6-PD deficiency. Patients with chronic, nonspherocytic hemolytic anemia (class I) G-6-PD deficiency must be differentiated from those with hereditary spherocytosis, hemoglobinopathies, and other enzymopathies.

ENZYMOPATHIES OF THE GLYCOLYTIC PATHWAY

The mature RBC beyond the reticulocyte stage lacks a nucleus, mitochondria, and other organelles and is unable to synthesize proteins and lipids or to perform oxidative phosphorylation. Its energy requirements are met by the generation of adenosine triphosphate through glycolysis; therefore, glycolysis is essential for the function and survival of the RBC (see Fig. 10–1). It is not surprising that enzyme deficiencies or abnormalities in the glycolytic pathway would result in hemolysis or other RBC abnormalities. The most common of these disorders is pyruvate kinase (PK) deficiency, but seven other defects of the RBC Embden-Meyerhof pathway have been described, including hexokinase, glucose phosphate isomerase, phosphofructokinase, aldolase, triosephosphate isomerase, phosphoglycerate kinase, and enolase deficiencies. In addition, deficiencies of 2,3-DPG mutase and phosphatase and lactate dehydrogenase have also been identified, but these do not result in hemolysis.[51] Several good reviews of these enzymopathies of the glycolytic pathway have appeared in the

literature.[51–53] All of these deficiencies are recessively transmitted, except that of phosphoglycerate kinase, which is X-linked, and enolase, which is presumably autosomal dominant.[51] Lactate dehydrogenase deficiency is not associated with hemolysis, and deficiencies of 2,3-DPG mutase and 2,3-DPG phosphatase are associated with mild erythrocytosis secondary to the near-absence of 2,3-DPG.[51] Table 17–4 summarizes the features associated with the glycolytic enzymopathies.

Pyruvate Kinase Deficiency

History and Mode of Inheritance

PK deficiency is the first-described defect and the most common one in the glycolytic pathway, accounting for about 90% of the defects of this pathway.[51] Dacie and coworkers first discussed a heterogeneous group of disorders that were referred to as *congenital nonspherocytic hemolytic anemias* in 1953.[54] In 1954, these disorders were classified as types I and II based on the results of their autohemolysis test.[55] Several groups presented evidence that some disorder of glycolysis existed in the erythrocytes in type II cases.[56] In 1961, the first deficiency of PK was documented. PK deficiency and class I type G-6-PD deficiency are equally common and together constitute most of the cases of chronic hemolytic anemia that result from erythrocyte enzymopathies.[51] PK deficiency is most common in people of Northern European ancestry but has been reported from many areas and appears to have a worldwide distribution.[53] An especially high prevalence of this disorder has been identified in the Mifflin County, Pennsylvania, Amish population.[52] PK deficiency is an autosomal recessive disorder with only rare exceptions; therefore both sexes are equally affected.[51] Usually, overt hemolytic disease occurs in homozygotes or compound heterozygotes; simple heterozygotes are not anemic, although their RBCs may show some enzyme alterations.[51]

Pathophysiology

PK is one of the rate-limiting key enzymes of the glycolytic pathway. It catalyzes the conversion of phosphoenolpyruvate to pyruvate with regeneration of adenosine triphosphate (see Fig. 10–1).[51] The exact mechanisms for hemolysis in PK-deficient cells are poorly understood. The adenosine triphosphate content is often decreased, as are the adenosine diphosphate and monophosphate contents of the RBC. The 2,3-DPG content is very often increased approximately twofold.[51] These alterations in the PK-deficient RBCs result in a rigid cell that is removed by the macrophages of the spleen and the liver.

Table 17–4. FEATURES ASSOCIATED WITH GLYCOLYTIC ENZYMOPATHIES

Enzyme	Incidence*	Inheritance	Hemolytic Anemia	Neurologic Abnormalities†	Myopathy†	Comments
Hexokinase (HK)	Rare	Autosomal recessive	Yes			Low 2,3-DPG level; suggestion of poor tolerance of anemia
Glucose phosphate isomerase (GPI)	Second to pyruvate kinase	Autosomal recessive	Yes	†	†	More than 45 cases reported; propensity for hemolytic crisis during infection
Phosphofructokinase (PFK)	Rare	Autosomal recessive	Variable		§	Hemolysis usually fully compensated; may have erythrocytosis; early onset gout
Aldolase (ALD)	Very rare	Autosomal recessive	Yes			Only three reported cases
Triosephosphate isomerase (TPI)	Rare	Autosomal recessive	Yes	§		Generalized disorder; most severe of glycolytic deficiencies; neurologic, infectious, and cardiac complications
Phosphoglycerate kinase (PGK)	Rare	X-linked recessive	Yes, usually	§	†	Mental retardation; neurologic defect most serious manifestation in affected men; multisystem disease
Diphosphoglycerate mutase (DPGM) and phosphatase (DPGP)	Very rare	Autosomal recessive	No			Both activities reside in the same enzyme protein; near-absence of 2,3-DPG; mild erythrocytosis
Enolase (ENO)	Very rare	Autosomal dominant?	Yes			Partial deficiency with spherocytic phenotype
Pyruvate kinase (PK)	Most common of group	Autosomal recessive	Yes			First-described and best-studied deficiency; more than 300 cases reported; prototype for group
Lactate dehydrogenase (LDH)	Very rare	Autosomal recessive	No		§	No hemolysis with lack of H-subunit; myopathy with lack of M-subunit

From Tanaka KR, Zeres CR: Red cell enzymopathies of glycolytic pathway. Semin Hematol 1990; 27(2):167.
* Rare indicates between 10 and 30 cases; very rare, fewer than five cases reported.
† Only in rare instances.
§ Usual manifestation of this deficiency.

Clinical and Laboratory Findings

Individuals with PK deficiency have a wide range of clinical presentations varying from severe neonatal anemia requiring exchange or multiple transfusions to a fully compensated hemolytic process in apparently healthy adults.[51] PK deficiency is generally more severe than hereditary spherocytosis. Except for those seriously affected during infancy, most PK-deficient patients have a stable hemoglobin level in the range of 8–12 g/dL.[51] PK-deficient patients may have a greater tolerance for anemia because of their increased 2,3-DPG levels, which decreases the oxygen affinity of their hemoglobin, therefore delivering more oxygen to the tissues even though lower amounts of hemoglobin are present.[51] Patients who present with the deficiency in infancy may require transfusions, and a splenectomy may be necessary during the first year of life.[52] Viral infections and pregnancy may exacerbate the chronic hemolytic process. Other rare complications include kernicterus, chronic leg ulcers, acute pancreatitis secondary to biliary tract disease, development of iron overload, splenic abscess, spinal cord compression by extramedullary hematopoietic tissue, and migratory phlebitis with arterial thrombosis.[52]

The RBC morphology is not a prominent factor in the diagnosis of PK deficiency. The RBCs are normochromic with only an occasional spiculated or irregularly contracted cell, except in children with severe anemia.[52] Reticulocytosis leads to a slight-to-marked macrocytosis. Postsplenectomy features include the usual Howell-Jolly bodies, siderocytes, and target cells. In addition, a characteristic finding suggestive of PK deficiency is many crenated RBCs of unusual form (shrunken echinocytes).[52] Frequently after splenectomy, a characteristic finding of PK deficiency is a very high percentage of reticulocytes in the range of 40–70%, which may persist.[53] The white blood cell (WBC) and platelet counts are normal or slightly increased. Patients usually display the characteristic

hallmarks of chronic hemolytic processes, such as variable degrees of jaundice, slight-to-moderate splenomegaly, and an increased incidence of gallstones.[53] Laboratory indications of hemolysis, including an increased indirect bilirubin level, a decreased haptoglobin level, and an increased fecal urobilinogen level, may be present. The osmotic fragility of fresh cells is usually normal, but the incubated osmotic fragility test may show some abnormality.[52, 53] The results of the incubated Heinz body test show increased numbers of Heinz bodies in the RBCs,[45] and the results of the direct antiglobulin test are negative. The autohemolysis test shows that many PK-deficient cells have increased hemolysis after 48 hours' incubation that is not corrected by glucose. However, the autohemolysis pattern is variable and is not very useful in the diagnosis of this disorder.[52, 53]

The diagnosis of PK deficiency depends on the specific demonstration of quantitatively reduced activity or qualitative abnormalities of erythrocyte PK.[52] Most homozygotes or compound heterozygotes have 5–25% of enzyme activity, and clinically normal heterozygotes have about half the normal activity.[52] The enzyme can be assayed by a spectrophotometric assay of a hemolysate prepared from RBCs with the WBCs carefully removed. Contaminating white cells may obscure the correct results because WBC/RBC PK activity is about 300:1.[52] The assay uses phosphoenolpyruvate (as substrate), crystalline lactate dehydrogenase, and NADH constituted in such a way so that the oxidation of NADH is followed at 340 nm, and optical density is decreased according to the amount of NADH oxidized to NAD[57] (Fig. 17–12). PK is an allosteric enzyme, and its activity at low phosphoenolpyruvate concentration is strongly dependent on the presence of fructose diphosphate.[48] More complex techniques may be necessary when a variant form of PK is suspected.[58] Screening tests for PK deficiency are based on the same principle as that described earlier, except that the hemolysate and reagents are absorbed onto filter paper and the

The enzyme pyruvate kinase catalyzes the following reaction:

1. ADP + Phosphoenolpyruvic acid $\xrightarrow[\text{Kinase}]{\text{Pyruvate}}$ ATP + Pyruvic acid

The pyruvic acid formed then takes part in the following reaction:

2. Pyruvic acid + NADH $\xrightarrow[\text{Dehydrogenase}]{\text{Lactic}}$ Lactic acid + NAD
   (high   (no fluorescence)
   fluorescence)

Figure 17–12 Principle of pyruvate kinase test. In the screening test, a red blood cell suspension made from blood with the plasma and buffy coat removed is incubated with the reagent that contains adenosine diphosphate (ADP), phosphoenolpyruvic acid, and nicotinamide-adenine dinucleotide, reduced form (NADH). Lactic dehydrogenase, which is also required for the reaction to proceed, is provided by the red blood cells. When pyruvate kinase is present, the NADH is destroyed, which results in a loss of fluorescence (spots made on filter paper are viewed under long-wave ultraviolet light). When pyruvate is deficient in the sample, the NADH remains intact, and no loss of fluorescence occurs. ATP, adenosine triphosphate; NAD, nicotinamide-adenine dinucleotide.

loss of fluorescence, rather than color, is visually evaluated to determine the oxidation of NADH to NAD.[48]

Therapy and Prognosis

No specific therapy is available for PK deficiency except supportive treatment and RBC transfusion as necessary. Splenectomy does not totally correct the hemolysis but usually raises the hemoglobin levels from 1 to 3 g/dL, which is enough to reduce or eliminate the need for transfusion.[52]

Differential Diagnosis

Because PK deficiency causes chronic hemolytic anemia, it must be differentiated from hemoglobinopathies, hereditary spherocytosis, and other enzymopathies.[59] The appropriate diagnostic strategy is to first eliminate the hemoglobinopathies (through electrophoresis and morphology) and hereditary spherocytosis (through morphology, osmotic fragility, and membrane protein studies), then proceed to tests for enzyme disorders as have been described.[48]

THE PORPHYRIAS

The porphyrias are a group of rare diseases that are usually hereditary. They result from errors in heme biosynthesis at different levels in the normal synthetic pathway (see Chapter 9). Each disorder is caused by a specific enzymatic defect, resulting in an overproduction of a specific porphyrin. Signs and symptoms vary, depending on which enzyme is reduced in function. Porphyrias may also be acquired as a result of drugs, chemicals, or heavy metals, such as lead.

The porphyrias include congenital erythropoietic porphyria, acute intermittent porphyria, porphyria cutanea tarda, erythropoietic protoporphyria, variegate porphyria, and hereditary coproporphyria. Table 17–5 summarizes the porphyrias, listing the missing enzyme, accumulated precursor, cutaneous signs, and systemic manifestations and suggesting treatment for each.[45]

PAROXYSMAL NOCTURNAL HEMOGLOBINURIA

History and Etiology

In the late 1800s, Gull published a case describing a patient with hematuria that was worse in the morning.[60] Strubing, in 1882, described a patient with hemoglobinuria after sleep.[61] He suggested that the RBCs were destroyed in the blood stream. He also found a fine-grain yellowish-brown sediment in the urine that may have been hemosiderin.

In 1911, van Den Berg showed that RBCs from a similar patient were lysed in normal serum as well as in the patient's serum.[62] Marchiafava and Micheli studied the disorder in detail, and for a time it was designated Marchiafava-Micheli syndrome.[63, 64]

Paroxysmal nocturnal hemoglobinuria (PNH) is regarded as a hemolytic anemia but is actually a myeloproliferative clonal disorder of the bone marrow that exhibits an intravascular hemolytic anemia resulting from increased susceptibility of the RBCs to complement.[65] The membrane defect is present not only in the erythrocytes but also in the platelets and granulocytes and possibly the lymphocytes.[65, 66] It is the only *acquired* hemolytic disorder caused by an abnormality of the RBC membrane. PNH results from a clonal somatic mutation that occurs at the pluripotential stem cell level.[65] The fact that PNH RBCs in G-6-PD heterozygous patients possess only one of the two enzyme variants, whereas both enzymes (G-6-PD-A and -B) are seen in the patient's normal cells, substantiates that this disorder is of a single-cell origin. In most patients, the abnormal clone coexists with normal hemopoiesis, which results in a dual population of blood cells.[67] This abnormal cell line appears to originate from a damaged marrow. Many PNH patients have a prior history of aplastic anemia or pancytopenia that may be either drug induced or idiopathic.[65]

Pathophysiology

The main defect in PNH is an acquired membrane abnormality that causes increased susceptibility of blood cells to complement.[65, 68] This abnormality of the RBC membrane causes intravascular, autologous, complement-mediated hemolysis, activated by either the classic or the alternative pathway. In addition, hemolysis due to complement occurs as a result of lowering of the pH or increasing of the Mg^{2+} levels of the blood plasma.[69] The characteristic membrane defects found in PNH erythrocytes as well as platelets, monocytes, and granulocytes result from missing proteins, all of which have been traced to a defective anchoring of the proteins to membrane glycophospholipids that contain phosphatidylinositol.[70, 71] Included in these missing proteins are the "decay-accelerating factor" and other complement regulatory proteins.[72, 73] The function of decay-accelerating factor is to accelerate the rate of destruction of erythrocyte-bound C3 convertase, which inhibits both classic- and alternative-pathway complement-mediated cell lysis.[74] The C3 activated by the alternative pathway attaches much more readily to PNH cell surfaces than to normal

Table 17–5. PORPHYRIAS

Disease	Missing Enzyme	Build-up	Cutaneous Signs	Systemic Manifestations	Treatment
Congenital erythropoietic porphyria (CEP)	Uroporphyrinogen III cosynthetase	Uroporphyrins II and III Coproporphyrin in marrow Uroporphyrin I in plasma, nucleated red cells, excreta	Exposure to daylight incurs photooxidation, mutilating photosensitivity, erythrodontia, scarring, alopecia, hypertrichosis of face	Splenomegaly, hemolytic anemia Most nucleated red cells, particularly metarubricytes, show intense red fluorescence in ultraviolet light Progressive disfigurement of exposed areas, leading to mutilation	Avoidance of sunlight Ingestion of beta carotene (antioxidant) to confer dermal tolerance to sunlight
Porphyria cutanea tarda (PCT)	Hepatic uroporphyrinogen decarboxylase	Hepatic accumulation and urinary excretion of uroporphyrin I and coproporphyrin	Photosensitivity of exposed skin; vesicles, bullae and erosions, moderate scarring, alopecia, milia formation, increased facial hair and periorbital pigmentation, hypertrichosis	Diabetes mellitus, occasional hepatic tumor, increased hepatic iron level Most common porphyria Occurs in alcoholic cirrhosis	Iron removal by phlebotomy or iron-chelating agents Decrease of alcohol consumption and estrogen hormones
Acute intermittent porphyria (AIP)	Porphobilinogen deaminase (impairs synthesis of uroporphyrinogen I synthetase)	Massive production of porphobilinogen δ-aminolevulinic acid in urine	None	Muscle paralysis, acute abdominal colic, hypertension, insomnia, polyneuropathy, depression	Avoidance of barbiturates, anticonvulsants, sulfonamide derivatives, sedatives
Hereditary coproporphyria	Coproporphyrinogen III oxidase	Coproporphyrin	Symptomless (50% of patients) Photosensitivity—less than in VP Abdominal colic—less than in VP Neurologic and mental manifestations	Similar to VP abdominal colic, neurologic and mental manifestations	Aggravated by barbiturates, anticonvulsants, and variety of sedatives
Erythropoietic protoporphyria	Heme synthetase	Free protoporphyrin IX	"Burning," erythema, edema, moderate scarring, "waxy" thickening of light-exposed areas; mild epidermal photosensitivity Test feces as well as urine for porphyrins	Cholelithiasis and occasional hepatic failure, protoporphyrin leaks out from erythroblasts into skin and tissues and is excreted in feces Common porphyria	Avoidance of sunlight Ingestion of beta carotene to confer dermal tolerance to sunlight
Variegate porphyria (VP)	Protoporphyrinogen oxidase	Coproporphyrin III in feces (vast increase) and urine	Photosensitivity to sunlight Chronic cutaneous involvement Bullae, erosions, hyperpigmentation scarring, hypertrichosis (but not as unsightly as in CEP)	Combinations of systemic manifestations of AIP and PCT, excrete increased coproporphyrin in feces Episodic attacks of abdominal colic, neuropsychiatric malfunction	Avoidance of barbiturates, sulfonamides, excess alcohol consumption

RBCs. The C3b activates terminal components C5 and C9, then easily penetrates the PNH cell surface because the membrane lacks decay-accelerating factor. PNH RBCs are also deficient in another membrane protein, homologous restriction factor, which inhibits complement-mediated transmembrane channel expression. Another abnormality found on PNH RBC membranes is a deficiency in C8 binding protein, which binds and inhibits C8. This lack makes PNH cells vulnerable to the autologous membrane attack of complex C5–C9 of complement. Also included in the abnormalities are deficiencies of membrane inhibitor of reactive lysis and lymphocyte function–associated antigen 3, increased susceptibility of glycophorin-α to proteolysis-122, and marked decreased activity of acetylcholinesterase in the RBC membranes.[70] The degree of acetylcholinesterase activity depression in the RBCs parallels the severity of the hemolysis in the disorder, but this deficiency is not of pathogenetic significance, because neither the hereditary deficiency of acetylcholinesterase nor its chemical inactivation leads to complement sensitivity or hemolysis, as occurs in PNH.[65]

The PNH erythrocytes have been classified into subpopulations according to their susceptibility to complement-mediated lysis. Two populations of RBCs have been identified by using monoclonal antibody immunofluorescence analysis for acetylcholinesterase activity. One subgroup is normally resistant to hemolysis in acidified serum and has normal membrane acetylcholinesterase activity; the other lacks acetylcholinesterase activity and is abnormally susceptible to lysis. In vitro, several cell populations can be identified because of differing sensitivity to lysis in acidified serum when graded amounts of complement are used. They are graded from PNH-I RBCs, which are nearly normal in their susceptibility to complement; to PNH-II, which are three to five times more sensitive; to PNH-III, which are extremely sensitive to complement (15 to 25 times more so than normal RBCs).[75] When a given quantity of serum complement is activated by either the classic or the alternative pathway, PNH cells fix many more molecules of activated C3 than normal RBCs do. The terminal lytic complex of complement components C5 through C9 creates membrane lesions. The membrane of a PNH-III cell looks like a sieve. The number of complement-sensitive RBCs varies from patient to patient; however, the percentage of PNH-III cells determines the intensity of the clinical symptoms. If a patient has fewer than 20% PNH-III cells, the hemolysis is mild, but if 20–50% PNH-III cells are present, the hemolysis is episodic (sleep induced), and if more than 50% PNH-III cells are present, there exist perpetual

hemoglobinemia and hemoglobinuria.[45, 75] The pathophysiology of PNH is summarized in Fig. 17–13.

Clinical and Laboratory Findings

PNH has an insidious onset, and 20% of cases have severe aplastic anemia for one to several years before diagnosis. It has been associated with middle age or young adulthood but can occur at any age.[45] It affects both sexes equally.

The anemia may be mild to severe, depending on the amount of hemolysis present. The nocturnal hemoglobinuria or the passage of reddish urine on arising from sleep, from which PNH derives its name, is present in only 25% of patients with PNH.[65] However, nocturnal hemoglobinemia is present in most patients. This condition is sleep induced and occurs during either daytime or nighttime sleep. The cause for the sleep hemoglobinemia has been disputed, but many explain that the phenomenon is caused by the lowered blood pH during sleep, facilitating complement binding to the PNH cells. Other causes also precipitate heightened hemolytic episodes, including infections, vaccinations, transfusions (which may increase the supply of complement available), x-ray contrast dye exposure, and possibly even strenuous exercise.[65]

Hemolytic Process

If the level of free hemoglobin in the plasma is less than 30–40 mg/dL, the hemoglobin is catabolized in the proximal tubules, and hemosiderinuria is present.[45] At levels greater than this, hemoglobinuria is present. Even in patients without classic hemoglobinuria, hemosiderinuria is usually present. This condition can be detected by performing a Prussian blue iron stain on the urine sediment and finding the sluffed tubular cells filled with iron (Fig. 17–14). Most patients develop iron deficiency anemia because of this heavy loss of iron in the urine. Infections are common because of defects in neutrophil function.[76] Patients with PNH have a predisposition to intravascular thrombosis, especially in the portal circulation or the venous circulation of the brain. Hepatic vein thrombosis or Budd-Chiari syndrome results in severe, colicky abdominal pain.[77] When the pain is fully developed, the prognosis is poor. Patients with PNH may have self-limited attacks of abdominal pain, presumably caused by intestinal infarction or bleeding. Severe headaches that present in some PNH patients may be caused by thrombi in small vessels of the brain. The thrombosis has been attributed to increased susceptibility of PNH platelets to complement activation.[78] The thromboplas-

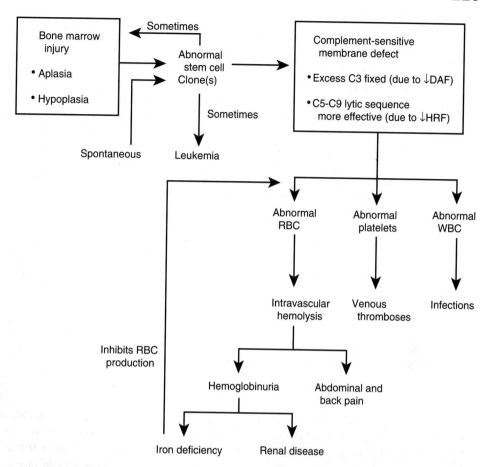

Figure 17–13 Pathophysiology of paroxysmal nocturnal hemoglobinuria (PNH). DAF, decay accelerating factor; HRF, homologous restriction factor. (From Beck WS (ed): Hematology, 5th ed. Cambridge, MA: MIT Press, 1991.)

tin material released by the intravascularly hemolyzed RBCs may also contribute to the hypercoagulable state.[79] Severely thrombocytopenic PNH patients may show bleeding tendencies.

Routine Hematologic Findings

Patients with PNH are usually pancytopenic with a mild-to-severe anemia, leukopenia, and thrombocytopenia. Hemoglobin levels vary from below 6 gm/dL to normal. Reticulocyte levels are mildly to moderately elevated but may be less than would be seen in other hemolytic anemias of the same magnitude. RBCs may appear slightly macrocytic because of this reticulocytosis. No shape abnormalities or spherocytosis is usually present. The osmotic fragility is normal and the results of the direct antiglobulin test are negative.[45] As the disease develops, if the patient does not undergo

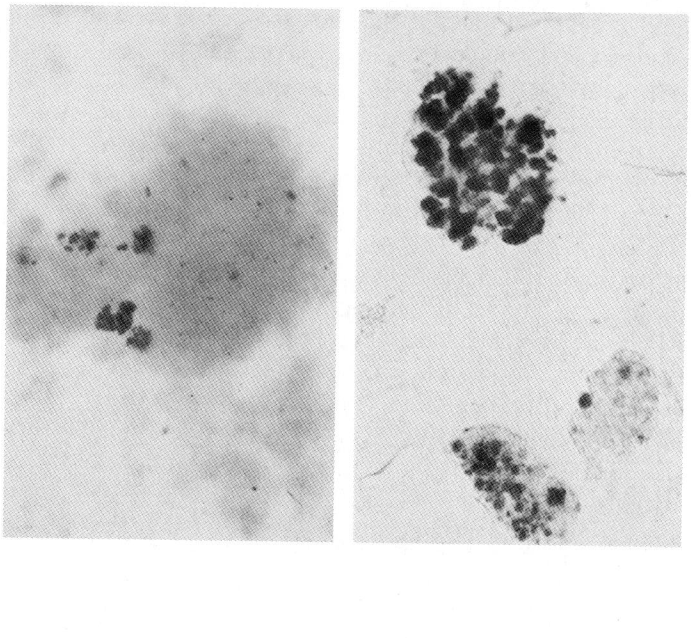

Figure 17–14 Renal tubular cells laden with hemosiderin and ferritin from a patient with paroxysmal nocturnal hemoglobinuria. (From Hoffbrand AV, Pettit JE: Clinical Haematology Illustrated: An Integrated Text and Colour Atlas. Edinburgh: Churchill Livingstone, 1987.)

transfusion, iron deficiency develops, and the RBCs become microcytic and hypochromic. At this point, the plasma iron and ferritin levels are usually low, and the total iron-binding capacity is elevated.[45] As is common in hemolytic disorders, folate deficiency often occurs if patients are not supplemented with folate.

A moderate neutropenia (causing leukopenia) is almost always present. Leukocyte alkaline phosphatase level is often very low.[80] Neutrophil life span appears normal. PNH granulocytes do have functional defects that cause decreased resistance to pyogenic organisms.[81] Infection causes 5–10% of fatalities in PNH patients. The platelet count may be moderately or markedly decreased (ranging from 50 to 100 × 10^9/L). Platelet life span also appears to be normal, but the platelets bind activated C3 excessively, causing the release of excess serotonin.[45, 65]

The bone marrow usually shows normal cellularity with RBC hyperplasia. However, some patients have aplasia or hypocellularity. Stainable iron is often absent unless the patient undergoes transfusion and then may be normal or even increased.[65]

Hemosiderinuria is an almost constant feature of PNH and is of great diagnostic importance. A Prussian blue stain of the urine sediment reveals blue-staining hemosiderin granules in the sluffed tubular cells (see Fig. 17–14). The presence of hemoglobinuria is variable, as discussed earlier. Hemoglobinuria may be distinguished from hematuria by a positive blood result on the reagent strip in urinalysis and by absence of intact RBCs on the urine microscopic examination. The hemoglobinuria may lead to formation and detection of hemoglobin casts. Renal problems due to the iron deposition may occur in PNH patients.[82]

Special Diagnostic Tests

The diagnosis of PNH should be suspected in any patient with idiopathic pancytopenia and an acquired nonspherocytic anemia accompanied by a reticulocytosis.[65] Screening tests should include urine hemosiderin determination and the sugar water test (sucrose hemolysis test). If the sugar water test result is positive, the Ham test (acidified serum lysis test) is used to confirm the diagnosis.[65]

Sugar Water Test (Sucrose Hemolysis Test). The sugar water test depends on the activation of complement at low ionic strengths.[83] When normal RBCs are suspended in an isotonic sucrose solution, osmotic lysis does not occur, because the sucrose does not penetrate the RBC membrane. If PNH RBCs are in this isotonic sucrose solution, the low ionic strength enhances the binding of complement components, especially C3 to the RBC membrane. The mechanism of hemolysis may be

that the complement-sensitive PNH RBCs develop membrane defects through which the sucrose can pass and produce osmotic lysis, or that complement may cause large enough defects to permit the loss of the RBC contents or hemolysis.

The sugar water screening test is performed by adding 0.2 mL of the patient's whole blood to 1.8 mL of an isotonic sucrose solution and incubating for 30 minutes at room temperature. A normal control should be run simultaneously. The percentage of hemolysis is calculated. Hemolysis of 5% is considered negative and within normal limits. Hemolysis of 6–10% is borderline. If more than 10% lysis is obtained, the diagnosis of PNH is almost certain. Some hemolysis may be seen in the absence of complement-sensitive PNH cells and may occur in megaloblastic anemia and AHA. If the patient's serum lacks complement, a false-negative result may be obtained. (See the Appendix for the complete procedure.)

Ham Test (Acidified Serum Lysis Test). The Ham test is used to establish a definitive diagnosis of PNH.[84] ABO compatible fresh normal serum (containing complement) is acidified to a pH of 6.8 with 0.15 N HCl and is added to both washed patient RBCs and washed normal RBCs for a control. The acidification of the serum activates complement by the alternative pathway and facilitates the binding of C3 to the RBC membrane. The PNH cell membrane defect renders them susceptible to the activated complement. Normal nonacidified serum and treated serum prepared by incubation at 56 °C for 30 minutes to inactivate complement activity are also added to the patient and control cells in separate tubes (Table 17–6). The test result is positive and the diagnosis of PNH probable if hemolysis occurs with the acidified serum but not with the heat-treated (complement-destroyed) serum. Some hemolysis may occur with the nonacidified serum. The percentage of lysis correlates to the percentage of complement-sensitive cells. The results of the acid hemolysis test may also be positive in some congenital dyserythropoietic anemias, but the sucrose hemolysis is normal.[75] (See Appendix for the complete procedure.)

Therapy and Prognosis

The treatment of PNH is mainly supportive with transfusions, antibiotics, and anticoagulants. Because both whole blood and packed red cells often contain enough activated complement components to increase hemolysis of the patient's own RBCs, the use of washed RBCs or frozen reconstituted RBCs prevents this.[85] Iron therapy is given to help alleviate the iron deficiency caused by the urinary loss of hemoglobin. Steroids given every

Table 17-6. ACIDIFIED SERUM LYSIS TEST (HAM TEST)

Reagent	Tube 1	Tube 2	Tube 3	Tube 4	Tube 5	Tube 6
Acidified serum	0.5 mL			0.5 mL		
Unacidified serum		0.5 mL			0.5 mL	
Heated acidified serum			0.5 mL			0.5 mL
Patient cells (50%, washed)	0.05 mL	0.05 mL	0.05 mL			
Normal cells				0.05 mL	0.05 mL	0.05 mL

The tubes are incubated for 60 minutes at 37 °C. If significant hemolysis occurs in tube 1 and no lysis occurs in tube 3, the diagnosis of paroxysmal nocturnal hemoglobinuria is probable. Slight hemolysis may occur in tube 3. Tubes 4 through 6 are controls.

other day may decrease the hemolysis in some patients. Anticoagulants are used in the treatment of thrombotic complications, such as Budd-Chiari syndrome associated with PNH. In suitable patients, bone marrow transplantation may be an option.[86]

The clinical course of PNH varies widely: rarely, a patient dies of the disorder within a few months, but most patients experience a chronic course, with the symptom severity changing from time to time as the amount of normal cells and the PNH clone change. The disease is very serious, and most patients die from its various complications, such as the thrombotic episodes or pancytopenia. Some PNH patients may develop acute leukemia as a terminal event.[87]

EXTRACORPUSCULAR (EXTRINSIC) ABNORMALITIES DAMAGING RED BLOOD CELLS

Microangiopathic Hemolytic Anemia

In 1962, Brain and colleagues[88] described microangiopathic hemolytic anemias as a group of clinical disorders characterized by RBC fragmentation in the circulation, resulting in intravascular hemolysis. The fragmentation occurred as a result of RBCs passing through fibrin deposits inside the lumens of arterioles and capillaries, or through damaged epithelium and vessel walls.[88] In vitro studies of RBC fragmentation demonstrate RBCs being forced through a fibrin clot, attaching to fibrin, folding around the strands, and fragmenting by the force of the flowing blood.[89] Two disorders with severe microangiopathic hemolytic anemia are thrombotic thrombocytopenic purpura (TTP) and hemolytic uremic syndrome (HUS), in which widespread microthrombi occur in arterioles and capillaries. These syndromes also have thrombocytopenia.

Microangiopathic hemolytic anemia may be observed in some patients with sepsis,[90] disseminated

carcinomatosis,[91] DIC,[88] after liver or kidney transplantation,[92] complications of pregnancy,[93] malignant hypertension,[94] and venoms and toxins.[95] Several antineoplastic drugs such as mitomycin[96] can cause a disorder similar to hemolytic uremic syndrome.

THROMBOTIC THROMBOCYTOPENIC PURPURA

History

TTP was first described by Moschcowitz[97] in 1925 in a 16-year-old girl with fever, weakness, malaise, anemia, purpura, petechiae, and renal involvement with hematuria. A postmortem examination provided evidence of hyaline thrombi in the terminal arterioles and capillaries of many organs. Moschcowitz suggested that the thrombi were composed of clumped RBCs. In 1936, Baehr and associates[98] reported on four TTP patients with thrombotic lesions in small arterioles and capillaries at autopsy; the thrombi were composed of agglutinated platelets and not RBCs. Studies of TTP by Gore[99] in 1950 revealed thrombi occluding capillaries and arterioles in all organs. The thrombi stained positively with periodic acid–Schiff (PAS), confirming that the hyaline material was of platelet and not of RBC origin.

Definition

TTP is a heterogeneous clinical syndrome characterized by the pentad of hemolytic anemia with RBC fragmentation, thrombocytopenia, fluctuating neurologic signs, fever, and progressive renal failure. Deposition of microthrombi that contain platelets and fibrin is observed in arterioles and capillaries of many organs.[45, 100, 101] Many patients may be cured with effective therapy, and remission may be induced in others. TTP is a rare, potentially fatal disorder, but the diagnosis can be made readily by examination of the blood smear and with clinical and laboratory procedures, and treatment can be life saving.[45, 100]

Pathogenesis

TTP is not a single disease but a syndrome with diverse etiologies and pathogenic mechanisms.[45, 100] Immunologic diseases, infectious diseases, pregnancy, and hereditary factors may be precipitating factors that influence this syndrome.[102] However, at times, predisposing factors may not be apparent.

An abnormality of the vascular endothelium may be present because TTP has been observed in association with lupus erythematosus, rheumatoid arthritis, and other disorders of autoimmune origin, thus suggesting an immunologic etiology for TTP.[102]

The deposition of platelet thrombi in capillaries and arteries is believed to be caused by endothelial cell injury with platelet adhesion; by aggregation and agglutination within the vessel, leading to endothelial cell damage; or by both processes occurring simultaneously.[103] In the gamma G immunoglobulin (IgG) fraction of normal plasma, an inhibitor of platelet aggregation is present.[101] A factor in the plasma of some patients with TTP is present that induces aggregation of normal platelets in vitro.[100] These observations must be taken into account in the pathogenic mechanism of TTP.

Recently, it has been reported that patients with TTP in remission may have abnormally large plasma von Willebrand's factor molecules, which probably result from endothelial cell damage, and these large molecules may aid in the formation of platelet thrombi when a patient relapses.[104] Normally, von Willebrand's factor molecules are larger in endothelial cells than in plasma but become smaller when circulating in plasma. The febrile nature of TTP is consistent with infection, such as with *Mycoplasma pneumoniae*,[90] and the disease has also occurred in association with viral infection.[94] Pregnancy has appeared to trigger the onset of TTP.[93] Because TTP has been reported in siblings, hereditary factors may play a role in the cause. Because of the varied causes given for TTP, this disorder may be the result of different conditions that affect the microcirculation.[103]

DIC may be present with similar clinical features, microangiopathic changes in erythrocytes, thrombocytopenia, and capillary lesions similar to those seen in TTP. However, hemolytic anemia with fragmented RBCs is not a common complication of DIC, and this disorder is not characterized by the severe hemolysis seen in TTP.[102]

Clinical and Laboratory Findings

TTP can occur at almost any age but is usually seen between 10 and 60 years of age.[102] Two forms exist: a chronic type, with symptoms persisting for months[105] or years, and an acute type, which is more common and is potentially fatal within a few days.[102]

Neurologic abnormalities with acute symptoms are the most common presenting complaints.[106] Central nervous system symptoms result from platelet thrombi in small vessels, which lead to small infarcts and hemorrhage. Central nervous system disturbances are headache, delirium, seizures, paresis, vertigo, and nerve palsy.[45, 102]

Hemorrhagic symptoms are the second most common complaint.[106] Severe hemolysis with jaundice and pallor may occur, and acute renal failure may be noted in some patients.[102]

Anemia is always present in TTP and may be severe.[102] Reticulocytes are increased, and nucleated RBCs are present on the peripheral smear. Erythrocytes reveal microangiopathic changes, such as fragmented, helmet, spherical, and small, bizarre shapes, which are pathognomonic of TTP, and the diagnosis is not made unless fragmented cells are present. Diffusely basophilic cells are prominent (Fig. 17–15).[106]

Severe thrombocytopenia is frequently present with platelet counts often below 20×10^9/L. Platelet survival is decreased because of consumption. Megakaryocytes are normal in number but do not often show platelet budding.[102]

The leukocyte count is often increased, and a shift to the left may occur in immature granulocytes.[106] Erythroid hyperplasia is noted in the bone marrow, and most of the cells are at the rubricyte stage.

Microthrombi in renal vessels may cause proteinuria, hematuria, and functional impairment in the kidney.[106] Coagulation procedures reveal a normal prothrombin time, a normal activated partial

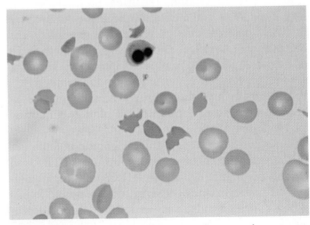

Figure 17–15 Thrombotic thrombocytopenic purpura (TTP).

thromboplastin time, a normal thrombin time, and a normal-to-increased fibrinogen level initially, but eventually the fibrinogen falls. Fibrin split products are increased.[106]

Prognosis and Treatment

About 80%[45] of patients respond dramatically to infusions of normal fresh-frozen plasma. Some patients respond immediately to infusion of two to three units of fresh-frozen plasma, but usually six to eight units are required for remission.[45] Plasma-exchange therapy or plasmapheresis on a cell separator and replacement with fresh-frozen plasma is recommended because of the increased survival rate that it confers.[102, 107] Reported response rates to plasma exchange and replacement therapy are 70–90%.[45, 107]

In some patients, plasma may supply a lacking substance. This substance might be able to depolymerize large von Willebrand's factor molecules or inhibit a platelet-aggregating factor. On the other hand, a toxic substance may be removed by plasma exchange.[102]

Oral anti-platelet agents, such as aspirin, dipyridamole, and sulfinpyrazone, should supplement the exchange if the main manifestations of TTP are thrombotic. Other agents used are prednisone and azathioprine.[45, 102]

Rarely, splenectomy produces amazing improvement when it is combined with anti-platelet drugs and high-dose corticosteroid therapy. To prevent early relapse, maintenance doses of anti-platelet drugs are recommended for about 6 months or for a longer period in patients with recurrent TTP.[105] Administration of platelet concentrates is not recommended in patients with thrombocytopenia, because the concentrates may be a potential hazard by aggravating the thrombotic process.[109]

Clearing of neurologic signs, decreased reticulocyte count, diminishing hemolysis, and rising platelet count are signs of improvement. Most patients now recover completely. In some patients, however, the neurologic abnormalities may be permanent, and a few patients may suffer relapses months or years after the first episode.[105]

Autopsy Findings

Autopsy findings include prominent microthrombotic lesions in vessels in the brain, heart, pancreas, and lymph nodes. Histopathologic examination shows accumulation of hyaline material with a strongly positive periodic acid–Schiff reaction in lumina of arterioles and capillaries as well as accumulation of fibrin in the lumen of vessels at the site of wall damage.[108] In electron microscopy, the microthrombi contain fibrinlike material, aggregates of platelets, and occasionally white cells and RBCs.

HEMOLYTIC UREMIC SYNDROME

History

HUS, an acquired disorder that resembles TTP, was described by von Gasser in 1955, 30 years after Moschcowitz's initial report on TTP.[97] Von Gasser reported on the triad of microangiopathic hemolytic anemia, thrombocytopenia, and acute renal failure in children. At first, this was considered to be a new syndrome because of the severity of renal failure. Later, it was noted that HUS was a heterogeneous syndrome with several clinical variants and that it resembled TTP but was different from TTP because of the severity of the renal failure.[45]

Pathogenesis

The typical HUS of childhood has many features that are observed in an enteric infectious disease.[102] A verocytotoxin produced by different serotypes of *Escherichia coli* has been commonly associated with HUS.[110, 111] Comparable toxins are produced by other organisms, such as *Shigella dysenteriae,*[112, 113] *Streptococcus pneumoniae,*[114] and *Campylobacter jejunii.*[115] The main target site for verocytotoxin appears to be the renal capillary endothelium. The establishment of a link between cytotoxin-producing *E. coli* and the clinical syndrome is an exciting development in the pathogenesis of HUS. The bacterial cytotoxin acts by inhibiting protein synthesis and leads directly to cell death.[110] One pathogenic mechanism for HUS may be an episode of DIC that is set off by an infection caused by a gram-negative endotoxin.[100] The macrophage system is not able to clear the circulating fibrin and large deposits are found in glomerular vessels. Local fibrinolysis does not lyse the fibrin deposits, which persist and produce damage to the glomerulus, renal failure, microangiopathic hemolytic anemia, and thrombocytopenia. Endothelial cell injury may also occur secondary to the thrombosis in the glomerulus.[45]

Abundant data support the presence of intravascular platelet activation, and possibly the most obvious mechanism is some form of endothelial insult in the kidney.[111] Glomerular lesions of varying severity are observed, as are thrombi in arterioles and capillaries of the glomerulus. Necrosis with proteinaceous material (similar to fibrin) in the glomerular arterioles is common. Fibrosis may also be present.[45, 116]

Clinical and Laboratory Findings

Clinical features of HUS resemble those found in TTP.[117] Typical HUS occurs in infants younger than 2 years of age, and the prognosis is usually good. The peak incidence of HUS occurs between 6 months and 4 years of age after a febrile illness, which is often associated with vomiting and diarrhea preceding renal failure, hemolysis, and purpura. In contrast to TTP, neurologic disturbances are rare.[117] HUS is characterized by the sudden onset of acute renal failure, intravascular hemolysis with RBC fragmentation, hemoglobinuria, abdominal pain with vomiting, and variable thrombocytopenia.[45, 116] HUS rivals TTP in its severity, suddenness, and vascular involvement.[117] Hypertension is present in more than half the patients with HUS.[102]

The hemolytic anemia is accompanied by microangiopathic changes in RBCs similar to the changes in TTP.[116, 117] Shortened RBC survival results from the hemolysis and sequestration in the spleen. Thrombocytopenia occurs in most patients, and platelet survival is reduced. Moderate neutrophilia is present. Nucleated RBCs may be present in the peripheral smear. Coagulation studies reveal that the activated partial thromboplastin time, prothrombin time, and thrombin time are usually normal to prolonged. Coagulation findings typical of DIC may occasionally be present. The urine contains protein, RBCs, and often RBC casts.[102]

Treatment

Therapy is directed at managing the acute renal failure and beginning dialysis early.[118] Dialysis helps most infants and children recover from HUS. The prognosis is worse in patients whose renal failure is longer than 2–3 weeks' duration. Therapy to control the hypertension is also important. Some children continue to have renal impairment and hypertension, and some may not recover from anuria.[45] With appropriate management and supportive care of the acute renal failure, the mortality in childhood has been reduced.[45]

Exchange transfusions, plasmapheresis, or plasma infusion may lead to hematologic and renal improvement. Some children who recover from the first attack may have a recurrence months later.[118]

HUS in Adults

Adult HUS is more closely related to TTP in severity and prognosis than to the classic HUS in infancy. In adult HUS, renal failure is more prominent, and neurologic dysfunction is less than that in TTP. Most of the patients with adult HUS are women in whom the condition develops after gram-negative infection, preeclampsia, and eclampsia, in the postpartum period, or after ingestion of oral contraceptives.[119] Microangiopathic hemolytic anemia is present in these disorders. Enteric infections are not often seen in adults. Recent reports have shown a link between HUS and malignant disease and HUS and chemotherapeutic agents (such as mitomycin C).[102]

Clinical features and laboratory findings in adult HUS are similar to those in childhood HUS.[102] Control of renal failure, hypertension, and anemia is the goal of the initial therapy, and hemodialysis is usually necessary. Some success has been obtained with plasmapheresis or plasma infusions.[120]

Adult HUS may respond to platelet inhibitors, such as aspirin and dipyridamole, if they are given early.[111] If DIC is present, heparin infusion combined with plasma exchange is given. If renal failure persists for weeks and function cannot be restored, renal transplantation may be an alternative to lifelong dialysis.[102]

MALIGNANT HYPERTENSION

Microangiopathic hemolytic anemia occurs in patients with malignant hypertension. The mechanical destruction of RBCs results from fibrin deposition in arterioles and from the forcing of RBCs through damaged endothelium of arterioles. When hypertension is brought under control, RBC fragmentation and hemolytic anemia disappear.[94]

DIFFUSE INTRAVASCULAR COAGULATION

RBC fragmentation, which occurs in approximately half the patients with DIC, is the result of fibrin strands in the microvasculature.[102] The hemolysis is not usually severe. Thrombocytopenia of varying degrees is observed, and platelet function is impaired by fibrin degradation products.[45] DIC accompanies many systemic disorders, such as obstetric complications, disseminated carcinoma, snake bite, and infections. (See Chapter 34 for discussion of DIC.)

DISSEMINATED CARCINOMA

A common complication of disseminated carcinoma, particularly metastatic carcinoma of the stomach, is microangiopathic hemolytic anemia.[91] Hemolytic anemia with RBC fragmentation, DIC, hemoglobinemia, increased levels of unconjugated bilirubin, absent haptoglobin, and increased lactate dehydrogenase, in addition to metastatic infiltration of marrow, may cause a very severe anemia. Fragmentation of RBCs results from fibrin deposition in small vessels and also from contact with tumor cell emboli. The infiltrating tumor releases mucin, which then causes fibrin deposition in the microvasculature, resulting in RBC fragmentation.[45, 91]

Macroangiopathic Hemolytic Anemia

TRAUMATIC CARDIAC HEMOLYTIC ANEMIA

History

After corrective cardiac surgery in the 1950s, patients with aortic valve replacement developed anemia. The anemia was caused by injury and fragmentation of RBCs exposed to high shear stresses on a foreign surface.[121] The construction of prosthetic valves and surfaces has been improved, and traumatic cardiac hemolytic anemia has almost disappeared.

Pathogenesis

The hemolysis that occurs in patients with valvular disorders is mild and rarely leads to hemolytic anemia, except in patients with severe aortic stenosis.[121] Turbulence in blood flowing around or through the valve may occur, the valve may be improperly positioned, or the valve may be spontaneously separated from the natural valve. RBC destruction in flowing blood results not only from turbulence and shear stresses on artificial prosthetic valves but also from turbulence on an artificial foreign surface, which is no longer covered by a layer of endothelial cells.[121, 122]

Clinical and Laboratory Findings (Fig. 17–16)

The anemia that occurs in patients with heart valve prosthesis is of variable severity, and usually

a mild compensated hemolysis occurs.[122] Rarely, a patient will have a severe anemia that requires transfusion.[121]

Blood films show helmet, triangular, and other types of fragmented RBCs. The reticulocyte count is increased in spite of a normal hematocrit and compensated hemolysis. Platelets may be decreased. Lactate dehydrogenase activity and plasma hemoglobin level are elevated. Haptoglobin concentration is decreased, resulting in hemosiderin in the urine and reduced serum ferritin levels due to loss of iron.[121]

Treatment

If severe anemia is present, the prosthesis should be replaced. If the anemia is mild or compensated, normal erythropoietic activity should be maintained, and administration of ferrous sulfate is recommended to replace urinary iron loss.[121, 122]

MARCH HEMOGLOBINURIA

Definition

March hemoglobinuria is the name for hemoglobinuria and hemoglobinemia that result from forceful impact of the feet or other parts of body on a hard surface.[123]

History

In 1881, a soldier in Germany complained of passing dark urine after strenuous marches.[123] His physician found hemoglobin in the urine. Eighty years later, Davidson[124] proposed that RBCs were destroyed in soles of feet during the long-distance running and stamping gait of track runners. He recommended that track runners wear soft linings in their shoes, and the hemoglobinuria disappeared. In spite of padded insoles, traumatic disruption of RBCs by pressure on soles during running and walking may occur.

Clinical and Laboratory Findings

The physical examination is normal in patients with march hemoglobinuria and sports anemia. Hematocrit and hemoglobin level are often at lower limits of normal. RBCs may be slightly macrocytic, and reticulocyte percentage may be increased after strenuous sports.[89] The urine may be red or dark after exertion and may show hemoglobin casts, hemosiderin, and hemoglobin but clears after 6 or 12 hours.[123, 124]

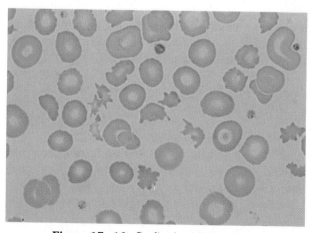

Figure 17–16 Cardiac hemolytic anemia.

Differential Diagnosis

March hemoglobinuria must be distinguished from paroxysmal cold hemoglobinuria or separated from hemoglobinuria that occurs after exposure to cold. Myoglobinuria can be distinguished from hemoglobinuria by solubility of urine in ammonium sulfate, by electrophoretic comparison with hemoglobin, and by muscle pain during exercise. Plasma is red or pink during hemoglobinuria but clear of pigment in myoglobinuria.[123, 124]

Treatment

The physician should reassure the patient that he or she does not have a serious problem. The condition will ameliorate when rubberized insoles are added to shoes or when the patient changes his or her gait.[123, 124]

Hemolytic Anemia Caused by Infection with Microorganisms

INTRACELLULAR MICROORGANISMS

Malaria

An infection of RBCs by malarial parasites is one of the most common causes of hemolytic anemia worldwide. More than 400 million individuals suffer from the disease. The yearly mortality of malaria is considered to be more than one million people.[125] Although malaria control measures have been implemented in numerous areas in the world for many years, in the past 25 years a resurgence of the disease has occurred as a result of resistance to many of the antimalarial drugs, particularly chloroquine. The *Anopheles* mosquito has also become resistant to insecticides.[126]

An increase in the disease has occurred in residents of the United States and other countries because of increased air travel to areas in which malaria is endemic.[126] Malaria may also be transmitted by blood transfusion, and the diagnosis should be considered in an individual with a febrile illness that occurs several weeks after a transfusion.[127]

Life Cycle

Malaria is a protozoan infection transmitted by the bite of the female *Anopheles* mosquito, which is the insect vector for the organism. Sporozoites in the salivary gland are injected into the human host. Sporozoites of the four species of the genus *Plasmodium* may cause malaria: *Plasmodium vivax, Plasmodium malariae, Plasmodium falciparum,* and *Plasmodium ovale.*

The sporozoites rapidly leave the circulating blood and invade hepatic parenchymal cells to begin exoerythrocytic schizogony, which occurs 6 to 12 days after exposure.[128] Hepatic cells rupture, releasing merozoites that invade circulating RBCs, and the erythrocytic life cycle schizogony begins. Inside the erythrocyte, the merozoite is nourished by the cell's contents, and it metabolizes the hemoglobin and grows intracellularly. The merozoite becomes a ring form, which grows into a late ring or ameboid trophozoite, then into an early schizont (chromatin dividing), and finally into a schizont that contains merozoites. The merozoites are released from the erythrocyte and invade other cells. The patient experiences chills and fever as the RBCs are ruptured.[128] It has been stated that some of the merozoites in *P. vivax* may reenter the liver to produce an exoerythrocytic cycle again, but this concept is not universally accepted. Other investigators state that some merozoites remain in the hepatocytes and may reappear in the circulation after a considerable length of time.[129]

Some of the merozoites form male and female gametocytes in the circulating blood. While taking a blood meal, gametocytes (sexual stages) are ingested by an *Anopheles* mosquito. The female gamete is fertilized by the male gamete in the stomach of the mosquito, resulting in a zygote, which establishes itself on the outer wall of the mosquito stomach and develops into an ookinete and then an oocyst. The oocyst produces sporozoites. As the abdomen enlarges by the force created by proteolysis of hemoglobin, the sporozoites become free and migrate to the salivary gland of the mosquito. When the mosquito takes a blood meal, the sporozoites inoculate the human host.[45]

Pathogenesis

The presence or lack of particular receptors on the surface of the RBC membrane determines the host range of the different plasmodia. RBCs lacking the Duffy determinants (Fya− b−) are not vulnerable to infection by *P. vivax.* The Duffy-negative phenotype has high frequency among West African blacks, and thus these individuals are resistant to vivax infection. The number of Duffy-negative individuals is lower and the incidence of *P. vivax* higher as one moves from West to East Africa. The development of the Duffy-negative population helped to prevent the spread of *P. vivax.* The missing or suppressed genes for the Duffy blood group seem to be a highly specific genetic adaptation to vivax malaria.[130, 131]

RBCs of patients with HPP are not invaded by malaria because the RBC cytoskeleton is altered and cells lack deformability.

The age of the cells somewhat determines what species of malaria infects the RBCs. *P. vivax* and *P. ovale* infect young RBCs and reticulocytes. *P.*

falciparum infects young and mature RBCs. *P. malaria* infects old RBCs.[132]

Having a hemoglobinopathy in some way guards against malarial infection and leads to an increased incidence of the hemoglobinopathy gene in the population. Hemoglobins S,[130-135] C,[136] and E[137]; a thalassemia[138]; and G-6-PD deficiency[138, 139] have been shown to benefit heterozygotes in combating malaria. The incidence of hemoglobin AS is greatest in areas where *P. falciparum* is prevalent.[45, 133] The specific physiologic benefit that hemoglobin AS provides is not clear. Further study is needed to elucidate the effect of sickle cell hemoglobin, other hemoglobinopathies, and G-6-PD on susceptibility to malaria.[133, 138, 139]

Growth of *P. falciparum* is low in fetal RBCs.[140] Adults with hereditary persistence of fetal hemoglobin have a low rate of parasite growth.

Clinical and Laboratory Findings

The clinical features of malaria vary with the species. The usual symptoms are fever, chills, rigors, sweating, headache, muscle pain, and prostration. About 25% of patients have a hemolytic anemia,[141] which may be accompanied by jaundice, splenomegaly, and hepatomegaly. In patients with chronic malaria or with repeated malarial infection, the spleen may be massively enlarged.

The main cause of anemia is the rupture of infected cells at the end of the asexual cycle; in addition, immune complexes may also play a role in the anemia. The amount of hemolysis is related to the number of RBCs parasitized; hemolysis is greatest in falciparum malaria because this species invades RBCs at all stages of development; hemolysis is less in vivax because the merozoites attach to reticulocytes.[141, 142] Hemolysis is characterized by spherocytosis, reticulocytosis, and shortened RBC survival. The spleen pits out the parasites from the infected RBCs, and the RBCs are often destroyed. At first, only parasitized RBCs succumb, but after several days, hemolysis becomes worse, and nonparasitized cells become spherical and are destroyed, possibly as a result of immunologic factors.[45, 142]

A few patients with malaria may have DIC,[143] which occurs with the release of thromboplastin material when RBCs are destroyed or as a result of immune complexes. Thrombocytopenia is found in about 75% of patients with resistance to chloroquine.[144]

During the infection, the white cell count is normal to slightly increased. Neutropenia may develop during chills and rigors. Monocytes and immature granulocytes may be observed if malaria persists. Malarial infection in patients with symptomatic infection is diagnosed by the presence of parasites in the peripheral blood smear stained with Wright-Giemsa. Smears should be made before the onset of chills and fever.[141] To concentrate parasites when few are present, a thick drop preparation should be prepared and stained with fresh diluted Giemsa (without fixing in methyl alcohol). RBCs are lysed with water-based Giemsa, and the parasite may be observed more frequently on this thick smear than on the thin smear; however, identification of the species is difficult. To identify the species, a thin smear must also be made. A platelet lying on top of a reticulocyte in a thick drop preparation may be confused with a malarial parasite (Fig. 17–17).

Malaria Species

Plasmodium vivax. *P. vivax* invades young RBCs, or reticulocytes.[141, 142] The early trophozoite has a small ring with a red chromatin dot and a blue-staining cytoplasmic circle. The RBC begins to grow larger and becomes pale and misshapen. Schüffner stippling is seen in the late ring stages and all other stages. In the growing trophozoite, the chromatin and cytoplasm increase in amount, and the ring shape is lost. The ameboid trophozoite almost fills the cell (Fig. 17–18). Yellow-brown pigment from digested hemoglobin appears. In an immature schizont, chromatin begins to divide into two or more masses. The mature schizont usually has 12–14 merozoites and yellow-brown hematin and hemosiderin in clumps (Fig. 17–19). The pale or decolorized RBC filled with merozoites soon releases the merozoites and disintegrates. A few merozoites prepare for sexual schizogony and transfer into large gametocytes with a bulky nucleus. Gametocytes are rounded with blue cytoplasm and pigment and either have a small, eccentrically placed, dispersed chromatin (male microgametocyte) or large, centrally located chro-

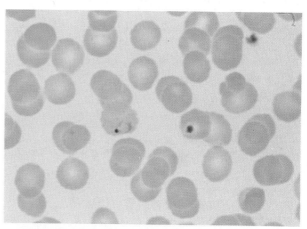

Figure 17–17 Platelet on top of a red blood cell, in comparison with *Plasmodium vivax*, ring form.

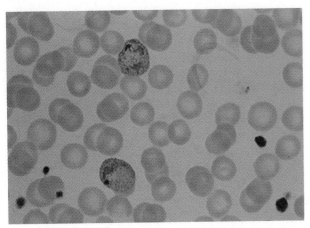

Figure 17–18 *Plasmodium vivax:* trophozoite.

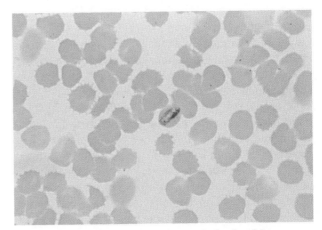

Figure 17–20 *Plasmodium malariae:* band form.

matin (female macrogametocyte). Erythrocytic cell cycle requires 44–48 hours.[45, 129, 132]

P. vivax has a worldwide distribution, especially in temperate climates and in the tropics. It is not as common in Africa as are other types.[129] *P. vivax* is difficult to eradicate, and relapses may occur. The schizont of *P. vivax* lies dormant for years in the liver and may become reactivated, causing a recurrence of infection.

Plasmodium ovale. Parasites invade young RBCs and reticulocytes. The young trophozoite resembles *P. vivax* and *P. malariae*. RBCs become enlarged, oval, and fringed and have Schüffner stippling. In the schizont stage, the RBCs are oval, and the parasite is round in the center of the cell. Merozoites can number four to eight or even more and are found in a rosette around a mass of pigment. Gametocytes are not able to be differentiated from *P. vivax*. The length of the asexual cycle is 48 hours.[129]

Plasmodium malariae. Parasites invade older RBCs, and the infection is usually mild. The ring stage has a single chromatin dot and a blue cyto-

plasmic ring that is often smaller and heavier than that of *P. vivax* but may not be distinguished from it. In growing trophozoites, chromatin is rounded or streaky; cytoplasm is in a narrow band form across the cell, and coarse brown pigment is noted. The band form is a characteristic feature of this species (Fig. 17–20). RBCs do not become enlarged, and no stippling occurs in the schizont stage (Fig. 17–21). Eight to 12 merozoites form a rosette around clumped pigment and are expelled from the cell. The asexual cycle is 72 hours, or every third day. Gametocytes are similar to those of vivax but smaller; pigment may be conspicuous, and few gametocytes are observed.[129]

P. malariae is found in tropical Africa, India, Burma, Malaysia, and Indonesia.[129, 135, 136] Infection with *P. malariae* is more amenable to chloroquine therapy than is that with *P. vivax*, but it also may be disabling. Rarely, patients may develop a nephropathy with albuminuria, hematuria, and edema that is likely a result of the deposition of immune complexes from parasite antigen in the kidney.[45]

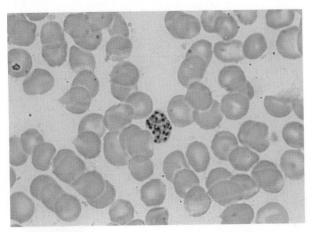

Figure 17–19 *Plasmodium vivax:* schizont.

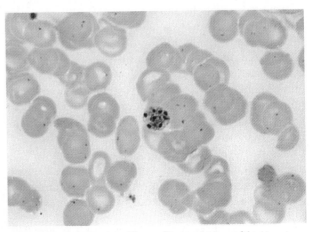

Figure 17–21 *Plasmodium malariae:* schizont.

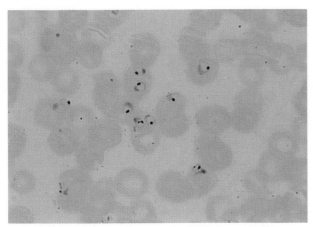

Figure 17–22 *Plasmodium falciparum:* ring form.

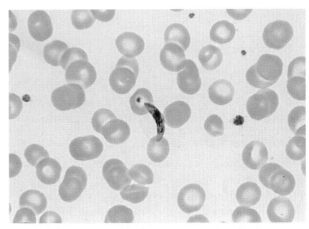

Figure 17–24 *Plasmodium falciparum:* gametocyte.

Plasmodium falciparum. Parasites invade old and young RBCs, which remain normal in size. Ring forms are numerous and may be missed because the ring is small with a small cytoplasmic circle and one or two little chromatin dots. One or more rings may be at the margin of the cell. The trophozoite grows somewhat and is usually the main form seen in circulation. Schizont stages occur in visceral organs and only rarely in peripheral blood, except in severe infections. Crescent- or banana-shaped gametocytes have deep blue cytoplasm with brownish pigment near the center and are easily recognized on thick preparations (Figs. 17–22 to 17–24). A cycle is 36–48 hours in length.[129]

P. falciparum is the most pathogenic human malaria, and it may run an acute fulminating course, ending in death if prompt treatment is not begun. It is important to make an early and rapid diagnosis. Massive intravascular hemolysis occurs with hemoglobinemia, hemoglobinuria, and jaundice. Acute renal failure may also occur. Mortality has been reported to be as high as 30%.[132] Erythrocytes with falciparum parasites plug up the microcirculation of many organs. DIC has been reported in patients with severe falciparum infection.[143] Cerebral malaria is caused by sludging of damaged RBCs in the microvasculature.[45]

Treatment

Therapy for malaria usually includes administration of chloroquine or quinine sulfate. Pyrimethamine and sulfonamides are also given. Chloroquine destroys all stages of malaria in erythrocytes except in drug-resistant falciparum infection: quinine sulfate is then often given in combination with pyrimethamine and sulfonamides.[45, 132, 144, 145]

Primaquine may be used to treat the hepatic stages of vivax malaria.[139] Patients with malaria and G-6-PD deficiency develop severe hemolysis after treatment with sulfones and primaquine.[139] When severe hemolysis develops in an individual with falciparum malaria, the patient should be checked for G-6-PD deficiency.[139] Because falciparum malaria has the potential for a rapid, fatal course, the infection should be treated as soon as possible after diagnosis. Drug-resistant strains of *P. falciparum* have required various combinations of antimalarial drugs.[139] Eventual cure for malaria lies in the development of a suitable vaccine.[139, 146, 147]

Babesia

Babesia are small ringlike protozoa (diameter less than 2 mm) within erythrocytes that resemble the ring stages of falciparum malaria.[129, 148] Babesiosis is an uncommon hemolytic disorder caused by a few of the 71 species of the small protozoan.[45] Most infections result from *Babesia microti,* which is transmitted from wild feral deer mice to humans by the tick *Ixodes dammini.*[143, 148] The disease is thought to be more severe in splenectomized indi-

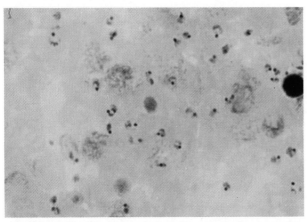

Figure 17–23 *Plasmodium falciparum:* thick preparation, ring forms.

viduals. Babesiosis has been transmitted by transfusion.

Geographic Distribution

Babesiosis occurs in Nantucket Island,[149] on coastal regions of the northeastern United States, and in California. It has been found in France, Ireland, Scotland, and other European countries.[45]

Laboratory Diagnosis

The diagnosis of babesiosis can be made by demonstration of the ring-shaped parasites on Wright-Giemsa–stained smears or by animal inoculation. Thick drop preparations are often preferred to thin smears because the parasites may be scarce.[129] Serologic tests for antibodies to *Babesia* have been described.[150]

Babesia are tiny rings with a minute chromatin dot and a minimal amount of cytoplasm. They may be round, oval, elongated, or ameboid. One or two chromatin dots, which stain dark purple, may be observed with practically no cytoplasm. More than one ring can be seen in an RBC.[45, 129, 151-153] Tetrad forms may be noted and aid in positively identifying babesia (Figs. 17–25 and 17–26).[153]

Treatment

The antibiotic clindamycin given in combination with quinine has been reported to be a highly effective treatment for babesiosis.[45] A cure should occur about a week after the institution of therapy, and consolidation therapy should continue for another week. The failure of chloroquine in human babesiosis has been reported.[154] Exchange transfusion has been used to treat transfusion-transmitted babesiosis.[155]

EXTRACELLULAR MICROORGANISMS

Clostridial Septicemia

Intravascular hemolysis, which is often fatal, is produced by the gram-positive, spore-forming ba-

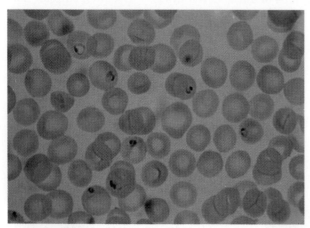

Figure 17–25 *Babesia microti:* rings.

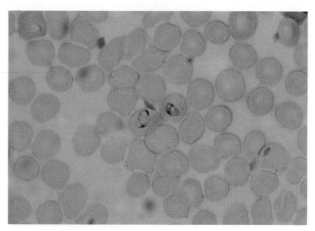

Figure 17–26 *Babesia microti:* tetrad.

cillus *Clostridium perfringens (welchii)*. Clostridial sepsis is a complication of septic abortion, deep wounds, and any condition that leads to destruction of RBCs and to lysis. Leukocytosis with a shift to the left and thrombocytopenia are often present.[45, 132, 156]

Swift therapy with transfusions, antibiotics, and other measures is required before the surgeon removes the infected organ. The prognosis is grave, and many patients die in spite of extensive treatment.[45, 132, 156, 157]

BARTONELLOSIS

Human bartonellosis (Carrión disease) is transmitted by the sand fly. The RBCs become infected with the organism *Bartonella bacilliformis*, which is thought to adhere to the exterior surface of the RBC. There are two clinical stages: acute hemolytic anemia (Oroya fever) is the early stage; the second stage, verruca peruviana, is characterized by eruptions on the face and extremities and by the development of bleeding, warty tumors.

Carrión disease was named for a medical student, Daniel A. Carrión, who in 1885 inoculated himself with blood from a verrucous node on the skin of a patient. He developed a fatal hemolytic anemia similar to the disease Oroya fever, which was first observed in railroad workers near the city of Oroya in the Peruvian Andes.[158, 159, 160]

Oroya fever responds to chloramphenicol, penicillin, streptomycin, and tetracyclines.[161]

Hemolytic Anemia Caused by Chemicals, Drugs, and Venoms

DRUGS AND CHEMICALS

RBCs may be hemolyzed in individuals who are deficient in RBC enzymes after an exposure to oxidative agents.[132, 162] Many oxidizing agents will interact with the hemoglobin molecule and produce

Heinz bodies either by denaturing globin chains or by oxidizing heme groups, thereby causing methemoglobinemia. Examples of such agents are dapsone (for leprosy) and salazopyrine (for ulcerative colitis).[132] High doses of dapsone chemically damage the RBC membrane, and bite RBCs may be observed. Nitrites are one of a group of chemicals that cause methemoglobinemia, particularly in young children who drink water contaminated with nitrites or eat vegetables in large amounts that contain nitrites.[132]

Exposure to high levels of arsenic, copper, and lead has caused intravascular hemolysis, as can the use of water irrigation during surgery. Spherocytes are seen on the blood film. In near-drowning, an individual may have severe hemolysis resulting from water inhalation.[162]

Aspirin, codeine, and phenacetin, when combined in high doses, may produce intravascular hemolysis and methemoglobinemia. Sodium chlorate, a weed killer, can produce acute intravascular hemolysis when exposure to high doses occurs.[132, 162]

VENOMS

The brown recluse spider (*Loxosceles reclusa*) injects a venom that leads to a severe hemolytic anemia with local pain, ischemic necrosis, and ulceration at the site of the bite. The venom contains enzymes that act directly on the RBC membrane and produce lysis.[162, 163] The venom of the black widow spider, the *Latrodectus mactans,* creates neurologic abnormalities, but no hemolysis or local necrosis occurs.[162] Bee and wasp stings have been reported to cause hemolysis in some patients.[162]

The venoms of certain snakes, such as the pit viper, contain hemolysins, thrombin-like enzymes, and activators and inactivators of complement. The amount of venom absorbed determines the intensity of the hemolysis. Sometimes the venom causes defibrination, but does not affect other coagulation factors.[45]

Hemolytic Anemia Caused by Thermal Injury (Fig. 17–27)

Patients with third-degree burns involving more than 20% of the body may have severe, acute hemolytic anemia. Direct thermal damage to RBCs circulating in the involved skin and tissues leads to hemolysis.[45, 164]

Morphologic RBC changes in widespread burns include globular fragmentation, budding, and microspherocytes, which are present for approximately 24 hours. These cells are rapidly removed from the circulation. Osmotic fragility at this time is increased.[164]

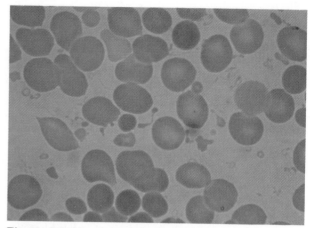

Figure 17–27 Fragmented red blood cells from severely burned patient.

Hemolysis abates within 48 hours after the burn incident, but tiny spherical fragments, spherocytes, methemalbumin, and hemosiderin in urine continue.[164]

Immune Hemolytic Anemia

In immune hemolytic anemias, damage to the RBCs is the result of an immunologic event occurring on the surface of the RBCs. Some immune hemolytic anemias directly involve the RBC membrane through action on the membrane by an antibody with or without complement. Some anemias indirectly involved the RBC membrane because an immune complex is adsorbed by the RBC and fixes complement, resulting in lysis of the RBC by monocytes.[45]

The immune hemolytic anemias are classified into autoimmune hemolytic anemias (AHAs), drug-induced immune hemolytic anemias, and alloimmune hemolytic anemias. The AHAs include warm-reactive autoantibody AHA, cold-reactive antibody AHA, and paroxysmal cold hemoglobinuria. The drug-induced immune hemolytic anemias consist of several types: immune complex–mediated, hapten-mediated, nonimmunologic protein reaction, and idiopathic autoimmune-mediated anemias. The alloimmune hemolytic anemias are the results of hemolytic disease of the newborn.[45, 165–167]

AUTOIMMUNE HEMOLYTIC ANEMIA

AHAs are probably secondary to an altered state if immunity is associated with a loss of immune tolerance. The result is the presence of autoantibodies that damage RBCs. Normally, the production of autoantibodies is kept in check by T suppressor lymphocytes. However, in AHA this check is lost, with the production of autoantibodies against RBC "self-antigens." This theory is supported by the association of the following altered states of immunity with AHA: chronic lymphocytic leukemia, lymphoma, immunoglobulin deficiency and autoimmune diseases (especially disseminated lupus erythematosus), drugs, and viral infection.[45, 166]

Diagnosis

The diagnosis of AHA depends on the demonstration of antibody, complement, or both, on the RBC surface. The general theory of Coombs' or the direct antiglobulin test is that the surface of RBCs has a net negative charge. This charge causes RBCs to repel one another, such that an IgG antibody does not bridge the gap between molecules and cause agglutination. Coombs' antiserum has antibodies against the Fc portion of human IgG and complement. When Coombs' antiserum is added to RBCs with IgG antibody or complement fixed to the surface, agglutination of RBCs occurs and can be seen macroscopically.[45, 165, 166]

Antibodies

Warm-Reactive

Two types of warm-reactive antibody exist: primary or idiopathic, in which the cause or underlying defect is not apparent, and secondary, which is associated with systemic autoimmune disease, chronic lymphocytic leukemia, lymphoma, occasionally viral infections, and, rarely, immune deficiency syndromes.[165]

The warm-reactive antibody is usually of the IgG type and is polyclonal because both κ and λ light chains are present. The immunoglobulin type is rarely IgM or IgA. The antibody or RBC reaction is maximum at 37 °C. There is no increase in antibody as the temperature falls. These antibodies were once thought not to fix complement but in some cases they do, particularly the subclasses IgG1 and IgG3. Complement-directed lysis and the resulting intravascular destruction of RBCs never occur in warm-reactive antibody AHA. The reason for the failure of complement-mediated lysis is that the antigen against which the antibody is directed is widely spaced on the RBC surface and the lytic sequence cannot be completed. Therefore, the destruction and removal of these RBCs is extravascular. Phagocytes in the spleen can fix to the IgG on the RBCs because these cells have Fc receptors. The presence of C3b may help in the splenic trapping of RBCs. A bit of a portion of the RBC membrane is removed and causes the formation of spherocytes, or the entire RBC may be engulfed. The presence of antibody and complement on the

RBC surface is particularly common in AHA that is secondary to systemic lupus erythematosus.[45, 165]

The clinical features of warm-reactive antibody are variable. The patient presents with a chronic hemolytic anemia, or occasionally jaundice may be a reason for seeking medical help. Sometimes, a patient may suddenly have symptoms of severe anemia and splenomegaly may be present. In very severe cases, the patient may have fever, pallor, splenomegaly, hepatomegaly, and tachycardia. An underlying lymphoproliferative disorder is suggested by massive splenomegaly and lymphadenopathy.[45, 165]

The anemia varies from mild to severe. The blood smear reveals an increase in polychromatophilic RBCs. Spherocytes are observed on the blood smear and suggest an immune hemolytic process after the diagnosis of hereditary spherocytosis has been eliminated. Nucleated RBCs and erythrocytosis can be observed in severe hemolysis. Reticulocyte count varies between 5 and 10%. The osmotic fragility test reveals increased hemolysis, and there is an erythroid hyperplasia in the bone marrow. Total bilirubin level is somewhat increased, as are urinary and fecal urobilinogen levels. Haptoglobin levels are low, yet hemoglobinuria is rarely encountered. Mild leukocytosis and neutrophilia are often noted. Platelets are normal in number.[165]

The demonstration of immunoglobulin or complement on the patient's RBCs is necessary to the diagnosis of AHA. Coombs' reagent, a broad-spectrum antiglobulin test with antibodies against human immunoglobulin and complement (mainly C3), is used as a screening procedure. If agglutination is demonstrated with the Coombs' reagent at 37 °C, then antisera that react with immunoglobulin or complement are used to detect the sensitization of the RBCs.[45, 165]

Nonimmune hemolytic anemias, such as hereditary spherocytosis, may be confused with AHA, but the results of the direct antiglobulin test are negative. However, patients with any type of hemolytic anemias may have spherocytosis and splenomegaly.[45]

Prednisone has improved the management and reduced the mortality in warm-reactive antibody AHA. A marked slowing down of hemolysis occurs in about two thirds of the patients. Complete remission occurs in about 20%, but 10% show no response to glucocorticoids. The treatment with prednisone should be administered for several months, and the drug should be tapered over 1 or 2 months. Relapses of AHA may occur, and patients should be followed up periodically.[45, 165]

Splenectomy may be performed in patients who require long-term, high-dose prednisone therapy to maintain the hemoglobin at a satisfactory level. With splenectomy, the primary organ trapping the RBCs is removed. However, splenectomy may not cure AHA, and immunosuppressive drugs are indicated.[45, 165]

Cold-Reactive

Cold-reactive antibody AHA occurs in two classes: primary, or idiopathic (also called cold agglutinin disease), and secondary. Cold agglutinins are usually IgM monoclonal antibodies and have κ light chains only. Cold agglutinins do not agglutinate RBCs above 30 °C. As the temperature decreases, the association of IgM with RBCs increases. Thermal amplitude is the highest temperature at which agglutination is detected. This amplitude varies from patient to patient and appears to influence the clinical picture. Cold agglutinins cause a chronic hemolytic anemia that is accentuated by exposure to cold.[45, 168]

Cold agglutinin disease refers to the somewhat rare chronic AHA in which the autoantibody agglutinates human RBCs directly below body temperature, usually at 0–5 °C. Complement fixed to RBCs by cold agglutinins occurs at temperatures usually between 20 and 25 °C. Patients who are usually middle-aged and elderly and have cold agglutinins have different combinations of hemolytic anemia, hemoglobinuria, and peripheral vaso-occlusive phenomena resulting from exposure to cold. Hematocrit and reticulocyte counts are variable. Hemolysis is extravascular but occasionally may be intravascular.

Secondary forms of cold-reactive antibody AHA are associated with infections (e.g., *M. pneumoniae*, infectious mononucleosis, and other viral infections), B cell malignancies (e.g., chronic lymphocytic leukemia and lymphoma), and autoimmune systemic disorders. Secondary cold-reactive antibody AHA is associated with the presence of polyclonal IgM antibodies. After 2 to 3 weeks of an acute infection, severe hemolytic anemia of 2 to 6 weeks' duration occurs. With the lymphoid malignancies, the condition is chronic.[45, 168]

Both types of cold-reactive antibody AHA involve the formation of IgM antibodies against the I-i system of antigens on the RBCs. The newborn has the i antigen, and it changes to the I antigen in the first few months of life.[168]

Fixation of complement can happen in several ways. Completion of the complement can occur with intravascular lysis of RBCs. On the other hand, the complement sequence may stop at C3b, and complement-mediated intravascular lysis may not occur, but extravascular hemolysis may occur in the spleen. Fixation of complement may occur when C3b is inactivated by transformation to C3d.

Phagocytes do not have C3d, which gives RBCs protection from further fixation of antibody and complement.[45, 168]

A screening test for cold-reactive antibody AHA involves immersing a tube of anticoagulated blood into an ice bath. If cold-reactive antibody is present, gross autoagglutination occurs. If the blood is warmed back to 37 °C, the agglutination disappears. The blood smears show agglutination of RBCs by cold-reactive antibody cooled to 20 °C (room temperature). If blood is warmed to 37 °C on a warm slide, no evidence of agglutination is present.[168]

The Coombs' test is positive at 15–32 °C and is usually positive only for complement. The cold agglutinin titer is positive and usually over 1:1000.[168]

Paroxysmal Cold Hemoglobinuria. Paroxysmal cold hemoglobinuria is an extremely rare form of cold-reactive antibody AHA. Paroxysmal cold hemoglobinuria is characterized by acute episodes of massive hemolysis that occur after exposure to cold. The IgG antibody attaches to RBCs only at temperatures of less than 15 °C and is directed against the P antigen. Complement is always fixed and binds to RBCs at low temperatures. The type of antibody is referred to as "biphasic" antibody–antibody attachment. Fixation of complement occurs at very low temperatures, but completion of complement sequence and RBC lysis occurs only after rewarming. This condition presents only infrequently as a severe, acute, self-limited hemolytic anemia because individuals are rarely chilled to less than 15°C. The cause of the autoantibody in paroxysmal cold hemoglobinuria is unknown.[168]

In 1904, Donath and Landsteiner were the first to describe the cold-reactive antibody, and paroxysmal cold hemoglobinuria is now called Donath-Landsteiner hemolytic anemia. It was formerly associated with congenital or tertiary syphilis, but now the disease occurs as a chronic idiopathic form and also as an acute, self-limited form after some types of viral syndromes. When the cells return to 37 °C in the circulation, they are rapidly lysed by the propagation of the terminal complement sequence through C9. At body temperature, the Donath-Landsteiner antibody is dissociated from RBCs.[168]

A short time after exposure to cold, the patient develops aching pains in the back and legs, abdominal cramps, and headaches, followed by chills and fever. Hemoglobinuria with dark red or brown urine is present after the symptoms develop.[168]

Chronic anemia, increase in reticulocytes, decreased hemoglobin, hemoglobinemia, and hyperbilirubinemia may be observed. Spherocytes are noted on the blood film, and monocytes and neutrophils may phagocytize RBCs. At first, leukopenia may be present, and later, leukocytosis.[168] The direct antiglobulin reaction is often positive during an attack and results from coating of surviving RBCs with complement (C3 fragments). The Donath-Landsteiner antibody, which binds only in the cold, is a nonagglutinating IgG, and it has specificity for the P blood group antigen. It can be detected by incubating the patient's fresh serum with RBCs at 4 °C and then warming the mixture to 37 °C. Intense hemolysis occurs after warming.[168]

DRUG-INDUCED HEMOLYTIC ANEMIA

Hemolytic anemias secondary to drug-mediated response are usually benign processes, but severe, even fatal, cases have occurred. After it is recognized, drug-induced immune hemolysis may be easily treated, and later episodes can be prevented by avoidance of the drug. Several types of drug-induced immune hemolytic anemia exist.[45, 167]

Immune Complex Type

The mechanism of the immune complex type involves the reaction of the antidrug antibody with the drug to form an immune complex. The complex is then adsorbed onto RBCs. The cell-bound complex may activate complement, and this results in acute intravascular hemolysis, often with renal failure or thrombocytopenia. RBCs have been considered the "innocent bystanders" in this reaction. The drugs responsible for this immunologic injury are quinidine, phenacetin, and stibophen. The hemolytic anemia occurs after small doses, after short periods of administration, or on readministration of a previously used drug. The direct Coombs' test shows only complement on the RBCs. In the indirect Coombs' test, the serum is reactive only in the presence of the drug. The RBC eluate is often nonreactive.[45, 167]

Hapten Type

The essential feature of the hapten type is that the drug is nonspecifically bound or adsorbed to RBCs and remains firmly adherent to the cells. If a patient develops an antidrug antibody, it reacts with the cell-bound drug. Complement is usually not fixed by an antibody reaction of this type. The drugs involved are penicillins and, rarely, cephalosporins. Large doses of penicillin (10–20 million U daily) produce a hemolytic reaction 7 to 10 days after the administration of the drug. The extravascular hemolysis is mild or moderate. The direct Coombs' test shows IgG or, rarely, IgG and complement on the RBCs. The indirect Coombs' test shows that the patient's serum is reactive with drug-treated RBCs but not with normal RBCs. The RBC eluate reacts only with the drug-treated RBCs.[45, 167]

Non-Immunologic Protein Adsorption

Cephalosporins alter the RBC membrane nonspecifically so that numerous proteins, including IgG and complement, are adsorbed to the RBC surface. This phenomenon results in a positive result on the direct Coombs' test, but only rarely has a hemolytic anemia been reported. The dose of the drug associated with a positive result on the antiglobulin test is high because IgG, complement, and other proteins are on the RBC surface. In the indirect Coombs' test, no serum antibodies are found.[45, 167]

Idiopathic Drug-Induced Immune Hemolytic Anemia

With exposure to the drug aldomet (alpha-methyldopa), a gradual onset of drug-induced AHA occurs over about 3 months of chronic extravascular hemolysis. This drug-induced anemia is different from the others in that the hemolytic state continues after administration of the drug is stopped. The drug does not have to be present for hemolysis to occur, possibly because of the effect of methyldopa on T suppressor lymphocytes. The result of the direct Coombs' test is strongly positive. IgG only is on the RBC surface, and complement is rarely present. Antibodies in the patient's serum or eluted from the RBC membranes react with unaltered homologous or autologous RBC in the absence of the drug in the indirect Coombs' test.[45, 167]

ALLOIMMUNE HEMOLYTIC ANEMIAS

Two types of alloimmune hemolytic anemias exist: hemolytic transfusion reactions and hemolytic disease of the newborn.

Transfusion Reactions

Hemolytic

Transfusion, even under ideal conditions, carries a risk of an adverse reaction. These reactions are associated with significant morbidity and sometimes a fatal outcome. Most of the reported fatalities involve human error: an ABO mismatch. Most reactions result from the administration of correctly cross-matched blood given to the wrong patient. Transfusion reactions may be immediate or delayed.[45, 166]

Immediate

Symptoms begin within minutes or hours and may include chills, fever, urticaria, tachycardia, nausea and vomiting, chest and back pain, shock, anaphylaxis, pulmonary edema, and congestive heart failure. These reactions may be hemolytic or febrile.

Hemolytic transfusion reactions result from intravascular breakdown, which is commonly due to an incompatibility in the ABO system or to destruction occurring in the macrophage system of the spleen, liver, and marrow. Abnormal bleeding resulting from consumptive coagulopathy or DIC may occur in patients who develop major intravascular hemolysis after an incompatible transfusion. In the clinical management of a hemolytic transfusion reaction, there should be immediate termination of the transfusion and institution of measures to correct the bleeding diathesis to correct shock and to maintain renal circulation to prevent acute tubular necrosis. The laboratory diagnosis of an acute hemolytic reaction is based on evidence of hemolysis and of a blood group incompatibility.[45] Hemoglobinemia, hemoglobinuria, or both are present. Bilirubin level is increased, and haptoglobin level is low. Urine should be examined for hemoglobin. The entire typing and cross-match procedures should be repeated to identify the blood group incompatibility.[45, 166] A febrile reaction associated with blood transfusion may result from a hemolytic reaction, sensitivity to leukocytes or platelets, bacterial contamination, or unidentifiable causes.[166]

Delayed

A delayed transfusion reaction may occur days or weeks after transfusion and may result in jaundice and anemia due to hemolysis. Also, transmission of infectious disease, such as malaria and babesia, hepatitis, human immunodeficiency virus, and cytomegalovirus, may occur. Development of undetected alloantibodies occurs 4 to 14 days after transfusion of apparently compatible blood. Often, the patient has been alloimmunized by a previous pregnancy or transfusion, and the antibody concentration at the time of transfusion was below the level of serologic detection. If the transfused blood has a corresponding antigen, a response ensues that consists of the formation of detectable antibody, which coats the transfused RBCs, leading to hemolysis. Jaundice and lack of increase in RBC mass are the principal clinical signs. The direct antiglobulin reaction with Coombs' test is positive.

These reactions are not as severe as the acute hemolytic reactions.[45, 166]

Rh Blood Group System and Erythroblastosis Fetalis

The D antigen in the Rh blood group system is the most important blood group antigen that may cause alloimmunization and hemolytic disease of the newborn, although other blood group antigens may also be responsible for erythroblastosis. Three pairs of genetically determined antigens exist: Cc, D(d), and Ee, according to the CDE nomenclature and Fisher and Race inheritance theory. The presence or absence of D antigen determines the Rh-positive or Rh-negative status of the individual. No antibody with the specificity of anti-d has ever been found. The production of anti-D in the Rh(D)–negative woman and the passage of anti-D across the placenta into the circulation of the Rh-positive fetus results in hemolytic disease of the newborn. If the Rh-positive husband is homozygous, the children will be D positive: if the husband is heterozygous, in each pregnancy, the chances are equal that the fetus will be D positive or D negative. Only the D-positive fetus can provoke Rh immunization, and only the D-positive fetus will be affected by the anti-D produced.[45, 166]

Erythroblastosis fetalis (alloimmune hemolytic disease) is a disease of the fetus and the newborn that is characterized by hemolytic anemia, hyperbilirubinemia, and extramedullary erythropoiesis. Neonatal or fetal death occurs in about one fourth of the cases. Severe jaundice with risk of brain damage occurs in about one fourth of the patients. The etiology and pathogenesis of hemolytic disease began with the rhesus monkey cell studies by Landsteiner and Wiener in 1940.[45, 166]

Hemolysis and Hydrops Fetalis. IgG anti-D crosses the placenta and coats the fetal Rh-positive RBCs. The coated RBCs form rosettes around macrophages, mainly in the spleen. The RBC membrane is invaginated by pseudopodia from the phagocyte; this phenomenon causes loss of membrane, sphering of RBCs, erythrophagocytosis, and eventually, lysis. The hemolysis causes anemia, splenomegaly, and hepatomegaly, with an outpouring of immature nucleated RBCs in the peripheral blood. Diffusely basophilic cells are present also. Thrombocytopenia may be common in severely affected babies and may lead to hemorrhagic problems.[45, 166]

In severe cases, venous pressure rises and ascites occurs. Hepatocellular damage and hypoalbuminemia are caused by further anemia and hepatic circulatory obstruction. The hydropic fetus either dies in utero (20–25% of cases) or, if born alive, dies soon after. The primary causes of hydrops fetalis are hepatocellular damage and hepatic obstruction.[45, 166]

Unconjugated bilirubin is the toxic product of hemolysis in utero. It is cleared across the placenta and conjugated to bilirubin. Levels of unconjugated bilirubin can be extremely high. After birth, large amounts of bilirubin from hemolysis cannot be conjugated by the infant's immature hepatic mechanism. Neuron cell death occurs, and evidence of kernicterus is present at autopsy.[45, 166]

Laboratory Findings

Maternal blood group antibody screening is essential during pregnancy. Optimal clinical management is possible only if alloimmunization is diagnosed early and followed up carefully. Rh grouping of the mother should be determined, and her plasma should be screened for alloantibodies. Testing of an unimmunized Rh-positive mother should be repeated at 20 weeks' gestation and thereafter every 6 weeks until delivery. The mother should have Rh prophylaxis at 28 weeks' gestation and after delivery if she remains unimmunized.[45, 166]

If the mother is alloimmunized, the specificity and titer of antibody should be determined by the indirect antiglobulin method. Antibody titers should be repeated at 18 weeks' gestation and every 2 to 4 weeks thereafter until delivery.[45, 166]

Determining the risk of hydrops and fetal death is based on the history and the antibody titer of the fetus. Titers of 1:16–1:32 indicate a risk of hydrops. Spectrophotometric measurement of bilirubin in amniotic fluid gives information on the severity of hemolytic disease.

Percutaneous umbilical venous fetal blood sampling using ultrasound equipment has enabled a very accurate profile of the severity of hemolytic disease. The Coombs' test, hemoglobin and bilirubin determinations, and other tests can be performed.[166]

Therapy

With the percutaneous umbilical venous fetal blood method, direct transfusions of compatible RBCs into fetal circulation can be carried out. Exchange transfusion (10–20 mL) after delivery is used to remove most coated hemolyzing RBCs and to prevent anemia and further bilirubin overproduction. Careful attention must be given to venous pressure.[45, 166]

Prevention of Rh Immunization

Rh immunization can be prevented by administration of Rh immune globulin to an Rh-negative, unimmunized mother carrying an Rh-positive fetus or delivering an Rh-positive baby. To be effective,

it should be given before the beginning of a primary Rh immune response, and in an adequate dose. With modern methods and skills, the perinatal mortality of alloimmune hemolytic disease has been reduced from 13% in 1960 to 2% in the middle 1980s. Successful Rh prevention programs are diminishing Rh erythroblastosis and are helping to decrease neonatal death.[45, 166]

Erythroblastosis Caused by Other Blood Group Antigens

ABO erythroblastosis is more common than Rh erythroblastosis serologically and usually occurs in first pregnancies. It produces hyperbilirubinemia and rarely anemia. ABO hemolytic disease usually occurs in babies with blood types A or B born to mothers with blood type O who produce IgG, anti-A, or anti-B rather than to mothers with blood types A or B with ABO incompatibility. The disease is milder than erythroblastosis due to Rh incompatibility because most anti-A and anti-B antibodies are IgM and do not cross the placenta. Antigens A and B are found on fetal tissue.[45, 166]

Hemolytic disease due to anti-c and anti-Kell is rarer than hemolytic disease due to anti-D. It does not differ in degree of severity or outlook from anti-D erythroblastosis. Disease due to anti-C or anti-E is usually mild and rarely produces hydrops. Mothers with these antibodies should be treated in the same way as mothers who are Rh immunized. Hydrops fetalis is rare in anti-A and anti-B hemolytic disease. Jaundice and possible kernicterus are the two clinical problems in anti-A, anti-B, anti-C, and anti-E hemolytic disease.[45, 166]

At delivery, cord blood may be collected for ABO and Rh testing; for Coombs' testing; for determination of hemoglobin level, unconjugated bilirubin level, and number of nucleated RBCs in peripheral blood; and for platelet and reticulocyte counts. The cord blood findings, plus the clinical appearance of the infant, determine treatment.[45, 166]

SUMMARY

Anemias resulting from increased destruction of erythrocytes may be subdivided into intracorpuscular, in which the hemolysis occurs because of a defect in the RBC itself, and extracorpuscular, which result from an event outside of the RBC that causes destruction.

Included in intracorpuscular RBC are membrane defects, such as HS and HE, and rarer defects, such as HPP. The two most common enzyme deficiencies that may lead to hemolysis are G-6-PD and PK deficiencies. The porphyrias are fairly rare disorders of heme biosynthesis that are caused by enzyme defects in the heme pathway. Many involve photosensitivity. PNH is a clonal myeloproliferative disease in which affected persons lyse RBCs when they sleep. In this disorder, the erythrocytes are abnormally sensitive to complement.

Extracorpuscular abnormalities include those resulting from microangiopathic hemolytic anemia, such as TTP and HUS, and macroangiopathic hemolytic anemia resulting from prosthetic heart valves and march hemoglobinuria, in which continuous pounding of the feet on hard surfaces causes destruction.

Intracellular microorganisms, including those that produce malaria and babesiosis, may be seen on thick drop preparations (stained with Giemsa) and on thin preparations stained with Wright-Giemsa. Infected RBCs rupture causing hemolytic anemia. Hemolytic anemias may also be caused by *C. perfringens,* drugs and chemicals, and severe burns.

Immune hemolytic anemias can be subdivided into autoimmune, drug-induced, and alloimmune. Within the autoimmune group are those caused by warm-reacting antibodies, cold-reacting antibodies, and paroxysmal cold hemoglobinuria. Drug-induced immune hemolysis may result from immune-complex-mediated, hapten-mediated, or nonimmunological protein reaction, or reactions of an idiopathic nature. Alloimmune hemolytic anemias are caused by transfusion reactions or by hemolytic disease of the newborn.

Case 1

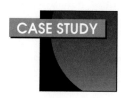

A 31-year-old white male sought medical attention for the onset of hematuria. Physical examination revealed hematuria, findings of petechiae on the palate, ecchymosis, slight abdominal distention, and a low-grade fever. The patient appeared healthy but was clearly quarrelsome and anxious. Lapsed memory was reported by the patient's wife. The following tests were ordered: complete blood cell count (CBC), reticulocyte count, urinalysis, chemistry profile, and measurements of prothrombin time (PT) and partial thromboplastin time (PTT).

Laboratory Data	Day 1	Day 5	Normal
WBC ($\times 10^9$/L)	10.6	25.9*	4.5–11.0
RBC ($\times 10^{12}$/L)	4.17	2.78	4.4–5.9
Hemoglobin (g/dL)	13.5	9.0	13.9–16.3
Hematocrit (L/L)	0.38	0.25	0.39–0.55
Platelet count ($\times 10^9$/L)	15.0	50.0	150–500
Reticulocytes (%)	3.5	11.3	0.5–2.0

The RBC indices were within normal limits. The peripheral blood smear on day 1 showed moderate anisocytosis, moderate microcytosis, slight polychromatophilia, slight poikilocytosis, few schistocytes, few spherocytes, and few teardrop-shaped RBCs. The smear contained essentially the same RBC picture on day 5 but greater degrees of anisocytosis, poikilocytosis with schistocytes, and a moderate macrocytosis. Also on day 5, 11 NRBCs were noted along with leukocytosis and a shift to the left. The urinalysis revealed a mahogany brown appearance with 3+ blood, 4+ protein, trace amounts of glucose, and microscopically TNTC (too numerous to count) RBCs, 10–25 WBCs/high-power field, with 10–25/low-power field each of hyaline and granular casts. The significant chemistry values included a blood urea nitrogen (BUN) level of 33 mg/dL (normal range, 0–26), a glucose level of 114 mg/dL (normal range, 70–110), a creatinine level of 2.0 mg/dL (normal range, 0.7–1.5), a total bilirubin level of 3.7 mg/dL (normal range, 0.2–1.2), and a lactate dehydrogenase (LDH) level of 2780 U/L (normal range, 100–190). The PT and PTT were within their normal ranges, but the plasma color was reported as being slightly lipemic and icteric.

A microangiopathic hemolytic anemia was evident from the presence of fragmented or injured erythrocytes, nucleated red blood cells, increased numbers of reticulocytes, increased total bilirubin level, and increased LDH, which reflected both

* Corrected for NRBCs.

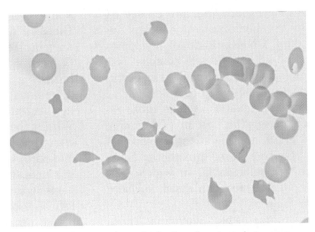

Figure 17–28 Thrombotic thrombocytopenic purpura.

erythropoietic stress and disruption of the marrow. The mechanism of hemolysis suggested by the blood morphology (Fig. 17–28) would be fragmentation caused by mechanical injury as RBCs are forced through partially occluded distal arterioles.

1. What conditions can cause hemolytic anemia by this mechanism?

2. What is the significance of the findings from the given blood films?

3. Can the diagnosis be made from the available data?

4. How can the improvement of this condition be measured?

Case 2

A 20-year-old female sought medical attention for an elevated temperature and a possible insect bite. Physical examination revealed a small bite wound on the right lateral area of the chest that was tender and contained a clear fluid with no pus. Necrosis was not evident. A diffuse erythematous rash on most of her body was also observed. The physician prescribed 40 mL of liquid acetaminophen (Tylenol), 1 g of intravenous ceftriaxone sodium (Rocephin), and 500 mg four times a day for 10 days of cephalexin (Keflex). A secretion from the lesion was subjected to culture, but there was no growth after 72 hours. Blood was drawn for cultures, which were reported as negative after 5 days. Four days later, the patient went to the emergency room, complaining of being unable to walk. A CBC, a urinalysis, urine and sputum cultures, and a chemistry profile were ordered.

Laboratory Data	Patient	Normal
WBC ($\times 10^9$/L)	5.9	4.5–11.0
RBC ($\times 10^{12}$/L)	1.14	4.3–5.9
Hemoglobin (g/dL)	3.8	13.9–16.3
Hematocrit (L/L)	0.10	0.39–0.55

The RBC indices and the platelet count were within normal ranges. The peripheral blood smear revealed a normochromic, normocytic RBC pattern with an abnormal increase in neutrophilic bands, few early WBCs, and 3 nucleated RBCs (Fig. 17–29). Her urinalysis yielded 3+ blood. Urine and sputum cultures were reported as negative. Significant values from her chemistry profile included elevated levels of total bilirubin, alkaline phosphatase, LDH, and aspartate amino transferase. Subsequently, the patient was typed and cross-matched for 1 unit of blood. A positive result of a direct Coombs' test was reported. The indirect Coombs' test result was negative. An eluate prepared from the patient's cells was negative with all panel cells tested.

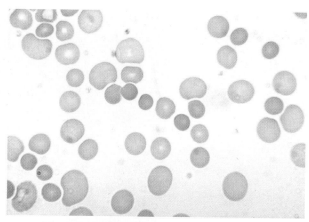

Figure 17–29 Drug-induced hemolytic anemia.

1. Is this type of anemia caused by intracorpuscular or extracorpuscular defects?

2. What does a positive result of a direct Coombs' test imply?

3. What mechanisms can lead to the development of drug-related antibodies and drug-induced immune hemolytic anemia?

4. Describe the mechanism that is the most probable etiology of this patient's anemia.

5. What is the treatment of choice?

Case 3

A 55-year-old male sought medical attention for the onset of chest pain. Physical examination revealed slight jaundice and splenomegaly. The past medical history included gallstones, and there was a family history of anemia. A CBC yielded the following results:

Laboratory Data	Patient	Normal
WBC ($\times 10^9$/L)	13.4	4.5–11.0
RBC ($\times 10^{12}$/L)	4.28	4.3–5.9
Hemoglobin (g/dL)	11.7	13.9–16.3
Hematocrit (L/L)	0.325	0.39–0.55
MCV (fL)	76	80–100
MCH (pg)	27.3	25.4–34.6
MCHC (g/dL)	36.0	31–37
RDW (%)	22.9	11.5–13.5

The peripheral blood smear revealed slight anisocytosis, slight polychromatophilia, and several microspherocytes that were dark and round and lacked a central pallor. The platelet count and platelet distribution on the smear were normal (Fig. 17–30).

1. From the data base just given, what is your initial diagnostic assessment of the anemia?

2. What additional laboratory tests would be of value in establishing the diagnosis, and what abnormalities in these tests would be expected in confirming your impression?

3. What is the cause of this type of anemia?

4. What form of treatment would be favorable?

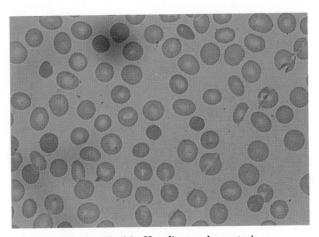

Figure 17–30   Hereditary spherocytosis.

Case 4

A 91-year-old white male sought medical attention for a progressive malaise. A CBC yielded the following results:

Laboratory Data	Patient	Normal
WBC (×10⁹/L)	4.3	4.5–11
RBC (×10¹²/L)	3.38	4.3–5.9
Hemoglobin (g/dL)	11.7	13.9–16.3
Hematocrit (L/L)	0.30	39–55
MCV (fL)	88.7	80–100
MCH (pg)	30.8	25.4–34.6
MCHC (g/dL)	34.7	31–37
RDW (%)	34.8	11.5–13.5
Platelet count (×10⁹/L)	194	150–500

The peripheral blood smear revealed marked anisocytosis and poikilocytosis; dimorphic and dichromic RBCs; many elliptocytes and schistocytes; and few spherocytes. The distribution of platelets was normal. Relative neutrophilia was noted (Fig. 17–31).

Additional tests yielded the following results: the total bilirubin level was 1.5 mg/ dL (normal range, 0.2–1.2); the LDH level was 320 U/L (normal range, 100–190);

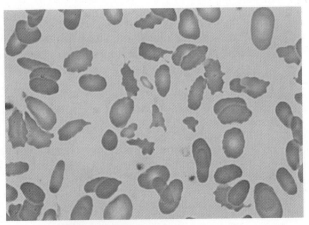

Figure 17–31   Hereditary elliptocytosis.

there was increased osmotic fragility; and there was increased autohemolysis, which was corrected by glucose.

1. What is your general assessment of the anemia of this patient?

2. What is responsible for the shape change in the erythrocytes? What is the inheritance?

3. On the basis of the classification according to the predominant morphology of this smear, what is the likely diagnosis?

4. What additional facts are needed for confirmation, and what are the treatment options?

References

1. Stephen BS, Beutler E: The red cell membrane. *In* Williams WJ, Beutler E, Erslev AJ, Lichtman MA (eds): Hematology, 4th ed. New York: McGraw-Hill, 1990:369–378.

2. Singer SJ, Nicholson GL: The fluid mosaic model of the structure of cell membranes. Science 1972; 175:720.

3. Vanlair CF, Masius JB: De la microcythemie. Bull R Acad Med Belg 5:515,1871.

4. Wilson C: Some cases showing hereditary enlargement of the spleen. Trans Clin Soc (London) 1890; 23:162.

5. Minkowski O: Ueber eine hereditare, unter dem Bilde eines chronischen Ikterus mit Urobilinurie, Splenomegalie und Neirenside-rosis verlaufende Affektion. Verh Dtsch Kongr Med 1900; 18:316.

6. Becher PS, Lux SE: Disorders of the red cell membrane. *In* Nathan DG, Oski FA (eds): Hematology of Infancy and Childhood, 4th ed. Philadelphia: WB Saunders, 1993:529–556.

7. Lux SE: Disorders of the red cell membrane skeleton: Hereditary spherocytosis and hereditary elliptocytosis. *In* Stanbury JB, Wyngaarden DS, Goldstein JL, Brown MS (eds): The Metabolic Basis of Inherited Disease, 5th ed. New York: McGraw-Hill, 1983:1573–1605.

8. Agre P, Orringer EP, et al: Deficient red cell spectrin in severe recessively inherited spherocytosis. N Engl J Med 1982; 306:1155.

9. Goodman SR, Shiffer KA, Casoria LK, et al: Identification of the molecular defect in the erythrocyte membrane skeleton of some kindreds with hereditary spherocytosis. Blood 1982; 60:772.

10. Costa FF, Agre P, Lux SE: Linkage of dominant hereditary spherocytosis to the gene for the erythrocyte membrane skeleton protein ankyrin. N Engl J Med 1990; 323:1046.

11. Savvides P, Shaler O, John KM, et al: Combined spectrin and ankyrin deficiency is common in dominant hereditary spherocytosis (abstract). Clin Res 1991; 39:313A.

12. Lux S, Bedrosian C, Shalev O, et al: Deficiency of band 3 in dominant hereditary spherocytosis with normal spectrin content (abstract). Clin Res 1990; 38:300a.

13. Wilkelmann JC, Marchesi SL, Watkins P, et al: Recessive hereditary spherocytosis is associated with an abnormal alpha spectrin subunit. Clin Res 1986; 34:474a.

14. Yawata Y, Ata K, Kanzaki A, et al: Membrane characteristics of membrane protein band 4.2 deficiency with congenital hemolytic anemia (abstract). Blood 1990; 76(Suppl 1):21a.

15. Jandl JH: Hemolytic anemias caused by primary defects of red cell membranes. *In* Jandl JH (ed): Blood. Boston: Little, Brown, 1987:237–264.

16. Mayman D, Zipursky A: Hereditary spherocytosis: The metabolism of erythrocytes in the peripheral blood and in the splenic pulp. Br J Haematol 1974; 27:201.

17. Lux SE, Becher PS: Hereditary spherocytosis and hereditary elliptocytosis. *In* Scriver CR, Beaudet AL, Sly WS, Valle D (eds): The Metabolic Basis of Inherited Disease, 6th ed. New York: McGraw Hill, 1989:2367–2408.

18. Palek P: Hereditary spherocytosis. *In* Williams WJ, Beutler E, Erslev AJ, Lichtman MA (eds): Hematology, 4th ed. New York: McGraw Hill, 1990:558–569.

19. Davidson RJ, Brown T, Wiseman D: Human parvo virus infection and aplastic crisis in hereditary spherocytosis. J Infect 1984; 9:298.

20. McKinney AA Jr, Morton NE, Kosower NS, et al: Ascertaining genetic carriers of hereditary spherocytosis by statistical analysis of multiple laboratory tests. J Clin Invest 1962; 41:554.

21. Emerson CP Jr, Shen SC, Haleham T, et al: Studies of the destruction of red blood cells: IX. Quantitative methods for determining the osmotic and mechanical fragility of red cells in the peripheral blood and splenic pulp: The mechanism of increased hemolysis in hereditary spherocytosis (congenital hemolytic jaundice) as related to the function of the spleen. Arch Intern Med 1956; 97:1–38.

22. Schwartz PE, Sterioff S, Mocha P, et al: Post splenectomy sepsis and mortality in adults. JAMA 1982; 248:2279.

23. Eraktis AJ, Kevy SV, Diamond LK, et al: Hazards of overwhelming infection after splenectomy in childhood. N Engl J Med 1967; 276:1225.

24. Buchanan GR, Holtkamp CA: Pocketed erythrocyte counts in patients with hereditary spherocytosis before and after splenectomy. Am J Hematol 1987; 25:253.

25. Dresbach M: Elliptical human red corpuscles. Science 1904; 19:469.

26. Cook PJL, Noades JE, Newton MS, et al: On the orientation of the Rh:El$_1$ linkage group. Ann Hum Genet 1977; 41:157.

27. Keats BJB: Another elliptocytosis locus on chromosome 1? Hum Genet 1979; 50:227.

28. Palek J: Hereditary elliptocytosis and related disorders. Clin Haematol 1985; 14:45.

29. Zarkowsky HS: Heat-induced erythrocyte fragmentation in neonatal elliptocytosis. Br J Haematol 1979; 41:515.

30. Mentzer WC, Turetsky T, Mohandus N, et al: Identification of the hereditary pyropoikilocytosis carrier state. Blood 1984; 63:1439.

31. Lande WM, Mentzer WC: Haemolytic anemia associated with increased cation permeability (review). Clin Haematol 1985; 14:89.

32. Kane JP, Havel RJ: Disorders of the biogenesis and secretion of lipoproteins containing the B apolipoproteins. *In* Scriver CR, Beaudet AL, Sly WS, Valle D (eds): Metabolic Basis of Inherited Disease, 6th ed. New York: McGraw-Hill, 1989:1139–1164.

33. Redman CM, Marsh WL, Scarborough A, et al: Biochemical studies on McLeod phenotype red cells and isolation of Kx antigen. Br J Haematol 1988; 68:131.

34. Udden MM, Umeda M, Hirano Y, et al: New abnormalities in the morphology of cell surface receptors, and electrolyte metabolism of *ln(Lu)* erythrocytes. Blood 1987; 69:52.

35. Arie THD: Pythagoras and beans. Oxf Med School Gaz 1959; 11:75–81.

36. Fermi C, Martinetti P: Studio sul favismo. Ann Ig Sper 1905; 15:75.

37. Carson PE, Flanagan CL, Ickes CE, Alving AS: Enzymatic deficiency in primaquine sensitive erythrocytes. Science 1956; 124:484.

38. Beutler E: The genetics of glucose-6-phosphate dehydrogenase deficiency. Semin Hematol 1990; 27:137.

39. Luzzatto L: G6PD deficiency and hemolytic anemia. In Nathan DG, Oski FA (eds): Hematology of Infancy and Childhood, 4th ed. Philadelphia: WB Saunders, 1993:674–695.

40. Luzzatto L, Mehta A: Glucose-6-phosphate dehydrogenase deficiency. In Scriver CR, Beaudet AL, Sly WS, Valle D (eds): The Metabolic Basis of Inherited Disease, 6th ed. New York: McGraw Hill, 1989:2237–2265.

41. Beutler E, Yoshida A: Genetic variation of glucose-6-phosphate dehydrogenase: A catalog and future prospects. Medicine (Baltimore) 1988; 67:311.

42. Beutler E: Glucose-6-phosphate dehydrogenase deficiency. In Williams WJ, Beutler E, Erslev AJ, Lichtman MA (eds): Hematology, 4th ed. New York: McGraw-Hill, 1990:591–606.

43. Beutler E: Glucose-6-phosphate dehydrogenase deficiency. N Engl J Med 1991; 324:169.

44. Borges A, Desforges JF: Studies of Heinz body formation. Acta Haematol 1967; 37:1.

45. Jandl JH: Blood, 1st ed. Boston: Little, Brown, 1987.

46. Biezle U, Lucas AO, Ayeni O, et al: Glucose-6-phosphate dehydrogenase and malaria. Greater resistance of females heterozygous for enzyme deficiency and of males with non-deficient variant. Lancet 1972; i:107–110.

47. Usanga EA, Luzzatto L: Adaptation of Plasmodium falciparum to glucose-6-phosphate dehydrogenase deficient host red cells by production of parasite-encoded enzyme. Nature 1985; 313:793–795.

48. Beutler E: Erythrocyte enzyme assays. In Williams WJ, Beutler E, Erslev AJ, Lichtman MA (eds): Hematology, 4th ed. New York: McGraw-Hill, 1990:591–606.

49. Brewer GJ, Tarlow AR, Alving AS, et al: The methemoglobin reduction for primaquine-type sensitivity of erythrocytes: A simplified procedure for detecting a specific hypersusceptibility to drug hemolysis. JAMA 1962; 180:386.

50. Jacob HS, Jandl JH: A simple visual screening test for glucose-6-phosphate dehydrogenase deficiency employing ascorbate and cyanide. N Engl J Med 1966; 274:1162.

51. Tanaka KR, Zerez CR: Red cell enzymopathies of the glycolytic pathway. Semin Hematol 1990; 27:165–186.

52. Valentine WN, Koyichi RT, Paglia DE: Pyruvate kinase and other enzyme deficiency disorders of the erythrocyte. In Scriver CR, Beaudet AL, Sly WS, Valle D (eds): The Metabolic Basis of Inherited Disease, 6th ed. New York: McGraw-Hill, 1989:1606–1628.

53. Mentzer WC Jr: Pyruvate kinase deficiency and disorders of glycolysis. In Nathan DG, Oski FA (eds): Hematology of Infancy and Childhood, 4th ed. Philadelphia: WB Saunders, 1993:634–673.

54. Dacie JV, Mollison PL, Richardson N, et al: Atypical congenital hemolytic anemia. Q J Med 1953; 22:79.

55. Selwyn JG, Dacie JV: Autohemolysis and other changes resulting from the incubation in vitro of red cells from patients with congenital hemolytic anemia. Blood 1954; 9:414.

56. Robinson MA, Loder PB, DeGrochy GC: Red cell metabolism in non-spherocytic congenital haemolytic anemia. Br J Haematol 1961; 7:327.

57. Valentine WN, Tanaka KR, Miwa S: A specific erythrocyte enzyme defect (pyruvate kinase) in three subjects with congenital non-spherocytic hemolytic anemia. Trans Assoc Am Physicians 1961; 74:100.

58. Blume KG, Arnold H, Löhr GW, Beutler E: Additional diagnostic procedures for the detection of abnormal red cell pyruvate kinase. Clin Chim Acta 1973; 43:443.

59. Keitt AS: Diagnostic strategy in a suspected enzymopathy. Clin Haematol 1981; 10:3.

60. Gull WP: A case of intermittent hematuria with remarks. Guys Hosp Rep 1866; 12:381.

61. Crosby WH: Paroxysmal nocturnal hemoglobinuria. A classic description by Paul Strubing in 1882, and a bibliography of the disease. Blood 1951; 6:270.

62. Hijmans Van Den Berg AA: Ictère hémolytique avec crises hémoglobinuriques fragilité globulaire. Rev Med 1911; 31:63.

63. Marchiafava E: Anemia emolitica con emosiderinuria perpituai. Policlinico (sez med) 1931; 18:241.

64. Micheli F: Anemia (splenomegalia) emolitica conemoglobinuria-emosiderinuria tipo Marchiafava. Hematologican 1931; 12:101.

65. Beutler E: Paroxysmal nocturnal hemoglobinuria. In Williams WJ, Beutler E, Erslev AJ, Lichtman MA (eds): Hematology, 4th ed. New York: McGraw-Hill, 1990:188–192.

66. Hillmen P, Bessler M, Crawford DH, Luzzatto L: Production and characterization of lymphoblastoid cell lines with the paroxysmal nocturnal hemoglobinuria phenotype. Blood 1993; 81:1, 193–199.

67. Rotoli B, Luzzatto L: Paroxysmal nocturnal hemoglobinuria. Semin Hematol 1989; 26:3, 201–207.

68. Dessypris EN, Clark DA, McKee LC, Krantz SB: Increased sensitivity to complement of erythroid and myeloid progenitors in paroxysmal nocturnal hemoglobinuria. N Eng J Med 1983; 309:690–693.

69. Jandl JH: Hemolytic anemias. In Jandl JH (ed): Blood: Pathophysiology, 1st ed. Oxford: Blackwell Scientific Publications 1991:145–181.

70. Rosse WF: Paroxysmal nocturnal hemoglobinuria. The biochemical defects and the clinical syndrome. Blood Rev 1989; 3:192.

71. Ferguson MAJ, William AF: Cell surface anchoring of proteins vis glycosylphosphatidylinositol structure. Annu Rev Biochem 1988; 57:285–320.

72. Rosse WF: Paroxysmal nocturnal hemoglobinuria and decay accelerating factor. Annu Rev Med 1990; 41:431.

73. Nicholson-Weller A, March JP, Rosenfeld SI, et al: Affected erythrocytes of patients with paroxysmal nocturnal hemoglobinuria are deficient in the complement regulatory protein, decay accelerating factor. Proc Natl Acad Sci U S A 1983; 80:5066.

74. Nicholson-Weller A, Spincer DB, Austen KF: Deficiency of the complement regulatory protein, "decay-accelerating factor" on membranes of granulocytes, monocytes and platelets in paroxysmal nocturnal hemoglobinuria. N Engl J Med 1985; 312:1091.

75. Schreiber AD, Gill FM, Manno CS: Autoimmune hemolytic anemia. In Nathan DG, Oski FA (eds): Hematology of Infancy and Childhood, 4th ed. Philadelphia: WB Saunders, 1993:507–508.

76. Craddock PR, Fehr J, Jacob HS: Complement-mediated granulocyte dysfunction in paroxysmal nocturnal hemoglobinuria. Blood 1976; 47:931.

77. Leibowitz AI, Hartmann RC: The Budd-Chiari syndrome and paroxysmal nocturnal haemoglobinuria [annotation]. Br J Haematol 1981; 48:1–6.

78. Blaas P, et al: Paroxysmal nocturnal hemoglobinuria. Enhanced stimulation of platelets by the terminal complement components is related to the lack of C8bp in the membrane. J Immunol 1988; 140:3045.

79. Newcomb TF, Gardner FH: Thrombin generation in paroxysmal nocturnal haemoglobinuria. Br J Haematol 1963; 9:84.

80. Kawakami Z, Ninomiya H, Tomiyama J, Abe T: Deficiency of glycosyl-phosphatidylinositol anchored proteins on paroxysmal nocturnal haemoglobinuria neutrophils and monocytes. Br J Haematol 1990; 74(4):508–513.

81. Craddock PR, Fehr J, Jacob HS: Complement-mediated granulocyte dysfunction in paroxysmal nocturnal hemoglobinuria. Blood 1976; 47:931.

82. Clark DA, Butler SA, Braren V, et al: The kidneys in paroxysmal nocturnal hemoglobinuria. Blood 1981; 57:83.

83. Hartmann RC, Jenkins DE Jr, Arnold AB: Diagnostic specificity of sucrose hemolysis test for paroxysmal nocturnal hemoglobinuria. Blood 1970; 35:462.

84. Ham TH: Studies on destruction of red blood cells. Arch Intern Med 1939; 64:1271.

85. Gockerman JP, Brouillard RP: RBC transfusions in paroxysmal nocturnal hemoglobinuria. Arch Intern Med 1977; 137:536.

86. Antin JH, Ginsburg D, Smith BR, et al: Bone marrow transplantation for paroxysmal nocturnal hemoglobinuria: Eradication of the PNH clone and documentation of complete lymphohematopoietic engraftment. Blood 1985; 66:1247.

87. Devine DV, Gluck WL, Rosse WF, Weinberg JB: Acute myeloblastic leukemia in paroxysmal nocturnal hemoglobinuria clone. J Clin Invest 1987; 79:314.

88. Brain MC, Dacie JV, Hourihane DO'B: Microangiopathic haemolytic anemia: The possible role of vascular lesions in pathogenesis. Br J Haematol 1962; 8:358–374.

89. Bull BS, Rubenberg ML, Dacie JV, Brain MC: Microangiopathic haemolytic anemia: Mechanisms of red cell fragmentation: in vitro studies. Br J Haematol 1968; 14:643–652.

90. McGehe WG, Rapaport SI, Hyort PF: Intravascular coagulation in fulminant meningococcemia. Ann Intern Med 1967; 67:250–260.

91. Carr DJ, Kramer BS, Dragonetti DE: Thrombotic thrombocytopenic purpura associated with metastatic gastric adenocarcinoma: Successful management with plasmapheresis. South Med J 1986; 79:476–479.

92. Kwaan HC: Miscellaneous secondary thrombotic microangiopathy. Semin Hematol 1987; 24:141–149.

93. Weiner CP: Thrombotic microangiopathy in pregnancy and the post-partum period. Semin Hematol 1987; 24:119–129.

94. Capelli JP, Wesson LG Jr, Erslev AJ: Malignant hypertension and red cell fragmentation syndrome. Ann Intern Med 1966; 64:128–136.

95. Fainara M, Eisenberg S, Manny N, Hershko C: The natural course of defibrination syndrome caused by Echis colorata venom in man. Thromb Diath Haemorrh 1974; 33:420–428.

96. Doll RC, Ringenberg QS, Yarbro JW: Vascular toxicity associated with antineoplastic agents. J Clin Oncol 1986; 4:1405–1417.

97. Moschcowitz C: An acute febrile pleochromic anemia with hyaline thrombosis of terminal arterioles and capillaries. An undescribed disease. Arch Intern Med 1925; 36:89–93.

98. Baehr G, Klemperer P, Schifrin A: An acute febrile anemia and thrombocytopenic purpura with diffuse platelet thrombosis of capillaries and arterioles. Trans Assoc Am Physicians 1936; 51:43–58.

99. Gore J: Disseminated arteriolar and capillary platelet thrombosis: A morphological study of its histogenesis. Am J Pathol 1950; 26:155–167.

100. Rapaport SI: Introduction to Hematology, 2nd ed. Philadelphia: JB Lippincott, 1987:500–504.

101. Kwaan HC: Clinicopathologic features of thrombotic thrombocytopenic purpura. Semin Hematol 1987; 24:71–81.

102. George JN, Aster RH: Thrombocytopenia due to enhanced platelet destruction by nonimmunologic mechanism. In Williams WJ, Beutler E, Erslev AJ, Lichtman MA (eds): Hematology, 4th ed. New York: McGraw-Hill, 1990:1355–1361.

103. Lian EC-Y: Pathogenesis of thrombotic thrombocytopenic purpura. Semin Hematol 1987; 24(2):82–100.

104. Moak JL, Rudy CK, Toll JH, et al: Unusually large plasma factor VIII: von Willebrand factor multimers in chronic relapsing thrombotic thrombocytopenic purpura. N Engl J Med 1982; 307:1432–1435.

105. Bowdler AJ: Chronic relapsing thrombotic thrombocytopenic purpura. South Med J 1987; 80:507–510.

106. Ridolfi RL, Bell WR: Thrombotic thrombocytopenic purpura. Report of 25 cases and review of the literature. Medicine 1981; 60:413–428.

107. Shepard KV, Bukowski RM: The treatment of thrombotic thrombocytopenic purpura with exchange transfusion, plasma infusion and plasma exchange. Semin Hematol 1987; 24:178–193.

108. Craig JM, Gitlin D: The nature of the hyaline thrombi in thrombotic thrombocytopenic purpura. Am J Pathol 1957; 31:251–265.

109. Harkness DR, Byrnes JJ, Lian EC-Y, et al: Hazard of platelet transfusion in thrombotic thrombocytopenic purpura. JAMA 1981; 246:1931–1933.

110. Karmali MA, Petrie M, Lim C, et al: The association between idiopathic hemolytic uremic syndrome and infection by verotoxin-producing Escherichia coli. J Infect Dis 1985; 151:775–782.

111. Beattie TJ: Recent developments in the pathogenesis of hemolytic uremic syndrome. Ren Fail 1990; 12(1):3–7.

112. Greenough WB: Hemolytic uremia syndrome after shigellosis. N Engl J Med 1975; 293:305.

113. Raghyupathy P, Date A, Shastry JCM, Sudarson A: Hemolytic-uremic syndrome complicating shigella dysentery in South Indian Children. BMJ 1978; 1(2):1518–1521.

114. Moorthy B, Makker SP: Hemolytic-uremic syndrome associated with pneumococcal sepsis. J Pediatr 1979; 95:558–559.

115. Delans RD, Binso JD, Saba SR: Hemolytic-uremic syndrome after Campylobacter-induced diarrhea in adult. Arch Intern Med 1984; 144:1074–1076.

116. Drummond KN: Hemolytic uremic syndrome—Then and now. N Engl J Med 1985; 312:116–118.

117. Brain MC, Beame PB: Thrombotic thrombocytopenic purpura and the hemolytic-uremic syndrome. Semin Thromb Hemost 1982; 8:186–187.

118. Seigler RL: Management of hemolytic-uremic syndrome. J Pediatr 1988; 122:1014–1020.

119. Nissenson AR, Krumlousky FA, del Grego F: Postpartum hemolytic-uremic syndrome: Late recovery after prolonged maintenance dialysis. JAMA 1979; 242:173–175.

120. Hakim RM, Schulman G, Churchill WH, Lazarus JM: Successful management of thrombocytopenia, microangiopathic anemia, and acute renal failure by plasmapheresis. Am J Kidney Dis 1985; 5:170–176.

121. Erslev AJ: Traumatic cardiac hemolytic anemia. In Williams WJ, Beutler E, Erslev AJ, Lichtman MA (eds): Hematology, 4th ed. New York: McGraw-Hill, 1990:654–656.

122. Marsh GW, Lewis SM: Cardiac hemolytic anemia. Semin Hematol 1969; 6:133–149.

123. Erslev A Jr: March hemoglobinuria and sports anemia. In Williams WJ, Beutler E, Erslev AJ, Lichtman MA (eds): Hematology, 4th ed. New York: McGraw-Hill, 1990:653–654.

124. Davidson RJL: Exertional hemoglobinuria. A report on three cases with studies on the haemolytic mechanism. J Clin Pathol 1964; 17:536–540.

125. Epitaph for global malaria eradication? [Editorial]. Lancet 1975; 2:15–16.

126. Wyler DJ: Malaria—Resurgence, resistance, and research. N Engl J Med 1983; 308:934–940.

127. Guerrero IC, Weniger BG, Scutz MG: Transfusion malaria in United States: 1972–1981. Ann Intern Med 1983; 99:221–226.

128. Dvorak JA, Miller LH, Whitehorse WC, et al: Invasion of erythrocytes by malaria merozoites. Science 1975; 187:748–750.

129. Ash LR, Orihel TC: Atlas of Human Parasitology, 2nd ed. Chicago, ASCP Press, 1984:14–17, 79–93.

130. Livingstone FB: The Duffy blood groups, vivax malaria, and malaria selection in human populations. A review. Hum Biol 1984; 56(3):413–425.

131. Miller LH, Mason ST, Clyde DF, et al: The resistance factor to Plasmodium vivax in blacks. The Duffy-blind-group phenotype FY-Fy. N Engl J Med 1976; 295:302–304.

132. Harmening DM: Clinical Hematology and Fundamentals of Hemostasis, 2nd ed. Philadelphia, FA Davis, 1991:210–215.

133. Allison AC: Protection afforded by sickle cell trait against subtertian malaria infection. BMJ 1954; 1:290–294.

134. Allison AC: The distribution of sickle cell trait in East Africa and elsewhere and its apparent relationship to subtertian malaria. R Soc Trop Med Hyg 1954; 48:312–318.

135. Fleming AF, Storey J, Molineaux L, et al: Abnormal haemoglobins in the Sudan savanna of Nigeria: I. Prevalence of haemoglobins and relationships between sickle cell trait, malaria and survival. Ann Trop Med Parasitol 1979; 73:161–172.

136. Storey J, Fleming AF, Cornille-Brogger R, et al: Abnormal haemoglobins in the Sudan savanna of Nigeria: IV. Malaria immunoglobulins and antimalarial antibodies in haemoglobin AC individuals. Ann Trop Med Parasitol 1979; 74:311–315.

137. Nagel RL, Raventos-Suarez C, Fabry ME, et al: Impairment of the growth of Plasmodium falciparum in Hb EE erythrocytes. J Clin Invest 1981; 68:303–305.

138. Siniscalco M, Bernini L, Felippi G, et al: Population genetics of hemoglobin variants, thalassemia and glucose-6-phosphate dehydrogenase deficiency, with particular reference to the malarial hypothesis. Bull WHO 1966; 34:379–393.

139. Luzzotto L, Bienzle V: The malaria/G-6-PD hypothesis (letter). Lancet 1979; 1:1183–1184.

140. Pasvol G, Weatherall DJ, Wilson RJM: The effects of fetal hemoglobin on susceptibility of red cells to Plasmodium falciparum. Nature 1977; 270:171–173.

141. Perrin LH, Mackey LJ, Miescher PA: The hematology of malaria in man. Semin Hematol 1982; 19:70–82.

142. Vryonis G: Observations on the parasitization of erythrocytes by Plasmodium vivax, with special reference to reticulocytes. Am J Hyg 1939; 30(Sect C):41–48.

143. Sheehy TW: Disseminated intravascular coagulation and severe falciparum malaria. Lancet 1975; 1(7905):516.

144. White NJ, Warrell DA: Clinical management of chloroquine-resistant Plasmodium falciparum malaria in Southeast Asia. Trop Doc 1983; 13:153–158.

145. Peters W: Plasmodium: Resistance to antimalarial drugs. Ann Parasitol Hum Comp 1990; 65(Suppl 1):103–106.

146. Howard RJ: Malaria. The search for vaccine antigens and new chemotherapeutic strategies. Blood 1989; 74(2):533–536.

147. Gordan DM: Malaria vaccines. Infect Dis Clin North Am 1990; 4(2):299–313.

148. Healy GR: Babesia infections in man. Hosp Pract 1979; 14:107–116.

149. Ruebush TK II, Cassaday PB, Marsh HJ, et al: Human babesiosis on Nantucket Island. Ann Intern Med 1977; 86:6–9.

150. Chisholm ES, Sulzer AJ, Ruebush TK II: Indirect immunofluorescence test for human Babesia microti infection. Antigenic specificity. Am J Trop Med Hyg 1986; 35:921–925.

151. Benach JL, Habicht GS: Clinical characteristics of human babesiosis. J Infect Dis 1981; 144:481.

152. Weinstein L: Two new diseases and a new tick: Babesiosis and Lyme disease. Infect Dis Pract 1980; 4(1):1–5.

153. Healy GR, Ruebush TK II: Morphology of Babesia microti in human blood smears. Am J Clin Pathol 1980; 73(1):107–109.

154. Miller LH, Neva FA, Gill F: Failure of chloroquine in human babesiosis (Babesia microti). Ann Intern Med 1978; 88:200–202.

155. Jacoby GA, Hunt JV, Kisinski KS, et al: Treatment of transfusion-transmitted babesiosis by exchange transfusion. N Engl J Med 1980; 303:1098–1100.

156. Mahn HE, Dantuono LM: Postabortal septicotoxemia due to Clostridium welchii. Am J Obstet Gynecol 1955; 70:604–610.

157. Beutler E: Hemolytic anemia due to infections with microorganisms. In Williams WJ, Beutler E, Erslev AJ, Lichtman MA (eds): Hematology, 4th ed. New York: McGraw-Hill, 1991:664.

158. Ricketts WE: Bartonella bacilliformis anemia (Oroya fever). A study of 30 cases. Blood 1948; 3:1025–1049.

159. Schultz MG: A history of bartonellosis (Carrión's disease). Am J Trop Med Hyg 1968; 17:503–512.

160. Reynafarje C, Ramos J: The hemolytic anemia of human bartonellosis. Blood 1961; 17:562–578.

161. Urteaga OP, Payne EM: Treatment of the acute febrile phase of Carrión's disease with chloramphenicol. Am J Trop Med Hyg 1955; 4:507–511.

162. Beutler E: Erythrocyte disorders: anemias related to erythrocyte damage mediated by chemicals, physical agents, or microorganisms. In Williams WJ, Beutler E, Erslev AJ, Lichtman MA (eds): Hematology, 4th ed. New York: McGraw-Hill, 1990:660–663.

163. Gorham R: The brown recluse spider Loxosceles reclusa and necrotic spider bite—A new public health problem in the United States. J Environ Health 1968; 31:138.

164. Shen SC: Studies on the destruction of red blood cells: III. Mechanism and complications of hemoglobinuria in patients with thermal burns: Spherocytosis and increased osmotic fragility of red blood cells. N Eng J Med 1943; 229:701–713.

165. Packman CH, Leddy JP: Acquired hemolytic anemia due to warm-reactive antibodies. In Williams WJ, Beutler E, Erslev AJ, Lichtman MA (eds): Hematology, 4th ed. New York: McGraw-Hill, 1990:666–673.

166. Bowman JM: Alloimmune hemolytic disease of the newborn. In Williams WJ, Beutler E, Erslev AJ, Lichtman MA (eds): Hematology, 4th ed. New York: McGraw-Hill, 1990:687–693.

167. Packman CH, Leddy JP: Drug-related immunologic injury of erythrocytes. In Williams WJ, Beutler E, Erslev AJ, Lichtman MA (eds): Hematology, 4th ed. New York: McGraw-Hill, 1990:681–686.

168. Packman CH, Leddy JP: Cryopathic hemolytic syndromes. In Williams WJ, Beutler E, Erslev AJ, Lichtman MA (eds): Hematology, 4th ed. New York: McGraw-Hill, 1990:675–680.

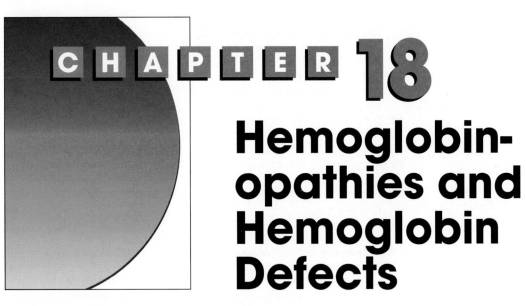

CHAPTER 18

Hemoglobin-opathies and Hemoglobin Defects

Doris McGhee and Martha Payne*

Outline

HEMOGLOBINOPATHIES
  Molecular Abnormality
  Abnormal States
  Definitions
  Hemoglobin S
  Hemoglobin C
  Hemoglobin C-Harlem (also
    called C-Georgetown)
  Hemoglobins D and G
  Hemoglobin E
  Hemoglobin O-Arab
  Interaction of Hemoglobin S
    with Other Hemoglobin
    Variants
  Hemoglobin M
  Unstable Hemoglobin Variants
  Hemoglobins with Increased
    and Decreased Oxygen
    Affinity
THALASSEMIAS
  Definition, History, and Etiology
  Genetic Control of
    Hemoglobin Synthesis
  Categories of Thalassemia
  Geographic Distribution

Objectives

AFTER COMPLETION OF THIS CHAPTER, THE READER WILL BE ABLE TO

1. Characterize the categories of the molecular abnormalities found in the various hemoglobinopathies.
2. Differentiate between the homozygous and heterozygous states, and qualitative and quantitative hemoglobin defects.
3. Define the pathologic basis of sickle cell disorder.
4. Describe the inheritance pattern of hemoglobin S variant.
5. State the amino acid substitution found in sickle cell disease.
6. Describe the solubility of hemoglobin S due to deoxygenation of erythrocytes containing hemoglobin S.
7. Describe the types of sickle cell crises.
8. Locate the geographic region, define the frequency of occurrence, and describe the impact of the incidence of *Plasmodium falciparum* malaria and G6PD deficiency on hemoglobin variants.
9. Describe the peripheral blood cell profile, chemistries, and other laboratory procedures in the diagnosis of hemoglobinopathies.
10. Define the treatment goal for hemoglobin S disease.
11. Name the amino acid substitution and electrophoretic mobility of hemoglobin C and hemoglobin C Harlem.
12. Explain the importance of identification of hemoglobins D and G and of differentiation from hemoglobin S.

* The authors wish to thank Ann Bell, Professor of Clinical Laboratory Sciences, for her invaluable advice, and the staff of the hematology laboratory at the Regional Medical Center in Memphis, Tennessee, for their assistance.

Pathophysiology
Genetic Defects Causing
    Thalassemia
Beta, Delta Beta, and Gamma
    Delta Beta Thalassemias
Alpha Thalassemias
Diagnosis of Thalassemia
Differential Diagnosis of
    Thalassemia and Iron
    Deficiency Anemia

13. Describe the hemoglobin substitution in hemoglobin E and the importance of genetic counseling.
14. Describe the laboratory findings in interactions of hemoglobin S with hemoglobin C, D, O Arab, and Korle Bu.
15. Identify the causes of methemoglobinemia.
16. Describe the inheritance patterns and causes of unstable hemoglobins.
17. Explain hemoglobins with increased and decreased oxygen affinities and how they differ from unstable hemoglobins.
18. Describe the hemoglobin defect found in thalassemias.
19. Name the chromosome that contains the beta gene cluster and the chromosome that contains the alpha genes.
20. Name the globin chains produced by the beta gene cluster.
21. Name the globin chains produced by the alpha gene cluster.
22. Explain the geographic distribution of thalassemia and its association with malaria.
23. Explain the pathophysiology caused by the imbalance of the globin chain synthesis in thalassemia.
24. List the thalassemias associated with genetic defects of the beta gene cluster and describe the clinical expression of each heterozygous and homozygous form.
25. Describe the peripheral blood condition, the indices, and the chemistries of heterozygous and homozygous beta thalassemias.
26. Describe the treatment of homozygous beta thalassemia, the risks involved, and list the laboratory tests to monitor the iron levels.
27. List the thalassemias associated with genetic defects of the alpha genes and describe the clinical expression associated with the number of alpha genes present.
28. Explain why genetic testing and counseling is important to those in Asian populations who have alpha thalassemia trait.
29. Describe the clinical syndromes of thalassemia associated with structural hemoglobin variants.
30. Name the red blood cell indices that are important in screening for thalassemia.
31. Describe the appearance of the bone marrow in the various thalassemia syndromes.
32. Explain how hemoglobin electrophoresis can be useful in diagnosing the various thalassemias.
33. Name the type of thalassemia for whose diagnosis quantitating hemoglobin A_2 is important, and describe the methods that can be used.
34. List the conditions in which the quantitation and distribution of hemoglobin F is important, and describe the methods that can be used.
35. Explain why globin chain testing and DNA analysis can be important in special cases in thalassemias.
36. Explain how thalassemia can be differentiated from iron deficiency anemia by laboratory methods.

Hemoglobinopathies are inherited disorders in which mutations in or near multiple globin genes alter either the structure or the rate of synthesis of a particular globin chain. These disorders are divided into hemoglobinopathies, in which the amino acid sequence is altered, and the thalassemia syndromes, which are inherited disorders caused by gene mutations that reduce or completely preclude the synthesis of one or more of the globin chains.

HEMOGLOBINOPATHIES

Molecular Abnormality

Approximately 400 hemoglobin (Hb) variants are known to exist throughout the world.[1] Molecular abnormalities that cause these various mutant hemoglobins may affect any adult hemoglobin (Hb) chain—alpha, beta, gamma, or delta. The molecular abnormalities are characterized as follows:[2]

1. The most common mutation substitutes one amino acid for another (e.g., valine for glutamic acid in hemoglobin S [HbS]).
2. Occasionally, more than one amino acid substitution takes place, as in glutamic acid for valine and asparate for asparagine in hemoglobin C Harlem.
3. The deletion of one or more amino acids is exemplified by glutamic acid's deletion in Hb Leiden.
4. There may be fusions of hemoglobin chains, as in delta-beta Hb Lepore.
5. The extension of chains exists, as in Hb Constant Spring, in which there are 31 additional residues.

The results of these substitutions depend on the type of amino acid and where it is located in the molecule. Most of them are clinically insignificant because they do not demonstrate any physiologic effect. Most abnormalities are associated with the beta-chain amino acids and more patients with these beta chain abnormalities present with abnormal physical conditions that result in clinical disease than patients with alpha-chain abnormalities. Involvement of the gamma and delta chains does occur but because of the small amount of hemoglobin involved, it is rarely detected and usually of no consequence.[3] Table 18–1 lists clinically significant abnormal hemoglobins. The most frequently occurring as well as the most severe of the abnormal hemoglobins is HbS.

Abnormal States

Abnormal hemoglobins are described as existing in either homozygous or heterozygous states.[4] In homozygous beta hemoglobinopathies, the variant hemoglobin is the major component and normal hemoglobin (HbA) is absent. Examples are sickle cell disease (HbSS) and hemoglobin C disease (HbCC).

In heterozygous beta hemoglobinopathies, the variant hemoglobin is usually present in a lesser amount than HbA. In some cases, however, they may be in equal amounts. Examples are hemoglobin C trait (HbAC) and hemoglobin S trait

Table 18–1. CLINICALLY IMPORTANT HEMOGLOBIN VARIANTS

I. Sickle syndromes
  A. Sickle cell trait
  B. Sickle cell disease
    1. SS
    2. SC
    3. SD-Los Angeles
    4. SO-Arab
    5. S-Thalassemia
II. Unstable hemoglobins → congenital Heinz body anemia (approximately 90 variants)
III. Hemoglobins with abnormal oxygen affinity
  A. High affinity → familial erythrocytosis (approximately 40 variants)
  B. Low affinity → familial cyanosis (Hbs Kansas, Beth Israel, St. Mandé)
IV. M hemoglobins → familial cyanosis (5 variants)
V. Structural variants that result in a thalassemic phenotype
  A. β-Thalassemia phenotype
    1. Lepore hemoglobins (δβ fusion)
    2. Hb E
    3. Hb Indianapolis
  B. α-Thalassemia phenotype
    Chain termination mutants (e.g., Hb Constant Spring)

From Nathan DG, Oski FA (ed): Hematology of Infancy and Childhood, 4th ed. Philadelphia: WB Saunders, 1993:714.

(HbAS). Hemoglobin F and HbA_2 are usually normal structurally.

In heterozygous alpha-hemoglobinopathies, the abnormality in the alpha chain will affect all three hemoglobin types (A, F, A_2); thus six different hemoglobin types are found. Three of these are normal and three are abnormal. Examples are HbD-Baltimore and HbM-Boston.

Definitions

Hemoglobinopathies and thalassemias are congenital (genetic) hereditary disorders in which a qualitative (structural) abnormality or a quantitative abnormality results from alterations of the deoxyribonucleic acid (DNA) genetic code for one or more globin chains.

Qualitative structural abnormalities involve a partial or complete replacement, an addition, or a deletion of one or more amino acids of the globin chains. The results of a change in the sequence will depend on the amino acids involved and their positions in the molecule. Fishleder and Hoffman[5] divided the structural abnormalities into four groups: (1) abnormal hemoglobins that result in hemolytic anemia, such as HbS and the unstable hemoglobins; (2) methemoglobinemia, such as hemoglobin M; (3) hemoglobins with either increased or decreased oxygen affinity; and (4) abnormal hemoglobins with no clinical or functional effect. Qualitative abnormalities are usually referred to when discussing hemoglobinopathies. Table 18–2

Table 18-2. FUNCTIONAL CLASSIFICATION OF HEMOGLOBIN VARIANTS

I. Homozygous: Hemoglobin polymorphisms: the variants that are most common

HbS	$\alpha_2\beta_2^{6Val}$	Severe hemolytic anemia; sickling	HbD-Punjab	$\alpha_2\beta_2^{121Gln}$	No anemia
HbC	$\alpha_2\beta_2^{6Lys}$	Mild hemolytic anemia	HbE	$\alpha_2\beta_2^{261Lys}$	Mild microcytic anemia

II. Heterozygous: Hemoglobin variants causing functional aberrations or hemolytic anemia in the heterozygous state

  A. Hemoglobins associated with methemoglobinemia and cyanosis

1. HbM-Boston	$\alpha_2^{58Tyr}\beta_2$	4. HbM-Milwaukee	$\alpha_2\beta_2^{67Glu}$	
2. HbM-Iwate	$\alpha_2^{87Tyr}\beta_2$	5. HbM-Hyde Park	$\alpha_2\beta_2^{92Tyr}$	
3. HbM-Saskatoon	$\alpha_2\beta_2^{63Tyr}$	6. HbFM-Osaka	$\alpha_2\gamma_2^{63Tyr}$	

  B. Hemoglobins associated with altered oxygen affinity

    1. Increased affinity and polycythemia

a. Hb Chesapeake	$\alpha_2^{92Leu}\beta_2$	f. Hb Ypsi (Ypsilanti)	$\alpha_2\beta_2^{99Tyr}$
b. HbJ-Capetown	$\alpha_2^{92Gln}\beta_2$	g. Hb Hiroshima	$\alpha_2\beta_2^{143Asp}$
c. Hb Malmo	$\alpha_2\beta_2^{97Gln}$	h. Hb Rainier	$\alpha_2\beta_2^{145Cys}$
d. Hb Yakima	$\alpha_2\beta_2^{99His}$	i. Hb Bethesda	$\alpha_2\beta_2^{145His}$
e. Hb Kemp	$\alpha_2\beta_2^{99Asn}$		

    2. Decreased affinity—may have mild anemia or cyanosis

a. Hb Kansas	$\alpha_2^{102Thr}\beta_2$	d. Hb Agenogi	$\alpha_2\beta_2^{90Lys}$
b. Hb Titusville	$\alpha_2^{94Asn}\beta_2$	e. Hb Beth Israel	$\alpha_2\beta_2^{102Ser}$
c. Hb Providence	$\alpha_2\beta_2^{82Asn,Asp}$	f. Hb Yoshizuka	$\alpha_2\beta_2^{108Asp}$

  C. Unstable hemoglobins

    1. Hb may precipitate as Heinz bodies after splenectomy; "congenital Heinz body anemia"

a. Severe hemolysis: no improvement after splenectomy		c. Mild hemolysis: intermittent exacerbations	
Hb Bibba	$\alpha_2^{136Pro}\beta_2$	HbL Ferrara	$\alpha_2^{47Gly}\beta_2$
Hb Hammersmith	$\alpha_2\beta_2^{42Ser}$	Hb Hasharon	$\alpha_2^{47His}\beta_2$
Hb Bristol	$\alpha_2\beta_2^{67Asp}$	Hb Leiden	$\alpha_2\beta_2^{6or7}$ (Glu deleted)
Hb Olmsted	$\alpha_2\beta_2^{141Arg}$	Hb Freiburg	$\alpha_2\beta_2^{23}$ (Val deleted)
b. Severe hemolysis: improvement after splenectomy		Hb Seattle	$\alpha_2\beta_2^{76Glu}$
Hb Torino	$\alpha_2^{42Val}\beta_2$	Hb Louisville	$\alpha_2\beta_2^{42Leu}$
Hb Ann Arbor	$\alpha_2^{80Arg}\beta_2$	Hb Zurich	$\alpha_2\beta_2^{63Arg}$
Hb Genova	$\alpha_2\beta_2^{28Pro}$	Hb Gun Hill	$\alpha_2\beta^{91-97}$ (5 a. a. deleted)
Hb Shepherd's Bush	$\alpha_2\beta_2^{74Asp}$	d. No disease	
Hb Köln	$\alpha_2\beta_2^{98Met}$	Hb Etobicoke	$\alpha_2^{84Arg}\beta_2$
Hb Wien	$\alpha_2\beta_2^{130Asp}$	Hb Dakar	$\alpha_2^{112Glu}\beta_2$
		Hb Sogn	$\alpha_2\beta_2^{14Arg}$
		Hb Tacoma	$\alpha_2\beta_2^{30Ser}$

    2. Tetramers of normal chains; appear in thalassemias

Hb Bart's	γ_4
Hb H	β_4
Hb (α_4^A)	α_4

From Henry JB: Clinical Diagnosis and Management by Laboratory Methods, 18th ed. Philadelphia: WB Saunders, 1991:650.
Modified from Winslow RM, Anderson WF: The hemoglobinopathies. *In* Stanbury JB, Wyngaarden JB, Fredrickson DS, Goldstein JL, Brown MS (eds): The Metabolic Basis of Inherited Disease, 5th ed. New York, McGraw-Hill, 1983, Chap. 76.

lists the functional classifications of some hemoglobin variants.

Quantitative abnormalities involve a partial or complete suppressed production of one or more structurally normal polypeptide chains. This imbalance is the basis for all thalassemia syndromes. Imbalanced chain production may also, in rare instances, be associated with a structurally abnormal chain, such as Hb Lepore, because of the reduced production of the abnormal chain,[6] as shown in Table 18-2.

Hemoglobin S

SICKLE CELL ANEMIA

History

Sickle cell anemia was first observed by a Chicago physician, James Herrick, in 1910, in a West Indian student suffering from severe anemia. Emmel (1917) recorded that sickling occurred in nonanemic patients as well as in those who were severely anemic. The pathologic basis of the disorder and its relationship to the hemoglobin molecule were described by Hahn and Gillespie in 1927. They showed that sickling occurred when a solution of red blood cells was deficient in oxygen and that the shape of the red cells was reversible when that solution was again oxygenated.[7, 8] In 1949, Pauling demonstrated that when HbSS is electrophoresed, it migrates differently than HbA. This difference was shown to be caused by an amino acid substitution in the globin chain. Pauling and coworkers defined the genetics of the disorder and clearly distinguished sickle trait, with its heterozygous state (HbAS) from the homozygous state (HbSS).[8]

Sickle cell diseases are the most common he-

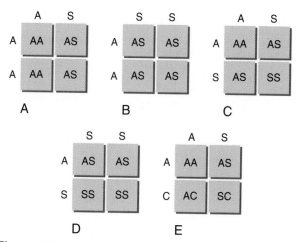

Figure 18–1 Punnett square illustrating the standard method for predicting the inheritance of abnormal hemoglobins. Each parent contributes one gene.

moglobinopathies and include a group of hereditary disorders characterized by the presence of only HbSS, or hemoglobin S in combination with another hemoglobin beta-chain mutation. The most common variants of the disease are HbS, sickle cell–hemoglobin C (HbSC), and sickle cell–beta thalassemia (HbS-β-thal).

Genetic Inheritance

Genes that carry genetic information for every normal and abnormal globin chain are located at specific loci on chromosomes 16 and 11. The alpha (α) genes are located on chromosome 16, which also contains the coding for zeta (ζ) chains for embryonic hemoglobin. The beta (β) gene coding is

located on the short arm of chromosome 11. Each chain has two loci; thus beta hemoglobin variants are inherited as autosomal codominants with two genes inherited from each parent.[6, 9]

Patients with sickle cell disease have inherited a sickle (S) gene from each parent; patients with sickle cell C disease have inherited a sickle gene from one parent and a HbC gene from the other parent; and patients with sickle cell–beta thalassemia have inherited a sickle gene from one parent and a beta thalassemia gene from the other. An individual with the sickle cell trait, or heterozygous state, has less severe disease, whereas an individual with sickle cell disease or homozygous state suffers from a more severe and often fatal disease. Figure 18–1 demonstrates inheritance of abnormal hemoglobins. Hemoglobins S and C are used as examples, but it applies to any hemoglobin variant.

Etiology and Pathophysiology

HbS is defined by the structural formula $\alpha_2\beta_2^{6\,Glu\rightarrow Val}$, which indicates that on the beta chain, at the sixth position, glutamic acid is replaced by valine. The highest frequency of the sickle cell state carrier is in Africa, where it is between 20 and 40%.[7] In the American black population, the occurrence of the heterozygous state of sickle cell trait is 8%, with the incidence of the homozygous state being 1 in 650 or 0.16%.[10] The sickle cell gene is also seen, to a lesser degree, in individuals from the Middle East and Greece (Fig. 18–2). Occasionally, the sickle gene can be found in whites in regions where admixture of races has

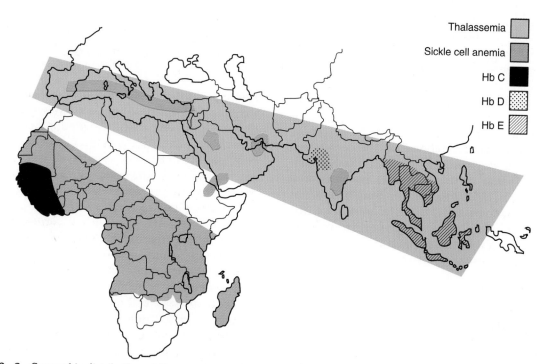

Thalassemia

Sickle cell anemia

Hb C

Hb D

Hb E

Figure 18–2 Geographic distribution of the more common inherited structural hemoglobin variants and the thalassemias. (From Hoffbrand AV, Pettit JE: Essential Haematology, 3rd ed. Oxford, England: Blackwell Scientific, 1993.)

occurred over the years.[8] Hemoglobin S is soluble in the erythrocyte and the cell remains a biconcave disc so long as it is oxygenated. Upon deoxygenation, however, the hemoglobin in the red cells becomes less soluble and cellular sickling occurs, which is associated with the formation of tactoids or liquid crystals of HbS. As sickle hemoglobin is deoxygenated, oxygen saturation drops below 85% and oxygen saturation in the heterozygote is decreased to 40%. The blood becomes more viscous and polymers are formed.[10] In addition to a decrease in oxygen tension, the pH is reduced and there is an increase in 2,3-diphosphoglycerate (2,3-DPG).

When the blood becomes de-oxygenated, viscosity increases as a result of the cellular rigidity that occurs with sickling. This, in turn, prolongs the exposure of erythrocytes to a hypoxic environment, and the lower tissue pH decreases the oxygen affinity, which further promotes sickling. The end result is occlusion of capillaries and arterioles and infarction of surrounding tissue.

Sickle cells are of two types:[11] reversible (RSC) and irreversible (ISC). The reversible sickle cells are those that undergo hemoglobin polymerization, show increased viscosity, and change shape upon deoxygenation. These cells have normal shape, normal viscosity, and no hemoglobin polymers when oxygenated. Viscosity parallels the presence of polymers. The vaso-occlusive complications of sickle cell disease are thought to be due to RSCs that are able to travel into the microvasculature because of their normal rheologic properties when oxygenated and then become distorted and viscous as they become deoxygenated in the vessel.

Irreversible sickled cells are cells that do not change their shape regardless of the change in hemoglobin polymerization. These cells are seen on the peripheral blood smear as elongated sickle cells with a point at each end.[12]

Clinical Features

The clinical manifestations of the sickle cell syndrome can vary from asymptomatic to a potentially lethal state as characterized by sickle cell disease (Table 18–3). Sickle cell disease does not manifest symptoms until the second half of the first year of life owing to the protective effect of HbF.[13] As beta chains of HbS replace gamma chains of HbF, erythrocytes containing S become susceptible to hemolysis and a progressive hemolytic anemia with splenomegaly becomes evident. The homozygous (SS) form of the disease, in some instances, is fatal by middle age.

Many patients with sickle cell disease undergo episodes termed *crises*. Sickle cell crises were described by Diggs[14] as "any new syndrome that de-

Table 18–3. CLINICAL FEATURES OF SICKLE CELL ANEMIA
I. Hematologic
1. Aplastic crisis
2. Hemolytic crisis
3. Vaso-occlusive crisis
II. Nonhematologic
1. Growth
2. Bone and joint abnormalities
a. Pain
b. *Salmonella* infection
c. Hand-foot dactylitis
3. Genitourinary
a. Renal papillary necrosis
b. Priapism
4. Spleen and liver
a. Autosplenectomy
b. Hepatomegaly
c. Jaundice
5. Cardiopulmonary
a. Enlarged heart
b. Heart murmurs
c. Pulmonary infarction
6. Eye
a. Retinal hemorrhage
7. CNS
8. Leg ulcers
9. Risky pregnancy

Abbreviation: CNS = central nervous system.
From Harmening D (ed): Clinical Hematology and Fundamentals of Hemostasis, 2nd ed. Philadelphia: FA Davis, 1992:148.

velops rapidly in patients with sickle cell disease, owing to the inherited abnormality." Various crises may occur: vaso-occlusive or infarctive (painful crises), aplastic crises, sequestration crises, and hemolytic crises.[15]

The vaso-occlusive crisis is the hallmark of sickle cell anemia and occurs most often in the bones, lungs, spleen, brain, and penis. The primary manifestation of this crisis is pain resulting from the obstruction of the blood vessels by rigid sickled red blood cells. The frequency of crises varies from almost daily to once yearly. Repeated splenic infarcts result in the spleen's diminishment by scarring (autosplenectomy). Patients with this condition have increased susceptibility to life-threatening bacterial infections, including sepsis, pneumonia, meningitis, osteomyelitis, and urinary tract infections. Infection is the most common cause of death in children with sickle cell anemia.[15]

Hemolytic crisis is characterized by a shortened red blood cell life span with a corresponding decrease in hematocrit and hemoglobin, an elevated reticulocyte count, and jaundice. Because other conditions may cause jaundice, such as hepatitis and gallstones, a hemolytic crisis is difficult to diagnose in sickle cell patients.[15]

Aplastic crisis presents clinical problems similar to those seen in hemolytic disorders, according to studies by MacIver and Parker-Williams.[16] These investigators found that sickle cell patients can usually compensate for the decrease in red blood cell survival by increasing bone marrow output. When the bone marrow is suppressed temporarily by bacterial or viral infections, however, the hematocrit drops substantially with no reticulocyte compensation. The spontaneous recovery phase is characterized by nucleated red cells and reticulocytosis. Most aplastic crises are short-lived and require no therapy. If anemia is severe and the bone marrow remains quiescent, transfusion(s) will be necessary.

Sequestration crisis occurs most often in infants and young children; however, it can occur in adults with splenomegaly. There is a sudden massive pooling of red cells in the spleen resulting in a hemoglobin level of less than 6 g/dL. This type of crisis is a main cause of death in infants with sickle cell anemia.[15]

Incidence with Malaria and G6PD Deficiency

The sickle gene occurs with greatest frequency in Central Africa, the Near East, the region around the Mediterranean, and in parts of India. The frequency of the gene parallels the incidence of *Plasmodium falciparum* and appears to offer some protection in young patients with cerebral falciparum malaria. Malarial parasites are living organisms within the red blood cells, which utilize the oxygen within the cells. This reduced oxygen tension causes the cells to sickle, resulting in injury to the cells. These injured cells tend to become trapped within the blood vessels of the spleen and other organs where they are easily phagocytized by scavenger white blood cells. Selective destruction of red blood cells containing parasites decreases the number of malarial organisms and increases the time for immunity to develop. One explanation for this phenomenon is that the infected cell is uniquely sickled and destroyed, probably in an area in the spleen or liver where phagocytic cells are plentiful and the oxygen tension is significantly decreased.[17]

Because of the high incidence of G6PD deficiency in patients with sickle cell disease, it was suggested that the G6PD deficiency had a protective effect on these patients.[18] This correlation has not been confirmed through studies, however. It has also been thought that hemolytic episodes are more frequent in these patients. This is said to be unlikely because studies have shown no relationship between the clinical severity of the disease and the presence or absence of G6PD deficiency. Because of the presence of young cells rich in G6PD, this increased hemolysis is thought to be more likely caused by the enzyme abnormality when the population is shifted to the oldest cell during the aplastic crisis.[19]

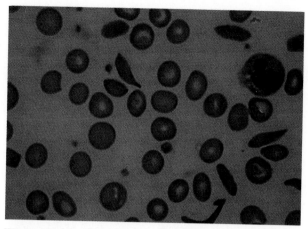

Figure 18–3 Cells from the peripheral blood smear of a patient with sickle cell disease. Anisocytosis, poikilocytosis, sickle cells, and a few spherocytes are present.

Laboratory Diagnosis*

The anemia of sickle cell disease is a chronic hemolytic anemia classified morphologically as normocytic, normochromic. The peripheral blood smear shows marked poikilocytosis and anisocytosis with normal, irreversibly sickled, target and nucleated red cells, a few spherocytes, basophilic stippling, and Howell-Jolly bodies. The characteristic cell present is a long, curved cell with a point at each end (Figs. 18–3 to 18–6). Because of their resemblance to a sickle, they were named sickle cells.[14] There is a moderate to marked amount of polychromasia corresponding to the hemolytic state or bone marrow response. The reticulocyte count is often between 10 and 25%. The red blood cell distribution width (RDW) is increased. The mean corpuscular volume (MCV), however, is not elevated to a degree commensurate with the in-

---

* Procedures referred to in this chapter are detailed in the Appendix.

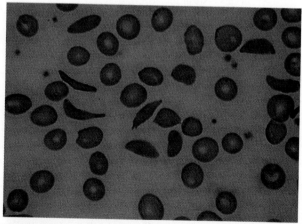

Figure 18–4 Cells from the peripheral blood smear of a patient with sickle cell disease. Several characteristic sickle cells with pointed ends are shown.

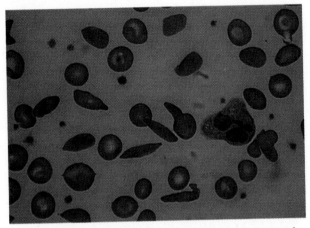

Figure 18–5 Cells from the peripheral blood smear of a patient with sickle cell disease. Note the presence of target cells and an elevated platelet count.

creased reticulocyte count. An aplastic crisis can be heralded by a decreased reticulocyte count. Moderate leukocytosis is usually present (sometimes as high as 40 to 50 $\times$ 10^9/L) with neutrophilia and a mild shift toward immature granulocytes. Thrombocytosis is usually present. The neutrophil alkaline phosphatase score is not elevated when neutrophilia is due to sickle cell crisis alone, and no underlying infection exists.[20] The marrow shows erythroid hyperplasia. Immunoglobulin levels, particularly IgA, are elevated in all forms of sickle cell disease. Serum ferritin levels of young patients are normal, but tend to be elevated later in life. Hemochromatosis is rare.

Diagnosis is made by testing to demonstrate the insolubility of S hemoglobin in the deoxygenated form and confirming its presence on electrophoresis. One very simple test employs the use of sodium metabisulfite. Red blood cells are exposed to an oxygen-poor environment where they become sickled. These sickled cells are identified by microscopy.

Testing can be accomplished with the use of several solubility testing reagents. The principle of solubility tests is based on turbidity occurring in a high-salt solution because of the selective insolubility of sickle hemoglobin. Other hemoglobins, however, can give a positive solubility test.[21] These are HbC-Harlem, HbC-Ziguinchor, HbS-Memphis, HbS-Travis, HbS-Antilles, HbS-Providence, HbS-Oman, Hb Alexander, and Hb Porto-Alegre.[16] All these hemoglobins have the same amino acid substitution, ($\beta^{6Glu \rightarrow Val}$), which is found in hemoglobin S in addition to a second substitution. HbS-Antilles is particularly important because it can cause sickling in the heterozygous state.

Alkaline electrophoresis is the first step in the definitive diagnosis of hemoglobinopathies. Because some hemoglobins have the same electrophoretic mobility patterns (e.g., HbS, D, and G have similar mobilities, and HbA$_2$, C, O, and E migrate together), separation at an acid pH may also be necessary. All hemoglobins that exhibit an abnormal electrophoretic pattern in an alkaline pH must be electrophoresed at an acid pH. Figure 18–7 shows electrophoretic patterns for abnormal hemo-

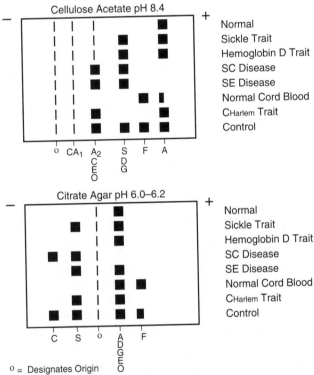

o = Designates Origin

Figure 18–7 Hemoglobin electrophoresis on cellulose acetate and citrate agar, showing relative mobilities of various samples. The relative amounts of hemoglobin are not necessarily proportional to the size of the band; e.g., in sickle cell trait (AS), the bands may appear equal, but the amount of HbA always exceeds that of HbS. (From Schmidt RM, Brosious EF: Basic Laboratory Methods of Hemoglobinopathy Detection, 6th ed [HEW publication no. (CDC)77-8266]. Atlanta: U.S. Department of Health, Education and Welfare, Centers for Disease Control, 1976.)

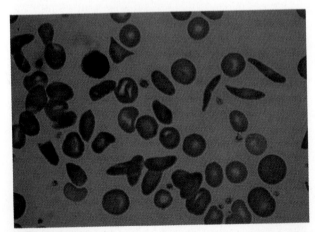

Figure 18–6 Cells from the peripheral blood smear of a patient with sickle cell disease. Polychromasia indicates bone marrow response to hemolysis.

globins. Because patients with sickle cell disease or SC disease lack normal beta-polypeptide chain genes, they have no A hemoglobin. Fetal hemoglobin is usually increased. When increased more than 20%, it has a tendency of moderating the severity of the disease, as in newborns and in the condition called hereditary persistence of fetal hemoglobin (HPFH).[22] Hemoglobin A_2 quantitation is useful in differentiating sickle cell anemia from sickle β° thalassemia. Hemoglobin A_2 is increased in the latter disease.

Treatment

There is no specific treatment for sickle cell anemia. Various drugs are administered to attempt to prevent fever or lessen the frequency of painful crises. The drugs of choice are those that inhibit polymerization of the abnormal hemoglobin with little effect on the oxygen affinity of the hemoglobin molecule. Hydroxyurea or butyrate therapy has offered some promise in relieving the sickling disorder by increasing the proportion of HbF in the erythrocytes of persons with sickle cell disease.[23] Because HbF does not copolymerize with HbS, it is believed that if the production of HbF could be sufficiently augmented, the complications of sickle cell disease might be avoided. It has been suggested that a threshold level of 20% hemoglobin F could alleviate recurrent painful crises and that 10% HbF may be required to relieve strokes or other single events.[22] The patient should be examined on a regular follow-up basis and routine testing should be done to establish normal values for the well patient. Continuous instruction about avoiding and treating painful episodes helps reduce morbidity and hospitalization. Children under the age of three years often have pain and swelling in hands and feet called the *Hand and Foot Syndrome*.[14] Treatment usually consists of increasing intake of fluids and giving analgesics for pain.

Serious infections from bacteria[24] such as *Streptococcus pneumoniae*, *Mycoplasma pneumoniae*, *Neisseria meningitidis*, *Haemophilus influenzae*, *Staphylococcus aureus*, and *Streptococcus pyogenes* are the major causes of morbidity and mortality with sickle cell anemia in childhood. The risk of bacterial infection probably increases in mature patients with hemoglobin SC disease as well as in those with homozygous sickle hemoglobin.[11]

Transfusions should be utilized *only* for the prevention of the complications of sickle cell disease. Transfusions should be used in sequestration and aplastic crisis to restore the red cell mass. In other circumstances such as CNS infarction, hypoxia with infection, and preparation for surgery, transfusions are used to decrease blood viscosity and thin the circulating sickle cells. Before surgery, HbSS patients are transfused with normal HbAA blood to bring the volume of HbS below 50% in an effort to prevent complications in surgery.[25] Maintenance transfusions in pregnancy should be done if the mother becomes symptomatic with either vaso-occlusive or anemia-related problems or if there is a sign of fetal distress or poor growth.[24]

Course and Prognosis

No accurate estimate of the life expectancy in sickle cell anemia is known. Many patients with sickle cell anemia live a full life with some reaching the sixth or seventh decades.[15] An individual with HbSS can pursue a wide range of vocations and professions. They are discouraged, however, from jobs that require strenuous physical exertion, exposure to high altitudes, or extreme environmental temperature variations.

Success with bone marrow transplantation has been reported in Europe. The procedure is currently being investigated in the United States as a cure for the disease.[25, 26]

SICKLE CELL TRAIT

The term sickle cell trait refers to the heterozygous state (HbAS) and describes a benign condition that does not generally affect mortality or morbidity. The trait occurs in approximately 8% of American blacks. It can also be found in Central Americans, Asians, and people from the region around the Mediterranean.[20]

Clinical Features

Individuals with sickle cell trait are generally asymptomatic and present with no significant clinical or hematologic manifestations. Under extreme hypoxic conditions, however, systemic sickling and vascular occlusion with pooling of sickled cells in the spleen, focal necrosis in the brain and even death can occur. In conditions such as severe respiratory infection, unpressurized flights at high altitudes, and anesthesia, in which pH and oxygen tension are sufficiently lowered to cause sickling, patients may develop splenic infarcts.[27] Failure to concentrate urine is the only consistent abnormality found in these patients.[28] This is caused by diminished perfusion of the vasa recta of the kidney, which impairs concentration of urine by the renal tubules.

Laboratory Diagnosis

The blood smear of a patient with sickle cell trait has normal red blood cell morphology. No abnormalities in the leukocytes and thrombocytes are seen. The solubility test is positive. The trait is diagnosed by detecting the presence of HbS and

HbA in the affected person. On electrophoresis, sickle cell trait has 20 to 40% of HbS and 60% or more of HbA. Hemoglobin A₂ and HbF are within normal limits. Levels under 40% HbS, however, can be seen in patients who also have alpha thalassemia or iron or folate deficiency.[11, 20]

Treatment and Prognosis

No treatment is required for this benign condition. The patient's life span is not affected by sickle cell trait.

Hemoglobin C

Hemoglobin C was the first hemoglobinopathy after HbS to be described. Spaet and Ranney reported this disease in the homozygous state (HbCC) in 1953.[7]

Etiology and Pathophysiology

Hemoglobin C is defined by the structural formula $(\alpha_2\beta_2{}^{6\text{Glu}\rightarrow\text{Lys}})$. Lysine is substituted for glutamic acid in the sixth position of the beta chain. Hemoglobin C occurs in the homozygous state (HbCC) and in the heterozygous state (HbAC).

Hemoglobin C is found in 17–28% of people of West African extraction. The disorder is found in 2–3% of American blacks. It is the second most common variant encountered in the United States and the third most common in the world.[4, 7, 25]

Clinical Features

Homozygous HbC disease is a mild chronic disorder characterized by fatigue, painful episodes, hemolytic anemia, and splenomegaly. The hemolytic state is attributed to dehydration with large efflux of potassium from red blood cells.[11] The heterozygous state is asymptomatic without anemia.

Laboratory Diagnosis

The blood picture of homozygous hemoglobin C presents as a normochromic, normocytic anemia. Occasionally, some microcytosis and mild hypochromia may also be present. Both the MCV and the mean corpuscular hemoglobin concentration (MCHC) are normal or increased. There is a marked increase in the number of target cells and reticulocytes. Nucleated red blood cells may or may not be present.

Intra-erythrocytic hemoglobin crystals may be seen on the smear (Figs. 18–8 to 18–11). Tetragonal crystals of HbC form within the erythrocyte. Many crystals appear free, with no evidence of a cell membrane.[29] In some cells, the hemoglobin is concentrated within the boundary of the crystal. The crystals are very densely stained and thus vary in size and appear oblong with pyramid-shaped or pointed ends. These crystals may be

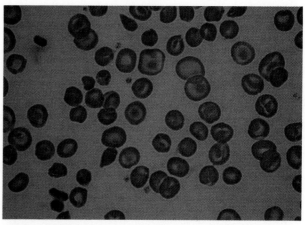

Figure 18–8 Cells from the peripheral smear of a patient with hemoglobin CC. Many target cells are present, along with several small tetragonal crystals.

demonstrated on wet preparation by washing red blood cells and resuspending them in a solution of sodium citrate.[9]

Definitive diagnosis is made with electrophoresis. No HbA is present in homozygous C. In the trait, about 60% of HbA and 30% of HbC are present. On cellulose acetate agar in an alkaline pH, hemoglobin C migrates in the same position as HbA₂, HbE, and HbO-Arab. Hemoglobin C is separated from other hemoglobins on citrate agar at an acid pH (see Fig. 18–7).

Treatment and Prognosis

No specific treatment is required. This disorder presents a problem only if infection occurs.

Hemoglobin C-Harlem[30–32]

This hemoglobin (also known as HbC-Georgetown) has a double substitution on the beta chain: The substitution at the sixth position of valine for glutamic acid is identical to the HbS substitution

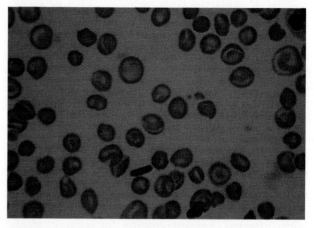

Figure 18–9 Cells from the peripheral smear of a patient with hemoglobin CC. The large polychromatophilic cells along with microcytes caused an elevated RDW in this patient.

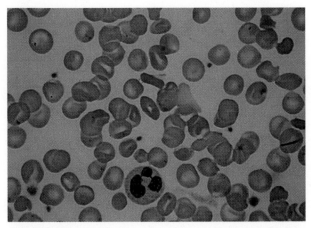

Figure 18–10 Cells from the peripheral smear of a patient with hemoglobin CC. One oblong crystal is seen just above the center.

and the substitution at the 73rd position of aspartic acid for asparagine is the same as that in the Korle Bu mutation.

Clinical Features

Patients with this anomaly are asymptomatic. Patients with double heterozygosity for HbS and HbC-Harlem have crises similar to those seen in HbSS disease.

Laboratory Diagnosis

A positive solubility test may occur with this hemoglobin. On cellulose acetate at pH 8.4, HbC-Harlem migrates as one band in the A position and another band in the C position. Agar gel electrophoresis at pH 6.2 shows migration in the A and S positions.

Treatment and Prognosis

Because so few cases have been identified, the clinical outcome of individuals affected with this abnormality is uncertain.[32]

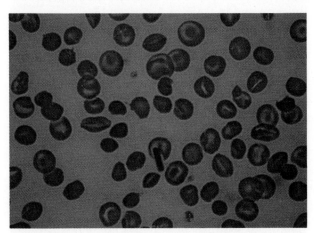

Figure 18–11 Cells from the peripheral smear of a patient with hemoglobin CC. Although this hemoglobin CC crystal is obvious, it is not always possible to find crystals in electrophoretically proven hemoglobin CC.

Hemoglobins D and G[7–9, 32]

Hemoglobins D and G are a group of at least 16 beta chain variants and six alpha chain variants that migrate in an alkaline pH at the same electrophoretic position as HbS. This is because their alpha and beta subunits have one less negative charge at an alkaline pH than does HbA. However, they do not sickle when exposed to reduced oxygen tension. Most variants are named for the place where they were discovered.

Hemoglobins D and G can be inherited as a homozygous (HbDD) or heterozygous (HbAD) condition.

Etiology and Pathophysiology

Hemoglobin D-Punjab and HbD-Los Angeles are identical hemoglobins, glycine being substituted for glutamic acid at the 121st position in the beta chain ($\alpha_2\beta_2^{121\text{Glu}\rightarrow\text{Gln}}$). Hemoglobin D-Los Angeles is the most common variant of HbD seen in America. This hemoglobin is usually seen in fewer than 2% of American blacks. Hemoglobin D-Punjab is seen in about 3% of the population in Northwest India.

Hemoglobin G-Philadelphia is an alpha variant of the D hemoglobins with a substitution of asparagine by lysine at the 68th position. The hemoglobin G-Philadelphia variant is the most common G variant encountered in American blacks and is seen with a greater frequency than other HbD variants. The HbG variant is also found in Ghana.

Clinical Features

Both HbD and HbG are asymptomatic in the heterozygous state. Hemoglobin DD has a mild hemolytic anemia and mild to moderate splenomegaly.

Laboratory Diagnosis

On alkaline electrophoresis HbD has the same mobility as HbS. Hemoglobin D is separated from HbS on citrate agar at a pH of 6.0. These hemoglobins do not sickle on the blood smear and yield a negative solubility test result. These variants should be suspected whenever a hemoglobin is encountered that migrates in the S position on cellulose and has a negative solubility.

Treatment and Prognosis

No treatment is required. These hemoglobins are benign.

Hemoglobin E

In 1954 HbE was described in independent studies by Itano[33] and by Chernoff et al.[34]

Etiology and Pathophysiology

Hemoglobin E is a beta-chain variant in which lysine is substituted for glutamic acid in the 26th position (HbE, $\alpha_2\beta_2^{26\ \text{Glu}\rightarrow\text{Lys}}$). The variant occurs with great frequency in Southeast Asia with the incidence up to 30% in some places. As a result of the influx of refugees from this area, HbE prevalence has increased in the U.S.[35] It occurs infrequently in blacks and whites.

Hemoglobin E trait (HbAE) is the heterozygous state, whereas HbEE is the homozygous state.

Clinical Features

The trait is asymptomatic. The disease, HbEE, resembles thalassemia trait. When HbE is combined with beta thalassemia, the disease becomes more severe than HbEE and more closely resembles beta thalassemia major.

The homozygous state (>90% E) presents as a mild anemia with microcytes and target cells (Figs. 18–12 and 18–13). The red blood cell survival time is somewhat shortened. The condition is not associated with icterus, hemolysis, or splenomegaly. The main concern of identifying homozygous HbE is differentiating it from iron deficiency, beta thalassemia trait, and HbE-β-thal.[34] (See the discussion in this chapter under Thalassemia). Hemoglobin E is thought to give protection against malaria. The highest incidence of the HbE gene is in those areas of Thailand where malaria is most common.[35]

[handwritten margin note: Icterus—jaundiced ↑ bilirubin from hemolysis]

Laboratory Diagnosis

In alkaline medium, HbE migrates with hemoglobins C, O, and A_2. On acid agar, it migrates with HbA. In the heterozygous state, approximately 30 to 40% of the hemoglobin is HbE on electrophoresis. Hemoglobin A is reduced or absent. The homozygous state presents with an MCV of about 67 fL, a normal MCHC, and erythrocyto-

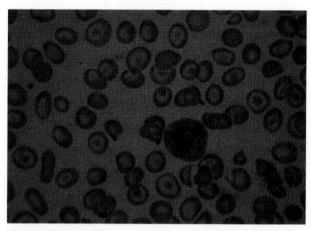

Figure 18–13 Cells from a patient with homozygous hemoglobin EE. Microcytosis is apparent compared with normal polymorphonuclear neutrophil.

sis. The reticulocyte count is normal. The blood film shows few to many target cells, irregularly contracted red cells, microcytosis, and hypochromia. The bone marrow has normocellularity or mild erythroid hyperplasia. Heinz bodies can be seen following drug therapy with an oxidant.

Treatment and Prognosis

No therapy is required because the patient's health is usually not affected. However, some patients may become fatigued and have an enlarged spleen.

Genetic counseling is recommended and HbE gene should be recognized as a mild thalassemia allele.[34]

Hemoglobin O-Arab[9, 15, 25]

Hemoglobin O-Arab ($\alpha_2\beta_2^{121\text{Glu}\rightarrow\text{Lys}}$) is a beta chain variant caused by the substitution of lysine for glutamic acid in the 121st amino position. It is a rare disorder found in Kenya, Israel, Egypt, and Bulgaria and in 0.4% of American blacks.

Clinical Features

No clinical symptoms are exhibited by individuals affected with this variant, except for a mild splenomegaly in homozygotes. When HbO-Arab is inherited with HbS, severe clinical conditions similar to those in HbSS result.

Laboratory Diagnosis

The peripheral smear of homozygous individuals demonstrates a mild hemolytic anemia with many target cells. Because HbO-Arab migrates with hemoglobins A_2, C, and E on cellulose acetate, citrate agar at an acid pH is required for differentiation. HbO-Arab is the only hemoglobin to move just slightly away from the point of application toward the cathode on citrate agar at an acid pH.

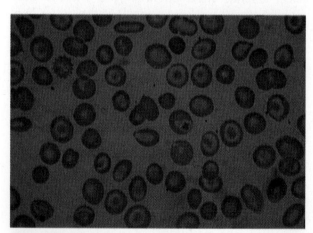

Figure 18–12 Cells from a patient with homozygous hemoglobin EE, demonstrating microcytes and target cells.

Treatment and Prognosis

No treatment is described for individuals affected with HbO-Arab.

Interaction of Hemoglobin S with Other Hemoglobin Variants[36-39]

In the double heterozygous state of beta hemoglobins where a different abnormal beta chain is inherited from each parent, the interaction of hemoglobins C, D, and O with HbS may occur. These interactions may produce hemolytic anemia of variable severity. Interactions with other hemoglobins such as HbE and Korle Bu cause disorders of no clinical consequence.

HEMOGLOBIN SC

Hemoglobin SC is a double heterozygous syndrome, which results from a structural defect in the hemoglobin molecule, wherein different amino acid substitutions are found on each of two beta-globin chains. Both abnormalities occur in the sixth position of the globin chain. In this substitution, glutamic acid is replaced by valine in HbS and lysine in HbC.

The frequency ranges to 25% in West Africa. The incidence in the United States is approximately 1 in 833 births.[40]

Clinical Features

The resulting disease is a mild, chronic hemolytic anemia associated with variable degrees of vaso-occlusive complications. Moderate splenomegaly is present in most patients. Unlike sickle cell disease, significant symptoms of HbSC usually do not occur until teenage years. The clinical symptoms are also milder and the complications much fewer.

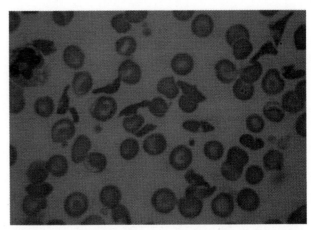

Figure 18-15 Cells from the peripheral blood of a patient with hemoglobin SC. Several sickle-like cells and target cells are evident.

Laboratory Diagnosis

The hemoglobin level is usually 11 to 13 g/dL and the reticulocyte count is 3 to 5%. HbF is normal. The peripheral smear has a few sickle cells, target cells, and intra-erythrocytic free crystalline structures. Crystalline aggregates of hemoglobin form in some cells where they protrude from the membrane[39] (Figs. 18-14 to 18-17). These have been denoted as HbSC crystals. The solubility test is positive. Electrophoretically, HbC and HbS migrate in almost equal amounts on cellulose acetate. HbC is confirmed on citrate agar at an acid pH, where it is separated from hemoglobins S, E, and O.

Hemoglobin A_2 migrates with HbC and its quantitation is of no consequence in HbSC. Determination of HbA_2 becomes vital, however, if a patient is suspected of having HbC concurrent with beta thalassemia. Beta thalassemia is discussed in detail in the thalassemia section later in this chapter.

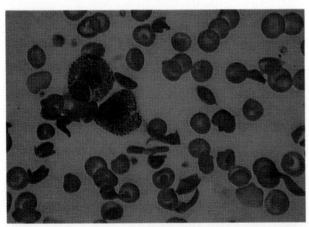

Figure 18-14 Cells from the peripheral blood of a patient with hemoglobin SC. Crystals protruding from the membrane are evident (*upper center and middle left*).

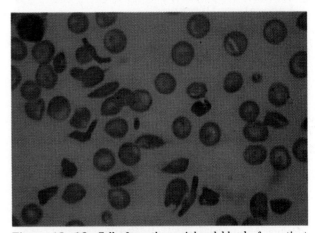

Figure 18-16 Cells from the peripheral blood of a patient with hemoglobin SC. One small hemoglobin C crystal is at the center. One stretched-out red blood cell with a hemoglobin concentration at each end is seen at the bottom center.

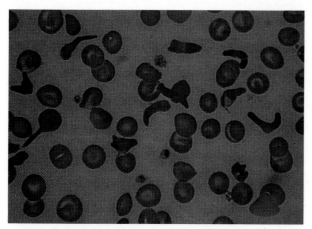

Figure 18–17 Cells from the peripheral blood of a patient with hemoglobin SC. Some cells appear to be both sickled and to contain a hemoglobin C crystal.

Treatment and Prognosis[32]

Therapy similar to that in sickle cell disease is applied to individuals with HbSC disorder. To prevent acidosis during childbirth, affected persons receive sodium bicarbonate. After childbirth, the mother might receive magnesium sulfate if thrombosis develops.

HEMOGLOBIN SD/SG-PHILADELPHIA[15, 32]

Both hemoglobins SD and SG-Philadelphia are double heterozygous syndromes. HbSG-Philadelphia is asymptomatic.

Clinical Features

HbSD syndrome, on the other hand, may cause a mild to severe hemolytic anemia. Some patients may have severe vaso-occlusive complications. The D hemoglobin syndrome in American blacks is usually due to the interaction of HbS with HbD-Los Angeles (HbD-Punjab).

Laboratory Diagnosis

The peripheral blood smear is comparable to that of HbSS. Hemoglobin S is separated on citrate agar from HbD and HbG. The clinical picture is of value to differentiate HbSD and HbSG.

Treatment and Diagnosis

The treatment is similar to that used in patients with sickle cell disease and is administered according to the severity of the clinical implications.

HEMOGLOBIN SO-ARAB[9, 15, 32]

Clinical Features

This disease is a rare double heterozygous hemoglobinopathy that causes severe chronic hemolytic anemia with vaso-occlusive episodes.

Laboratory Diagnosis

HbSO-Arab can be mistaken for HbSC on routine electrophoresis, but differentiation is easily made on citrate agar at acid pH. Electrophoresis at 8.6 on cellulose acetate does not differentiate HbC from HbO-Arab because they migrate together; therefore, citrate agar should be done in patients with severe symptoms who are SC suspects.

Treatment and Prognosis

Therapy for these patients is similar to that given to individuals affected with sickle cell disease.

HEMOGLOBIN S-KORLE BU[15]

Hb Korle Bu is a rare mutated hemoglobin. When inherited with HbS, it interferes with lateral contact between HbS fibers by blocking the critical receptors for β_6 valine; therefore, the double heterozygote, HbS-Korle Bu, is asymptomatic.

HEMOGLOBIN SC-HARLEM

Another double heterozygous hemoglobin is SC-Harlem. Hemoglobin C-Harlem has two substitutions on the beta chain: the sickle mutation and the Korle Bu mutation. Patients heterozygous for only HbC-Harlem are asymptomatic. The double heterozygous HbSC-Harlem resembles HbSS clinically. HbC-Harlem yields a positive solubility test result, migrates to the HbC position on cellulose acetate electrophoresis at an alkaline pH, and to the HbS position on acid citrate agar electrophoresis.

HEMOGLOBIN SE

Hemoglobins S and E can also be inherited as a double heterozygous hemoglobinopathy. Individuals with this inheritance pattern are asymptomatic.

Treatment and Prognosis

No treatment is required for this disorder.

Hemoglobin M[32, 41]

Hemoglobin M is caused by a structural abnormality in the globin portion of the molecule. The majority of the M hemoglobins involve a substitution of a tyrosine amino acid for either the proximal (F_8) or the distal (E_7) histidine amino acid in the alpha or beta chains. These substitutions prevent the iron in hemoglobin from being oxidized, which results in the presence of methemoglobin. Thus HbM has iron in the ferric state (Fe^{3+}) and is unable to carry oxygen. Five hemoglobin variants have been classified as M hemoglobins: HbM-Hyde Park, HbM-Boston, HbM-Iwate, HbM-Saskatoon, and HbM-Milwaukee. The hemoglobin variants are named for the locations in which they were discovered.

Clinical Features

Hemoglobin M variants have altered oxygen affinity and are inherited as autosomal dominant disorders. When HbM is exposed to certain oxidants, such as sulfonamides or phenacetin, a chocolate brown color develops. Patients appear cyanotic due to the chocolate color of circulating hemoglobin. Affected persons have 30–50% methemoglobin.

Laboratory Diagnosis

The blood sample is usually brown. Heinz bodies may be seen on wet preparations because methemoglobin causes globin chains to precipitate. All hemoglobin should be converted to methemoglobin by adding potassium cyanide before electrophoresis, so that any migration differences observed are due to an amino acid substitution instead of to differences in iron states. On cellulose acetate, HbM migrates slightly slower than HbA. The electrophoresis should be performed at a pH of 7.1.

Diagnosis is made by use of spectral absorption of hemolysate or by hemoglobin electrophoresis. The absorption spectrum peaks are determined at various wavelengths. The unique absorption range of each HbM variant is identified when these are compared with the spectrum of normal blood. Further confirmation with amino acid chain studies must be done.

Treatment and Prognosis

No treatment is necessary. Diagnosis is essential to prevent inappropriate treatment to the patient for other ailments such as cyanotic heart disease.

Unstable Hemoglobin Variants[32, 42]

Over 100 variants of unstable hemoglobins exist. Most of these are beta-chain variants and the others are alpha-chain variants. Most unstable hemoglobin variants have no clinical significance, although the majority have an increased oxygen affinity. About 25% of unstable hemoglobins are responsible for hemolytic anemia, varying from compensated mild anemia to severe hemolytic episodes.

At one time the anemia was referred to as congenital non-spherocytic hemolytic anemia (CNSHA) or congenital Heinz body anemia. The syndrome appears at or just after birth depending on the alpha or beta chains involved. The syndrome is inherited as an autosomal dominant pattern. All patients are heterozygous for the disorder; the homozygous condition is apparently incompatible with life.

The instability of the hemoglobin molecule can be caused by several things: (1) substitution in the interior of the molecule of the polar for non-polar amino acids, (2) substitution around the heme pocket, (3) substitution of the alpha and beta chains at the contact point, (4) replacement with proline, and (5) deletion or elongation of the primary structure.

Clinical Features

The unstable hemoglobin disorder is usually detected in early childhood in patients with hemolytic anemia concurrent with jaundice and splenomegaly. Elevated fever or ingestion of an oxidant exacerbates the hemolysis. The severity of the anemia depends on the degree of stability of the hemoglobin molecule. The unstable hemoglobin precipitates in vivo and in vitro because of exposure factors that do not affect normal hemoglobin, e.g., drug ingestion and exposure to heat or cold.

Because of the large degree of instability in these hemoglobins, the extent of hemolysis varies greatly. In some unstable hemoglobins, such as Hb Zurich, an oxidant is required for any significant degree of hemolysis to occur.

Laboratory Diagnosis

The hemoglobin precipitates in the red blood cell as Heinz bodies. The precipitated hemoglobin attaches to the cell membrane, thus decreasing its flexibility and shortening its survival. The oxygen affinity of these cells is abnormal.

The red blood cell morphology is somewhat variable. It may be normal or demonstrate slight hypochromia and prominent basophilic stippling, which is possibly caused by excessive clumping of ribosomes. Heinz bodies can be demonstrated by using a supravital stain. After splenectomy Heinz bodies are more numerous and larger. Many patients excrete dark urine that contains dipyrrole.

Many of the unstable hemoglobins migrate in the normal AA pattern and so are not detected by electrophoresis. Other tests used to detect unstable hemoglobins include the isopropanol precipitation test, which is based on the principle that an isopropanol solution at 37 °C weakens the bonding forces of the hemoglobin molecule. If unstable hemoglobins are present, rapid precipitation occurs in 5 minutes and heavy flocculation occurs after 20 minutes. Normal hemoglobin does not begin to precipitate until approximately 40 minutes. The heat denaturation test can also be used. In this test, many unstable hemoglobins are heat sensitive, and the appearance of a flocculent precipitate occurs within 1 hour when incubated at 50°C. Normal blood shows little or no precipitation. The Heinz body staining technique reveals significant numbers of Heinz bodies when incubated with supravital stain. This is especially true after splenectomy, but even the blood of persons with spleens who have unstable hemoglobins forms more Heinz bodies with longer incubation and the addition of oxidative substances such as acetylphenylhydrazine than does the blood of those with normal hemoglobin.

Treatment and Prognosis

Patients are treated to prevent hemolytic crises. In certain cases, the spleen must be removed to reduce hemolysis. Because unstable hemoglobins are rare, prognosis in these affected individuals is not clear.

Hemoglobin with Increased and Decreased Oxygen Affinity[32, 43]

The transition of the three-dimensional conformation that accompanies the addition and removal of oxygen determines the functional behavior of normal hemoglobin. When normal hemoglobin is fully deoxygenated (tense state), it has low affinity for oxygen and other heme ligands and high affinity for allosteric effectors, such as Bohr protons and 2,3-DPG. In the oxygenated (relaxed state), hemoglobin has a high affinity for heme ligands, such as oxygen, and a low affinity for Bohr protons and 2,3-DPG. The transition from the tense to the relaxed state involves a series of structural changes that have a marked effect on hemoglobin function. If an amino acid substitution lowers the stability of the tense structure, the transition to the relaxed state occurs at an earlier stage in ligation, and the hemoglobin will have increased oxygen affinity and decreased heme-heme intensity (see Chapter 9). Some examples of these beta-chain hemoglobin variants are Hb Chesapeake and Hb Kempsey. These hemoglobins have amino acid substitutions at sites crucial to hemoglobin function.

HEMOGLOBINS WITH INCREASED OXYGEN AFFINITY

The high affinity variants, like other structurally abnormal hemoglobins, are inherited as through autosomal dominance. Affected persons have equal volumes of HbA and the abnormal variant. Exceptions to this are double heterozygotes for Hb Abruzzo and beta thalassemia and for Hb Crete and beta thalassemia, in which abnormal Hb is greater than 85%.

Approximately 50 variant hemoglobins with high oxygen affinity have been discovered. Such hemoglobins produce increased erythropoietin; affected patients have compensatory erythrocytosis. These variants differ from unstable hemoglobin, which may also have abnormal oxygen affinity, in that they do not have any hemolysis or abnormal red cell morphology.

Clinical Features

Most individuals are asymptomatic and present with no physical symptoms except a ruddy complexion. Erythrocytosis is usually detected during routine examination because the patient generally has high red blood cell count, and high hemoglobin and hematocrit test results.

Laboratory Diagnosis

The white blood cell count, platelet count, and peripheral smear are generally normal. The hemoglobin electrophoresis may establish a diagnosis. An abnormal band that separates from the A band is present on cellulose acetate in some variants; therefore, if a band is not found, the diagnosis of increased oxygen affinity is not ruled out. Some cases can be separated by using citrate agar (pH of 6.0) or by gel electrofocusing.

Treatment and Prognosis

Patients with high oxygen affinity live normal lives and require no treatment. Diagnosis should be made to avoid unnecessary treatment of the erythrocytosis as a myeloproliferative disorder or a secondary erythrocytosis.

HEMOGLOBIN WITH DECREASED OXYGEN AFFINITY

Several hemoglobins with decreased oxygen affinity that quickly releases oxygen to tissue, resulting in normal to decreased hemoglobin concentration and slight anemia, have been identified. The best known is Hb Kansas, which has an amino acid substitution of asparagine by threonine at the 102nd position of the beta chain. Other patients are anemic because of the increased release of oxygen resulting from the decreased oxygen affinity. These hemoglobins may be present when cyanosis and a normal arterial oxygen tension are present together, and most may be detected by starch gel electrophoresis.

THALASSEMIAS

Definition, History, and Etiology

Cooley and Lee first described a severe form of anemia associated with splenomegaly and bone

Table 18-4. NORMAL PERCENTAGES OF HEMOGLOBINS IN ADULTS	
HbA ($\alpha_2\beta_2$)	95–97%
HbA$_2$ ($\alpha_2\delta_2$)	2–3%
HbF ($\alpha_2\gamma_2$)	2%

changes occurring in young children.[44] The condition was later named thalassemia (*thalassa* is Greek for *sea*) because the first cases were in individuals whose ancestors traced to the lands bordering the Mediterranean. During the 1940s, the true genetic character of this disorder became known. The disease described by Cooley and Lee is the homozygous state for the abnormal autosomal gene for beta-globin chain synthesis that has become known as thalassemia major. The heterozygous state associated with much milder hematologic changes is known as thalassemia minor.[45]

The thalassemias are a heterogeneous group of hereditary anemias caused by absent or defective synthesis of one or more of the polypeptide chains of globin for hemoglobin. The milder mostly heterozygous forms are the most frequent genetic defect in humans, whereas the more severe forms can cause significant morbidity and mortality. Thalassemia is not a single disease but a group of disorders that can be defined as a condition in which a reduction in the rate of synthesis of one or more of the globin chains leads to imbalanced globin chain synthesis, defective hemoglobin production, and

damage to the red blood cells or their precursors by the build-up of the globin chain that is produced in excess.[46, 47] Usually the synthesis of either the alpha or beta chains of HbA ($\alpha_2\beta_2$) is impaired; the thalassemias are named according to the chain with reduced or absent synthesis.

Genetic Control of Hemoglobin Synthesis

The normal hemoglobin molecule is a tetramer (double dimer) of two alpha-like chains (either α or ζ) with two beta-like chains (either β, γ, δ, or ϵ). Combination of these chains produce six normal hemoglobins. Three are embryonic hemoglobins: Hb Gower-1 ($\zeta_2\epsilon_2$), Hb Gower-2 ($\alpha_2\epsilon_2$), and Hb Portland ($\zeta_2\gamma_2$). The others are fetal hemoglobin: HbF ($\alpha_2\gamma_2$), and two adult hemoglobins: HbA ($\alpha_2\beta_2$), and HbA$_2$ ($\alpha_2\delta_2$)[4] (Fig. 18–18). By the tenth week of gestation, zeta and epsilon chain production ceases and gamma chain synthesis begins, which combines with alpha chains to make HbF, the predominant Hb of fetal life. After birth, gamma chain synthesis decreases and beta chains are the predominant chain produced. This transition from gamma chain to beta chain is called the gamma-to-beta switch.[47] (see Fig. 9–3 and Table 18–4 for a representation of the normal percentages of each hemoglobin after the first year of life.) The alpha genes are located on the short arm of chromosome 16 and the cluster of beta-like genes is broadly distributed on the short arm of chromo-

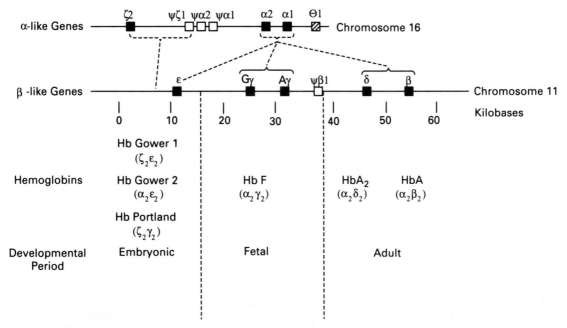

Figure 18–18 Chromosome organization of globin genes and their expression during development. The solid boxes indicate functional globin genes; the open boxes indicate pseudogenes. The scale of the depicted chromosomal segments is in kilobases (kb) of DNA. The switch from embryonic to fetal hemoglobin occurs between 6 and 10 weeks of gestation, and the switch from fetal to adult hemoglobin occurs at approximately the time of birth. (From Nathan DG, Oski FA [eds]: Hematology of Infancy and Childhood, 4th ed. Philadelphia: WB Saunders, 1993.)

some 11. The cluster contains five functional genes (ζ, $^G\gamma$, $^A\gamma$, δ, and β), which are arranged on the chromosome with an order that corresponds to their developmental stage of expression. Two peptides that differ by a single amino acid (glycine or alanine) are coded for by the gamma genes and are designated as $^G\gamma$ and $^A\gamma$. The alpha gene loci are duplicated on each chromosome 16 and are denoted as $\alpha 1$ and $\alpha 2$. Interspersed between the functional genes on these chromosomes are four functionless gene-like loci or pseudogenes that are designated by the prefixed symbol ψ. The organization of these genes on chromosomes 16 and 11 and the hemoglobins produced are shown in Figure 18–18.

Categories of Thalassemia

The thalassemias are divided into beta thalassemias, which include all the disorders of reduced globin chains affecting the beta cluster of genes on chromosome 11, and alpha thalassemias, which involve the $\alpha 1$ and $\alpha 2$ loci on chromosome 16. Various deletion and nondeletion defects can cause each of these disorders. Even those that appear the same clinically are heterogeneous at the genetic level. The beta thalassemias affect mainly the beta chain production but also may involve the δ, $^A\gamma$, $^G\gamma$, and ϵ chains. Included in this group is β^0 thalassemia, in which no beta chains are produced from the beta gene locus on one chromosome 11, and β^+ thalassemia, in which the production is reduced but present. In addition β^{++} (β^+s) thalassemia has been designated for the defect in which the deficiency of the beta chain production is very mild. The $(\delta\beta)^0$ thalassemias are those where no delta or beta chains are produced. In the homozygous state these are included in the heterogeneous hereditary persistence of fetal hemoglobin (HPFH) thalassemic disorders. Alpha thalassemia involves either the $\alpha 1$ or the $\alpha 2$ gene on chromosome 16 (α^+ thalassemia), or both the $\alpha 1$ and the $\alpha 2$ gene on chromosome 16 (α^0 thalassemia).[46] These are summarized in Table 18–5.

Geographic Distribution

Even though thalassemias are found all over the world, certain forms occur with higher frequencies in certain populations.[48, 49] Beta thalassemia is more common in populations from Mediterranean regions, such as those from southern Italy and Greece where 5 to 10% of the population is heterozygous for beta thalassemia. It also occurs in the Middle East, parts of India, Pakistan, and throughout Southeast Asia. It is less common in Africa but does exist in isolated pockets. Alpha

Table 18-5. THE MAIN GROUPS OF THALASSEMIAS

β Thalassemia and Related Disorders

β^0 (NO β CHAINS PRODUCED)

Deletion
Nondeletion

β^+ (10-50% OF NORMAL β CHAINS PRODUCED)

High HbA$_2$
Normal HbA$_2$
Normal HbA$_2$; High HbF

β^+(β^{+s}) (SMALL REDUCTION IN β CHAIN PRODUCTION; NEARLY NORMAL α to β CHAIN RATIO)

Normal HbA$_2$

$\delta\beta$ Thalassemia

$\delta\beta^0$	(No β or δ chains produced; only $^A\gamma$ and $^G\gamma$ chains produced from the β cluster)
$(^A\gamma\delta\beta)^0$	(Only $^G\gamma$ chains produced from the beta gene cluster)
Hb Lepore(s)	(Non-α chain composed of the first 50 to 80 amino acids residues of the δ chain and the last 60 to 90 of the C-terminal β chain)

Hereditary Persistence of Fetal Hemoglobin: High HbF in Adults

DELETION

($\delta\beta$)

NONDELETION

Linked to the β-globin gene cluster
$^G\gamma\beta^+$, $^A\gamma\beta^+$
Unlinked to β-globin gene cluster

α Thalassemia

α^0 (α-thal-1)	(no globin is produced from the α gene complex)
Deletion	(both chromosomes from the α gene complex; – –)
α^+ (α-thal-2)	(decreased production of the α chains from α gene complex)
Deletion	(one chromosome from the α gene complex; –α)
Nondeletion (nonfunctional α gene; $\alpha\alpha^T$)	
α globin structural variants	

thalassemia is more common in Thailand, China, the Philippines, and other Asian countries. In Thailand, the gene frequency for various forms of alpha thalassemia reaches 25%. It also occurs widely throughout Africa. The distribution of thalassemia seems to follow a belt along the tropics where malaria is prevalent[47] (see Fig. 18–2). Even in these areas the prevalence of the gene is higher at lower altitudes where there is greater risk of malaria than in the mountains where malaria is rarely present.[50] It has been suggested that the frequency of thalassemia in these areas might be because of the selective advantage of heterozygous thalassemias that enhance resistance to malaria.[51] Despite much research it has not been possible to define the mechanism whereby thalassemic red blood cells might provide protection from malaria.

Pathophysiology

The pathophysiology of all the thalassemias is almost entirely due to the imbalance of globin chain synthesis.[45-48] In beta thalassemia, this results in a lack of hemoglobin produced in the erythroid precursors, and therefore small, hypochromic, red blood cells are present. More important, however, are the excess unpaired globin chains, which precipitate in the developing cells, causing damage to the surface membranes in both developing and mature blood cells, which can cause ineffective erythropoiesis (cells being destroyed in the bone marrow) or premature hemolysis of peripheral red blood cells by removal by the macrophages. In alpha thalassemia non–alpha-chain production has quite different consequences. Because the alpha chains are shared by both fetal and adult hemoglobins, defective alpha-chain production produces excess chain production in both fetal and adult life. In the fetus there is excess gamma-chain production, which produces γ_4 tetramers or Hb Bart's, and in the adult there is an excess of beta-chain production, which produces the β_4 tetramers of HbH. Because these tetramers are soluble, they do not precipitate to any significant degree in the marrow and therefore do not cause severe ineffective erythropoiesis. These tetramers do precipitate as the mature red blood cells age in the blood and form inclusion bodies (Heinz-like bodies). The spleen removes these cells with inclusions and a hemolytic process generally develops. The red blood cells are also microcytic, and hypochromic due to the lack of hemoglobin synthesis. Both HbH and Hb Bart's have a very high affinity for O_2 and therefore are ineffective oxygen carriers.

Genetic Defects Causing Thalassemia

Applying recombinant DNA technology to the study of the globin producing genes has revealed many different types of defects at the molecular level.[48, 52] Among the types of genetic defects that cause a decrease of a particular globin chain and therefore thalassemia are the following:

- a point mutation in the noncoding part of the gene that produces inefficient splicing from pre-mRNA to mRNA (messenger RNA) causing the amount of mRNA to be decreased
- a mutation in the promoter area decreasing the rate of expression of the gene
- a partial or total deletion of a globin gene
- a mutation at the end of a gene that causes a lengthening of the amino acids or
- a nonsense mutation leading to early termination of the globin synthesis[51] (Fig. 18–19)

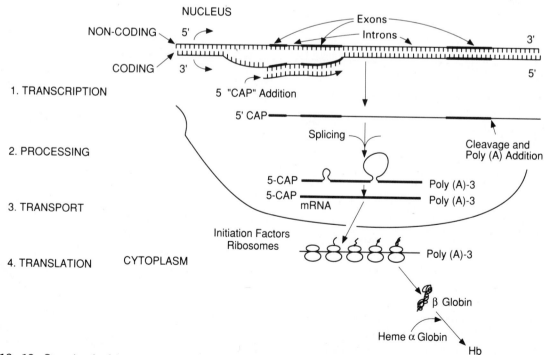

Figure 18–19 Steps involved in gene expression include gene transcription, RNA processing, nuclear-to-cytoplasmic RNA transport, and translation of mRNA into protein. (From Nienhuis AW, Maniatis T: Structure and expression of globin genes in erythroid cells. *In* Stamatoyannopoulos G, Nienhuis AW, Majerus PW, Varmus F [eds]: The Molecular Basis of Blood Diseases. Philadelphia: WB Saunders, 1987.)

All of these genetic defects cause a decrease or lack of synthesis of one globin chain, which causes the thalassemia syndromes.

Beta, Delta Beta, and Gamma Delta Beta Thalassemias

Using recombinant DNA technology to study the molecular pathology of the beta thalassemias has determined that the disorder is heterogeneous.[45-47, 52] Over 50 different mutations have been found in association with the beta thalassemia phenotype including both deletions and nondeletions that affect the transcription, processing, and translation of messenger RNA (see Fig. 18–19). The most common genetic defect in β^0 thalassemia, wherein no beta chains are synthesized, is the production of nonfunctional mRNA, which results from a point mutation within the beta gene and prevents the translation of the globin chain. In β^+ thalassemias, wherein the beta chain synthesis is reduced, other point mutations occur that affect the processing step of globin mRNA (pre-mRNA) which results in unstable mRNA. Altogether there are over 30 point mutations causing beta-thalassemia, which are single base substitutions (or occasionally small insertions or deletions within the beta-globin gene). Of these many forms of beta thalassemia identified at the level of DNA mutation, only about 10 to 15 variants account for the vast majority of patients affected. Within a single ethnic or geographic area, a much smaller number are responsible for the disorder. This has made prenatal testing for homozygous thalassemia easier by DNA hybridization methods. Deletions of entire genes are rare in beta thalassemia as opposed to alpha thalassemia.

CLINICAL SYNDROMES OF BETA THALASSEMIA

Historically, beta thalassemia has been divided into three clinical syndromes: beta thalassemia minor (heterozygous), a mild microcytic, hypochromic hemolytic anemia; beta thalassemia major (homozygous), a severe transfusion-dependent anemia; and beta thalassemia intermedia with symptoms of severity between the other two.[45-47, 53] Recently a fourth syndrome designated as a silent carrier has been described (Table 18–6). Because there are only two loci for the beta gene, these syndromes can be explained not by the number of genes but by the interaction of specific mutations that variably affect beta-globin gene expression. A good portion of the mutations cause the beta gene not to be expressed at all (designated as the β^0 gene), whereas others cause a variable decrease in production of the beta chain (designated as the β^+ gene).[53] The amount of production by the various β^+ genes also varies, ranging from 10–50% of normal beta-chain synthesis. Genes that produce over 50% have been associated with the beta thalassemia silent carrier (β^{++} [β^{+s}] thalassemia).

Table 18–6. CLINICAL SYNDROMES OF BETA-THALASSEMIAS

Genotype	HbA	A₂	F	Lepore
NORMAL (NORMAL HEMATOLOGIC PARAMETERS)				
$\beta\beta$	nl	nl	nl	—
SILENT CARRIER (USUALLY NORMAL)				
β^{++s} thalassemia (β^{++s}/β)	nl	nl	nl	—
THALASSEMIA MINOR (MILD HEMOLYTIC ANEMIA, MICROCYTIC, HYPOCHROMIC)				
β^+ thalassemia (β^+/β)	↓	↑	nl to sl ↑	—
β^0 thalassemia (β^0/β)	↓	↑	nl to sl ↑	—
$\delta\beta^0$ thalassemia ($\delta\beta^0/\delta\beta$)	↓	↓	5–20%	—
Hb Lepore thalassemia (Hb Lepore/β)	↓	↓	↑	5–15%
THALASSEMIA MAJOR (SEVERE TRANSFUSION-DEPENDENT HEMOLYTIC ANEMIA; MICROCYTIC, HYPOCHROMIC)				
β^+ thalassemia				
β^+/β^+	↓↓	v	↑	—
β^+/β^0	↓↓↓↓	v	nl to ↑	—
β^0 thalassemia ($\beta^0\beta^0$)	—	v	75%	—
Hb Lepore (Hb Lepore/Hb Lepore)	—	—		25%
THALASSEMIA INTERMEDIA (MODERATE HEMOLYTIC ANEMIA WITH FEW TRANSFUSION REQUIREMENTS; MICROCYTIC, HYPOCHROMIC)				
Homozygous				
β^{+s} thalassemia (β^{+s}/β^{+s})	↓	↓	↑	—
$\delta\beta^0$ thalassemia ($\delta\beta^0/\delta\beta^0$)	—	—	100%	—

Abbreviations: nl = normal; sl = slight; v = variable; usually thalassemia major depends on how many beta chains are produced.

Silent Carrier State of Beta Thalassemia

The silent carriers are the various heterogeneous beta mutations that produce only a small decrease in production of the beta chains and that result in a nearly normal alpha/beta chain ratio and no hematologic abnormalities. The silent carrier state was recognized through a study of families in which affected children had a more severe beta thalassemia syndrome than a parent with the typical beta thalassemia trait.[45, 52, 54] These silent carriers when studied often revealed a slight impairment in beta-chain synthesis on radiolabeling of the globin chains in peripheral blood reticulocytes. Sometimes the red blood cell sizing revealed a very slight microcytosis.[54] These individuals have normal levels of HbA$_2$. Several patients who are homozygous for the silent carrier thalassemia gene have been described.[45, 47, 54] They have a moderate microcytic, hypochromic anemia with a hemoglobin level in the range of 6–7 g/dL. The HbF values range from 10–15% and the HbA$_2$ level is elevated to the range which is normally seen in individuals with thalassemia trait.

Beta Thalassemia Minor

Beta thalassemia minor is caused by the heterozygous mutations that affect the beta-globin synthesis. It usually presents as a mild, asymptomatic, hemolytic anemia.[45-47] One beta gene is affected by a mutation that decreases or abolishes its function, whereas the other beta gene is normal. The peripheral blood count reveals a hemoglobin level in the 10–13 g/dL range and the red blood cell count is normal or slightly elevated. The anemia is microcytic and hypochromic with the patient usually showing some degree of poikilocytosis, including target cells and elliptocytes. An increased number of stippled red blood cells may be seen on the Wright-Giemsa stained smear. (Fig. 18–20). Tests on bone marrow reveal mild to moderate erythroid hyperplasia, with slight ineffective erythropoiesis. Hepatomegaly and splenomegaly are seen in a small percentage of patients. The most common beta thalassemia syndromes characteristically have a high HbA$_2$ level which can vary from 3.5–8.0%. HbF levels usually range from 1–5%. Less common variants of beta thalassemia traits exist; one has a HbA$_2$ level elevated as just described but with the HbF in the 5–20% range.[55] This form may result from a deletion of the beta-globin gene that leaves both the delta and gamma genes intact. Another variant has the same red blood cell conditions as above but has a normal HbA$_2$ level. This phenotype is thought to represent the inheritance of two mutations, one that decreases beta-globin chain production and the other that decreases delta-globin chain production.[56]

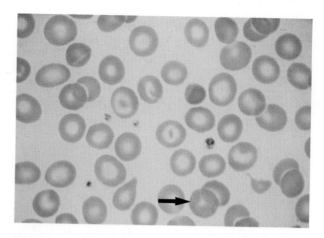

Figure 18–20 Red blood cells from a patient with beta thalassemia minor, demonstrating microcytic, hypochromic red blood cells with target cells, other poikilocytes, and a stippled red blood cell (*arrow*).

Beta Thalassemia Major

Beta thalassemia major is characterized by a severe anemia first detected in early childhood as the gamma to beta switch takes place.[45-48] Patients with severe beta thalassemia are usually diagnosed between 6 months and 2 years of age. As the child matures, if not treated by hypertransfusion, increasing hepatosplenomegaly occurs along with jaundice and marked bone changes due to an expanded marrow cavity caused by extreme erythroid hyperplasia. Radiography demonstrates the typical "hair on end" appearance (Fig. 18–21). The long bones may become rarefied from marrow expansion and are subject to pathologic fracture. A typical facies results with prominence of the forehead, cheekbones, and upper jaw (Fig. 18–22). Physical growth and development are delayed. The hemoglobin level falls very low to 3 or 4 g/dL. The red blood cells are markedly hypochromic with extreme poikilocytosis such as target cells, teardrop cells, and elliptocytes. There are also both stippled and many nucleated red blood cells on the blood smear (Fig. 18–23). The MCV is in the range of 50 to 60 fL. A characteristic red blood cell finding is enlarged, and very thin, often wrinkled and folded cells containing clumps of hemoglobin. A reticulocyte count of 2–8% is noted which is low in relationship to the amount of red blood cell hyperplasia and hemolysis present. This is probably explained by the intramedullary destruction (ineffective erythropoiesis) due to the excess alpha-chain production. Electrophoresis shows most of the hemoglobin present is HbF with a slightly increased HbA$_2$. Hemoglobin F is shown to be heterogeneously distributed among the red blood cells by the acid elution technique. The bone marrow shows marked erythroid hyperplasia with a erythroid:myeloid (E:M) ratio of approximately 20:1

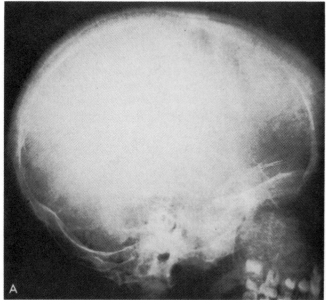

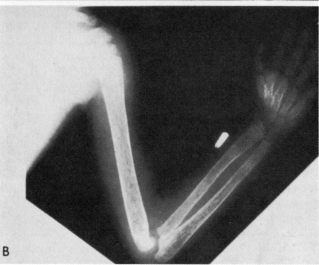

Figure 18–21 Bone changes in severe beta thalassemia major. *A,* Skull radiograph. (From Beck WS [ed]: Hematology, 2nd ed. Boston: MIT Press, 1976.) *B,* Radiograph of forearm and hand. (From Nathan DG: Thalassemia. N Engl J Med 1972; 286:586.)

(M:E ratio of 0.05:1). HbA is present only if a β^+ gene is present. The prognosis of untreated beta thalassemia major is usually grave. In early studies performed before therapy existed, death usually occurred in infancy or early childhood.

Transfusions are necessary to prevent early death and are usually initiated in the first year of life in the United States.[47, 57] Until 15 years ago, transfusions were given only when symptoms of severe anemia (fatigue, weakness, and irritability) occurred because of the fear of the consequences of transfusion-induced hemosiderosis. The children still had extreme hypertrophy of erythroid marrow due to the hemolysis and severe anemia. Life expectancy was below 20 years. Beginning in about 1975, it became the practice to give regular transfusions to prevent the anemia and bone changes.

The hemoglobin level is usually maintained above 9 to 10 g/dL. These transfusion regimens are termed *hypertransfusion.* Growth patterns become normal and excessive erythropoiesis is effectively, although partially, suppressed as the number of reticulocytes and nucleated red blood cells decrease. Enlargement of the liver and spleen (hepatosplenomegaly) does not occur. As the children are transfused, an excessive iron burden and transfusional hemosiderosis occur, resulting in parenchymal organ toxicity and becoming the basis of morbidity and mortality in thalassemia major.[58] Without iron chelation, cardiac disease due to cardiac hemosiderosis will end the life of a transfused thalassemia patient during the teenage years.

There is no physiologic way to induce significant excretion of iron. Several drugs with chelating properties have been tried and deferoxamine (DFO) has been found the most effective. DFO is used in daily 10- to 12-hour subcutaneous injections of about 30–40 mg/kg with the use of a small battery-driven pump. The results are very encouraging in children begun on chelation therapy before 8 to 10 years of age. The onset of cardiac disease may be prevented and the life expectancy may increase to the fourth decade. Bone marrow transplantation has been successful, but must still be considered highly experimental because it involves mortality rates of 10–25%.[62] Thalassemia has also been treated with drugs that cause the gamma gene to switch on so that the patients' red blood cells contain higher levels of HbF.[63] In the future, thalassemia may be treated by gene replacement.[64]

Thalassemia Intermedia

Thalassemia intermedia is a term used to describe patients who are able to maintain a minimum hemoglobin of approximately 7 g/dL or greater without transfusion.[45–47] Their imbalance in the alpha- and beta-chain synthesis falls between that observed in the thalassemia trait and thalassemia major, and, thus, their general clinical phenotype falls between the extremes of transfusion-dependent thalassemia major and asymptomatic trait. Patients with thalassemia intermedia may be homozygous for mutations that cause a mild decrease in beta-globin expression, or they may be doubly heterozygous for these mild mutations and a mutation that causes a more significant reduction in beta-globin expression.[65] (Table 18–7). Coinheritance of alpha thalassemia may permit homozygotes for more severe beta thalassemia mutation to remain transfusion independent because the alpha/beta–chain ratio is more even.[66] An enhanced capacity for gamma-globin chain production, from a nondeletion or deletion mecha-

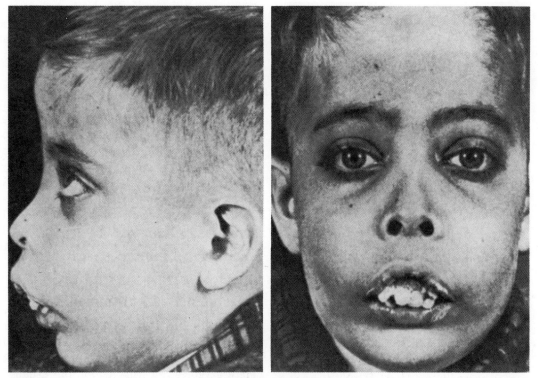

Figure 18–22 Typical facial appearance of a child with untreated homozygous beta thalassemia major. (From Jurkiewicz MJ, Pearson HA, Furlow LT Jr: Reconstruction of the maxilla in thalassemia. Ann N Y Acad Sci 1972; 165:586–594.)

nism, with a resulting increase of HbF, will give the thalassemia intermedia picture. (See the sections discussing delta beta thalassemia and HPFH.) The deletion forms of delta beta thalassemia fall into this category, and individuals homozygous for these mutations, or compound heterozygotes for delta beta thalassemia and a beta-thalassemia mutation, have thalassemia intermedia. Co-inheritance of a triplicated alpha-globin locus ($\alpha\alpha\alpha$) (see alpha thalassemia) is also a cause of thalassemia intermedia in individuals heterozygous for beta thalassemia.[67]

The red blood cell morphology of thalassemia intermedia is similar to that previously described for thalassemia major. Electrophoresis may reveal 20–100% HbF, up to 7% HbA$_2$, and 0–80% HbA depending on the exact phenotype of the individual.[47] The HbF is heterogeneously distributed among the circulating cells. The clinical course is variable from those that have mild disease, despite moderately severe anemia (especially among the black population), to those with severe exercise intolerance and pathologic fractures.[47] Patients with thalassemia intermedia may also suffer from prob-

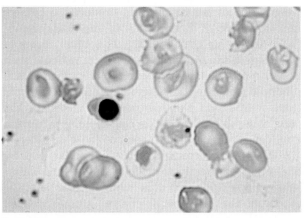

A

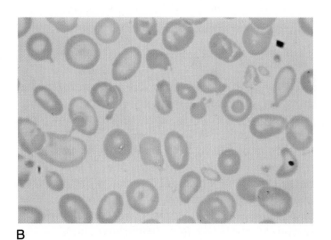

B

Figure 18–23 Red blood cells from a patient with beta thalassemia major. (Reprinted with permission from the American Society for Hematology slide bank.)

Table 18-7. GENOTYPES ASSOCIATED WITH THE β-THALASSEMIA SYNDROMES

Normal
β/β

Silent Carrier
β^{++}/β ($\beta^{+}s/\beta$)

β Thalassemia Minor
β/β^{0}
β/β^{+}
$\beta/(\delta\beta)^{0}$
$\beta/(\delta\beta)^{Lepore}$

Thalassemia Major
β^{0}/β^{0}
β^{+}/β^{+} (in blacks)
β^{0}/β^{+}
$(\delta\beta)^{Lepore}/(\delta\beta)^{Lepore}$

Thalassemia Intermedia
β^{+}/β^{+}
β^{0}/β^{++}
β/β^{+} with coinheritance of α-thalassemia
$(\delta\beta)^{Lepore}/(\delta\beta)^{Lepore}$
$(\delta\beta)^{0}/(\delta\beta)^{0}$
$\beta^{0}/(\delta\beta)^{0}$
$\beta^{+}/(\delta\beta)^{0}$
$\beta^{0}/(\delta\beta)^{Lepore}$
$(\delta\beta)^{0}/(\delta\beta)^{Lepore}$
β^{0}/β with coinheritance of ($\alpha\alpha\alpha$) (α triplicated)

lems of iron overload even though they are not transfused. The markedly accelerated, though ineffective, erythropoiesis with the resulting increase in plasma iron turnover, provokes an increase in gastrointestinal iron absorption.[47] For this reason cardiac and endocrine complications present 10 to 20 years later in thalassemia intermedia patients than in patients who are regularly transfused.

Prenatal Diagnosis

Beta-thalassemia mutations can usually be detected by direct analysis of DNA obtained from the fetus by either chorionic villus biopsy or amniocentesis. The DNA is analyzed by molecular hybridization methods for the presence of thalassemia mutations.[68]

OTHER THALASSEMIAS CAUSED BY DEFECTS IN THE BETA-CLUSTER GENES: DELTA BETA THALASSEMIA

Delta beta thalassemias are a heterogeneous group of disorders due to either a deletion that removes or inactivates only the delta and beta genes, designated $(\delta\beta)^{\circ}$ in which only $^{A}\gamma$ and $^{G}\gamma$ chains are produced from the beta-gene cluster, or a deletion that also inactivates the $^{A}\gamma$ gene designated $(^{A}\gamma\delta\beta)^{\circ}$ in which only $^{G}\gamma$ chains are produced from the beta-gene cluster.[47] Heterozygous delta beta thalassemia is similar to beta thalassemia minor but with the fetal hemoglobin level in the 5–20% range distributed heterogeneously in the

red blood cells and with HbA_2 values normal or slightly reduced. The doubly heterozygous state for the high A_2 beta thalassemia gene and delta beta thalassemia gene is usually associated with clinical thalassemia intermedia (see Table 18–7). The rare homozygous state for delta beta thalassemia is clinically milder than beta thalassemia major and is also one form of thalassemia intermedia.[47] Only HbF is present; HbA and HbA_2 are not produced.[46]

Thalassemia intermedia caused by homozygous delta beta thalassemia has moderate anemia and rarely requires transfusions. Growth and development are nearly normal and even though the red blood cells may have striking thalassemic features, splenomegaly is modest.[46] No HbA or HbA_2 is found. These patients do well with 100% HbF even with its higher affinity for oxygen.

GAMMA DELTA BETA THALASSEMIA

Mutations that cause deletion of all the gamma delta beta cluster genes have been identified and are signified as gamma delta beta thalassemia. Heterozygotes for this condition usually present with transient hemolytic anemia that is microcytic and hypochromic in the perinatal period and converts to a phenotype of beta-thalassemia trait with low HbA_2 after the completion of the hemoglobin switching.[69] This diagnosis should be considered in any infant with hemolysis and microcytic, hypochromic red blood cells. Homozygosity for these mutations is presumably lethal.

HEREDITARY PERSISTENCE OF FETAL HEMOGLOBIN

Hereditary persistence of fetal hemoglobin (HPFH) is closely related to delta beta thalassemia.[70] It refers to a group of rare conditions characterized by continued synthesis of high levels of HbF in adult life in the absence of the usual clinical and hematologic features of thalassemia even when 100% of the hemoglobin produced is HbF in homozygotes.[45–48, 52] These are of very little significance except as they interact with other forms of thalassemia or structural hemoglobin variants such as sickle cell anemia. The additional gamma chains produced balances the uneven chain ratio in beta thalassemias and the increased HbF reduces the percentage of HbS in sickle cell anemia, producing a milder clinical course in each of these disorders.

HPFH is characterized at the molecular level by a deletion or inactivation of the beta- and delta-gene complex. Before detailed molecular analysis to define the differences, clinical studies divided adult individuals with high HbF into two different categories based on the morphologic difference of the distribution of HbF in the red blood cells and the amount of HbF present (Table 18–8). HPFH heterozygotes have normal size red blood cells that are fully hemoglobinized, whereas delta beta-thalassemia heterozygotes have hypochromic, microcytic cells. Many HPFH heterozygotes have up to 30% HbF with a uniform or pancellular distribution in the red blood cells, whereas delta beta-thalassemia heterozygotes have a lower HbF level and an uneven or heterocellular distribution among the red cells. Rare individuals are homozygous for HPFH and have 100% HbF. These individuals have slightly hypochromic, microcytic red cells and globin synthesis is modestly imbalanced. Homozygous delta beta–thalassemia individuals have a mild β^0-thalassemia intermedia phenotype.[47] These two clinical entities represent specific deletions that effect the multiple regulatory elements that are present within the gamma delta beta–gene cluster.

Several types of heterocellular HPFH have also been described including British, Georgia, Swiss, Atlanta, and Seattle heterocellular or, less commonly, pancellular HPFH.[71] It appears that gene promoters are present outside the cluster and a point mutation here presumably causes the gamma genes to capture the regulatory apparatus of the beta-globin cluster in adulthood with increased amount of HbF being produced and are thus classified as HPFH.

The total percentage of HbF is moderately increased in all types with individuals having HbF values ranging from only slightly elevated to over 20%, typically in a heterocellular distribution, but a few have also had a pancellular distribution.[47]

HEMOGLOBIN LEPORE AND KENYA (CROSSOVER GLOBINS)

Another rare class of delta beta thalassemias results in structural hemoglobin variants called Le-

pore that have as the non–alpha-globin chain, a delta beta fusion chain that is composed of the first 50 to 80 amino acid residues of the delta chain and the last 60 to 90 residues of the normal C-terminal amino acid sequence of the beta chain.[45-47] These have probably resulted from non-homologous crossing over between the delta locus on one chromosome and the beta locus on the complementary chromosome (Fig. 18–24). Lepore globin is synthesized in small amounts because it is under the control of the delta-globin promoter, which normally sustains transcription at only 2.5% of the level of the beta-globin gene. Heterozygotes have mainly HbA, 2–4% Hb Lepore and 3–5% HbF. Homozygotes for Hb Lepore have 90% HbF and approximately 10% Hb Lepore but neither HbA nor HbA₂. Hb anti-Lepore has also been described. Individuals with this Hb also have two normal beta-globin genes; therefore, their red blood cells do not show any thalassemic changes.

Another crossover globin, Hb Kenya, has been described that contains a non-alpha-chain composed of the N-terminal sequence of the gamma globin and the C-terminal sequence of the beta globin.[45-47] The crossover point is close to the 100th amino acid. Heterozygotes are clinically well and have approximately 10% Hb Kenya and 6 to 10% HbF of the $^G\gamma$ type.

Alpha Thalassemias

In contrast to the beta-globin cluster, in which point mutations are the most common cause of thalassemia, large deletions in the alpha-globin genes are the predominant cause of alpha thalassemia.[45-48] The degree of decreased production of the alpha chain depends on the specific mutation, the number of alpha genes affected and whether an $\alpha2$ or $\alpha1$ gene is affected. The $\alpha2$ gene appears to produce approximately 75% of the alpha-globin chains in normal red blood cells. No-

Table 18–8. HEREDITARY PERSISTENCE OF FETAL HEMOGLOBIN (HPFH)			
	HbF Distribution	RBC Morphology	Amount of Hemoglobin
HPFH (Deletion)			
Heterozygous	Pancellular	Normal	15–30%
Homozygous		Slightly hypochromic, microcytic	100%
$\delta\beta$			
Heterozygous	Heterocellular	Hypochromic, microcytic	5–15%
Homozygous		Hypochromic, microcytic	100%
HPFH (point mutations gene promoter)	Pancellular or heterocellular	Normal	Variable with different mutations: 1–4% in one type of mutation, 30% in another

Abbreviations: HbF = fetal hemoglobin; RBC = red blood cell.

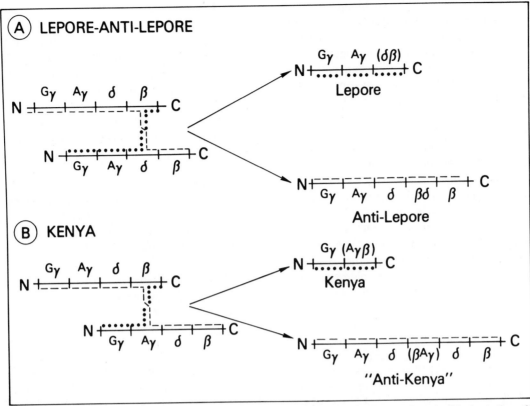

Figure 18–24 Representation of the unequal crossover events that occurred during meiosis and resulted in formation of the Lepore and anti-Lepore *(A)* and Kenya *(B)* genes. (From Nienhuis AW, Benz EJ Jr: Regulation of hemoglobin synthesis during the development of the red cell [part 1]. N Engl J Med 1977; 297:1318–1328.)

tation for the normal alpha gene complex or haplotype is expressed as $\alpha\alpha$ signifying the two normal genes ($\alpha2$ and $\alpha1$) on one chromosome 16 that produces alpha chains; therefore a normal genotype is $\alpha\alpha/\alpha\alpha$. The alpha thalassemias can then be divided into α^+ thalassemias (haplotype $-\alpha$), which have a decreased production from the alpha-chain complex (originally named α-thal-2) and α^0-thalassemias (originally named α-thal-1) in which no alpha globin is produced from the alpha-gene complex (haplotype $--$).

The most common deletions are those that generate chromosomes bearing a single gene, α^+ ($-\alpha$). The most common two deletions resulting in α^+ are ones with 3.7 kilobases (kb) deleted from the complex (designated as $-\alpha^{3.7}\alpha$) and another which deletes 4.3 kb (designated as $-\alpha^{4.3}\alpha$). The first is most common and caused by misalignment and crossing over, which creates a single fused gene from which 3.7 kb of DNA are missing. This single gene complex is the product of an $-\alpha^{3.7}$ "rightward deletion." It is found in all populations where alpha thalassemia is found. About 30% of American blacks are heterozygous for the deletion $\alpha^{3.7}\alpha/\alpha\alpha$, and 2% are homozygous ($\alpha^{3.7}\alpha/\alpha^{3.7}\alpha$). The second, a less common crossing over, causes a "leftward deletion" of 4.2 kb of DNA producing the $-\alpha^{4.2}$. As the majority of alpha globin is encoded by the alpha-2 gene, loss of mutation affect-

ing the α-2 locus, which is common in Asians, creates a more serious imbalance in the α/β-synthetic ratio and a higher percentage of Hb Bart's γ_4 than loss or mutation of the $\alpha1$ locus.

The above deletions also produce a triplicated haplotype $\alpha\alpha\alpha^{anti3.7}$ or $\alpha\alpha\alpha^{anti4.2}$. The third gene is also expressed leading to a slight increase in the alpha- to beta-chain ratio in homozygotes for the triplication, but no clinical consequences are observed. If this haplotype is inherited with a beta-thalassemia gene, however, a thalassemia intermedia clinical picture may be present because of the more unequal alpha-to-beta-globin chain production.[72]

Point mutations rather than deletions that affect the predominant $\alpha2$ gene (haplotype designated as $\alpha^T\alpha$ may also produce the alpha-thalassemia trait ($\alpha\alpha/\alpha^T\alpha$). Point mutations that decrease the expression from the $\alpha2$ gene ($\alpha^T\alpha$) result in an α^+ thalassemia which generates fewer alpha-globin chains than does deletion α^+ haplotype ($-\alpha/$). The homozygote for point mutations in both $\alpha2$ genes ($\alpha^T\alpha/\alpha^T\alpha$) phenotypically produces HbH disease and not the alpha-thalassemia trait. Also a nondeletion α^+ haplotype with α^0-thalassemia ($--/\alpha^T\alpha$) produces a more severe HbH disease than the α^0 interaction with an α^+ haplotype ($--/-\alpha$).[4]

Eleven deletions have been described that involve both the alpha genes (α° or α-thal-1) that cause no production of alpha chains from that chromosome. Genes for α^0-thalassemia are found frequently (as high as 3%) in Southeast Asia (haplotype $--^{\text{SEA}}$), less frequently in the Mediterranean area (haplotype $--^{\text{MED}}$), and sporadically in other parts of the world.[45-48] It is found infrequently in Africa and in persons of African ancestry.

Other more uncommon molecular lesions that affect expression of the alpha-globin gene include mutations in the termination codon resulting in several variant hemoglobins, the most common being Constant Spring. Others are Hb Koya Dora, Hb Seal Rock, and Hb Icaria. Hb Quong Sze and Hb Suan Dok have a single amino acid change in the alpha chain, resulting in the same blood study analysis.[46-51] These structural alpha chain mutants also result in a decreased output of chains due either to a degradation of the chain or to an instability of the corresponding mRNA.

CLINICAL SYNDROMES

Four clinical syndromes are present in alpha thalassemia depending on the gene number and *cis* or *trans* pairing, and the amount of alpha chains produced.[45-47, 53] The four syndromes are: silent carrier, alpha thalassemia trait (α-thal minor), HbH disease, and homozygous (hydrops fetalis) alpha thalassemia (Table 18-9).

Silent Carrier

The deletion of one alpha-globin gene leaving three functional alpha-globin genes causes the silent carrier syndrome. The α/β chain ratio is nearly normal and no hematologic abnormalities are present. At birth, Hb Bart's (γ_4) is in the range of 0-2%. There is no reliable way to diagnose silent carriers by hematologic criteria. When necessary for genetic counseling, gene studies can be done by restriction-endonuclease mapping.

Alpha Thalassemia Trait

Alpha thalassemia trait can be caused by the homozygous α^+ ($-\alpha/-\alpha$) or heterozygous α^0 ($--/\alpha\alpha$).[45-47] This syndrome exhibits a mild anemia with microcytic, hypochromic red blood cells. At birth Hb Bart's (γ_4) is in the range of 2-10%. No HbH (β_4) is usually present in the adult.

Hemoglobin H Disease

Hemoglobin H disease is usually caused by the presence of only one gene producing alpha chains ($--/-\alpha$).[45-47] It can also be caused by the combination of α^0 and Hb Constant Spring ($--/\alpha^{\text{CS}}\alpha$) and other more rare alpha thalassemia gene combinations found in Mediterranean area and Saudi Arabian populations. This genetic abnormality is particularly common in Asians because the α^0 gene (haplotype $--$) is prevalent and is characterized by the accumulation of excess unpaired beta chains, which form the unstable tetramers (β_4) called

Table 18-9. CLINICAL SYNDROMES OF ALPHA-THALASSEMIA

Genotype	HbA	Hb Barts (in Newborn)	HbH (in Adult)	Constant Spring
NORMAL (NORMAL HEMATOLOGIC PARAMETERS)				
$\alpha\alpha/\alpha\alpha$	97-98%	0	0	0
SILENT CARRIER (NORMAL HEMATOLOGIC PARAMETERS)				
$-\alpha/\alpha\alpha$	97-98%	0-2	0	0
$\alpha\alpha\text{CS}^*/\alpha\alpha$	96%	0	0	2
ALPHA-THALASSEMIA MINOR (NORMAL TO MILD HEMOLYTIC ANEMIA; MICROCYTIC, HYPOCHROMIC)				
$--/\alpha\alpha$	90-95%	5-10%	0	0
$-\alpha/-\alpha$	90-95%	5-10%	0	0
$\alpha\alpha\text{CS}/\alpha\alpha\text{CS}$	85-90%	5-10%	0	6
HBH DISEASE (MODERATE HEMOLYTIC ANEMIA WITH FEW TRANSFUSION REQUIREMENTS; MICROCYTIC, HYPOCHROMIC)				
$--/-\alpha$	↓	25-40%	2-40%	0
$--/\alpha\alpha\text{CS}$	↓	25-40%	2-40%	1.5-2.6
HYDROPS FETALIS (LETHAL: INFANTS STILLBORN OR DIE WITHIN HOURS OF BIRTH; SEVERE ANEMIA)				
$--/--$	0	80 (with 20% Hb Portland)	0-20%	0

* Constant Spring.

HbH. (See the section on electrophoresis.) In the newborn, 10–40% of the hemoglobin is Hb Bart's (γ_4) with the remainder being HbF and HbA. After the γ to β switch, HbH (β^4) replaces the Hb Bart's. The hemoglobin percentages are then 30–50% HbH, reduced amount of HbA_2, and traces of Hb Bart's, with the remainder being HbA.[46]

In the Constant Spring variant, a small amount of Hb Constant Spring is also present. The alpha-chain synthesis is usually 40% of the beta-chain production, which is higher than the number of alpha genes would indicate. HbH disease is characterized by a mild to moderate, chronic, hemolytic anemia with Hb concentrations averaging 7–10 g/dL and reticulocytes from 5–10%.[46, 47] The bone marrow exhibits erythroid hyperplasia and the spleen is usually enlarged. As with most chronic hemolytic states, infection, pregnancy, or exposure to oxidative drugs may cause a hemolytic crisis.

These crises may cause the detection of the syndrome because individuals with HbH disease can otherwise lead normal lives. The red blood cells are microcytic, hypochromic with marked poikilocytosis, especially in deformed and target red blood cells. The HbH is vulnerable to oxidation and will gradually precipitate in vivo to form Heinz-like bodies of this denatured Hb.[46] Many of these HbH inclusions are removed by the culling mechanisms of the spleen and are much more prevalent post-splenectomy. These inclusions alter the shape and viscoelastic properties of the red blood cells contributing to the decreased red blood cell survival. Splenectomy is often beneficial.[73] The red blood cells of a patient with HbH, which are incubated in brilliant cresyl blue acquire fine, evenly dispersed, granular inclusions. Before splenectomy only a portion of the cells will have this characteristic, but afterward the majority of the red blood cells are so full of these inclusions that they have been described as resembling a golf ball or raspberry (Fig. 18–25).

In rare instances HbH disease has been associated with mental retardation.[47] There appears to be a locus or loci near the alpha-gene cluster on chromosome 16 that when mutated or co-deleted with the alpha-gene cluster can lead to mental retardation in association with alpha thalassemia.[74] An acquired HbH disease has also been associated with myeloproliferative disorders such as erythroleukemia, acute myeloid leukemia, and sideroblastic anemia.[75]

Hydrops Fetalis Alpha Thalassemia

Homozygous alpha thalassemia (−−/−−), which is incompatible with life, results in the absence of all alpha-chain synthesis.[45–47] The baby is born with hydrops fetalis, which is edema and ascites caused by accumulation of serous fluid in

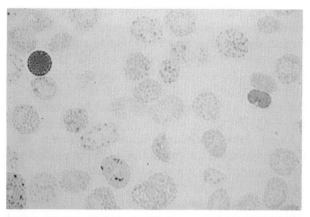

Figure 18–25 Red blood cells from a patient with hemoglobin H, incubated with brilliant cresyl blue, that have acquired fine, evenly dispersed granular inclusions. (Courtesy of Ann Bell.)

the fetal tissues as a result of the severe anemia. The predominant hemoglobin is Hb Bart's ($\gamma 4$), along with 5–20% Hb Portland and traces of HbH.[46, 76] Hb Bart's has a high O_2 affinity so that it cannot transport O_2 to the tissues. The fetus survives to the third trimester because of the Hb Portland, but this Hb cannot support the later stages of fetal growth, and the affected fetus dies of anoxia. The fetus is delivered prematurely and is stillborn or dies shortly after birth. In addition to anemia, edema, and ascites, the fetus has gross hepatosplenomegaly and cardiomegaly.[45–47] The blood test results of the baby at delivery show a severe microcytic, hypochromic anemia with numerous nucleated red blood cells in the peripheral blood. The bone marrow cavity is expanded, and marked erythroid hyperplasia is present, as is extramedullary erythropoiesis.

Hydropic pregnancies are hazardous to the mother, resulting in toxemia and severe postpartum hemorrhage.[45, 46] These changes can now be detected in midgestation by means of ultrasound testing. If both parents carry the alpha thalassemia minor gene, prenatal diagnosis of homozygosity can be made by restriction endonuclease analysis of DNA obtained from chorionic villi sampling or amniotic fluid. Absence of the alpha-globin genes establishes the diagnosis. Early termination of the pregnancy prevents toxemia and postpartum hemorrhage in the mother.

Thalassemia Associated with Structural Hemoglobin Variants

HbS-THALASSEMIA

HbS-thalassemia is a double heterozygous genetic abnormality in which the abnormal genes for both HbS and thalassemia are inherited by a single individual. HbS-alpha thalassemia is fairly common because both the gene for HbS and α^+ thalassemia are common in populations of African descent. These individuals have less HbS than those with only sickle cell trait. They are usually asymptomatic.[77] The clinical expression of HbSS-alpha thalassemia is milder than sickle cell anemia. There is an increased percentage of HbF, which reduces the severity of the sickling process. The amount of F is proportional to the number of alpha genes affected. Patients with α^0 thalassemia have approximately 16% HbF, and those with α^+ have approximately 8%.

HbS–beta thalassemia results from the inheritance of a beta thalassemia gene from one parent and a HbS gene from the other. This syndrome has been reported in the populations of Africa, the Mediterranean area, the Middle East, the West Indies, and in the black population of North America.[45] The clinical expression of S-beta thalassemia depends upon the type of beta thalassemia mutation inherited.[78] The interaction of either β^0 or β^+ thalassemia, which produces only a small amount of beta chains with sickle cell, causes a clinical syndrome similar to sickle cell anemia. The electrophoresis shows mostly HbS with slightly elevated HbA_2 and variable amounts of HbF and HbA (depending on the specific gene inherited). These patients are often from the Mediterranean area and can be distinguished from those with sickle anemia because they have microcytosis and splenomegaly. One parent will have sickle cell trait and the other beta thalassemia minor.[78] The interaction of mild β^+, which produced more beta chains, results in a condition that may be only a little more severe than sickle cell trait. The individual has a mild anemia with splenomegaly. These patients can be distinguished from those with sickle cell trait because the hemolytic anemia, the splenomegaly, and the amounts of microcytosis and HbS are greater than those in patients with HbAS. The hemoglobin percentages are approximately 30% HbS, 65% HbA, 4–5% HbA_2, and HbF in the range found in sickle cell anemia.[73]

Beta thalassemia can also be inherited with HbC. A moderately severe hemolytic disorder associated with splenomegaly, hypochromia, and microcytosis with numerous target cells on the blood test results. The hemoglobin pattern varies depending on the type beta thalassemia gene inherited. HbC makes up 65–95% of the total hemoglobin.[47]

Hemoglobin E-thalassemia is common in Southeast Asia where both genetic mutations are prevalent. Because hemoglobin E is synthesized at a reduced rate as are beta chains in beta thalassemia, when both are inherited together there is a marked deficiency of beta chain production and

the clinical picture may range from thalassemia intermedia to a transfusion-dependent condition indistinguishable from homozygous beta thalassemia.

Diagnosis of Thalassemia

HISTORY AND CLINICAL EXAMINATION

The patient's individual and family histories are important in the diagnosis of thalassemia, because it is an inherited genetic abnormality. The race or ethnic background of the individual should be investigated because of the increased frequency of different abnormal genes in certain populations. In the clinical examination, pallor indicating anemia, jaundice indicating hemolysis, splenomegaly due to pooling of the abnormal cells, and skeletal deformity especially in beta thalassemia major due to expansion of the bone marrow cavities are important findings that suggest thalassemia (Fig. 18–26).

LABORATORY FINDINGS

Complete Blood Count (CBC) with Differential and Reticulocyte Count

Most of the thalassemia syndromes are characterized by a microcytic, hypochromic anemia. These are routinely detected on all modern electronic cell analyzers.[51] The MCV, MCH, hemoglobin, and hematocrit values are low, but the red blood cell count is usually normal or elevated relative to the degree of anemia. The MCHC may be slightly decreased and the red blood cell distribution width (RDW) is usually normal except in untreated thalassemia major, in which it is elevated as a result of the tremendous anisocytosis. In most thalassemias, the MCV is markedly decreased while the red blood cell count is high. This fact differentiates thalassemia from iron deficiency anemia, wherein the MCV value is less striking and the red blood cell count decreased. The reticulocyte count is elevated, indicating the bone marrow is responding to a hemolytic process. In HbH disease, the reticulocyte count may be up to 10% and in homozygous beta thalassemia, it is approximately 5%. It is disproportionately low in relation to the degree of anemia in beta thalassemia major probably as a result of the ineffective erythropoiesis.[51]

The red blood cells on a Wright's stained smear are microcytic and hypochromic in most thalassemia syndromes except the silent carrier phenotypes in which the red blood cells appear normal. In heterozygous beta thalassemia and HbH disease, the cells are microcytic with mild to moderate poikilocytosis and in heterozygous α^0 thalassemia,

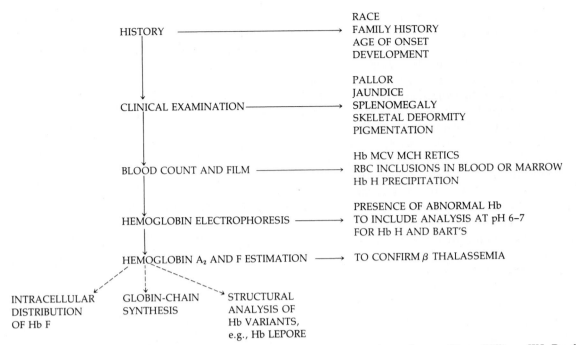

Figure 18–26 Flowchart showing the approach to the diagnosis of the thalassemia syndromes. (From Williams WJ, Beutler E, Erslev AJ, Lichtman MA [eds]: Hematology, 4th ed. New York: McGraw-Hill, 1990:533.)

there is a mild hypochromia and microcytosis but less poikilocytosis. In homozygous and double heterozygous beta thalassemia, extreme poikilocytosis may be present including target cells and elliptocytes as well as polychromasia, basophilic stippling, and nucleated red blood cells.

BONE MARROW

The bone marrow in untreated homozygous beta thalassemia is markedly hypercellular with extreme red blood cell hyperplasia. Extramedullary hematopoiesis is prominent. HbH disease shows less bone marrow red blood cell hyperplasia. The heterozygous thalassemias show slight erythroid hyperplasia.

OSMOTIC FRAGILITY

The microcytic, hypochromic red blood cells of the thalassemias have a decreased osmotic fragility. This trait has been used as a basis for a one-tube variation of the osmotic fragility test to screen for the thalassemia carrier state in populations in which thalassemia is frequent.[79] Because iron deficiency anemia also has a decreased osmotic fragility, it does not differentiate between the two.

BRILLIANT CRESYL BLUE STAIN

In alpha thalassemia trait, HbH disease, and silent alpha thalassemia, the brilliant cresyl blue test

for HbH inclusion can be used to induce precipitation of the intrinsically unstable HbH.[80] The hemoglobin H inclusions which are denatured beta-globin chains typically appear as small, multiple, irregularly-shaped, greenish-blue bodies with a pitted pattern similar to that of a golfball or a raspberry (see Fig. 18–25). They are usually fairly uniformly distributed throughout the erythrocyte. In HbH disease, almost all the red blood cells contain these inclusions, whereas in alpha thalassemia trait only a few cells may contain these inclusions, and in silent carrier alpha thalassemia, only a rare cell does. These inclusions appear different from Heinz body inclusions, which are larger and fewer in number and most often appear eccentrically along the membrane of the red blood cell. A negative result on this examination for HbH inclusions does not necessarily exclude the trait or silent forms of alpha thalassemia. To facilitate the finding of these inclusions, the top portion of the red blood cells in a centrifuged sample may be used to isolate the younger red blood cells, which contain more HbH and are more buoyant.[81]

ELECTROPHORESIS

Hemoglobin electrophoresis on cellulose acetate at alkaline pH is important in the diagnosis of thalassemia to screen for HbH, Hb Bart's, Hb Constant Spring, Hb Lepore, and other hemoglobin variants that may interact with thalassemia. HbH and Hb Bart's are fast-moving on cellulose acetate at an alkaline pH but are the only Hb variants that migrate anodally at an acid pH (6.5–7.0)[82] (Fig. 18–27). It may also be used to screen for the elevated HbA_2 associated with beta thalassemia trait, which can then be quantitated by microchromatography. Increased HbF can be detected on electrophoresis, which is important in delta beta thalassemia, HPFH, and other beta thalassemia variants. It, too, should be quantitated by other methods. Citrate agar gel electrophoresis performed at an acid pH can be used in the diagnosis of thalassemia by differentiating between HbS and Hb Lepore.

HbA₂ AND HbF ESTIMATION

Quantitation of HbA₂ by Microchromatography

Values for HbA_2 determined by microchromatography in normal subjects may be up 3.0%. Values elevated to 8% generally indicate beta thalassemia trait.[82] HbA_2 may also be slightly elevated in association with sickle cell trait (1.7–4.5%) or sickle cell anemia (1.7–5.9%). The overlap in the ranges of HbA_2 for these groups is influenced by the amount of HbF present with high levels of HbF usually resulting in lower levels of HbA_2. Decreased levels of HbA_2 can be seen in iron deficiency anemia, sideroblastic anemia, or certain thalassemia syndromes, such as HbH disease, carrier states of alpha thalassemia, delta beta thalassemia, Hb Lepore syndromes, or in hereditary persistence of fetal hemoglobin.[82]

This test is based on ion exchange chromatography in which a hemolysate of whole blood is absorbed onto a chromatography column of positively charged diethylaminoethyl cellulose. The pH of the buffer present determines the net charge of the different hemoglobins, which then bind to the positively charged cellulose resin. A 0.05 M *tris*-HCl buffer at pH 8.3 is used to elute HbA_2 from a column. At this pH and ionic strength, HbA adheres more strongly to the ion exchange resin than does HbA_2, resulting in rapid separation and elution of HbA_2. The percentage of A_2 can be calculated based on the optical density of the eluate compared with that of the total amount of Hb present.

Another method to quantitate HbA_2 is to elute the HbA_2 band from cellulose acetate membrane following electrophoresis.[83] This generally gives satisfactory results and is fast and simple. The results of HbA_2 with this method will tend to be high in the presence of HbS because HbA_2 is often incompletely separated from HbS.

Quantitation of HbF

High amounts of HbF are present in homozygous β^0 and β^+ thalassemia, delta beta thalassemia, Hb Lepore, and pancellular HPFH. A moderate or slight elevation in HbF can be seen in beta thalassemia minor and the heterocellular forms of HPFH.

The alkali denaturation test is accurate and precise for the quantitation of HbF especially in the 2–40% range. Radioimmunoassay is more accurate when HbF concentration is under 2%, and column chromatography is more accurate when it is greater than 40%.[84]

The principle of the alkali denaturation test is that most human hemoglobins are denatured upon exposure to a strong alkali, but HbF is not. The denaturation is stopped by the addition of saturated ammonium sulfate, which precipitates the denatured hemoglobin. The HbF remains soluble and can be filtered from the precipitate, measured, and expressed as the percentage of alkali-resistant hemoglobin.[82]

Acid Elution Slide Test for HbF

As has been mentioned, the intracellular distribution of the HbF is used to differentiate thalassemias with increased HbF from pancellular HPFH. In thalassemia, there is a nonuniform, heterogeneous pattern, meaning that some red blood cells contain F and others do not; and in deletion HPFH, all the red blood cells contain F (a homogeneous pattern).[80] The heterogeneous distribution of HbF is also found in other disorders with a high HbF such as sickle cell anemia, and other hemoglobinopathies.

The principle of this procedure is that when blood smears are immersed in an acid buffer, adult hemoglobin is eluted from the erythrocytes, whereas fetal hemoglobin is resistant to acid elu-

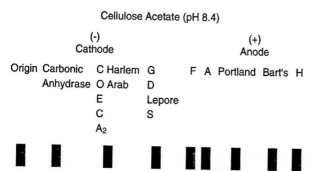

Figure 18–27 Relative electrophoretic mobilities on cellulose acetate, pH 8.4, of various hemoglobins that are important in the diagnosis of thalassemia syndromes and hemoglobinopathies.

tion and is not eluted. If the smears are subsequently stained, erythrocytes having HbF will take up the stain, whereas those containing only adult hemoglobin will appear as "ghosts."

OTHER SPECIAL PROCEDURES

Other special procedures can be used to identify specific genotypes for research purposes, to differentiate an alpha thalassemia carrier from beta thalassemia carrier, to identify a silent carrier gene, or to examine for family inheritance patterns with multiple genes. This further testing is done in more specialized laboratories. It must be decided whether the benefit of a complete diagnosis warrants the expense.

Globin Chain Testing

Globin chain testing determines the ratio of the globin chains being produced.[85] A patient's reticulocytes from the peripheral blood or nucleated red blood cells from the bone marrow are incubated in the presence of radioactively labeled leucine. The red blood cells are lysed and the chains produced with the radioactive amino acid are separated by column chromatography. The radioactivity of each fraction is counted and the rate of synthesis for each of the chains is calculated to obtain the alpha/beta globin ratio.

DNA Analysis

Gene or DNA analysis is accomplished by using restriction endonucleases and hybridization with complementary DNA probes to detail the specific defect at the molecular DNA level.[85] This results in restriction-fragment–length polymorphism analysis that is characteristic of the specific haplotype associated with various thalassemias. This technique is used in difficult cases to diagnose for proper treatment and more importantly for genetic counseling purposes. It is also used in antenatal diagnosis of thalassemia from chorionic villus sample at 9 to 11 weeks gestation.[47]

Testing in the Chemistry Section

An increased indirect bilirubin level is present in thalassemias with a hemolytic component. It is usually a mild increase in the thalassemia traits, but moderate in thalassemia intermedia and HbH disease. Thalassemia major also shows an increase, however, it is less elevated because of the inability to produce hemoglobin.

The iron status of an individual with microcytic, hypochromic anemia is important in the differential diagnosis of a thalassemia trait and iron deficiency anemia. It is also useful in the assessment of the iron load in a patient with transfused thalassemia major or thalassemia intermedia. Patients who have a large iron load will have an increased level of serum iron and the total-iron-binding capacity will approach 100% saturation. The serum ferritin level, which indicates the amount of iron deposited in the tissues, will be elevated.[87]

Differential Diagnosis of Thalassemia and Iron Deficiency Anemia

Because the heterozygous thalassemias are microcytic and hypochromic they must be differentiated from iron deficiency anemia and other microcytic, hypochromic anemias. The precise, automated cell counters of the modern hematology laboratory detect asymptomatic microcytosis in a good number of patients.[88] Almost all of these cases are caused by either iron deficiency or thalassemia. A differential diagnosis is important so that unnecessary iron therapy or analysis for the source of undetected blood loss indicated by iron deficiency can be avoided in thalassemia. Iron deficiency is often the first condition considered by the physician because it is more common.

A mild erythrocytosis (high red blood cell count) and marked microcytosis (low MCV) are characteristic of thalassemia trait and are important in the differential diagnosis.[47, 48] The red blood cell count is usually decreased in patients with iron deficiency and the MCV may be normal or decreased, depending on whether the iron deficiency anemia is acute or chronic but is usually not as decreased as it is in thalassemia.[47] The RDW, a parameter on automated counters, may be helpful in the differential diagnosis, but has been found by some investigators to be useless by itself.[89] Several formulas have been developed to help define the two disorders[47] (Table 18–10). None are infallible but all can be useful. The evaluation of the color of the patient's serum may provide a clue because in iron deficiency, it is pale and watery whereas in thalassemia it is normal or slightly icteric.

The free erythrocyte protoporphyrin (FEP) is an additional useful screening test because it is elevated in iron deficiency anemia but normal in thalassemia.[90] The measured zinc protoporphyrin/ heme (ZnPP/H) ratio is similar to the FEP. Both are present in excess of that used for hemoglobin synthesis and are increased in iron deficiency caused by various conditions. The ZnPP can be measured directly with a hematofluorometer, whereas the FEP requires an acid extraction.[80] Of course, measurement of transferrin saturation or ferritin may also be used to verify or exclude the diagnosis of iron deficiency. Thalassemia may also have to be differentiated from other microcytic anemias.

Table 18-10. FORMULAS FOR DIFFERENTIATION OF THALASSEMIA TRAIT FROM IRON DEFICIENCY

	Thalassemia Trait	Iron Deficiency
Mentzer index MCV/RBC	< 13	> 13
Shine and Lal (MCV)2 × MCH	< 1530	> 1530
England and Fraser MCV − RBC − (5 × Hb) − 8.4	Negative values	Positive values

Abbreviations: MCV = mean corpuscular volume; RBC = red blood cell; MCH = mean corpuscular hemoglobin; Hb = hemoglobin.
From Nathan DG, Oski FA (eds): Hematology of Infancy and Childhood, 4th ed. Philadelphia: WB Saunders, 1993:832.

SUMMARY

Hemoglobinopathies include both structurally abnormal hemoglobins, which result from mutations that alter the amino acid sequence of the molecule, and the thalassemia syndromes, in which the synthesis of one or more of the globin chains is diminished or absent.

Hemoglobin S is the most common hemoglobinopathy resulting from an amino acid substitution in the beta-globin chain. HbS polymerizes inside the red blood cell because of abnormal interaction with adjacent hemoglobin tetramers when it is in the deoxygenated form. In sickle cell anemia (homozygous SS), this polymerization of hemoglobin causes sickling of cells, resulting in a hemolytic anemia caused by the early removal of these cells and a compromised microcirculation as the abnormally shaped cells obstruct blood flow into the tissues. Persons with sickle cell trait (heterozygous AS) show no clinical symptoms. Sickle cell anemia is a normochromic, normocytic anemia characterized by a single band in the S position on cellulose acetate and a positive tube solubility.

The second two most common hemoglobinopathies are HbC and HbE. Both are asymptomatic in the heterozygous state and cause mild hemolysis in the homozygous state. HbE results in a microcytic blood picture.

There are hundreds of other variant hemoglobins, most of which cause no clinical symptoms. Some are unstable, and other variants have an abnormal affinity for oxygen.

The many laboratory procedures used to diagnose the hemoglobinopathies include peripheral blood smear (for studying red blood cell morphology); hemoglobin electrophoresis under alkaline condition on cellulose acetate or under acid conditions on agar; the solubility test; HbA$_2$ and HbF quantitation; Heinz body stain; and the isopropanol precipitation test and heat denaturation for the unstable hemoglobins.

The thalassemias are a group of heterogeneous disorders in which one or more globin chains are reduced or absent, resulting in an imbalance of globin chains and a hypochromic, microcytic hemolytic anemia. The beta thalassemias are usually caused by mRNA abnormalities. The abnormal gene can produce some beta chains (β^+) or no beta chains (β^0). The decreased production of beta chains results in an excess of alpha chains that precipitate, causing the red blood cells to be subsequently removed by the spleen, resulting in hemolysis. The decreased production of hemoglobin leads to a microcytic anemia. Heterozygous beta thalassemia minor usually has an elevated HbA$_2$ level, which aids in the diagnosis. Homozygous beta thalassemia major is a severe anemia that leads to hepatosplenomegaly and expansion of bones as a result of marrow hyperplasia. Severe anemia with growth retardation and delayed sexual development occurs unless the patient undergoes transfusion. Beta thalassemia intermedia manifests with abnormalities whose level of severity is between those of beta thalassemias major and minor. Other thalassemia syndromes involving the beta-globin cluster on chromosome 11 are Hb Lepore, hereditary persistence of fetal hemoglobin, delta beta thalassemia, and associations with hemoglobinopathies such as HbS-beta thalassemia.

The alpha thalassemias are usually caused by deletion of one or both of the alpha genes on chromosome 16, resulting in reduced or absent production of alpha chains. Tetramers of gamma chains may precipitate as Hb Bart's, or tetramers of beta chains may precipitate as HbH. Clinically, alpha thalassemias are characterized in four categories. The first, hydrops fetalis, in which all four of the alpha genes are deleted, is incompatible with life. HbH disease is the result of the deletions of three of the four alpha genes. The excess beta chains precipitate, causing a hemolytic anemia. Alpha thalassemia trait is the result of the deletion of two alpha genes and is clinically similar to beta thalassemia minor. Of course, there is no increase in HbA$_2$ because it also contains alpha chains.

Alpha thalassemia silent carrier status is the result of the deletion of one of four alpha genes and is totally asymptomatic.

Diagnosis of thalassemia is made from the red blood cell morphology, hemoglobin electrophoresis, Heinz body test, and HbA$_2$ and F quantitation. In rare instances, DNA analysis and alpha beta–globin chain synthesis may be done. Thalassemia must be differentiated from other microcytic, hypochromic anemias, especially iron deficiency anemia. Iron studies are important for this differentiation.

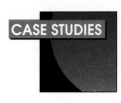
CASE STUDIES

Case 1

An 18-year-old black female was seen in the emergency room for fever and abdominal pain. A blood count was performed and the following results were obtained:

Hematocrit:	0.32 L/L
Hemoglobin:	10.5 g/dL
Red blood cell count:	3.87×10^{12}/L
Reticulocyte count:	2.9%
Indices:	Normal
Red blood cell distribution width:	19.5
Platelet count:	389×10^9/L
WBC	12.3×10^9/L
Segmented neutrophils:	78%
Lymphocytes:	13%
Monocytes:	4%
Eosinophils:	4%
Basophils:	1%

On hemoglobin electrophoresis at alkaline pH, one band migrated in the S position and the other in the C position.

1. What confirmatory tests should be performed? Discuss the migration pattern.

2. Identify and describe the most typical abnormal red blood cell seen on the peripheral smear.

3. What diagnosis is suggested based on the electrophoretic pattern?

4. Considering the Mendelian laws of heredity and with each parent having the trait form of HbC and HbS, what would be the expected genotype of each of four children?

Case 2

A 24-year-old male medical student in a southern area of the United States was found to have a hematocrit of 0.35 L/L in a hematology laboratory class. A hematologist at the university discovered during a family history of this student that his mother had always been anemic, had periodically been given iron shots, and had had several gall bladder "attacks." Both of her parents had been born in Sicily, Italy. A cousin on the student's mother's side had two children who had died at the ages of 4 and 5 of thalassemia major and had a third young daughter who also received a diagnosis of thalassemia major and was being treated by frequent blood transfusions. The student's laboratory results were as follows:

Hematocrit:	0.352 L/L
Hemoglobin:	10.2 g/dL
Red blood cell count:	5.74×10^{12}/L
Mean corpuscular volume:	61.3 fL
Mean corpuscular hemoglobin:	17.78 pg
Mean corpuscular hemoglobin concentration:	28.9%

The peripheral red blood cell morphology exhibited moderate anisocytosis with microcytic red blood cells, slight hypochromia, slight poikilocytosis with occasional target cells, and several red blood cells with basophilic stippling. Hemoglobin A_2: 4.9 percent by column chromatography.

1. Why was the family history so important in this case, and what diagnosis did it suggest?

2. What laboratory value helped confirm the diagnosis?

3. What other disorders should this anemia be differentiated from, what laboratory test would be helpful, and why is differentiation important?

4. If this individual were planning to have children, what genetic counseling should be done?

References

1. Jandl JH: Abnormal hemoglobins and hemoglobinopathies. *In* Jandl JH (ed): Blood: Textbook of Hematology. Boston: Little, Brown, 1987.
2. Fishleder AJ, Hoffman GC: A practical approach to the detection of hemoglobinopathies: part I. The introduction and thalassemia syndrome. Lab Med 1987; 18(6):368–372.
3. Bauer JD: Clinical Laboratory Methods, 6th ed. St. Louis: CV Mosby, 1982:72–74.
4. Nelson DA, Davey FR: Erythrocytic disorders. *In* Henry JB (ed): Clinical Diagnosis and Management by Laboratory Methods, 18th ed. Philadelphia: WB Saunders, 1991:649–655.
5. Fishleder AJ, Hoffman GC: A practical approach to the detection of hemoglobinopathies: part II. The sickle cell disorders. Lab Med 1987; 18:441–443.
6. Miale JB: Anemia due to decreased erythrocyte survival—the hemoglobinopathies. *In* Miale JB (ed): Laboratory Medicine: Hematology, 6th ed. St. Louis: CV Mosby, 1982:603.
7. Beutler E: Erythrocyte disorders: Anemias related to abnormal globin. The sickle cell diseases and related disorders. *In* Williams WJ, Beutler E, Erslev AJ, Lichtman MA (eds): Hematology, 4th ed. New York: McGraw-Hill, 1990:615–627.
8. Conley CL: Sickle cell anemia, the first molecular disease. *In* Wintrobe MM (ed): Blood, Pure and Eloquent. New York: McGraw-Hill, 1980:319.
9. Zeringer H, Harmening DM: Hemolytic anemias: intracorpuscular defects, the hemoglobinopathies. *In* Harmening DM (ed): Clinical Hematology and Fundamentals of Hemostasis, 2nd ed. FA Davis, 1992:142–160.
10. Phillips III JA, Kazazian HH Jr: Hemoglobinopathies and thalassemias. *In* Spivak JL (ed): Fundamentals of Clinical Hematology, 2nd ed. Philadelphia, Harper & Row, 1984:57.
11. Platt OS, Nathan DG: Disorders of hemoglobin, sickle cell disease. *In* Nathan DG, Oski FA (eds): Hematology of Infancy and Childhood, 3rd ed. Philadelphia: WB Saunders, 1987: 663–666,687.
12. Nagel RL, Fabry ME, Paul DK: New insights on sickle cell anemia. Diagn Med, 1984; 7:26.
13. Noguuchi CT, Rodgers GP, Serjeant G, Schechter AN: Levels of hemoglobin necessary for treatment of sickle cell disease: N Engl J Med 1988; 318:96.
14. Diggs LW: Sickle cell crises. J Clin Pathol, 1965; 44:1–19.
15. Platt OS, Dover GJ: Sickle cell disease. *In* Nathan DG, Oski FA (eds): Hematology of Infancy and Childhood, 4th ed. Philadelphia: WB Saunders, 1993:746–776.
16. MacIver JE, Parker-Williams EJ: Aplastic crisis in sickle cell anemia. J Lab Clin Med 1950; 35:721.
17. Luzzatto L: Genetics of red cells and susceptibility to malaria. Blood 1979; 54(5):961.
18. Beutler E, Johnson C, Powars D, West C: Prevalence of glucose-6-phosphate dehydrogenase deficiency in sickle cell disease. N Engl J Med 1974; 80:217.
19. Steinberg MH, Dreiling BJ: Glucose-6-phosphate dehydrogenase deficiency in sickle cell anemia. Ann Int Med 1974; 80:217.
20. Bain BJ: Interpretation—red cells, and platelets. *In* Bain BJ (ed): Blood Cells, A Practical Guide. Philadelphia: JB Lippincott, 1989:269.
21. Zeringer H, Pittiglio HD: Hemolytic anemias: intracorpuscular defects III: the hemoglobinopathies. *In* Pittiglio DH, Sacher RA (eds): Clinical Hematology and Fundamentals of Hemostasis. Philadelphia: FA Davis, 1987:111.
22. Powars DR, Weiss JN, Chan LS, Schroeder WA: Is there a threshold level of fetal hemoglobin that ameliorates morbidity in sickle cell anemia? Blood 1984; 63:921.
23. Platt OS, Thorington BD, Brambilla DJ, et al: Pain in sickle cell disease. Rates and risk factors. N Engl J Med 1991; 325(1):11–16.
24. Charache S, Lubin B, Reid CD: Management and Therapy of Sickle Cell Disease. Washington: U.S. Dept. of Health, NIH publication no. 84-2117, 1984:6.
25. Bunn FH, Forget BG: Sickle Cell Disease—Clinical and Epidemiological Aspects. *In* Bunn FH, Forget BG (eds): Hemoglobin: Molecular, Genetic and Clinical Aspects. Philadelphia: WB Saunders, 1986: 503–510.
26. Kadish E, Lantos J, Stocking C, Singer PA, et al: Bone marrow transportation for sickle cell disease. N Engl J Med 1991; 325(19):1349–1353.
27. McCormick WE: Abnormal hemoglobins II: the pathology of sickle cell trait. Am J Med Sci 1961; 241:329.
28. Schlitt LE, Keital HG: Renal manifestations of sickle cell disease. A review. Am J Med Sci 1960; 239:773.
29. Bell, A: Homozygous Hemoglobin C Disease, Hematology Tech Sample H-71. Chicago: ASCP, 1974.
30. Bunn FH, Forget BG: Human hemoglobin variants. *In* Bunn FH, Forget BG (eds): Hemoglobin: Molecular, Genetic and Clinical Aspects. Philadelphia: WB Saunders, 1986: 421.
31. Bookchin RM, Nagel RL, Ranney NM: Structure and properties of HbC Harlem. A human hemoglobin variant with amino acid substitutions in 2 residues of the β-chain. J Biol Chem 1967; 242:248–255.
32. Pearce CJ, Dow P: Anemia of abnormal globin development—hemoglobinopathies. *In* Lotspeich-Steininger CA, Stiene-Martin EA, Koepke JA (eds.): Clinical Hematology, Principles, Procedures, Correlation. Philadelphia: JB Lippincott, 1990:185–211.
33. Rabinovitch A (Chair): Hemoglobinopathy survey, Set HG-B. Northfield, MN: CAP, 1992:2–3.
34. Fairbanks VF, Gilchrist GS, Brimhall B, et al: Hemoglobin E trait reexamined: a cause of microcytosis and erythrocytosis. Blood 1979; 53:109–115.
35. Anderson HM, Ranney HM: Southeast Asian immigrants: the new thalassemias in America. Semin Hematol 1990; 27:239–246.
36. Diggs WL, Bell A: Intraerythrocytic hemoglobin crystals in sickle cell-hemoglobin C disease. Blood 1965; 25(2):218–223.
37. Hoffman GC: The sickling disorders. Lab Med 1990; 21:797–807.
38. Moewe C: Hemoglobin SC: A brief review. Clin Lab Sci 1993; 6(3):158–159.

39. Nagel RL, Lawrence C: The distinct patholobiology of sickle cell–hemoglobin C disease. Hematol Oncol Clin North Am 1991; 5:433–451.

40. Lawrence C, Fabry ME, Nagel RI: The unique red cell heterogeneity of SC disease: Crystal formation, dense reticulocytes and unusual morphology. Blood 1991; 78(8):2104–2112.

41. Bunn FH: M hemoglobins. *In* Bunn FH, Forget BG (eds): Hemoglobin: Molocular, Genetic and Clinical Aspects. Philadelphia: WB Saunders, 1986:623–631.

42. Bunn FH: Unstable Hemoglobin Variants—Congenital Heinz Body Hemolytic Anemia. Philadelphia: WB Saunders, 1986:565–587.

43. Bunn FH: Hemoglobinopathy due to abnormal oxygen binding. *In* Bunn FH, Forget BG (eds): Hemoglobin: Molecular, Genetic and Clinical Aspects. Philadelphia: WB Saunders, 1986:595–616.

44. Cooley TB, Lee P: A series of cases of splenomegaly in children with anemia and peculiar bone changes. Trans Am Pediatr Soc 1925; 37:29.

45. Weatherall DJ, Clegg JB: The Thalassemia Syndromes, 3rd ed. Oxford: Blackwell Scientific, 1981.

46. Weatherall, DJ: The thalassemias. *In* Williams WJ, Beutler E, Erslev AJ, Lichtman MA (eds): Hematology, 4th ed. New York: McGraw-Hill, 1990.

47. McDonagh KT, Nienhuis AW: The thalassemias. *In* Nathan DG, Oski FA (eds): Hematology of Infancy and Childhood, 4th ed. Philadelphia: WB Saunders, 1993.

48. Weatherall DJ, Clegg JB, Higgs DR, Wood WG: The hemoglobinopathies. *In* Scriver CR, Beaudet AL, Sly WS, Valle D (eds): The Metabolic Basis of Inherited Disease, 6th ed. New York: McGraw-Hill, 1989.

49. Livingstone, FB: Frequencies of Hemoglobin Variants. New York: Oxford University Press, 1985.

50. Siniscalco M, Bernini L, et al: Population genetics of haemoglobin variants, thalassemia and glucose 6-phosphate dehydrogenase deficiency with particular reference to malaria hypothesis. Bull WHO 1966; 34:379.

51. Harrison CR: Hemolytic anemias: intracorpuscular defects, thalassemia. In Harmening DM (ed): Clinical Hematology and Fundamentals of Clinical Hemostasis, 2nd ed. Philadelphia: FA Davis, 1992.

52. Bunn HF, Forget BG: Hemoglobin: Molecular, Genetic and Clinical Aspects. Philadelphia: WB Saunders, 1986.

53. Kazazian HH, Jr: The thalassemia syndromes: molecular basis and prenatal diagnosis in 1990. Semin Hematol 1990; 27:209.

54. Schwartz E: The silent carrier of beta thalassemia. N Engl J Med 1969; 281:1327.

55. Gelman JG, Huisman TH, et al: Dutch beta°-thalassemia: a 10 kilobase DNA deletion associated with significant gamma-chain production. Br J Haematol 1984; 56:339.

56. Oggiano L, Pirastu M, et al: Molecular characterization of a normal Hb A_2 beta-thalassemia determinant in a Sardinian family. Br J Haematol 1987; 67:225.

57. Fosburg MT, Nathan DG: Treatment of Cooley's anemia. Blood 1990; 76:435.

58. Fink H: Transfusion hemochromatosis in Cooley's anemia. Ann N Y Acad Sci 1964; 119:680.

59. Engle MA: Cardiac involvement in Cooley's anemia. Ann N Y Acad Sci 1964; 119:694.

60. Hershko C, Weatherall DJ: Iron-chelating therapy. Crit Rev Clin Lab Sci 1988; 26:303.

61. Matthew R, Brain M, et al: Thalassemia. *In* Brain MC, Carbone PP (eds): Current Therapy in Hematology/Oncology-3. Philadelphia: BC Decker, 1988.

62. Lucarelli G, Galimberti M, et al: Bone marrow transplantation in patients with thalassemia. N Engl J Med 1990; 322:417.

63. Perrine SP, Miller BA, et al: Sodium butyrate enhances fetal globin gene expression in erythroid progenitors of patients with Hb SS and β thalassemia. Blood 1989; 74:454.

64. Friedmann T: Progress toward human gene therapy. Science 1989; 224:1275.

65. Wainscoat JS, Thein SL, et al: Thalassemia intermedia. Blood Rev 1987; 1:273.

66. Kanavakio K, Wainscoat JS, et al: The interaction of alpha thalassemia with beta thalassemia. Br J Haematol 1982; 52:465.

67. Kulozik AE, Thein SL, et al: Thalassemia intermedia: interaction of the triple alpha-globin gene arrangement and heterozygous beta-thalassemia. Br J Haematol 1987; 66:109.

68. Cai SP, Chang CA, et al: Rapid prenatal diagnosis of beta thalassemia using DNA amplification and nonradioactive probes. Blood 1989; 73:372.

69. Kan YW, Forget BG, et al: Gamma-beta thalassemia: a cause of hemolytic disease of newborns. N Engl J Med 1972; 286:129.

70. Wood WG, Clegg JB, Weatherall DJ: Hereditary persistence of fetal haemoglobin (HPFH) and $\delta\beta$ thalassemia. Br J Haematol 1979; 42:509.

71. Gilman JG, Mishima NEA: Upstream promoter mutation associated with a modest elevation of fetal hemoglobin expression in human adults. Blood 1988; 72:78.

72. Kulozik AE, Thein SJ, et al: Thalassemic intermedia: interaction of the triple alpha globin gene arrangement and heterozygous beta-thalassemia. Br J Haematol 1987; 66:109.

73. Rigas DA, Koler RD: Decreased erythrocyte survival in hemoglobin H disease as a result of the abnormal properties of hemoglobin H: The benefit of splenectomy. Blood 1961; 18:1.

74. Weatherall DJ, Higgs DR, Bunch C, et al: Hemoglobin H disease and mental retardation; a new syndrome or a remarkable coincidence? N Engl J Med 1981; 305:607.

75. Higg DR, Wood WG, Barton C, Weatherall DJ: Clinical features and molecular analysis of acquired hemoglobin H disease. Am J Med 1983; 75:1813.

76. Weatherall DJ, Clegg JB, et al: The hemoglobin constitution of infants with haemoglobin Bart's hydrops foetalis syndrome. Br J Haematol 1970; 18:357.

77. Steinberg MH, Adams JG, et al: Alpha thalassemia in adults with sickle cell trait. Br J Haematol 1975; 30:3.

78. Platt OS, Dover GJ: Sickle cell disease. *In* Nathan DG, Oski FA (eds): Hematology of Infancy and Childhood, 4th ed. Philadelphia: WB Saunders, 1993.

79. Rowley PT, Fisher L, Lipkin M: Screening and genetic counseling for beta thalassemia trait. Am J Hum Genet 1979; 31:781.

80. LeCrone CN: Anemias of abnormal globin development-thalassemias. *In* Lotspeich-Steininger CA, Stiene-Martin EA, Koepke JA, (eds): Clinical Hematology. Philadelphia: JB Lippincott, 1992.

81. Jones JA, Broszeit HK, Le Crone CN, Detter JC: An improved method for detection of red cell hemoglobin H inclusions. Am J Med Tech 1981; 47:94.

82. Brown BA: Special hematology procedures. *In* Brown BA (ed): Hematology: Principles and Procedures, 6th ed. Philadelphia: Lea & Feiger, 1993.

83. Hamilton SR, Miller ME, Jessop M, et al: Comparison of microchromatography and electrophoresis with elution of hemoglobin (Hb A_2) quantitation. Am J Clin Pathol 1979; 71:388.

84. National Committee For Clinical Laboratory Standards: Solubility test for confirming the presence of sickling hemoglobins: approved standard (NCCLS Publication H10-A). Villanova, PA: NCCLS, 1986.

85. Weatherall DJ: The thalassemias. *In* Weatherall DJ (ed): Methods in Hematology, Vol. 6. New York: Churchill Livingstone, 1983.

86. Kazazian HH, Boehm CD: Molecular basis and prenatal diagnosis of β-thalassemia. Blood 1988; 72:1107.

87. Harrison DR: Hemolytic anemias: intracorpuscular defects: thalassemia. *In* Harmening DM (ed): Clinical Hematology and Fundamentals of Hemostasis, 2nd ed. Philadelphia: FA Davis, 1992.

88. Pearson HA, O'Brien RR, et al: Screening for thalassemia trait by electronic measurement of mean corpuscular volume (MCV). N Engl J Med 1973; 288:35.

89. Flynn MM, Reppon TS, et al: Limitation of red blood cell distribution with (RDW) in evaluation of microcytosis. Am J Clin Pathol 1986, 85:445.

90. Meloni T, Gallisai D, et al: Free erythrocyte porphyrin (FEP) in the diagnosis of beta thalassemia trait and iron deficiency anemia. Haematologica 1982; 67:34.

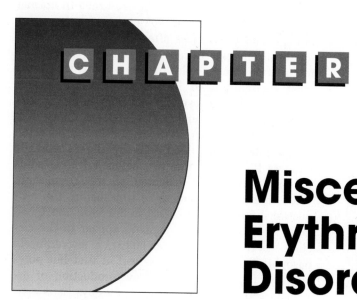

CHAPTER 19

Miscellaneous Erythrocyte Disorders

Karen Clark and Teresa Hippel

Outline

Objectives

AFTER COMPLETION OF THIS CHAPTER, THE READER WILL BE ABLE TO

1. Discuss the pathophysiology of anemia due to acute blood loss.
2. List the characteristics of anemia due to chronic renal failure.
3. Discuss the pathophysiology or mechanisms of anemia caused by chronic renal failure.
4. Discuss treatment of anemia due to chronic renal failure.
5. List hormone deficiencies that may lead to anemia.
6. Discuss characteristics of anemia due to viral infections.
7. Discuss the effects of azidothymidine (AZT) on erythrocytes.
8. Define chronic disease.
9. List the characteristics of anemia caused by chronic disease.
10. Differentiate anemias resulting from chronic disease from other hypochromic, microcytic anemias.
11. Discuss mechanisms of anemias caused by chronic disease.
12. List characteristics of anemia associated with liver disease.
13. Explain the mechanism that results in anemia caused by alcoholism.

The anemias discussed in this chapter are those that have multiple etiologies, questionable or unknown etiologies, and those for which there was no "clear fit" in another chapter.

ACUTE BLOOD LOSS ANEMIA

Acute blood loss anemia occurs when sufficient damage causes red blood cells to escape from intravascular spaces. With severe blood loss, the decreasing blood volume leads to cardiovascular collapse, shock, and death. The sudden depletion of the total blood volume is the important finding in this situation rather than the loss of circulating red blood cells. If the blood loss is more gradual, blood volume may be restored by expanding plasma volume; however, the depletion of the circulating red blood cell mass may impair oxygen delivery to the tissues. To try to compensate for the severe or gradual blood loss, adjustments have to be made in blood volume, red blood cell production, oxygen transport of red blood cells, and cardiovascular dynamics.

CLINICAL FEATURES

A normal individual may lose up to 20% of total blood volume without developing signs or symptoms of anemia or cardiovascular problems. The hematocrit may not reflect the quantity of blood lost. The physician uses clinical signs and symptoms to estimate the depletion of blood volume. If the blood loss exceeds 20%, there are signs of cardiovascular stress (e.g., tachycardia with exercise or hypotension when standing). If the blood loss exceeds 30–40%, there is gradual onset of shock whereby the patient becomes immobile, needs air, and has a rapid pulse and cold skin. With greater than 50% blood loss there is a high risk of death.[1]

REPLACEMENT THERAPY FOR VOLUME LOSS

In managing a patient with acute blood loss, it is first necessary to maintain an adequate blood volume and to prevent shock. Intravenous infusion of electrolyte solutions (isotonic saline, Ringer's lactate, crystalloid solution) and solutions of plasma protein and albumin are given to restore blood volume and circulation. The use of whole blood to treat acute blood loss is discouraged and should be reserved only for massive hemorrhage where there is tissue hypoxia caused by low red blood cell mass.[1]

REPLACEMENT THERAPY FOR RED CELL LOSS

When total blood volume has returned to normal by expansion of plasma volume, the depletion of the red blood cell mass after blood loss may then manifest anemia. Because there is no reserve of mature red blood cells, oxygen supply to tissues must be maintained by adjusting cardiovascular dynamics. Plasma levels of erythropoietin increase within 6 hours after anemia appears. This hormone is then responsible for the increase in the production of red blood cells by the marrow. It requires 2–5 days, however, before effective adult red blood cells are delivered to the circulation. Thus there is a considerable time before the production of red blood cells can increase the blood mass and reticulocytes begin to appear in the circulation. In the peripheral smear, a few diffusely basophilic cells may be observed at first but polychromasia increases as marrow production of erythroid cells increases. After 8–10 days, it is estimated that marrow production and increased reticulocyte production are fully functional. If the erythropoietin response is normal, and the amount of iron available to the erythroid marrow determines that the level of marrow production stores remain diminished, the patient is unable to increase red blood cell production and the marrow response is severely impaired. The presence of iron deficiency may then be noted. When iron is recovered from degraded hemoglobin after large amounts of red blood cells have been destroyed, marrow production proceeds rapidly because of return of iron to erythroid marrow. Marrow production of erythroid elements may be three times normal or greater with improved iron delivery. Supplements of oral iron may be given but should be reserved for those situations where a rapid response is necessary, such as in preparation for surgery or in prolonged hemorrhage.

Blood transfusion should be reserved for situations in which normal marrow response and iron supplements are insufficient to maintain an adequate red blood cell mass or when an acute situation necessitates an immediate response.

ANEMIA OF CHRONIC RENAL FAILURE

Damage to the erythropoietin-generating apparatus in the kidney can cause an anemia caused by decreased erythropoietin stimulation. The association of anemia with renal failure was first documented by Richard Bright more than 150 years ago. The nature of this anemia was poorly understood until Erslev proved that erythropoietin was the hormone that regulates erythropoiesis.[2] L.O. Jacobson then demonstrated that erythropoietin originated in the kidney.[3]

Anemia resulting from renal disease can best be categorized as hypoproliferative. The diagnosis of a hypoproliferative anemia can be based on the following characteristics: the red blood cells are normocytic and normochromic; the reticulocyte count, when corrected for the degree of anemia, is usually less than two times normal; the circulating red blood cells are often irregular in shape (burr cells or echinocytes); the erythroid:myeloid (E:M) ratio in the bone marrow is slightly decreased or normal; renal insufficiency is present (as defined by a serum creatinine above 2–3 mg/dL); and serum erythropoietin levels, measured by radioimmunoassay, are generally within a normal range.[4]

The pathophysiology of this anemia has been postulated by four mechanisms. These include erythropoietin deficiency,[5] hemolysis,[6] retained inhibitors or toxic metabolites that inhibit erythropoiesis,[7] and blood loss.

Erythroid colony-forming units (CFU-E) are under the control of the hormone erythropoietin. This hormone causes the proliferation and maturation of the red blood cells. Erythropoietin's action on the bone marrow, however, is disrupted by renal disease and results in a submaximal response. This is not surprising because 90% of the hormone is produced in the kidney and only 10% in the liver.[8]

Red blood cell hemolysis, although mild, may contribute to the anemia. Radioisotopic studies have proved the presence of mild hemolysis. Studies have suggested that some intravascular substance retained in patients with advanced renal failure shortened red blood cell survival; when red blood cells from a patient with advanced renal failure are infused into a normal subject, red blood cell life span is restored to normal.[9]

Observations made from the care of dialysis patients have provided indirect support for the existence of inhibitors or toxic factors that accumulate in the sera of uremic patients. These toxic factors are removed in part by dialysis therapy. These factors have been proposed to be parathyroid hormone, polyamines, and a protein with a relative mass of more than 1500 D.[10]

Polyamines are organic cations that play a role in normal cellular proliferation and differentiation. A study performed by J.W. Fisher demonstrated that a polyamine, putrescine, was capable of inhibiting noncompetitively the biologic activity of erythropoietin at the cellular level. Elevated levels of polyamines may inhibit erythropoiesis by binding irreversibly to a site on erythroid cells at the level of the bone marrow and block the response of erythropoietin. Polyamines may also interact with the enzyme at the chromosomal level and affect the expression of genes.[10]

Patients with progressive renal failure can have significant blood loss caused by platelet dysfunction, which prolongs the bleeding time. Several mechanisms can explain this platelet dysfunction: decreased platelet factor 3 activity, decreased platelet levels of thromboxane A_2, and increase in prostacyclin (an inhibitor of platelet aggregation derived from the vascular endothelium), and suboptimal Factor VIII: von Willebrand complex activity.[4]

Treatment of anemia caused by renal failure has included administration of androgens and transfusions if severe hypoxic symptoms occur. Patients who are on dialysis are also given folic acid and iron to help replenish loss resulting from the dialysis. Androgens can improve the anemia by stimulating the erythroid marrow or possibly by stimulating renal or liver erythropoietin production.[4]

ENDOCRINE DISORDER ANEMIA

In addition to erythropoietin, other hormones participate in the regulation of erythropoiesis. Some hormones influence erythropoietin production indirectly by affecting oxygen equilibrium. Hormones may also affect enzymes and protein synthesis so that the synthesis of hemoglobin and the production of red cells are affected. The hormones most often associated with anemia of endocrine disorders are those of the pituitary and thyroid glands, adrenal cortex, and gonads.

Pituitary

Patients with hypopituitarism or pituitary ablation develop a normochromic, normocytic anemia. The pituitary is responsible for the secretion of adenohypophysial hormones. These hormones include the thyroid-stimulating hormone and gonadotropins, which control the production of androgens. Replacement therapy of the thyroid hormone and androgens, along with steroid therapy, usually reverses the anemia.

Thyroid

Myxedema or other hypothyroid disorders decrease erythropoiesis by decreasing the demand for oxygen. In hypothyroidism, the red cell life span is normal, and ferrokinetics indicates hypoactive but effective marrow function. The anemia in hypothyroid patients is mild to moderate, with a hemoglobin concentration less than 8–9 g/dL. Although this anemia is normocytic, normochromic, it can be complicated by nutritional deficiencies of iron, vitamin B_{12}, and folic acid. A microcytic, hypochromic anemia may be observed as a result of iron deficiency resulting from menorrhagia, achlorhydria, or intestinal malabsorption of iron.

Patients with hyperthyroidism have an above normal erythroid activity of the marrow caused by increased erythropoiesis, in turn caused by increased demand for oxygen. These subjects, however, have an increase in plasma volume that helps keep the hematocrit within normal limits.

Adrenal Cortex

The adrenal cortex secretes several hormones called corticosteroids. Insufficiency of these hormones, especially the glucocorticoids, may result in a mild normocytic, normochromic anemia. The cause of this anemia is not known.

Gonads

Androgens are a group of hormones that exert profound influence on the male genital tract. They also are associated with the development and maintenance of secondary male sex characteristics. They are secreted by the adrenals, the testes, and the ovaries. The effect of androgens can be seen in the difference in hemoglobin concentrations between men and women. Androgens influence erythropoiesis by promoting stimulation of the bone marrow along with erythropoietin and by increasing the production of erythropoietin.

Patients with refractory anemia have been treated with androgens because the androgens are potent stimulators of red blood cell production. A mild normocytic, normochromic anemia develops in the mature male with gonadal hypofunction. This can also be seen in elderly men and boys. The administration of androgens usually reverses this condition.

ANEMIA OF VIRAL INFECTIONS

It is well documented that viral infections can induce white blood cell changes. The changes in red blood cells are not so clearly defined. Confusion enters when patients with prior evidence of normal iron status have changes induced by the viral process that are clinically indistinguishable from iron deficiency.

Measles

A study performed by Olivares and colleagues used the measles vaccine as a model to define the hematologic changes during a mild viral infection.

Ninety-three infants who were immunized with live attenuated measles virus were found to have hemoglobin concentrations decreased significantly by days 9 and 14. The reticulocyte production index was found to be decreased at 9 days but increased slightly after 30, heralding the recovery of hemoglobin levels after the decrease induced by the infection. No changes were detected in the mean corpuscular volume (MCV), total iron-binding capacity, and free erythrocyte protoporphyrin. Iron and transferrin saturation values were found to be decreased.[11]

The origin of this anemia is likely multifactorial. Iron sequestration in the monocyte/macrophage system correlates with decreased serum iron concentration and increased serum ferritin levels. Decreased iron availability for erythropoiesis coupled with the decrease of iron absorption in febrile persons could cause a decrease in red cell production.

Parvovirus B19

Another virus that has been well studied is parvovirus B19. Cossart in 1975 discovered a parvovirus-like particle in a sample encoded B19 while searching for a possible viral agent of hepatitis B.[12] This virus is now known to be the causative agent responsible for several aplastic crises in diverse chronic hemolytic anemias, compensated hemolytic processes, and certain hematopoietically unstable situations. A variety of cells can be invaded by B19 but it has a marked proclivity for invading erythroid precursors. Studies show a reticulocytopenia and a slight drop in the hemoglobin. Although this infection can be life-threatening with the formation of adequate antibodies, reticulocytes re-emerge in 7 to 14 days and the bone marrow is completely reactivated by 3 weeks. Administration of intravenous gamma globulin can evoke a dramatic correction of the anemia.[13]

Acquired Immune Deficiency Syndrome

The etiologic agent of acquired immune deficiency syndrome (AIDS) is linked to the human immunodeficiency virus (HIV). A hallmark finding in AIDS is the decrease in CD4-T lymphocytes, as well as decreases in red cell counts.

Anemia that develops in AIDS patients suggests that it is a hypoproliferative anemia caused by the low reticulocyte response. The causes of this anemia may be considered multifactorial owing to nutritional factors, infections, tumors, immunologic impairment, cytokine-induced suppression, or inhibition of progenitor cells. Any of these may contribute to inadequate erythropoiesis.

Anemia is usually normocytic, normochromic. Several studies have shown that between 70 and 95% of AIDS patients are anemic at presentation, with mean hemoglobin levels ranging between 9.7 and 11.7 g/dL.[14]

Unlike the anemia caused by other viral infections that induce changes indistinguishable from iron deficiency, microcytosis is an uncommon finding in the anemia of AIDS patients.[15] Patients with advanced HIV disease will have at least mild changes in red blood cell size and shape, reflected by an increased red blood cell distribution width. Macrocytosis is rarely seen in the non-azidothymidine (AZT) treated patients; macrocytosis may be seen, however, in up to 70% of patients with a mean corpuscular volume (MCV) exceeding 110 fL after 2 weeks of AZT therapy.[16]

ANEMIA OF CHRONIC DISEASE

Definition

Anemia of chronic disease (ACD) is the term used for anemia associated with chronic infection, inflammation, or malignancy. ACD is second only to iron deficiency anemia (IDA) as the most common cause of anemia.[17]

Characteristics of ACD include

1. Mild to moderate hypoproliferative anemia[18]
   a. Hematocrit, 0.30–0.40 L/L
   b. Reticulocyte count decreased
   c. Indices (normocytic, normochromic [usually] and microcytic, hypochromic [occasionally])
   d. Serum iron level decreased
   e. Total iron-binding capacity decreased
   f. Tissue iron stores normal to increased
   g. Serum ferritin level increased
2. Presence of "acute phase" reactants[17]
   a. Fibrinogen
   b. Ceruloplasmin
   c. Haptoglobin
   d. Complement C3
   e. C-reactive protein
   f. Amyloid A protein
   g. Increased white blood cell count
   h. Increased erythrocyte sedimentation rate (ESR)

Differentiation

Patients with a slightly decreased MCV (78–80 fL) and a low total-iron-binding capacity (TIBC) may be difficult to distinguish from those with IDA. Treatment of ACD with iron is not helpful and may be harmful;[17] therefore, it is important to differentiate this anemia from IDA. A bone

marrow iron stain (Prussian blue) is most useful; patients with ACD have normal to increased stores, whereas those with IDA demonstrate reduced iron stores. Serum ferritin level correlates well with marrow iron stores and can be used as an alternative test. Serum ferritin levels, however, are increased in inflammation, leukemias, and in liver disease; they may mask a coexisting IDA (see Table 16–2).

Mechanisms

Several mechanisms have been proposed to explain ACD. These include

Hemolysis[18]
Reduced availability of iron in the monocyte/macrocyte system caused by the inflammatory response[18]
Decreased erythropoietin production[18]
Inhibited erythroid colony formation by interleukin-1[18]

Interleukin-1 is a polypeptide produced by the monocyte/macrophage system and it is directly related to many of the findings in ACD. Some effects of interleukin-1 are

Fever[17]
Neutrophilic leukocytosis[17]
Production of acute phase reactants[17]
Release of lactoferrin (iron-binding protein)[17]
Inhibition of erythropoietin production[17]

Research continues to further define the role that interleukin-1, as well as other monokines and lymphokines, play in the development and treatment of ACD.

Treatment

Only treatment of the underlying disease will affect the anemia of chronic disease. The degree of anemia present is related to the severity of the underlying disease. If the condition worsens, or remains severe for a long period, the anemia is more pronounced and may require transfusion. When the underlying disease is treated, the patient's hematologic status may improve.

ANEMIA ASSOCIATED WITH LIVER DISEASE

The anemia associated with liver disease may present as ACD with normocytic, normochromic indices, or as a macrocytic anemia (MCV of 110–115 fL) that is not caused by folate or vitamin B_{12} deficiency. An IDA caused by blood loss may also be present.

The macrocytes in liver disease are round, not the oval macrocytes characteristically found in megaloblastic anemia. The bone marrow of a patient with liver disease does not demonstrate megaloblastic changes (see Chapter 16). This macrocytic anemia does not respond to vitamin B_{12} nor to folate therapy.

Morphologically, codocytes or target cells are often present. These thin red cells with a "bull's eye" appearance are deformed because the red blood cell membrane is altered by changes in the composition of plasma. In liver disease, plasma cholesterol and phospholipids are increased and the reticulocyte count is often increased.

Another morphologic finding in patients with severe liver disease is the presence of acanthocytes. Hemolytic anemia may be present because the red blood cell membranes are so rigid that they are destroyed by the reticuloendothelial system (RES). Acanthocytes correlate with a poor prognosis.[19]

Patients with liver disease should be evaluated for gastrointestinal blood loss and resultant iron deficiency, folate and vitamin B_{12} deficiencies, hypoproteinemia, alcohol-related deficiencies, bone marrow suppression, viral suppression of erythropoiesis, and coagulopathies due to liver damage.[20]

ANEMIA CAUSED BY ALCOHOLISM

ACD is common in alcoholics; however, chronic disease is seldom the only cause of anemia in alcoholism. Hemolytic anemias and megaloblastic anemias are also seen. A hemolytic anemia occurs primarily because the red blood cells (which have increased cholesterol) have decreased deformability and are removed by, or torn as they pass through, the spleen. Megaloblastic anemia probably results from a folate deficiency caused by malnutrition and the interference of ethanol with folate metabolism. Reticulocytosis can be suppressed by ethanol ingestion; in alcoholic patients, the withdrawal of alcohol increases the reticulocyte count.[19]

SUMMARY

The anemias discussed in this chapter are those that have multiple etiologies, unknown or questionable etiologies, and those that do not clearly fit into another category.

Anemia caused by chronic renal failure is a normocytic, normochromic, hypoproliferative anemia that often demonstrates echinocytes on the peripheral blood smear. Pathophysiologies responsible for this anemia include erythropoietin deficiency, hemolysis, retained inhibitors or toxic metabolites that inhibit erythropoiesis, and blood loss.

Hormones associated with anemia of endocrine disorders include those of the pituitary and thyroid glands, adrenal cortex, and gonads. Most of these anemias are normocytic, normochromic.

Changes in erythrocytes caused by a virus are not as clearly defined as those in leukocytes. Parvovirus has been shown to cause aplastic crises. HIV causes a normocytic, normochromic, hypoproliferative anemia. When AZT is administered, up to 70% of AIDS patients will show increased MCVs.

The phrase *anemia of chronic disease* refers to anemias caused by chronic infection, inflammation, or malignancy. ACD is the second most common cause of anemia; IDA is first. ACD is most often normocytic, normochromic, but may be microcytic, hypochromic and requires differentiation from IDA. Anemia of chronic disease may be caused by hemolysis, reduced availability of iron in the monocyte/macrophage system, decreased erythropoietin levels, and inhibited erythroid colony formation by interleukin-1.

Anemia associated with liver disease may be either normocytic, normochromic or macrocytic and normochromic. Vitamin B_{12} and folate levels are normal. Macrocytes are round, not oval as they are in pernicious anemia. Codocytes may be present.

Alcoholism results in an anemia caused by chronic disease, hemolysis, folate deficiency, malnutrition, or a combination of several of these.

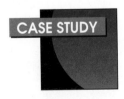
CASE STUDY

A 79-year-old woman with a history of chronic renal failure and multiple metastases from adenocarcinoma of the lung was admitted to the hospital. She had had a fluctuating mental status and now had become lethargic. On admission, her laboratory results revealed the following:

Hematology

WBC: 9.7×10^9/L
RBC: 3.85×10^{12}/L
Hemoglobin: 11.6 g/dL
Hematocrit: 0.35 L/L
Mean corpuscular volume: 90.9 fL

Chemistry

Urea nitrogen: 31 mg/dL
Creatinine: 7.7 mg/dL
Lactic dehydrogenase: 269 u/L
Creatine kinase: 20 u/L
Blood urea nitrogen/creatinine ratio: 4

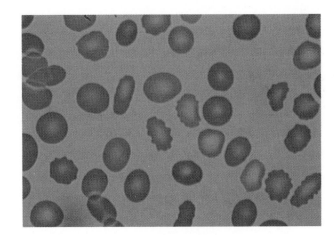

Figure 19–1 Peripheral blood smear from patient in case study. Note the echinocytes characteristic of chronic renal failure.

Mean corpuscular hemoglobin:
30.1 pg
Mean corpuscular hemoglobin concentration: 33.1 g/dL
Red blood cell distribution width:
18.8
Platelet count: $46.0 \times 10^9/L$

Coagulase negative *staphylococcus* was recovered from blood cultures drawn at the time of admission. Blood cultures drawn the next day were negative. A CT scan was performed to rule out a left cerebral infarction occurring from a hypercoagulable state or possibly carcinomatous meningitis. The CT scan revealed no metastatic disease but found evidence of inflammatory disease.

Her admission CBC revealed a mild anemia with red blood cell morphology as shown in Figure 19–1.

1. What are the characteristic erythrocytes seen in Figure 19–1?

2. Give several mechanisms for the anemia in this patient.

References

1. Hillman RS: Erythrocyte disorders: anemias due to acute blood loss. *In* Williams WJ, Beutler E, Ersler AJ, Lichtman MA (eds): Hematology; 4th ed. New York: McGraw-Hill, 1990:700–704.

2. Erslev AJ: Humoral regulation of red blood cell production. Blood 1953; 8:349–387.

3. Jacobson LO, Goldwasser E, Fried W, Plzak L: Role of the kidney in erythropoiesis. Nature 1957; 179:633–634.

4. Eschbach JW: The anemia of chronic renal failure: pathophysiology and the effects of recombinant erythropoietin. Kidney Int 1989; 35:134–148.

5. Pavlovic-Kentera V, Clemons GK, Djukanovic L, Biljanovoic-Paunovic L: Erythropoietin and anemia in chronic renal failure. Exp Hematol 1987; 15:785–789.

6. Shaw AG: Hemolysis in chronic renal failure. Br Med J 1967; 213–244.

7. Kushner DS, Beckman BS, Fisher JW: Do polyamines play a role in the pathogenesis of the anemia of end-stage renal disease? Kidney Int 1989; 36:171–174.

8. Fried W: The liver as a source of extrarenal erythropoietin production. Blood 1973; 40:671–677.

9. Chaplin H, Mollison PL: Red cell life-span in nephritis and in hepatic cirrhosis. Clin Sci 1953; 40:671–677.

10. Kushner DS, Beckman BS, Fisher JW: Polyamines in the anemia of end-stage renal disease. Kidney Int 1991; 39:725–732.

11. Olivares M, Walter T, Osorio M, et al: Anemia of a mild viral infection: the measles vaccine as a model. Pediatrics 1989; 84:851–855.

12. Cossart YE, Field AM, Cant B, Widdows D: Parvovirus-like particles in human sera. Lancet 1975; 1:72–73.

13. Kurtzman G, Frickhofen N, Kimball J, et al: Pure red cell aplasia of 10 years' duration due to persistent parvovirus B19 infection and its cure with immunoglobulin therapy. N Engl J Med 1989; 321:519–523.

14. Weber JN, Walker D, Engelkins M, et al: The value of hematologic screening for AIDS in an at-risk population. Genitourin Med 1985; 61:325–329.

15. Castella A, Croxson TS, Mildvan D, et al: The bone marrow in AIDS: A histologic, hematologic and microbiologic study. Am J Clin Pathol 1985; 84:425.

16. Richman DD, Fischl MA, Grieco MH, et al: The toxicity of azidothymidine (AZT) in the treatment of patients with AIDS and AIDS-related complex. N Engl J Med 1987; 317:192.

17. Lee GR: The anemia of chronic disease. Semin Hematol 1983; 20:60–80.

18. Roodman GD: Mechanisms of erythroid suppression in the anemia of chronic disease. Blood Cell. 1987; 13:171–184.

19. Cooper R: Hemolytic syndromes and red cell membrane abnormalities in liver diseases. Semin Hematol 1980; 17:103.

20. Gwaltney-Krause S: Anemias associated with other disorders. *In* Harmening DM (ed): Clinical Hematology and Fundamentals of Hemostasis, 2nd ed. Philadelphia: FA Davis, 1992:224–237.

PART V

Hemato-pathology: Leukocyte Disorders and Ancillary Studies

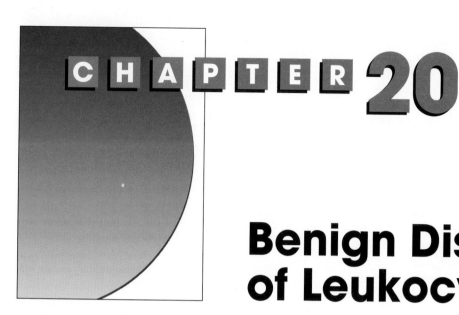

CHAPTER 20

Benign Disorders of Leukocytes

Susan J. Leclair

Outline

Objectives

AFTER COMPLETION OF THIS CHAPTER, THE READER WILL BE ABLE TO

1. Compare and contrast nonmalignant changes in granulocytes, using criteria such as method of acquisition, location, potential cellular dysfunction, and clinical significance.
2. Explain the biochemical or ultrastructural origins (if known) for each of the changes seen in granulocytes.
3. Correlate the presence of nonmalignant granulocytic changes with possible diagnoses or prognoses.
4. List the nonmalignant morphologic changes observed in monocytes and macrophages.
5. Correlate the presence of nonmalignant lymphocytic changes with possible diagnoses or prognoses.
6. Compare and contrast nonmalignant changes in lymphocytes, using criteria such as method of acquisition, location, potential cellular dysfunction, and clinical significance.
7. Explain the biochemical or ultrastructural origins (if known) for each of the morphologic changes seen in lymphocytes.

Benign disorders of leukocytes are unusual inherited or acquired alterations that do not possess the characteristics of dysplasia or malignancy. Although many of the inherited conditions may be asymptomatic and of interest only to morphologists, others are life-threatening. Acquired changes are seen with changes in response to a specific set of circumstances and are interpreted as indicators of those disease states. These conditions can be distinguished by many different means such as mode of transmission (inherited or acquired), frequency (common or rare), location (nuclear or cytoplasmic), or microscopic manifestation (morphologic or nonmorphologic). An assumption common to each of these separation methods is comparison with its opposite manifestation rather than the presence of a characteristic unique to a cell type. While providing these typical descriptors, each discussion of an unusual cellular manifestation includes a description of the underlying structural or functional aberration.

NUCLEAR/MORPHOLOGIC ALTERATIONS OF GRANULOCYTES

Pelger-Huët Anomaly

A common (1/6000) inherited nuclear aberration found in granulocytes is hyposegmentation of the nucleus. Known as the Pelger-Huët anomaly,[1] it is clinically insignificant because there is no loss of cellular function. Inherited through autosomal dominance, the keys to identification are (1) nuclei that are round, oval, or bilobed with a characteristic pinched or pince-nez appearance; (2) clumping of the chromatin is overly mature for the overall shape of the nucleus; and (3) most cells look alike

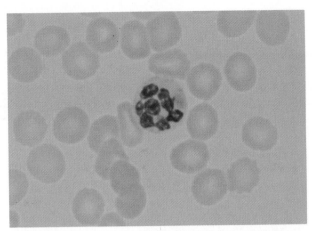

Figure 20–2 Megaloblastic hypersegmentation. Usually consisting of more than five lobes, these polymorphonuclear neutrophils have twisted and distorted nuclei, which sometimes appear rounded or swollen.

(Fig. 20–1). The rare homozygote has rounded nuclei. Inexperienced morphologists may incorrectly report these cells as myelocytes, metamyelocytes, or bands. An appropriate procedure would be to report these cells as mature cells, remarking on the possibility of the Pelger-Huët anomaly. It is usually an incidental finding, and so there is a need to differentiate these cells from pseudo–Pelger-Huët cells. Pseudo–Pelger-Huët cells are acquired phenomena that may be clinically significant. These cells have nuclei that are less dense than those of normal cells or true Pelger-Huët cells, and they may have hypogranular cytoplasm. Pseudo–Pelger-Huët cells are found in high-stress situations (such as burns, drug reactions, and infections), myelodysplastic syndromes, chronic granulocytic leukemia, and acute leukemia (see Chapter 23).

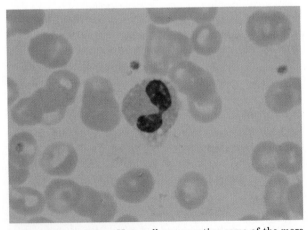

Figure 20–1 Pelger-Huët cell, representing some of the more important features of such cells: bilobed appearance, incomplete formation of the nuclear segment, and intensely dense heterochromatin content of the nucleus.

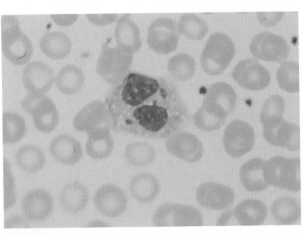

Figure 20–3 Twinning. This type of mirror image is seen in a variety of conditions and may or may not be significant.

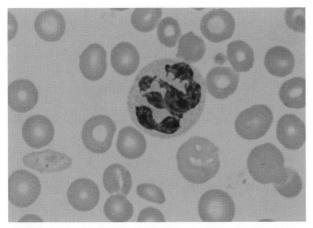

Figure 20-4 Nuclear extrusions. Although also hypersegmented, the nucleus shows multiple extrusions of nuclear material that are not drumsticks but are usually singular and are believed to be the inactivated X chromosome found frequently in women.

Hereditary Hypersegmentation

Hereditary hypersegmentation of granulocyte nuclei, inherited through autosomal dominance, is clinically insignificant. This manifestation must be distinguished from the hypersegmentation seen in the megaloblastic anemias (vitamin B_{12} or folate deficiency or point mutations affecting DNA replication) (Fig. 20-2) and from acquired hypersegmentation (also known as twinning deformity). Twinning is clinically significant in stress situations, malignancies, and treatment with some oncologic regimens[2] (Fig. 20-3).

Less common than hyposegmentation or hypersegmentation, increases in drumstick or small extrusions of nuclear material may be found in persons with trisomy of group E chromosomes, with extra "X" chromosomes, or with other aneuploidy states (Fig. 20-4).

CYTOPLASMIC/MORPHOLOGIC ALTERATIONS OF GRANULOCYTES

Alder-Reilly Anomaly

Alder-Reilly anomaly[1] may be transmitted as a possible recessive disorder in which decreased mucopolysaccharide degradation results in deposition of mucopolysaccharides (lipids) in the cytoplasm of most, if not all, cells. When stained, these deposits appear as metachromatic (deep purple to lilac) granules. The penetrance of this inheritance can range from abnormal granulation found only in neutrophils to abnormal granulation in all white blood cells. In the extreme manifestation, eosinophils and basophils may possess highly unusual granulation, which makes it difficult to distinguish between them.[3]

Chédiak-Higashi Syndrome

Chédiak-Higashi syndrome is a rare autosomal recessive state in which abnormally large peroxidase-positive lysosomes[4] are seen in most cells of the body. This fusion of granules is seen in many sites, such as melanosomes, the disturbance of which results in albinism. Apparently, uncontrolled activity of the granular membrane creates large primary, secondary, and mixed primary/secondary granules[5] (Fig. 20-5). An increased rate of precursor cell death in the marrow causes moderate peripheral blood neutropenia, which, when taken into consideration with the granulocyte's normal phagocytosis but prolonged inefficient bactericidal function, seems to explain the increased susceptibility to infections.[6] Affected patients also demonstrate bleeding problems caused by thrombocytopenia and abnormal platelets with large granules, resulting in increased bleeding time, decreased clot retraction, a positive result of a tourniquet test, and small vessel bleeding.[7] The syndrome progresses through peripheral neuropathy, pancytopenia, systemic infections associated with lymphocytic proliferation, hepatosplenomegaly, and lymphadenopathy to death.[8]

May-Hegglin Anomaly

The May-Hegglin anomaly is a rare autosomal dominant condition in which patients are at risk for infections and bleeding. This anomaly is characterized by the presence of large, Döhle body–like formations (described in the section on acquired alterations) in all cells, thrombocytopenia, and giant platelets with abnormal platelet function and lifespan. The rods seen in the May-Hegglin anomaly are similar to Döhle bodies in that they are a combination of rods and granules which are ribo-

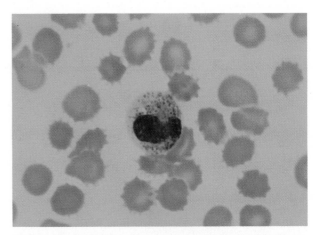

Figure 20-5 Chédiak-Higashi syndrome. Notice that the cytoplasm contains Döhle bodies, and the granules are both larger in size and fewer in number than normal.

Table 20-1. INHERITED GRANULOCYTE ALTERATIONS AND ANOMALIES*
Nucleus Pelger-Huët anomaly Hereditary hypersegmentation
Cytoplasm Chédiak-Higashi syndrome May-Hegglin anomaly Alder-Reilly granulation

* Inherited morphologic anomalies of granulocytes occur in both the nucleus and cytoplasm. Both of the inherited nuclear anomalies are without clinical significance and need only be differentiated from similar manifestations that are both acquired and significant. Inherited morphologic cytoplasmic anomalies are always significant.

somal in origin; however, they tend to be larger and more spindle-shaped than oval, are permanent features of the cells, and can be found in monocytes and lymphocytes as well.[9] The inherited granulocyte alterations and anomalies are summarized in Table 20-1.

Toxic Granulation

The acquired demonstration of abnormally large or dominant primary granules is called toxic granulation and is a stress response to infection or inflammation. Cellular stimulation, particularly in the younger cells, may cause alteration in the membrane, which in turn causes granules to appear visibly larger and darker with the common staining procedures. Toxic granulation is clinically significant because it appears to reflect a poorer prognosis[10] (Fig. 20-6). Artifactual heavy granulation caused by poor staining is seen homogeneously spread within each cell and in all granulocytes, whereas toxic granulation is unevenly spread throughout the cytoplasm of certain cells.

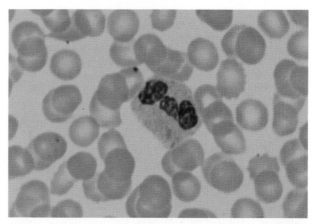

Figure 20-7 May-Hegglin anomaly. Although similar in structure to Döhle bodies that are realigned RNA segments found in occasional cells in patients experiencing bacterial or other stress, the homogeneously blue inclusion seen in the cytoplasm of this cell is found in every white blood cell; however, electron microscopic techniques are usually needed for visualizing this phenomenon.

Döhle Bodies

Döhle bodies develop in the cytoplasm of granulocytes of patients with infections or in stress states, are round to oval, are approximately 1-5 μm in diameter, and are composed of parallel rows of ribosomal RNA (Fig. 20-7). When stained, they vary in color from gray to light blue. Döhle bodies appear shortly after stress induction, which suggests that they affect storage pool cells. Although no clear mechanism for their production is known, they are associated with a wide range of chemical and physical insults such as burns, infections, and surgery and with pregnancy.

Vacuolization

Phagocytic vacuoles may be found in neutrophils as a result of various situations. Autophagocytosis

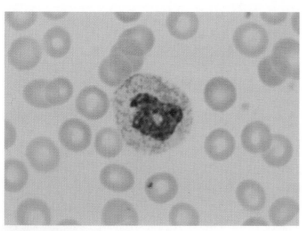

Figure 20-6 Toxic granulation. Notice that the number and size of the primary granules give the cell a bluish appearance.

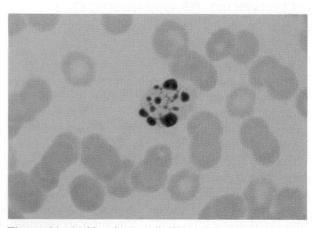

Figure 20-8 Necrobiotic cell. This cell's nucleus has been degraded into small, round, featureless droplets and can be found in dead or dying white blood cells.

Table 20-2. ACQUIRED GRANULOCYTE ALTERATIONS AND ANOMALIES*
Nucleus
Pseudo Pelger-Huët anomaly
Megaloblastic hypersegmentation
Nuclear distortions (projections/ring forms)
Pyknotic or necrobiotic forms
Twinning deformity
Cytoplasm
Toxic granulation
Döhle bodies
Degranulation
Vacuolization
Pseudopodia

* The majority of the acquired morphologic cytoplasmic anomalies are seen in severe stress situations such as burns and infections. Acquired morphologic nuclear anomalies other than megaloblastic hypersegmentation are seen in infections and malignancies.

(phagocytosis of self) is usually seen with prolonged exposure to drugs such as antimicrobial agents and to toxins such as alcohol and radiation.[11] Vacuoles caused by the ingestion and degradation of bacteria or fungi are larger than those seen in autophagocytosis, are not as evenly distributed, and are considered clinically significant, especially when associated with toxic granulation, degranulation, and/or Döhle bodies.[12]

Necrobiosis

Granulocytes eventually die, and large numbers of dead granulocytes in the peripheral blood smear indicate a severe strain in the granulocyte development pools. These cells appear to have exploded nuclei and pale or nongranular cytoplasm (Fig. 20-8). The acquired granulocyte alterations and anomalies are summarized in Table 20-2.

CYTOPLASMIC/ NONMORPHOLOGIC ALTERATIONS OF GRANULOCYTES

Chronic Granulomatous Disease of Childhood

Chronic granulomatous disease of childhood (CGD) is a collection of genetic disorders in which the intracellular kill mechanism of the granulocyte is defective.[13] At least two patterns of inheritance may govern this disease; the two most common are sex-linked and autosomal recessive. A rare disorder in which the ratio of affected males to affected females is 6:1, CGD results in death from bacterial infection, usually at 5-7 years of age. The manifestations of this disease are biochemically variable, resulting from combinations of defective/ absent respiratory burst, membrane nicotinamide-

adenine dinucleotide (NADH) or reduced nicotinamide-adenine dinucleotide phosphate (NADPH) oxidase, reduced cytosolic factor, and/or cytochrome B defects.[14, 15] In normal systems, hydrogen peroxide is concentrated in the phagosome containing microorganisms. This peroxide, together with activity from cytochrome B and NADPH oxidase, kills the ingested microorganism. Because of failure to metabolize oxygen to superoxide anion and hydrogen peroxide, CGD cells cannot kill catalase-positive or non-H_2O_2-producing microorganisms such as *Staphylococcus,* Enterobacteriaceae, or *Candida.* As a result of the increased susceptibility and subsequent cellular protection for the ingested microorganism, chronic pyogenic infections of all systems, abscess formation, lymphadenopathy, and hepatosplenomegaly are common findings. The secondary anemia of chronic disease is seen with normal to elevated serum iron and transferrin levels, with a typical infective white blood cell picture of toxic granulation, degranulation, vacuoles, Döhle bodies, and immature cells. The measurement of intracellular kill mechanisms is determined by measuring superoxide generation via the rarely performed chemiluminescence method[16] or by the more commonly seen nitroblue tetrazolium reduction,[17] which detects peroxide formation by the reduction of the dye to a black formazan deposit.

Miscellaneous Deficiencies

Other manifestations of neutrophilic dysfunction can be characterized as humoral or cellular abnormalities. Disorders of complement activation, for example, can be described as humoral abnormalities, whereas impaired chemotaxis or enzymopathies can be considered cellular abnormalities.

Congenital C3 deficiency is a rare autosomal recessive trait in which carriers have approximately half the normal C3 activity, which is adequate enough for carriers to be considered asymptomatic. Homozygotes get repeated bacterial infections as a result of poor opsonization. Deficiencies of serum opsonic activity result in recurrent pyogenic infections.[18]

Disorders of movement such as Job syndrome (hyperimmunoglobulin E syndrome) and lazy leukocyte syndrome are rare. Their mode of inheritance is unknown. They are differentiated by motility studies and clinical manifestations. In patients with Job syndrome, cells have poor directional motility, and boils are persistent.[19] In patients with lazy leukocyte syndrome, cells have poor directional and random movement, and there is a history of recurrent mucous membrane infections.

Myeloperoxidase deficiency was discovered as a result of the use of peroxidase indicators in automated differential instruments.[20] It is a relatively mild disorder with minimal symptoms, and compensation for the deficiency occurs through the increased use of respiratory bursts.

The World Health Organization has clustered a group of disorders characterized by poor leukocyte adherence. These cells have a defect in surface glycoproteins designated CD11/CD18. Neutrophilic and monocytic cells demonstrate abnormalities in adherence, aggregation, and complement receptor 3 (CR3) activities, and lymphocytes may have lessened natural killer function.[21]

CYTOPLASMIC/MORPHOLOGIC ALTERATIONS OF THE MONOCYTE/MACROPHAGE

The monocyte/macrophage is responsible for the disposal of unwanted materials. Monocytes/macrophages store materials that are unsatisfactorily degraded, regardless of whether this partial degradation is due to intrinsic cellular enzyme defects, overaccumulation of substrate, or unsuitability of the material to the cell's degradative processes.

In the normal course of events, cellular structures are built up and broken down. The breakdown requires a strict sequential enzymatic degradation in the secondary lysosomes with the phagocytic vacuole containing the ingested material. Hereditary absence or dysfunction of any enzyme in the pathway causes an increase in substrate concentration and a decrease or absence of the product. Commonly known as storage cell diseases, these are hereditary disorders in which one or more tissues are engorged with a substance whose type and distribution have a characteristic pattern. These abnormalities are discussed briefly in this chapter. A more detailed discussion of storage diseases, as well as a table summarizing the abnormalities, is in Chapter 30.

Syndromes in which there is a defect in the degradation of mucopolysaccharides result in enlarged cytoplasm with clear areas that are filled with mucopolysaccharides. On occasion, granulocytes from affected patients manifest with Alder-Reilly bodies.

Lipid storage diseases parallel mucopolysaccharide disorders in that a missing enzyme results in the long-term storage of incompletely processed material. The most common lipid storage disease is Gaucher disease, in which there is an inability to degrade glucocerebroside. Gaucher disease has three manifestations: Type I, or chronic adult type; type II, or acute infantile neuronopathic type; and type III, which is a less defined subacute neuro-

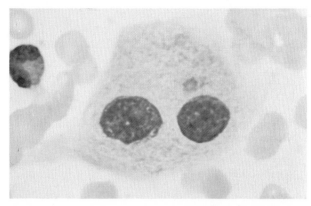

Figure 20–9 Gaucher cell. Notice the characteristic parallel striations within the cytoplasm. This cell is from a bone marrow aspirate from a patient with chronic myelogenous leukemia.

nopathic type.[22] Type I is found primarily in Ashkenazi Jews. The characteristic Gaucher cell is large and has an eccentric nucleus and a cytoplasm that has been described as "crumpled tissue paper" or "chicken scratch," the latter because it appears as if a chicken walked across it and made scratch marks (Fig. 20–9).

Patients with Niemann-Pick disease have an inability to degrade sphingomyelin. "Typical," or type A, Niemann-Pick disease includes visceral involvement, cerebral manifestations, and massive somatic wasting. In type B there is visceral involvement and massive somatic wasting but no cerebral manifestations. Inherited through rare autosomal recessiveness, Niemann-Pick disease is also seen in Ashkenazi Jews.

The pathophysiologic process results from a sphingomyelinase disorder in which there is an accumulation of sphingomyelin and a secondary pigment, ceroid, along with a subsequent decrease in ceramides.[23] Demonstrated in foam histiocytes found in lymphoid tissue, there is widespread phagocyte and parenchymal cell involvement (Fig. 20–10).

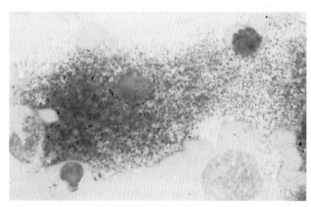

Figure 20–10 Niemann-Pick cell. Notice the characteristic bubble pattern of storage deposit in the cytoplasm.

Other inherited storage cell diseases such as gangliosidosis, Tay-Sachs disease, and Fabry disease do not have significant hematologic implications. The acquired hyperlipidemias occur when a condition produces an abnormal amount of lipids for monocyte/macrophage cells to process. These may be a primary disease, such as hypercholesterolemia, or a disease secondary to such conditions as diabetes mellitus or chronic leukemia.[24, 25]

MORPHOLOGIC ALTERATIONS OF LYMPHOCYTES

Nonmalignant morphologic variants is lymphocytes are neither as frequent nor as dramatic as those seen in neutrophils. Most changes seen in lymphocytes are directly related to antigenic stimulation and can be considered as normal activity. Lymphocytes with these changes are pleomorphic and, as a group, are more correctly referred to as "reactive," "stimulated," or "committed" rather than the older term "atypical." Differentiation of B cells can occur independently of antigen stimulation. These mature B cells are capable of expressing surface immunoglobulins of one specificity. After maturing, B lymphocytes migrate to lymphoid organs, in which they may contact antigens. Until antigenic stimulation occurs, these B lymphocytes remain in the G_0, or resting, stage. Once an antigen particle binds to the surface immunoglobulin receptor, the lymphocytes proliferate. Morphologic changes include both enlarged nuclei containing more euchromatin and possibly visible nucleoli with increased cytoplasmic basophilia. These morphologic features become apparent and then regress over time, and thus it is possible to see a wide range of manifestations on the themes of altered euchromatin/heterochromatin ratios and increasing basophilia with increased sophistication of the rough endoplasmic reticulum. These proliferating cells mature into plasma cells that synthesize and secrete copious quantities of immunoglobulin whose binding specificity is that present on the initially stimulated cell.

Antigenic stimulation of T cells is more varied because of the range of activity expressed by T cells. Upon stimulation, T cells undergo a clonal expansion and pass through a series of stages detectable from gene rearrangements and the presence of specific cluster designation surface markers. During clonal expansion, the nuclei of the cells appear younger and contain more euchromatin. At the cellular level, this metamorphosis is reflected in cells that are larger in size and that contain azurophilic granulation (Figs. 20–11, 20–12).

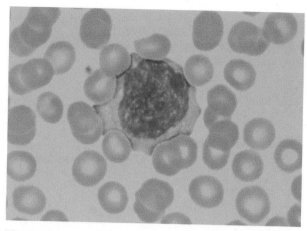

Figure 20–11 Reactive lymphocyte. Notice that although the overall size of this cell is larger than usual, the nucleus-to-cytoplasm ratio, chromatin pattern, and cytoplasm can be characterized as within acceptable limits for nonmalignant but reactive lymphocytes.

Nuclear Abnormalities

Clefting of the nucleus is sometimes seen in malignancies, especially lymphomas, and is discussed in greater detail in Chapter 25. Abnormal nuclei with a peculiar cerebriform pattern of heterochromatin are seen in patients with Sézary syndrome (see Chapter 23).

Cytoplasmic Abnormalities

Vacuolization of the cytoplasm can be seen in the genetic mucopolysaccharidoses, Gaucher disease, Tay-Sachs disease, Niemann-Pick disease, and Pompe disease. Azurophilic granulation can be seen in response to antigenic stimulation and in Hunter syndrome, a genetic disease. Increased amounts of nonstaining materials such as Golgi

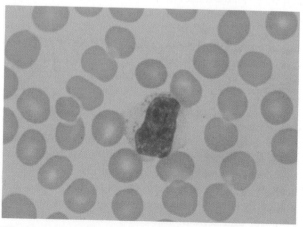

Figure 20–12 Reactive lymphocyte. This cell is from the same peripheral blood smear as that in Figure 20–11 but appears different, and yet it nonetheless has the major characteristics of a lymphocyte with distortions in granulation instead of size.

Table 20-3. Lymphocyte Morphologic Abnormalities*

Abnormalities in the Nucleus
CLEFTING
Some malignancies
Especially lymphomas
CEREBRIFORM HETEROCHROMATIN
Sezary syndrome

Abnormalities in the Cytoplasm
VACUOLIZATION
Genetic mucopolysaccharidosis
Tay-Sachs disease
Pompe disease
Niemann-Pick disease
Gaucher disease
AZUROPHILIC GRANULATION
Response to antigenic stimulation
Hunter syndrome
INCREASED AMOUNTS OF NONSTAINING MATERIALS†
Response to antigenic stimulation
Increased activity of cell as result of
    Multiple myeloma
    Waldenström's macroglobulinemia
    Immune system malignancies

* Unusual morphologic presentations of lymphocytes can be expected as in the case of reactivity, inherited as in the storage diseases, or as a result of malignancy.
† E.g., polypeptides in rough endoplasmic reticulum in a plasma cell.

apparatus or polypeptides are a result of increased activity of cells in response to antigenic stimulation or malignancy. See Table 20-3 for a summary of morphologic alterations in lymphocytes.

NONMORPHOLOGIC ALTERATIONS OF LYMPHOCYTES

Most of the nonmorphologic alterations are seen in diseases of immunologic function. The alterations result from either a lack of the specific cell type itself or a failure of a cell to act in a mature manner. Alterations in B cells are responsible for a large list of hypogammaglobulinemias, agammaglobulinemias, and dysgammaglobulinemias; quantitative and qualitative defects in T cells can be described by cell marker phenotypes.

T Cell Abnormalities

Patients with Wiskott-Aldrich syndrome, a rare X-linked recessive disorder, have platelet defects in number, size, and function in addition to defects in both B and T cell function. Caused by an abnormality in CD43,[26] this condition results in lessened humoral and cellular immunity with increased susceptibility to infection.

DiGeorge first described a condition that included parathyroid, cardiac, and skeletal abnormalities, and patients with this condition have been shown to have a signifiant decrease (to less than 10% of normal) of circulating T cells.[27]

B Cell Abnormalities

Sex-linked agammaglobulinemia[28] may show an absence of B cells, although some pre-B cells may be demonstrated. This condition differs from congenital agammaglobulinemia, in which the defect is either in the pre-B cell or in a qualitative interaction between the mature B cell and its counterpart T cells.[29]

SUMMARY

Many of the morphologic alterations seen in leukocytes are significant indicators of disease. They must be recognized and differentiated from staining artifacts and insignificant findings. Rarely does one alteration occur alone, and it is important to be able not only to recognize the various changes but also to synthesize an explanatory report that is timely, concise, and appropriate to the situation.

REVIEW QUESTIONS

1. A patient whose peripheral blood smear is exhibiting immaturity of the granulocytes with toxic granulation and Döhle bodies may have been admitted to the hospital for
   a. viral infection
   b. bacterial infection
   c. parasitic infection
   d. malignancy

2. The presence of hyposegmented granulocytes
   a. might be of no clinical significance
   b. is always seen in bacterial infections
   c. may be associated with first- and second-degree burns
   d. always implies a poor prognosis

3. Hypersegmentation of the neutrophilic granulocyte is seen in
   a. vitamin B_{12} deficiency or iron deficiency
   b. iron deficiency or viral infections
   c. folate deficiency or as an inherited anomaly
   d. an inherited anomaly or as a result of third-degree burns

4. Monocyte changes are usually seen in
   a. parasitic infections
   b. agammaglobulinemia
   c. chronic granulomatous disease
   d. lipid storage diseases

5. The defect seen in chronic granulomatous disease is

a. a failure of the nucleus to segment
b. a ringed form nucleus
c. an inability to produce superoxide
d. increased vacuolization

6. The May-Hegglin anomaly and Chédiak-Higashi syndrome can be differentiated by the presence of
a. hypersegmented polymorphonuclear cells
b. lymphocytes and azurophilic granules

c. decreased numbers of enlarged granules
d. cytochemical staining

7. The inability of a cell to produce a formazan deposit is seen in
a. May-Hegglin anomaly
b. Chédiak-Higashi syndrome
c. Job syndrome
d. CGD

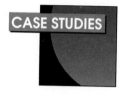

A 4-year-old girl was admitted to the hospital with second-degree burns over 40% of her body. Her complete blood count (CBC) on admission revealed elevated hemoglobin, elevated hematocrit, and leukocytosis with the preponderance of polymorphonuclear leukocytes. Two days later, she had a fever of 40 °C and positive findings from wound culture. Her CBC data at that time revealed a mild anemia and leukocytosis with 45% polymorphonuclear cells, 40% bands, 2% metamyelocytes, 1 myelocyte, 10 lymphocytes, and 2 monocytes. Comments concerning the white blood cells were 2+ toxic granulation and 2+ Döhle bodies. Appropriate antimicrobial treatment was initiated. Three days later, her CBC showed a mild anemia, a leukocyte count of 15 × 10⁹/L, and a differential of 69% polymorphonuclear cells, 20% lymphocytes, and 1 monocyte.

1. How would you explain the initial CBC results?

2. Why did her values change after 2 days?

3. What is the explanation of the last CBC data?

References

1. Brunning RD: Morphologic alterations in nucleated blood and marrow cells in genetic disorders. Hum Pathol 1970; 1:99.
2. Eichacker P, Lawrence C: Steroid-induced hypersegmentation in neutrophils. Am J Hematol 1985; 18:41.
3. Reilly WA, Lindsay S: Gargoylism (lipochondrodystrophy): a review of clinical observations in eighteen cases. Am J Dis Child 1948; 75:595.
4. Higashi O: Congenital gigantism of peroxidase granules: first case ever reported of qualitative abnormality of peroxidase. Tohoku J Exp Med 1954; 59:315.
5. White JG, Clawson CC: The Chédiak-Higashi syndrome: the nature of the giant neutrophil granules and their interactions with cytoplasm and foreign particulates. Am J Pathol 1980; 98:151.
6. Blume RS, Bennett JM, Yankee RA, Wolff SM: Defective granulocyte regulations in the Chédiak-Higashi syndrome. N Engl J Med 1968; 279:1009.
7. Boxer GJ, Holmsen H, Robkin L, et al: Abnormal platelet function in Chédiak-Higashi syndrome. Br J Haematol 1977; 35:521.
8. Rubin CM, Burke BA, McKenna RW, et al: The accelerated phase of Chédiak-Higashi syndrome: an expression of the virus-associated hemophagocytic syndrome. Cancer 1985; 56:524.
9. Cawley JJ, Hayhoe FGJ: The inclusions of the May-Hegglin anomaly and Döhle bodies of infection: an ultrastructural comparison. Br J Haematol 1972; 22:491.
10. Kugel MA, Rosenthal N: Pathological changes in polymorphonuclear leukocytes during progress of infection. Am J Med Sci 1932; 183:657.
11. Ponder E, Ponder RV: The cytology of the polymorphonuclear leukocyte in toxic conditions. J Lab Clin Med 1942; 28:316.
12. Solberg CO, Hellum KB: Neutrophil granulocyte function in bacterial infections. Lancet 1972; 2:727.
13. Gallin JI, Buscher ES: Recent advances in chronic granulomatous disease. Ann Intern Med 1983; 99:657.
14. Boxer LA, Baehner RL: Defects in neutrophil leukocyte function. In Franklin EC (ed): Clinical Immunology Update. New York: Elsevier North-Holland, 1981:357.
15. Seligmann BE, Gallin JI: Use of lipophilic probes of membrane potential to assess human neutrophil activation abnormality in chronic granulomatous disease. J Clin Invest 1980; 66:493.
16. Gallin JI, Buscher ES: Recent advances in chronic granulomatous disease. Ann Intern Med 1983; 99:657.
17. Gifford RH, Malawista SE: A simple rapid micromethod for detecting chronic granulomatous disease of childhood. J Lab Clin Med 1970; 75:511.
18. Alper CA, Rosen FS: Complement deficiencies in humans. In Franklin EC (ed): Clinical Immunology Update. New York: Elsevier North-Holland, 1981:59.
19. Leung DY, Geha RS: Clinical and immunologic aspects of the hyperimmunoglobulin E syndrome. Hematol Oncol Clin North Am 1988; 2:81.
20. Parry M, Root RK, Metcalf JA, et al: Myeloperoxidase deficiency: prevalence and clinical significance. Ann Intern Med 1981; 95:293.
21. Todd RF, Freyer DR: The CD11/CD18 leukocyte glycoprotein deficiency. Hematol Oncol Clin North Am 1988; 2:13.
22. Beutler E: Gaucher's disease. Blood Rev 1988; 2:59.

23. Brady RO, Find FM: Neimann-Pick disease. *In* Hers HG, van Hoof F (ed): Lysosomes and Storage Disease. New York: Academic Press, 1973:439.

24. Kattlove HE, Williams JC, Gaynor E, et al: Gaucher cells in chronic myelocytic leukemia: an acquired abnormality. Blood 1969; 33:379.

25. Fox H, McCarthy P, Andre-Schwartz J, et al: Gaucher's disease and chronic lymphocytic leukemia. Clin Lab Haematol 1986; 8:321.

26. Parkman R, Remold-O'Donnell E, Kenney DM, et al: Sur-

face protein abnormalities in the lymphocytes and platelets from patients with Wiskott-Aldrich syndrome. Lancet 1981; 2:1387.

27. DiGeorge AM: Congenital absence of thymus and its immunologic consequences: concurrence with congenital hypoparathyroidism. Birth Defects 1968; 4:116.

28. Bruton OC: Agammaglobulinemia. Pediatries 1952; 9:722.

29. Paul WE, Ohar J: B cell stimulatory factor 1/interleukin 4. Annu Rev Immunol 1987; 5:429.

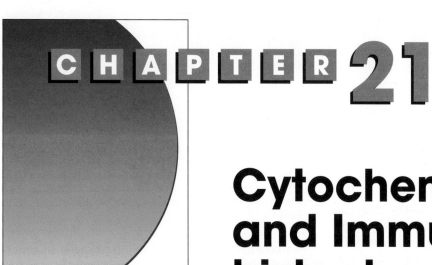

CHAPTER 21

Cytochemistry and Immuno- histochemistry

Jeff Bailey and Karla John

Outline

CYTOCHEMISTRY
  Principle
  Acceptable Specimens and
    Fixatives
  Controls and Troubleshooting
IMMUNOHISTOCHEMISTRY
  Principle
  Antibody Production
  Immunologic Methodology
  Immunohistochemical
    Techniques
  Chromogens
  Tissue Types
  Controls

Objectives

AFTER COMPLETION OF THIS CHAPTER, THE READER WILL BE ABLE TO

1. Discuss the purpose for performing cytochemical stains.
2. Determine appropriate specimen types and fixatives for cytochemical stains.
3. Discuss the principles and cell staining patterns for the following tests: myeloperoxidase, Sudan black B, esterases, periodic acid Schiff (PAS), leukocyte alkaline phosphatase, and leukocyte acid phosphatase.
4. Justify the use of controls in cytochemical and immunohistochemical staining.
5. Describe routine troubleshooting in cytochemical techniques.
6. Explain how polyclonal and monoclonal antibodies are manufactured.
7. Describe the direct and indirect immunohistochemical procedures.
8. Compare and contrast labeled and unlabeled antibody techniques.

CYTOCHEMISTRY

Principle

Cytochemistry is the study of chemical elements found in cells. These elements may be enzymatic (e.g., peroxidase) or non-enzymatic (e.g., lipids and glycogen).

Since the early 20th century, cytochemical staining of cells has been found to be a useful tool in differentiating hematopoietic diseases. Over the years, these stains have been a, if not *the,* most important laboratory test for the differentiation of acute and chronic leukemias. With the development of new technologies such as the evaluation of cell surface markers by flow cytometry and improved high-resolution techniques for cytogenetics, however, cytochemistry studies are used mostly in conjunction with these new technologies and not as the sole diagnostic tool. (Leukemias are discussed in Chapter 23; cytogenetics in Chapter 22; flow cytometry in Chapter 29.)

Acceptable Specimens and Fixatives

Many specimen types are adequate for cytochemical studies. Smears and imprints made from bone marrow, lymph nodes, the spleen, or peripheral blood are preferred. For the best results in enzymatic techniques, fresh smears should be used whenever possible to ensure optimal enzyme activity. Smears for non-enzymatic stains such as periodic acid Schiff or Sudan black B may remain stable for months if stored at room temperature.

Certain elements may be inhibited during the fixation of smears and imprints; therefore, it is important to use the proper fixative for the cytochemical stains. Fixatives containing alcohol (methanol or ethanol), acetone, formaldehyde, or a combination of these are commonly used for most cytochemistry studies.

PEROXIDASE

Peroxidase (Fig. 21–1) is an enzyme found in the primary granules of neutrophils, eosinophils, and, to a certain extent, monocytes. Lymphocytes do not exhibit peroxidase activity. This stain is useful for differentiating acute myeloid leukemia (AML) from acute lymphoblastic leukemia (ALL).

Principle. When hydrogen peroxide is present, peroxidase oxidizes dye substrates, creating black to red-brown (depending on the substrate) at the site of the activity. Benzidine used to be the substrate most often used, but because of its carcinogenic properties, other substrates such as 3,3'-di-

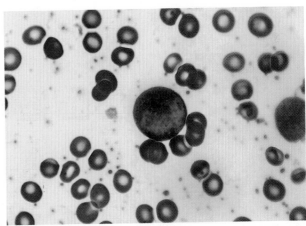

Figure 21–1 Myeloperoxidase showing positivity in early myeloid cell.

aminobenzidine (DAB) or p-phenylenediamine dihydrochloride and catechol are currently used.[1, 2]

Interpretation. Peroxidase is present in the primary granules of myeloid cells, beginning at the promyelocyte stage and continuing throughout maturation. Leukemic myeloblasts are also usually positive. In many cases of the acute myeloid leukemias—without maturation (FAB M1), with maturation, and promyelocytic leukemia (M3)—it has been found that more than 80% of the blasts demonstrate peroxidase activity. Aüer rods found in the leukemic blasts and promyelocytes are very strongly peroxidase positive. Because of their strong peroxidase positivity, many Aüer rods that could not be seen with just a Wright-Giemsa stain can be seen with the peroxidase stain.

Monocytes are peroxidase negative to weak or diffusely positive. In contrast, lymphoblast and lymphoid cells are peroxidase negative; in patients with ALL, fewer than 3% of the blasts show peroxidase positivity.[3]

It is important that the reaction in only the *blast* cells be used as the determining factor for the differentiation of acute leukemias. This is true for peroxidase as well as the other cytochemical stains that are mentioned in this chapter. The fact that maturing granulocytes are peroxidase positive is normal and has little or no diagnostic significance.

SUDAN BLACK B

Sudan black B (Figs. 21–2, 21–3) is another useful staining technique for the differentiation of AML from ALL. The staining pattern is quite similar to that of peroxidase for the most part; Sudan black B is possibly a little more sensitive for the early myeloid cells.

Principle. Sudan black B stains lipids, such as sterols, neutral fats, and phospholipids because of the solubility of the dye in lipid particles. These

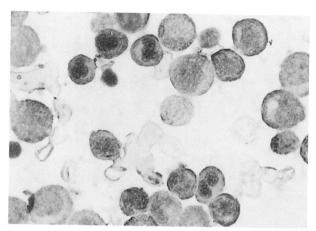

Figure 21-2 Sudan black B reaction. Note that the positivity increases with the maturity of the myeloid cell.

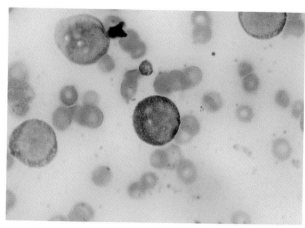

Figure 21-4 AS-D chloroacetate esterase demonstrating positivity in two myeloid cells.

lipids are found in the primary and secondary granules of neutrophils and in the lysosomal granules of monocytes.[4]

Interpretation. Granulocytes (neutrophils) are Sudan black B positive from the myeloblast through the maturation series. The staining is more intense the more mature the cell becomes, as a result of the increase in the numbers of the primary and secondary granules.

Monocytic cells can be negative to weakly positive, showing diffuse activity.

Lymphoid cells are generally negative. In ALL, fewer than 3% of the blast cells demonstrate positivity.[3]

ESTERASES

Esterase reactions are used to differentiate myeloid cells from cells of monocytic origin. To do this, different substrates are used, such as naphthol AS-D chloroacetate (specific), alpha-naphthyl acetate, or alpha-naphthyl butyrate (nonspecific).

Principle. Esterases hydrolyze an ester. A naphthol compound is released and combines with a diazonium salt (in general, hexazotized pararosaniline, hexazotized new fuchsin, or fast blue BB), producing a brightly colored compound at the site of the enzyme activity.[5]

Interpretation. Esterases can be used to distinguish acute leukemias that are myeloid (M1, M2, M3) from those that are made of mostly cells of monocytic origin (M5). When naphthol AS-D chloroacetate is used as a substrate, the reaction shows positivity in the myeloid cells and negativity to weak activity for the monocytic cells (Fig. 21-4). Chloroacetate esterase is present in the primary granules of neutrophils. Leukemic myeloblasts are generally positive. Aüer rods demonstrate positivity as well.

The reaction of alpha-naphthyl acetate esterases produces strong positive activity in monocytes which can be inhibited with the addition of sodium fluoride.[6] Myeloid and lymphoid cells are generally negative (Figs. 21-5, 21-6).

The reaction of alpha-naphthyl butyrate is posi-

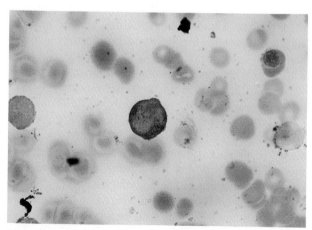

Figure 21-3 Sudan black B demonstrating positivity in an early myeloid cell.

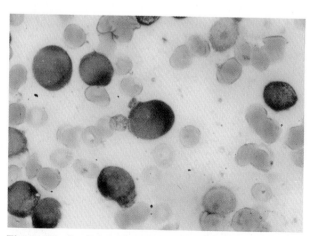

Figure 21-5 Alpha-naphthyl acetate esterase reaction showing positivity in monocytes.

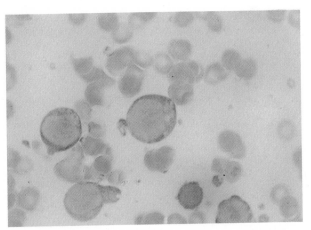

Figure 21-6 Same specimen as in Figure 21-5 with sodium fluoride. Note that the reaction in the monocytes is inhibited.

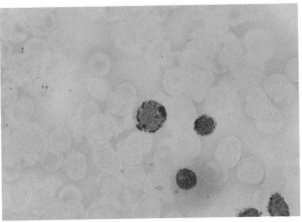

Figure 21-8 Periodic acid Schiff reaction demonstrating coarse (block) positivity, from a child with acute lymphoblastic leukemia.

tive in monocytes. Alpha-naphthyl butyrate is less sensitive than the alpha-naphthyl acetate but is more specific. Myeloid and lymphoid cells are generally negative (Fig. 21-7).

AML (M4) should demonstrate both positive AS-D chloroacetate activity and positive alpha-naphthyl butyrate or alpha-naphthyl acetate activity because in this leukemia, both myeloid and monocytic cells are present.

PERIODIC ACID SCHIFF

PAS staining (Fig. 21-8) may be helpful in the diagnosis of some ALLs and the FAB M6 type of AML.

Principle. Many different cell types contain glycogen. Periodic acid oxidizes glycogen, mucoproteins, and other high-molecular-weight carbohydrates to aldehydes. These aldehydes react with the colorless Schiff reagent, staining them a bright red-pink. The intensity of the staining depends on the number of aldehyde groups liberated by the

periodic acid. The PAS stain pattern may be fine and diffuse, coarse and granular (block), or a mixture of both.

Interpretation. Granulocytes are PAS positive; the intensity of staining increases as the cell matures. Megakaryocytes exhibit finely diffuse staining, whereas platelets turn intensely red-pink. Normal erythrocyte precursors do not turn color.

In ALL, cells demonstrate a varied staining pattern. Lymphoblasts of ALL may show a coarse, block pattern of activity, a finely diffuse pattern, or a combination of the two patterns. Lymphoblasts of ALL may also be PAS negative, especially for the subtype L3 (Burkitt).[7]

In subtype M6 of AML, erythroid precursors are strongly PAS positive, whereas erythroid precursors in normal bone marrow demonstrate no PAS activity.

A simplified cytochemistry reaction chart intended for quick reference is shown in Table 21-1.

LEUKOCYTE ALKALINE PHOSPHATASE

Leukocyte alkaline phosphatase (LAP) enzyme activity is useful for differentiating chronic myelogenous leukemia from a leukemoid reaction, which may be seen in severe infections.

Principle. LAP is an enzyme found in the secondary granules of neutrophils. The substrate naphthol AS-BI phosphate is hydrolyzed by the enzyme at an alkaline pH. This hydrolyzed substrate in combination with a dye such as fast red-violet LB or fast blue BB produces a colored precipitate at the site of the enzyme activity.

Scoring. LAP activity is scored in the mature polymorphonuclear cells and bands only. The activity scores range from 0 to 4+ (Fig. 21-9). The scores of 100 mature polymorphonuclear cells and

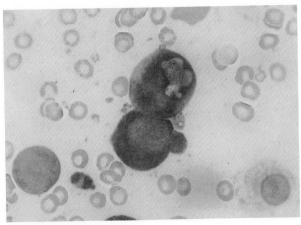

Figure 21-7 Alpha-naphthyl butyrate esterase positivity in two cells of monocytic origin.

Table 21-1. ACUTE LEUKEMIA REACTION CHART SIMPLIFIED*

Condition	Myeloperoxidase	Sudan Black B	Naphthol AS-D Chloroacetate Esterase	α-Naphthyl Butyrate Esterase (NBE)	PAS
ALL (L1-3)	−	−	−	−	Varied; usually positive in L1 & L2
AML (M1-3)	+	+	+	−	Varied
AMML (M-4)	+	+	+	+	Varied
AmoL (M-5)	−	±	−	+	Varied
Erythroid (M-6)	−	−	−	−	Positive in RBC precursors

Abbreviations: PAS, periodic acid Schiff; ALL, acute lymphoblastic leukemia; AML, acute myelogenous leukemia; AMML, acute myelomonocytic leukemia; AmoL, acute monocytic leukemia; RBC, red blood cell.

* This simplified chart is intended for quick reference. For more complete explanations, refer to discussion in this chapter or to cytochemical atlases.

bands are added for the LAP score. Because scoring is so subjective, it is recommended that two slides from an individual patient be scored by two people. These scores should agree within 10% of each other. If the scores do not agree, a third slide from the patient must be scored. For example:

Score	Number of Cells	Score × Number of Cells
0	20	0
1	45	45
2	25	50
3	5	15
4	5	20
Total	100	130 = LAP score

Eosinophils do not demonstrate alkaline phosphatase activity and must not be mistaken for mature neutrophils with a score of zero.

Interpretation. A normal LAP score should be between 20 and 100, but because of the scoring subjectivity, it is very important that every laboratory establish its own normal values.

Persons with untreated chronic myelogenous leukemia have decreased LAP scores; those with leukemoid reactions have scores ranging from high normal to increased. Other conditions producing higher scores include the third trimester of preg-

Table 21-2. RESULTS OF LEUKOCYTE ALKALINE PHOSPHATASE STAIN

Finding	Score
Normal	20–100
Chronic myelogenous leukemia	<13
Leukemoid reaction	>100
Polycythemia vera	100–200
Secondary polycythemia	10–100

nancy and polycythemia vera. The score is normal in cases of secondary polycythemia. Conditions in which decreased scores are found include paroxysmal nocturnal hemoglobinuria, sideroblastic anemia, and myelodysplastic disorders. A summary of LAP interpretation is shown in Table 21-2.

ACID PHOSPHATASE (TARTRATE RESISTANT)

Almost all blood cells contain seven nonerythroid isoenzymes of acid phosphatase: 0, 1, 2, 3, 3b, 4, and 5.[8] Hairy cells produce isoenzyme 5 in abundance. This makes the acid phosphatase stain (Fig 21-10; Table 21-3) a useful diagnostic tool for confirmation of hairy cell leukemia (leukemic reticuloendotheliosis).

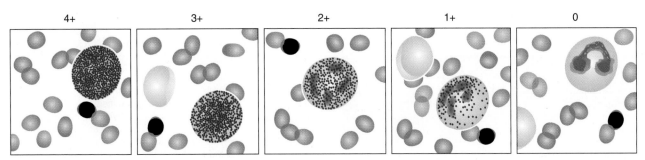

Figure 21-9 Drawing of leukocyte alkaline phosphatase (LAP) reaction demonstrating reactivity from 0 to 4 +.

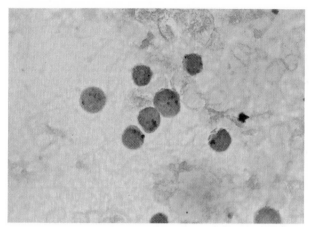

Figure 21–10 Positive acid phosphatase stain. If hairy cells are present, the stain will remain positive after the addition of tartaric acid to the incubation mixture.

Principle. Acid phosphatase hydrolyzes the substrate naphthol AS-BI phosphoric acid. Once hydrolyzed, this substrate couples with a dye such as fast garnet GBC and produces a red precipitate at the site of the enzyme activity. When L(+)-tartaric acid is added, all isoenzymes except isoenzyme 5 are inhibited. Isoenzyme 5 is tartrate resistant.

Interpretation. Most hematopoietic cells demonstrate acid phosphatase activity. Granulocytes, lymphocytes, and monocytes all show positivity to some extent until the addition of L(+)-tartaric acid. The activity is inhibited because isoenzyme 5 is lacking. Hairy cells, which contain isoenzyme 5, remain positive with the addition of L(+)-tartaric acid in that at least two or more cells contain 40 or more red granules.[1]

Controls and Troubleshooting

For most cytochemical stains mentioned in this chapter, a normal blood smear containing neutrophils, lymphocytes, and monocytes is sufficient as a control sample. A few normal hematopoietic cells contained in the marrow aspirate or imprint can serve as an internal control for staining. For hairy cell leukemia, a normal smear can be used to demonstrate inhibition by L(+)-tartaric acid, but it is more difficult to obtain a control for demonstrat-

ing resistance. Only a smear from a patient known to have hairy cell leukemia could be used.

When the control slides do not exhibit the proper staining pattern, such as showing no activity when they should be positive or exhibiting the wrong color precipitate, certain aspects should be investigated. Possibly a wrong reagent, no reagent, or an expired reagent was added to the test system. A reagent may have been contaminated; if this is the case, the examiner should make or open a new reagent. If the reagent is acceptable, the examiner should go over the procedure to make sure that all steps were followed correctly. Another aspect that might need investigating is the age of the smear and how it was stored. Some enzymes diminish in activity over time. Fresh smears are always best.

If the controls are not acceptable, the cytochemical stain in question must be repeated.

IMMUNOHISTOCHEMISTRY

Principle

The science of immunohistochemistry involves the use of antibodies to identify antigens within a cell suspension or a tissue section. The main goal is to classify the cells in question by a means more specific than nonimmunologic histochemical staining. Visualization of the antigen-antibody bond is achieved by tagging the antibody with an indicator, such as a fluorochrome or an enzyme, that can be observed under the microscope.

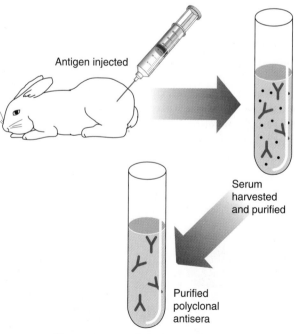

Antigen injected

Serum harvested and purified

Purified polyclonal antisera

Figure 21–11 Polyclonal production.

Table 21–3. RESULTS OF LEUKOCYTE ACID PHOSPHATASE STAIN		
Cell Type	**Without Tartrate**	**With Tartrate**
Lymphocytes	+	–
Hairy cells	+	+

Antibody Production

POLYCLONAL[9]

To make polyclonal antisera (Fig. 21–11), antigens are injected into the animal in which the antibody reaction is desired. Rabbits are frequently the animal of choice, but goats, sheep, horses, and guinea pigs may also be chosen. When the antibody titer is high enough, the blood is harvested. First, cellular components are removed; this procedure is followed by salt precipitation and affinity chromatography to purify the antisera of any cross-reacting antibodies. Polyclonal antibodies are produced by different cells, and so they are immunochemically dissimilar to one another, reacting with different epitopes on the same antigen.[10]

MONOCLONAL[9]

Production of a monoclonal antibody (Fig. 21–12) is achieved in much the same manner as described for polyclonal antibody; the difference is that monoclonal antibodies are by-products of a single cloned cell, not a group of similar cells (polyclonal). The animal of choice is usually the mouse. After achieving an immune response, the B cells are harvested from either the lymph nodes or the spleen. B cells (which secrete the appropriate antibody) are then fused with myeloma cells (which

keep the cell culture alive) to form a hybridoma cell. The unhybridized cells are removed, which results in a culture specific for one particular antigen. The reactivity of the hybrid cell line is then tested and allowed to propagate in culture media.[10] After the culture has grown sufficiently, a single hybridoma cell is cloned and recloned over and over to achieve a cell line that produces the exact same antibody. Through this method, large quantities of antisera can be produced. The hybridoma cells can also be stored in liquid nitrogen for later use.

Monoclonal antibodies produce less nonspecific background than do polyclonal antibodies, but monoclonal antibodies can also be too specific to be effective, inasmuch as they react with only one epitope on only one antigen. If a monoclonal antibody is used on a particular tissue section that is lacking a specific epitope, the antibody does not react. For example, if a case is being reviewed for the possibility of multiple myeloma, the immunoglobulins produced may be defective or missing parts of their chains. If the portion of the missing chain is the part that normally reacts with the antibody, a false negative reaction results. The only way to solve this problem is to use a polyclonal antibody or a mixture of three or four monoclonal antibodies, each reactive with a different epitope but specific to the same antigen.

Early monoclonal nomenclature tended to vary from manufacturer to manufacturer, and no two terminologies were the same. Two designations found to be identical did not imply that a similar antigen was being used. To combat this problem, each monoclonal antibody was appointed a differentiation or cluster designation (CD) number by the Fourth International Workshop and Conference on Human Leucocyte Differentiation Antigens[11] (Table 21–4). Within each of these groups, there are antibodies with major and minor differences, each sharing a similar reactivity. Most manufacturers today give an antibody its own nomenclature (specific to each manufacturer) and also assign the antibody a known CD classification.

Immunologic Methodology[12]

For years laboratory professionals have been demonstrating antigen-antibody reactions in vitro. At present, new methods of visualizing these reactions have been found. The most commonly used procedures are the fluorochrome-conjugated and the enzyme-conjugated immunohistochemical methods. These procedures are covered in detail in immunochemistry texts. One general procedure is included in this chapter as an example.

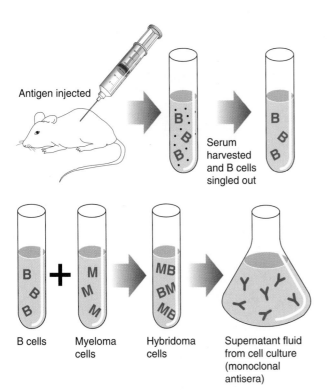

Antigen injected

Serum harvested and B cells singled out

B cells

Myeloma cells

Hybridoma cells

Supernatant fluid from cell culture (monoclonal antisera)

Figure 21–12 Monoclonal production.

Table 21-4. CLUSTERS OF DIFFERENTIATION

Antibody	Clone	Common Names	Reactivity
CD3	(poly)	Leu4	Early T cells
CD4	OPD4	Leu3	Helper T cells
CD8	DK25	Leu2	Suppressor T cells
CD10	SS2/36	Common acute lymphoblastic leukemia antigen (CALLA)	Lymphocyte progenitor
CD15	C3D-1	LeuM1	Mature granulocytes/Reed-Sternberg cells/monocytes/histocytes
CD20	L-26	L-26	Majority of B cells
CD30	BerH$_2$	BerH$_2$	Reed-Sternberg cells/large-cell lymphoma
CD43	DF-T1	Leu22/MT1	T cells/myeloid cells
CD45RB	PD7/26	Leukocyte common antigen (LCA)	Leukocytes
CD45RO	UCHL-1	UCHL-1	Majority of T cells
CD68	KP1	Macrophage	Macrophages
CD74	LN2	LN2	B cells/Reed-Sternberg cells/histocytes/monocytes
CDw75	LN1	LN1	B cells (germinal center)
EMA	E29	Epithelial membrane antigen	Glandular epithelial
Factor VIII	(poly)	von Willebrand's factor	Endothelium/megakaryocytes
Hemoglobin	(poly)	Hemoglobin	Red blood cells (hemoglobins A$_1$, A$_2$, F)
Immunoglobulin G	(poly)	Gamma heavy chain	Plasma cells secreting gamma chains
Kappa	(poly)	Kappa light chain	Plasma cells secreting kappa chains
S-100	(poly)	S-100	S-100 (alpha and beta chains)
Myeloperoxidase	(poly)	Mpx	Primary granules (neutrophils, monocytes)
Lysozyme	(poly)	Muramidase	Neutrophils/eosinophils/mast cells/histocytes/epithelial cells

Data from Knapp W, Dörken B, Gilks WR, et al (eds): Leucocyte Typing IV: White Cell Differentiation Antigens. New York: Oxford University Press, 1989.

FLUOROCHROME-CONJUGATED IMMUNOHISTOCHEMISTRY[12-16]

Fluorochrome-conjugated antibodies are added to a cell suspension or tissue section, forming an immune complex that can then be observed through flow cytometry or fluorescent microscopy, respectively (Fig. 21-13). The fluorochromes most commonly used include fluorescein isothiocyanate and tetramethylrhodamine isothiocyanate.

ENZYME-CONJUGATED IMMUNOHISTOCHEMISTRY[15]

Enzyme-conjugated antibodies are added to a cell smear or tissue section, forming an immune complex that is then colorized by the addition of a chromogen and is observed under a light microscope (Fig. 21-14). Virtually any enzyme can be used as long as it is soluble, stable, and not present in quantities that would interfere with immunohistochemical interpretations. Enzymes most frequently used include horseradish peroxidase (HRP) and alkaline phosphatase (AP).

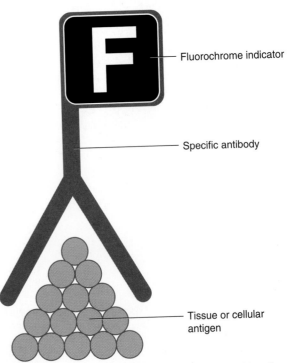

Fluorochrome indicator

Specific antibody

Tissue or cellular antigen

Figure 21-13 Fluorochrome-conjugated immunohistochemistry study.

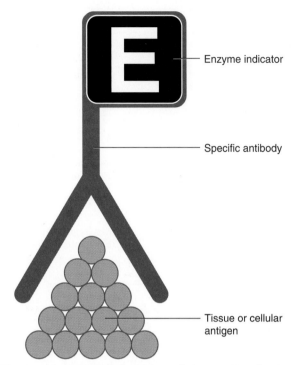

Figure 21–14 Enzyme-conjugated immunohistochemistry study.

Immunohistochemical Techniques

These techniques involve the use of either fluorochrome-conjugated or enzyme-conjugated antisera.[9, 10, 16–18]

DIRECT IMMUNOCHEMICAL PROCEDURE (ONE-STEP METHOD)

An enzyme- or fluorochrome-conjugated primary antibody is initially made to react with a tissue or cellular antigen. Visualization of the reaction is accomplished with the aid of a chromogen, and the results are viewed under a microscope (Fig. 21–15). Although this procedure is easy, it is the least sensitive: strong specific antigen-antibody staining usually accompanies large amounts of nonspecific background, making interpretations difficult.

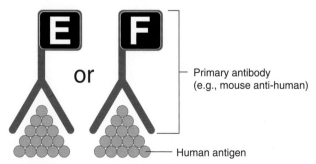

Figure 21–15 Direct immunochemical procedure (one-step procedure). E, enzyme; F, fluorochrome.

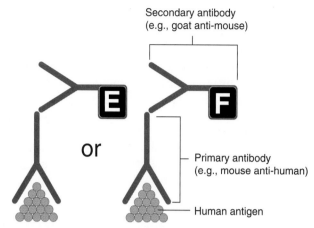

Figure 21–16 Indirect immunochemical procedure (two-step procedure). E, enzyme; F, fluorochrome.

INDIRECT IMMUNOCHEMICAL PROCEDURE (TWO-STEP METHOD)

An unconjugated primary antibody is made to react with a tissue or cellular antigen. An enzyme- or fluorochrome-conjugated secondary antibody (which is specific for the host and immunoglobulin class of the primary) is then allowed to react. After colorization with a chromogen, the results are viewed under a microscope (Fig. 21–16).

Further elaboration of the indirect procedure is the three-step method. A tertiary conjugated antibody is attached to the secondary conjugated antibody (Fig. 21–17). Through the use of a secondary or a tertiary antibody, a higher number of enzyme molecules are available to react with the chromogen and ultimately produce a more intense immunohistochemical reaction.

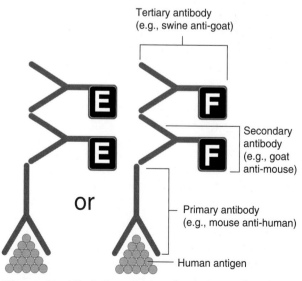

Figure 21–17 Indirect immunochemical procedure (three-step method). E, enzyme; F, fluorochrome.

UNLABELED ANTIBODY PROCEDURE

This method, also called the soluble enzyme immune complex method, entails the use of an enzyme and the antibody specific for that enzyme. The soluble enzyme immune complex and the primary antibody must be made from the same host; otherwise, the secondary antibody will not bind them together. The peroxidase–anti-peroxidase (PAP) and alkaline phosphatase–anti-alkaline phosphatase (APAAP) methods, discussed as follows, are two well-known examples.

PAP.[10, 15, 18–20] The PAP complex (Fig. 21–18) is a large molecule consisting of three peroxidase molecules and two anti-peroxidase antibodies.

APAAP.[10] The APAAP complex (Fig. 21–19) is made up of two molecules of alkaline phosphatase and one anti-alkaline phosphatase antibody.

LABELED ANTIBODY PROCEDURE[15, 18, 20, 21] (AVIDIN-BIOTIN METHOD)

In nature, avidin has a very strong affinity for biotin. Because of this property, Streptavidin (from the culture broth of *Streptomyces avidinii* can be made to react with biotin (vitamin H) to form a complex that, when used in immunohistochemical staining procedures, invokes a very strong and highly sensitive antigen-antibody reaction. The specific reactions are intensely colorized, whereas nonspecific background is usually minimal or absent. Currently, two avidin-biotin methods are in use: the avidin-biotin complex (ABC) method (Fig.

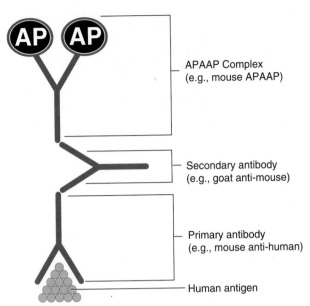

Figure 21–19 Unlabeled antibody procedure (APAAP complex). AP, alkaline phosphatase.

21–20) and the labeled avidin-biotin (LAB) technique (Fig. 21–21). A typical ABC method for immunoperoxidase is detailed in Table 21–5.

IN-SITU HYBRIDIZATION AND IMMUNOCHEMISTRY

This technique (also called hybridization histochemistry) allows specific DNA or RNA sequences at the single cell level to be labeled by immunohistochemical methods.[22] Single-stranded fragments of DNA or RNA complementary to target sequences (probes) are labeled with an antigenic compound (e.g., digoxigenin or biotin). These probes hydro-

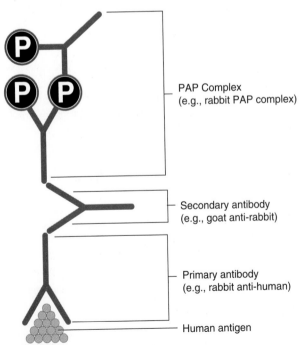

Figure 21–18 Unlabeled antibody procedure (PAP complex). P, peroxidase.

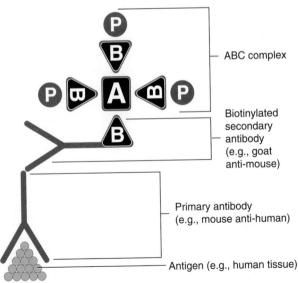

Figure 21–20 Labeled antibody procedure (ABC complex). P, peroxidase; B, biotin; A, avidin.

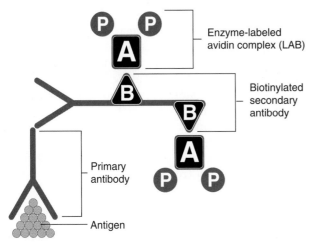

Figure 21–21 Labeled antibody procedure (LAB complex). P, peroxidase, A, avidin; B, biotin.

Table 21–5. GENERAL IMMUNOPEROXIDASE STAINING PROCEDURE*
1. Deparaffinize and rehydrate sections
2. Block with 3% hydrogen peroxide
3. Rinse in phosphate buffered saline (PBS)
4. Block with normal serum (from same host as secondary antibody) (e.g., normal goat serum)
5. Apply primary antibody (e.g., mouse anti-human leukocyte common antigen antibody)
6. Rinse in PBS
7. Apply secondary antibody (e.g., goat anti-mouse biotinylated antibody)
8. Rinse in PBS
9. Apply ABC solution (e.g., Streptavidin-biotin-peroxidase complex)
10. Rinse in PBS
11. Apply chromogen (e.g., DAB)
12. Rinse in tap water
13. Counterstain and coverslip (e.g., Harris hematoxylin)

Abbreviations: ABC, avidin-biotin complex; DAB, 3,3'-diaminobenzidine tetrahydrochloride.
* Based on the ABC method.

gen-bond (hybridize) to single-stranded cellular DNA or RNA under the appropriate conditions to form stable hybrids. An antibody or Streptavidin conjugate is then added to localize the hybrids. The antigen-antibody reactions can then be amplified with osmium tetroxide (or other heavy metals), and this results in a cell that is labeled by its chromosome (Fig. 21–22). Currently, cytomegalovirus-, human papillomavirus–, and Epstein-Barr virus–positive cells are detected in this manner.

Chromogens

A chromogen is an electron donor that, upon being oxidized, becomes a colored product. Of all the potential chemicals that could act as chromogens, the two most often chosen are 3-3′ diaminobenzidine tetrahydrochloride (DAB) and 3-amino-9-ethylcarbazole (AEC).

DAB.[15] DAB produces a dark brown, granular reaction product that is insoluble in alcohol. The intensity of the DAB reaction may be increased by the addition of osmium tetroxide or a heavy metal such as gold chloride, cobalt chloride, or silver sulfide[9] (Fig. 21–23). DAB coupled with osmium tetroxide not only increases the staining intensity but increases the electron density as well; thus it is a good chromogen for immunoelectron microscopy.

AEC. AEC produces a brick-red reaction product that is soluble in alcohol. The AEC reaction product eventually fades, and thus this chromogen is slightly inferior to DAB.

Tissue Types[10, 23, 24]

There are three basic tissue types used in immunohistochemical staining: fresh, frozen, and fixed. Fresh tissues include touch imprints, cytocentrifuge and buffy coat preparations, and cytologic smears obtained from body fluids, fine needle aspirates, and so forth. Frozen tissues are cryostat sections. Both fresh and frozen tissues are generally used to localize lymphocyte markers, because surface antigens are better preserved in these specimens than in fixed tissue.

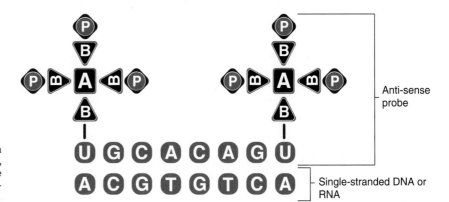

Figure 21–22 In situ hybridization (DNA and RNA probes). E, enzyme; U, uracil, G, guanine (DNA) or guanosine (RNA); C, cytosine; A, adenine; T, thymine.

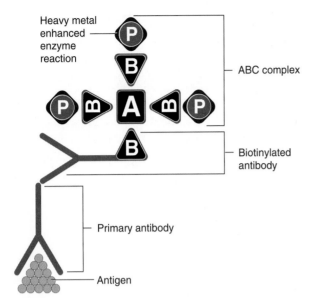

Figure 21–23 Heavy metal enhancement. P, peroxidase; B, biotin; A, avidin.

Fixed tissues include paraffin- and plastic-embedded preparations obtained from lymph nodes, bone marrow biopsy specimens, and so forth. Morphologically and immunochemically fixed tissues are superior to unfixed tissues. Cellular antigens tend to diffuse out of the membrane and into the spaces upon cell death. Fixing the tissue causes the membranes to become rigid, disallowing antigen diffusion and thus sharpening immunohistochemical staining.

Controls

Reagent controls and procedural controls are needed for validating the results of any chemical staining.[9, 10, 17, 25] With the use of both positive and negative controls with each different antibody tested, all procedures and reagents can be validated as reproducible and functional, respectively.

Serum Controls. The positive serum control is the primary antibody. The negative serum control should be an affinity-absorbed serum from the same species as the primary antibody and used in place thereof. For example, if the primary antibody is mouse anti-human, the negative control should be a nonimmune serum from a mouse (i.e., normal mouse serum).

Tissue Controls. A positive tissue control is any tissue known to contain the antigen desired.

For example, if B cells are the desired antigen, the positive control might be normal lymph node. Positive controls are needed to ensure that the primary antibody is working properly. The negative control is needed for validating specific staining from nonspecific staining and should be a tissue in which the desired antigen is not found. For example, a negative control could be the patient's tissue. Any staining found on the negative control represents nonspecific background staining and should be disregarded as a true positive finding.

SUMMARY

Cellular morphology alone can sometimes be misleading or confusing. Cytochemical stains can aid in differentiation of disease by identification of enzymes, lipids, or glycogen in cells. Immunocytochemical stains can identify cells by means of antigen/antibody reactions.

Cytochemical reactions may be either enzymatic or non-enzymatic. Fresh smears should be used to detect enzymatic activity, whereas non-enzymatic procedures may be performed on specimens that have been stored at room temperature.

Peroxidase and Sudan black B are useful in differentiating myeloid from lymphoid cells. Esterases help differentiate myeloid from cells of monocytic origin. PAS stains are positive in specimens of patients with many ALLs and with erythroid precursors of M6 leukemia.

LAP is most useful in distinguishing chronic myelogenous leukemia from leukemoid reactions. Acid phosphatase with tartrate inhibition is positive in specimens from patients with hairy cell leukemia.

Either polyclonal or monoclonal antibodies may be used in immunohistochemical reactions. An antigen/antibody reaction may be visualized in many ways. Of these methods, the ABC method produces superior results. Chromogens commercially available to aid in this visualization differ in their solubility in organic solvents and in slide permanency. As with all special staining, positive and negative controls are an important part of quality control in the immunohistochemical laboratory.

Both cytochemistry and immunohistochemistry provide valuable adjuncts to morphology, flow cytometry, and cytogenetics in establishing a diagnosis.

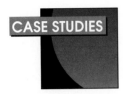
CASE STUDIES

Case 1

A 5-year-old boy was admitted to the hospital on the advice of the family physician. His mother said that he had complained of leg pain, seemed to be "paler" than normal, and had some unexplained bruising. The complete blood cell count on admission included a white blood cell (WBC) count of $15.0 \times 10^9/L$, hemoglobin (Hb) of 6.5 g/dL, and platelet count of $17.0 \times 10^9/L$. Fifty-eight percent of the mononuclear cells on the differential were abnormal. Similar cells composed 93% of the bone marrow. The cytochemical characteristics of these cells were as follows:

Myeloperoxidase:	Negative
Sudan black:	Negative
AS-D chloroacetate esterase:	Negative
Alpha-naphthyl acetate esterase:	Negative
Alpha-naphthyl butyrate esterase:	Negative
PAS:	60% coarsely positive

What is a possible diagnosis?

Case 2

A 48-year-old woman had the following results from procedures performed in her physician's office: WBC count, $45.0 \times 10^9/L$; Hb, 9.5 g/dL; platelet count, $158 \times 10^9/L$. The differential revealed 5 promyelocytes, 9 metamyelocytes, 18 bands, 55 polymorphonuclear cells (polys); 3 lymphocytes, 7 eosinophils, and 3 basophils. Her physician sent her to the hospital for more tests. An LAP test was ordered, and the score after counting 100 bands and polys was found to be as follows:

0 = 89
1 = 10
2 = 1
3 = 0
4 = 0

A. What is the total LAP score?

B. With what diagnosis are the results consistent?

C. If the LAP score were 135, what would the probable diagnosis be?

Case 3

A 16-year-old girl was sent to the hospital with a WBC count of $27.0 \times 10^9/L$, an Hb of 7.7 g/dL, and a platelet count of $110.0 \times 10^9/L$. Sixty-seven percent of mononuclear cells were abnormal; some cells appeared to be immature monocytes. A bone marrow examination revealed that 78% of the cells were the abnormal mononuclear cells. The cytochemical findings of these cells were as follows:

Myeloperoxidase:	Positive
Sudan black:	Positive
Alpha-naphthyl butyrate esterase:	Positive
Alpha-naphthyl acetate esterase:	Positive
Alpha-naphthyl acetate esterase with sodium fluoride:	Partial inhibition

What is the probable diagnosis?

Case 4

A 52-year-old man was admitted to the hospital with severe hepatosplenomegaly, a WBC count of $38.0 \times 10^9/L$, and an Hb of 9.3 g/dL. His peripheral blood smear showed a population of abnormal mononuclear cells in which the cytoplasm had fine projections. A bone marrow examination showed the same type abnormal mononuclear cells. The results of tartrate-resistant acid phosphatase staining were as follows:

Slide without tartrate: Abnormal cells are positive
Slide with tartrate: Abnormal cells are positive

A. What is the probable diagnosis?

B. Which isoenzyme makes these abnormal cells tartrate resistant?

Case 5

A 72-year-old man came to the emergency room complaining of fatigue, malaise, and easy bruising. Physical examination revealed splenomegaly, along with extensive ecchymosis on his left leg. Laboratory results were as follows:

WBC count	2.4×10^9/L
Red blood cell count	2.88×10^{12}/L
Hb	9.0 g/dL
Hematocrit	0.27 L/L
Platelet count	46.0×10^9/L
Polys	52%
Bands	1%
Myelocytes	2%
Blasts	1%
Lymphocytes	44%

A bone marrow performed at time of admission to the hospital revealed a hypercellular marrow composed primarily of erythroid precursors, of which many were megaloblastic and a few were binucleated. The non-erythroid blast population constituted more than 30% of the total cellularity. In the biopsy section, there were increased mitotic figures and decreased megakaryopoiesis. The results of immunohistochemical staining were as follows:

Myeloperoxidase:	Scattered positivity
Hb:	90% of cells positive
Terminal deoxynucleotidyl transferase:	Negative
Glycophorin C:	90% of cells positive
Lysozyme:	Negative
LeuM1:	Negative
CD68:	Negative
Factor VIII:	Scattered positivity

Preliminary diagnosis was determined to be acute nonlymphocytic leukemia (FAB M6). On the basis of morphologic findings and immunochemical staining, substantiate the preliminary diagnosis.

Case 6

A 54-year-old man was admitted with fever, night sweats, mild anemia, and unexplained weight loss. Laboratory values were as follows:

WBC	35.0×10^9/L
Hb	6.0 g/dL
Hematocrit	0.19 L/L
Platelet count	521×10^9/L
Polys	90%
Bands	1%
Lymphocytes	7%
Monocytes	2%

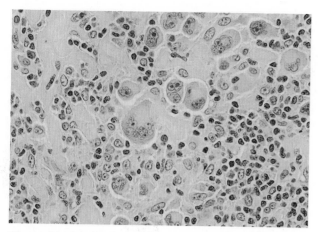

Figure 21–24 Section of a lymph node stained with hematoxylin and eosin (400X).

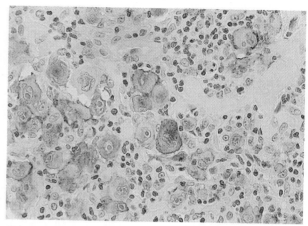

Figure 21–25 Lymph node reaction with CD30 (Ber H₂) antibody.

Further examination revealed a cluster of enlarged cervical lymph nodes. Fine-needle aspirate showed abnormal cells suggestive of malignancy. Tissue sections of the excised nodes contained scattered nodules of large cells mixed with small lymphocytes, plasma cells, and occasional eosinophils. Figure 21–24 is a section of lymph node stained with hematoxylin and eosin. Immunohistochemical staining revealed the following:

CD30 (Ber H₂) (Fig. 21–25)	
CD15 (LeuM1):	Positivity in the Golgi complex of large cells
CD20 (L-26):	Negative in large cells
CD45RB (LCA):	Negative in large cells
CD45RO (UCHL-1):	Negative in large cells
CD74 (LN2):	Positive in large cells

According to the immunohistochemical staining, what is the most likely diagnosis? What morphologic feature contributed to your diagnosis?

Case 7

A 37-year-old man complained of lethargy and irregular heart beat. Laboratory values revealed hypercalcemia and proteinemia. Hematology values were as follows:

WBC count	5.5×10^9/L
Red blood cell count	1.57×10^{12}/L
Hb	5.3 g/dL
Hematocrit	0.17 L/L
Platelet count	165×10^9/L
Polys	61%
Bands	15%
Metamyelocytes	1%
Promyelocytes	1%
Lymphocytes	16%
Monocytes	6%

On the bone marrow biopsy there was decreased erythropoiesis, granulopoiesis, and megakaryopoiesis. Ninety percent of the cells were composed of immature and atypical plasma cells. Figure 21–26 is Wright's stain of the bone marrow aspirate.

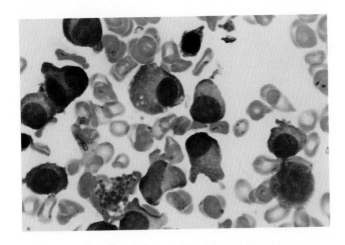

Figure 21–26 Bone marrow aspirate stained with Wright's stain (1000×).

Immunohistochemical results were as follows:

Immunoglobulin G (poly)	Negative
Immunoglobulin A (poly)	Negative
Immunoglobulin M (poly)	Negative
Kappa cells (poly)	Positive in most plasma cells
Lambda cells (poly)	Negative
CD45RO (UCHL-1)	Negative
CD20 (L-26)	Negative

What disease process is most likely? Support your decision.

References

1. Sun T, Li Cy, Yam LT: Atlas of Cytochemistry & Immunochemistry of Hematologic Neoplasms. Chicago: American Society of Clinical Pathology Press, 1985.
2. Kaplow LS: Substitute for benzidine in myeloperoxidase stain. Am J Clin Pathol 1975, 63:451.
3. Bennett JM, Catovsky D, Daniel MT, et al: Proposed revised criteria of acute myeloid leukemia. A report of the French-American-British (FAB) Cooperative Group. Ann Intern Med 1985, 103:620.
4. Hayhoe FJG: The cytochemical demonstration of lipids in blood and bone marrow cells. J Pathol Bacteriol 1953, 65:413–421.
5. Li CY, Lam KW, Yam LT: Esterases in human leukocytes. J Histochem Cytochem 1973, 21:1–12.
6. Wachstein M, Wolf G: The histochemical demonstration of esterase activity in human blood and bone marrow smears. J Histochem Cytochem 1958, 6:457.
7. Humphrey GB, Nesbit ME, Brunning RD: Prognostic values of the periodic acid-Schiff (PAS) reaction in acute lymphoblastic leukemia. Am J Clin Pathol 1974, 61:393.
8. Li CY, Yam LT, Lam KW: Acid phosphatase isoenzyme in human leukocytes in normal and pathologic conditions. J Histochem Cytochem 1970, 18:473–481.
9. True LD (ed): Atlas of Diagnostic Immunohistopathology. New York: Gower Medical, 1990.
10. Naish SJ (ed): Handbook of Immunochemical Staining Methods. Carpinteria, CA: DAKO Corporation, 1989.
11. Knapp W, Dörken B, Gilks WR, et al (eds): Leucocyte Typing IV: White Cell Differentiation Antigens. New York: Oxford University Press, 1989.
12. Stites DP, Stites DP, Stobo JD, et al: Basic & Clinical Immunology, 4th ed. Los Altos, CA: Lange Medical, 1982.
13. Pease RW (ed): Webster's Medical Desk Dictionary. Springfield, MA: Merriam-Webster, 1986.
14. Unanue ER, Benacerraf B: Textbook of Immunology, 2nd ed. Baltimore: Williams & Wilkins, 1984.
15. Sheehan DC, Hrapchak BB: Theory and Practice of Histotechnology, 2nd ed. Columbus, OH: Battelle, 1980.
16. Bauer J: Clinical Laboratory Methods, 9th ed. St. Louis: CV Mosby, 1982.
17. Heyderman E: Immunoperoxidase technique in histopathology: applications, methods, and controls. J Clin Pathol 1979, 32:971–978.
18. Bancroft J, Stevens A (eds): Theory and Practice of Histological Techniques, 3rd ed. New York: Churchill Livingstone, 1990.
19. Sternberger LA, Hardy PH, Cuculis JJ, Meyer HG: The unlabelled antibody enzyme method of immunohistochemistry: preparation and properties of soluble antigen-antibody complex (horseradish peroxidase-antiperoxidase) and its use in identification of spirochaetes. J Histochem Cytochem 1970, 18:315.
20. Naritoku WY, Clive RT: A comparative study of the use of monoclonal antibodies using three different immunohistochemical methods: an evaluation of monoclonal and polyclonal antibodies against human prostatic acid phosphatase. J Histochem Cytochem 1982, 30:253–260.
21. Hsu SM, Raine L, Fanger H: Use of avidin-biotin-peroxidase complex (ABC) in immunoperoxidase techniques: a comparison between ABC and unlabeled antibody (PAP) procedures. J Histochem Cytochem 1981, 29:577–580.
22. Regional Educational Course by American Society of Clinical Pathologists (ASCP): Immunohistology: Techniques and Interpretation for Immunoperoxidase, Immunofluorescence and In situ Hybridization. Chicago: ASCP, August 1990.
23. Miller RT: Immunohistochemistry in the community practice of pathology: part I. Lab Med 1991; 22:457–464.
24. Miller RT: Immunohistochemistry in the community practice of pathology: part II. Lab Med 1991; 22:527–532.
25. Nadji M, Morales AR: Immunoperoxidase: part I. The techniques and its pitfalls. Lab Med 1983, 14:767.

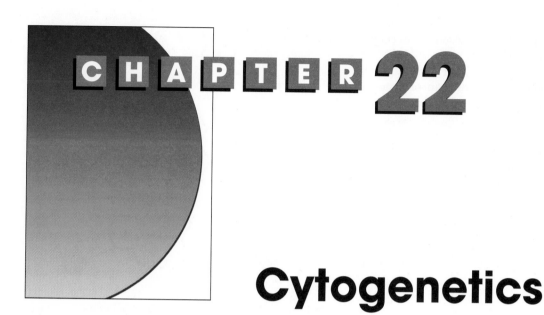

CHAPTER 22

Cytogenetics

Objectives

AFTER COMPLETION OF THIS CHAPTER, THE READER WILL BE ABLE TO

1. Describe chromosome structure and the methods used in chromosome identification.
2. Explain the basic laboratory techniques for preparing chromosomes for analysis.
3. Differentiate between numerical and structural chromosome abnormalities.
4. Identify clinical genetic syndromes associated with specific chromosome abnormalities.
5. Discuss the importance of a karyotype in diagnosis and prognosis in cancer.

Cytogenetics is the study of chromosomes, their structure, and their inheritance. There are more than 50,000 genes in the human genome, most of which reside on the 46 chromosomes normally found in each somatic cell.

Chromosome disorders are either structural or numerical and involve the loss or gain of either a piece of a chromosome or the entire chromosome. Because each chromosome contains thousands of genes, a chromosomal abnormality that is observable by light microscopy causes the disruption of the action and interaction of hundreds of genes. Such disruptions often have a profound clinical effect. Chromosomal abnormalities are observed in approximately 0.6% of all live births.[1] The gain or loss of an entire chromosome other than a sex chromosome is usually incompatible with life and accounts for 50% of first trimester spontaneous abortions.[2]

REASONS FOR CHROMOSOME ANALYSIS

Chromosome analysis is an important diagnostic procedure in clinical medicine. Not only are chromosomal anomalies a major cause of reproductive loss and birth defects, but also certain nonrandom chromosome abnormalities are recognized in many forms of cancer.

Physicians who care for patients of all ages may order karyotyping for analysis of mental retardation, infertility, ambiguous genitalia, short stature, fetal loss, risk of genetic or chromosomal disease, and cancer. In the following discussion, basic cytogenetic concepts and procedures are presented. This field is in a period of tremendous growth; therefore, supplementation of the text with molecular methods is recommended.

CHROMOSOME STRUCTURE

Chromosome Architecture

A chromosome is formed from a single, long DNA molecule that contains a series of genes. The complementary double-helix structure of DNA was established in 1953 by Watson and Crick.[3] The backbone of this structure consists of a sugar-phosphate-sugar polymer. The sugar is deoxyribose. Attached to the backbone and filling the center of the helix are four nitrogen-containing bases. Two of these, adenine (A) and guanine (G), are purines, and the other two, cytosine (C) and thymine (T), are pyrimidines (Fig. 22–1).

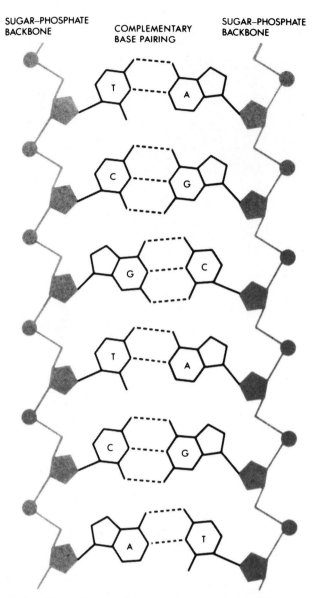

Figure 22–1 The two DNA chains are held together by the pairing of bases on the interior of the helix. Hydrogen bonds unite a purine base with a pyrimidine base. (From Watson JD, Tooze J, Kurtz DT: Recombinant DNA: A Short Course. New York: WH Freeman, 1983.)

The chromosomal DNA of the cell resides in the cell nucleus. This DNA and protein are referred to as chromatin. During the cell cycle at a stage called mitosis, the nuclear chromatin condenses approximately 10,000-fold to form chromosomes.[4] Each chromosome represents a folding and compaction of the entire nuclear chromatin. This compaction is achieved through multiple levels of helical coiling and supercoiling (Fig. 22–2).

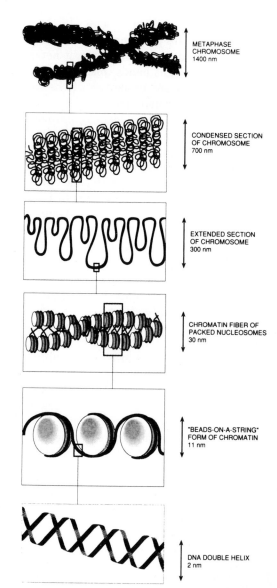

Figure 22–2 Chromosome structure. The folding and twisting of the DNA double helix. (From Gelehrter TD, Collins FS: Principles of Medical Genetics. Baltimore: Williams & Wilkins, 1990.)

Metaphase Chromosomes

Electron micrographs of metaphase chromosomes have provided models of chromosome structure. In the "beads on a string" model of chromatin folding, the DNA helix is looped around a core histone protein.[5] This packaging unit is known as a nucleosome and measures approximately 11 nm in diameter.[6] Nucleosomes are then packed together in regular twisting arrays to form an approximately 30-nm chromatin fiber. This fiber, called a solenoid, is further condensed and bent into a loop configuration. These loops extend at an angle from the main chromosome axis[7] (Fig. 22–3).

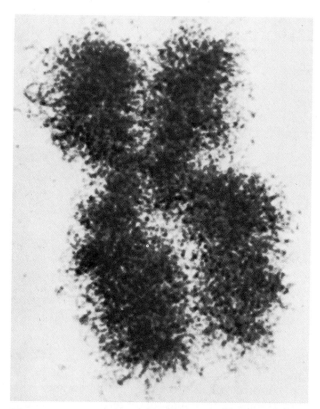

Figure 22–3 Electron microscopy of a human metaphase chromosome demonstrating the looped chromatin attached to a central scaffold. (From Bahr GF: In Yunis JJ [ed]: Molecular Structure of Human Chromosomes. New York: Academic Press, 1977:143.)

CHROMOSOME IDENTIFICATION

Cell Cycle

The cell cycle is divided into four stages: G_1, the period before DNA synthesis; S, DNA synthesis; G_2, the period after DNA synthesis; and M, the shortest phase of the cell cycle, mitosis or cell division. During mitosis, chromosomes are maximally condensed. While in mitosis, cells are chemically treated to arrest cell progression through the cycle so that the chromosomes can be analyzed (Fig. 22–4).

Chromosome Banding

Analysis of each individual chromosome is made possible by staining the mitotic chromosome with dye. In fact, the name chromosome is derived from Greek: *chroma,* meaning color, and *soma,* meaning body; hence *chromosome* means colored body. Caspersson in 1969[8] was the first investigator to successfully stain chromosomes with a fluorochrome dye. Using quinicrine mustard, which binds to adenine-thymine (AT)–rich areas of the chromosome,

DNA Synthesis

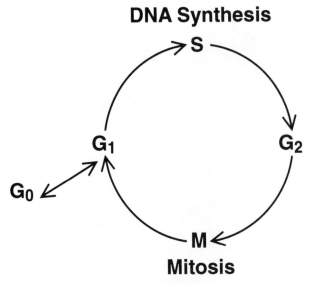

Figure 22–4 Cell cycle.

4 and the acrocentric chromosomes (13, 14, 15, 21, and 22). Humans are polymorphic (i.e., their chromosomes contain differing amounts of heterochromatin) for these bright bands, just as they are for the size and fluorescent properties of the satellites of the acrocentric chromosomes.

Other stains are used to identify chromosomes, but unlike Q-banding, these methods normally necessitate some pretreatment of the slide to be analyzed. Giemsa (G) bands can be obtained by pretreating the chromosomes with the proteolytic enzyme trypsin. GTG banding means G-banding by Giemsa with the use of trypsin. Giemsa positively stains AT-rich areas of the chromosome. These dark bands are called G+ bands. Guanine-cytosine (GC)–rich areas of the chromosome have little affinity for the dye and are referred to as G− bands. G+ bands correspond to the brightly fluorescing bands of Q-banding (Fig. 22–6).

R-banding (reverse Giemsa or G− bands) requires pretreatment of the chromosomes with hot (80–90 °C) alkali and subsequent staining with Giemsa. As the name implies, this banding pattern is the opposite of Giemsa staining: that is, the G+ bands by Giesma are light with R-banding, and the G− bands by Giemsa are dark with R-banding. R-banding is often useful for the study of structural changes of the ends of the chromosomes or telomeres. By G-banding, these areas are often

he was able to distinguish a banding pattern unique to each individual chromosome. This banding pattern, called Q-banding, differentiates the chromosome into bands of differing lengths and relative brightnesses (Fig. 22–5). The most brightly fluorescent bands of the 46 human chromosomes are the distal end of the Y chromosome and the centromeric regions of chromosomes 3 and

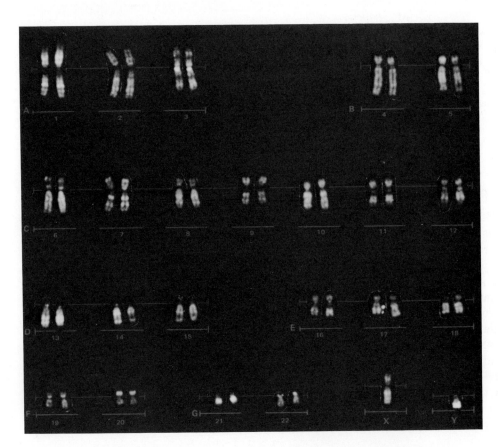

Figure 22–5 Q-banded preparation. Note the intense brilliance of Yq. (Courtesy of the Cytogenetic Laboratory, Indiana University School of Medicine.)

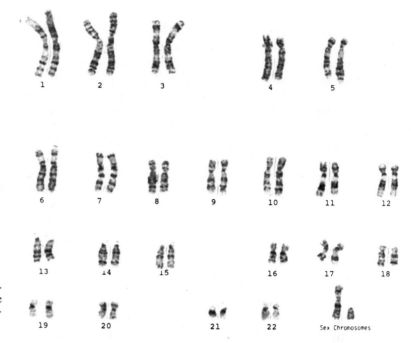

Figure 22–6 Normal male karyotype: G-banded preparation. (Courtesy of the Cytogenetic Laboratory, Indiana University School of Medicine.)

light (G–), and so with R-banding they would be stained positively and be dark.

C-banding stains the centromere (primary constriction) of the chromosome and the surrounding heterochromatin. Constitutive heterochromatin is a special type of repetitive DNA that is located primarily at the centromere of the chromosome. In C-banding, the chromosomes are treated first with an acid and then with an alkali (barium hydroxide) before Giemsa staining. C-banding is most intense in human chromosomes 1, 9, and 16 and the Y chromosome. Polymorphisms are also observed in the C bands from different individuals. These polymorphisms have no clinical significance (Fig. 22–7).

Specific chromosomal regions that are associated

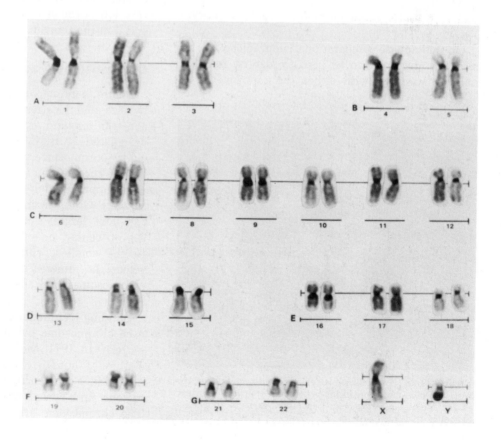

Figure 22–7 C-banded male karyotype. (Courtesy of the Cytogenetic Laboratory, Indiana University School of Medicine.)

with the nucleoli in interphase cells are called nucleolar organizer regions (NORs). NORs contain tandemly repeated ribosomal RNA genes. NORs can be differentially stained in chromosomes by a silver stain that is referred to as AG-NOR banding.

Chromosome banding is visible after chromosome condensation, and the banding pattern observed depends on the degree of condensation. By examining human chromosomes very early in mitosis, it has been possible to estimate that the total haploid genome (23 chromosomes) contains approximately 2000 AT-rich (G+) bands.[9] The later the stage of mitosis, the more condensed the chromosome and the fewer total G+ bands.

Nonradioactive in Situ Hybridization

Use of new molecular methods coupled with standard karyotype analysis is improving chromosomal detection capability beyond that of the light microscope. DNA or RNA probes labeled with either fluorescent or enzymatic detection systems are being hybridized directly to metaphase or interphase cells on the microscopic glass slide. These probes usually belong to one of three classes: (1) probes for repeated DNA sequences, primarily generated from centromeric DNA; (2) whole chromosome probes, which include segments of an entire single chromosome; and (3) specific loci or single copy probes. The first two types of probes are typically generated from chromosome-specific libraries.

On metaphase preparations, nonradioactive in situ hybridization can be used to identify individual chromosomes with either the centromeric or whole chromosome "paint" probes (Fig. 22–8). Marker chromosomes represent chromatin material that has been structurally rearranged and sometimes cannot be identified by a typical band pattern. Fluorescent in situ hybridization (FISH) has been helpful in marker identification.[10]

Specific loci probes can be used to map anonymous segments of DNA to individual chromosomes. FISH has been applied to the detection of deletions of specific gene loci, as in the Miller-Dieker syndrome,[11] as well as to the detection of amplification or increased gene copy number.[12]

Nonradioactive in situ hybridization can also be performed on interphase cells. The use of interphase cells avoids the necessity of culturing and harvesting cells for metaphase preparation.

Chromosome Number

In 1956, Tijo and Levan[13] identified the correct number of human chromosomes as 46. This is the diploid chromosome number and is determined by counting the chromosomes in dividing somatic cells. The term representing the diploid number is 2n. Gametes (ovum and sperm) have half the diploid number (23). This is called the haploid number of chromosomes and is designated n.

Different species have different numbers of chromosomes. The reindeer has a relatively high chromosome number for a mammal (2n = 76), whereas the Indian muntjac, or barking deer, has a very low chromosome number (2n = 7 in the male and 6 in the female).[14]

Chromosome Size and Type

Before banding, chromosomes were categorized by size and location of the centromere (primary constriction) and assigned to one of seven groups designated A, B, C, D, E, F, or G. Group A includes chromosome pairs 1, 2, and 3. These are the largest chromosomes, and their centromeres are located approximately in the middle (i.e., are metacentric). Group B chromosomes, pairs 4 and 5, are the next largest chromosomes; their centromeres are off-center, or submetacentric. Group G refers to the smallest chromosomes, pairs 21 and 22, whose centromeres are located at the ends of the chromosomes and are designated acrocentric (Fig. 22–9).

Banding techniques enabled scientists to identify each chromosome pair by a characteristic banding pattern. In 1971, the Paris conference for nomenclature of human chromosomes was convened to designate a nomenclature system to describe the regions and specific bands of the chromosomes. The chromosome arms were designated p (petite)

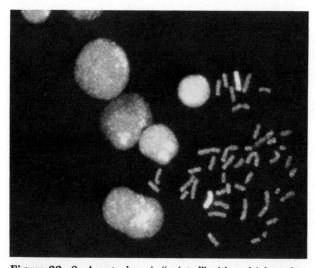

Figure 22–8 A metaphase is "painted" with multiple probes from chromosome 7, producing a fluorescent signal. (Courtesy of the Molecular Cytogenetic Laboratory, Indiana University School of Medicine.)

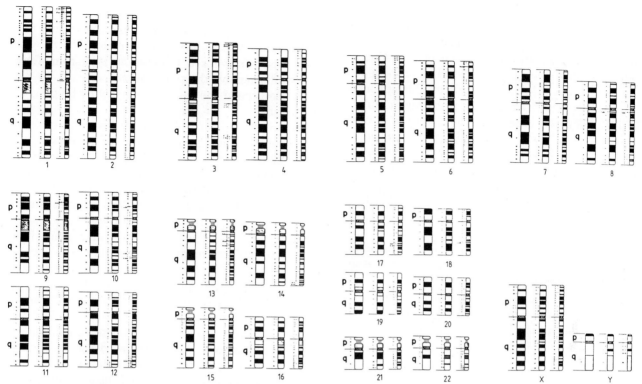

Figure 22–9 International System for Human Cytogenetic Nomenclature. (From Report of the Standing Committee on Human Cytogenetic Nomenclature. Basel, Switzerland: S. Karger AG, 1985.)

for the short arm, and q for the long arm. The regions in each arm as well as the bands contained within each region were numbered consecutively from the centromere toward the telomere. Therefore, to designate a specific region of the chromosome, the number is written first, followed by location on the short or long arm, then the region of the arm, and finally the specific band. For example Xq21 is the X chromosome, the long arm, region 2, band 1. To designate a sub-band, a decimal point is placed after the original band designation, followed by the number assigned to the sub-band: for example, Xq21.1 (Fig. 22–10).

TECHNIQUES OF CHROMOSOME ANALYSIS

Tissues used for chromosome analysis are composed of cells that either exhibit an inherently high mitotic rate (bone marrow cells) or can be stimulated to divide in culture (blood lymphocytes). Special harvesting procedures are established for each tissue. The method that follows is for blood leukocytes and represents the standard procedure from which various modifications are made. This is the method used in the cytogenetic laboratory at Indiana University School of Medicine.

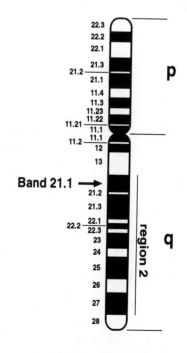

X Chromosome

Figure 22–10 Banding pattern of the human X chromosome at the 550-band level.

Preparation of Blood

Peripheral blood leukocytes can be stimulated to divide in culture by the addition of the mitogens such as phytohemagglutinin (PHA) or pokeweed mitogen. PHA primarily stimulates T lymphocytes to divide,[15] whereas pokeweed primarily stimulates B lymphocytes.[16] After short-term culture of mitogen-stimulated white blood cells, cell growth is arrested during metaphase by the addition of colcemide, which inhibits formation of the mitotic spindle. The specimen is treated with a hypotonic solution to swell the cells. Then cells are fixed in a 3:1 mixture of methanol and acetic acid and dropped onto cold, wet slides to achieve optimal dispersal of the chromosomes. Peripheral blood is a tissue frequently used for postnatal chromosome studies. It is easy to obtain, and culture is simple. Blood is collected in sodium heparin (green top) tubes, and cultures are prepared with either whole blood (microculture) or isolated leukocytes (macroculture).

MACROCULTURE METHOD

The macroculture method for culture of leukocytes, as performed in the cytogenetics laboratory of the Indiana University School of Medicine, is as follows:

1. Allow blood (7–10 mL) to settle for 1–3 hours at room temperature or centrifuge at 100 g for 5–10 minutes.
2. Using a pipette, dispense 10 mL of culture medium (McCoy's 5A with 20% heat-activated Rehatuin and 0.1% antibiotics plus glutamine) into a sterile 25-cm² culture flask.
3. Add 0.2 mL (9 mg/mL) of PHA.
4. With a pipette, siphon off 0.7 mL to include the plasma, the buffy coat, and a small amount of red blood cells. Place into the 25-cm² culture flask containing media and PHA.
5. Place culture in a 5% CO_2 incubator at 37 °C with caps loosened.
6. Incubate cultures at 37 °C for 66–72 hours.
7. Add 60 μL (10 mg/mL) of colcemide.
8. Re-incubate culture at 37 °C for 35 minutes.
9. At the end of 35 minutes, decant the contents of the culture flask into a 15 mL conical centrifuge tube.
10. Centrifuge for 5 minutes at 1400 rpm.
11. Using a pipette, siphon off supernatant, and mix pellet by flicking the bottom of the tube with a finger. Add 10 mL of 0.075M KCL while holding conical tube at a 45-degree angle.
12. Invert conical tube to mix. Place the tube in a 37 °C incubator for 13 minutes.

13. After 13 minutes, invert tube to mix. Add 2 mL of cold 3:1 methanol and acetic acid fixative. Invert to mix.
14. Centrifuge for 8 minutes at 1000 rpm. Carefully remove the supernatant.
15. Resuspend the pellet completely by tapping the tube.
16. Add 10 mL of 3:1 fixative. Invert to mix. Incubate at room temperature for 20 minutes.
17. Spin at 1000 rpm for 8 minutes. Carefully remove the supernatant.
18. Add 4 mL of fixative. Cap tightly and invert gently. Spin at 1000 rpm for 8 minutes. Aspirate the supernatant. Repeat once.
19. Tightly cap the conical tube, and place it in the refrigerator overnight or for up to 3 days. Alternatively, two more rounds of fixative-centrifugation will prepare cells for slide dropping.
20. After the last round of fixative-centrifugation, the pellet of cells should be diluted in fresh 3:1 fixative to give an adequate suspension for dropping, one that is not so dense that metaphase cells overlap one another or so sparse that only a few metaphase cells are seen on the entire slide.
21. The fixed cell suspension is dropped onto cold, wet, ethanol-cleaned slides. The technician reviews the slide under phase microscopy for the quality of metaphase cell preparation.
22. Slides are dried on a 65 °C hotplate and then placed in a 65 °C oven for 18–24 hours.
23. Slides are ready for GTG banding.

MICROCULTURE METHOD

If the blood sample is from an infant or a small child, 0.5 mL of whole blood is used instead of the buffy coat. The whole blood is added to a 25-cm² culture flask containing media and PHA and is processed in the same way as in the macroculture method.

PROCEDURE FOR G BANDING

As stated earlier, G bands are produced by pretreatment of slides with mild salt, or proteolytic enzymes (trypsin), followed by staining with one of the Romanowsky dyes (Giemsa, Wright's, or Leischmann's stain). G+ bands correspond to late-replicating DNA, and the G− bands correspond to early-replicating DNA.

Solutions

1. Trypsin (1:250) 0.1 g of powdered trypsin in 100 mL of isotonic buffered saline (or Isoton).
2. Phosphate buffer, pH 6.8: one Gurr buffer tablet, pH 6.8, per 1 L of triple-distilled H_2O.

3. Isoton with serum: 1 mL of bovine serum/50 mL of Isoton.
4. Working stain solution with Giemsa: 1 mL of Giemsa stain in 49 mL of phosphate buffer, pH 6.8.

Procedure

1. Place working solutions in Coplin jars in the following sequence:
   A. trypsin
   B. isotonic saline with 1 mL of fetal calf serum
   C. isotonic saline
   D. stain
   E. phosphate buffer
   F. triple distilled water
2. Immerse a dried slide in trypsin. The time in trypsin varies, depending on the length of baking of the slide, the humidity conditions, and the type of specimen. Slides prepared from peripheral blood are immersed for approximately 4–5 seconds.
3. Rinse in Isoton with serum.
4. Rinse in Isoton.
5. Stain for 2.5 minutes in working stain solution. Stain times may vary.
6. Rinse in phosphate buffer, pH 6.8.
7. Rinse in triple-distilled H_2O.
8. Blow the slide dry, and wipe excess stain off the back of the slide with alcohol.

METAPHASE ANALYSIS

After banding, slides are scanned under a light microscope with a low-power objective lens ($10\times$). When a metaphase has been selected for analysis, a $63\times$ or $100\times$ oil immersion objective lens is used. Each metaphase is analyzed first for chromosome number. Then each individual chromosome is analyzed for its banding pattern. A normal cell contains 46 chromosomes, which include 2 sex chromosomes. Any variation in number and banding pattern is recorded by the technician. At least 20 metaphase cells are analyzed from leukocyte cultures. If abnormalities are noted, the technician may need to analyze additional cells.

Photography is used to confirm and record the technician's microscopic analysis. Metaphase cells are selected for photography on the bases of (1) containing the modal number of chromosomes, (2) having sharply banded chromosomes, (3) containing no artifacts, and (4) having little or no chromosome overlap.[9]

Prenatal Diagnosis

Prenatal diagnosis involves the use of ultrasonography and cytogenetics in the determination of birth defects. Amniotic fluid is the tissue most commonly used for prenatal diagnosis and is obtained by transabdominal amniocentesis, usually after the 14th week of gestation. However, early amniocentesis can be performed at approximately 11 weeks of gestation.

Amniotic fluid contains cells derived mainly from fetal skin and genitourinary, alimentary, and respiratory tracts, as well as the conjunctivae and amnion. Amniocytes are preferentially cultured on coverslips by in situ harvesting techniques for a more rapid diagnosis.

Chorionic villus sampling involves the removal of a small sample of placental tissue (chorion) for prenatal diagnosis, usually by aspiration biopsy with a thin plastic catheter inserted transabdominally or transcervically into the uterus.[17, 18]

Cytogenetic analysis of the villi can be accomplished either by direct analysis or by culturing the cells on coverslips. Results from direct analysis are available in 24 hours. Cytogenetic results from cultured cells are available in 7–10 days.

CANCER CYTOGENETICS

Cancer cytogenetics is a field that has been built upon the finding of nonrandom chromosome abnormalities in many types of cancer. For example, the Philadelphia chromosome, which represents a reciprocal translocation between the long arm of chromosome 9 and the long arm of chromosome 22, is found in the majority of cases of chronic myelogenous leukemia. Bone marrow is the tissue most frequently used to study the cytogenetics of hematologic malignancies. Cytogenetics of cancer involving other organ systems can be analyzed from solid tissue obtained during surgery or by needle biopsy.

CHROMOSOME DEFECTS

There are many types of chromosome defects, such as deletions, inversions, ring formation, trisomies, and polyploidy. All these defects can be grouped into two major types: those involving an abnormality in the *number* of chromosomes and those involving *structural* changes in one or more chromosomes.

Numerical Abnormalities

Numerical abnormalities are subclassified into aneuploidy and polyploidy. Aneuploidy refers to any number of chromosomes that is not a multiple of the haploid number (23 chromosomes). The common forms of aneuploidy in humans are trisomy (the presence of an extra chromosome) and monosomy (the absence of a single chromosome). Aneuploidy is the result of nondisjunction, the failure of chromosomes to separate normally during cell division. Nondisjunction can occur during meiosis or mitosis. When nondisjunction occurs after fertilization (mitotic nondisjunction), mosaicism occurs. Mosaicism describes the existence of two or more populations of chromosomally different cell lines.

There are two kinds of cell division: mitosis and meiosis. During mitosis, a cell divides once to produce two cells that are identical to the parent cell. Meiosis is a special type of cell division that is used to generate male and female gametes (sperm and oocytes). Unlike mitosis, meiosis entails two cell divisions, meiosis I and meiosis II. The end result is a cell with 23 chromosomes, which is the haploid number (n).

In the first meiotic division, homologous chromosomes, each of which has two chromatids, synapse (pair) and then move toward opposite poles, providing daughter cells with one chromosome of each pair. During the second meiotic division, each chromosome splits longitudinally into individual sister chromatids, which move to opposite poles (dysjunction). As an end result, each of the daughter cells of meiosis that form the gametes contains a haploid number (n) of chromosomes, whereas somatic cells have a diploid number (2n) (Fig. 22–11).

In polyploidy, a chromosome number is greater than 46 but is always an exact multiple of the haploid chromosome number of 23. Triploidy is a karyotype with 69 chromosomes (Fig. 22–12). A karyotype with 92 chromosomes is called tetraploidy.

Structural Aberrations

Structural rearrangements result from breakage of a chromosome region with subsequent rejoining

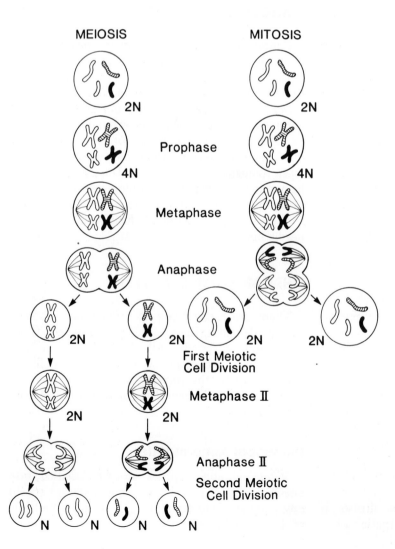

Figure 22–11 In the mitotic cell cycle, there is duplication of nuclear DNA and one cell division, resulting in two daughter cells each with 46 chromosomes. In meiotic division, there is also one replication of nuclear DNA but two cell divisions, resulting in four gametes each with 23 chromosomes. (Modified from Watson JD, Tooze J, Kurtz DT: Recombinant DNA: A Short Course. New York: WH Freeman, 1983.)

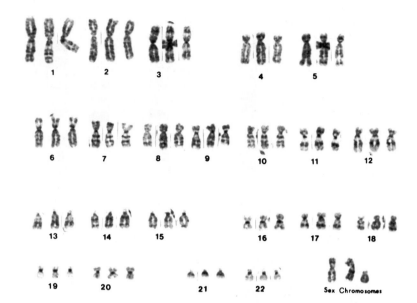

Figure 22-12 A triploid karyotype, 69,XXY. (Courtesy of the Cytogenetic Laboratory, Indiana University School of Medicine.)

in an abnormal combination. Structural rearrangements are defined as balanced (no loss or gain of genetic chromatin) or unbalanced (addition or loss of genetic material).

Structural rearrangements of single chromosomes include inversions, deletions, isochromosomes, ring formations, insertions, translocations, and duplications. Inversions involve one or two breaks in a single chromosome. If the chromosomal material involves the centromere, the inversion is called pericentric. If the material that is inverted does not include the centromere, the inversion is called paracentric (Fig. 22-13).

Interstitial deletions arise after two breaks in the same chromosome and loss of the segment between the breaks. Terminal deletions (loss of chromosomal material from the end of a chromosome) and interstitial deletions involve the loss of genetic material. The clinical consequence to the person with a deletion depends on the extent of the deletion (Fig. 22-14).

Isochromosomes arise from abnormal division of the centromere, which divides perpendicular to the long axis of the chromosome rather than parallel to it. Each resulting daughter cell has a chromosome in which either the short arm or the long arm is duplicated.

Ring chromosomes can result from breakage and reunion of a single chromosome with loss of chromosomal material outside the break. Alternatively, both telomeres may join to form a ring chromosome without significant loss of chromosomal material.

Insertions involve movement of a segment of a chromosome from one area of the chromosome to another area of the same chromosome or movement to another chromosome. The segment is re-

leased as a result of two breaks, and the insertion occurs at the site of another break; thus there are usually three chromosome breaks for an insertion to occur, unless the material inserted is from a terminal segment.

Translocations occur when there is breakage in two chromosomes and each of the broken pieces reunites with another chromosome. If chromatin is neither lost nor gained, the exchange is called reciprocal translocation. A parent with a reciprocal translocation is normal because all chromatin material is present. However, a child of this person may have an unbalanced translocation (usually either monosomy or trisomy for a segment of the chromosome) and therefore be abnormal.

Another type of translocation involving breakage and reunion near the centromeric regions of two acrocentric chromosomes is known as a Robertsonian translocation. These translocations are one

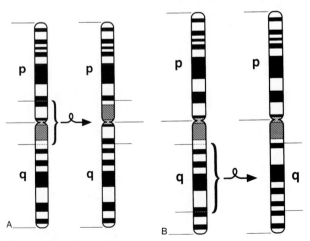

Figure 22-13 *A*, Pericentric inversion. *B*, Paracentric inversion.

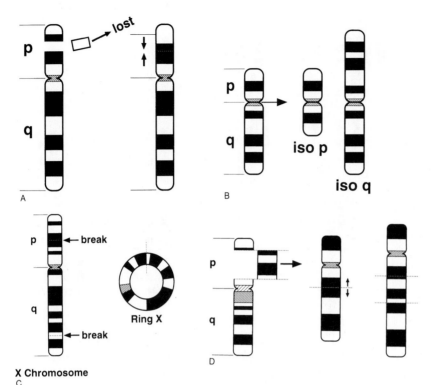

Figure 22–14 *A,* Interstitial deletion. *B,* Isochromosome. *C,* Ring chromosome. *D,* Insertion.

of the most common balanced structural rearrangements seen in the general population, with a frequency of 0.09–0.1%.[19] All five human acrocentric autosomes (13, 14, 15, 21 and 22) are capable of forming a Robertsonian translocation. In this case the resulting balanced karyotype has only 45 chromosomes, which include the translocated chromosome (Fig. 22–15). The carrier of a Robertsonian translocation is phenotypically normal; however, unbalanced offspring result from meiotic

segregation of the translocated chromosome with one of the homologous chromosomes involved in the translocation (e.g., 14;21,+21) or loss of one homologous chromosome (e.g., monosomy 14) (Fig. 22–16).

Duplication means partial trisomy for part of a chromosome. This can result from an unbalanced insertion or unequal crossing over in meiosis or mitosis.

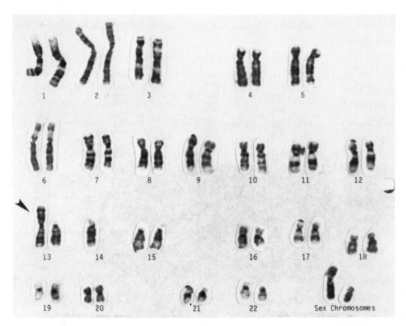

Figure 22–15 A balanced Robertsonian translocation between chromosomes 13 and 14. (Courtesy of the Cytogenetic Laboratory, Indiana University School of Medicine.)

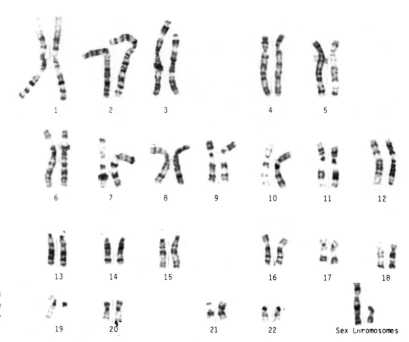

Figure 22–16 An unbalanced Robertsonian translocation, 46,XY,t(21q21q). (Courtesy of the Cytogenetic Laboratory, Indiana University School of Medicine.)

CHROMOSOME SYNDROMES

Down Syndrome and Trisomies 13 and 18

Down syndrome was the first medical condition demonstrated to result from a chromosome abnormality (trisomy 21).[20] Down syndrome is present in approximately 1 in 700 liveborn children and is the most common chromosomal syndrome.[21] About 95% of cases of Down syndrome are due to trisomy 21 (47,XY, or XX,+21), which results from nondisjunction at meiosis I or II in either parent. Most cases arise as a result of an error in segregation in maternal meiosis I.[22] The incidence of nondisjunction increases with maternal age. A 30-year-old mother has a 1/900 risk of giving birth to a child with Down syndrome; a 35-year-old mother has a 1/350 risk; and a 40-year-old mother has a 1/100 risk.[23]

A Robertsonian translocation involving chromosome 21 [t(14;21), t(21;21)], can also result in Down syndrome (see Fig. 22–16). Approximately 4% of individuals with Down syndrome have an extra chromosome 21 as a result of a translocation. This is not age dependent, and persons with trisomy 21 resulting from a translocation cannot be distinguished clinically from those with trisomy 21 resulting from an extra (47th) chromosome.

Clinical features in Down syndrome include growth retardation, mental retardation, and typical facial features that include a flattened face and occiput, upslanting of the eyes, and a protruding tongue. The hands are short and broad, often with a single transverse palmar crease known as a "simian crease." Medical complications occurring at birth and during childhood include congenital heart disease, tracheoesophageal fistula, duodenal atresia, an increased risk of leukemia, and thyroid disease.

Trisomy 13 was first described by Patau and associates in 1960.[24] Like most other trisomies, it is associated with late maternal age. The extra chromosome usually arises from nondisjunction. Trisomy 13 is present in about 1 of 15,000 newborns.[25] These children have severe growth and mental retardation and a shortened life span. Forebrain malformations, such as arhinencephaly and holoprosencephaly, and cleft lip or cleft palate or both are often present, as are a sloping forehead, microphthalmia, and iris coloboma. Also characteristic of trisomy 13 is postaxial polydactyly (extra digits) and cutis aplasia of the scalp. Different types of heart anomalies are common (Fig. 22–17).

Trisomy 18 (Edward's syndrome)[26] is present in approximately 1 in 8000 liveborn infants.[25] As in trisomy 13, prolonged postnatal survival is rare, and like the other trisomies, it is associated with advanced maternal age. The clinical features of trisomy 18 include mental retardation, failure to thrive, microcephaly, prominent occiput, short sternum, overriding clenched fingers, and rocker-bottom feet. Facial features such as small, low-set ears, prominent tip of the nose, small mouth, and micrognathia are common. Like the other trisomies, trisomy 18 can result from meiotic nondisjunction or an unbalanced translocation (see Fig. 22–16).

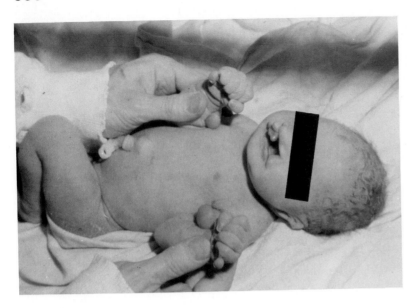

Figure 22–17 An infant with trisomy 13. Note the cleft palate and lip, sloping forehead, and bilateral polydactyly.

Sex Chromosome Disorders

X and Y chromosome aneuploidy is relatively common, and sex chromosome abnormalities are among the most common of all human genetic disorders. The primary clinical abnormality associated with numerical anomalies or structural defects in sex chromosomes is abnormal gonadal development.

X CHROMOSOME TRISOMY (47,XXX)

Trisomy for the X chromosome (47,XXX) is compatible with life, whereas trisomy of an autosome of a size comparable to the X chromosome would not be compatible with life. Affected females may show relatively few abnormal clinical features; however, many have learning disabilities and may be infertile. The relatively mild phenotypic expression of this sex chromosome aneuploidy is thought to be secondary to X chromosome inactivation, in which two X chromosomes would be inactive and late replicating. The theory of X chromosome inactivation was hypothesized by Lyon[27] in an attempt to explain the equalization of expression of X-linked genes in the two sexes. Lyon proposed that one of the X chromosomes in female tissues is inactivated and that inactivation may occur randomly for either the maternal or paternal X chromosome in embryonic development. The X inactivation center has been localized to Xq13.

Although X inactivation is normally random in female somatic cells, nonrandom inactivation is observed in patients with structural abnormalities of the X chromosome or an X;autosome translocation. In an X;autosome translocation, the normal X is preferentially inactivated, and the two parts of the translocated chromosome remain active, selecting against loss of expression or inactivation of autosomal genes.

KLINEFELTER SYNDROME (47,XXY)

The most common disorder of sex chromosome number occurring in males is Klinefelter syndrome (47,XXY). The incidence of this disorder is reported at 1 per 1000 liveborn males. Clinically, affected males are usually physically normal until late childhood or early puberty, at which time they express evidence of hypogonadism. The testes remain small and fail to produce normal amounts of sperm. Secondary sexual characteristics often remain underdeveloped (Fig. 22–18). Almost all Klinefelter patients are infertile. These males may also show breast development (gynecomastia). Klinefelter males may have an average or a below-average IQ and demonstrate behavior problems and personality disturbances.

It has been reported that the nondisjunctional error responsible for approximately 50% of the cases results from errors in paternal meiosis I, one third from errors in maternal meiosis I, and the remainder from errors in meiosis II or from postzygotic mitotic error that leads to mosaicism.[28] About 15% of Klinefelter patients have mosaic karyotypes.

TURNER SYNDROME (45,X)

Unlike the previously mentioned sex aneuploidies, Turner syndrome (45,X) has a very high in utero lethality, peaking around 12–15 weeks. Turner syndrome is characterized by a person who

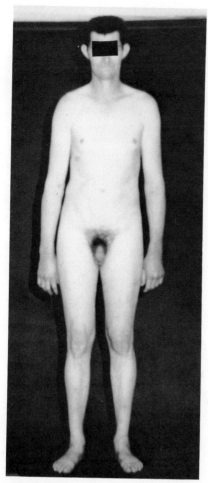

Figure 22–18 A patient with Klinefelter syndrome, 47,XXY.

combination (crossover) from a parent with a balanced translocation. Deletions may involve large amounts of DNA and may be visible by light microscopy, or the deleted segment may be smaller, not visible under the light microscope but detectable by molecular techniques.

PRADER-WILLI SYNDROME

The Prader-Willi syndrome is characterized by hypotonia in infancy, mental retardation, obesity, short stature, small hands and feet, and hypogonadism. Sixty percent of affected patients have an associated deletion of chromosome 15 involving bands q11–q13. Prader-Willi syndrome is present in 1 in 25,000 liveborn infants,[29, 30] and its occurrence is generally sporadic. Prader-Willi syndrome is an example of genetic imprinting. Imprinting implies that genes are modified differently depending on parental origin. Prader-Willi syndrome results from loss of the paternal allele on chromosome 15.[31]

MILLER-DIEKER SYNDROME

The Miller-Dieker syndrome includes lissencephaly (smooth brain), microcephaly, and characteristic facial features such as bitemporal hollowing, a long philtrum with a thin upper lip, and anteverted nares. These patients have mental retardation, and most have seizures. This syndrome results from monosomy of (17) (p13.3).[32]

Molecular probes localized to the Prader-Willi or Miller-Dieker region on the chromosome are routinely used in some laboratories to supplement traditional metaphase analysis for deletions.

CRI DU CHAT (5p—) SYNDROME

The loss of the short arm of chromosome 5, primarily the region of 5p14–5p15, results in a syndrome that includes severe growth retardation, mental retardation, and microcephaly but is characterized particularly by an abnormal cry, which is weak and sometimes high-pitched and sounds like that of a cat. This cry normalizes with age.

is a phenotypic female with gonadal dysgenesis and sexual immaturity. These girls have short stature with generally normal intellectual development. Other characteristic clinical findings are low posterior hairline, webbing of the neck, hypoplastic and widely spaced nipples, increased carrying angles of the elbows, a shield-shaped chest, short fourth metacarpals, and cardiovascular and renal anomalies (Fig. 22–19).

Loss of one entire X chromosome or loss of the short arm of the X chromosome results in Turner syndrome. Chromosomal rearrangements that may yield a Turner phenotype could include an X;autosome translocation with loss of material on Xp, a ring X chromosome, an isochromosome Xq, and X chromosome mosaicism.

Deletion Syndromes

Chromosomal deletions result in partial monosomy of genetic material. Deletions may arise de novo (normal chromosomes in the parents) or result from loss secondary to abnormal meiotic re-

CHROMOSOME DEFECTS IN NEOPLASIA

Unique and recurring chromosomal abnormalities are characteristic of human malignant disease. In hematologic neoplastic disease, specific structural rearrangements are associated with distinct subtypes of leukemia that have certain morphologic and clinical features. Cytogenetic analysis of

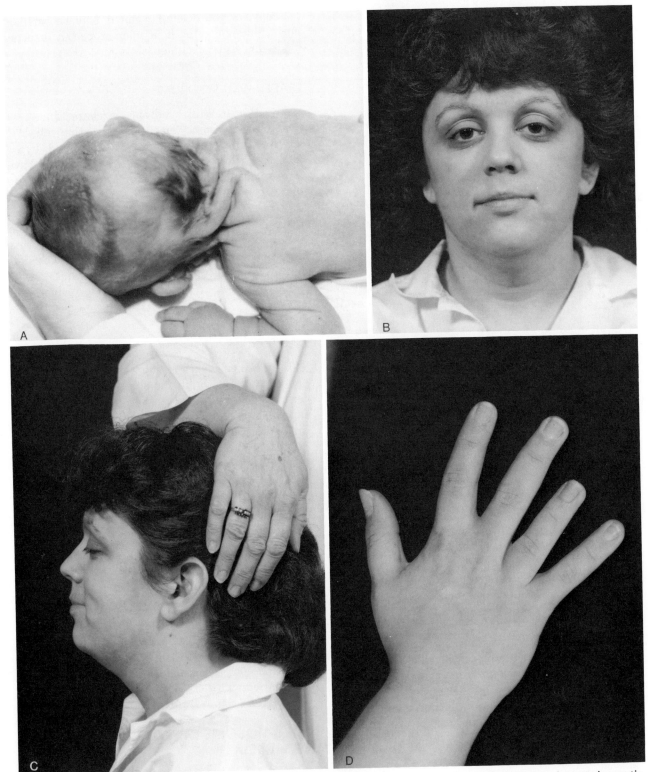

Figure 22–19 *A,* Infant with a 45,X karyotype and redundant neck skin after reabsorption of fluid from an intrauterine cystic hygroma. *B* and *C,* Anteroposterior and lateral views of a 24-year-old woman with three cell lines: 45X/46,X,r(X)/46,X,i(Xq). *D,* right hand with a short fourth metacarpal. (From Davee MA, Weaver DD: Turner syndrome. *In* Buyse ML (ed): Birth Defects Encyclopedia. Cambridge, UK: Blackwell Scientific, 1990:117–118.)

malignant cells can help determine the diagnosis of a hematologic neoplasm and assist the oncologist in the selection of the appropriate therapy, as well as aid in the monitoring of the effects of therapy. Chromosomal defects observed in neoplasia include aneuploidy, polyploidy, and numerous types of structural abnormalities.

Chronic Myelogenous Leukemia

The first malignancy associated with a specific chromosome defect was chronic myelogenous leukemia, in which approximately 90% of patients were found to have a Philadelphia chromosome, t(9;22)(q34;q11).[33, 34] The Philadelphia chromosome represents a balanced translocation between the long arms of chromosome 9 and 22. At the molecular level, the gene for c-abl, which is a proto-oncogene, joins a gene on chromosome 22 named BCR. The result of the fusion of these two genes is a new protein of about 210 kD that is thought to have growth-promoting capabilities that may overcome the normal cell regulatory mechanisms[35] (Fig. 22–20) (see Chapter 27).

Acute Leukemia

The Philadelphia chromosome is also observed in acute leukemia. It is seen in about 20% of adults with acute lymphocytic leukemia (ALL), 2–5% of children with ALL, and 1% of patients with acute myeloid leukemia.[36–38] In childhood ALL, chromosome number is particularly important for predicting the severity of the leukemia. Children whose leukemic cells contain more than 50 chromosomes and who do not have structural abnormalities have the best prognosis for complete recovery with therapy.

The acute myelogenous leukemias are subdivided primarily into seven morphologic classifications ranging from M1 to M7[39] (see Chapter 23). Characteristic chromosome translocations are associated with each classification. A translocation between the long arm of chromosome 8 and the long arm of chromosome 21, t(8;21)(q22;q22), is representative of M2 (acute myeloid leukemia with maturation). M3 (acute promyelocytic leukemia) is associated with a translocation between the long arms of chromosomes 15 and 17, t(15;17)(q22;q12). These recurring translocations have enabled researchers to localize genes critical to cell growth and regulation.

Solid Tumors

Like the recurring structural and numerical chromosome defects observed in the hematologic malignancies, a wide range of abnormalities have been found in a large number of tumors. Some of these abnormalities confer a proliferative advantage on the malignant cell and serve as useful prognostic indicators.

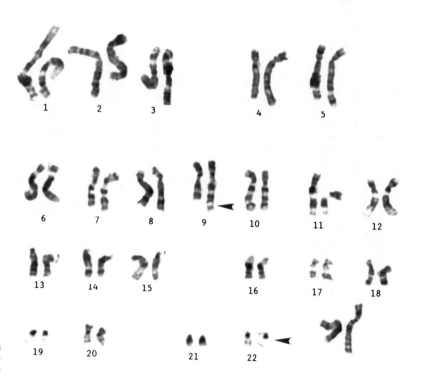

Figure 22–20 Karyotype from a patient with chronic myelogenous leukemia with a Philadelphia chromosome. (Courtesy of the Cytogenetic Laboratory, Indiana University School of Medicine.)

46,XX,t(9;22)(q34;q11)

SUMMARY

Cytogenetic analysis of fetal cells, peripheral blood, bone marrow, and tumor tissue is an integral part of the clinical diagnosis of disease and malformation.

Molecular cytogenetic techniques have considerably broadened the diagnostic capability of cytogenetic laboratories in both the clinical and research settings. In the future, more and more molecular techniques will become part of routine cytogenetic laboratory procedure.

REVIEW QUESTIONS

1. Give two reasons for chromosome analysis.

2. What does the "beads-on-a-string" appearance represent in chromosome structure?

3. What does the nomenclature 1q21 designate?

4. Give two characteristics of tissues used for chromosome analysis.

5. What is the purpose of adding potassium chloride and colcemid to cell cultures?

6. Differentiate between aneuploidy and polyploidy, and give examples of each defect.

7. Define translocation. What is the common translocation found in CML?

8. Name the syndrome that is associated with loss of chromatin from the short arm of chromosome 5. What are the clinical features of this syndrome?

References

1. Buckton KE, O'Riordan ML, Ratcliffe G, et al: A G-band study of chromosomes in liveborn infants. Ann Hum Genet Lond 1980; 43:227–239.
2. Boué J, Boué A, Lazar P: Retrospective and prospective epidemiological studies of 1500 karyotyped spontaneous human abortions. Teratology 1975; 12:11–26.
3. Watson JD, Crick FHC: Molecular structure of nucleic acids: a structure for deoxyribose nucleic acid. Nature 1953; 171:737–738.
4. Earnshaw WC: Meiotic chromosome structure. Bioassays 1988; 9(5):47–150.
5. Olins AL, Olins DE: Spheroid chromatin units. Science 1974; 183:333.
6. Oudit P, Gross-Ballard M, Chamben P: Electron microscope and biochemical evidence that chromatin structure is a repeating unit. Cell 1973; 4:281.
7. Rattner, JB: Chromatin hierarchies and metaphase chromatin structure. In Adolph KW (ed): Chromosomes and Chromatin, vol 3. Boca Raton, FL: CRC Press, 1988:30.
8. Caspersson T, Zech L, Modest EJ, et al: Chemical differentiation with fluorescent alkylating agents in Vicia faba metaphase chromosomes. Exp Cell Res 1969; 58:128–140.
9. Yunis JJ: Cytogenetics. In Henry JB (ed): Clinical Diagnosis and Management by Laboratory Methods, 16th ed. Philadelphia: WB Saunders, 1979:825.
10. Plattner R, Heerema NA, Yurov YB, Palmer CG: Efficient identification of marker chromosomes in 27 patients by stepwise hybridization with alpha satellite DNA probes. Hum Genet 1993; 91:131–140.
11. Kuwano A, Ledbetter SA, Dobyns WB, et al: Detection of deletions and cryptic translocations in Miller-Dieker syndrome by in situ hybridization. Am J Hum Genet 1991; 49:707–714.
12. Trask B, Hamlin J: Early dihydrofolate reductase gene amplification events in CHO cells usually occur on the same chromosome arm as the original locus. Genes Dev 1984; 3:1913–1925.
13. Tijo JH, Levan A: The chromosome number of man. Hereditas 1956; 42:1–6.
14. Hsu TC: Human and Mammalian Cytogenetics. New York: Springer-Verlag, 1979:6–7.
15. Nowell PC: Phytohemagglutinin: an initiator of mitosis in culture of normal human leukocytes. Cancer Res 1960; 20:462–466.
16. Farnes P, Barker BE, Brownhill LE, Fanger H: Mitogenic activity of Phytolacca americana (pokeweed). Lancet 1964; 2:1100–1101.
17. Jackson LG: Prenatal genetic diagnosis by chorionic villus sampling. In Porter IH, Hatcher NH, Willey AM (eds):

Perinatal Genetics: Diagnosis and Treatment. New York: Academic Press, 1986:95–113.
18. Jackson LG, Gibas LM, Coutinho W: Chorionic villus sampling. In Verma RS, Babu A (eds): Human Chromosomes: Manual of Basic Techniques. New York: Pergamon Press, 1989:19.
19. Turleau C, Chavin-Colin F, de Grouchy J: Cytogenetic investigation in 413 couples with spontaneous abortions. Eur J Obstet Gynecol Reprod Biol 1979; 9:65.
20. Lejeune J, Gautier M, Turpin R: Etude des chromosomes somatiques de neuf enfant mongoliens. Compt Rend 1959; 248:1721–1722.
21. Mikkelson M: Down syndrome: cytogentic epidemiology. Hereditas 1977; 86:45–50.
22. Autonarakis SE, Down Syndrome Collaborative Group: Parental origins of the extra chromosome in trisomy 21 as indicated by analysis of DNA polymorphisms. New Engl J Med 1991; 324:872–876.
23. Hook EB: Rates of chromosome abnormalities at different maternal ages. Obstet Gynecol 1981; 58:282–285.
24. Patau KA, Smith DW, Therman EH, et al: Multiple congenital anomalies carried by an extra autosome. Lancet 1960; 1:790–793.
25. Harper PS: Practical Genetic Counseling, 3rd ed. Oxford, England: Butterworth Heinemann, 1988:53.
26. Edwards JH, Harnden DG, Cameron AH, et al: A new trisomic syndrome. Lancet 1960; 1:787–790.
27. Lyon MF: Gene action in the X-chromosome of the mouse. Nature 1961; 190:372–373.
28. Jacobs PA, Hassold TJ, Whittington E, et al: Klinefelter's syndrome: an analysis of the origin of the additional sex chromosome using molecular probes. Am J Hum Genet 1988; 52:93–109.
29. Prader A, Labhart A, Willi H: Ein syndrome von adipositas kleinwucks, kryptochismus and oligophrenie nach myatonieartigen zustard in neugeboren-enalter. Schweiz Med Wochenschr 1956; 86:1260–1261.
30. Butler MG: Prader-Willi syndrome: current understanding of cause and diagnosis. Am J Med Genet 1990; 35:319–322.
31. Nicholls RD, Knoll JHM, Butler MG, et al: Genetic imprinting suggested by maternal heterodisomy in non-deletion Prader-Willi syndrome. Nature 1989; 342:281–288.
32. Stratton RF, Dobyns WB, Airhart SD, Ledbetter DH: New chromosomal syndrome: Miller-Dieker syndrome and monosomy 17p13. Hum Genet 1984; 67:193–200.
33. Nowell PC, Hungerford DA: A minute chromosome in human chronic granulocytic leukemia. Science 1960; 132:1497.
34. Rowley JD: A new consistent chromosomal abnormality in

chronic myelogenous leukemia identified by quinacrine fluorescence and Giemsa staining. Nature 1973; 243:290–293.

35. Ben-Neriah Y, Daley GQ, Mes-Masson A, et al: The chronic myelogenous leukemia-specific P210 protein is the product of the bcr/abl hybrid gene. Science 1986; 233:212–214.

36. Third International Workshop on Chromosomes in Leukemia: Chromosomal abnormalities in acute lymphoblastic leukemia: structural and numerical changes in 234 cases. Cancer Genet Cytogenet 1981; 4:101–110.

37. Riberio RC, Abromowitch M, Raimondi SC, et al: Clinical and biologic hallmarks of the childhood ALL. Blood 1987; 70:948–953.

38. Crist W, Carroll A, Shuster J, et al: Philadelphia chromosome positive ALL: clinical and cytogenetic characteristics and treatment outcome. A pediatric oncology group study. Blood 1990; 76:4892–4894.

39. Bennett JM, Catovsky D, Daniel MT, et al: Proposals for classification of the acute leukaemias. French-American-British (FAB) Co-operative Group. Br J Haematol 1976; 33:451–458.

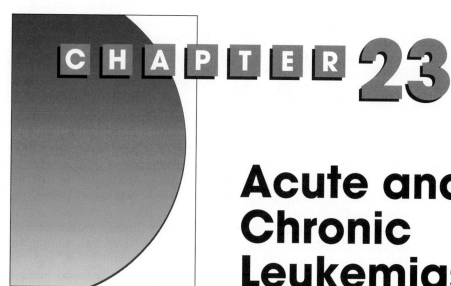

CHAPTER 23

Acute and Chronic Leukemias

Ann T. Moriarty

Objectives

AFTER COMPLETION OF THIS CHAPTER, THE READER WILL BE ABLE TO
1. Clinically and morphologically distinguish acute and chronic leukemias.
2. Characterize blasts of lymphoid and myeloid origin.
3. Explain the subclassification of acute myeloid and lymphoblastic leukemias.
4. Discuss the manifestations of a variety of chronic leukemias.

The leukemias are a group of diseases in which the common manifestation is a malignant unregulated proliferation of cells endogenous to the bone marrow. Leukemia may involve any of the blood-forming cells or their precursors. Although each type of leukemia progresses differently, the unregulated proliferating cells (1) usually replace normal marrow, (2) eventually interfere with normal marrow function, (3) may invade other organs, and (4) eventually cause death if not treated.

The leukemias were first described in 1845. The chronic leukemias were first to be characterized. Bennett[1] and Virchow[2] noticed large spleens and "white blood" at autopsy of patients who had died of an uncharacterized chronic disease of 1–2 years' duration. Virchow's description of "white blood" was subsequently translated into the Greek word *leukemia*.[3] Acute leukemia was described about 25 years later when patients with "white blood" were noted to die rapidly, not after a long debilitating illness.[4, 5] It was not until 1877, when Ehrlich developed a stain that allowed microscopic evaluation of white blood cells,[6] that it was realized that "white blood" was caused by increased numbers of white corpuscles. Later, in 1900, it was established that acute and chronic leukemias involved different types of white blood cells.[3] In the chronic leukemias, "white blood" was made up of mature cells; acute leukemias involved immature cells, or "blasts."

Since the 1900s, leukemias have been studied with the microscope, cytochemical stains, electron microscopy, immunologic nuclear and surface markers, and cytogenetic techniques. By subclassification and directed treatments, it is hoped that better treatment and cures will be developed for both acute and chronic leukemias.

GENERAL CLASSIFICATION OF LEUKEMIAS

Despite continued studies and subclassification, the leukemias can still be generally divided into acute and chronic diseases.

Acute leukemias are characterized by abrupt onset of clinical symptoms (fever, hemorrhage, weakness), and death occurs within months if treatment is not instituted.[7, 8] Acute leukemias occur both in children and in adults. Blasts (immature cells of myeloid or lymphoid origin) populate the bone marrow and constitute at least 30% of all nucleated bone marrow cells.[9] Thrombocytopenia is usually found in patients with acute leukemia; in contrast, normal or increased platelet counts are initially seen in patients with chronic leukemia. Anemia and neutropenia are also hallmarks of the acute leukemias.

Chronic leukemias are characterized by the insidious onset of symptoms (weakness, pallor, enlargement of spleen and liver), and death occurs years after the diagnosis.[10] Chronic leukemias usually occur in adults. White blood cell counts are usually elevated in the peripheral blood, and the bone marrow is infiltrated by an increased number of mature cells or cells with recognizable counterparts of normal maturation. Thrombocytopenia is rare until late in the course of the disease. Anemia is often present in the chronic leukemias. In Table 23–1, the clinical and laboratory data of acute and chronic leukemias are compared.

Subclassification of Acute Leukemia

LYMPHOID VERSUS MYELOID

Historically, acute leukemias have also been divided cytomorphologically into acute myeloid (AML) and acute lymphoblastic leukemia (ALL) on the basis of the blasts' morphologic resemblance to myeloblasts or immature lymphocytes (lymphoblasts). AML may also be referred to as acute nonlymphocytic leukemia (ANLL). The cornerstone of the diagnosis has been morphologic features of well-prepared Romanowsky-stained bone marrow specimens.[9, 11, 12] Cytochemistry studies, cytogenetics, and immunophenotyping have recently supplemented the microscopic evaluation of these blasts (see Chapters 21 and 22).

Distinguishing morphologic features are subtle. Lymphoblasts are usually smaller than myeloblasts

Table 23–1. ACUTE AND CHRONIC LEUKEMIAS: COMPARISON OF CLINICAL AND LABORATORY MANIFESTATIONS		
Presentation	**Acute Leukemia**	**Chronic Leukemia**
Onset	Abrupt	Insidious
Death	Months	Years
Ages	All	Adults
White cell counts	Elevated/normal/low	Elevated
Appearance of cells	Blasts (immature)	Mature
Neutropenia	Present	Absent
Anemia	Present	Present
Platelets	Low	Normal/increased
Organomegaly	Mild	Severe

but two to three times the size of normal lymphocytes. When counted by an impedance-type cell counter, their volume overlaps with the that of normal lymphocyte and "monocyte" distribution regions (Fig. 23–1). They usually have scant blue cytoplasm with uniformly coarse chromatin. Their nuclei usually contain few nucleoli.

Myeloblasts are larger cells with larger nuclei. When counted by an impedance-type particle counter, their volume overlies the monocytic or immature granulocytic region (see Fig. 23–1). The cytoplasm is moderate and more grey than that of a lymphoblast. The chromatin is homogeneous and finely granular. Myeloblasts often have two or more prominent nucleoli. Auer rods (spindle-shaped pink-red inclusions composed of azurophilic granule derivatives) may be seen in the cytoplasm of any subtype of AML.[13]

The use of microscopy alone is the initial step in distinguishing AML from ALL. However, flow cytometry, cytogenetics, and cytochemistry studies have increased the accuracy of classification and contributed critically to the final diagnosis in most cases.[14, 15, 16] The effect of treatment protocols will only be meaningful if we accurately classify acute leukemia. As Frederick Gunz has so aptly stated: "Although the simple act of looking at a cell has never lost its importance, it is from the combined use of all tools now available that progress is likely to come."[8]

ACUTE LYMPHOBLASTIC LEUKEMIA

ALL is a disease of childhood; the majority of cases occur between the ages of 2 and 10 years. Although it is rare in adults, a second peak in incidence does occur among elderly patients.[13] Treatment of childhood ALL is a triumph of modern hematology. A uniformly fatal disease before 1970, "good prognosis" ALL has a 90% rate of complete remission, and 60% of the patients are cured.[17] Unfortunately, adults with the disorder have a bleaker outlook: a 74% rate of complete remission and a 37% cure rate.[18]

Only half of patients with ALL have leukocytosis and may not have circulating lymphoblasts.[17] Neutropenia, thrombocytopenia, and anemia are usually present. Because of this pancytopenia, the patients have symptoms of fatigue (caused by anemia), fever (caused by neutropenia and infection), and bleeding (a result of thrombocytopenia). There often is accompanying lymph node enlargement (lymphadenopathy), and a mediastinal mass is present in 5–10% of patients.[17] Enlargement of the spleen (splenomegaly) and of the liver (hepatomegaly) may be seen. Bone pain often results from infiltration of leukemic cells into the bone covering (periosteum). Infiltration of malignant cells into

the meninges occurs in 50% of patients, and lymphoblasts are found in the cerebrospinal fluid (CSF).[19] Intrathecal (instilled into the spinal column) chemotherapy is often given to these patients to prevent central nervous system relapse (see Chapter 28 for treatment) In addition, lymphoblast infiltration into the testes and ovaries is common, especially in relapse.[17]

Prognosis in ALL is dependent primarily on age at the time of diagnosis, on lymphoblast "load" (tumor burden), and on immunophenotype.[8] Patients 2–10 years of age have the best prognosis. Children less than 1 year of age do poorly;[20] children between 1 and 2 have an intermediate prognosis, as do teenagers and young adults.[21] Elevated peripheral blood lymphoblast counts greater than $20-30 \times 10^9$/L, hepatosplenomegaly, and lymphadenopathy all adversely affect outcome and are considered high-risk factors.[8, 22] The T cell and B cell immunophenotypes are associated with a worse outcome in both children and adults, in contrast to the immature B cell phenotypes.[8] In addition, the presence of an aberrant myeloid surface marker found in ALL is associated with a poor outcome in adults.[23]

Other variables possibly associated with poorer prognosis are race (African-American children have a worse prognosis than do whites),[24] the presence of karyotypic abnormalities,[25] and male sex.[26]

Three morphologic subtypes of "blasts" have been identified in ALL according to the French-American-British (FAB) classification system. Although there is much disparity among observers[12] and little prognostic information is gained from the system,[27] it is helpful to understand the range of morphology encountered in ALL[11] (Fig. 23–2).

The FAB-L1 blast is a small lymphoblast (one to two and one-half times the size of a normal lymphocyte). It has scant, blue cytoplasm and indistinct nucleoli and is the most common type of blast encountered in ALL; 71% of cases have the L1 morphology.[13]

The FAB-L2 blast is larger (two to three times the size of a lymphocyte) and has prominent nucleoli and nuclear membrane irregularities. Bone marrow specimens of patients with L2 type of ALL display variation in cell size (a heterogeneous population), as opposed to the specimens of patients with FAB-L1, whose blasts appear monotonous. L2 morphology is seen second most commonly in ALL and accounts for approximately 27% of ALL cases.[28] The FAB-L2 blast may be confused with the blasts of acute myeloid leukemia. Morphologic scoring systems have been developed to help distinguish cases of FAB-L1 from FAB-L2.[12] Unfortunately, from morphology alone, the immunophenotype of L1 or L2 blasts cannot be determined.

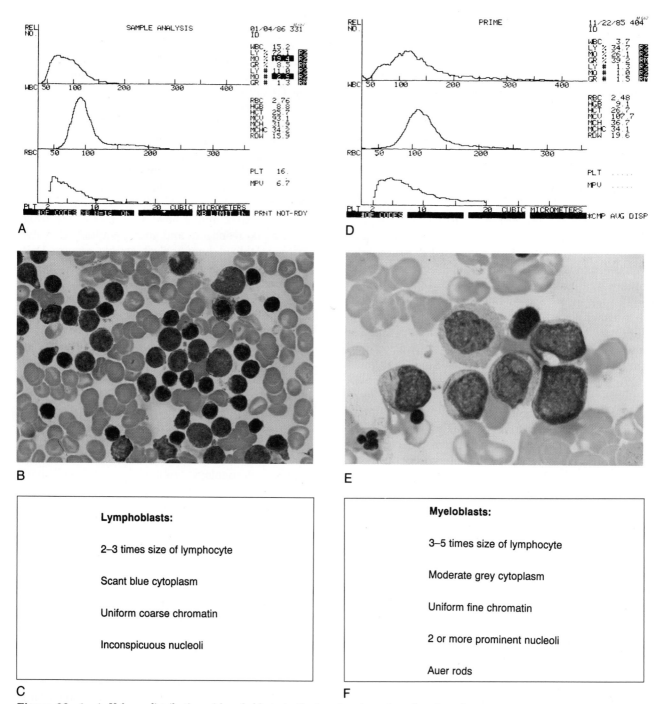

Figure 23–1 *A*, Volume distribution of lymphoblasts in the lymphocyte region of an impedance counter. *B*, Lymphoblasts (bone marrow, Wright's stain; original magnification, 220×). *C*, Description of lymphoblasts. *D*, Volume distribution of myeloblasts. *E*, Myeloblasts (bone marrow, Wright's stain; original magnification, 330×). *F*, Description of myeloblasts.

The FAB-L3 lymphoblasts are very large, have three to five prominent nucleoli and midnight blue cytoplasm, and often contain cytoplasmic vacuoles. The L3 blast resembles the malignant lymphocyte seen in undifferentiated lymphoma (Burkitt's lymphoma) (see Chapter 25). This subtype accounts for a small number of cases of ALL.[13]

Although morphology is the first tool in distinguishing ALL from AML, immunophenotyping is

often the only reliable indicator of a cell's origin. Because it has such prognostic implications, immunologic characterization of ALL should be performed in all cases. In general, four types of ALL are identified immunologically: CALLa(CD10) expressing immature B cell ALL; pre–B cell ALL without CALLa(CD10); T cell ALL; and B cell ALL.[29]

In the most common type of immature B cell

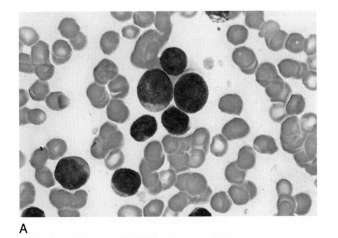

A

L1 Lymphoblast:

Small

Scant blue cytoplasm

Round nuclei

Indistinct nucleoli

Most common type

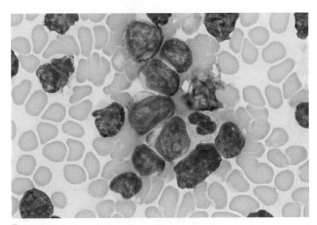

B

L2 Lymphoblast:

2–3 times size of lymphocyte

Moderate cytoplasm

Irregular nuclear membrane

Prominent nucleoli

May overlap with AML

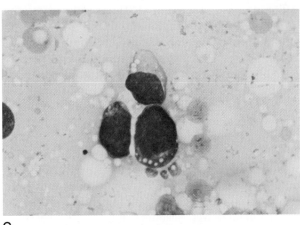

C

L3 Lymphoblast:

Large

Midnight blue cytoplasm

Cytoplasmic vacuoles

3–5 nucleoli

Figure 23–2 Morphologic variants of lymphoblasts according to the French-American-British (FAB) classification. *A*, L1 lymphoblast (bone marrow, Wright's stain; original magnification, 250×). *B*, L2 lymphoblast (bone marrow, Wright's stain; original magnification, 250×). *C*, L3 lymphoblast (bone marrow, Wright-Giemsa stain; original magnification, 250×).

ALL, the marker CALLa (common ALL antigen) or CD10 is expressed on the cell surface. Other immature B cell markers are expressed, but not cytoplasmic immunoglobulin (CIg) or surface immunoglobulin (SIg). This type constitutes 80% of pre–B cell ALLs. Pre–B cell ALL, in which immature B cell markers but not CD10 are expressed, is the second most common ALL; and CIg but not SIg is expressed. Immature B cell ALL is associated with the best prognosis.[8, 13]

B cell ALL is the most uncommon ALL, and SIg as well as kappa or lambda light chain restriction is expressed. Morphologically, a large number of B cell ALLs correspond to FAB-L3.[30] This condition carries a very poor prognosis; death occurs within 1 year of diagnosis.[31]

In T cell ALL, a variety of T cell surface antigens are expressed. The cells may be terminal deoxyribonucleotidyl transferase– (Tdt-) positive. T cell ALL is most often seen in teenage males with a mediastinal mass, elevated peripheral blast counts, meningeal involvement, and infiltration of extramarrow sites. Although this immunophenotype has classically been associated with a poor outcome, aggressive chemotherapy has resulted in improved prognosis with an outcome intermediate between those of B cell ALL and pre–B cell ALL.[27]

A fifth subtype of ALL is the so-called null ALL. It is probably a variety of diseases. It is associated with a poor prognosis and is now considered to be very rare. No lymphocyte surface antigens or cytoplasmic immunoglobulin are present. No myeloid antigens are expressed; Tdt may be expressed. As investigators become better able to classify ALL, this "wastebasket" subset will probably be invalidated.[27]

ACUTE MYELOID LEUKEMIA

AML is the most common leukemia in children less than 1 year of age. It is rare in older children and adolescents, and a second peak of incidence occurs among adults 40 years of age. This leukemia is rapidly fatal if not treated.[13] There are seven types of AML, which are discussed in detail.

The clinical presentation of a patient with AML is nonspecific and reflects the decreased production of normal bone marrow elements. The patient with AML usually has an elevated white blood cell count, and myeloblasts are present.[32] Anemia, thrombocytopenia, and neutropenia give rise to the clinical findings of pallor, fatigue, bruising and bleeding, and fever with infections. In addition, disseminated intravascular coagulation (DIC) and other bleeding abnormalities are noted, especially with the promyelocytic (M3) and monocytic (M5) types of AML.[33] Infiltration of malignant cells into the gums and other mucosal sites, as well as skin, are commonly seen in the myelomonocytic (M4) and monocytic (M5) types.[34]

Bone pain and joint pain are seen as the first symptoms in 25% of patients. Splenomegaly is seen in half of all AML patients, but lymph node enlargement is rare. CSF involvement in AML is rare and does not seem to be as ominous as in ALL. Patients with AML tend to have few symptoms related to the central nervous system when it is infiltrated by blasts.[32]

Other laboratory abnormalities commonly seen in patients with AML are elevated lysozyme levels (especially in monocytic subtypes), hyperuricemia (caused by increased cellular turnover), hyperkale-

mia (caused by cell breakdown), hyperphosphatemia, and hypocalcemia. When cell counts are elevated and these findings are pronounced, this condition is called the "tumor-lysis syndrome,"[35] and renal failure, tetany, and lethal heart arrhythmias may develop.

The FAB cooperative group has defined seven subtypes of AML. These subtypes are based on bone marrow morphology and cytochemical reactions.[9] A 500-cell differential count of Romanowsky-stained films of bone marrow should be performed. The myeloid-to-erythroid ratio (M:E) should be established first. When the myeloid cells outnumber the erythroid precursors (M:E ratio > 1), 30% or more of all nucleated cells of the marrow must be blasts in order to render a diagnosis of AML. If fewer than 30% are blasts, a diagnosis of myelodysplastic syndrome (see Chapter 26) should be considered.

If the erythroid precursors outnumber the myeloid cells (M:E ratio < 1), myeloblasts must constitute 30% of non-erythroid cells to qualify for a diagnosis of AML. This specific type of AML is FAB-M6, or erythroleukemia, and is discussed in greater detail later in this chapter.

Two types of myeloblasts have been described by the FAB group: type I blasts have a typical blast morphology and do not have azurophilic granules; type II blasts may contain a small number of primary granules.[36]

The seven subtypes of AML as defined by the FAB are described as follows.[9]

M1: Acute Myeloblastic Leukemia Without Maturation. This subtype displays minimal myeloid differentiation (Fig. 23–3). Myeloblasts must constitute more than 30% of the marrows' nucleated cells, and the M:E is greater than 1. Ninety percent of the non-erythroid cells are myeloblasts. Three percent of the myeloblasts must show positivity when stained for myeloperoxidase or Sudan black B. This subtype is easily confused with ALL (usually the L2 type), and immunophenotyping is often helpful in assigning lineage to this leukemia. M1 accounts for 20% of cases of AML.

M2: Acute Myeloblastic Leukemia with Maturation. Again, 30% of all nucleated cells must be blasts in a bone marrow, and myeloid cells outnumber nucleated red blood cells. Blasts constitute fewer than 90% of non-erythroid cells, and there is maturation beyond the promyelocyte stage in more than 10% of non-erythroid cells (Fig. 23–4). Monocytes must constitute fewer than 20% of non-erythroid cells. The majority of blasts show positivity when stained with myeloperoxidase or Sudan black B.[13] This subtype accounts for approximately 30% of cases of AML.

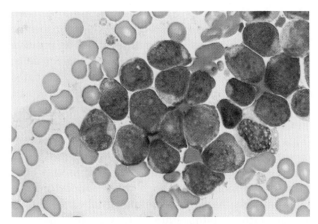

Figure 23–3 Acute myeloblastic leukemia without maturation (FAB-M1). Blasts constitute 90% of the non-erythroid cells; there is less than 10% maturation of the granulocytic series beyond the promyelocyte stage. (Bone marrow, Wright's stain; original magnification, 250×).

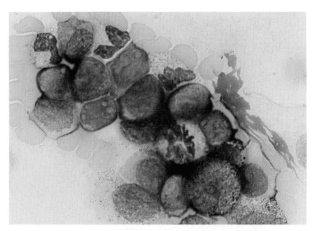

Figure 23–4 Acute myeloblastic leukemia with maturation (FAB-M2). Blasts constitute 30% of the nucleated cells of the marrow, and there is maturation beyond the promyelocytic stage in more than 10% of non-erythroid cells. Notice the band forms, myelocytes, and metamyelocytic cells in association with myeloblasts. (Bone marrow, Wright's stain; original magnification, 250×.)

M3: Acute Promyelocytic Leukemia. There are two types of M3 AML. The more common is the hypergranular variant. In hypergranular M3, more than 30% of cells are myeloblasts, and abnormal promyelocytes with extremely heavy granularity of the cytoplasm are present (Fig. 23–5A). There are numerous Auer rods, often stacked like cords of wood (so-called faggot cells). Nuclei are frequently reniform or bilobed. The cells are strongly positive for myeloperoxidase and Sudan black. The second type of M3 AML, the microgranular promyelocytic leukemia (M3V), is promyelocytic leukemia whose granules are so small as to be unresolved (cannot be distinguished from one another) by the light microscope. Numerous granules are visible by electron microscopy.[37] These cells have the same reniform or bilobed nuclear features as those in the hypergranular variant,

with abundant clear cytoplasm and rare dust-like granules seen in an eccentric location next to the nucleus (see Fig. 23–5B). The abnormal cells likewise are strongly positive for myeloperoxidase. This subtype is often confused with acute monocytic leukemia (M5).

Additional information, not considered in the FAB classification, that may be helpful in the diagnosis of AML M3 is the absence of human leukocyte antigen DR(1a) (HLA-DR1a), as detected by flow cytometry,[38] and the presence of a characteristic chromosome translocation, t(15;17)[39] (see Chapters 22 and 27).

It is extremely important to recognize both types of M3 AML because a bleeding diathesis may occur when these patients are treated and the

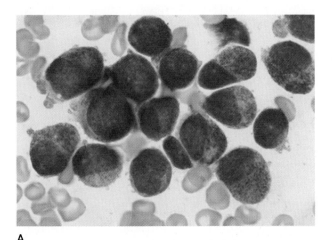

A

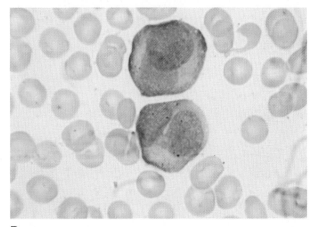

B

Figure 23–5 Acute promyelocytic leukemia (FAB-M3). *A,* A low-power view of the more common granular variant. (Peripheral blood smear, Wright's stain; original magnification, 330×.) *B,* A high-power view showing bilobed nuclear features of the microgranular variant. (Bone marrow, Wright-Giemsa stain; original magnification, 250×.)

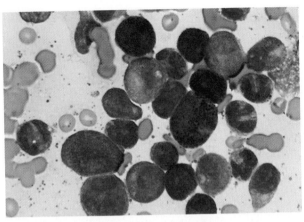

Figure 23–6 Acute myelomonocytic leukemia with eosinophilia (FAB-M4E). Monocytic cells constitute more than 20% of the marrow cells, but fewer than 80%. The hybrid eosinophilic cells with large basophilic granules are apparent in this figure. (Bone marrow, Wright's stain; original magnification, 250×.)

granules are released. DIC may occur in patients with either hypergranular M3 or M3V, and patients are often treated with heparin before the institution of chemotherapy.[33] M3V and hypergranular M3 together account for approximately 15% of all AML.

M4: Acute Myelomonocytic Leukemia. Acute myelomonocytic leukemia is characterized by malignant cells with both granulocytic and monocytic features. In a marrow specimen in which more than 30% of all nucleated cells are blasts, when the M:E ratio is greater than 1, more than 20% of non-erythroid cells are of monocytic origin. The proportion of monocytic cells cannot exceed 80% of the non-erythroid cells. If the absolute monocyte count in the peripheral blood is 5×10^9/L or higher, the diagnosis is M4. If there is no

absolute monocytosis in the peripheral blood, then in order to make the diagnosis of M4, a nonspecific esterase stain of the bone marrow must be positive in more than 20% of bone marrow precursor cells, or serum or urine lysozyme levels must be three times higher than normal.

A small proportion (4%) of myelomonocytic leukemias are characterized by moderate eosinophilia. This subtype is referred to as myelomonocytic leukemia with eosinophilia (M4E) (Fig. 23–6). Bone marrow specimens from affected patients may contain 5% or more eosinophils with monocytoid nuclei and large basophilic granules that stain abnormally with chloroacetate esterase and periodic acid–Schiff (PAS). These M4E leukemias are also associated with a characteristic inversion of chromosome 16 (inv [16][p13 q22]).[40] AML-M4E patients are more likely to have CSF involvement[41] and, paradoxically, to have a better remission rate and better rate of response to chemotherapy. Recognition of this subtype is therefore extremely important.[42]

M5: Acute Monocytic Leukemia. Acute monocytic leukemia accounts for 12% of AML cases. The diagnosis is based solely on the bone marrow morphology. More than 30% of cells are blasts in a marrow with more myeloid than erythroid precursors. More than 80% of the cells must be of monocytic morphology; less than 20% are granulocytic cells. Two subtypes of M5 are recognized: M5a and M5b.

M5a is acute monocytic leukemia, poorly differentiated; more than 80% of the monocytic cells are monoblasts. Monoblasts have delicate chromatin, prominent nucleoli, and dark blue to grey budding cytoplasm (Fig. 23–7A). Because of the undifferentiated appearance, this subtype may be confused

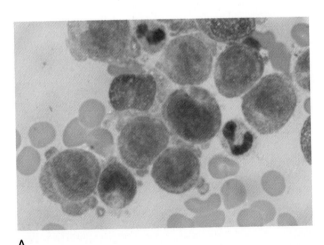

A

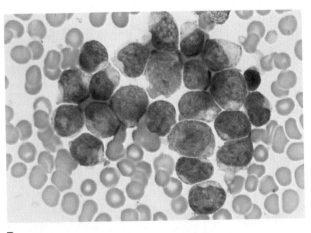

B

Figure 23–7 Acute monocytic leukemia (FAB-M5). A, Poorly differentiated monocytic leukemia (M5a) consists of 80% monoblasts. These are undifferentiated cells with prominent central nucleoli and, often, budding cytoplasm. B, Acute monocytic leukemia with differentiation (M5b). Less than 80% of the monocytic component is composed of monoblasts. There is monocytic differentiation with cerebriform nuclei and abundant cytoplasm. (Bone marrow, Wright's stain; original magnification, 250×.)

with M1. Patients with M5a tend to be younger, to have elevated peripheral blast counts, and to have a poorer prognosis.[34]

M5b is acute monocytic leukemia, differentiated. Fewer than 80% of the monocytic cells are monoblasts, and the preponderance of cells are recognizable monocytes and promonocytes, with large cerebriform nuclei that may have nucleoli and abundant translucent grey cytoplasm that may contain fine pink granules (Fig. 23–7B). The peripheral blood in patients with M5b usually has a high percentage of more mature monocytes. This subtype is associated more often with gingival hypertrophy (gum infiltration). Skin involvement is seen in both subtypes, and DIC is also seen in M5 (like M3), but heparin therapy is not necessary (unlike M3).

In both subtypes, more than 80% of leukemic cells are stained with nonspecific esterase. Myeloperoxidase and Sudan black stains may not reveal any cytoplasmic positivity.

M6: Acute Erythroleukemia. Acute erythroleukemia is a rare type of AML (3% of cases) and is the only AML with hyperplasia of erythroid precursors. More than 50% of the bone marrow cells are nucleated red blood cells (a reversed M : E ratio). Of the remaining (non-erythroid) cells, 30% are myeloblasts. The erythroid cells are often bizarre and show megaloblastoid features; multinucleation is common. There may be perinuclear vacuoles in pronormoblasts and basophilic normoblasts (Fig. 23–8). PAS stains are frequently positive in the erythroid cells; early precursors have "block" positivity, whereas later erythroblasts exhibit diffuse PAS staining. Ringed sideroblasts may also be prominent.

A myelodysplastic syndrome often precedes AML-M6[43] and has been referred to as "erythemic myelosis." During this phase of the disease, the patient has progressive anemia with erythroid hyperplasia of the bone marrow with dyserythropoiesis, but the blasts are less than 30% of nonerythroid cells. Ringed sideroblasts may be seen, as are prominent peripheral basophilic stippling.

M7: Acute Megakaryocytic Leukemia. Acute megakaryocytic leukemia is the rarest of AML, constituting 1% or fewer cases of AML, and is the variant most recently defined by the FAB.[44] The incidence of this disorder may be underestimated because of the difficulty in defining the megakaryoblast cytochemically, and it may actually represent as much as 10% of cases of AML.[45] The diagnosis of M7 depends on the presence of 30% blasts in the marrow (all nucleated cells); 30% of these blasts are megakaryoblasts.

Morphologically megakaryoblasts are heterogeneous in size; some blasts are the size of L1 lymphoblasts with scant cytoplasm, whereas others are three times that size. Chromatin is delicate with prominent nucleoli. Immature megakaryocytes may be seen, and cells may have light blue cytoplasmic blebbing (Fig. 23–9). Megakaryoblasts do not react with Sudan black stain, myeloperoxidase, or alpha-naphthyl butyrate esterase, but they may stain with alpha-naphthyl acetate esterase. The blasts must be identified with platelet peroxidase activity detected by electron microscopy[46] or, preferably, from positive staining with antibodies to platelet glycoprotein IIb/IIIa, Ib or factor VIII:related antigen (VIIIR:Ag).[47]

In adults, M7 has a varied clinical manifestation. Many patients with M7 have a preceding myeloproliferative disorder with pancytopenia or myelofibrosis.[48] In children, M7 is seen more frequently

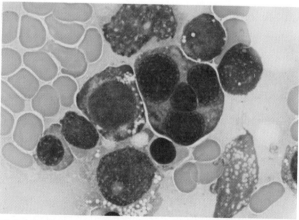

Figure 23–8 Acute erythroleukemia (FAB-M6). Dyserythropoeisis is present with megaloblastoid chromatin. Note the abnormal vacuolated pronormoblast centrally. The vacuoles would stain with periodic acid–Schiff. The blast count in M6 is 30% of non-erythroid cells. (Bone marrow, Wright's stain; original magnification, 250×.)

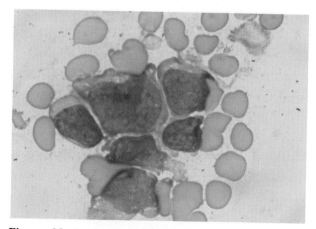

Figure 23–9 Acute megakaryocytic leukemia (FAB-M7). Variable blast size and cytoplasmic blebbing are present. These cells expressed glycoprotein IIb/IIIa. (Bone marrow, Wright's stain; original magnification, 330×.)

among patients less than 3 years old and with Down syndrome.[47] Response to therapy is relatively poor.[48]

OTHER ACUTE MYELOID-LIKE LEUKEMIAS

Acute undifferentiated leukemia, minimally differentiated (M0) AML, and hybrid leukemias are often treated as AML and are therefore mentioned briefly.

Undifferentiated acute leukemia is a heterogeneous group of disorders in which the lineage of malignant blasts cannot be determined. The blasts are unreactive with cytochemical studies, express no cell antigens that can be detected, and are Tdt-negative.[49]

M0 AML is AML in which the blasts are cytochemically unreactive but myeloid or monocytic cell antigens are detectable on cell surfaces. Some patients with M0 may express Tdt, an enzyme usually associated with ALL.[50]

Hybrid leukemias are leukemias with both lymphoid and myeloid characteristics.[51] They may be bilineal (a mixed population of cells expressing either myeloid or lymphoid features) or biphenotypic (individual cells showing both myeloid or lymphoid features in the same cells). The bilineal hybrid leukemias may occur synchronously (at the same time) or metachronously (one leukemia followed by a relapse with a different type).[14, 52, 53]

Most of these unusual types of acute leukemias are treated on the basis of traditional morphologic and cytologic data.[49] However, as the understanding of acute leukemia expands and investigators are better able to identify and delineate these malignant cells, treatment regimens and prognoses may change. The laboratory will be challenged to remain abreast of this evolution.

Subclassification of Chronic Leukemia

Just as in the acute leukemias, chronic leukemias can be divided into those of lymphoid and myeloid origin.

LYMPHOCYTIC DISORDERS

There are two major types of chronic lymphoid leukemias: chronic lymphocytic leukemia (CLL) and hairy cell leukemia. A variety of rarer forms of chronic lymphoid leukemias are also mentioned briefly.

Chronic Lymphocytic Leukemia. CLL is the most common type of leukemia and usually occurs in older patients; it is rare in patients less than 40 years of age.[54] It affects twice as many males as females.[55] The clinical course is variable. Most patients live at least 1–2 years after the diagnosis; median length of survival is 6 years, and some patients live many more years with the disease and die of other causes.[13, 56]

The disease is often discovered incidentally when other medical problems are being investigated. If symptoms are present, they are usually nonspecific, such as weakness, fatigue, and weight loss. Lymphadenopathy and marked hepatosplenomegaly are frequently seen in patients with this disease. In fact, well-differentiated lymphocytic lymphoma (WDLL) (see Chapter 25) is a lymph node–based disease composed of the same malignant cells as seen in CLL. These two disease processes are indistinguishable morphologically and immunophenotypically.

The malignant cell in CLL is usually a small, mature-appearing lymphocyte with a B cell immunophenotype (Fig. 23–10A) The diagnosis of

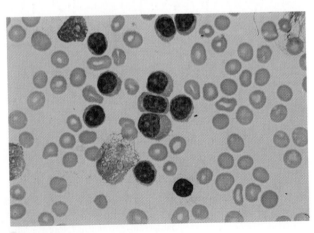

A   B

Figure 23–10   *A,* Chronic lymphocytic leukemia (CLL) characterized by small round, mature-appearing lymphocytes. *B,* Prolymphocytoid "transformation" in CLL. Cells have prominent nucleoli and more cytoplasm than in typical CLL. (Peripheral blood smear, Wright's stain; original magnification, 250×.)

CLL depends on a sustained lymphocyte count greater than 10×10^9/L. All other causes of lymphocytosis must be ruled out. More than 30% of all nucleated blood cells in the bone marrow are lymphocytes with a weak expression of SIg with light chain expression. Typically, these cells express both CD5 (usually thought of as a T cell marker) and characteristic B cell antigens.

If the patient's lymphocyte counts are sustained at greater than 10×10^9/L, documenting either bone marrow or the typical phenotype is acceptable for diagnosis. If lymphocyte counts are less than 10×10^9/L, both bone marrow involvement and immunophenotype must be present in order to render a diagnosis of CLL.

Anemia and thrombocytopenia usually appear late in the course of the disease and are associated with a later stage of CLL. Two staging systems are currently used for CLL (Table 23–2), and integrating both systems is recommended.[57]

CLL is often associated with autoimmune phenomena. Autoimmune hemolytic anemia occurs in 15–35% of patients.[58] Immune-associated neutropenia, thrombocytopenia, and in rare instances, pure red blood cell aplasia[59-61] have been seen.

CLL may remain stable or undergo morphologic "transformation." Over several years, some patients' lymphocytes may gradually undergo a prolymphocytoid transformation. There is usually increasing anemia, thrombocytopenia, splenomegaly, and lymphadenopathy. The circulating cells have more finely granular chromatin and prominent nucleoli and occur as a second population among the smaller, more mature-appearing cells. The patients who have undergone prolymphocytoid transformation usually are less responsive to treatment.[55]

Richter's syndrome is a transformation of CLL to a large-cell lymphoma, a rapidly progressing lethal disease that occurs in 3–15% of patients with CLL.[62] On rare occasions (fewer than 1% of the cases), acute blast crisis occurs in CLL; the blasts usually resemble L2 lymphoblasts of ALL.[63]

Hairy Cell Leukemia. Hairy cell leukemia is a rare malignant disorder accounting for 2% of all leukemias. It usually occurs in middle-aged patients; median age is 50 years.[13] It has an insidious onset characterized by weakness and lethargy. Splenomegaly is present in 80% of patients.[64] Pancytopenia is characteristic of this disorder, and bone marrow aspirates result in a "dry tap" as a result of infiltration of the bone marrow and reticuloendothelial organs of the body by hairy cells.

Hairy cells have reniform to oval nuclei with finely granular chromatin and delicate grey cytoplasm with projections (filipodia), which give the cells their "hairy" appearance (Fig. 23–11). These cells are stained with acid phosphatase, which is not destroyed by preincubation with tartrate (so-called tartrate-resistant acid phosphatase [TRAP] staining).[65]

Because a "dry tap" occurs frequently in the procurement of bone marrow samples, hairy cell leukemia is most often evaluated with bone marrow biopsy, in which the hairy cells are widely spaced and have oval to indented centrally placed nuclei, which give them a "fried egg" appearance.

Immunologically, the hairy cell is a mid- to late B cell with SIg and cytoplasmic immunoglobulin as well as the antigen PCA-1 but not PC-1.[66]

Like patients with other chronic leukemias, patients with hairy cell leukemia may live for years with the disease; the median length of survival is 7 years.

Table 23-2. THE TWO STAGING SYSTEMS FOR CHRONIC LYMPHOCYTIC LEUKEMIA	
Stage	**Presentation**
RAI STAGING SYSTEM	
0	Lymphocytosis in blood and bone marrow
I	Lymphocytosis and enlarged lymph nodes
II	Lymphocytosis with organomegaly
III	Lymphocytosis and anemia (Hb < 11.0 g/dL)
IV	Lymphocytosis and thrombocytopenia (platelet count < 100 × 10⁹/L)
BINET STAGING SYSTEM	
A	Hb > 10.0 g/dL Platelet count > 100 × 10⁹/L < 3 Lymph node areas enlarged
B	Hb > 10.0 g/dL Platelet count > 100 × 10⁹/L > 3 Lymph node areas enlarged
C	Hb < 10.0 g/dL or Platelet count < 100 × 10⁹/L

Abbreviation: Hb, hemoglobin.

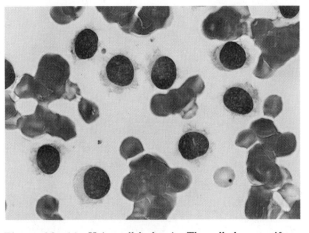

Figure 23–11 Hairy cell leukemia. The cells have reniform to oval nuclei with delicate grey cytoplasmic projections. (Peripheral blood smear, Wright-Giemsa stain; original magnification, 400×.)

Other Chronic Leukemias of Lymphoid Origin. Other chronic leukemias of B lymphoid cells are prolymphocytic leukemia, Waldenström's macroglobulinemia, and lymphosarcoma cell leukemia. Prolymphocytic leukemia is a de novo B cell leukemia characterized by cells resembling the prolymphocytoid cells of CLL. Clinically, the leukocyte level is greatly elevated (higher than 100×10^9/L), and there is severe splenomegaly and, in rare instances, lymphadenopathy.[67] Waldenström's macroglobulinemia is characterized by plasmacytoid lymphocytes with both surface and intracytoplasmic IgM. Secretion of IgM results in a monoclonal protein with hyperviscosity syndrome.[55] Lymphosarcoma cell leukemia is a leukemic phase of a malignant lymphoma, usually a small cleaved-cell lymphocytic lymphoma.[68]

Chronic leukemias of T cell origin are rare. Fewer than 5% of patients with CLL have a T cell phenotype. (T cell CLL is more aggressive than B cell CLL and often infiltrates the skin.[55] Sézary syndrome, or cutaneous T cell lymphoma, occurs in middle-aged patients who have skin rashes or dermatitis (a disease called mycosis fungoides) characterized by Sézary cells that invade the dermis. These cells are mature T cells that express CD4. Late in the course of the skin disease, these cells may circulate and infiltrate lymph nodes and other organs. Sézary cells have cerebriform nuclei, coarse chromatin, and inconspicuous nucleoli[69] (Fig. 23–12A). Adult T cell leukemia/lymphoma syndrome is an aggressive T cell disorder characterized by lytic bone lesions, leukocytosis (leukocyte counts higher than 50×10^9/L), hypercalcemia, and skin infiltration and infection by the human T cell leukemia/lymphoma virus 1 (HTLV-1). The cells are cerebriform but more variable in size than those seen in T cell CLL or Sézary syndrome[70] (Fig. 23–12B).

CHRONIC MYELOGENOUS LEUKEMIA

CML is best considered a chronic myeloproliferative disorder and is discussed in Chapter 24. Like all the other myeloproliferative disorders, CML is characterized by panmyelosis with a predominance of the myeloid component in the bone marrow, peripheral blood, and other organs.

CML can occur at any age but is most common after the age of 45 years. Weight loss and fatigue are often the initial symptoms (as in most chronic leukemias). There is usually massive splenomegaly as a result of the myeloid infiltration. This splenomegaly may cause left upper abdominal pain.

There is anemia, markedly elevated levels of leukocytes (50 to 500×10^9/L or greater), thrombocytosis, eosinophilia, basophilia, and a spectrum of granulocytic maturation with a predominance of myelocytes in the peripheral blood. Myeloblasts constitute fewer than 10% of circulating leukocytes. Occasional nucleated red blood cells are seen; in fact, when the peripheral blood resembles a bone marrow aspirate specimen, CML is usually the diagnosis (Fig. 23–13).

Leukocyte alkaline phosphatase is usually close to zero, and the Philadelphia chromosome (Ph¹), a translocation of the long arm of chromosome 22 to chromosome 9, t(9;22), is present in virtually all cases of CML when sensitive molecular probes are used.[71]

Patients with CML usually undergo a chronic phase that lasts 3 years (median). An accelerated phase then ensues characterized by worsening clinical features that are less responsive to therapy.[72]

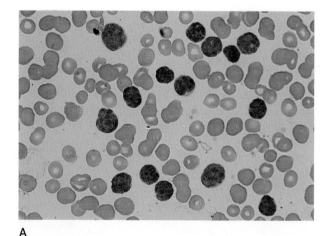

A

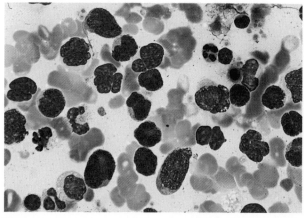

B

Figure 23–12 *A*, Sézary cells of mycosis fungoides with cerebriform, clefted nuclei and coarse chromatin. (Peripheral blood smear, Wright's stain; original magnification, 220×.) *B*, Adult T cell leukemia/lymphoma cells in a patient who was infected by HTLV-1. The cells are cerebriform and vary more in size than do Sézary cells. (Peripheral blood smear, Wright's stain; original magnification, 250×.)

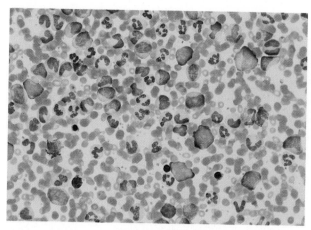

Figure 23–13 Peripheral blood smear from a patient with chronic myelogenous leukemia. At low power, the peripheral blood resembles bone marrow. Nucleated red cells and the entire spectrum of granulocytic maturation are represented. (Wright's stain; original magnification, 100×.)

Approximately one third of patients enter "blast crisis," in which their disease resembles acute leukemia; the proportion of blasts exceeds 30% of cells in blood and bone marrow. One third of patients experiencing blast crisis have ALL, and two thirds have AML blast crisis.[73]

SUMMARY

Leukemia is a group of disorders that has been recognized only since the mid-1800s. Leukemias can be either acute (rapid clinical course) or chronic (prolonged disease process). Leukemias can also be divided into those of lymphoid or myeloid origin. There are morphologic, cytochemical, immunologic, and sometimes cytogenetic characteristics of each of the leukemias that allow them to be distinguished from one another.

Regardless of the subtype, the malignant cells of leukemias proliferate in the bone marrow, interfere with normal marrow function, may invade the blood and other organs, and eventually cause death if left untreated.

By better defining the leukemias, better treatment and better prognoses for patients with the disease will become available.

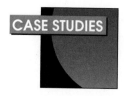

CASE STUDIES

Case 1

A 70-year-old man was seen by his physician for fatigue, decreased exercise tolerance, and left upper quadrant abdominal pain. He had always been in good health, walked several miles a day, and lived alone.

Physical examination revealed that he was a well-developed, slightly pale patient who had splenomegaly and three enlarged nontender lymph nodes in his neck. Laboratory studies showed a white blood cell count of 37.9 × 10⁹/L, a hemoglobin level of 9.7 g/dL, an MCV of 91.2 fL, and a platelet count of 130 × 10⁹/L.

1. Given the patient's age, the physical examination findings, and the laboratory data, what is the most likely diagnosis?

2. Would you expect this to be a T cell or B cell disorder?

3. What would the blast count be in the bone marrow?

4. Would you expect this patient to live for more than 5 years, die rapidly after treatment, or be treated with bone marrow transplantation?

Case 2

A five-year-old female was seen by her family doctor because of weakness and headaches. She had been in good health except for the usual communicable diseases of childhood.

Physical examination revealed a pale, listless child with multiple bruises. The white blood cell count was 15 × 10⁹/L, the hemoglobin count was 8.0 g/dL, and the platelet count was 90 × 10⁹/L. She had "abnormal cells" in her peripheral blood (Fig. 23–14).

1. What is the most likely diagnosis: chronic lymphocytic leukemia, essential thrombocythemia, chronic granulocytic leukemia, or acute lymphoblastic leukemia?

2. What are the best prognostic features of this disease?

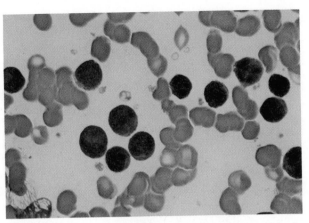

Figure 23–14 Case 2: "abnormal cells" in peripheral blood.

3. Which would be considered a "good" phenotype for these cells: CD10 and TDT positivity, surface immunoglobulin positivity, the presence of T cell phenotype, or cytoplasmic immunoglobulin?

Case 3

A 48-year-old male was seen by his primary care physician for a fever of 3 days' duration. He complained of mouth sores, bleeding gums, and a sore throat. He noticed that he had been tired and bruised easily in the past week.

When examined, he had oral ulceration, oozing gums, pallor, and bruises on his lower extremities. He was febrile, with increased heart and respiratory rates. His liver and spleen were not enlarged, and he had no lymphadenopathy. The white blood cell count was $142 \times 10^9/L$, the hemoglobin level was 11.6 g/dL, and the platelet count was $30 \times 10^9/L$. Cells seen on his peripheral blood are pictured in Figure 23–15.

1. What is the most likely diagnosis, in view of the clinical picture, the blood counts, and the blood smear findings?

2. Which subtypes of this disorder are most likely to cause gum infiltrates?

3. Why does the patient have bruises?

4. What would the bone marrow findings be?

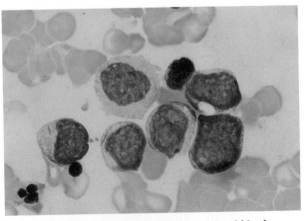

Figure 23–15 Case 3: cells in peripheral blood.

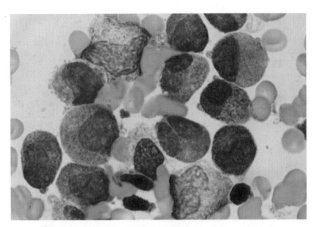

Figure 23–16 Case 4: cells in peripheral blood.

Case 4

A 20-year-old female was admitted to the emergency room with fever and chills. She complained of "not feeling well" for 2 days.

Upon examination, she was very pale but had no localized findings. The white blood cell count was 80×10^9/L, the hemoglobin level was 9.0 g/dL, and the platelet count was 65×10^9/L. A peripheral blood smear contained cells shown in Figure 23–16. A bone marrow aspiration and a biopsy specimen were obtained. The M:E ratio was 2:1, and more than 30% of the cells resembled those seen on the peripheral blood smear.

1. What immunophenotypic findings might be present?

2. What characteristic chromosome abnormality might be seen?

3. What subtypes of AML might be considered in the differential diagnosis?

References

1. Bennett JH: Two cases of disease and enlargement of the spleen in which death took place from the presence of purulent matter in the blood. Edinb Med Surg J 1845; 64:413–423.
2. Virchow R: Weisses Blut und Milztumoren. Med Ztg 1846; 15:151–163.
3. Gunz FW: The dread leukemias and their prospects. *In* Wintrobe MM (ed): Blood Pure and Eloquent: A Story of Discovery, of People, and of Ideas. New York: McGraw-Hill, 1980:511–516.
4. Friedreich N: Ein neuer fall von leukamie. Arch Pathol Anat 1857; 12:37–58.
5. Ebstein W: Ueber die acute leukamie und pseudoleukamie. Deutsches Arch Klin Med 1889; 44:343–358.
6. Ehrlich P: Farbenanalyttische untersuchungen zur histologie und klinik des blutes. Berlin: Hirschwald, 1891:141.
7. Tivey H: The natural history of untreated acute leukemia. Ann N Y Acad Sci 1954; 60:322.
8. Henderson ES: Treatment terminology and overview. *In* Henderson ES, Lister TA (eds): Leukemia, 5th ed. Philadelphia: WB Saunders, 1990:385.
9. Bennett JM, Catovsky D, Daniel MT, et al: Proposed revised criteria for the classification of acute myeloid leukemia. Ann Intern Med 1985; 103:626–629.
10. Perkins ML: Introduction to leukemia and the acute leukemias. *In* Pittiglio DH, Sacher RA (eds): Clinical Hematology and Fundamentals of Hemostasis. Philadelphia: FA Davis, 1987:227–243.
11. Bennett JM, Catovsky D, Daniel MT, et al: Proposals for the classification of acute leukaemias. Br J Hematol 1976; 33:451–458.

12. Bennett JM, Catovsky D, Daniel MT, et al: The morphological classification of acute lymphoblastic leukaemia: concordance among observers and clinical correlations. Br J Hematol 1981; 47:553–561.
13. Davey FR, Nelson DA: Leukocytic disorders. *In* Henry JB (ed): Clinical Diagnosis and Management by Laboratory Methods, 18th ed. Philadelphia: WB Saunders, 1991:693.
14. Del Vecchio L, Schiavone EM, Ferrarra F, et al: Immunodiagnosis of acute leukemia displaying ectopic antigens: proposals for a classification of promiscuous phenotypes. Am J Hematol 1989; 31:173–180.
15. Chan LC, Pegram SM, Greaves MF: Contribution of immunophenotyping to the classification and differential diagnosis of acute leukemia. Lancet 1985; 1:475–479.
16. Neame PB, Soamboonsrup P, Browman GP, et al: Classifying acute leukemia by immunophenotyping: a combined FAB-immunologic classification in AML. Blood 1986; 68:1355–1362.
17. Poplak DG, Reaman G: Acute lymphoblastic leukemia in childhood. Pediatr Clin North Am 1988; 35:903–936.
18. Hoelzer D, Theil E, Loffler H, et al: Prognostic factors in a multicenter study for treatment of acute lymphoblastic leukemia in adults. Blood 1988; 711:123–131.
19. Jacobs AD, Gale RP: Recent advances in the biology and treatment of acute lymphoblastic leukemia in adults. N Engl J Med 1984; 311:1219–1231.
20. Reaman GH, Steinherz PG, Gaymon PS, et al: Improved survival of infants less than 1 year of age with acute lymphoblastic leukemia treated with intensive multiagent chemotherapy. Cancer Treat Rep 1987; 71:1033–1038.

21. Sather HN: Age at diagnosis of childhood acute lymphoblastic leukemia. Med Pediatr Oncol 1986; 14:166–172.
22. George S, Fernbach D, Viette J, et al: Factors influencing survival in pediatric acute leukemia. Cancer 1973; 32:1542–1553.
23. Drexler H, Theil E, Ludwig W: Review of the incidence and clinical relevance of myeloid antigen–positive acute lymphoblastic leukemia. Leukemia 1991; 5:637–645.
24. Walters TR, Bushmore M, Simone J: Poor prognosis in Negro children with acute lymphoblastic leukemia. Cancer 1972; 29:210–214.
25. Cimino MC, Rowley JD, Kinnealey A, et al: Banding studies of chromosome abnormalities in patients with acute lymphocytic leukemia. Cancer Res 1979; 39:227–238.
26. Miller DR: Prognostic factors in childhood acute lymphoblastic leukemia. J Pediatr 1975; 87:672–676.
27. Henderson ES, Hoelzer D, Freeman AI: The treatment of acute lymphoblastic leukemia. *In* Henderson ES, Lister TA (eds): Leukemia, 5th ed. Philadelphia: WB Saunders, 1990:468.
28. Bororwitz MJ: Acute lymphoblastic leukemia. *In* Knowles DA (ed): Neoplastic Hematopathology. Baltimore: Williams & Wilkins, 1992:1297.
29. Greaves MF, Janossy G, Peto J, Kay H: Immunologically defined subclasses of acute lymphoblastic leukaemia in children: their relationship to presentation features and prognosis. Br J Haematol 1981; 48:179–197.
30. Van Eys J, Pullen J, Head D, et al: The French-American-British (FAB) classification of leukemia. The Pediatric Oncology Group experience with lymphocytic leukemia. Cancer 1986; 57:1046–1051.
31. Henderson ES, Afshani E: Clinical manifestation and diagnosis. *In* Henderson ES, Lister TA (eds): Leukemia, 5th ed. Philadelphia: WB Saunders, 1990:327.
32. Miller KB: Clinical Manifestations of acute nonlymphocytic leukemia. *In* Hoffman R (ed): Hematology: Basic Principles and Practice. New York: Churchill Livingstone, 1991:720.
33. Goldberg MA, Ginsburg D, Mayer R, et al: Is heparin administration necessary during induction chemotherapy for patients with acute promyelocytic leukemia? Blood 1987; 69:187–191.
34. Tobelem G, Jacquillot C, Chaastana C, et al: Acute monoblastic leukemia: a clinical and biologic study of 74 cases. Blood 1980; 55:71–76.
35. Thomas MR, Robinson WA, Mughal TI, Glode LM: Tumor lysis syndrome following VP16-213 in chronic myelogeneous leukemia in blast crisis. Am J Hematol 1984; 16:185–188.
36. Bennett JM, Catovsky P, Daniel MT, et al: Proposals for the classification of the myelodysplastic syndromes. Br J Haematol 1982; 5551:189–199.
37. Golomb HM, Rowley JD, Vardiman JW, et al: "Microgranular" acute promyelocytic leukemia: a distinct clinical ultrastructural and cytogenetic entity. Blood 1980; 55:253–259.
38. DeRossi G, Avvisati G, Coluzzi S, Fenu S: Immunological definition of acute promyelocytic leukemia (FAB M3): a study of 39 cases. Eur J Haematol 1990; 45:168–172.
39. Berger R, Bloomfield CD, Sutherland G: Report of the Committee on Chromosome Rearrangements in Neoplasia and on Fragile Sites. Cytogenet Cell Genet 1985; 40:490–535.
40. Le Beau MM, Larson RA, Bitter MA, et al: Association of an inversion of chromosome 16 with abnormal marrow eosinophils in acute myelomonocytic leukemia. N Engl J Med 1983; 309:630–636.
41. Holmes R, Keating MJ, Cork A: A unique pattern of central nervous system involvement in acute myelomonocytic leukemia associated with inv (16) (p13q22). Blood 1985; 65:1071–1078.
42. Neri G, Daniel A, Hammond N: Chromosome 16 eosinophilia and leukemia. Cancer Genet Cytogenet 1985; 14:371–372.
43. Van Rhenen DJ, Langenhuijsen MMAC: Clinical and laboratory data related to maturation in acute leukemia. Cancer 1984; 53:1923–1926.
44. Bennett JM, Catovsky D, Daniel MT, et al: Criteria for the

diagnosis of acute megakaryocytic lineage (M7): A report of the French-American-British cooperative group. Ann Intern Med 1985; 103:460–462.
45. Gerwitz AM: Acute megakaryocytic leukemia. Mayo Clin Proc 1989; 64:1447–1451.
46. Bain BJ, Catovsky D, O'Brien M, et al: Megakaryoblastic leukemia presenting as acute myelofibrosis—a study of four cases with the platelet-peroxidase reaction. Blood 1981; 58:206–213.
47. Windebank KP, Tefferi A, Smithson WA, et al: Acute megakaryocytic leukemia (M7) in children. Mayo Clin Proc 1989; 64:1339–1351.
48. San Miguel JF, Gonzales M, Canizo MS, et al: Leukemia with megakaryoblastic involvement: clinical hematologic and immunologic characteristics. Blood 1988; 72:402–407.
49. Chesom B, Cassileth PA, Head DR, et al: Report of the National Cancer Institute–sponsored workshop on definitions of diagnosis and response in acute myeloid leukemia. J Clin Oncol 1990; 8:813–819.
50. Parreira A, Pombo de Oliviera MS, Matutes E, et al: Terminal deoxynucleotidyl transferase–positive acute myeloid leukemia; an association with immature myeloblastic leukemia. Br J Haematol 1988; 69:219–224.
51. Hurwitz CA, Mirro J: Mixed lineage leukemia and asynchronous antigen expression. Hematol Oncol Clin North Am 1990; 4:767–794.
52. Lee EL, Schiffer CA: Leukemias of indeterminant lineage. Clin Lab Med 1990; 10:737–754.
53. Gale RP, Bassat IB: Hybrid acute leukemia. Br J Haematol 1987; 65:261–264.
54. Spier CM, Kjeldsberg CR, Head DR, et al: Chronic lymphocytic leukemia in young adults. Am J Clin Pathol 1985; 84:675–678.
55. Gale RP, Foon KA: Chronic lymphocytic leukemia: recent advances in biology and treatment. Ann Intern Med 1985; 103:101–120.
56. Champlin R, Gale RP, Foon KA, Golde DW: Chronic leukemias: oncogenes, chromosomes and advances in therapy. Ann Intern Med 1986; 104:671–688.
57. Binet JL, Catovsky D, Dighiero G, et al: Chronic lymphocytic leukemia: recommendations for diagnosis, staging and response criteria. Ann Intern Med 1989; 110:236–238.
58. Bergsagel DE: The chronic leukemias: a review of disease manifestations and the aims of therapy. Can Med Assoc J 1967; 96:1615–1620.
59. Carey RW, McGinnis A, Jacobson BM, Carvalho A: Idiopathic thrombocytopenic purpura complicating chronic lymphocytic leukemia. Arch Intern Med 1976; 136:62–66.
60. Rustagi P, Han T, Ziolowski L, et al: Antigranulocyte antibodies in chronic lymphocytic leukemia and other chronic lymphoproliferative disorders [Abstract]. Blood 1983; 62(Suppl 1):106.
61. Abeloff MD, Waterbury L: Pure red cell aplasia and chronic lymphocytic leukemia. Arch Intern Med 1974; 134:721–724.
62. Long JC, Aisenberg AC: Richter's syndrome: a terminal complication of chronic lymphocytic leukemia with distinct clinical pathologic features. Am J Clin Pathol 1975; 63:786–795.
63. Frenkel EP, Ligler FS, Graham MS, et al: Acute lymphocytic leukemic transformation of chronic lymphocytic leukemia: substantiation by flow cytometry. Am J Hematol 1981; 10:391–398.
64. Dalal BI, Fitzpatric LA: Hairy cell leukemia: an update. Lab Med 1991; 22:31–36.
65. Yam LT, Li CCY, Lam KW: Tartrate resistant acid phosphatase isoenzyme in the reticulum cells of leukemic reticuloendotheliosis. N Engl J Med 1971; 284:357–360.
66. Jansen J, Der Ottohander GJ, Schmit HRE, et al: Hairy cell leukemia: its place among the chronic B cell leukemias. Semin Oncol 1984; 11:386–393.
67. Galton DAG, Goldman JM, Wiltshaw E, et al: Prolymphocytic leukemia. Br J Haematol 1974; 27:7–23.
68. Mintzer DM, Hauptman SP: Lymphosarcoma cell leukemia and other non-Hodgkin's lymphomas in leukemic phase. Am J Med 1983; 75:110–120.

69. Lutzner M, Edelson R, Schein P, Cutaneous T-cell lymphomas: the Sézary syndrome, mycosis fungoides, and related disorders. Ann Intern Med 1975; 83:534–552.
70. Bunn PA, Schechter GP, Jaffe E, et al. Clinical course of retrovirus associated adult T-cell lymphoma in the United States. N Engl J Med 1983; 309:2257–2264.
71. Fitzgerald PH, Beard MEJ, Morris CM, et al: Ph-negative chronic myeloid leukemia. Br J Haematol 1987; 66:311–314.
72. Canellos GP: Chronic granulocytic leukemia. Med Clin North Am 1976; 60:1001–1035.
73. Griffin JD, Todd RF, Ritz J, et al: Differentiation patterns in the blastic phase of chronic myeloid leukemia. Blood 1983; 61:85–91.

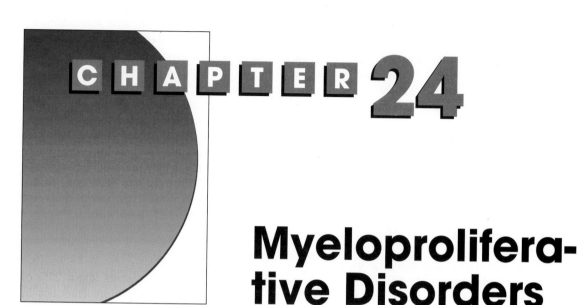

CHAPTER 24

Myeloprolifera-tive Disorders

John Griep

Outline

Objectives

AFTER COMPLETION OF THIS CHAPTER, THE READER WILL BE ABLE TO
1. Define myeloproliferative disorders (MPD).
2. List the most common diseases included in the classification of myeloproliferative disorders.
3. Define chronic myelogenous leukemia (CML).
4. Discuss the theory of pathogenesis of CML.
5. Describe the peripheral blood and bone marrow in CML.
6. Discuss the cytogenetics of CML.
7. List the clinical phases of CML.
8. Define polycythemia rubra vera (PRV or PV).
9. Discuss clinical symptoms commonly observed in patients with PV.
10. Identify major morphologic changes in the bone marrow and peripheral blood in patients with PV.
11. List diagnostic criteria for PV.
12. Discuss the progression of PV.
13. Define essential thrombocythemia (ET).
14. List the diagnostic criteria for ET.
15. List the morphologic changes in the peripheral blood in patients with ET.
16. List two complications that may occur in patients with ET.
17. Define agnogenic myeloid metaplasia (AMM).
18. Describe the key pathologic features of AMM in bone marrow, peripheral blood and tissues.
19. Describe the course of disease of AMM.

The myeloproliferative disorders (MPD) are considered clonal hematopoietic stem cell diseases that result in excessive production and overaccumulation of erythrocytes, granulocytes, and platelets in some combination in the bone marrow, peripheral blood, and body tissues.[1, 2, 3, 4] They are grouped as myeloproliferative diseases because they may express common clinical features, laboratory changes, and pathogenetic similarities.[5]

Depending upon the predicted length of the disease they may be classified as chronic, subacute, or acute myeloproliferative diseases. The subacute group of diseases are now considered as myelodysplastic processes even though in certain patients a clear separation from the chronic diseases may be difficult from clinical and morphologic perspectives. The acute diseases are generally placed as one of the variants in the acute myelogenous or nonlymphocytic leukemia phenotypic classification scheme (see Chapter 23).

By convention, the myeloproliferative disorders, as classified in most studies, reflect the chronic processes and include the distinct clinical diseases of chronic myelogenous leukemia (CML), polycythemia vera, also known as polycythemia rubra vera (PV or PRV), essential (primary) thrombocythemia(ET), and agnogenic myeloid metaplasia (AMM). CML and PV usually express overproduction of erythrocytes, granulocytes and platelets to varying degrees.[2, 6, 7] AMM may exhibit a combination of overproduction of hematopoietic cells and ineffective hematopoiesis with resultant peripheral blood cytopenias.[8] ET manifests with increased megakaryocytopoiesis and peripheral blood thrombocytosis.[9]

In general, patients with MPD present in a clinically stable phase that may transform to an aggressive cellular growth phase such as acute leukemia, or manifest a depleted cellular phase such as bone marrow hypoplasia, or exhibit clinical symptoms and morphologic patterns resembling a more aggressive cellular expression of a chronic myeloproliferative disorder. During the transition to acute leukemia, some patients may show progressive clinical symptoms and proceed to morphologic patterns similar to those observed in subacute myeloproliferative disease processes.

CHRONIC MYELOGENOUS LEUKEMIA

Chronic myelogenous leukemia (CML) is a myeloproliferative disorder arising as a clonal process in a pluripotential hematopoietic stem cell and manifesting with a chronic clinical phase, which in 3 to 4 years often terminates as an accelerated or acute phase resembling acute leukemias. The main clinical features of this disorder are anemia, bleeding, and splenomegaly, which are secondary to massive pathologic accumulations of myeloid progenitor cells in bone marrow, peripheral blood, and extramedullary tissues. Granulocyte immaturity, generally composed of cells in the later maturational stages, basophilia, eosinophilia, and often thrombocytosis are present in peripheral blood.

Verification of the clonal origin of hematopoietic cells in CML is apparent from studies of female patients with mosaicism for glucose-6-phosphate dehydrogenase, in which only one isoenzyme is active in affected cells, whereas two isoenzymes are active in nonaffected cells of these women.[10]

Incidence

CML occurs at all ages, represents about 20% of all cases of leukemia, is slightly more frequent in men than women, and manifests a mortality rate of 1.5/100,000 per year.

Symptoms associated with clinical onset of the disease may be of minimal intensity. Ease of fatigue, decreased tolerance to exertion, anorexia, abdominal discomfort, weight loss and symptomatic effects from splenic enlargement are commonly encountered. A variety of other complaints are less common.

Cytogenetics

A unique chromosome, the Philadelphia chromosome (Ph[1]), is present in proliferating hematopoietic cells. This chromosome is formed most commonly from a reciprocal translocation of gene segments between chromosomes 22 and 9[11] (see Chapter 22). This acquired somatic mutation specifically reflects the translocation of an abl protooncogene from band q34 of chromosome 9 to band q11 of chromosome 22 resulting in a unique chimeric gene, bcr-abl.[12] This new gene is translated and transcribed to a 210-kD protein, P210, which manifests enhanced tyrosine kinase activity when compared with its natural enzymatic counterpart. P210 catalyses the transfer of the terminal phosphate of adenosine triphosphate to proteins. This increased tyrosine kinase activity may induce clonal cell proliferation secondary to a reduction or loss of sensitivity to protein regulators.[13] The mutation affects maturation and differentiation of hematopoietic and lymphopoietic cells whose progeny eventually dominate in the affected individual. Progeny cells, which exhibit this chromosome, include neutrophils, eosinophils, basophils, monocytes, nucleated erythrocytes, megakaryocytes, and B-lymphocytes.[6, 14]

Although the cause for this gene translocation or rearrangement is unknown, it appears more frequently in populations exposed to ionizing radiation.[15, 16] In most patients a cause cannot be identified. Appearance of the Ph[1] chromosome in donor cells after allogeneic bone marrow transplantation implicates a possible transmissible agent.[17]

Peripheral Blood and Bone Marrow

Morphologically there are usually dramatic changes in the peripheral blood and bone marrow that reflect the dominance of the expansion of the granulocyte pool, particularly in the later maturational stages of cell development.

In Table 24–1 the common major changes at time of diagnosis in the peripheral blood, bone marrow, and extramedullary tissues are listed and qualitatively indicated. Extramedullary granulopoiesis may involve both sinuses and medullary cords in the spleen and sinusoids, portal tract zones, and solid areas of the liver.

Table 24-1. COMMON MORPHOLOGIC CHANGES IN CHRONIC MYELOGENOUS LEUKEMIA

Peripheral Blood	
Erythrocytes	N or D
Reticulocytes	N
Nucleated RBC	P
Total WBC	I
Lymphocytes	N or I
Neutrophils	I
Basophils	I
Eosinophils	I
Myelocytes	I
LAP	D
Platelets	N or I
Cytologic anomaly	P
Bone Marrow	
Hypercellular	
Granulopoiesis	I
Erythropoiesis	D
Megakaryopoiesis	I or N
Reticulin	I
Macrophages	I
Gaucher-like	
Sea-blue	
Green-grey crystals	
Megakaryocytes	I
Small	
CFU	I
Extramedullary Tissue	
SPLENOMEGALY	
Sinusoidal	
Medullary	
HEPATOMEGALY	
Sinusoidal	
Portal tract	
LOCAL INFILTRATES	

Abbreviations: N = normal; D = decreased; P = present; I = increased; RBC = red blood cells; WBC = white blood cells; LAP = leukocyte alkaline phosphatase; CFU = colony forming unit.

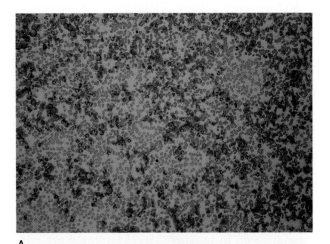

A

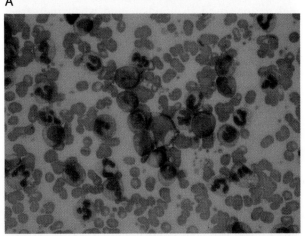

B

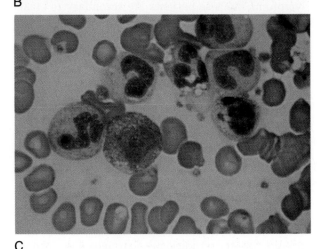

C

Figure 24–1 Peripheral blood smears in chronic phase CML. *A,* Leukocytosis is evident at scanning power (magnification, 10×). *B,* Bimodal population of segmented neutrophils and myelocytes (magnification, 40×). *C,* Immature eosinophil and basophil (magnification, 100×).

Figure 24–1 illustrates a common pattern in the peripheral blood of chronic phase CML at the time of diagnosis. There is an obvious leukocytosis readily apparent at scanning microscopic powers. Segmented neutrophils and myelocytes predominate in the white blood cell differential, and immature and mature eosinophils and basophils are easily discovered. Myeloblasts and promyelocytes are usually present between 1–5%. Lymphocytes and monocytes are present and often increased. Nucleated erythrocytes are rare. Platelets are normal or increased in frequency and some may exhibit abnormal morphology.

Bone marrow changes are illustrated in Figure 24–2. An intense hypercellularity is comprised of granulopoiesis, which exhibits broad zones of immature granulocytes, usually perivascular or periosteal, differentiating into more centrally placed mature granulocytes. Nucleated erythrocytes appear reduced in number. Megakaryocytes are normal or increased in number, and when increased, may appear in clusters and exhibit dyspoietic cytologic changes. When present in normal numbers, they often appear small. Reticulin fibers are increased in most patients.

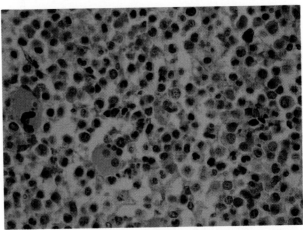

Figure 24–2 Bone marrow biopsy specimen in chronic stable phase CML, demonstrating hypercellularity with increased granulocytes and megakaryocytes (magnification, 40×).

Other Laboratory Findings

Clinical problems, which may cause complications in these patients, include hyperuricemia and hyperuricosuria that may be associated with secondary gout, urinary uric acid stones, and uric acid nephropathy.[18] Hyperleukocytosis occurs in approximately 15% of patients who exhibit total white blood cell counts greater than 300×10^9/L.[19] Symptoms in these patients are secondary to stasis of vascular flow and possible intravascular consumption of oxygen by the blood leukocytes. Symptoms are reversible with the lowering of the total white blood cell count.[20]

Progression

Most patients eventually transform to acute leukemia.[21] Before complete transformation, some patients proceed through a more aggressive phase referred to as metamorphosis or accelerated phase. There is an increase in frequency and type of clinical symptoms, adverse changes in laboratory values and less response to therapy than in the chronic phase. Additional chromosome abnormalities may appear, associated with enhanced dyshematopoietic cell maturation patterns and increases in morphologic and functional abnormalities in blood cells. There is often an increasing degree of anemia, and in the peripheral blood, fewer mature leukocytes, increased basophilia, more severe thrombocytopenia including greater proportions of abnormal platelets, and the appearance of micromegakaryocytes and megakaryocyte fragments. Usually the circulating blast count increases to between 15% and 29%. This total blast percentage, or a combination of 30% blast and promyelocytes, are proposed as diagnostic criteria for the accelerated phase.[22]

Blast crisis phase may involve the peripheral blood, bone marrow, and extramedullary tissues. Blasts comprising more than 30% of total bone marrow cellularity is considered a transformation to blast crisis, and the peripheral blood usually exhibits increased blasts.[21] Blast crisis leukemia usually is of acute myelogenous or acute lymphocytic phenotypes, but origins from other hematopoietic cells are possible. Extramedullary growth may occur as lymphocytic or myelogenous cell proliferations; the latter are often referred to as granulocytic sarcoma. Extramedullary sarcoma is observed at many sites or locations in the body, and may precede a marrow blast crisis. The clinical onset of marrow blast crisis simulates that of acute leukemia with severe anemia, leukopenia, and thrombocytopenia. New chromosome abnormalities observed in cells during accelerated phases or blast crisis include additional Ph[1] chromosome, isochromosome 17, trisomy 8, loss of Y chromosome, and trisomy 19.[23, 24]

Related Diseases

Some patients, who manifest diseases similar to CML, exhibit cells negative for the Ph[1] chromosome. Chronic neutrophilic leukemia manifests with peripheral blood, bone marrow, and extramedullary infiltrative patterns similar to those of CML, except that only neutrophilic granulocytes are represented in these proliferations.[25] Similarly, chronic monocytic leukemia appears to involve a similar expansion of monocytes including functional monocytes.[26]

Juvenile chronic myelomonocytic leukemia is observed in children less than 4 years of age and is accompanied by an expansion of monocytes and granulocytes, including immature granulocytes, and manifestations of dyserythropoiesis.[27] Chronic myelomonocytic leukemia in adults is better viewed as a myelodysplastic disorder and is discussed with that group of disorders (see Chapter 26). Some of the cases of Ph[1] chromosome–negative CML are likely examples of chronic myelomonocytic leukemia.

A puzzling group of patients exhibit Ph[1] chromosome–positive acute leukemia. Studies reveal 2% of AML cases exhibit the presence of Ph[1] chromosome in a significant proportion of blasts, whereas 5% of childhood-onset ALL and 20% of adult-onset ALL are positive.[28, 29] The proper alignment of these cases within the spectrum of CML is somewhat speculative.

Therapy

Therapy for CML involves myelosuppression by alkylating agents, hydroxyurea, or an attempt to eliminate Ph[1]–positive cell clones by multidrug regimens. In approximately 75% of patients in chronic phase CML, alpha interferon will normalize blood counts (see Chapter 28).

POLYCYTHEMIA VERA

Polycythemia vera (PV) is a neoplastic clonal myeloproliferative disorder, which most commonly expresses with panmyelosis in the bone marrow and increases in erythrocytes, granulocytes, and platelets in the peripheral blood.[2] Splenomegaly is common. This clonal neoplastic transformation arises in a pluripotential hematopoietic stem cell, and the hypothesis of a clonal origin for PV is supported by molecular level studies of X-linked restriction–fragment-length DNA polymorphism, which exhibits a monoclonal pattern of X chromosome inactivation in all cellular elements in the blood.[30]

In PV, neoplastic clonal stem cells are exquisitely sensitive to erythropoietin for cell growth. Trace levels of erythropoietin in serum stimulate growth of these erythroid progenitor cells in in vitro colony forming growth systems. There is, however, preservation of both hypersensitive and normosensitive erythroid colony forming units indicating that some level of normal hematopoiesis is characteristic of this disorder.[31] The adverse clinical progression observed in these patients over time seems to correlate with the propagation of colony forming units, which are exquisitely sensitive to erythropoietin.[32]

Approximately 80% of patients manifest bone marrow panmyelosis and up to 100% of bone marrow volume may exhibit hematopoietic cellularity. Although the bone marrow pattern may simulate other myeloproliferative disorders, the increased peripheral blood cytology tends to appear normal with normocytic, normochromic erythrocytes, mature granulocytes, and normal-sized, granulated platelets. The other 20% of patients with PV exhibit lesser degrees of cellularity in the bone marrow and peripheral blood. Splenomegaly and hepatomegaly as well as generalized vascular engorgement and circulatory disturbances may increase a patient's risk for the complications of hemorrhage, tissue infarction, or thrombosis.

Diagnosis

The clinical diagnosis of PV includes an increased red blood cell mass of 36 mL/kg or greater in males and 32 mL/kg or greater in females, an arterial O_2 saturation at 92% (normal) or greater, and splenomegaly. Lacking any one of these three parameters, the presence of two of the following parameters is considered diagnostic: thrombocytosis of greater than 400×10^9/L, leukocytosis of greater than 12×10^9/L without fever or infection, or increases in leukocyte alkaline phosphatase, serum vitamin B_{12} or unbound vitamin B_{12} binding capacity.[33, 34]

It is not always easy to assign an early diagnosis of PV. Persons with erythrocytosis secondary to hypoxia or erythropoietin-producing neoplasms are the most difficult to diagnose correctly. In these persons, the bone marrow exhibits only erythroid hyperplasia without granulocytic or megakaryocytic hyperplasia. Patients with stress or spurious erythrocytosis exhibit increased hemoglobin and hematocrits without increased erythrocyte volume or splenomegaly.

Peripheral Blood and Bone Marrow

Common qualitative peripheral blood, bone marrow, and tissue findings are listed in Table 24–2 for patients with the early or proliferative phase of PV. Figures 24–3 and 24–4 reflect common morphologic patterns of peripheral blood and bone marrow morphologic and cellular changes.

Therapy and Prognosis

PV stable phase progresses to a spent phase in a small proportion of patients. Usually patients experience progressive splenomegaly (palpable spleen) and/or hypersplenism (large spleen with bone marrow hyperplasia and peripheral blood cy-

Table 24-2. COMMON MORPHOLOGIC CHANGES IN POLYCYTHEMIA VERA	
Peripheral Blood	
Hemoglobin	I
Hematocrit	I
RBC volume	I
Erythrocytes	
Normocytic	
Normochromic	
Total WBC	I
Granulocytes	I
Platelets	I
LAP	N or I
Bone Marrow	
Normoblasts	I
Granulocytes	I
Megakaryocytes	I
Reticulin	I
Extramedullary Tissue	
SPLENOMEGALY	
Sinusoidal	
Medullary	
HEPATOMEGALY	
Sinusoidal	

Abbreviations: I = increased; N = normal; RBC = red blood cells; WBC = white blood cells; LAP = leukocyte alkaline phosphatase.

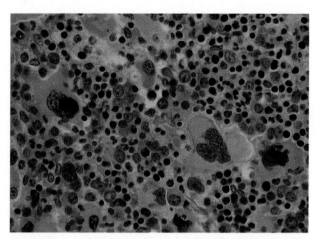

Figure 24-4 Bone marrow biopsy specimen in stable phase polycythemia vera, demonstrating panmyelosis (magnification, 40×).

topenias), and pancytopenia, or the triad of bone marrow fibrosis, splenomegaly, and anemia with teardrop-shaped poikilocytes. The latter pattern is referred to as postpolycythemic myeloid metaplasia (PPMM) because the morphologic features are similar to AMM. Peripheral blood counts for erythrocytes and leukocytes vary widely and nucleated erythrocytes, immature granulocytes, and large platelets are present. Usually, splenomegaly is secondary to extramedullary hematopoiesis.[35] Myelofibrosis occurs within the bone marrow and may come to occupy a significant proportion of bone marrow volume with subsequent ineffective hematopoiesis.[36]

The disease progresses to acute leukemia in up to 15% of patients. Patients receiving myelosuppressive therapy such as ^{32}P or alkylating agents appear at increased risk.[34] Some patients may manifest with a temporary disease pattern similar to myelodysplasia, and cytologically, the cell morphology in transformation to acute leukemia may be difficult to classify.

Patients with both early and advanced phases of PV may present with clinical features, peripheral blood features, bone marrow features, and extramedullary features that simulate those possible in patients with other myeloproliferative disorders.

ESSENTIAL THROMBOCYTHEMIA

Essential (primary) thrombocythemia (ET) represents a clonal myeloproliferative disorder involving increased megakaryopoiesis with thrombocytosis greater than $600 \times 10^9/L$, commonly above $1000 \times 10^9/L$.[37] Generally appearing in an older age group, ET must be differentiated from secondary or reactive causes for thrombocythemia, or from other myeloproliferative disorders. Secondary causes include thrombocythemia associated with chronic active blood loss, with active hemolytic anemia, concurrent to chronic inflammation or infection, or in the presence of nonhematogenous neoplasia.

Diagnosis

The diagnostic criteria for ET proposed by the Polycythemia Vera Study Group (PVSG) are intended to distinguish ET from other MPDs and include a platelet count of greater than $600 \times 10^9/L$, hemoglobin less than 13 g/dL or a normal eryth-

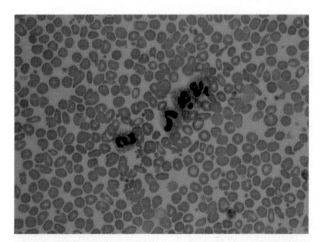

Figure 24-3 Peripheral blood smear in stable phase polycythemia vera. Note increase in all cell lines with essentially normocytic, normochromic erythrocytes (magnification, 40×).

rocyte mass, stainable iron in the bone marrow or a failure of iron therapy, a negative study for the Philadelphia chromosome, absent marrow collagen fibrosis or less than one third of a biopsy proving fibrous, no splenomegaly, no leukoerythroblastotic reaction, nor any known cause of reactive thrombocytosis.[38] The major qualitative morphologic peripheral blood, bone marrow, and extramedullary findings are listed in Table 24–3.

Peripheral Blood and Bone Marrow

Illustrating the peripheral blood film in the early phase, Figure 24–5 exhibits thrombocytosis with a greater than normal variation in platelet size and shape including changes such as giantism, agranularity, pseudopod formation, and atypical shapes. Commonly, platelets are present in clusters and tend to accumulate near the thin edge of the blood film. Neutrophils may be increased but are present as segmented neutrophils, and basophils are not increased. Erythrocytes are normocytic and normochromic unless iron deficiency is present secondary to excessive clinical bleeding.

The bone marrow morphology in the early phase usually demonstrates marked megakaryocytic hypercellularity, clustering of megakaryocytes, and increases in average megakaryocytic size with associated nuclear hyperlobulation and density (Fig. 24–6). Special studies reveal increased smaller and less mature megakaryocytes.[39] Increased granulopoiesis and erythropoiesis may contribute to bone

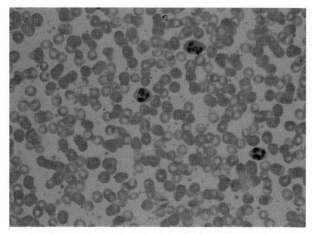

Figure 24–5 Peripheral blood smear in stable phase essential thrombocythemia, showing increased numbers of platelets and mature neutrophils (magnification, 40×).

marrow hypercellularity, and, in a minority of patients, reticulin fibers may be increased.

Therapy and Prognosis

Patients with ET experience relatively long survival rates provided they remain free from serious thromboembolic or hemorrhagic complications. Clinical symptoms associated with thromboembolic vaso-occlusive events include the syndrome of erythromelalgia (throbbing and burning pain in the hands and feet, accompanied by mottled redness of areas), transient ischemic attacks, seizures, and cerebral or myocardial infarction. Other symptoms include headache, dizziness, visual disturbances, and dysesthesias (decreased sensations). Hemorrhagic complications include bleeding from oral and nasal mucous membrane or gastrointestinal mucosa, and the appearance of cutaneous ecchymoses.

Table 24–3. COMMON MORPHOLOGIC PATTERNS IN ESSENTIAL THROMBOCYTHEMIA	
Peripheral Blood	
Hemoglobin	D (slight)
Hematocrit	D (slight)
RBC volume	N
Total WBC	I (slight)
Neutrophils	I (slight)
Platelets	I
Platelet function	D
Bone Marrow	
Normoblasts	N or I
Granulocytes	N or I (slight)
Megakaryocytes	I
Clusters	
Large	
Hyperlobulated	
Dense nuclei	
Variability in size	
Reticulin	N or I (slight)
Extramedullary Tissue	
SPLENOMEGALY	
Sinusoidal	
Medullary	
MEGAKARYOCYTIC PROLIFERATION	

Abbreviations: D = decreased; N = normal; I = increased; RBC = red blood cells; WBC = white blood cells.

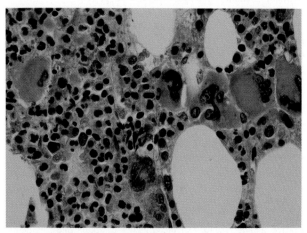

Figure 24–6 Bone marrow biopsy specimen in essential thrombocythemia, with marked megakaryocytic hypercellularity.

Treatment involves prevention or early alleviation of hemorrhagic or vaso-occlusive complications. These tend to occur as the platelet count rises, and the production of platelets must be reduced by suppressing marrow megakaryocyte production with ^{32}P or one of several alkylating agents. As observed with PV, ET patients so treated may incur an increased risk for disease transformation to acute leukemia or myelofibrosis. ET occurs in younger patients, in whom treatment with hydroxyurea may achieve a desired reduction of peripheral platelets without the risk of complications experienced with myelosuppressive agents, because the normal risk of leukemic transformation appears relatively low.

Median survivals of greater than 10 years for population groups with ET is common, including the instances in which the process arises in younger patients.

AGNOGENIC MYELOID METAPLASIA

Agnogenic myeloid metaplasia (also known as myelofibrosis with myeloid metaplasia) is a clonal myeloproliferative disorder[4] in which there is ineffective hematopoiesis manifesting with marrow hypercellularity, marrow fibrosis, immature granulocytes and erythroblasts in peripheral blood, poikilocytosis (including teardrop-shaped erythrocytes), and splenomegaly.

The clonal character for this disorder is manifest from studies in which cytogenetic abnormalities are detected in erythroblasts, neutrophils, macrophages, basophils and megakaryocytes, and from studies of female patients heterozygous for glucose-6-phosphate dehydrogenase isoenzymes A and B, in whom blood cells were of a single enzyme isotype and tissue cells, including marrow fibroblasts, contained both enzyme isotypes.[4]

Myelofibrosis

The myelofibrosis in this disease comprises three of the five major types of collagen: types I, III, and IV. Increases in type III are detected by silver impregnation techniques, in type I by staining with trichrome, and in type IV by the presence of osteosclerosis, which may be diagnosed by an increased bone density during radiographic studies.[40] Increases in these collagens are not a part of the clonal proliferative process, but are considered secondary to an increased release of fibroblastic growth factors such as platelet-derived growth factor, transforming growth factor–beta from megakaryocyte alpha granules, tumor necrosis

factor–alpha and interleukin-1–alpha and –beta. Consequences arising from increased marrow fibrosis include an expansion of marrow sinuses and vascular volume with an increased rate of blood flow.

Bone marrow fibrosis is not the sole criterion for a diagnosis of AMM as increases in marrow fibrosis may reflect a reparative response to injury from benzene or ionizing radiation, as a consequence of immunologic-mediated injury, or as a reactive response to other hematologic conditions.

Extramedullary Hematopoiesis

Extramedullary hematopoiesis, clinically recognized as hepatomegaly or splenomegaly, appears to originate from an increased release of clonal stem cells into circulation[41] with excess accumulation of these cells in the spleen, liver, or other organs including adrenals, kidney, lymph nodes, bowel, breast, lungs, mediastinum, mesentery, skin, synovium, thymus, or lower urinary tract.

Body cavity effusions containing hematopoietic cells may arise from extramedullary hematopoiesis in the cranium, the intraspinal epidural space, or the serosal surfaces of pleura, pericardium, and peritoneum. Portal hypertension, with its attendant consequences of ascites, esophageal and gastric varices, gastrointestinal hemorrhage and hepatic encephalopathy, arises from a combination of a massive increase in splenoportal blood flow and a decrease in hepatic vascular compliance secondary to fibrosis around the sinusoids and hematopoietic cells within the sinusoids.[42]

Peripheral Blood and Bone Marrow

AMM patients present with a broad range of changes in laboratory test values, and peripheral blood film and bone marrow biopsy examination provides most of the information for diagnosis. A summary of changes commonly observed during peripheral blood and bone marrow examination are listed in Table 24–4.

Abnormalities in erythrocytes noted on peripheral blood films include poikilocytosis, teardrop-shaped erythrocytes, nucleated erythrocytes, and polychromatophilia. Granulocytes are increased, normal, or decreased and may include immature granulocytes, blasts, and cells with nuclear or cytoplasmic anomalies. Platelets may be normal, increased, or decreased with a mixture of normal or abnormal morphology (Fig. 24–7). Megakaryocyte nuclei may be observed.

The bone marrow biopsies exhibit intense fibrosis, granulocytic and megakaryocytic hypercellularity, dysmegakaryopoiesis, dysgranulopoiesis, and

Table 24-4. COMMON MORPHOLOGIC CHANGES IN AGNOGENIC MYELOID METAPLASIA

Peripheral Blood	
Hemoglobin	N or D
Anisocytosis	I
Poikilocytosis	I
Teardrop-shaped erythrocytes	P
NRBC	P
Polychromasia	N or I
Total WBC	N, D, or I
Immature granulocytes	I
Blasts	P
Basophils	P
Leukocyte anomaly	P
LAP	I, N, or D
Platelets	I, N, or D
Abnormal platelets	P
Megakaryocytes	P
Bone Marrow	
Hypercellular	
Granulopoiesis	I
Megakaryocytes	I
Erythropoiesis	N or I
Myelofibrosis	I
Sinuses	I
Dysmegakaryopoiesis	P
Dysgranulopoiesis	P
Extramedullary Tissue	
SPLENOMEGALY	
Sinusoidal	
Medullary	
HEPATOMEGALY	
Sinusoidal	
Portal tract	
Local infiltrates	
OTHER TISSUES	

Abbreviations: N = normal; D = decreased; I = increased; P = present; NRBC = nucleated red blood cells; WBC = white blood cells; LAP = leukocyte alkaline phosphatase.

numerous dilated sinuses containing luminal hematopoiesis.

Neutrophils from patients with AMM may exhibit impairment of physiologic functions, such as phagocytosis, oxygen consumption, and hydrogen peroxide generation, and decreased myeloperoxi-

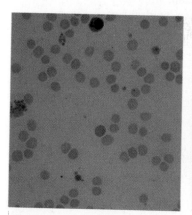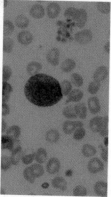

Figure 24-7 Peripheral blood smear in agnogenic myeloid metaplasia, illustrating an nRBC, a giant platelet, and a myelocyte (magnification, 40×).

dase and glutathione reductase activities. Platelets have impaired aggregation in response to epinephrine, decreased adenosine diphosphate concentration in dense granules, and decreased activity of platelet lipoxygenase.

Immune Response

Humoral immune responses are altered in approximately 50% of patients and include the appearance of autoantibodies to erythrocyte antigens, nuclear proteins, gamma globulins, phospholipids, and organ-specific antigens.[43] Circulating immune complexes as evidence for complement activation, increased proportions of marrow reactive lymphocytes, and the development of amyloidosis represent evidence for the presence of active immune processes in these patients. Collagen disorders have coexisted with myelofibrosis suggesting that immunologic processes may stimulate marrow fibroblast activity.

Incidence

The disease occurs in older patients, may be diagnosed in asymptomatic patients, and generally presents with symptoms of fatigue, weakness, shortness of breath, palpitations, weight loss, and discomfort or pain in the left upper quadrant associated with splenomegaly.

Therapy and Prognosis

Average survival from time of diagnosis is about 5 years, but patients have lived up to 15 years. Adverse prognostic indicators include the severity of anemia and thrombocytopenia, the magnitude of hepatomegaly, unexplained fever, and evidence for hemolysis. Mortality is associated with infection, severe hemorrhage, post-splenectomy complications, and transformation to acute leukemia.

A diverse spectrum of therapies has been applied to alleviate symptoms or modify clinical problems in these patients. Severe anemia has been treated with androgen therapy and hemolytic anemia with glucocorticosteroids. Reduction of myelofibrosis and of marrow and tissue hypercellularity has been accomplished with busulfan and other alkylating agents, hydroxyurea, and, in a few patients, alpha and gamma interferon. Radiotherapy is considered for patients with severe splenic pain, for those with massive splenomegaly who are not clinical candidates for splenectomy, for those with ascites secondary to serosal implants, and for those with localized bone pain and other localized extramedullary fibrohemopoietic masses, especially in the epidural space. Splenectomy is generally performed to end severe pain, excessive transfusion requirements, or severe thrombocytopenia, and also to correct severe portal hypertension.

SUMMARY

MPD are clonal hematopoietic stem cell disorders that result in excessive production and over-accumulation of erythrocytes, granulocytes, and platelets in some combination in bone marrow, peripheral blood, and body tissues. Within this classification are CML, PV, ET, and AMM.

In CML there are large numbers of myeloid precursors in the bone marrow, peripheral blood, and extramedullary tissues. The peripheral blood exhibits leukocytosis with increased myeloid series, particularly the later maturation stages, often with increases in basophils and eosinophils. The leukocyte alkaline phosphatase is dramatically decreased. Ph[1] is present in most cases. The bone marrow exhibits intense hypercellularity composed of myeloid precursors. Megakaryocytes are normal to increased. Patients with CML progress from a chronic stable phase through an accelerated phase into transformation to acute leukemia.

Polycythemia vera expresses with panmyelosis in the bone marrow with increases in erythrocytes, granulocytes, and platelets. The clinical diagnosis requires an increased red blood cell mass, normal or increased arterial O_2 saturation, and splenomegaly. If only two of these criteria are present, however, the diagnosis can be made if two of the following are present: platelet count $> 400 \times 10^9/L$, WBC $> 12.0 \times 10^9/L$ in the absence of infection, increased leukocyte alkaline phosphatase, or B_{12} or B_{12} binding capacity.

ET involves increased megakaryocytes with platelet count $> 600 \times 10^9/L$. Other diagnostic criteria include normal RBC mass, stainable iron in bone marrow, absence of Ph[1], absent marrow collagen fibrosis, no splenomegaly or leukoerythroblastic reaction, nor known cause of reactive thrombocytosis.

In the early phases of the disease, peripheral blood shows increased platelets with abnormalities in size and shape. Bone marrow megakaryocytes are increased in number and in size. Complications include thromboembolism and hemorrhage.

AMM expresses with ineffective hematopoiesis, marrow hypercellularity, bone marrow fibrosis, splenomegaly, and hepatomegaly. The peripheral blood exhibits immature granulocytes and nRBC. Dacryocytes (teardrop cells) are a common finding. Platelets may be normal, increased, or decreased with abnormal morphology. Micromegakaryocytes may be present. Immune responses are altered in about 50% of patients.

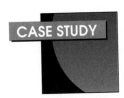

Case 1

A 34-year-old female presented with a 2-month history of increasing weakness, persistent nonproductive cough, fever and chills accompanied by night sweats, and a 13-pound weight loss over a 6-month period. Chest radiographs and purified protein derivative (PPD) test (for tuberculosis) were negative. The patient was treated with Ciprofloxacin with improvement in her cough, but she continued to grow weaker and was able to consume only small quantities of food. On physical examination her weight was 112 pounds, temperature 99.7°F, blood pressure 120/70, pulse rate 120/minute, and respiration rate 20/minute. The patient appeared pale and cachectic. There was tenderness and fullness in the left upper quadrant with the spleen palpable below the umbilicus. No hepatomegaly or peripheral adenopathy was noted.

Her laboratory results were as follows:

White blood cell count: $248 \times 10^9/L$
Hemoglobin: 9.5 g/dL
Hematocrit: 0.263 L/L
Platelet count: $449 \times 10^9/L$
Segmented neutrophils: 44%
Band neutrophils: 4%
Lymphocytes: 10%
Eosinophils: 3%
Basophils: 7%
Myelocytes: 30%
Promyelocyte: 1%

Myeloblast: 1%
Nucleated red blood cells: 2/100 WBC
Reticulocyte count: 3.0%
Leukocyte alkaline phosphatase (LAP) score: 20(control, 40–130)
Prothrombin time: 14.5 seconds (control, 11.7)
Activated partial thromboplastin time: 34.9 seconds (control, 26.5)
Lactate dehydrogenase: 692 IU (normal, 140–280)
Alkaline phosphatase: 125 U/L (normal, 25–125)
Uric acid: 8.1 mg/dL (normal, 4–6)

Blood urea nitrogen, creatinine, glucose, and electrolytes were in normal ranges. Urinalysis exhibited 1+ protein, 1+ bilirubin, and 1+ ketone. Bacterial cultures of blood and stool were negative. Urine cultures were positive for a *Staphylococcus* species, coagulase test result was negative, and beta-lactamase test result was positive. Bone marrow was diagnostic for *chronic myelogenous leukemia*.

The patient was treated with allopurinol, cyclophosphamide (Cytoxan), and hydroxyurea (Hydrea) with ondansetron HCl_2 (Zofran). Six weeks later, her white blood cell count was 1.0×10^9/L, platelet count 2.0×10^9/L, and hemoglobin was 7.2 g/dL.

Case 2

A 64-year old male was admitted to the hospital for repair of an incarcerated right inguinal hernia. The patient experienced increasing pain in the right scrotum for 3 days without gastrointestinal or gastric ulceration symptoms. The patient had been diagnosed with essential thrombocytosis 5 years previously, and subsequently had experienced no symptoms, including no excessive bleeding. His appetite remained good, his weight was steady, and he had not noted blood in his urine.

Laboratory values were as follows:

White blood cell count: 12.5×10^9/L
Red blood cell count: 4.63×10^{12}/L
Hemoglobin: 13.8 g/dL
Hematocrit: 0.414 L/L
Platelet count: 1345×10^9/L
Segmented neutrophils: 79%
Band neutrophils: 2%
Lymphocytes: 10%
Monocytes: 5%
Eosinophils: 2%
Basophils: 2%
LAP score: 50 (control, 40–130)
Prothrombin time: 13.0 seconds (control, 11.6)
Activated partial thromboplastin time: 23.3 seconds (control, 26.4)
Bleeding time: 6 minutes (normal, 2–10)
Urinalysis: Normal, except for 6–10 red blood cells per high power field
Clinical chemistry screen: Essentially normal

This patient presented a picture typical of *essential thrombocytosis, stable phase*.

References

1. Fialkow PJ, Jacobson RJ, Papayannopoulou T: Chronic myelocytic leukemia; clonal origin in a stem cell common to the granulocytic, erythrocytic, platelet and monocyte/macrophage. Am J Med 1977; 63:125.
2. Adamson JW, Fialkow PJ, Murphy S, et al: Polycythemia vera: stem-cell and probable clonal origin of the disease. N Engl J Med 1976; 295:913.
3. Fialkow PJ, Faguet GB, Jacobson RJ, et al: Evidence that essential thrombocythemia is a clonal disorder with origin in a multipotent stem cell. Blood 1981; 58:916.
4. Jacobson RJ, Salo A, Fialkow PJ: Agnogenic myeloid metaplasia: a clonal proliferation of hematopoietic stem cells with secondary myelofibrosis. Blood 1978; 51:189.
5. Dameshek W: Editorial. Some speculations on the myeloproliferative syndromes. Blood 1951; 6:372.
6. Whang J, Frei E III, Tijo JH, et al: The distribution of the

Philadelphia chromosome in patients with chronic myelogenous leukemia. Blood 1963; 22:664.

7. Spiers ASD, Bain BJ, Turner JE: The peripheral blood in chronic granulocytic leukemia; study of 50 untreated Philadelphia-positive cases. Scand J Hematol 1977; 18:25.

8. Ward HP, Block MH: The natural history of agnogenic myeloid metaplasia (AMM) and a critical evaluation of its relationship with the myeloproliferative syndrome. Medicine 1971; 150:357.

9. Mitus AJ, Schafer AI: Thrombocytosis and thrombocythemia. Hematol Oncol Clin North Am 1990; 4:157.

10. Barr RD, Fialkow PJ: Clonal origin of chronic myelocytic leukemia. N Engl J Med 1973; 289:307.

11. Rowley JD: A new consistent chromosome abnormality in chronic myelogenous leukemia identified by quinacrine fluorescence and Giemsa banding. Nature 1973; 243:290.

12. Stam K, Heisterkamp N, Grosveld G, et al: Evidence of a new chimeric bcr/c-abl mRNA in patients with chronic myelocytic leukemia and the Philadelphia chromosome. N Engl J Med 1985; 313:1429.

13. Epner DE, Koeffler HP: Molecular genetic advances in chromic myelogenous leukemia. Ann Intern Med 1990; 113:3.

14. Douer D, Levine AM, Sparkes RS, et al: Chronic myelocytic leukemia: a pluripotent haemopoietic cell is involved in the malignant clone. Br J Haematol 1981; 49:615.

15. Bizzozzero OJ, Johnson KG, Ciocco A: Radiation-related leukemia in Hiroshima and Nagasaki, 1946–1964. I. Distribution, incidence, and appearance time. N Engl J Med 1966; 274:1095.

16. Court Brown WM, Doll R: Mortality from cancer and other causes after radiotherapy for ankylosing spondylitis. Br Med J 1965; ii:1327.

17. Marmont A, Frassoni F, Bacigalupo A, et al: Recurrence of Ph¹-positive leukemia in donor cells after marrow transplantation for chronic granulocytic leukemia. N Engl J Med 1984; 310:903.

18. Klineberg JR, Bluestone R, Schlosstein L, et al: Urate deposition disease. How it is regulated and how can it be modified? Ann Intern Med 1973; 78:99.

19. Lichtman MA, Rowe JM: Hyperleukocytic leukemias: rheological, clinical and therapeutic considerations. Blood 1982; 60:279.

20. Lichtman MA, Heal J, Rowe JM: Hyperleukocytic leukemia. Balliére's Clin Haematol 1987; 1:725.

21. Muehleck SD, McKenna RD, Arthur DC, et al: Transformation of chronic myelogenous leukemia: clinical, morphologic and cytogenetic features. Am J Clin Pathol 1984; 82:1.

22. Kantarjian HM, Dixon D, Keating MJ, et al: Characteristics of accelerated disease in chronic myelogenous leukemia. Cancer 1988; 61:1441.

23. Bernstein R: Cytogenetics of chronic myelogenous leukemia. Semin Hematol 1988; 25:20.

24. Sandberg AA: Chromosomes in the chronic phase of CML. Virchous Arch [B] 1978; 29:51.

25. Bareford D, Jacobs P: Chronic neutrophilic leukemia. Am J Clin Pathol 1980; 73:837.

26. Bearman RM, Kjeldsburg CR, Pangalis GA, et al: Chronic monocytic leukemia in adults. Cancer 1981; 48:2239.

27. Thomas WJ, North RB, Poplack DG, et al: Chronic myelomonocytic leukemia in childhood. Am J Hematol 1981; 10:181.

28. Bloomfield CD, Lindquist LL, Brunning RD, et al: The Philadelphia chromosome in acute leukemia. Virchows Arch [Cell Pathol] 1978; 29:81.

29. Catovsky D: Ph¹-positive acute leukemia and chronic granulocytic leukaemia: One or two diseases? Br J Haematol 1979; 42:493.

30. Gilliland DG, Blanchard KL, Levy J, et al: Determination of clonality in myeloproliferative disorders: analysis by means of the polymerase chain reaction. Proc Natl Acad Sci (USA) 1991; 88:6848.

31. Prechal JF, Adamson JW, Murphy S, et al: Polycythemia vera: The in vitro response of normal and abnormal stem cell lines to erythropoietin. J Clin Invest 1978; 61:1044.

32. Adamson JW, Singer JW, Catalano P, et al: Polycythemia vera: further in vitro studies of hematopoietic regulation. J Clin Invest 1980; 66:1363.

33. Berlin N: Diagnosis and classification of the polycythemias. Semin Hematol 1975; 12:339.

34. Berk PD, Goldberg JN, Donovan PB, et al: Therapeutic recommendations in polycythemia vera based on Polycythemia Vera Study Group protocols. Semin Hematol 1986; 23:132.

35. Wolf BC, Bank PM, Mann RB, Nieman RS: Splenic hematopoiesis in polycythemia vera: a morphologic and immunohistologic study. Am J Clin Pathol 1988; 89:69.

36. Ellis JT, Peterson P, Geller SA, Rappaport H: Studies of the bone marrow in polycythemia vera and the evolution of myelofibrosis and second hematologic malignancies. Semin Hematol 1986; 23:14.

37. Mitus AJ, Schafer A: Thrombocytosis and thrombocythemia. Hematol Oncol Clin North Am 1990; 4:157.

38. Murphy S, Iland H, Rosenthal D, Laszlo J: Essential thrombocythemia: an interim report from the Polycythemia Vera Study Group. Semin Haematol 1986; 23:177.

39. Kuecht H, Streuli RA: Megakaryopoiesis in different forms of thrombocytosis and thrombocytopenia: Identification of megakaryocyte precursors by immunostaining of intracytoplasmic factor VIII-related antigen. Acta Haematol 1985; 74:208.

40. McCarthy DM: Annotation: Fibrosis of the bone marrow, content and causes. Br J Haematol 1985; 59:1.

41. Wang JC, Cheung CP, Fakhiuddin A, et al: Circulating granulocyte and macrophage progenitor cells in primary and secondary myelofibrosis. Br J Haematol 1983; 54:301.

42. Jacobs P, Maze S, Tayob F, et al: Myelofibrosis, splenomegaly, and portal hypertension. Acta Haematol 1985; 74:45.

43. Vellenga E, Mulder N, The T, et al: A study of the cellular and humoral immune response in patients with myelofibrosis. Clin Lab Haematol 1982; 4:239.

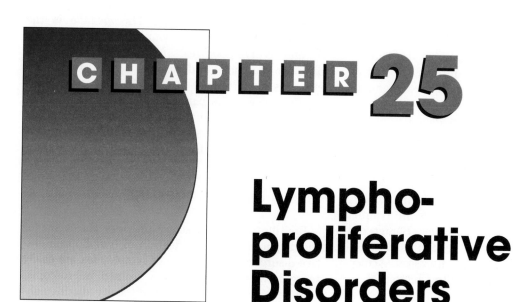

CHAPTER 25

Lympho-proliferative Disorders

Patricia K. Kotylo, Kimberly Gatzimos, and John Krause

Outline

NORMAL LYMPH NODE
  MORPHOLOGY
LYMPH NODE PROCESSING
BENIGN LYMPHOID
  PROLIFERATIONS
MALIGNANT DISORDERS
  Hodgkin's Disease
  Non-Hodgkin's Lymphoma
  Plasma Cell Dyscrasia

Objectives

AFTER COMPLETION OF THIS CHAPTER, THE READER WILL BE ABLE TO

1. List and define several lymphoproliferative disorders.
2. Name four major subtypes of Hodgkin's lymphoma.
3. Describe the clinical, morphologic, and immunologic characteristics of low-, intermediate-, and high-grade non-Hodgkin's lymphoma.
4. Discuss the clinical findings and immunologic origin of Hodgkin's disease and the features that distinguish this entity from non-Hodgkin's malignant lymphoma.
5. Discuss the clinical features and prognosis of lymphoproliferative disorders that arise in the immunocompromised host.
6. Compare and contrast the typical clinical and laboratory findings observed in plasma cell dyscrasias, including multiple myeloma, Waldenström's macroglobulinemia, plasma cell leukemia, and monoclonal gammopathy of uncertain significance.

The term *lymphoproliferative disorders* refers to a large group of benign and malignant lesions of the lymphoid system. Included in this category are Hodgkin's disease, non-Hodgkin's lymphomas, plasma cell dyscrasias, chronic lymphocytic leukemia, and other lymphoid proliferations that may behave in an aggressive fashion. The malignant lesions are thought to be derived from a clone of cells and may demonstrate immunologic or molecular features of a clonal proliferation. Although these disease states involve lymphocytes and related cells, they differ in clinical presentation, organ involvement, and biologic behavior.

The disorders presented in this chapter include malignant proliferations that originate in lymph nodes or other lymphoid related tissues. Benign or reactive disorders, which may be confused with malignant proliferations, are also discussed. Acute and chronic leukemias are covered in Chapter 23.

NORMAL LYMPH NODE MORPHOLOGY

Lymphoid tissues scattered throughout the body serve as sites for antigen recognition and processing and for lymphopoiesis. Normal lymph nodes are small (1–2 cm in diameter), round-to-oval, soft, tan nodules found along lymphatic channels that drain different areas of the body; aggregates of lymphoid tissues may also be found along mucosal tissues of the respiratory and gastrointestinal tracts (mucosal-associated lymphoid tissues). Lymph nodes or lymphoid aggregates are composed of loosely arranged cells, including lymphocytes, plasma cells, macrophages, and other cells, which are supported by a meshwork of delicate connective tissue fibers. A lymph node is normally surrounded by a thin, fibrous tissue capsule. Three anatomically distinct regions are present in lymph nodes: cortex, medulla, and paracortex (see Fig. 6–10).

The *cortex* is located in the outer rim of the node and contains round structures called lymphoid follicles. These follicles are composed primarily of B cells with a smaller component of T cells and are sites of immunologic response to antigens. The microscopic appearance of these follicles varies with antigenic stimulation or exposure. *Primary follicles* are composed of small, round, mature lymphocytes. Exposure of these primary follicles to a foreign antigen may result in the development of *secondary follicles,* which are characterized by a clear, centrally placed germinal center that contains enlarged activated lymphocytes, macrophages, plasma cells, and dendritic cells; mitotic activity is also present in the germinal center.

Both primary and secondary follicles are surrounded by a rim of small, compact B lymphocytes called a mantle zone. The *medulla* is the central-most portion of a lymph node and contains T and B lymphocytes, plasma cells, lymphatic drainage channels, and vascular spaces. Lymphoid elements are arranged in cords around these medullary sinuses. The *paracortical zone* is located between the cortex and the medulla and is composed primarily of T lymphocytes, postcapillary venules, and antigen-presenting cells.[1]

LYMPH NODE PROCESSING

Routine light microscopy provides the basis for the diagnosis and classification of lymphoproliferative disorders. Many types of lymphomas are easily recognized; however, even a trained microscopist may occasionally experience difficulty distinguishing florid reactive disorders from malignant lymphomas when subclassifying different types of lymphoma. Careful processing of lymph node tissue preserves the histologic features that are the major criteria for the classification of lymphomas. Ancillary studies, such as flow cytometry, cytogenetics, or electron microscopy, may also provide valuable diagnostic information.

A physician performing a lymph node biopsy should schedule this procedure after having careful communication with the laboratory to ensure that appropriate technical support services are available for processing the tissue sample. The surgeon then removes an intact lymph node most likely to be involved with the disease process. The node is covered with gauze moistened with sterile saline and is immediately transported to the pathology laboratory. No fixatives of any type should be placed on a lymph node before it undergoes pathologic evaluation in a laboratory. Once in the laboratory, the exterior of the node is measured and described. A clean scalpel is used to cut the biopsy into thin sections, 1–2 mm thick. The color and the consistency of the interior of the node are evaluated, and areas of hemorrhage or necrosis are noted. Frozen-section studies, which have been traditionally used to immediately evaluate tissue samples for the presence of malignancy, are usually not performed on a lymph node biopsy specimen, because freezing artifact often obscures morphologic features used to diagnose lymphoma. Touch imprints, which are morphologically superior to frozen sections, are routinely used instead. With this technique, a glass slide is gently touched to the cut surface of a node, and cells are physically affixed to the slide and air dried. Several touch imprints may be easily obtained and quickly stained with a

Wright-Giemsa stain for immediate morphologic review. Additional slides may be saved for other special stains, including immunohistochemical studies for cell surface antigens or stains for microorganisms. Once several touch imprints have been obtained, a portion of thinly sliced node is placed in 10% buffered formalin for routine tissue processing; formalin-fixed tissue sections are helpful in the assessment of overall architectural features of the node. Additional tissue samples should be placed in a mercuric fixative, such as B5, which preserves nuclear detail. Thin sectioning of a lymph node is critical to allow permeation of these fixatives throughout tissue sections. Any remaining fresh tissue may then be submitted for additional studies. If an infectious etiology of lymph node enlargement (lymphadenopathy) is suspected, microbiologic cultures may be obtained. Fresh tissue may also be processed for flow cytometric analysis to identify the presence of a clonal proliferation of cells or to determine the lineage of a cellular population. Another sample may be used for cytogenetic studies, molecular diagnostics (gene rearrangement studies), or electron microscopy. If appropriate facilities and space are available, a portion of the biopsy may be quickly frozen at −70°C and placed in storage for future studies or research.[2]

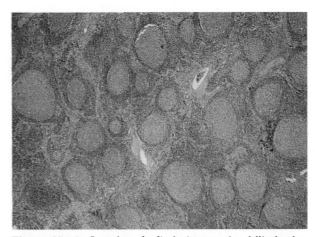

Figure 25–1 Lymph node displaying reactive follicular hyperplasia. Lymphoid follicles vary in shape and size. A rim or mantle of small, round lymphocytes surrounds benign follicles (hematoxylin-eosin, 10X).

centers; their shape and size vary considerably (Fig. 25–1).[3]

Other types of lymphadenopathy may be associated with the acquired immunodeficiency syndrome (AIDS) and are discussed later in this chapter.

BENIGN LYMPHOID PROLIFERATIONS

Lymphadenopathy does not always represent a malignant proliferation of lymphoid tissue. Benign lymphadenopathy may occur in patients of all ages and may result from antigenic stimulation with bacteria, viruses, or drugs. Autoimmune disorders, such as rheumatoid arthritis or systemic lupus erythematosus, may also be associated with benign lymphadenopathy.

Reactive enlargement of a lymph node is termed *hyperplasia* and involves the expansion and proliferation of normal lymphoid tissues. Various anatomic areas of the lymph node may be affected, and the histologic appearance of hyperplasia varies with the zone of the node involved in the proliferative process. Microscopic patterns that are observed include *follicular, diffuse, sinusoidal,* or *mixed hyperplasia.* The most common hyperplastic pattern is follicular hyperplasia and typically results from B cell proliferation occurring in response to one of the forms of antigenic stimulation described earlier. Microscopically, follicular hyperplasia is characterized by prominent proliferation of lymphoid follicles throughout the cortex and the medulla of the node. Lymphoid follicles are typically enlarged and have prominent germinal

MALIGNANT DISORDERS

Hodgkin's Disease

GENERAL FEATURES

Hodgkin's disease was first described in 1832 by the British physician Thomas Hodgkin. Sixty years later, C. Sternberg and colleagues described a characteristic giant cell seen in this newly described disease but considered the disorder to be a variant of tuberculosis. In 1902, Dorothy Reed distinguished this binucleate giant cell from the multinucleate giant cell of tuberculosis and believed the etiology of Hodgkin's disease resulted from an unidentified infectious agent.

Hodgkin's disease encompasses a group of heterogeneous disorders and is characterized morphologically by a proliferative background of benign inflammatory cells, such as lymphocytes, histiocytes, plasma cells, and eosinophils interspersed with relatively fewer numbers of large malignant cells and their variants (Reed-Sternberg cells). Hodgkin's disease accounts for approximately one third of all malignant lymphoproliferative disorders, and 7500 new cases are diagnosed each year.[4] It may occur in patients of all ages but is one of the most common types of malignancy in children. Two disease incidence peaks (bimodal age distribution) may be observed: one disease peak occurs in young adults aged 14 to 40 years, and the second disease peak occurs in adults aged 50 years and older. Hodgkin's disease, however, is generally considered a "young person's disease" and the median age at the time of presentation is 32 years. Patients with Hodgkin's disease typically present with a single, firm, enlarged lymph node, often a cervical lymph node. This lymphadenopathy may be associated with fever, night sweats, weight loss, and peripheral blood eosinophilia. Hodgkin's disease may begin in a single lymph node but usually spreads in an orderly manner (contiguous spread) along a lymph node chain that is centrally located in the body. Extranodal Hodgkin's disease may also occur and may involve such organs as the liver, the spleen, the lungs, or the bone marrow. Several different histologic types of Hodgkin's disease have been clearly described and are characterized by the presence of Reed-Sternberg cells or their variants.

REED-STERNBERG CELLS AND THEIR ASSOCIATED VARIANTS

Hodgkin's disease is characterized by a large malignant cell termed a *Reed-Sternberg cell*, or a related cell. A classic Reed-Sternberg cell or one of its variants must be present in an appropriate cellular environment for the diagnosis of Hodgkin's disease to be made. Application of the morphologic criteria presented later is necessary to correctly identify this disease and to distinguish it from other benign conditions, including viral disorders, such as infectious mononucleosis, which may be associated with large cells that mimic Reed-Sternberg cells. Immunologic and molecular diagnostic techniques suggest these heterogeneous cells, at least in lymphocyte-predominant Hodgkin's disease, are lymphoid in origin. Reed-Sternberg cells and associated variants seen in Hodgkin's disease include the following four basic cell types:

1. The classic *Reed-Sternberg cell* is a large cell with a bilobated or polylobated nucleus and a thick nuclear membrane. Each nucleus contains a large, prominent eosinophilic nucleolus, which is surrounded by a clear zone, or halo (Fig. 25-2). A binucleate Reed-Sternberg cell with two prominent eosinophilic nucleoli has been described as resembling "owl eyes." The cytoplasm associated with these cells may be clear or acidophilic (pink). Classic Reed-Sternberg cells are present in all histologic subtypes of Hodgkin's disease but are observed in the greatest numbers in the mixed cellularity subtype. A Hodgkin's cell is a large cell with a single nucleus that has a prominent eosinophilic nucleolus and pale,

pink cytoplasm. A Hodgkin's cell is considered to be a mononuclear variant of the Reed-Sternberg cell (Fig. 25-2).

2. *Lacunar cells* are usually seen in nodular sclerosis Hodgkin's disease. A lacunar cell is a large cell with a multilobated or polylobated nucleus and inconspicuous nucleoli; twisted, pale-staining nuclei may be associated with ample pale cytoplasm. These cells are best seen in formalin-fixed tissue and are surrounded by a space or lacunae.

3. *Polylobated* or *lymphocyte-histiocyte variants* are large cells with multilobated nuclei ("popcorn cells") that have pale cytoplasm; nucleoli are inconspicuous. This cell variant is most commonly observed in lymphocyte-predominant Hodgkin's disease.

4. *Pleomorphic* or *anaplastic Reed-Sternberg variants* are large cells with angular, variably sized, hyperchromatic nuclei and scant cytoplasm. These cells resemble malignant epithelial or sarcoma cells and may be mistaken for metastatic tumor. They are most frequently observed in the lymphocyte-depletion subtype of Hodgkin's disease.[5]

HISTOLOGIC CLASSIFICATION OF HODGKIN'S DISEASE

The Rye classification scheme divides Hodgkin's disease into four major subtypes: (1) lymphocyte predominance, (2) nodular sclerosis, (3) mixed cellularity, and (4) lymphocyte depletion. Each subtype demonstrates characteristic histologic features and differing clinical prognoses and may be observed in different patient populations.

Lymphocyte Predominance. This histologic subtype is not especially common and accounts for

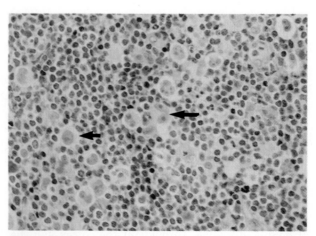

Figure 25-2 Lymph node displaying Hodgkin's disease: Reed-Sternberg cell (*large arrow*) and Hodgkin's cell (*small arrow*) (hematoxylin-eosin, 100×).

approximately 5% of all cases of Hodgkin's disease. It is usually observed in younger males; lymphocyte-predominance Hodgkin's disease has the best prognosis of all subtypes and is associated with an indolent clinical course. A lymph node involved with this subtype is typically replaced by a diffuse background of small, mature lymphocytes. Clusters of histiocytes (tissue macrophages) may also be observed and may resemble infectious granulomatous inflammation. Areas of necrosis are unusual, and eosinophils and plasma cells should not be prominent. The characteristic malignant cell of lymphocyte predominance Hodgkin's disease is the multilobated lymphocyte-histiocyte variant. The finding of a rare Reed-Sternberg cell confirms the diagnosis of Hodgkin's disease.

The lymphocytic background of lymphocyte predominance Hodgkin's disease is composed of benign, mature B lymphocytes; the lymphocyte-histiocyte Reed-Sternberg variants usually express the B cell surface antigen CD20 (L26) but do not display a marker usually present on classic or lacunar Reed-Sternberg cells (CD15/LeuM1). These observations are especially interesting because lymphocyte predominance Hodgkin's disease is immunologically related to other B cell lymphoproliferative disorders and may, in some cases, progress to a malignant large cell lymphoma of B cell origin.

Nodular Sclerosis. This is one of the most common subtypes and accounts for approximately 60% of all cases of Hodgkin's disease. Like the lymphocyte predominance variant, nodular sclerosis Hodgkin's disease tends to occur in young patients; these individuals may be asymptomatic at the time of diagnosis or may present with a mediastinal mass. Nodular sclerosis Hodgkin's disease is associated with an intermediate prognosis that lies between that of the indolent lymphocyte predominance subtype and the poor prognosis of the lymphocyte depletion Hodgkin's disease discussed later. It is characterized by varying degrees of lymph node fibrosis and lacunar Reed-Sternberg cells. The lymph node capsule is typically thickened and fibrotic; interlacing bands of collagenous tissue subdivide the node into cellular nodules. These nodules are composed predominantly of benign lymphocytes associated with varying numbers of granulocytes, macrophages, and eosinophils. Numerous lacunar Reed-Sternberg cells are typically observed in groups or clusters at the centers of these cellular islands. Occasionally, mummified cells and relatively fewer numbers of classic Reed-Sternberg cells may also be seen. Unlike lymphocyte predominance Hodgkin's disease, the background lymphocytes in nodular sclerosis are predominantly CD4 T helper cells rather than B lymphocytes. Lacunar cells usually do not display

B lymphocyte surface antigens, such as CD45 and L26 (CD20) but do express CD15 (LeuM1).

Mixed Cellularity. After nodular sclerosis, mixed cellularity is the most frequently observed subtype (20%) of Hodgkin's disease. Like nodular sclerosis Hodgkin's disease, mixed cellularity Hodgkin's disease has an intermediate clinical prognosis. It may be seen in both men and women and is frequently associated with such clinical symptoms as fever, weight loss, or night sweats. Mixed cellularity Hodgkin's disease may present in any clinical stage at the time of diagnosis. Lymph nodes involved with the mixed cellularity subtype have a variable microscopic appearance but are usually replaced with a heterogeneous infiltrate of neutrophils, mature lymphocytes, macrophages, and eosinophils. The eosinophilic component may be especially prominent. In contrast to the other subtypes previously described, classic binucleate Reed-Sternberg cells are common and are easily observed in mixed cellularity Hodgkin's disease.

Lymphocyte Depletion. The lymphocyte depletion subtype is unusual and accounts for fewer than 5% of all forms of Hodgkin's disease. It most frequently occurs in older patients who typically have advanced disease at the time of clinical presentation. Lymphocyte depletion Hodgkin's disease has the poorest prognosis and the shortest survival of any type of Hodgkin's disease. A lymph node involved with the lymphocyte depletion subtype is characterized by loss or depletion of background lymphocytes and other cells and the presence of variable diffuse fibrosis. Reed-Sternberg cells are prominent and may have a highly atypical or anaplastic appearance.[6]

EXTRANODAL HODGKIN'S DISEASE

Hodgkin's disease may be found in body sites other than lymph nodes; organs such as bone marrow, liver, spleen, or lung may be involved with tumors. Nodular sclerosis and mixed cellularity subtypes are most frequently seen in liver and bone marrow; the lymphocyte predominance subtype, in contrast, is rarely observed in these sites. Gastrointestinal tract, skin, or other body tissues are usually not involved with extranodal Hodgkin's disease. A surgical pathologist frequently evaluates tissues from organs, such as bone marrow, liver, or spleen, for the presence of extranodal disease. However, the primary diagnosis and subclassification of this lymphoproliferative disorder should be determined only after microscopic evaluation of lymph node tissues is performed. Subtyping or diagnosis of Hodgkin's disease should not be attempted based solely on histologic features observed in extranodal tissues.[6]

PROGNOSIS

Before current treatment protocols, the survival rate in Hodgkin's disease was extremely low. Combined chemotherapy and irradiation therapy regimens now result in overall survival and cure rates of at least 80% at major medical centers. Among patients with localized disease, a 90% survival and cure rate may be expected.

The clinical course of Hodgkin's disease varies with age, stage of disease, and histologic subtype. Patient age of greater than 50 years; the presence of clinical symptoms, such as night sweats, fever, or weight loss; or the presence of extensive disease (advanced stage) (Table 25-1) are considered to be poor prognostic indicators. As previously described, patients with lymphocyte predominance Hodgkin's disease have a favorable prognosis; those with nodular sclerosis or mixed cellularity subtype, an intermediate prognosis; and those with lymphocyte depletion subtype a poor prognosis and an aggressive clinical course. Patients with Hodgkin's disease are also at risk for developing various types of secondary malignancies, including solid tumors of breast, lung, bone, and soft tissue, as well as acute leukemia, several years after an apparent cure. These secondary tumors are commonest in individuals treated with combination irradiation therapy and chemotherapy.[7] Treatment is discussed in Chapter 28.

Non-Hodgkin's Lymphoma

GENERAL FEATURES

Non-Hodgkin's lymphoma is a neoplastic proliferation of lymphoid tissue. It is more common than Hodgkin's disease: 40,000 new cases are diagnosed each year. It is the commonest neoplasm in patients between 20 and 40 years of age, and a linear increase in disease incidence occurs with increasing age. Malignant lymphoma occurs in a wide variety of individuals who have altered immune function, including transplant patients treated with immunosuppressive drugs; those with autoimmune disorders, such as systemic lupus erythematosus, rheumatoid arthritis, or Sjögren's syndrome; those with inherited primary immunodeficiencies, or those with AIDS. Lymphomas may also develop in association with pre-existing Hodgkin's disease.[4]

Malignant lymphomas are a heterogeneous group of disorders that differ in microscopic appearance, immunologic cell of origin, and biologic behavior. Classic malignant lymphoma arises in peripheral lymph nodes throughout the body and is characterized by prominent lymphadenopathy. However, in contrast to Hodgkin's disease, the lymph node sites involved with malignancy are variable, and malignant lymphoma may be observed in anatomically distinct lymph node sites (noncontiguous spread of disease). *Extranodal malignant lymphoma* refers to malignant lymphoma that originates in any lymphoid tissue in the body outside of lymph nodes. Typical sites for extranodal malignant lymphoma include mucosa-associated lymphoid tissue of the gastrointestinal and respiratory tracts, skin, liver, or spleen. Different subtypes of lymphoma, especially low-grade follicular lymphomas, may be present in the bone marrow. Lymphoma cells usually are not found circulating in the peripheral blood, and if present, they may represent advancing or progressive disease.

Subclassification of malignant lymphomas has been controversial, and several classification schemes have been proposed over the past several decades. These classifications are often based on microscopic or immunologic features of cells comprising the neoplastic process; other groupings are based on biologic behavior. Histologic criteria commonly used in subclassification of malignant lymphoma may include such features as growth pattern (nodular or diffuse), cell type (small cell, large cell), or nuclear shape (cleaved or noncleaved nucleus).

The original Rappaport classification subdivided lymphomas based on tumor growth pattern observed in the lymph node (nodular or diffuse); this system was later revised to include further subtypes based on cell size or shape. The Rappaport system, however, was developed in the early 1960s, before a comprehensive understanding of the immunologic features of lymphoid cells was reached. The Kiel (Lennert) system also classified lymphomas based on histologic features of lymph nodes and further subdivided these lesions based on clinical behavior into low- and high-grade lymphomas.

Stage	Extent of Disease
	Table 25-1. CLINICAL STAGING FOR HODGKIN'S AND NON-HODGKIN'S LYMPHOMAS (ANN ARBOR CLASSIFICATION)
I	Disease confined to one lymph node site
II	Disease confined to lymphatic tissue in more than one site but on only one side of the diaphragm
III	Disease confined to lymphatic tissue or spleen but on both sides of diaphragm
IV	Bone marrow involvement, liver involvement, and widespread lymphoma at any other site of extranodal disease

Modified from Carbone P, Kaplan HS, Mushoff K, et al: Report of the Committee on Hodgkin's Disease Staging Classification. Cancer Res 1971; 31:1707.

Lukes and Collins incorporated both morphologic and immunologic characteristics in their description of malignant lymphoma and subdivided malignant lymphoma into tumors of B or T cell origin.

The Working Formulation was proposed based on a large multi-institutional study of malignant lymphoma and is now the most commonly used classification scheme (Table 25–2). This system subdivides malignant lymphoma into three major groups based on clinical behavior: low-, intermediate-, and high-grade lymphomas. Within these subgroups, further classification was based on growth pattern (nodular or diffuse), cell size (small, large, or mixed small and large cells), or other cytologic features (cleaved or noncleaved nucleus). Immunologic features of malignant lymphomas have not been consistently integrated with morphologic findings in this system. However, major institutions now examine malignant lymphomas by using a panel of antibodies to determine the cell lineage and to identify a clonal proliferation of lymphoid cells when possible. Molecular diagnostics may also provide a valuable adjunct to these studies and may help identify a clonal proliferation of T or B cells by using gene rearrangement studies. Cytogenetic studies are commonly performed because specific chromosomal abnormalities have been reported in some subtypes of malignant lymphoma.[4]

Finally, nuclear DNA content and proliferative fraction have been studied in malignant lymphoma. Low-grade lymphomas typically demonstrate diploid DNA stemlines, whereas high-grade lymphomas typically have an aneuploid or aberrant DNA content. S-phase or proliferative fraction also parallels lymphoma grade, with lowest S-phase fractions seen in low-grade lesions ($<5\%$) and higher S-phase fractions ($>15\%$), in aggressive or high-grade lymphomas.[8]

LOW-GRADE LYMPHOMAS

Low-grade malignant lymphomas are characterized by a malignant proliferation of small lymphoid cells and include small lymphocytic lymphoma and two forms of follicular lymphoma. These tumors occur predominantly in adults. Follicular lymphomas are indolent, slowly growing lesions of B cell origin. They are frequently associated with mild lymphadenopathy and enlarged cervical or inguinal lymph nodes. Clinical signs of systemic disease, such as night sweats, fevers, or weight loss, are not usually observed. Although follicular lymphomas are frequently disseminated to several lymph node chains and bone marrow, extranodal tumor involving sites such as skin, gastrointestinal tract, gonads, or other solid organs is unusual. Low-grade malignant lymphomas may be controlled with chemotherapy and are associated with survival times of several years but are difficult to cure.[9]

Small Lymphocytic Lymphoma and Chronic Lymphocytic Leukemia. Small lymphocytic lymphoma and chronic lymphocytic leukemia are variants of the same disease process. If the proliferation of small, malignant lymphoid cells is limited to peripheral blood and bone marrow, it is classified as *chronic lymphocytic leukemia*. When this proliferation primarily involves lymph nodes without circulating malignant lymphoid cells in peripheral blood, it is termed *small lymphocytic lymphoma*. Patients with small lymphocytic lymphoma usually present with generalized lymphadenopathy and splenomegaly. Bone marrow involvement with this lymphoma may occur, but lymph node disease predominates. Small lymphocytic lymphoma is characterized by a proliferation of small, round lymphocytes that diffusely efface normal lymph node structures (Fig. 25–3). These malignant lymphocytes may be distinguished from normal lymphoid elements by their coarse, irregular nuclear chromatin. Prominent nucleoli or mitotic activity is not observed. Ninety-five percent of small lymphocytic lymphomas are of B cell origin, and the remaining cases are T cell in derivation. The B cells of small lymphocytic lymphoma usually display pan-B antigens, such as CD19, CD20, and CD23, along with HLA-DR. These neoplastic lymphocytes also coexpress the pan-T marker CD5 (CD19/CD5 coexpression), which is characteristic of small lymphocytic lymphoma and chronic lymphocytic leukemia. Weak surface immunoglobulin, including IgM or IgD, may be observed in associa-

---

Table 25-2. WORKING FORMULATION CLASSIFICATION OF MALIGNANT LYMPHOMAS

Low Grade
Small lymphocytic lymphoma and chronic lymphocytic leukemia
Follicular lymphoma, small cleaved-cell type
Follicular lymphoma, mixed, small cleaved- and large-cell type

Intermediate Grade
Follicular lymphoma, large-cell type
Diffuse lymphoma, small cleaved-cell type
Diffuse lymphoma, mixed, small- and large-cell type
Diffuse lymphoma, large-cell type

High Grade
Large-cell, immunoblastic lymphoma
Lymphoblastic lymphoma
Small noncleaved-cell lymphoma, Burkitt's and non-Burkitt's types

Modified from Rosenberg SA, Berard CW, Brown BW, et al: National Cancer Institute sponsored study of classification of non-Hodgkin's lymphomas: Summary and description of a working formulation for clinical usage. Cancer 1982; 49:2112.

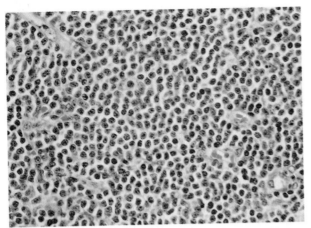

Figure 25-3 Lymph node displaying small lymphocytic lymphoma (hematoxylin-eosin, 100X).

tion with κ or λ light chain restriction; CD10 (common acute lymphoblastic leukemia antigen [CALLA]) is not present. Although small lymphocyte lymphoma may be associated with a survival of several years, approximately 10–15% of these lymphomas develop into a large-cell lymphoma (Richter's syndrome).[10]

Follicular Small Cleaved-Cell Lymphoma. This lymphoma is one of the most common varieties of malignant lymphoma and is characterized by a nodular growth pattern. The neoplastic nodules are uniform in size and shape, and they typically replace the entire lymph node and extend into perinodal adipose tissue. The neoplastic cells within nodules are relatively small and have angular, twisted, or indented nuclei (small, cleaved cells). Nucleoli are not especially prominent, and mitoses are rarely observed. Most small-cell cleaved lymphomas are of B cell origin and arise from germinal centers of lymphoid follicles. In contrast to small lymphocytic lymphomas, the neoplastic cells express bright monoclonal surface immunoglobulin, usually IgG-κ or IgG-λ, in association with prominent CD10 (CALLA). Although B cell markers such as CD19 and CD20 are also present, CD5 coexpression is not observed. Cytogenetic studies may be helpful because a t(14;18) anomaly is observed in approximately 80% of follicular lymphomas. The t(14;18) translocation is also associated with *bcl*-2 oncogene deregulation and prolonged survival of tumor cells.[11]

Follicular Mixed Small Cleaved- and Large-Cell Lymphoma. This lymphoma is composed of a mixture of malignant cells of varying size. Mann and Berard have established criteria to distinguish small cleaved from mixed small cleaved- and large-cell lymphomas as follows: if zero to five large malignant lymphoid cells are present per microscopic high-power field, the lesion

is classified as a small cleaved-cell lymphoma; if five to 15 large cells are present per high-power field, the lesion is "mixed" small- and large-cell lymphoma; and if more than 15 large malignant cells are present, the lesion is a large-cell lymphoma.[12]

INTERMEDIATE-GRADE LYMPHOMAS

Intermediate-grade malignant lymphomas include follicular large-cell malignant lymphoma and three forms of diffuse lymphoma. Both follicular and diffuse malignant lymphoma arise in germinal centers of lymphoid follicles and are typically B cell in origin. The lymphoma cells may be small, large, or a mixture of both. Unlike follicular or nodular lymphomas, which occur predominantly in adults, diffuse malignant lymphoma may be seen in children and adults. Diffuse lymphomas are also frequently associated with systemic symptoms, such as night sweats, weight loss, and fever. Involvement of extranodal sites is more common in diffuse than in follicular varieties of malignant lymphoma. Intermediate-grade lymphomas are associated with a relatively worse prognosis than are low-grade lymphomas.[13]

Follicular Large-Cell Lymphoma. This lymphoma is one of the less common varieties of malignant lymphoma. It is characterized by replacement of the normal lymph node architecture with uniformly sized, round nodules of large lymphoma cells; the mantle zone, or rim of normal lymphocytes that typically surrounds benign lymphoid follicles, is absent. The malignant large cells within the follicles have round or oval nuclei with open chromatin and several nucleoli closely apposed to a thick nuclear membrane. Most of these lesions are B cell in origin and demonstrate cytogenetic and immunophenotypic features of follicular lymphomas described previously. Nodular large-cell lymphoma is associated with a relatively worse prognosis than are other subtypes of follicular malignant lymphoma.

Diffuse Small Cleaved-Cell Lymphoma. This lymphoma replaces lymph nodes with pleomorphic, small lymphoid cells that have angular, indented nuclei and thick nuclear membranes. Nucleoli are readily observed; mitotic figures are also occasionally present. A few residual lymphoid nodules may be present, but the overall pattern is that of a diffuse process. Variable survival rates have been reported in this form of malignant lymphoma.

Diffuse Mixed Small Cleaved-Cell and Large-Cell Lymphoma. This lymphoma is uncommon. Lymph nodes are replaced with a diffuse proliferation of approximately equal numbers of small cleaved and large malignant lymphoid cells.

Variable survival rates have been described in this subtype.[14]

Diffuse Large-Cell Lymphoma. This lymphoma is one of the more commonly observed forms of malignant lymphoma (Fig. 25–4). It frequently involves extranodal sites, such as the gastrointestinal tract, lungs, skin, or other body organs; however, bone marrow dissemination is unusual and occurs late in the disease process. Lymph nodes are replaced with a diffuse population of large malignant cells with oval, noncleaved, or cleaved nuclei. Multiple nucleoli are readily observed adjacent to a thickened nuclear membrane. Unlike small-cell lymphomas, the large lymphoma cells demonstrate ample amounts of clear cytoplasm. Mitoses are readily observed in this rapidly proliferating malignant neoplasm, and focal necrosis may also occur. Most diffuse malignant lymphomas, including diffuse large-cell lymphoma, are B cell in origin, and the remaining cases demonstrate T cell differentiation or a null cell pattern.

Diffuse large-cell lymphomas display aggressive biologic behavior if left untreated. However, some patients may respond favorably to chemotherapy. The prognosis of this lymphoma is complex and depends on several factors, including age, extent of dissemination, and stage of disease. Approximately 80–90% of individuals with localized large-cell lymphoma may be cured with combination chemotherapy. However, elderly patients with advanced disease may experience a cure rate of only 30% and an overall survival of 1 to 2 years.[15, 16]

HIGH-GRADE LYMPHOMAS

High-grade malignant lymphomas include immunoblastic, lymphoblastic, and Burkitt's malignant lymphomas. These lymphomas are associated with characteristic clinical features and aggressive biologic behavior. Each subtype of high-grade malignant lymphoma is treated with a different chemotherapeutic protocol; therefore, lymphoblastic lymphoma and Burkitt's lymphoma must be correctly identified when possible.[17]

Large-Cell Immunoblastic Lymphoma. This lymphoma is typically observed in adults and is associated with a history of pre-existing autoimmune disease, such as systemic lupus erythematosus, rheumatoid arthritis, or AIDS. Current research suggests that prior immune dysfunction may result in defective immune surveillance and the subsequent development of this high-grade lymphoma. Immunoblastic lymphoma is characterized by prominent lymphadenopathy, and lymphomatous involvement of extranodal sites, such as the gastrointestinal tract, lungs, and skin may also be observed.

Histologic sections of lymph node demonstrate diffuse sheets of large, malignant cells with abundant eosinophilic or clear cytoplasm; mitotic activity is markedly increased. Nuclear features of immunoblastic lymphoma include the presence of a prominent, centrally located eosinophilic nucleolus within an oval-shaped nucleus that has a thick nuclear membrane and cleared chromatin. The proliferation of large malignant cells is frequently associated with varying numbers of plasma cells and a background of benign proliferating vessels. Some immunoblastic lymphomas may demonstrate plasmacytic differentiation and may have an eccentrically placed nucleus and a clear perinuclear Golgi zone or hof.

Most immunoblastic lymphomas are of B cell origin and express pan-B markers, such as CD19, CD20, or CD21; CD10 (CALLA) expression is variable. Monoclonal cytoplasmic or surface immunoglobulin may be observed in half of immunoblastic lymphomas, and in the remaining cases, surface immunoglobulin is weak or absent. Immunoblastic lymphoma may occasionally be of T cell origin; these tumors are associated with large, clear tumor cells that demonstrate multilobated, folded, or convoluted nuclei. Patients with immunoblastic lymphoma usually present with prominent lymphadenopathy and advanced disease. Immunoblastic lymphoma is an aggressive neoplasm with a median survival of approximately 21 months.[18]

Lymphoblastic Lymphoma. This lymphoma is characterized by a proliferation of immature lymphoid cells that are similar in appearance to the lymphoblasts of acute lymphoblastic leukemia. This tumor is commonly seen in children and accounts for approximately 30% of all childhood non-Hodgkin's lymphomas. It may also arise in adults and accounts for 3% of adult non-Hodgkin's lymphomas. Lymphoblastic lymphoma is typically

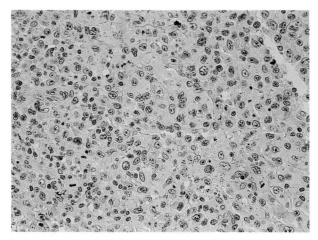

Figure 25–4 Lymph node displaying large-cell lymphoma (hematoxylin-eosin, 100×).

associated with a large, fleshy mediastinal tumor mass and supradiaphragmatic lymphadenopathy. Rapid growth of mediastinal or thoracic lymph nodes may result in tracheal compression and life-threatening airway obstruction. Central nervous system lymphoma may be present at the time of diagnosis in 20% of these cases. Lymphoblastic lymphoma infiltrates may also occur at body sites that are not typically involved in other subtypes of malignant lymphoma, such as the eye, the gonad, or the kidney; abdominal lymphadenopathy is unusual. The bone marrow is typically free of lymphoblastic lymphoma infiltrates. However, the presence of lymphoblasts in both bone marrow and peripheral blood in a young patient with a mediastinal mass may obscure the differentiation of acute lymphoblastic leukemia from disseminated lymphoblastic lymphoma. Lymphoblastic lymphoma is currently defined as a supradiaphragmatic mass, or adenopathy, or both, often with a mediastinal mass; fewer than 25% of blasts are in the bone marrow. Morphologically, lymphoblastic lymphoma cells resemble the blasts seen in acute lymphoblastic leukemia. The tumor mass is composed of sheets of uniform cells with scant cytoplasm, fine nuclear chromatin, and small, inconspicuous nucleoli. The nuclear membrane is frequently described as indented or convoluted, and mitotic activity is readily observed.

Lymphoblastic lymphoma is a neoplasm of immature lymphoid origin. Eighty percent of lymphoblastic lymphomas are of T cell derivation and express immature thymic markers, including nuclear terminal deoxynucleotidyl transferase (TdT) and surface antigens CD1, CD7, CD2, CD3, and CD5. The remaining cases demonstrate an immature B phenotype that is usually seen in childhood acute lymphoblastic leukemia (TdT/CD19/CD20/CD10 positive). Nuclear TdT expression in most subtypes of malignant lymphoma is unusual, and TdT positivity is a characteristic feature of lymphoblastic lymphoma. The t(11;14) translocation may be observed in lymphoblastic lymphoma of T cell origin. Lymphoblastic lymphoma is associated with an aggressive clinical course. Although these patients may experience a good initial response to therapy, remissions are of short duration, and the long-term prognosis is poor (overall survival is 1 to 2 years).[19]

Small Noncleaved-Cell Malignant Lymphoma. This class includes the high-grade Burkitt's lymphoma. This tumor is usually seen in children but may occur in adults with AIDS. Two clinical variants of Burkitt's lymphoma have been described and include the African (endemic) and the American (sporadic) forms. The African variety, originally described in 1958, included young children (average age, 7 years) who presented with a large jaw mass. Abdominal lymphadenopathy also occurred in these children, but peripheral lymph node enlargement was not especially prominent, and mediastinal, splenic, or bone marrow infiltrates were rare. The sporadic Burkitt's lymphoma, reported in the United States, typically occurred in slightly older children or in young adults and was associated with a large abdominal mass as well as localized cervical lymphadenopathy. Jaw lesions were not reported in the American form. Bone marrow or circulating leukemic cells were unusual in both variants but occurred more commonly in the American variety. Central nervous system infiltrates were reported in both variants. All forms of Burkitt's lymphoma are morphologically identical and consist of a diffuse proliferation of small neoplastic lymphoid cells intermingled with lighter-staining histiocytes, creating a diagnostic "starry-sky" pattern (Fig. 25–5). Malignant cells demonstrate round, noncleaved nuclei with clumped chromatin, multiple nucleoli, and numerous mitoses. A thin rim of basophilic cytoplasm is usually associated with Burkitt's cells. Touch imprints may be useful and often reveal cytoplasmic vacuoles that are not easily seen in routine histologic sections. The Epstein-Barr virus is associated with the pathobiology of Burkitt's lymphoma. Although viral particles have not been observed in Burkitt's cells, multiple copies of the Epstein-Barr virus genome have been detected using molecular diagnostic techniques in approximately 80% of patients with Burkitt's lymphoma. Burkitt's lymphoma is of mature B cell derivation and expresses B cell surface antigens, such as CD19, CD20, or CD22. Monoclonal surface IgM-κ or IgM-λ is also present. CD10 (CALLA) may be positive, but nuclear TdT is weak or absent. Cytogenetic studies frequently demonstrate the pres-

Figure 25–5 Lymph node with Burkitt's lymphoma and prominent "starry sky" pattern (hematoxylin-eosin, 25X).

ence of t(8;14), t(2;8), or t(8;22) translocations. Inappropriate *c-myc* oncogene expression may also be observed in Burkitt's lymphoma in association with these cytogenetic anomalies.[17]

PERIPHERAL T CELL LYMPHOMAS

Peripheral T cell lymphomas (PTCLs) consist of a large group of heterogeneous tumors that are not currently included in the Working Formulation classification scheme. PTCLs are derived from mature, post thymic lymphocytes that express pan-T surface antigens but lack nuclear TdT and surface marker CD1.

PTCLs usually occur in older adults and are associated with clinical symptoms, such as fever, night sweats, and weight loss. Approximately one third of these patients may have a prior history of autoimmune disorders, such as Sjögren's syndrome, rheumatoid arthritis, Hashimoto's thyroiditis, or polyclonal hypergammaglobulinemia. Peripheral lymphadenopathy is the predominant clinical finding in PTCL, but extranodal involvement of spleen, skin, bone marrow, or liver may also occur. PTCLs are associated with nodular or ulcerating skin lesions; circulating malignant T cells in peripheral blood are rarely observed.[20]

PTCLs are morphologically diverse and are usually associated with diffuse replacement of lymph nodes with large malignant cells. The multinucleated neoplastic cells are irregularly shaped and are associated with ample eosinophilic or clear cytoplasm. Lymphoblastic nuclear features are not observed. Lymphoid tissues with tumor infiltrates may also demonstrate a prominent vascular proliferation and a background of eosinophils; plasma cells; small, benign lymphocytes; and macrophages. PTCLs express varying combinations of mature pan-T antigens, such as CD2, CD3, CD4, CD5, CD7, and CD8. Immature thymic markers, including nuclear TdT and surface CD1, are absent. Patients with PTCL often present with advanced stage III or IV disease at the time of the initial clinical diagnosis. PTCLs are currently considered high-grade aggressive lymphomas, and median survival of 9 to 18 months has been reported in some series.[21, 22]

CUTANEOUS T CELL LYMPHOMAS

Cutaneous T cell lymphomas are another diverse group of mature T lymphoproliferative lesions that primarily involve the skin. The two commonest forms of cutaneous T cell lymphomas include mycosis fungoides and Sézary syndrome. Mycosis fungoides is defined as a mature T cell lymphoma with characteristic skin lesions that progress over

time. Lymphadenopathy and involvement of other body organs occur later during the disease course. When significant numbers of malignant T cells circulate in peripheral blood in association with skin lesions and lymphadenopathy, the disease is then called Sézary syndrome. Thus, mycosis fungoides and Sézary syndrome are related forms of cutaneous T cell lymphoma, and these two terms are frequently used interchangeably.

Mycosis fungoides/Sézary syndrome, like PTCL, is a disease of older adults and is typically associated with clinical symptoms, such as fever and weight loss. Distinctive skin lesions characterize this disease and are divided into three major stages. The initial *erythematous stage* consists of red, scaly, weeping skin changes that may resemble psoriasis or eczema. These lesions may regress or develop into a *plaque stage,* in which the lesions are disk-shaped, white elevations with circumscribed borders. The final *tumor stage* consists of large, nodular, fungating bulky tumors that ulcerate and are frequently associated with infection and bleeding. These skin lesions typically progress through these stages over a period of several years. Neoplastic cells may eventually spread to lymph nodes as well as other body organs, including the lung, the spleen, the liver, and the kidneys. Bone marrow involvement, however, is unusual. Although occasional circulating cerebriform cells may be noted in mycosis fungoides, the term Sézary syndrome is used only when lymphocytosis with many circulating malignant cells is present in peripheral blood.

The skin and lymph nodes involved with mycosis fungoides/Sézary syndrome are infiltrated with a mixture of large and small lymphoid cells with darkly staining, folded, or cerebriform nuclei and prominent nucleoli (Fig. 25–6). Scant cytoplasm is

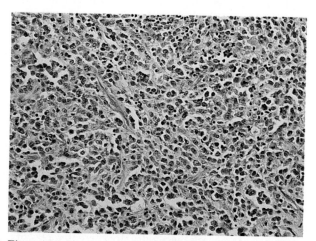

Figure 25–6 Lymph node replaced with T cell lymphoma, mycosis fungoides. Note irregularly shaped and cerebriform nuclei of malignant lymphoid cells. (hematoxylin-eosin, 63×).

associated with these cells. Like in PTCL, these malignant T cells may be admixed with other benign elements, including plasma cells, eosinophils, benign lymphocytes, and macrophages. Lymphadenopathy is frequently observed in both mycosis fungoides and Sézary syndrome. However, reactive lymphadenopathy may occur early in the disease course in association with eczematous skin lesions. When neoplastic adenopathy occurs, malignant infiltrates may be subtle and consist of small numbers of mycosis fungoides/Sézary syndrome cells in interfollicular T cell zones. As the disease evolves, the entire node is diffusely replaced with sheets of malignant cells.

Immunophenotyping of involved skin or lymph node reveals a mature T cell pattern with several pan-T markers, such as CD2, CD3, and CD5; CD7 expression is variable, and some patients with mycosis fungoides/Sézary syndrome may lack the pan-T antigen CD7. The helper cell antigen CD4 is usually present, but CD8 is absent. Nuclear TdT, CD1, or CD4/CD8 coexpression is unusual.

Mycosis fungoides and Sézary syndrome are indolent but progressive lymphoproliferative disorders. Patients may initially display skin lesions; neoplastic infiltrates often involve other body organs later in the disease course. The prognosis is poor once organ involvement is present; the average survival is only several months.[23]

TRUE HISTIOCYTIC LYMPHOMA

A true histiocytic lymphoma (THL) is a proliferation of malignant cells derived from macrophages. Before the development of modern immunologic studies, these lesions were frequently confused with large-cell lymphomas of T cell origin. THL is considered a disease of adults but may also occur in children. It is associated with prominent lymphadenopathy and extranodal involvement of organs, including skin, bone, and gastrointestinal tract. Skin lesions frequently occur and consist of nodular pink or blue tumors that may ulcerate and bleed. Circulating malignant histiocytic cells are not usually observed in peripheral blood. Microscopically, THL is composed of large cells with lobulated nuclei, finely reticular nuclear chromatin, and occasional nucleoli. Malignant histiocytic cells are also associated with abundant pale cytoplasm and distinct cell borders. THL typically infiltrates and expands sinuses of involved lymph nodes. The histologic features of THL may closely resemble T cell leukemia or lymphoma, and, in many cases, both immunologic and cytochemical stains are necessary to correctly classify this unusual lymphoma. Cytochemical stains that identify cells of macrophage or monocytic lineage,

such as alpha-naphthyl butyrate, lysozyme, and alpha-1 antitrypsin, are positive in patients with THL. THL may also demonstrate macrophage-associated markers, including HLA-DR, CD15, CD11B, and CD14; the specific histiocytic marker CD68 may be useful and should be positive in most patients with THL. B or T cell surface markers should not be observed in this disease. The prognosis of true histiocytic lymphoma is difficult to assess because many of these lesions were misdiagnosed before the development of current immunologic studies. However, one recent report of a limited number of patients with well-characterized THL suggested that this tumor may grow aggressively, and patients with it have a clinical survival of 2 years or less. Additional studies are necessary to confirm these findings.[24, 25]

COMPOSITE LYMPHOMA

Composite lymphoma is rare and is defined as the coexistence of two or more distinct cytologic forms of non-Hodgkin's lymphoma at one or more sites in a single patient. The commonest type of composite lymphoma consists of the simultaneous presence of follicular and diffuse large-cell lymphomas. Hodgkin's disease may also coexist with non-Hodgkin's lymphoma, especially the lymphocyte predominance variant in combination with a large-cell lymphoma. The overall prognosis is generally that of the most aggressive histologic type observed.[26]

MALIGNANT LYMPHOMA IN THE IMMUNOCOMPROMISED PATIENT

Malignant lymphomas may arise in association with various immune deficiency states.

Patients with AIDS may demonstrate benign or malignant lymphadenopathy. Benign AIDS-related lymphadenopathy may have several different histologic appearances that develop sequentially as the disease progresses. The *type A* AIDS-related change is characterized by marked follicular hyperplasia, focal areas of lymph node hemorrhage, and multinucleated giant cells (Warthin-Finkeldey bodies). The *type B* stage adenopathy is associated with regression of the initial dramatic follicular hyperplasia, loss of lymphocytes, and proliferation of plasma cells and interfollicular vessels. In the *type C* stage, the lymph node demonstrates depletion of lymphocytes, atrophic follicles, and fibrosis, with prominent plasma cell infiltrates. Reactive vascular proliferation is also readily observed. Kaposi sarcoma, which is a malignant proliferation of blood vessels, may also occur in lymph nodes of patients with type C adenopathy.[19]

Individuals with AIDS experience a 60-fold increased risk for lymphoproliferative disorders over that of the general population and may develop either non-Hodgkin's or Hodgkin's lymphoma. Most of the non-Hodgkin's lymphomas that occur in this population are B cell in origin and include diffuse large-cell, immunoblastic, or Burkitt's lymphomas. AIDS-related lymphomas are also associated with a high incidence of involvement of extranodal sites and frequently display areas of necrosis, prominent mitotic activity, and nuclear atypia. When Hodgkin's disease occurs in patients with AIDS, it is usually of the mixed cellularity or lymphocyte depleted type. Lymphoproliferative disorders in this patient population are associated with aggressive biologic behavior, rapid disease spread, and short survival.[19]

Lymphoproliferative disorders arise in transplant patients who are being treated with immunosuppressive agents. The incidence of lymphomas in this patient group is 350 times that of the general population and affects approximately 2% of all organ transplant recipients. Post-transplant lymphoproliferative disorders (PTLD) include a spectrum of histologic appearances that have been described as "polymorphous" or "monomorphous." PTLD is related to Epstein-Barr virus infection and is associated with the immunosuppressive drug therapy used to preserve grafted organs. These patients may develop lymphadenopathy or localized tumor masses. Extranodal lymphomas may occur in the gastrointestinal tract, brain, or transplanted organ. Lymph nodes demonstrate architectural effacement and capsular or vascular invasion with heterogeneous cellular proliferations. Many individuals may have a polymorphous PTLD and a proliferation of several cell types, including small lymphocytes, immunoblasts, and plasma cells. Other patients have a monomorphous PTLD, characterized by a proliferation of monotonous large cells, often with plasmacytic features. Both polymorphous and monomorphous variants are B cell in origin and may be polyclonal, monoclonal, or both. The prognosis of PTLD is variable, but most polyclonal and approximately half of the monoclonal proliferations regress with reduction of the immunosuppressive drug regimen. Monoclonal, monomorphous proliferations may grow aggressively and are frequently treated with therapeutic regimens used in malignant lymphomas.[19, 27]

Plasma Cell Dyscrasia

Plasma cell dyscrasia is a group of disorders that arise from clonal proliferations of plasma cells or associated B cells. Many of these disorders are associated with the production of significant quantities of abnormal immunoglobulin, which may be detected in serum or urine. These diseases include multiple myeloma, plasma cell leukemia, Waldenström's macroglobulinemia, and MGUS (monoclonal gammopathy of uncertain significance).

The distinction between polyclonal and monoclonal gammopathy is a central concept in the study of plasma cell dyscrasias. *Polyclonal gammopathy* refers to an increase in several different types of immunoglobulin in the serum that are produced by different clones of plasma cells, usually in response to antigenic stimulation. Polyclonal immunoglobulins are not detected in the urine and are not associated with an underlying malignant disorder. *Monoclonal gammopathy* is defined as the production of a homogeneous immunoglobulin of a single type (paraprotein) produced by a single cell line or clone of cells. This paraprotein is observed in association with underlying malignancies, such as plasma cell dyscrasias, malignant lymphoma, or carcinoma. Unlike polyclonal gammopathy, monoclonal gammopathies are associated with abnormal protein in the urine as well as in the serum. Paraprotein production is also associated with a reduction of the other normal immunoglobulin fractions.

MULTIPLE MYELOMA

Multiple myeloma is a malignant proliferation of plasma cells in bone marrow in association with osteolytic bone lesions and a monoclonal immunoglobulin in serum and/or urine. Multiple myeloma is found in older adults at a median age of 63 years; it is rarely observed in individuals younger than 40 years of age, and the incidence increases with increasing age.

The clinical findings observed in this disease are closely related to the protein products produced by the malignant clone of plasma cells. Multiple myeloma is associated with bone lesions or pathologic bone fractures, which may be detected by radiographic studies. Proliferating plasma cells in the marrow secrete an osteoclast-activating factor, which causes increased bone resorption and the resultant lytic bone lesions and fractures. These lytic lesions are associated with significant morbidity and mortality and most frequently occur in the vertebrae, ribs, skull, pelvis, and femur. Increased bone turnover results in an elevated serum calcium level and the destructive deposition of calcium in normal tissues. Myelomatous infiltrates in bone may proliferate, erode through bone cortex, and damage adjacent spinal nerves or spinal cord.

Malignant plasma cells typically produce a monoclonal immunoglobulin, usually greater than 3 g/dL. With the use of serum protein electrophoresis (M-spike), this homogeneous immunoglobulin of a single type may be detected as a single band. IgG is the most commonly produced monoclonal protein, followed by IgA or, rarely, IgD or IgE. The heavy chain in the monoclonal protein is associated with a single light chain, either κ or λ subtype, but not both. In approximately 25% of multiple myelomas, plasma cells secrete only κ or λ light chains without an associated heavy chain. These free light chains may be detected in serum or in urine and are called Bence Jones protein. Proteinuria occurs in at least 50% of patients with multiple myeloma. Excretion of monoclonal proteins, especially light chains in urine, may cause obstruction or damage of nephrons, resulting in renal insufficiency. Malignant plasma cells also synthesize soluble factors, which results in suppression of normal plasma cells that produce a spectrum of normal immunoglobulins of different isotypes. The subsequent decrease in normal serum immunoglobulin levels results in an increased susceptibility to infection, which is a major cause of death in these patients.

Monoclonal protein in the serum may polymerize and cause increased viscosity, poor circulation, and the formation of red blood cell rouleaux. It may also bind to platelets and clotting factors and may interfere with the coagulation cascade. Amyloidosis is also associated with multiple myeloma and consists of tissue deposits of protein composed of light chains or their fragments. This material may be deposited in organs such as the kidney, the heart, or the lungs and may result in tissue damage or dysfunction. A normocytic normochromic anemia is typically present; rare circulating plasma cells may also be observed in the peripheral blood.

The bone marrow in multiple myeloma demonstrates an increased number of mature or abnormal plasma cells. Abnormal plasma cells should account for at least 10% of the nucleated marrow elements and frequently grow in sheets or clusters (Fig. 25–7). Cytologic features observed in malignant plasmacytosis include immature plasmablasts with multiple nucleoli, mitotic figures, or intranuclear inclusions. An increased nuclear:cytoplasmic ratio, abnormal condensation of nuclear chromatin, or loss of perinuclear hof may also be observed. Myeloma infiltrates typically involve bone marrow. Although they may also proliferate in other body sites, they do not usually result in lymphadenopathy or hepatosplenomegaly.[28]

Immunophenotypic studies of myeloma cells demonstrate monoclonal cytoplasmic immunoglobulin; however, surface immunoglobulin or pan-B antigens, such as CD19, CD20, or CD22, are absent. Multiple myeloma may express plasma cell–affiliated antigens, such as CD38 or PCA. Some

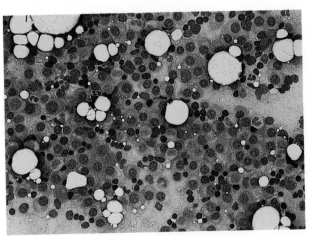

Figure 25–7 Bone marrow aspirate with multiple myeloma. Note sheets of plasma cells and plasmablasts replacing normal hematopoietic tissue (Wright-Giemsa, 100×).

myelomas demonstrate surface CD10 (CALLA), which is associated with a poor prognosis.[29]

The clinical course in multiple myeloma is determined by overall tumor burden. Early-stage disease is associated with a survival of greater than 60 months, whereas advanced multiple myeloma is associated with a survival of approximately 23 months. The median survival for CD10-negative multiple myeloma is 56 months; the median survival of CD10-positive myeloma is poor, only 6 months.[30]

PLASMA CELL LEUKEMIA

Plasma cell leukemia occurs when greater than 2×10^9/L circulating cells are present in peripheral blood. Plasma cell leukemia may occur at the time of initial diagnosis of multiple myeloma (primary type) or may be the terminal event in patients with leukemic transformation of a previously diagnosed myeloma (secondary plasma cell leukemia).[31]

WALDENSTRÖM'S MACROGLOBULINEMIA

Waldenström's macroglobulinemia is an unusual immunoproliferative disorder that displays features of both malignant lymphoma and multiple myeloma. Like multiple myeloma, Waldenström's macroglobulinemia occurs in older adults at a median age of 63 years. Clinical findings observed in Waldenström's macroglobulinemia include normocytic, normochromic anemia; hepatosplenomegaly; lymphadenopathy; and peripheral neuropathy. Waldenström's macroglobulinemia is characterized by the presence of greater than 3 g/dL of IgM monoclonal antibody in the serum. This paraprotein is detected as a serum spike in the beta-gamma zone in serum protein electrophoretic studies and may be associated with cold agglutinin anti-I activity. This large molecule is associated with prominent hyperviscosity; it may also coat platelets and inhibit several coagulation factors, resulting in a bleeding diathesis. The IgM paraprotein is present in the serum, but Bence Jones protein or free light chains are not necessarily noted in urine. Lytic bone lesions, hypercalcemia, or renal dysfunction are not typical clinical features of Waldenström's macroglobulinemia.

Malignant cellular infiltrates involve primarily bone marrow, which is typically hypercellular and demonstrates a lymphoplasmacytic infiltrate. Waldenström's macroglobulinemia is considered an indolent low-grade lesion; patients with it have a median survival of 50 months.[32]

MONOCLONAL GAMMOPATHY OF UNCERTAIN SIGNIFICANCE

MGUS is defined as the presence of a circulating monoclonal protein without an associated plasma cell dyscrasia or other neoplasm. MGUS has been observed in 3% of all adults over 70 years of age. The monoclonal protein may be of any isotype but is usually less than 3 g/dL. Levels of other normal serum immunoglobulins are not decreased; serum calcium level is not elevated. Anemia, increased erythrocyte sedimentation rate, hypercalcemia, and

proteinuria are not observed. Lytic bone lesions, which are seen in multiple myeloma, are absent. A mild plasmacytosis of the bone marrow may be observed. However, these reactive plasma cells are evenly dispersed throughout the marrow and should constitute less than 10% of all nucleated marrow elements. It is currently theorized that monoclonal protein produced in MGUS is synthesized by a stable clone of plasma cells or leukocytes. Patients with MGUS are monitored with repeat serum immunoglobulin level determinations, which are usually stable for several years. Approximately 15% of patients with MGUS have been reported to progress to multiple myeloma after a period of approximately 10 years.[33, 34]

SUMMARY

The lymphoproliferative disorders include a large group of benign and malignant lesions involving the lymphoid system. The malignant processes are frequently derived from a single clone of cells and often demonstrate immunologic or molecular features of a clonal proliferation. Appropriate recognition and classification of these disorders is best accomplished through the integration of clinical and morphologic disease features by immunophenotypic, cytogenetic, and molecular studies.

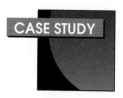

Case 1

A 16-year-old white woman presented to her physician complaining of fever (101°F), night sweats, and a 15-lb weight loss. On physical examination, several enlarged, rubbery, right supraclavicular and cervical lymph nodes were noted. No other lymphadenopathy was present; the spleen and liver were not enlarged. Laboratory findings were unremarkable and demonstrated a mild normocytic, nor-

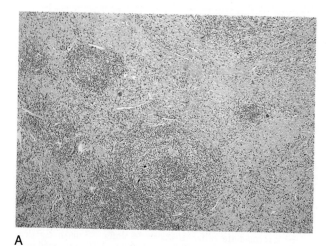

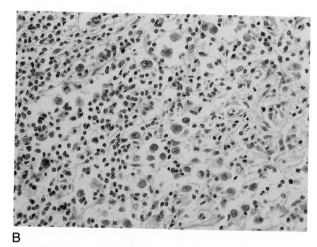

A   B

Figure 25–8 *A,* Lymph node displaying nodular sclerosis Hodgkin's disease, low power. Dense collagenous bands divide lymph node into cellular islands (hematoxylin-eosin, 16×). *B,* Lymph node with nodular sclerosis Hodgkin's disease. Large cells in this field include classic Reed-Sternberg cells and associated variants (hematoxylin-eosin, 100×).

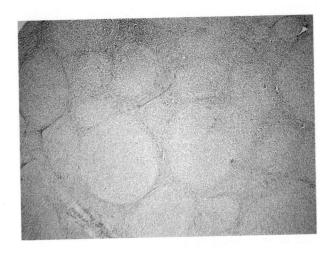

Figure 25–9 Lymph node with follicular malignant lymphoma. The neoplastic nodules are relatively uniform in size and lack a mantle of small lymphocytes (hematoxylin-eosin, 10×).

mochromic anemia (11.0 g/dL). A review of the patient's peripheral blood smear revealed a mild eosinophilia without circulating malignant cells. The patient's lymph node biopsy is shown in Figure 25–8, *A* and *B*).

1. On the basis of these findings, what is the most likely diagnosis?

2. Describe the tissue pattern present in the biopsy and the diagnostic cells in the cellular areas of the lymph node.

Case 2

A 53-year-old black woman complained of malaise and abdominal pain. On physical examination, her physician noted prominent distention of her abdomen with ascites and an abdominal mass. Ultrasound studies of the abdomen revealed the presence of an 8-cm mass of matted lymph nodes in mesenteric fat. A generalized lymphadenopathy was also present. A biopsy was performed on an enlarged right anterior cervical lymph node (Fig. 25–9).

1. Describe the histologic features of the tissue biopsy; are these findings those of a benign reactive or a malignant process?

2. What additional studies may be helpful in this case?

References

1. Roitt I, Brostoff J, Male D: Immunology, 2nd ed. Philadelphia: JB Lippincott, 1989.
2. Banks PM: Technical aspects of specimen preparation and special studies. *In* Jaffe ES (ed): Surgical Pathology of the Lymph Nodes and Related Organs. Philadelphia: WB Saunders, 1985:1–21.
3. Schnitzer B: Reactive lymphoid hyperplasia. *In* Jaffe ES (ed): Surgical Pathology of the Lymph Nodes and Related Organs. Philadelphia: WB Saunders, 1985:22–56.
4. Freedman AS, Nadler LM: Malignant lymphomas. *In* Isselbacher KJ, Braunwald E, Wilson JD (eds): Harrison's Principles of Internal Medicine, 13th ed. New York: McGraw-Hill, 1994:1784–1788.
5. Grogan TM: Hodgkin's disease. *In* Jaffe ES (ed): Surgical Pathology of the Lymph Nodes and Related Organs. Philadelphia: WB Saunders, 1985:92–96.
6. Burke JS: Hodgkin's disease: histopathology and differential diagnosis. *In* Knowles DM (ed): Neoplastic Hematopathology. Baltimore: Williams & Wilkins, 1992:497–533.
7. Berliner N, Smith BR: The pathobiology of lymphoproliferative disease. *In* Hoffman R, Benz EJ, Shattil SJ, et al (eds): Hematology: Basic Principles and Practice. New York: Churchill Livingstone, 1991:897–911.

8. Duque RE, Braylan RC: Applications of flow cytometry to diagnostic hematopathology. *In* Coon JS, Weinstein RS (eds): Diagnostic Flow Cytometry. Baltimore: Williams & Wilkins, 1991:89–102.
9. Jaffe ES: An overview of the classification of non-Hodgkin's lymphomas. *In* Jaffe ES (ed): Surgical Pathology of the Lymph Nodes and Related Organs. Philadelphia: WB Saunders, 1985:92–96.
10. Ben-Ezra J: Small lymphocytic lymphoma. *In* Knowles DM (ed): Neoplastic Hematopathology. Baltimore: Williams & Wilkins, 1992:603–616.
11. Hardy R, Horning S: Molecular biologic studies in the clinical evaluation of non-Hodgkin's lymphoma. Hematol Oncol Clin North Am 1991; 5:891–900.
12. Harris N, Ferry J: Follicular lymphoma and related disorders. *In* Knowles DM (ed): Neoplastic Hematopathology. Baltimore: Williams & Wilkins, 1992:645–674.
13. Mann RB: Follicular lymphoma and lymphocytic lymphoma of intermediate differentiation. *In* Jaffe ES (ed): Surgical Pathology of Lymph Nodes and Related Organs. Philadelphia: WB Saunders, 1985:165–202.
14. Weisenburger D, Chan W: Lymphomas of follicles. Am J Clin Pathol 1993; 99:409–420.

15. Stein H, Dallenbach F: Diffuse large cell lymphomas of B and T cell type. *In* Knowles DM (ed): Neoplastic Hematopathology. Baltimore: Williams & Wilkins, 1992:675–687.
16. Davey FR, Nelson DA: Leukocytic disorders. *In* Henry JB (ed): Clinical Diagnosis and Management by Laboratory Methods. Philadelphia: WB Saunders, 1991:705–707.
17. Bierman PJ, Vose JM, Armitage JO: Clinical manifestations, staging and treatment of non-Hodgkin's lymphoma. *In* Hoffman R, Benz EJ, Shattil SJ, et al (eds): Hematology: Basic Principles and Practice. New York: Churchill-Livingstone, 1991:963–982.
18. Cossman J: Diffuse aggressive non-Hodgkin's lymphomas. *In* Jaffe ES (ed): Surgical Pathology of Lymph Nodes and Related Organs. Philadelphia: WB Saunders, 1985:203–217.
19. Ioachim HL: Lymph Node Pathology, 2nd ed. Philadelphia: JB Lippincott, 1994.
20. Weiss LM, Crabtree GS, Rouse RV, et al: Morphologic and immunologic characterization of 50 peripheral T-cell lymphomas. Am J Pathol 1985; 118:316–324.
21. Pinkus G, Said JW: Peripheral T cell lymphomas. *In* Knowles DM (ed): Neoplastic Hematopathology. Baltimore: Williams & Wilkins, 1992:837–867.
22. Winberg C: Peripheral T-cell lymphoma. Am J Clin Pathol 1993; 99:426–435.
23. Barcos M: Mycosis fungoides: Diagnosis and pathogenesis. Am J Clin Pathol 1993; 99:452–458.
24. Ben-Ezra JM, Koo CH: Langerhans' cell histiocytosis and malignancies of the M-PIRE system. Am J Clin Pathol 1993; 99:464–471.
25. Ben-Ezra J, Bailey A, Azumi N, et al: Malignant histiocytosis X. Cancer 1991; 68:1050–1060.
26. Kim H: Composite lymphoma and related disorders. Am J Clin Pathol 1993; 99:445–451.
27. Ferry JA, Jacobson JO, Conti D, et al: Lymphoproliferative disorders and hematologic malignancies following organ transplantation. Mod Pathol 1989; 2:583–592.
28. Grogan TM, Spier CM: The B cell immunoproliferative disorders including multiple myeloma and amyloidosis. *In* Knowles DM (ed): Neoplastic Hematopathology. Baltimore: Williams & Wilkins, 1992:1235–1265.
29. Durie BG, Grogan TM: CALLA-positive myeloma: An aggressive subtype with poor survival. Blood 1985; 66:229–232.
30. Kyle RA: Plasma cell proliferative disorders. *In* Hoffman R, Benz EJ, Shattil SJ, et al (eds): Hematology: Basic Principles and Practice. New York: Churchill-Livingstone, 1991:1021–1038.
31. Kyle RA, Maldonado JE, Bayrd ED: Plasma cell leukemia. Arch Intern Med 1974; 133:813–818.
32. Pilarski LM, Andrew EJ, Serra HM, et al: Abnormalities in lymphocyte profile and specificity repertoire of patients with Waldenström's macroglobulinemia, multiple myeloma, and IgM monoclonal gammopathy of undetermined significance. Am J Hematol 1989; 30:53–60.
33. Kyle RA, Garton JP: The spectrum of IgM monoclonal gammopathy in 430 cases. Mayo Clin Proc 1987; 62:719–731.
34. Keren D, Morrison N, Gulbranson R: Evolution of a monoclonal gammopathy. Lab Med 1994; 25:313–317.

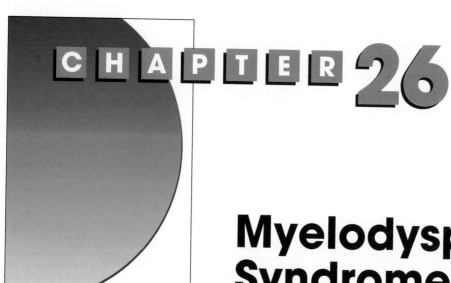

CHAPTER 26

Myelodysplastic Syndromes

Bernadette F. Rodak and
Jacqueline Carr

Objectives

AFTER COMPLETION OF THIS CHAPTER, THE READER WILL BE ABLE TO
1. Define myelodysplastic syndromes.
2. Describe the incidence of myelodysplastic syndromes (MDS).
3. Explain the sequence of events thought to lead to MDS.
4. Recognize morphologic features of dyspoiesis in bone marrow and peripheral blood.
5. Discuss abnormal functions of granulocytes, erythrocytes, and thrombocytes in MDS.
6. Correlate peripheral blood and bone marrow findings in MDS with the French-American-British (FAB) classification.
7. Discuss prognostic indicators in MDS, including FAB classification, Bournemouth score, chromosome analysis, and monoclonal antibodies.
8. List common causes of death in MDS.
9. Discuss modes of treatment for MDS.

For decades, laboratorians have observed a group of morphologic abnormalities in peripheral blood and bone marrow smears of elderly patients. Because some of these disorders progressed to acute leukemia, it was thought that these abnormalities represented a preleukemic condition.[1-3] The findings are heterogeneous in nature, affect all cell lines, and may remain stable for years or progress rapidly to death. As a result, a wide variety of names have been used to describe the presence of these cellular abnormalities. In 1982, the French-American-British (FAB) Cooperative Leukemia Study Group proposed terminology and a specific set of morphologic criteria to describe what are now known as myelodysplastic syndromes (MDS).[4] These are a group of acquired clonal hematologic disorders characterized by progressive cytopenias in the peripheral blood that reflect defects in erythroid, myeloid, and/or megakaryocytic maturation.[5, 6]

MDS are diseases primarily of the older population, occurring most frequently among people over age 50.[1] MDS occur less frequently among young adults and are uncommon among children, but documented cases have been reported.[7, 8] The incidence of these disorders appears to be increasing, but this apparent increase may be attributable, in part, to improved techniques for identifying these diseases and to improved classification.[9] At this time, the fastest growing segment of the population is over 60 years of age; thus MDS is becoming a more common finding in the hematology laboratory and an essential part of the body of knowledge of all medical technologists.

ETIOLOGY

Although MDS appear to be a group of heterogeneous diseases, all are the result of proliferation of abnormal pluripotential stem cells.[5, 6, 10, 11] It is proposed that the abnormal pluripotential stem cell is the result of a somatic mutation. The mutation may be caused by chemical insult, radiation, or viral infection.[12] The mutated stem cell then produces a pathologic clone of cells that expands in size at the expense of normal cell production.[13] Because each mutation produces a unique clone with a specific cellular defect, MDS has a multitude of expressions. However, two morphologic findings are common to all types of MDS: the presence of progressive cytopenias and dyspoiesis in one or more cell lines. The progressive cytopenia is caused by expansion of the abnormal clone, and the dyspoiesis (abnormal development) is the result of the specific cellular mutation.

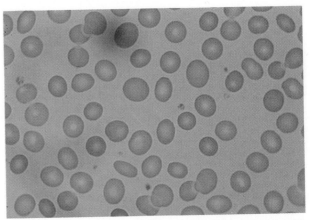

Figure 26–1 Oval macrocytes in peripheral blood. (Magnification, 500×.)

MORPHOLOGIC ABNORMALITIES IN PERIPHERAL BLOOD AND BONE MARROW

Each of the three major myeloid cell lines has dyspoietic morphologic features. The following sections are descriptions of the more common abnormal morphologic findings.[4, 14] These descriptions, however, are not all-inclusive, because of the large number of possible cellular mutations and combinations of mutations.

Dyserythropoiesis

In the peripheral blood, the most common morphologic finding in dyserythropoiesis is the presence of oval macrocytes (Fig. 26–1). When these cells are seen in the presence of normal vitamin B_{12} and folate values, MDS should be included in the differential diagnosis. Hypochromic microcytes with adequate iron stores are also seen in MDS. A dimorphic red blood cell (RBC) population (Fig. 26–2) is another indication of the clonality of this

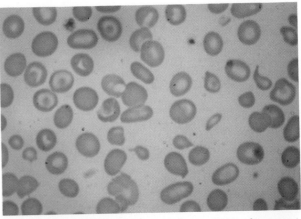

Figure 26–2 Dimorphic erythrocyte population, demonstrating both hypochromic and normochromic cells, in peripheral blood. (Magnification, 500×.)

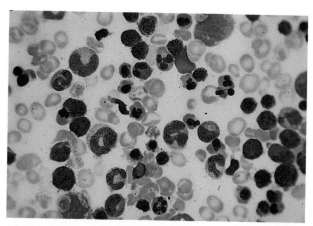

Figure 26–3 Bone marrow specimen demonstrating erythroid hyperplasia and nuclear budding in erythroid precursors. (Magnification, 500×.)

Table 26-1. MORPHOLOGIC EVIDENCE OF DYSERYTHROPOIESIS
Oval macrocytes
Hypochromic microcytes
Dimorphic RBC population
RBC precursors with >1 nucleus
RBC precursors with abnormal nuclear shapes
RBC precursors with uneven cytoplasmic staining
Ringed sideroblasts

Abbreviation: RBC, red blood cell.

disease. The presence of poikilocytosis, basophilic stippling, Howell-Jolly bodies, and/or siderocytes are also indications that the erythrocyte has undergone abnormal development.

Dyserythropoiesis in the bone marrow is evidenced by RBC precursors with more than one nucleus and/or abnormal nuclear shapes. The normally round nucleus may have lobes or buds. Nuclear fragments may be present in the cytoplasm (Fig. 26–3). The abnormal cytoplasmic features may include basophilic stippling or heterogeneous staining (Fig. 26–4). Ringed sideroblasts are a common finding. Megaloblastoid cellular development in the presence of normal vitamin B$_{12}$ and folate values is another indication of MDS. These bone marrows may have erythrocytic hyperplasia or hypoplasia (Table 26–1).

Dysmyelopoiesis

Dysmyelopoiesis in the peripheral blood is suspected when there is a persistence of basophilia in the cytoplasm of otherwise mature white blood cells (WBCs), indicating nuclear/cytoplasmic asynchrony (Fig. 26–5). Abnormal granulation of the cytoplasm of WBCs is a common finding, in the form of granules larger than normal, hypogranulation, or the absence of granules. Agranular bands can be easily misclassified as monocytes (Fig. 26–6). Abnormal nuclear features may include hyposegmentation, hypersegmentation, or nuclear rings (Fig. 26–7).

In the bone marrow, dysmyelopoiesis may be represented by nuclear/cytoplasmic asynchrony. Cytoplasmic changes may include uneven staining, such as a dense ring of basophilia around the periphery with a clear unstained area around the nucleus or whole sections of cytoplasm unstained with the remainder of the cytoplasm stained normally (Fig. 26–8). There may be abnormal granulation of the cytoplasm in which promyelocytes and/or myelocytes are devoid of primary granules (Fig. 26–9), primary granules may be larger than normal, or secondary granules may be reduced in number or absent, and there may be an occasional Auer rod. (Agranular promyelocytes may be mistaken for blasts. This could lead to misclassification of the disease as acute nonlymphocytic leukemia [ANLL].) Abnormal nuclear findings may

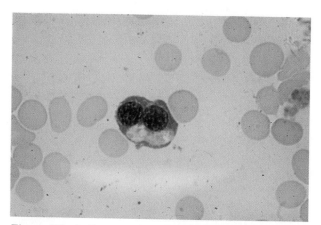

Figure 26–4 Bone marrow specimen demonstrating heterogeneous staining in a bilobed erythroid precursor. (Magnification, 500×.)

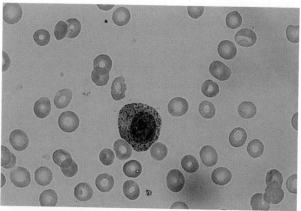

Figure 26–5 This myelocyte in peripheral blood has a nucleus with clumped chromatin and a basophilic immature cytoplasm, demonstrating asynchrony. Note the larger-than-normal granules. (Magnification, 500×.)

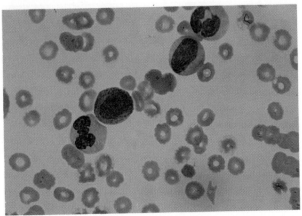

Figure 26–6 Agranular myeloid cells in peripheral blood. (Magnification, 500×.)

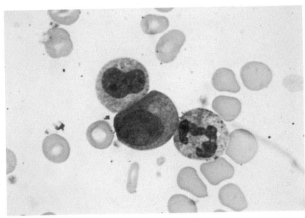

Figure 26–8 Uneven staining of white blood cell cytoplasm in bone marrow specimen. (Magnification, 500×.)

include hypersegmentation or hyposegmentation and possibly ring-shaped nuclei (Table 26–2).

The bone marrow may exhibit granulocytic hypoplasia or hyperplasia. Monocytic hyperplasia is a common finding in dysplastic marrows.

Abnormal localization of immature precursors (ALIP) is a characteristic finding in bone marrow biopsy specimens from patients with MDS.[15] Normally, myeloblasts and promyelocytes reside along the endosteal surface of the bone marrow. In some cases of MDS, these cells tend to cluster centrally in marrow sections.

Platelets also exhibit dyspoietic morphology in the peripheral blood. Common changes include giant platelets and abnormal platelet granulation, either hypogranulation or agranulation (Fig. 26–10). Some platelets may possess large fused granules. Circulating micromegakaryocytes have been described in peripheral blood from patients with MDS.

Dysmegakaryopoiesis

The megakaryocytic component of the bone marrow may exhibit abnormal morphology: large mononuclear megakaryocytes, micromegakaryocytes, or micromegakaryoblasts. The nuclei in these cells may be bilobed or have multiple small separated nuclei (Fig. 26–11; Table 26–3).

ABNORMAL CELLULAR FUNCTION

The cells produced by abnormal maturation have not only abnormal appearance but also abnormal function.[16] The granulocytes may have decreased adhesion,[17, 18] deficient phagocytosis,[18] decreased chemotaxis,[17, 18] and/or impaired microbicidal capacity.[13] The RBCs may exhibit shortened survival,[13] and the platelets may have defective aggregation.[19] The type and degree of dysfunction is dependent on the somatic mutation or mutations present in the pluripotent stem cell.

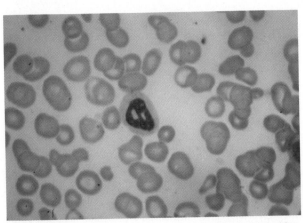

Figure 26–7 Nuclear ring in peripheral blood. (Magnification, 500×.)

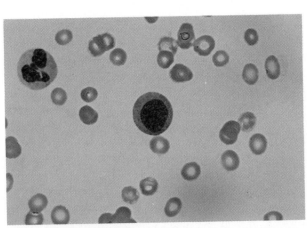

Figure 26–9 Promyelocyte or myelocyte, devoid of granules, and an agranular neutrophil in bone marrow. (Magnification, 500×.)

Table 26-2. MORPHOLOGIC EVIDENCE OF DYSMYELOPOIESIS
Persistent basophilic cytoplasm
Abnormal granulation
Abnormal nuclear shapes
Uneven cytoplasmic staining

FAB CLASSIFICATION OF MYELODYSPLASTIC SYNDROMES

In an effort to standardize the diagnosis of MDS, the FAB created five classes of MDS, each with a specific set of hematologic criteria:

1. Refractory anemia.
2. Refractory anemia with ringed sideroblasts (RARS).
3. Refractory anemia with excess blasts (RAEB).
4. Chronic myelomonocytic leukemia (CMML).
5. Refractory anemia with excess blasts in transformation (RAEB-t).

The diagnostic criteria for peripheral blood and bone marrow for each of these categories is discussed as follows.[20]

Refractory Anemia

Patients with refractory anemia usually have symptoms of anemia. Reticulocytopenia is present, and oval macrocytes are a common finding. Neutropenia and/or thrombocytopenia may be present, but rarely is dysmyelopoiesis or dysmegakaryopoiesis. Blasts, if present in the periphery, constitute fewer than 1% of the nucleated cells. The bone marrow is normocellular to hypercellular with erythroid hyperplasia and/or dyserythropoiesis. Iron stores are increased. The granulocytes and megakaryocytes are usually morphologically normal. Fewer than 5% of the nucleated cells are blasts.

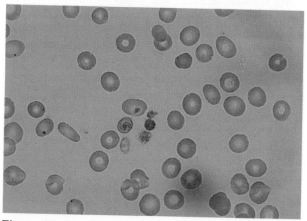

Figure 26-10 Abnormal platelet granulation in peripheral blood. (Magnification, 500×.)

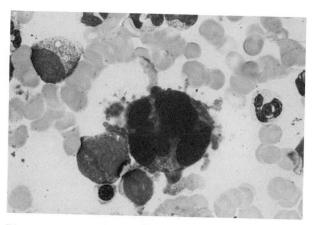

Figure 26-11 Megakaryocyte with small separated nuclei, in bone marrow. (Magnification, 500×.)

Refractory Anemia with Ringed Sideroblasts

Patients with RARS have all of the signs and symptoms of refractory anemia; in addition, more than 15% of nucleated bone marrow cells are ringed sideroblasts. These cells often appear in clusters.

Refractory Anemia with Excess Blasts

In many patients with RAEB, oval macrocytes are present in the peripheral blood. Trilineage cytopenias are commonly present, as are significant dysmyelopoiesis and/or dysmegakaryopoiesis. The morphologic abnormalities of WBCs may include hypogranular neutrophils or pseudo–Pelger-Huët cells. The platelets may have abnormal numbers of granules, which may exhibit abnormalities in size. If present, there are fewer than 5% circulating blasts.

The bone marrow is normocellular to hypercellular with granulocytic and/or erythroid hyperplasia. Trilineage dyspoiesis is present, and 5–20% of the nucleated bone marrow cells are blasts. It is no surprise that these patients present with a wide variety of complaints. The symptoms vary from those of anemia to fever, bleeding, and infection.

Table 26-3. MORPHOLOGIC EVIDENCE OF DYSMEGAKARYOPOIESIS
Giant platelets
Platelets with abnormal granulation
Circulating micromegakaryocytes
Large mononuclear megakaryocytes
Micromegakaryocytes and/or micromegakaryoblasts
Abnormal nuclear shapes in the megakaryocytes/blasts

Chronic Myelomonocytic Leukemia

The peripheral blood in patients with CMML may have characteristics similar to those in the refractory anemias, such as oval macrocytes and reticulocytopenia. The presence of dyserythropoiesis and dysmegakaryopoiesis is variable. Thrombocytopenia may be present. In contrast to other classes of MDS, CMML manifests with leukocytosis. The peripheral WBC concentration may be as high as $100 \times 10^9/L$. Absolute monocytosis ($>1.0 \times 10^9/L$) is always present. Blasts constitute fewer than 5% of peripheral WBCs. The bone marrow demonstrates granulocytic hyperplasia with dysmyelopoiesis. Monocytosis and dysmegakaryopoiesis are present, and 5–20% of nucleated bone marrow cells are blasts. Clinical features include symptoms of anemia, fever, bleeding, and infection.

Refractory Anemia with Excess Blasts in Transformation

The peripheral blood morphology is the same in RAEB-t as in RAEB except that there are more than 5% of circulating blasts, and Auer rods may be present. The bone marrow has the same characteristics as that in RAEB except there are between 20% and 30% blasts, and Auer rods may be visible. (The presence of ≥30% blasts in the bone marrow implies a diagnosis of acute leukemia; see Fig. 26–12 for diagrammatic relationship of MDS to ANLL. The clinical picture is the same as that of RAEB.)

The criteria for each of the five classes of MDS are summarized in Table 26–4.

PROGNOSIS

The life expectancy of patients with MDS varies from less than 1 year to more than 6 years; mean length of survival is 15 months. Some patients require only supportive therapy, such as blood transfusions, whereas in others the disease is much more aggressive and death occurs within a year of diagnosis. Acute leukemia is the most common sequela of MDS; however, death is not always caused by a transformation into acute leukemia. More often it results from severe cytopenias, bleeding, bone marrow failure, or organ failure.[21] Patients with a favorable prognosis must be identified, because certain therapies, even in low dosages, may exacerbate existing cytopenia and increase the risk of morbidity and mortality.[10, 13]

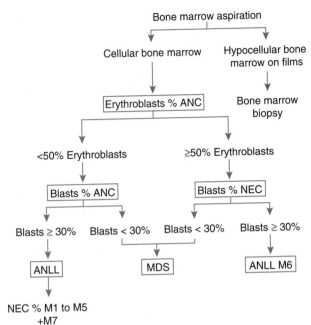

Figure 26–12 Differential diagnosis of myelodysplastic syndrome (MDS) vs. acute nonlymphocytic leukemia (ANLL), based on bone marrow aspirate. *Other abbreviations:* ANC, all nucleated cells; NEC, non-erythroid cells. (Adapted from Bennett JM, Catovsky D, Daniel MT, et al: Proposed revised criteria for the classification of acute myeloid leukemia. Ann Intern Med 1985; 103:626–629.)

Prognosis According to FAB Classification

It has been shown that patients with refractory anemia and RARS have a much better survival rate than those with RAEB, RAEB-t, or CMML.[22] The best prognosis is for patients with refractory anemia or RARS who have a normal karyotype, no neutropenia, and no thrombocytopenia. In this group, median length of survival is 70 months, and there is only a 5–10% risk that the disease will transform into acute leukemia. In fact, an unrelated problem, such as cerebrovascular accident or heart disease, is often the cause of death in these patients.[10, 13] At the other end of the spectrum are the patients with RAEB-t: they have the worst prognosis, and in 55% the disease transforms into acute leukemia.[21]

Within the other FAB subgroups, there is wide variation in length of survival. A research group from Bournemouth, United Kingdom, devised a simple scoring system to increase predictability of survival. A score of 1 was assigned to each of the following:

1. Bone marrow blasts, >5%.
2. Platelet count, $<100 \times 10^9/L$.
3. Neutrophils, $<2.5 \times 10^9/L$.
4. Hemoglobin, <10.0 g/dL.

Table 26-4. FEATURES OF PERIPHERAL BLOOD AND BONE MARROW IN MYELODYSPLASTIC SYNDROME

	Refractory Anemia	Refractory Anemia with RS	Refractory Anemia with Excess Blasts	Refractory Anemia with Excess Blasts in Transformation	Chronic Myelo-monocytic Leukemia	Acute Nonlympho-blastic Leukemia
% peripheral blood blasts	<1	<1	<5	≥5	<5	na*
% bone marrow blasts	<5	<5	5–20	>20, <30	5–20	≥30
Other significant findings	Oval macro-cytes Cytopenias	>15% RS Dimorphic RBC population Oval macrocytes Cytopenias	Cell dysfunction evident Oval macrocytes Cytopenias	Absolute mono-cytosis (>1.0 × 10⁹/L) Oval macrocytes	Absolute mono-cytosis (>1.0 × 10⁹/L) Oval macrocytes	

Abbreviation: RS, ringed sideroblast.
* Diagnosed on bone marrow only.

In accordance with this system, patients were classified into three groups:

group A (score, 0–1)
group B (score, 2–3)
group C (score, 4)

The mean lengths of survival were 62 months for patients in group A, 22 months for patients in group B, and 8.5 months for patients in group C. These findings seemed to correlate well for all the subgroups except the patients with CMML. Their courses varied from benign to aggressive, regardless of Bournemouth score. In 1987, the scoring system for neutrophils was modified to include neutrophilia of more than 16.0×10^9/L. With this modification, it was found that patients with CMML with scores of 2 or higher had a clinical course similar to that of patients with RAEB, with poor survival. Those with scores of less than 2 reacted more like patients with refractory anemia, with long survival.[23]

Several other scoring systems have been developed.[24, 25] However, no single system can predict survival or transformation of MDS into ANLL as well as a combination of all prognostic indicators. Most investigators believe that the most important prognostic features are the percentage of bone marrow blasts, severity of cytopenias, and cytogenetic abnormalities.[13, 14, 26]

Other Negative Prognostic Factors

Several other negative prognostic factors have been identified:

1. Chromosomal abnormalities, especially complex ones, or karyotypic evolution during the course of the disease.
2. Defective incidence of CFU-GM in bone marrow culture.
3. History of previous alkylating agent chemotherapy and/or ionizing radiation (secondary MDS).
4. Presence of ALIP in the bone marrow.[15]
5. Presence of certain antigenic markers (e.g., CD34).

CD34, also known as human progenitor cell antigen (HPCA), is found on pluripotential stem cells and immature precursor cells but is not present on normal mature peripheral blood cells. The presence of this marker in MDS had been associated with both progression to ANLL and poor survival rates.[27]

Chromosome abnormalities are found in 40–70% of MDS patients.[13] According to results of high-resolution chromosome analysis, up to 80% of MDS patients are found to have abnormalities.[10] Translocations, which are common among patients with ANLL, are rarely found in patients with MDS. The most common abnormalities are −5, 5q−, −7, 7q−, and trisomy 8. Less common abnormalities in MDS are 12p−, 20q−, iso 17, −22, and loss of the Y chromosome.[28–31]

In patients who have only the deletion of 5q (5q−), the disease represents a fairly well-defined syndrome, affecting predominantly females. These patients typically have refractory macrocytic anemia, thrombocytosis, hypolobulated megakaryocytes, and erythroid hypoplasia.[10, 13, 28] Patients with the 5q− syndrome have long-term stable disease, and often only supportive therapy is needed.[10, 13, 26, 28]

Syndromes characterized by several other single-chromosome abnormalities (including monosomy 7, iso 17) have been suggested to be distinct MDS subclassifications, because of the characteristic clinical and hematologic features that they have in common.[14, 32] However, none has been as widely studied or accepted as the 5q− syndrome.

The presence of monosomy 7, 7q−, trisomy 8, or complex chromosome aberrations (abnormalities in three or more chromosomes) is associated with a poor prognosis.[31, 33] Single-chromosome abnormalities provide a better prognosis. Patients with a normal karyotype tend to do best.[13, 30, 34–36]

Complex abnormalities appear to reflect a poor prognosis, even for patients with low Bournemouth scores. Toyama and associates devised a scoring system based on scoring both cytogenetic abnormalities and the Bournemouth score (hematologic values). The results of their study suggest that these systems in combination provide a more accurate prognosis, which in turn enables determination of appropriate therapy, including cytokines, chemotherapy, and bone marrow transplantation.[33]

TREATMENT

Although the only "cure" for MDS is bone marrow transplantation, several other therapies are useful, depending on FAB type and other prognostic indicators. Among these are supportive therapy only, vitamins and hormones, chemotherapy (low-dose and aggressive), and inducers of differentiation or biologic response modifiers (see Chapter 28).

Supportive therapy is often all that is needed by patients who do not have an excess of bone marrow blasts, bleeding problems, or infections. They are carefully monitored with periodic blood cell counts, bone marrow examinations, and physical examinations. If severe anemia develops with cardiopulmonary problems or severe bleeding, blood products (RBC and/or platelets) should be given. However, the physician must be careful to avoid hemochromatosis as a result of iron overload.

Younger patients with refractory anemia and RARS may be given iron chelation therapy to avoid organ failure resulting from hemochromatosis.[13, 37]

Vitamins and hormones have been tried in patients with MDS, usually with less than satisfactory results. However, in a small percentage of patients, these measures do appear to have some success. Among the agents used are folic acid, vitamin B_{12}, pyridoxine, heme arginate, androgens, and danazol.[3, 10, 13]

Corticosteroids in general have not been successful, because of the potential toxicity of the drug when given in doses large enough to elicit a response.[3, 10, 13, 37]

Chemotherapy has been used, both in low-dosage and aggressive protocols. Low-dosage cytosine arabinoside has not prolonged survival and has produced myelotoxicity.[13, 37] Aggressive chemotherapy has been successful in treating acute myeloid leukemias, and so it was hoped that it would also induce remission in MDS. However, patients with MDS do not respond as well as do those with de novo acute myeloid leukemia. Remissions are often brief and mortality is high, especially among elderly patients, who die of severe infections, especially from opportunistic organisms.

Aggressive chemotherapy is usually indicated in younger patients with severe cytopenias or an excess of blasts and in patients with more than 20% blasts who are to receive a bone marrow transplant.[13]

Biologic response modifiers are theoretically the most desirable treatment for MDS, as well as for other malignancies (see Chapter 28). Whereas "traditional" chemotherapy destroys normal cells along with the leukemic ones ("crusader" approach), biologic response modifiers convert the abnormal clone to normal behavior ("missionary" approach).[37] Some such modifiers that have been tried in MDS include

colony simulating factor (CSF)
interleukins
13-*cis*-retinoic acid (isotretinoin) (Accutane)
vitamins A and D and their analogues
dimethylsulfoxide (DMSO)
interferons
antithymocyte globulin (ATG)

Although use of these agents has met with disappointing or limited success, continued research, especially with the growth factors, interleukins, and interferons, may someday bring success.

Bone marrow transplantation is, at present, the only real cure for MDS. Allogeneic transplantation is the therapy of choice for the 10–15% of patients less than 50 years old with progressive disease or poor prognostic markers.[9, 13] In patients with fewer than 20% bone marrow blasts, transplantation can be used as first-line therapy; those with more than 20% blasts probably benefit from aggressive ANLL induction therapy before bone marrow transplantation.[13] Bone marrow transplantation is discussed in detail in Chapter 28.

SUMMARY

Myelodysplastic syndromes are a group of clonal disorders characterized by progressive cytopenias and dyspoiesis of the myeloid, erythroid, and megakaryocytic cell lines. The dyspoiesis is evidenced by abnormal morphologic appearance and abnormal function of the cell lines affected. Currently, the classification of these syndromes is determined by a strict set of morphologic guidelines. As the knowledge of molecular biology expands, cell surface markers and gene rearrangement information presumably will become an integral part of the diagnosis of MDS.

Prognosis in MDS depends on several indicators, including FAB classification, percentage of bone marrow blasts, cytopenias, and karyotypic abnormalities. Other factors, although less prognostic, are useful in predicting outcome. Treatment for MDS depends on the prognosis. Patients with favorable prognosis may receive only supportive therapy. Other treatments that have met with limited success include chemotherapy and biologic response modifiers. Currently the only cure for MDS is bone marrow transplantation.

REVIEW QUESTIONS

1. Myelodysplastic syndromes (MDS) are most common in which age group?
   a. 2–10
   b. 15–20
   c. 25–40
   d. >50

2. What type of maturation is evident in myelodysplastic syndromes?
   a. hypohemopoietic
   b. hyperhemopoietic
   c. dyshemopoietic
   d. no hemopoietic maturation

3. Which of the following is one of the major indications of MDS in the peripheral blood and bone marrow?
   a. leukocytosis with left shift
   b. dyspoiesis
   c. normal bone marrow with abnormal peripheral blood picture
   d. thrombocytosis

4. The alert technologist in the Hematology laboratory should recognize which of the following peripheral blood abnormalities as diagnostic clues in myelodysplastic syndromes?
   a. oval macrocytes
   b. agranular neutrophils
   c. circulating micromegakaryocytes
   d. all of the above

5. One criterion for classification of RAEB-t is the presence of which percentage of blasts in the bone marrow?

   a. <5
   b. 5–20
   c. 20–30
   d. >60

6. It is theorized that the somatic mutation in MDS occurs in which of the following?
   a. the pluripotent stem cell
   b. CFU-E
   c. CFU-GM
   d. the committed stem cell

References

1. Layton DM, Mufti GJ: Myelodysplastic syndromes: their history, evolution and relation to acute myeloid leukemia. Blut 1986; 53:423–436.
2. Mufti GJ, Galton DAG: Myelodysplastic syndromes: natural history and features of prognostic significance. Clin Haematol 1986; 15:953–971.
3. Koeffler HP: Preleukemia. Clin Haematol 1986; 15:829–850.
4. Bennett JM, Catovsky D, Daniel MT, et al: Proposals for the classification of the myelodysplastic syndromes. Br J Haematol 1982; 51:189–199.
5. Janssen JWG, Buschle M, Layton M, et al: Clonal analysis of myelodysplastic syndromes: evidence of multipotential stem cell origin. Blood 1989; 73:248–254.
6. Greenberg PL: Biologic nature of the myelodysplastic syndromes. Acta Haematol 1987; 78 (Suppl 1):94–99.
7. Jackson GH, Carey PJ, Cant AJ, et al: Myelodysplastic syndromes in children [Letter]. Br J Haematol 1993;84:185–186.
8. van Wering ER, Kamps WA, Vossen JM, et al: Myelodysplastic syndromes in childhood: three case reports. Br J Haematol 1985; 60:137–142.
9. Hoelzer D: Cytobiology and clinical findings of myelodysplastic syndromes. Recent Results Cancer Res 1988; 106:172–179.
10. Beris P: Primary clonal myelodysplastic syndromes. Semin Hematol 1989; 26:216–233.
11. Tsukamoto N, Morita K, Maehara T, et al: Clonality in myelodysplastic syndromes: demonstration of pluripotent stem cell origin using X-linked restriction fragment length polymorphisms. Br J Haematol 1993;83:589–594.
12. Jacobs A, Clark RE: Pathogenesis and clinical variations in the myelodysplastic syndromes. Clin Haematol 1986; 15:925–951.
13. Tricot G: The myelodysplastic syndromes. In Hoffman R, Benz EJ, Shattil SJ, et al (eds): Hematology: Basic Principles and Practice. New York: Churchill Livingstone, 1991:805–817.
14. Bick RL, Laughlin WR: Myelodysplastic syndromes. Lab Med 1993; 24:712–716.
15. Tricot G, De Wolf-Peeters R, Vlietinck R, Verwilghen RL: Bone marrow histology in myelodysplastic syndromes. Br J Haematol 1984; 58:217–225.
16. Barbui T, Cortelazzo S, Viero P, et al: Infection and hemorrhage in elderly acute myeloblastic leukemia and primary myelodysplasia. Hematol Oncol 1993; 11(Suppl 1):15–18
17. Mazzone A, Ricevuti G, Pasotti D, et al: The CD11/CD18 granulocyte adhesion molecules in myelodysplastic syndromes. Br J Haematol 1993;83:245–252.
18. Mittelman M, Karcher D, Kammerman L, Lessin L: High Ia (HLA-DR) and low CD11b (Mo1) expression may predict early conversion to leukemia in myelodysplastic syndromes. Am J Hematol 1993; 43:165–171.
19. Lintula R, Rasi V, Ikkala E, et al: Platelet function in preleukemia. Scand J Haematol 1981;26:65–71.
20. Bennett JM, Catovsky D, Daniel MT, et al: Proposed revised criteria for the classification of acute myeloid leukemia. Ann Intern Med 1985; 103:626–629.
21. Mufti GJ, Stevens JR, Oscier DG, et al: Myelodysplastic syndromes: a scoring system with prognostic significance. Br J Haematol 1985;59:425–433.
22. Tricot G, Vlietinck MA, Boogaerts MA, et al: Prognostic factors in the myelodysplastic syndromes: importance of initial data on peripheral blood counts, bone marrow cytology, trephine biopsy and chromosomal analysis. Br J Haematol 1985; 60:19–32.
23. Worsley A, Oscier DG, Stevens J, et al: Prognostic features of chronic myelomonocytic leukaemia: a modified Bournemouth score gives the best prediction of survival. Br J Haematol 1988; 68:17–21.
24. Goasguen JE, Garand R, Bizet M, et al: Prognostic factors of myelodysplastic syndromes—a simplified 3-D scoring system. Leuk Res 1990; 14:255–262.
25. Sanz GF, Sanz MA, Vallespi T, et al: Two regression models and a scoring system for predicting survival and planning treatment in myelodysplastic syndromes: a multivariate analysis of prognostic factors in 370 patients. Blood 1989; 74:395–408.
26. Nimer SD, Golde DW: The 5q− abnormality. Blood 1987; 70:1705–1712.
27. Sullivan SA, Marsden KA, Lowenthal, et al: Circulating CD34+ cells: an adverse prognostic factor in the myelodysplastic syndromes. Am J Hematol 1992; 39:96–101.
28. Geddes AD, Bowen DT, Jacobs A: Clonal karyotype abnormalities and clinical progress in the myelodysplastic syndrome. Br J Haematol 1990; 76:194–202.
29. Jotterand-Bellomo M, Parlier V, Schmidt PM, Beris P: Cytogenetic analysis of 54 cases of myelodysplastic syndromes. Cancer Genet Cytogenet 1990; 46:157–172.
30. Musilova J, Michalova K: Chromosome study of 85 patients with myelodysplastic syndrome. Cancer Genet Cytogenet 1988; 33:39–50.
31. Tricot GJ: Prognostic factors in the myelodysplastic syndromes. Leuk Res 1992; 16:109–115.
32. Solé F, Torrabadella M, Granada I, et al: Isochromosome 17q as a sole anomaly: a distinct myelodysplastic syndrome entity? Leuk Res 1993; 17:717–720.
33. Toyama T, Ohyashiki K, Yoshida Y, et al: Clinical implication of chromosomal abnormalities in 401 patients with myelodysplastic syndromes: a multicentric study in Japan. Leukemia 1993; 499–508.
34. Suciu S, Kuse R, Weh HJ, Hossfeld DK: Results of chromosome studies and their relation to morphology, course, and prognosis in 120 patients with de novo myelodysplastic syndrome. Cancer Genet Cytogenet 1990; 44:15–26.
35. Jacobs RH, Cornbleet MA, Vardiman JW, et al: Prognostic implication of morphology and karyotype in primary myelodysplastic syndromes. Blood 1986; 67:1765–1772.
36. Yunis JJ, Lobell M, Arnesen MA, et al: Refined chromosome study helps define prognostic subgroups in most patients with primary myelodysplastic syndrome and acute myelogenous leukaemia. Br J Haematol 1988; 68:189–194.
37. Boogaerts MA: Progress in the therapy of myelodysplastic syndromes. Blut 1989; 58:265–270.

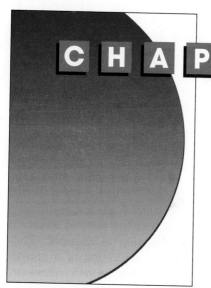

CHAPTER 27

Origins of Leukocyte Neoplasia

Robert Hromas and Dean Putt

Outline

Objectives

AFTER COMPLETION OF THIS CHAPTER, THE READER WILL BE ABLE TO

1. Describe the types of oncogenic DNA changes.
2. Describe how a point mutation can change the reading frame.
3. List the different types of oncogenes.
4. Describe how a tumor suppressor gene can cause neoplasia.
5. List the environmental agents implicated in causing the DNA structural abnormalities that result in acute lymphocytic and myelogenous leukemia.
6. List the inherited genetic abnormalities that predispose to acute lymphocytic leukemia (ALL) and acute myelogenous leukemia (AML). State whether ALL or AML is the more common result.
7. Name the viruses implicated in ALL and lymphoma.
8. Describe how *myc* is activated in Burkitt leukemia or lymphoma.
9. Describe how *Lyl*1, *Tal*1, *Tal*2, and *Hox*11 are activated in ALL.
10. Describe how the two E2A fusion transcripts produce B cell ALL.
11. Describe the two diseases that different fusion *bcr-abl* transcripts can produce.
12. Name the two abnormalities of the retinoic acid receptor alpha that can occur in acute promyelocytic leukemia.
13. Name the gene involved in follicular lymphomas. Describe how it immortalizes lymphocytes.
14. Name the gene activated by point mutations in some myelodysplasias and AMLs.
15. Name the type of gene deleted at 5q31 in myelodysplasias.
16. Describe how therapy of leukocyte neoplasia can be made less toxic.

GENETIC CHARACTERISTICS OF LEUKOCYTE MALIGNANCIES

The white blood cell malignancies, leukemia and lymphoma, are acquired genetic diseases. They are acquired in that most patients are not born with the illness but acquire it sometime later.

The majority of leukocyte malignancies are not localized. The bone marrow, in which leukemias arise, and the lymphatic system, in which lymphomas originate, have passages throughout the body. A single leukemia cell arising in the marrow can pass via the blood stream to any location that blood vessels reach. Therefore, leukemias and most lymphomas are systemic diseases. Treatment given only at a certain location of the body, such as radiation or surgery, will not cure most leukocyte malignancies. These diseases affect the whole person, and the whole person must be systemically treated; that is why intravenous chemotherapy is so commonly used to treat these disorders.

IMPORTANCE OF DNA MUTATION

The disorders are genetic by virtue of their ability to pass on to their progeny the malignant phenotype; that is, they divide without stopping, and their progeny do the same. They replicate this proliferative phenotype and transmit it across cell division; thus this phenotype must be imprinted physically in the DNA of the malignant cell. This structural change in the cancer cell's DNA must occur, or the DNA replicating enzymes will not recognize it.

In this chapter, "structural changes in DNA" is referred to many times as the root cause of many leukocyte malignancies. The types of malignancies whose etiology is not certain will, in the end, when they have been defined, be found to have a structural change in their DNA that they can pass on to their progeny. Indeed, many of the environmental insults that cause leukocyte cancer are known to damage or rearrange DNA.

TYPES OF ONCOGENIC DNA CHANGES

Four major types of permanent DNA changes are oncogenic in white blood cells: chromosomal translocations, amplifications, deletions, and point mutations.[1]

Chromosomal Translocations

Given a certain genetic predisposition, and a certain environment, chromosomes break and relegate to one another. Infrequently, one chromosome relegates to a different chromosome, and that structural change can cause a malignancy. When that happens, the site of the breakage has translocated, or moved, a gene from its normal situation into one in which its function is changed. That change in function may be activation of a growth stimulator or inactivation of a growth repressor. This translocation and the subsequent deregulation of a gene are permanent, and can be passed on to progeny.

In fact, these chromosomal translocations can be seen with special stains and a microscope. They can serve as markers that help examiners diagnose a given leukocyte neoplasia and follow its treatment. Just as important, these cancer-causing gene rearrangements are targets of specific therapy. Oncologists are just beginning to study these potential areas for treatment (Fig. 27–1).

Deletions of Tumor Suppressor Genes

In some leukocyte cancers, only a small piece of chromosome is missing. In chromosomal translocations, one chromosome breaks and ligates to another, producing an abnormal chromosome that is part one and part another. In deletions, there is a small piece missing (deletion) in a single chromosome that is often barely visible under a microscope. Such deletions can also cause white blood cell malignancies.

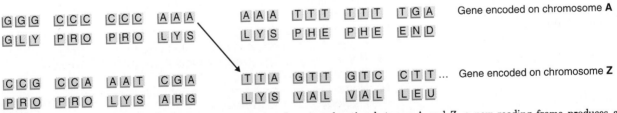

Figure 27–1 How translocations produce fusion proteins. In a translocation between A and Z, a new reading frame produces a longer protein that has a new function. In translocations that cause cancer, this new function is often to stimulate cell growth. Translocations are almost always acquired and thus affect only certain tissues. *Abbreviations:* G, guanine; C, cytosine; A, adenine; T, thymine; GLY, glycine; PRO, proline; LYS, lysine; PHE, phenylalanine; ARG, arginine; VAL, valine; LEU, leucine.

When a portion of DNA is deleted and malignancy results, a tumor suppressor gene must have been within that DNA segment. These genes are important negative regulators of cell division. When they are not present, cell growth and division takes place without stopping.

Amplifications of Oncogenes

Sometimes segments of DNA can be copied many times during DNA replication, instead of just once. This leads to an amplification of that segment of DNA, and the genes in that segment are thereby expressed many more times than in the normal situation. If a gene that stimulates a cell to divide is amplified and thus overexpressed, cancer may result.

Amplifications can be seen under the microscope. They take two main forms. In one, the homogeneously staining region (HSR), the amplified segment of DNA, has remained in the chromosome, and thus a large portion of that chromosome is stained the same, instead of the usual complex pattern of banding. This type of amplification is very stable across cell division. DNA amplifications can also occur outside of any chromosome, on miniature chromosomal segments called double minutes. These do not replicate very well on their own, away from a chromosome. Therefore, they often do not last very long, as opposed to the HSRs.

Point Mutations

Some leukocyte malignancies have point mutations, or changes in just a few nucleotides of a given gene. These mutations are enough to alter the function of the gene and make it cause a malignancy. These nucleotide alterations obviously cannot be seen within whole chromosomes under a microscope. These changes can be identified only by cloning and sequencing the gene isolated in a patient with a given cancer.

Three types of point mutations can occur. The most common is a substitution, in which one nucleotide is exchanged for another. Because there is no net gain or loss of nucleotides, the amino acid reading frame does not change. Thus this type of mutation affects only the amino acid to which the codon has been mutated. However, such a change in a crucial amino acid in a growth regulatory protein is enough to make the cell neoplastic. Another type of point mutation is an insertion, in which a nucleotide is added to the DNA sequence. Because there is a loss or an addition to the DNA sequence, the amino acid reading frame, and therefore the protein, changes markedly over long stretches. The

third type of point mutation is a deletion. In this type, a given nucleotide is deleted from the DNA.

Although point mutation by definition implies a change in only a single nucleotide, each of these types can occur more than once, separately or in stretches, in any given mutated protein (Table 27–1).

TYPES OF GENES THAT CAUSE LEUKOCYTE NEOPLASIA

As discussed, the changes that make a blood cell malignant are inherited across cell division. Thus these changes must be changes in DNA structure. The structural changes in DNA just described affect genes that govern how a cell grows and divides. There are two major groups of these genes. The first group is the oncogenes,[2] which generally stimulate a cell to grow and divide. Constitutive activation of oncogenes by one of the DNA mutations mentioned earlier produces neoplasia. The second group is the tumor suppressor genes,[3] which cause a cell to slow growth and stop dividing. Inactivation of tumor suppressor genes by deletion or point mutation produces the neoplasia.

Oncogenes

Oncogenes get their name from the fact that they were first described as the genes in viruses that were crucial in causing cancer in animals. These genes would also give normal mouse fibroblasts grown in a culture dish malignant characteristics. The transformed fibroblasts would then cause tumors if they were injected into mice. By definition, therefore, a gene that transformed a normal fibroblast into a malignant one was called an oncogene. As scientists have learned more about the genes that cause human cancer, the definition of an oncogene has expanded. Some of the human

Table 27–1. HOW POINT MUTATIONS CHANGE THE AMINO ACID READING FRAME						
Original	AGC	GAG	AGA	CAG	GTC	AAA ACC
	SER	PHE	ARG	GLN	VAL	LYS THR
Substitution	AGC	GAG	A**TA**	CAG	GTC	AAA ACC
	SER	PHE	**ILE**	GLN	VAL	LYS THR
Insertion	AGC	GAG	AG**T**	ACA	GGT	CAA AAC
	SER	PHE	**SER**	**THR**	**GLY**	**GLN ASN**
Deletion	AGC	GAG	A**AC**	AGG	TCA	AAA CCT
	SER	PHE	**ASN**	**ARG**	**SER**	**LYS PRO**

Abbreviations: A, adenine; G, guanine; C, cytosine; T, thymine; SER, serine; PHE, phenylalanine; ARG, arginine; GLN, glutamine; VAL, valine; LYS, lysine; THR, threonine; ILE, isoleucine; GLY, glycine; ASN, asparagine; PRO, proline.

oncogenes do not necessarily transform mouse fibroblasts, but they surely play a role in the development of human cancer.

There are three major types of oncogenes. The first type is *growth factors*. They are cell-to-cell signals that diffuse through the environment to signal all the cells in the area to divide. Examples of these genes include *sis,* which is related to platelet-derived growth factor, and *hst* and *int*-2, which are related to basic fibroblast growth factor. These altered genes produce their growth factor product in an autocrine mechanism; that is, they stimulate the growth and division of the very tumor cells that produce the growth factors.

The second type of oncogenes is *signal transducers*. In the normal cell, they obtain a signal from the environment from, for example, a growth factor, and relay (transduce) that signal to the nucleus of the cell. Then the cell begins the work of division. The oncogenic signal transducers are mutated in such a way that they relay a signal to grow and divide all the time. They do not depend on whether the proper environment is there. In general, they reside in the cell's membrane or in the cytoplasm close to the membrane. There are several forms of oncogenic signal transducers, including tyrosine and serine/threonine kinases, which relay growth signals by passing along a phosphate molecule. This phosphate molecule finally reaches a protein that directly activates growth and division. A list of oncogenes that are kinases appears in Table 27–2. Another group of oncogenic signal transducers is called G proteins. A group of proteins called the *ras* family make up most of the G proteins. They probably end up activating kinases.

Transcriptional activators are the third type of oncogene.[4] A list of genes that belong in this category is in Table 27–3. In general, they reside in the nucleus. They activate the transcription of the entire group of genes needed for the actual work of growth and division. They are generally composed of a DNA-binding domain, which designates which genes they activate, and an activating domain. The DNA-binding domains are categorized into families

on the basis of shared amino acid sequences.[4] These families include basic-region-helix-loop-helix proteins, leucine zipper proteins, zinc finger proteins, homeobox proteins, cysteine-rich LIM proteins, ETS proteins, and Forkhead proteins. Most, but not all, of these transcription factor classes are involved in human leukocyte neoplasia. When they are mutated in such a way that they are active all the time, not just when an appropriate signal transducer has turned them on, the cell divides without stopping.

As mentioned later, most oncogenes active in human leukocyte neoplasias are transcription factors.

One oncogene important in human tumors, *bcl*-2, does not fit any of the functional classes just described.[5] It appears to immortalize lymphocytes by preventing them from undergoing programmed cell suicide (apoptosis) as they differentiate. Normal lymphocytes have a finite lifespan. When they reach that endpoint, they die spontaneously, without environmental influence. When *bcl*-2 is activated, lymphocytes undergo this programmed cell death but keep on dividing.

A normal cell is influenced by the environment around it not to grow and divide. Other cells are

---

Table 27–3. TRANSCRIPTION FACTOR ONCOGENES ACTIVATED BY CHROMOSOMAL ABNORMALITIES IN HUMAN LEUKOCYTE NEOPLASIA[4, 11]

DNA Binding Domain	Translocation	Affected Gene
ALL		
Helix-loop-helix	t(8:14)	*myc*
	t(2:8)	*myc*
	t(8:22)	*myc*
	t(7:19)	*Lyl1*
	t(1:14)	*Tal1/Scl/Tcl5*
	t(7:9)	*Tal2*
LIM	t(11:14)	*Rhombotin1/Ttg1*
	t(11:14)	*Rhombotin2/Ttg2*
Homeobox	t(10:14)	*Hox11*
	t(7:10)	*Hox11*
	t(1:19)	*E2a-Pbx1**
Leucine zipper	t(17:19)	*E2A-Hlf**
BIPHENOTYPIC/ALL/AML		
Zinc Finger	11q23 disruptions	*MLL†*
AML		
Zinc Finger	t(15:17)	*PML-RAR**
	t(11:17)	*PLZF-RAR**
Unclassified putative	t(6:9)	*Dek-Can**
Transcription factors	t(8:21)	*AML1-Eto**

* Fusion transcript with the 5′-most portion of the fusion transcript first.

† *MLL* takes part in multiple fusion transcripts (as the 5′ portion) beyond the scope of this chapter that are just now being described.

Abbreviations: ALL, acute lymphocytic leukemia; AML, acute-myelogenous leukemia.

Table 27–2. VIRAL ONCOGENES ACTIVE IN HUMAN TUMORS CLASSIFIED BY FUNCTION

Tyrosine Kinases
abl

G Proteins
ras

Transcription Activators
myc
ets

too close, no essential growth hormone is present, or there is not enough nutrition. However, a mutation anywhere along this signal pathway, from an environmental growth factor to a signal transducer to a nuclear transcription factor, can produce a malignancy. Again, that mutation must be a structural change in DNA, or it will fade out as the cell divides, and its effects will become diluted.

Tumor Suppressor Genes

Sometimes cancer is caused by the absence of function of certain genes, as opposed to activation. These genes are called tumor suppressor genes. For a cell to be malignant because of one of these genes, its DNA must be deleted or mutated in such a way that the encoded protein does not work. An example of these genes include *Rb,* which helps stop a cell from dividing when it is not supposed to. When it is missing, retinoblastoma (an eye tumor in children) can develop. Another important example of this type of gene is P53, which may also act to slow cell division, although not directly. It probably activates transcription of a series of genes that do the actual work. P53 has point mutations in a wide variety of human tumors, from lung and bone cancer to chronic myelogenous leukemia.

In some families, a mutated P53 gene is inherited. The resulting disorder is called the Li-Fraumeni syndrome, after the two physicians who described it. This germ line mutation leaves members of these families very susceptible to many forms of neoplasia. They get colon cancer, breast cancer, and bone cancer at rates many times higher than normal. In fact, they sometimes have more than one tumor at the same time. This situation is different from that of a mutation in a certain tissue, acquired from environmental insults that result in sporadic cases of P53-induced solid tumors.

ETIOLOGY OF LEUKOCYTE NEOPLASIA

In the following sections, the causes of leukocyte neoplasia are surveyed. These causes range from environmental toxins to the actual gene that is structurally changed to become oncogenic.

Acute Lymphoblastic Leukemia (ALL)

Environment. The risk of ALL is increased after exposure to organic solvents such as benzene[6] and also after exposure to radiation. Thus the survivors of atomic explosions in Japan in World War

II had an increased chance of acquiring ALL.[7] In addition, cancer survivors whose therapy included alkylating agents have an increased chance of acquiring ALL. However, in all these cases, the risk of acquiring acute myelogenous leukemia (AML) is much greater than the risk of ALL. Note that all of these environmental agents can mutate DNA.

Viruses. There are two types of ALL in which viruses may play a role.[8] The first is ALL subtype L3, which is similar to Burkitt lymphoma. In both Burkitt lymphoma and ALL L3, Epstein-Barr virus (EBV) has been implicated as an etiology. There is an especially strong association of EBV with the African form of Burkitt lymphoma. In some cases of Burkitt lymphoma, the EBV genome has been recovered from the tumor. However, it is also clear that other factors, including a chromosomal translocation, play important parts in the development of Burkitt lymphoma.

The human T cell lymphotropic virus type 1 (HTLV-1) is the cause of a rare T cell leukemia, adult T cell leukemia/lymphoma (ATLL) syndrome. This type of ALL is much more common in Japan and in the Caribbean islands than in North America. The virus is not very infectious; in fact, some family members living with an infected person do not catch the virus. It is transmitted through body fluids, like the hepatitis B and the human immunodeficiency viruses. Although it is not clear exactly how HTLV-1 causes ATLL, a viral transcription factor that can activate growth genes called *TAT* probably is important.

Inherited Genetic Abnormalities. People with inherited chromosomal abnormalities such as Down syndrome (trisomy 21), Klinefelter syndrome (XXY), and neurofibromatosis (point mutations in *NF*1) have a higher chance of getting ALL.[9] People with inherited disorders of DNA repair, such as Bloom syndrome, Fanconi anemia, and ataxia-telangiectasia, also have an increased risk of ALL. The fact that these disorders are greatly predisposed to DNA mutations from their defect in DNA repair is consistent with the hypothesis that DNA structural change is essential in the development of neoplasia. Monozygotic twins also have a higher than expected incidence of ALL, which also indicates an important genetic component to this disease. AML is much more common than ALL in inherited genetic abnormalities.

Acquired Chromosomal Abnormalities. In ALL, many of the chromosome abnormalities occur in the regions of the immunoglobulin genes in B cells and antigen receptor genes in T cells. These segments of DNA undergo rearrangement during the course of normal B or T cell development. A mistake in rearrangement can result in the insertion of an oncogene into one of these regions, causing improper expression. Thus these regions are prone to producing the permanent DNA structural change needed for oncogenesis. Three chromosomal translocations result in the development of ALL L3 subtype, also called Burkitt leukemia: t(8;14), t(8;22), and t(2;8). This disease is caused by a similar cell, and the translocations are similar to those in Burkitt lymphoma. These different translocations all produce the same phenotypic leukemia, a B cell with surface immunoglobulin present; this is because in each case the transcription factor *myc* is translocated away from its normal location and put next to one of the immunoglobulin genes. *myc* is overexpressed in these translocations, producing growth and division when there should not be any. This is because during this stage of B cell development, the immunoglobulin genes are highly expressed. Thus *myc* is caught in that regulatory domain and overexpressed also.

Similar to *myc* are a number of genes that are activated in T cells by translocation to one of the T cell antigen receptor genes instead of to the immunoglobulin loci. When these antigen receptor genes are turned on during T cell development, the translocated gene is also activated. These translocated genes are transcription factors. Like *myc*, they turn on the transcription of other growth-related genes. When they are activated at the wrong time, they cause the T cells to divide instead of to mature. *Lyl*1 is involved in the t(7;19). *Tal*1 is involved in the t(1;14), and *Tal*2 in t(7;9). They are all structurally similar to *myc*: they all have a basic region that binds DNA, followed by a helix-loop-helix that allows them to dimerize with other transcription factors of this class, including themselves. They all cause aggressive T cell leukemias because they are activated as a T cell develops.

*Hox*11 belongs to a different class of transcriptional activators called the homeobox family. It is involved in two translocations that cause ALL: t(10;14) and t(7;10). It is also translocated to a T cell antigen receptor gene. When the T cell receptor region is activated during T cell maturation, this gene is also turned on, like the ones mentioned earlier, and causes the T cell to divide instead of to mature.

*Ttg*1 and *Ttg*2, involved in the t(11;14), are in the LIM family of transcription factors. LIM molecules have a cysteine-rich DNA binding domain. Like the *Hox*11, *Lyl*1, *Tal*1, and *Tal*2 genes, they are also translocated to a T cell receptor locus, thereby producing T cell leukemias. In fact, *myc* itself can in rare instances be translocated to a T cell antigen receptor gene, t(8;14) instead of to one of the immunoglobulin genes, and thereby produce a T cell leukemia.

Another pair of translocations that produces a specific type of B cell ALL are (t1;19) and t(17;19). These translocations fuse the transcriptional activating N-terminal domain of E2A to the C-terminal DNA binding domain of a gene called *Pbx*1 or *Hlf*, respectively. E2A is normally expressed at high levels during pre–B cell development, when it helps turn on the immunoglobulin (antibody) genes. However, the fusion E2A/*Pbx*1 or E2A/*Hlf* molecule activates growth genes instead because the *Hlf* or *Pbx*1 portion makes E2A bind to different genes than it would normally. E2A is not able to perform its normal job of activating the antibody genes; instead, it activates genes that induce the cell to divide. Thus the developing B cell is stimulated to continue dividing at a time when it should be maturing into a nondividing antibody-producing cell.

The t(9;22) also produces a specific aggressive ALL syndrome. This results in a fusion oncogene, called *bcr-abl*, that is 190 kD in size. This *bcr-abl* fusion gene has excessive tyrosine kinase activity. The kinase signals the cell to divide continuously. This translocation is very similar to one that has a part in the development of chronic myelogenous leukemia (CML). However, the translocation in CML results in a *bcr-abl* kinase that is 210 kD in size. This larger protein has less kinase activity, resulting in less growth signaling and a slower growing leukemia. Another signal transducer involved in T cell ALL is *lck;* it is activated by the t(1;7) translocation, which signals the T cell to keep growing when it should instead mature.

All of the chromosomal abnormalities involving the transcription factors described in this chapter are summarized in Table 27–3.[5, 10]

Biphenotypic Leukemias

Some leukemias share characteristics of both ALL and AML. These are called biphenotypic leukemias. One type of biphenotypic leukemia that occurs both in adults and in children shares a common chromosomal translocation. This leukemia has a tendency to have both lymphocytic and monocytic characteristics. These translocations involve chromosome 11q23.[11, 12] The gene at 11q23 is rearranged and fused to a number of other genes, depending on the translocation; it was first called *MLL* (also called *Trx*). This gene product is also a transcription factor of the zinc finger class. It is related to an essential fruitfly developmental control gene called trithorax.

It is important to mention that sometimes leukemias with 11q23 aberrancies have mainly monocytic or mainly lymphocytic characteristics. They are not always completely biphenotypic, even though the same gene is disrupted. However, they behave the same way even if the cell surface characteristics are more myeloid or more lymphoid or both. They all develop very fast and are hard to treat effectively.

Acute Myelogenous Leukemia

Environmental Agents. The organic solvents such as benzene and radiation, mentioned earlier as causes of ALL, also cause AML.[6, 7] In fact, they are more likely to cause AML than ALL. Often these agents cause a prodrome of poor blood cell production called myelodysplasia before AML occurs.

Inherited Genetic Abnormalities. The inherited genetic abnormalities, mentioned earlier as causes of ALL, also cause AML.[13] Indeed, Bloom syndrome, ataxia-telangiectasia, Fanconi anemia, Down syndrome, Klinefelter syndrome, and neurofibromatosis are all associated with AML at a higher rate than with ALL.[9, 13]

Acquired Chromosomal Abnormalities. As in ALL, there are several acquired chromosomal abnormalities that result in AML. Again, these abnormalities involve transcription factor genes. Indeed, all of the chromosomal abnormalities in the acute leukemias except one—ALL t(9;22) *bcr-abl*—involve abnormal activation of transcription factor genes, whereas chromosomal abnormalities in chronic leukemias involve signal transduction.

A significant chromosomal abnormality involves the retinoic acid alpha-receptor gene on chromosome 17. Both the t(15;17) and the t(11;17) result in acute promyelocytic leukemia. Retinoic acid from the environment is essential for a promyelocyte to develop into a mature granulocyte. Thus when the receptor for retinoic acid is modified, promyelocytes fail to develop because they cannot sense the retinoic acid environmental signal. Administering excess retinoic acid is effective treatment for this type of leukemia.

Two other chromosomal aberrancies that produce AML are t(6;9) and t(8;21). Both result in the disruption and abnormal expression of transcription factor genes. The t(6;9) produces the fusion of two genes called *Dek* and *Can;* the t(8;21) produces the fusion of two genes called *AML*1 and *Eto.* In one case of AML, immortalized by the HL60 cell line, *myc* was found to be amplified many times on chromosome 14. Thus amplification of a growth gene can also produce leukemia in humans.

Chronic Myelogenous Leukemia

CML can be a late effect of radiation, although this is quite rare. Few environmental or inherited disorders are known to cause CML. In almost every case of CML, there is a characteristic chromosomal translocation: the Philadelphia chromosome, a t(9;22) that results in the 210 kD (also called p210) *bcr-abl,* as described in the section on ALL. Some patients with CML do not have the classic Philadelphia chromosome, but a *bcr-abl* fusion transcript is nevertheless present at the molecular level. Thus just a small fragment that contained the appropriate genes, not the whole chromosome, has rearranged. This is excellent evidence for the fact that the *bcr-abl* fusion transcript produces CML. In addition, a CML-like disease can be recapitulated in mouse marrow forced to express *bcr-abl.*

When further chromosomal abnormalities result, the slow-growing CML can transform into a rapidly fatal phase called blast crisis. For example, another Philadelphia chromosome can occur within a cell that already has one. This addition produces more impetus for cell division than just the one p210 *bcr-abl.*

Lymphoma

Burkitt Lymphoma. Burkitt lymphoma, a rapidly growing B cell lymphoma similar to the FAB L3 subtype of ALL, also involves translocations in which the *myc* oncogene is placed near one of the highly expressed immunoglobulin genes. This proximity produces a high level of *myc* expression, which stimulates lymphocyte growth. The actual chromosomal translocations are the same as those described for ALL L3. Burkitt lymphoma is also associated with EBV infection. The EBV does not cause lymphoma on its own, but it can stimulate B cells to transiently proliferate, thus providing more opportunity for the chromosomal translocation that deregulates *myc* to take place.

Follicular Lymphoma. Patients with a slow-growing lymphoma called follicular lymphoma also have a chromosomal translocation involving an immunoglobulin gene, t(14;18). In this translocation, the *bcl*-2 gene is placed next to the immunoglobulin heavy chain gene.[5] During B cell development, the heavy chain gene is highly expressed. The *bcl*-2 gene also becomes highly expressed and immortalizes these B cells. It appears to work not by stimulating division but by preventing programmed cell death. When B cells mature, they are programmed to eventually die. Overexpression of *bcl*-2, however, prevents this, and these lymphocytes slowly accumulate, giving rise to follicular lymphoma.

Myelodysplasia

Myelodysplasias probably have many causes. Indeed, within a given patient, several steps may lead to the production of the disease.

In about 30% of myelodysplasias and AMLs, point mutations inappropriately activate the *ras* gene.[15] Putting one of these activated *ras* genes into a growth factor–dependent blood cell line can make that cell line grow without the growth factor. This transformation indicates that *ras* activation may play a role in the genesis of these diseases. However, because not all myelodysplasias or AMLs involve these mutations, they are not sufficient to cause these diseases on their own. They may, however, contribute to their development.

Myelodysplasias that develop after treatment with drugs such as VP-16 have abnormalities in chromosome 11q23. These abnormalities produce changes in the MLL gene (mentioned earlier) in biphenotypic leukemias. There are also myelodysplasias in which 11q23 abnormalities are not a result of VP-16 treatment but have developed de novo.

In addition, a distinct set of myelodysplasias involves a deletion of 5q31. Many affected patients are middle-aged women whose platelet counts are higher than normal. The fact that there is a consistent deletion at this region implies that a tumor suppressor gene is missing from these patients' marrow cells, which leads to the myelodysplasia. A transcription factor called *IRF*2 has been described as possibly being this tumor suppressor gene.

SUMMARY

Current technology has demonstrated that most leukocyte neoplasia is caused by structural DNA abnormalities. These DNA abnormalities produce deregulated growth-stimulatory genes, which direct a cell to divide instead of to mature into a functional blood cell. The majority of deregulated genes are transcriptional activators of other genes. Most acute leukemias and aggressive lymphomas are caused by inappropriate expression of a transcriptional activator. Most slow-growing leukemias and lymphomas are caused by other types of oncogenes, such as signal transducers.

The products of these genetic lesions are targets of future therapy. Use of these lesions as targets will result in truly specific therapeutic agents with the possibility of curing the majority of these cancers without substantial toxicity.

REVIEW QUESTIONS

1. Why is DNA mutation essential for the development of cancer?

2. What is the difference between an oncogene and a tumor suppressor gene?

3. What are the environmental agents that can cause acute lymphoblastic or acute myelogenous leukemia?

4. What are the inherited genetic abnormalities that can predispose to acute lymphoblastic or acute myelogenous leukemia?

5. What viruses can cause leukemia or lymphoma?

6. What type of leukemia is produced by translocations at chromosome 11q23? What anticancer drug can produce 11q23 translocations, leading to leukemia?

7. What translocations and cancer types is the oncogene *myc* involved in?

8. What are the two diseases that the 9;22 translocation can produce? Why do these diseases have different manifestations and courses?

9. What are the different types of oncogenes? Give examples of each type.

10. What is the unique way that *bcl*-2 produces follicular lymphoma?

11. What is the retroviral oncogene that is often mutated in myelodysplasia and AML?

References

1. Lewin B: Genes III. New York: J Wiley, 1987:17–36.
2. Varmus H: Cellular and viral oncogenes. *In* Stamatoyannopoulos G, Nienhuis A, Leder P, Majerus P (eds): The molecular basis of blood diseases. Philadelphia: WB Saunders, 1987:271–346.
3. Weinberg RA: Tumor suppressor genes. Science 1991, 254:1138–1145.
4. Hromas R, Zon L, Friedmen AD: Hematopoietic transcriptional regulators and the origins of leukemia. Crit Rev Oncol Hematol 1992, 12:167–190.
5. Williams GT: Programmed cell death: apoptosis and oncogenesis. Cell 1991, 65:1097–1098.
6. Askoy M, Erdem S, Dincol G: Types of leukemia in chronic benzene poisoning: a study of 34 patients. Acta Haematol (Basel) 1976, 55:65–75.
7. Heath CW: Leukemogenesis and low dose exposure to radiation and chemical agents. *In* Yohn DS, Blakeslee JR (eds): Advances in Comparative Leukemia Research. Amsterdam: Elsevier/North-Holland, 1982:23.
8. Nowell PC: Origins of human leukemia: an overview. *In* Bruce J, et al (eds): Origins of Human Cancer: A Comprehensive Review. Cold Spring Harbor, NY: Cold Spring Harbor Laboratory Press, 1991:513–520.
9. McKinney PA, Alexander FE, Cartwright RA, Ricketts TJ: The Leukemia Research Fund Data Collection Study: descriptive epidemiology of acute lymphoblastic leukemia. Leukemia 1989, 3:880.
10. Rabbitts TH: Translocations, master genes, and the differences between acute and chronic leukemias. Cell 1991, 67:641–644.

11. Tkachuk D, Kohler S, Cleary ML: Involvement of a homo-logue of *Drosophila trithorax* by 11q23 chromosomal trans-locations in acute leukemias. Cell 1992, 71:691–700.

12. Gu Y, Nakamura T, Prasad A, et al: The t(4;11) chromo-some translocation of human acute leukemias fuses the ALL-1 gene, related to *Drosophila trithorax* to the AF-4 gene. Cell 1992, 71:701–708.

13. Sandler D: Epidemiology of acute myelogenous leukemia. Semin Oncol 1987, 14:359.

14. Clark S, Crist W, Witte O: Molecular pathogenesis of Ph-positive leukemias. Ann Rev Med 1989, 40:113.

15. Bos JL: *Ras* oncogenes in human cancer: a review. Cancer Res 1989, 49:4682–4689.

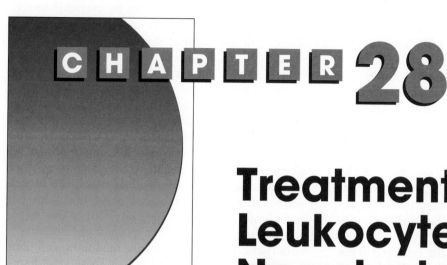

CHAPTER 28

Treatment of Leukocyte Neoplasia

Dean Putt and Robert Hromas

Outline

Objectives

AFTER COMPLETION OF THIS CHAPTER, THE READER WILL BE ABLE TO

1. Address briefly the psychologic and ethical concerns related to treatment of leukocyte disorders.
2. Contrast treatment protocols as they relate to cure vs. remission.
3. Describe alternatives to traditional therapy.
4. Define chemotherapy.
5. Explain the mechanisms for the actions of (a) alkylating agents, (b) plant alkaloids, (c) anti-tumor antibiotics, (d) anti-metabolites, (e) glucocorticoids, and (f) miscellaneous agents.
6. Discuss the limiting factor of treating leukocyte neoplasia with radiotherapy.
7. List the types of biologic response modifiers and describe their potential roles in the management of leukocyte neoplasms.
8. Explain the differences among syngeneic, allogeneic, and autologous bone marrow transplantation.
9. Discuss the role for bone marrow transplantation in the outlook of future cancer treatment.
10. List the risks associated with bone marrow transplantation.
11. Discuss the three phases of chemotherapy in the management of acute leukemias.
12. List the various chemotherapy regimens commonly used to treat acute leukemia and the expected toxic effects.
13. Define the role of bone marrow transplantation as it relates to chronic myelogenous leukemia.
14. Describe the typical treatment management of chronic lymphocytic leukemia.
15. Discuss the importance of staging in Hodgkin's disease as it relates to treatment.
16. Recognize the various four-drug regimens used in the treatment of Hodgkin's and non-Hodgkin's lymphomas.
17. Explain the role of tumor load management in the treatment of plasma cell dyscrasias.

Because of the complexity of leukocyte neoplasms, treatments are diverse and constantly changing. Before the medical decision of which type of therapy to institute, the goals and objectives for therapy must be established. Some important criteria used to decide course of action include age, physical condition, the patient's preference, expense, availability of donors (transplants), progression or stage of disorder, and experimental drugs available.

In order to accurately assess a treatment protocol, a reliable diagnosis must be established. Even the most effective therapies will not work if the wrong disorder is being treated. Each patient must be treated as an individual with regard for not only physical state but also for his or her feelings, emotions, financial status, and family support. Diagnostic variables for establishing the type and stage of leukocyte disorders are discussed elsewhere in this book (see Chapters 23 and 25). Once these parameters are determined, the physician must weigh all the alternatives and discuss these with the patient and family. As research has continued to progress, cure has become an option for some disorders. If a cure is realistically attainable, it is the goal of therapy. Patients in the early stages of Hodgkin's disease and non-Hodgkin's lymphomas have a realistic chance for cure. Children with acute lymphoblastic leukemia have a higher-than-50% chance of long-term disease-free survival at this writing. Also, for patients with chronic myelogenous leukemia, acute myeloid leukemia, acute lymphoblastic leukemia and other malignancies, for which bone marrow transplantation has been successful, cure is a goal. However, for patients with many of the leukocyte neoplasms, despite promising medications and techniques on the horizon, complete remission is the only realistic goal for therapy. For most of these conditions, cure is unlikely; thus the steps taken to attain complete remission are quite rigorous. Supportive care during these rigorous treatments make essential differences in survival. The various chemotherapeutic drugs most commonly used to treat leukemias and related disorders are discussed in more detail later in this chapter.

Unfortunately, even the most intensive chemotherapy protocols do not always attain or sustain a remission. Alternatives are made available at each stage of the process as the patient's condition and prognosis are continuously assessed. If side effects of therapy appear to be responsible for more morbidity than the original neoplasm would carry without offering a high probability of remission, it may be more humane to discontinue therapy in favor of supportive care only. Supportive care might involve blood products, pain killers, and other amenities to make life more comfortable. The importance of these decisions involving the future of a patient's life cannot be overemphasized. All the options and risks must be discussed in detail with the patient amidst very narrow time constraints. The sooner the treatment can be started after diagnosis, the better. At some point, to ensure a semblance of quality of life, the aggressive therapy must be abandoned. The treatment should never be worse than the disease. At the same time, if the treatment is not likely to offer any short- or long-term benefits, no treatment at all may be more beneficial.

Despite setbacks in individual cases, the overall outlook for treatment of leukocyte neoplasia has been bright. There are basically four major methods of treating leukocyte neoplasms: chemotherapy, radiotherapy, biologic response modifiers, and bone marrow transplantation. Each of these treatments is discussed in turn in the first section of this chapter. In the second section, the specific treatments for many of the specific leukocyte neoplasias are discussed.

CHEMOTHERAPY

The very sound of the words "leukemia" and "chemotherapy" for most people conjure a scenario of hopelessness, morbidity, and eventual death. Before 1960, this scenario was frequently real. Vast improvements have been made since then in the use of chemotherapy and its role in the treatment of leukocyte neoplasia. No longer is treatment rendered merely to represent the last attempt to prolong a life for several months or to demonstrate to the patient and family that the physician is doing all that can be done. Aggressive steps now are taken to realistically cure the disease or at the very least induce a complete remission or disease-free state. This more aggressive stance requires sophisticated supportive care for the patient to withstand the marked to total immunosuppression and myriad complications that may follow. The most common life-threatening complications after chemotherapy are infection and bleeding. The key to successful chemotherapy is the ability to control these complications; otherwise, the patient may die from treatment-related causes even though the original neoplasm has been controlled. Aggressive chemotherapy requires close monitoring of all blood cells by the use of laboratory tests. Total leukocyte, neutrophil, and platelet counts and hemoglobin levels are closely followed in order to institute strict isolation, to administer blood and/or platelet transfusions, or to decide whether to continue or discontinue the current treatment. A standard regimen of antibiotics (which differs depending on treatment protocol) is often infused prophylactically before blood count nadirs (lowest counts) are reached. By this preventative measure, many infectious processes are avoided. Close monitoring of the serum drug levels by the laboratory also prevents the side effects and pathologic processes of drug toxicity. The laboratory plays a major role in the diagnostic treatment processes associated with leukocyte neoplasia.

Chemotherapy can be defined as the treatment of cancer with the use of compounds with anti-tumor properties, administered either orally or parenterally. The methods of action of the chemotherapy drugs vary considerably. Chemotherapy agents can be classified in two ways: by their effects on the cell cycle and by their biochemical mechanism of action. Chemotherapy drugs can affect specific phases of the cell cycle (phase specific). Other drugs act without regard to the cell cycle (phase nonspecific). (See Figure 6–11).

Phase-nonspecific agents affect any phase of the cell cycle. Agents in this category usually have a linear-dose response curve (i.e., the higher the dose, the more cells are killed). There are two subgroups:

1. Cycle-specific agents, which kill cells that are moving through the cell cycle, independently of whether the cells are in G_1, G_2, S, or M phase (e.g., alkylating agents, cisplatin).
2. Cycle-nonspecific agents, which kill nondividing cells or cells in the resting state (e.g., steroids and anti-tumor antibiotics).

Phase-specific agents are effective only if present during a certain phase in the cell cycle. Within a certain dose range, agents of this category show no increase in killing of cells with a further increase in dosage. Examples include L-asparagine amidohydrolase (G_1 phase), anti-metabolites such as methotrexate (S phase), and vinca alkaloids (M phase).[1]

Chemotherapeutic agents affect normal as well as neoplastic cells. The effect is most pronounced with rapidly dividing cells such as those of the mucosa of the gastrointestinal (GI) tract and the bone marrow. This limits the dosage and usually determines the maximum tolerated dose for a patient.

Chemotherapy agents (Table 28–1) can be categorized in the following manner:

Alkylating Agents. The mechanism of alkylating agents is to ionize within cells, forming highly reactive free radicals that damage DNA. These agents act on any phase of the cell cycle. They include such drugs as nitrogen mustard, cyclophosphamide, chlorambucil, busulfan, and melphalan (Alkeran).

Plant Alkaloids. Plant alkaloids, or stathmokinetic agents, affect microtubules and interrupt the process of mitotic spindle formation during the metaphase stage of mitosis. These agents include vincristine and vinblastine.

Anti-Tumor Antibiotics. Compounds derived from living microorganisms are termed antibiotics, and some have anti-tumor effects. Antibiotics inhibit RNA or DNA synthesis and interfere with the G_2 phase of the cell cycle. Some commonly used tumor antibiotics are daunorubicin and doxorubicin (Adriamycin).

Anti-Metabolites. These compounds interfere with the normal functions of various essential metabolites. Examples in this class include methotrexate, folate antagonists, and the purine analogues such as 6-mercaptopurine and 6-thioguanine, which most often affect cells in S phase.

Glucocorticoids. The synthetic or natural steroids include compounds such as hydrocortisone, prednisone, dexamethasone, and prednisolone. The steroids have a lympholytic effect and affect nonproliferating cells as well as those in cycle. Protein synthesis and mitosis may also be inhibited.[2]

RADIOTHERAPY

Shortly after the discovery of x-rays, their usefulness in the treatment of Hodgkin's disease and lymphoma was described. Radiation kills cells by producing unstable ions that damage DNA and may thereby cause instant or delayed death of the cell.

The toxic effects of radiotherapy can occur either during therapy or much later. Complications can be reduced through the use of combined anterior and posterior treatment ports and of maximal shielding techniques. The hematopoietic system, the GI tract, and the skin are most often affected during radiotherapy. The toxic effects are usually reversible when radiation is stopped.

The epithelium of the entire GI tract is a rapidly dividing cellular system that is very sensitive to irradiation. There may be drying up of saliva and loss of taste. If the stomach is irradiated, anorexia, nausea, and vomiting may occur. Intestinal radiation may result in malabsorption and diarrhea. Radiated skin becomes erythematous and tender. Permanent loss of body hair and hyperpigmentation may also occur in irradiated areas. Spinal and pelvic irradiation can cause marrow suppression, sometimes lowering blood counts to the life-threatening range.

Table 28–1 CHEMOTHERAPY AGENTS

Agent	Other Names	Uses	Toxic Effects
ALKYLATING AGENTS			
Busulfan	Myleran	CML, pretransplantation	Myelosuppression, infertility
Cyclophosphamide	Cytoxan	Lymphoma, MM, pretransplantation	Marrow suppression, N&V, cystitis
Nitrogen mustard	Mechlorethamine	Hodgkin's disease, NHL	Myelosuppression N&V, infertility
Chlorambucil	Leukeran	CLL, Waldenström's macroglobulinemia, NHL, Hodgkin's disease	Myelosuppression, hair loss
Melphalan	Alkeran	MM	Myelosuppression
Carmustine	BCNU	Hodgkin's disease, NHL	Myelosuppression
Dacarbazine	DTIC	Hodgkin's disease	Myelosuppression, N&V
PLANT ALKALOIDS			
Vincristine	Oncovin	ALL, NHL, Hodgkin's disease, CLL, MM	Neurotoxicity, hair loss
Vinblastine	Velban	ALL, NHL, Hodgkin's disease, CLL, MM	Myelosuppression
Etoposide	VP-16	NHL, pretransplantation	Myelosuppression, hair loss
ANTI-TUMOR ANTIBIOTICS			
Daunorubicin	Daunomycin	AML, ALL	Myelosuppression, cardiotoxicity, N&V, hair loss
Doxorubicin	Adriamycin	Hodgkin's disease, NHL, CLL, MM	Similar to those of daunorubicin
Bleomycin	Bleo	Hodgkin's disease, NHL	Lung toxicity, gastrointestinal toxicity
Idarubicin	—	AML	Myelosuppression
ANTI-METABOLITES			
Methotrexate	Amethopterin, MTX	ALL, NHL	Myelosuppression, gastrointestinal toxicity
Ara-C	Cytosine arabinoside, cytarabine	AML, NHL, Hodgkin's disease	Myelosuppression, gastrointestinal toxicity, hair loss
Mercaptopurine	6-MP	ALL	Hepatotoxicity, myelosuppression
Thioguanine	6-TG	AML	Myelosuppression
Pentostatin	—	Hairy cell leukemia, CLL, lymphomas	Neurotoxicity, myelosuppression
Fludarabine	—	Hairy cell leukemia, CLL, lymphomas	Neurotoxicity, myelosuppression
2-CDA	CDA, 2-chlorodeoxyadenosine	Hairy cell leukemia, CLL, lymphomas	Neurotoxicity, myelosuppression
GLUCOCORTICOIDS			
Prednisone	—	ALL, CLL	Fluid retention, muscle weakness
Methylprednisolone	—	Hodgkin's Disease, NHL, AMM	Fluid retention, muscle weakness
Hydrocortisone	—	Hodgkin's Disease, NHL, AMM	Fluid retention, muscle weakness
Decadron	Dexamethasane	MM	Fluid retention, muscle weakness
OTHERS			
Hydroxyurea	Hydrea	CML, PV, AMM	Leukopenia, N&V
Asparaginase	L-asparagine amidohydrolase	ALL, refractory NHL	Nephrotoxicity, N&V
Cisplatin	*Cis*-platinum	—	Nephrotoxicity, ototoxicity
Procarbazine	—	Hodgkin's disease, NHL	Myelosuppression

Abbreviations: CML, chronic myelogenous leukemia; ALL, acute lymphoblastic leukemia; AML, acute myeloid leukemia; AMM, agnogenic myeloid metaplasia; CLL, chronic lymphocytic leukemia; MM, multiple myeloma; NHL, non-Hodgkin's lymphoma; N&V, nausea and vomiting.

Radiation is used most commonly in the treatment of localized malignancies, whereas chemotherapy is the treatment of choice for diffuse malignancies.

BIOLOGIC RESPONSE MODIFIERS

Substances that are produced naturally in the human body and are used to help treat cancer are termed biologic response modifiers (BRM).

One type of BRM used in the support of chemotherapy patients is the colony stimulating factor (CSF). G-CSF (granulocyte) and GM-CSF (granulocyte/monocyte) are used to stimulate rapid production and maturation of the white blood cell lines important in fighting infection. These substances are most often used when post-therapy recovery of granulocytes is slow and the patient is at increased risk of contracting infections. Rapid increases in neutrophil counts as high as 100,000/mm^3 (100 × 10^9/L) in a period of a few days have been witnessed. CSFs are thought to be stimuli for the proliferation of committed progenitor cells and their progeny. For even better clinical responses, it would be desirable to stimulate stem cells to generate additional stem cells.[3] The CSFs can also be used to increase the effectiveness of chemotherapy.

Granulocyte/monocyte stimulating factor has been shown to stimulate leukemic myeloblasts to follow an active cell cycle. This may increase the cytotoxic effectiveness of certain S-phase specific drugs such as ara-C and hydroxyurea.[4]

Factors that contribute to useful monoclonal antibodies for immunotoxins include both high tissue specificity and high affinity for cell surface antigens that are rapidly internalized into the cell. Such a combination has been demonstrated for several lymphoid antigens commonly expressed on lymphoid leukemias and lymphomas.[5]

Another important BRM is alpha-interferon. Clinical experience has shown that alpha-interferon can induce remissions in hairy cell leukemia, B cell leukemia and lymphoma, and chronic myelogenous leukemia (CML).[6]

Interleukin-2 (IL-2) is a cytokine that activates cytotoxic T cells. IL-2 administration induces tumor necrosis factor (TNF), alpha-interferon, interleukin-6, and GM-CSF from activated T cells. These various BRMs could play a role in the prevention of leukemic relapses by inhibiting the proliferation of leukemic cells or by inducing differentiation of the leukemic stem cell.[6] IL-2 is somewhat effective in treating thymoma and renal cell carcinoma.

In theory, BRMs would be the most desirable of cancer treatments: they could selectively attack malignant cells without encroaching upon the normal cell lines. Because these biologic compounds are derived from human and other animal sources, they could greatly minimize life-threatening and uncomfortable side effects. The problem has been that the BRMs used to treat cancer are not toxic enough to the tumor, and so the tumor returns. Many difficulties have surfaced during research on BRMs, but the future still holds promise with regard to interferons, interleukins, and growth factors.

BONE MARROW TRANSPLANTATION

Bone marrow transplantation has a somewhat poor reputation because patients initially treated were already extremely ill and frequently did not survive. Transplantation is now a curative treatment for selected disorders. The National Bone Marrow Donor Program has improved the odds of finding an unrelated donor with matching cell types for allogeneic transplantation. The more closely matched the donor's cells are to those of the recipient, the lower the odds that the recipient will experience severe graft vs. host disease (GVHD). Controlling GVHD and other complications of transplantation improves the outlook for bone marrow transplantation.

Transplantation still remains an expensive and rigorous treatment alternative. Once the decision to transplant has been made and a donor has been found, an extensive hospital stay is required. The pretransplantation conditioning reduces the body's immunity to dangerously low levels, which necessitates special protective isolation. Granulocyte counts approaching 0 are commonly seen immediately before and after transplantation. After the infusion of donor or autologous marrow, the recipient remains in a severely immunosuppressed condition for 2 weeks or more. The return of granulocytes, reticulocytes, and platelets to normal levels is monitored closely in the peripheral blood. Hematology laboratory evaluation and management of red blood cells and platelet transfusions are critical components of bone marrow transplantation. After the patient's release from hospitalization, the blood counts, along with bone marrow aspirate and core biopsies, continue to be monitored to measure the progress of engraftment of the donor marrow.

Bone marrow transplantation, once reserved for end-stage patients, is now recommended as the treatment of choice early in the course of certain nonmalignant and malignant diseases.[7] Bone marrow transplantation should no longer be thought of as salvage therapy. It should be consid-

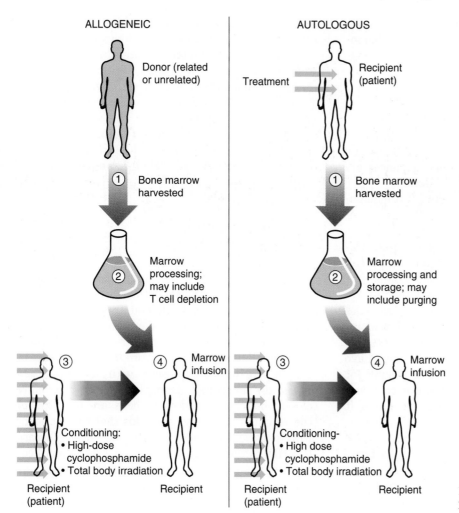

Figure 28–1 Bone marrow transplantation schematic.

ered early in the course of disease, when, because of poor prognostic findings or because of relapse after first-line therapy, the possibility of cure with more conventional treatment is low or remote.[8]

The procedure for successful transplantation involves conditioning of the recipient by eradicating malignant cells and suppressing host immunity. This is accomplished by high doses of cyclophosphamide and total body irradiation. Busulfan is occasionally used in place of total body irradiation[9] (Fig. 28–1). The conditioning process takes 7–10 days and results in extreme pancytopenia. Strict isolation of the patient at this point is of the utmost importance. Prophylactic antibiotics and intravenous nutrition are also essential in keeping the patient alive until the marrow engrafts.

Donor bone marrow is obtained in the operating room with the donor under general anesthesia by aspirating from multiple sites along the posterior iliac crests. The risk to the donor is minimal. The amount of donor marrow necessary depends on the size of the recipient. After processing, marrow from a donor is infused intravenously into the recipient, usually on the same day that it is harvested.[10]

Marrow transplantations for malignant disease have come from donors of three general types: (1) an identical twin donor (a syngeneic transplant), (2) a donor genetically different from the recipient (an allogeneic transplant) or (3) the patient's own marrow (an autologous transplant).[11]

Syngeneic transplants are most desirable because of the perfect match of cells. They are very uncommon, for obvious reasons, and therefore are not discussed further.

Allogeneic Transplantation

Most marrow donors are genetically different from the recipient. The intent is to match as many of the human leukocyte antigens (HLAs) as possible. Within any given family, there can be only four HLA haplotypes (two from the mother and two from the father), and every patient has one chance in four of having an HLA-identical sibling. In addition to HLA-identical grafts, HLA-mismatched donors within families have been used.[9]

A major complication of an allogeneic marrow graft is the immunologic reaction of donor T cells

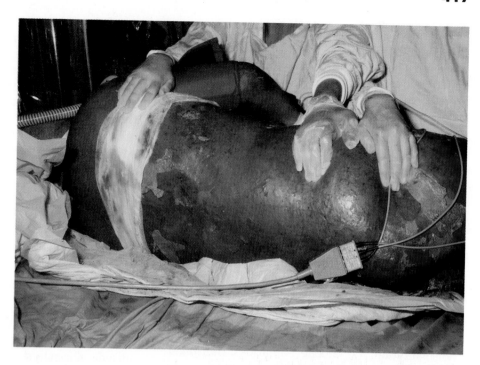

Figure 28–2 A 34-year-old female allogeneic transplant patient with severe graft vs. host disease. (Courtesy of Dr. E. Randolph Broun, Indiana University Medical Center, Indianapolis, Indiana.)

against the tissues of the recipient, resulting in GVHD (Figs. 28–2, 28–3).[11] Two forms of GVHD are recognized: acute and chronic. Acute GVHD develops in the immediate post-transplantation period or shortly thereafter. It is characterized by a skin rash, liver dysfunction, and diarrhea. Chronic GVHD, by definition, develops more than 100 days after transplantation. It is frequently generalized, in the form of a multisystem autoimmune disease. Skin lesions, joint contractures, chronic hepatitis, malabsorption, and chronic obstructive pulmonary disease are frequent features of the chronic GVHD

syndrome.[10, 11] Clinically significant GVHD is associated with a risk of fatality that is 25 times higher than that in patients without GVHD.

T cell depletion of donor bone marrow is the most effective means of preventing acute and chronic GVHD, but this benefit has been offset by the substantial increase in the risk of leukemic relapse and infections.[12] There is considerable clinical evidence that allogeneic grafts lower the risk of leukemic relapse. This anti-leukemia effect is most pronounced in the presence of chronic GVHD.

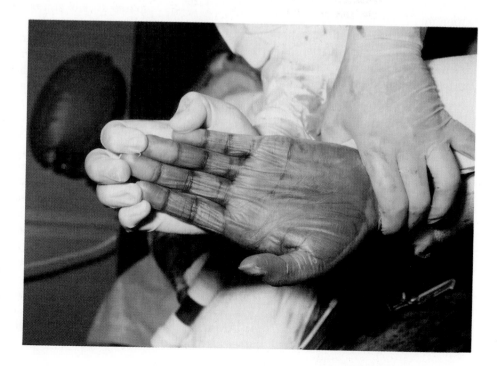

Figure 28–3 The palm of the hand from the patient with severe graft vs. host disease shown in Figure 28–2. (Courtesy of Dr. E. Randolph Broun, Indiana University Medical Center, Indianapolis, Indiana.)

Autologous Transplantation

In autologous bone marrow transplantation, marrow is harvested from the patients and, after conditioning, transplanted back into them. Harvested remission marrow, presumably contaminated with malignant cells, is purged in vitro through the use of anti-leukemic monoclonal antibodies or cytotoxic drugs.[10] After conditioning of the patient with cyclophosphamide and total body irradiation to eradicate remaining malignant cells, the purged autologous marrow is reinfused. Requirements for success in autologous transplants are the presence of normal multipotent stem cells and reduction in number of malignant cells to a level insufficient to cause recurrence from reinfused marrow.

A comparison of autologous transplants with matched allogeneic transplantation demonstrates that (1) in contrast to allogeneic transplantation, almost every patient is eligible for autologous transplantation; (2) among autologous transplant recipients, post-transplantation morbidity and mortality are lower and hospital stays are shorter; and (3) the relapse rate is higher among autologous recipients than among allogeneic recipients.[13]

Some of the apparent cures of leukemia may have been due to a graft-vs-leukemia effect directed against normal and perhaps leukemia-associated antigens present on leukemic cells.[9] Prevention or reduction of GVHD involves the use of immunosuppressive drugs after grafting, a combination of methotrexate/cyclosporine. T cell depletion appears to have substantially reduced the incidence of acute and possibly also chronic GVHD, but, however, at the risk of increases in graft rejection and leukemic relapse.[12]

Even with the continued improvement in technique and supportive care, bone marrow transplantation carries many risks. Death from transplant is most likely caused by

1. Complications of conditioning such as infections or bleeding from bone marrow suppression.
2. Complications of GVHD.
3. Relapse (regrowth of malignant cells).
4. Failure of donor cells to engraft.

THERAPY FOR ACUTE LEUKEMIA

Treatment for acute leukemia can basically be divided into two groups: therapy for acute myeloid leukemia (AML) vs. acute lymphoblastic leukemia (ALL). The diagnostic criteria for these types of leukemias designed by the French-American-British (FAB) classification M1–M7 for AML and L1–L3 for ALL, respectively are discussed in more detail in Chapter 23. The treatment of AML is essentially the same regardless of the FAB classification, with the exception of M3 promyelocytic leukemia. Without effective therapy, victims of AML traditionally lived an average of 2.5 months after diagnosis, and only rarely did they live more than a year.[14] Since 1970, chemotherapy has become the treatment of choice for acute leukemias. Average survival rates are generally in the range of 2–4 years. The goal of chemotherapy is to achieve complete remission and extend the patient's life; cure of AML is not yet a realistic goal in most cases. As discussed in this section, transplantation is an option for cure once complete remission is achieved.

Acute Myeloid Leukemia

Induction therapy is the initial treatment of AML designed to induce remission. Standard criteria for complete remission have been defined and include normalization of peripheral blood counts with fewer than 5% blasts in the bone marrow.[15] To induce remission, various combinations of drugs may be used, depending on the institution, the physician, and the patient's situation. One of the more common combinations shown to be effective includes cytosine arabinoside (ara-C), one of the anthracyclines (either daunorubicin or doxorubicin), and sometimes an additional third drug, such as 6-thioguanine.[16]

Remission can be obtained in 70–80% of patients with AML under the age of 60; success rates are lower for those over 60. About 60% of patients under 60 achieve complete remission after a single course of this combination. A further 20% achieve remission after treatment with a second course. The failure rate is about 20% and includes patients in four main categories: (1) those whose leukemic cells are eradicated but who do not recover from the hypoplastic state, (2) those whose leukemia seems to be resistant to the full course of cytotoxic drugs, (3) those who die of infection or hemorrhage before treatment can be evaluated, and (4) those in whom relapse (return of leukemia blasts) is rapid.[17]

Consolidation refers to one or more courses of therapy, administered soon after achieving remission, that produces severe myelosuppression (suppression of bone marrow cells). The purpose of this phase of therapy is to destroy malignant cells that may have survived induction and may eventually proliferate into a relapsed state. If therapy is at a higher dose than the induction dose, consolidation is called *intensification*. Patients can tolerate intensification because they are not as sick as when the leukemia is in relapse. Late intensification involves one or more courses of similarly intensive chemotherapy but given after a delay of 6–12 months. Maintenance chemotherapy is generally conceived of as frequent courses resulting in less severe myelosuppression, given over several months or years.[16]

In recent years, advances have been made in supportive care to improve remission rates attained by chemotherapy. Effective platelet support, development of newer antibiotics, and standardization of clinical approaches to the use of antibiotics and antifungal agents have meant that patients with AML generally live long enough for chemotherapeutic agents to work.[16]

For patients under the age of 50 with AML, an option for cure is bone marrow transplantation. Many studies have been conducted in this area with regard to allogeneic vs. autologous transplantation. For patients with AML in first remission after a course of chemotherapy and with an identically matched sibling donor, the probability of disease-free survival at 4 years is about 40%.[17] If only consolidation chemotherapy is given instead of bone marrow transplantation, the 4-year survival rate is about 20%. Patients undergoing transplantation in later remissions or in relapse have a 20–30% chance of survival. Autologous transplantations have been attempted in AML with a higher risk of relapse and the absence of the graft-vs.-leukemia effect seen with allogeneic transplantation. As more experience is gained in this area of transplantation, the chances of complications will decrease, and disease-free survival rates will continue to improve.

Approximately half of AML patients are over 60 years old. The treatment of the elderly remains controversial because they do not respond as well as younger patients to traditional chemotherapy. The incidence of infection and relapse is high among elderly patients. The use of growth factors may decrease the overall toxicity of more intensive consolidation treatments once patients are in remission and thereby improve their survival.[4]

Patients with AML preceded by myelodysplastic syndrome (MDS), or preleukemia, have a poorer prognosis than do patients with de novo AML. A study at the University of California, Los Angeles, showed that the remission rate among patients with AML and MDS was 41%, in comparison with a 73% complete remission rate among patients with de novo AML given the same therapy.[18] Leukemias that develop from MDS often are characterized by cytogenetic changes and by a low growth fraction. It may be possible to improve the cytotoxic effects of chemotherapy by use of growth factors.

One of the AMLs has responded to a type of therapy not used for the other myeloid leukemias. Patients with acute promyelocytic leukemia FAB M3, characterized by chromosomal aberration t(15;17) and a disseminated intravascular coagulation–(DIC-) type bleeding disorder, have shown long disease-free survival after ara-C and daunorubicin combinations. A more recent treatment has consisted of all-transretinoic acid, a compound that turns the leukemic promyelocyte cells into mature nondividing cells instead of killing them. DIC generally disappears, and the patients can be treated with consolidation chemotherapy; the cure rate is about 50%.[18]

Acute Lymphoblastic Leukemia

ALL, the most common childhood malignancy, can be cured in over 50% of the cases, cure being defined as being in remission 4 years or more without therapy. The first objective is to induce remission. A combination of vincristine, prednisone, and asparaginase is fairly standard for induction therapy. Intensification to reduce any residual leukemia follows up the induction therapy. Intrathecal therapy (injection of chemotherapy agents into the central nervous system) is used prophylactically to destroy residual leukemia cells in the cerebrospinal fluid. The drugs used for this purpose are generally ara-C and methotrexate. Intracranial irradiation may also be required in patients who have elevated leukocyte counts. Maintenance therapy may be continued over 3 years with low doses of methotrexate and 6-mercaptopurine. Patients with high-risk features such as being in an older age group; having marked leukocytosis, structured chromosome abnormalities, and certain immunophenotypes; and especially having failed chemotherapy should be candidates for allogeneic bone marrow transplantation.

ALL accounts for only 15% of adult acute leukemias, but the incidence rises among persons over the age of 60. Different chemotherapy regimens have been tried, with remission rates as high as 84% (M.D. Anderson Center).[18] A regimen of vincristine, doxorubicin (Adriamycin), and dexamethasone (VAD) and VAD plus cyclophosphamide has been most successful. In these more intensive protocols, multiple drugs in various combinations and doses for inductions, consolidation, and maintenance therapy are used for a total of 2–3 years.[18]

Poor prognostic factors include age of over 30, more than 30,000/mm³ (30 × 10⁹/L) white blood cells at presentation, extramedullary disease, Burkitt-type leukemia, chromosomal abnormalities such as the Philadelphia chromosome, and the need for more than 6 weeks of induction to achieve a remission. As with childhood ALL, patients with these poor risk factors should be considered for allogeneic bone marrow transplantation early in remission.[18]

Experimental protocols involving new immunotherapeutic approaches with cytokines, antibodies, and antibodies linked to isotopes or toxins are increasingly being used for patients who suffer relapse and those whose disease is resistant to traditional chemotherapy drugs.[13]

With the advent of improved therapy leading to cures, in ALL and Hodgkin's disease in particular but also post–bone marrow transplantation survivors, consideration must be given to the readjustments to life for these survivors. Support of a social, psychological, and economic nature must be provided to ensure that quality of life is not overly compromised. This facet of treatment is fairly new but is very much welcomed.

THERAPY FOR CHRONIC LEUKEMIA

Chronic Myelogenous Leukemia

CML is a disorder that affects fairly young people; nearly half of those affected in the United States are under the age of 40.[2] Among patients with CML, the median length of survival is about 3.5 years. The chronic phase of CML is somewhat benign, but it may abruptly terminate in blast transformation, a disease that is usually refractory to conventional chemotherapy. In the chronic phase, chemotherapy with busulfan (Myleran) or hydroxyurea can alleviate symptoms in patients but has not led to an increase in length of survival.[9]

Busulfan and hydroxyurea bring the leukocyte counts down to nearly normal levels and decrease the size of the spleen. Most patients are asymptomatic at this point but may nonetheless show signs of leukemia, such as residual splenomegaly and basophilia or persistent immature granulocytes in the blood. Attempts have been made to cure the disease by use of chemotherapy to eliminate Philadelphia chromosome–positive cells. Various drugs have been used in addition to splenic irradiation and splenectomy. No appreciable improvement over the effects of traditional chemotherapy has been observed with these curative attempts.

Although CML may be controlled by busulfan or hydroxyurea, the disease is essentially never cured by chemotherapy. Bone marrow transplantation is the only chance for cure. Bone marrow transplantation results in a survival rate of 50%–70% of patients undergoing transplantation in the chronic phase of the disease. A small fraction of patients with accelerated or blastic phase can be cured, but the best results are achieved when patients undergo transplantation while still in the chronic phase.[11]

CML has become an important indication for allogeneic bone marrow transplantation since 1980. It seems highly probable that most patients who are alive and free of leukemia 4 years after transplantation are genuinely cured. It is useful to design a recommended approach to the new CML patient even though the precise clinical details differ from patient to patient. For a patient under 50 years of age with a matched sibling donor, allogeneic transplantation within 1 year of diagnosis is probably the best treatment. For the younger patient under 50 without a sibling donor, a trial of alpha-interferon followed by autologous transplantation or allogeneic transplantation from a matched unrelated donor[19] are being investigated. A patient over 50 years of age might best be treated with alpha-interferon or busulfan/hydroxyurea. As with therapies for other leukocyte neoplasms, many variables affect treatment decisions, including the prevailing academic consensus of the institution.

Chronic Lymphocytic Leukemia

The aim of the classic treatment of chronic lymphocytic leukemia (CLL) is to prolong survival, without attempting to eradicate the disease. No treatment short of bone marrow transplantation cures CLL. Because CLL occurs primarily in an elderly population and is so slow growing, transplantation is rarely used. A large number of antineoplastic agents, alone or in combination, are active in CLL. The combination of chlorambucil and steroids (such as prednisone) is the therapy of choice because of its effectiveness and tolerance by the patient. Radiotherapy has also been successful in treating CLL. Good results have been achieved in certain instances by using a combination of total body irradiation, total nodal irradiation, extracorporeal blood irradiation, low-dose splenic irradiation, and thymic irradiation.[20]

Treatment for CLL is not recommended in patients who are asymptomatic and whose blood cell counts are near normal limits. An elevated lymphocyte count or enlarged lymph nodes do not necessarily indicate need for therapy until bone marrow involvement is evident. Treatment should be started for painful nodes or spleen, decreased blood counts, persistent infections, and autoimmune problems. Complications attributed to inappropriate antibody formation or hypogammaglobulinemia are responsible for most cases of morbidity and death associated with CLL. Infections must be responded to quickly with antibiotic therapy. Autoimmune hemolytic anemia is a complication seen in 5–10% of CLL patients and is generally treated with prednisone with support from blood transfusions as needed.

THERAPY FOR LYMPHOPROLIFERATIVE DISEASE

Hodgkin's and Non-Hodgkin's Lymphomas

The treatments for Hodgkin's disease and non-Hodgkin's lymphoma (NHL) vary considerably, depending on the clinical staging and type of lymphoma. (Lymphomas are discussed in Chapter 25.) Detailed descriptions of chemotherapy regimens and radiotherapy for Hodgkin's disease and NHL are beyond the scope of this book, but the more commonly used protocols are summarized.

Therapy with the intent to cure should be undertaken in most cases of Hodgkin's disease. The clinical stages IA, IB, and IIA are generally treated with radiotherapy; the long-term disease-free survival rate is 75%.[21] Excellent results such as these require the services of a skilled radiation oncologist to administer the radiation.

Patients with stage IIB Hodgkin's disease with an elevated sedimentation rate, multiple sites of disease, and other pathologic processes are treated with one of the four-drug regimens of chemotherapy, with excellent results (Table 28–2). The presence of massive mediastinal disease (>⅓ chest diameter) necessitates one of these regimens with the addition of local radiotherapy.

After all staging procedures, approximately 60% of patients receive the diagnosis of advanced disease (stage III or IV). Chemotherapy is considered the treatment of choice for advanced-stage disease. Any of the protocols listed in Table 28–2 induces complete remissions in 70–90% of patients.[21] If chemotherapy fails, salvage therapy includes treatment with a different regimen; if resistance continues, allogeneic or autologous bone marrow transplantation may be the treatment of choice. Because of the large number of Hodgkin's disease survivors, complications of therapy may surface more frequently than relapse of the disease itself. Infections and second cancers (AML, MDS, lymphoma)[21] are the most severe complications and may produce fatal consequences.

Therapy for NHL is based on many prognostic factors and the stage of the lymphoma. The staging of the disease is of the utmost importance in determining appropriate therapy. NHL occurs in a wide variety of age groups but is more frequently seen in persons over 50 years of age. The age of the patient may determine the management op-

tions for therapy. Frequently, younger patients are able to withstand more aggressive chemotherapy than are the elderly.

NHL is divided into three groups: low-, intermediate-, and high-grade, on the basis of how rapidly the tumor cells are dividing. The diffuse low-grade lymphomas cannot be cured with treatment, but

Table 28–2 CHEMOTHERAPY DRUG COMBINATIONS

Hodgkin's Disease

MOPP

Mechlorethamine
Vincristine (Oncovin)
Prednisone
Procarbazine

ABVD

Doxorubicin (Adriamycin)
Bleomycin
Vinblastine
Dacarbazine

MVPP

Mechlorethamine
Vinblastine
Procarbazine
Prednisone

CHlVPP

Chlorambucil
Vinblastine
Procarbazine
Prednisone

MOPP-ABV

Mechlorethamine
Vincristine (Oncovin)
Prednisone
Procarbazine
Doxorubicin (Adriomycin)
Bleomycin
Vinblastine

Non-Hodgkin's Lymphoma

CHOP

Cyclophosphamide
Adriamycin
Vincristine (Oncovin)
Prednisone

CAP-BOP

Cyclophosphamide
Doxorubicin (Adriamycin)
Procarbazine
Bleomycin
Vincristine (Oncovin)
Prednisone

COP

Cyclophosphamide
Vincristine (Oncovin)
Prednisone

MACOP-B

Mechlorethamine
Doxorubicin (Adriamycin)
Cyclophosphamide
Vincristine (Oncovin)
Prednisone
Bleomycin

the patient can live quite long because the tumor grows slowly. The intermediate- and high-grade lymphomas can be cured with treatment, but if they are not cured, the average patient's life span after diagnosis is short: perhaps less than 1 year.

LOW-GRADE LYMPHOMA

Radiotherapy is most effective with localized lymphoma, and a cure is possible in stages I or II with radiotherapy only; however, most patients present with diffuse disease. A standard protocol for diffuse low-grade lymphoma is cyclophosphamide or chlorambucil, or a combination of cyclophosphamide, doxorubicin (Adriamycin), vincristine, and prednisone. A "watch and wait" attitude is taken with elderly patients; no chemotherapy is given unless there are clinical signs or laboratory signs (decreased hemoglobin, decreased platelet count, or increased numbers of circulating lymphoma cells) of disease progression. Low-grade lymphomas often transform to higher grade, more aggressive lymphomas.

INTERMEDIATE-GRADE LYMPHOMA

In the different histologic types of intermediate-grade lymphoma, radiotherapy alone is not usually effective unless extensive staging has been performed to confirm that the malignancy is localized. Aggressive chemotherapy may cure disseminated intermediate-grade lymphoma. There is no best treatment regimen. A typical treatment modality would be as depicted in Figure 28–4.

If there is complete remission (no evidence of disease in bone marrow or nodes), the patient should undergo two more cycles of chemotherapy, and blood counts should be maintained until relapse. If disease is still present, the patient should undergo two or more chemotherapy cycles (up to a total of 7) with reassessment if residual disease exists. Alpha-interferon may help improve chemotherapy remission rates.

HIGH-GRADE LYMPHOMA

High-grade lymphoma progresses more rapidly than the other types and must be dealt with more aggressively. High-risk factors to watch for include central nervous system involvement, bone marrow involvement (as determined by core biopsy), and lactate dehydrogenase levels higher than 500 U/L (which may indicate diffuse disease). Cure is possible with high-grade lymphoma if the patient can tolerate aggressive high-dose chemotherapy. A case of advanced-stage high-grade lymphoma with high-risk factors is attacked with a chemotherapy regimen such as CHOP or CAP-BOP (see Table 28–2) with central nervous system prophylaxis as seen with ALL therapy. Autologous bone marrow transplantation is an option at first remission or after the first best response. If transplantation is not possible, relapse with a more refractory lymphoma is probable. Different types of salvage chemotherapy are instituted if the lymphoma is drug resistant or if the patient is unable to tolerate the toxic effects of high-dose chemotherapy. In cases of relapse or refractory lymphoma, autologous bone marrow transplantation is the treatment of choice. Five-year disease-free survival rates range from 20–40% with autologous transplantation for lymphoma.[1] There remains the potential for other forms of treatment for lymphoma. Research into monoclonal antibodies, interferon, and interleukins continues.

Multiple Myeloma

The plasma cell dyscrasias include multiple myeloma and Waldenström's macroglobulinemia. Multiple myeloma can be a severe, acute disorder that, if untreated, is fatal within 6 months of diagnosis, whereas Waldenström's macroglobulinemia tends to be slower growing. Both tumors produce a clonal immunoglobulin, which can be observed to follow the effectiveness of treatment. Most cases of multiple myeloma are systemic and are treated with chemotherapy. A standard protocol of mel-

3 cycles (21- or 28-day cycle)

	Day	1	2	3	4	5	6	7	8	9	10	11	12	13	14	15	16	17	18	19	20	21
Cyclophosphamide	(C)	X																				
Doxorubicin (hydroxydaunorubicin)	(H)	X																				
Vincristine (Oncovin)	(O)	X																				
Prednisone	(P)	X	X	X	X	X																

Restage after recovery from third cycle

Figure 28–4 A typical aggressive chemotherapy protocol (CHOP) for intermediate-grade lymphoma involves three cycles of either 21 or 28 days, with drugs given on the days indicated. After recovery from the third cycle, the patient should be restaged.

phalan and prednisone is commonly used to decrease the tumor load of the disorder and extend the patient's life. Chemotherapy is initiated after consideration of clinical symptoms (such as bone pain, weakness, spots on radiographs, and renal problems) and laboratory data (including platelet counts, hemoglobin, and protein levels). Median length of survival for patients with most types of multiple myeloma with therapy ranges from 30 to 40 months.[1] If the myeloma cells become resistant to the standard therapy of melphalan and prednisone, vincristine and doxorubicin may be instituted. There has also been success with five-drug regimens (e.g., melphalan, cyclophosphamide, carmustine, vincristine, and prednisone). These protocols tend to be more toxic than melphelan-prednisone but may be effective for myelomas with high tumor loads (increased numbers of plasma cells).

Chemotherapy for myeloma is generally continued for 1–2 years and discontinued when immunoglobulin levels in serum and urine have been stable for 6 months, with fewer than 5% plasma cells in the bone marrow and no other evidence of active disease. Another risk from extensive chemotherapy is the chance that a secondary acute leukemia (usually monocytic) or MDS will develop. The use of alpha-interferon has been used with some success in prolonging disease-free states after chemotherapy. An option to consider once the myeloma is controlled is bone marrow transplantation.

Waldenström's macroglobulinemia is not treated as aggressively as is multiple myeloma. Treatment is initiated only if the disease causes problems such as anemia, weight loss, fatigue, night sweats, hyperviscosity, hepatosplenomegaly, or lymphadenopathy. The therapy is directed against the abnormal plasma cells. A combination of chlorambucil and prednisone is used and discontinued when a plateau of effect is achieved. An average 5-year survival rate is expected with this disease. If hyperviscosity (measured by serum viscosity test) causes clinical problems, it may be controlled by plasmapheresis and replacement by normal albumin. Few data are available concerning bone marrow transplantation for victims of Waldenström's macroglobulinemia.

Hairy Cell Leukemia

Hairy cell leukemia, a disorder generally found in the elderly, rarely requires very aggressive treatment. Patients generally are monitored with blood counts and physical examinations, and there is no indication for therapy unless cytopenia, marked splenomegaly, or recurrent infections occur. Splenectomy is considered the treatment of choice. Alpha-interferon is frequently used and causes improvements in approximately 90% of the cases.[1] The mechanism of action of alpha-interferon has not been established, but the drug remains the treatment of choice for the future. Pentostatin and 2-CDA have been effective in achieving complete remissions in more than 60% of patients with hairy cell leukemias when the treatment plans just described fail.

SUMMARY

The treatment of leukocyte neoplasia involves a wide variety of drugs and technologies that are constantly changing. Chemotherapy is frequently the treatment of choice, because hematologic neoplasia is most often disseminated on presentation. The use of bone marrow transplantation continues to become more prevalent in treating all types of disorders. As purging techniques become more sophisticated, autologous transplantation will find its niche in the treatment of acute leukemias and myelomas, as well as in the treatment of the various stages of solid tumors. With supportive care becoming more successful, more intensive chemotherapy has been used with greater success. Prophylactic antibiotics, strict isolation techniques, hyperalimentation, and CSFs have revolutionized drug dosing. Now patients who were formerly unable to tolerate aggressive chemotherapy can receive potentially curative drug combinations. CSFs are being upgraded all of the time, with improved spectrums of activity. They too will allow dose intensification to proceed even further.

However, few new successful drugs have been introduced since 1980. The BRMs that directly attack tumor cells have been a disappointment, as has immunotherapy against neoplasia. The revolution in supportive care has clearly not been matched by advances in treatment. Future advances in the treatment of hematologic neoplasia will result from identification of the molecular lesions that produce the neoplasia and targeting them with specifically designed drugs.

References

1. Hoffman R, Benz E, Shattil SJ, et al: Hematology: Basic Principles and Practice. New York: Churchill Livingstone, 1991:669–670.
2. Wintrobe MM, Lee GR, Boggs DR, et al: Clinical Hematology, 8th ed. Philadelphia: Lea & Febiger, 1981:1869.
3. Metcalf D: Haemopoietic growth factors 2: clinical applications. Lancet 1989; 1:885–887.
4. Geller B, Larson A: Therapy for acute myeloid leukemia and acute lymphoblastic leukemia in adults. Curr Opin Oncol 1991; 3:30–38.

5. Hertler AA, Frankel AE: Immunotoxins in the therapy of leukemias and lymphomas. Cancer Invest 1991; 9(2):211–219.

6. Sosman JA, Sondel P: The graft vs. leukemia effect: possible mechanisms and clinical significance to the biologic therapy of leukemia. Bone Marrow Transplant, 1991; 7(Suppl 1):33–37.

7. Kaehler SL, Goodwin JM, Young LD: Bone marrow transplantation—mastering the experience despite psychological risk factors. Psychosomatics 1989; 30:337.

8. Santos GW: Bone marrow transplantation in hematologic malignancies. Cancer 1990; 65:786–791.

9. Storb R: Bone marrow transplantation for the treatment of chronic myelogenous leukemia. Am J Med Sci 1988; 296:87–94.

10. Trigg, ME: Bone marrow transplantation for treatment of leukemia in children. Pediat Clin North Am 1988; 35(4):934–943.

11. Thomas ED: Marrow transplantation for malignant diseases. Am J Med Sci 1987; 294(2):75–79.

12. Champlin R: Immunobiology of BMT as treatment for hematologic malignancies. Transplant Proc 1991; 23:2124–2125.

13. Ramsay, NKC, Kersey, J: Indications for marrow transplantation in acute lymphoblastic leukemia. Blood 1990; 75:815–818.

14. Boggs DR, Wintrobe MM, Cartwright GE: To treat or not to treat acute granulocytic leukemia. II. Arch Intern Med 1969; 123:568–570.

15. Stein RS: Review: Advances in the therapy of acute non-lymphocytic leukemia. Am J Med Sci 1989; 297:27.

16. Champlin R, Gale RP: Acute myelogenous leukemia: recent advances in therapy. Blood 1987; 69:1551–1562.

17. Goldman JM: Review: Prospects for cure in leukaemia. J Clin Pathol 1987; 40:985–994.

18. Gajewski JL, Ho WG, Nimer SD, et al: Efficacy of intensive chemotherapy for acute myelogenous leukemia associated with a preleukemic syndrome. J Clin Oncol 1989; 7:1637–1645.

19. Goldman JM: Bone marrow transplantation for chronic myeloid leukaemia. Bone Marrow Transplant 1991; 7(Suppl 2):62–63.

20. Bandini G, Michallet M, Rosti G, Tura S: Bone marrow transplantation for chronic lymphocytic leukemia. Bone Marrow Transplant 1991; 7:251–253.

21. Urba, WJ, Longo DL: Hodgkin's disease. N Engl J Med 1992; 326:678–687.

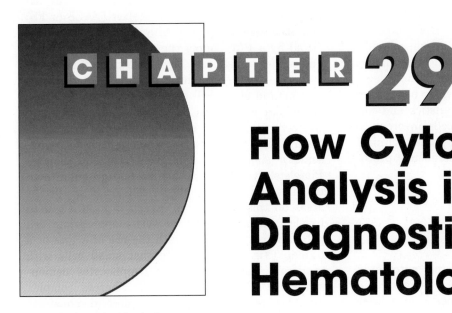

CHAPTER 29

Flow Cytometric Analysis in Diagnostic Hematology

Patricia K. Kotylo

Objectives

AFTER COMPLETION OF THIS CHAPTER, THE READER WILL BE ABLE TO

1. Describe the basic components and operation of a flow cytometer.
2. Describe the expected maturation sequence of different cell lines, and relate the immunophenotypic features to the classification of leukemias and lymphomas.
3. Identify aberrant antigenic patterns that may be observed in hematopoietic disorders and surface marker characteristics of a clonal lymphoid proliferation.
4. Define and recognize the clinical significance of nuclear DNA content (cell cycle analysis) in hematopoietic neoplasia.
5. Discuss the clinical relevance of lymphocyte subset analysis in the immunocompromised patient.

Pathologic evaluation of hematopoietic disorders has traditionally consisted of microscopic examination of stained smears of peripheral blood, bone marrow, or other lymphoid tissues. Unfortunately, significant interobserver variation in the classification and diagnosis of leukemias and lymphomas has been reported among experienced pathologists.[1] Flow cytometry technology is currently being used to study surface antigenic characteristics and nuclear DNA content of neoplastic cells in order to accurately classify these lesions, predict clinical outcome, and determine optimal therapeutic protocols.

FLOW CYTOMETRY INSTRUMENTATION

A flow cytometer is a sophisticated, automated instrument that measures physical or antigenic characteristics of single cells by means of a laser light source.

A laser is an enclosed tube filled with an inert gas such as argon, helium, or neon. Laser light is produced by passing an electrical current through this gas-filled tube, which excites the inert gaseous molecules to a higher level. When these excited ions drop back to their natural low-entropy state, energy is released in the form of a photon of light. This light is intensified in the laser tube through a series of mirrors and is finally emitted as a narrow light beam of a single, specific wavelength (monochromatic light). The wavelength of the monochromatic light is characteristic of the gas within the laser tube.

A sample is aspirated into tubing that has a peripheral moving stream of fluid (the *sheath*) and a central stream of fluid (the *sample*). The sample stream is *hydrodynamically focused* into a single file line of particles by altering the diameter of the sheath. The pressure and velocity exerted on the sheath fluid are adjusted so that the cells move single file, like beads on a string, in the center of the liquid stream. The term for the movement of two liquids past one another without mixing is *laminar flow* (Fig. 29–1).

The laser beam is focused on the single cells with the use of a series of lenses and prisms. This light can be measured as it is reflected or *scattered* off cells, or it can excite fluorescent particles attached to cells.

A series of sensitive light detectors called photomultiplier tubes (PMTs) collect light scattered around and through cells in the line of the laser beam. Light collected from cells that have not been treated with exogenous chemicals or dyes reflects intrinsic cellular characteristics—that is, native cellular features. Intrinsic cellular features are detected by forward-angle light scatter (FALS or FS) and side scatter (SS). FALS refers to light collected by a PMT along the axis of the laser beam and relates to cell size. Light deflected off cells at a 90-degree angle to the laser beam is SS and reveals information about cell density, nuclear complexity, or cellular granularity. The light deflected off native cells is then converted to a dot plot or scattergram of FALS against SS, wherein each dot represents a single cell of a given size and density. Platelets, lymphocytes, monocytes, granular neutrophils, and other neoplastic cells occur in specific areas on this scattergram, which is routinely used to electronically isolate or select appropriate cell populations for analysis with the use of a gate or a bitmap (Fig. 29–2A). Note that small cells with minimal cytoplasm such as lymphocytes demonstrate low FALS and low SS, whereas complex granular cells such as neutrophils demonstrate high FALS and high SS. Other cellular characteristics such as surface or nuclear antigens and nuclear DNA content must be evaluated with exogenous reagents or dyes and are termed extrinsic cellular characteristics. These extrinsic parameters are quantitated through the use of another series of filters and photomultiplier tubes designed to detect light of a specific wavelength emitted from fluorescent dyes excited by the laser beam. A computer system then converts the emitted light signal to a histogram, which plots increasing intensity of cellular fluorescence on the X axis (LFL 1:log green fluorescence) against cell count on the Y axis (LFL 2:log red fluorescence) (see Fig. 29–2B). This graph of immunofluorescence may be further analyzed with computer programs to determine the relative percentage of cells that are stained with a specific probe.[2] Several dyes are currently available for clinical use and may be excited by a monochromatic laser beam, but they emit light of distinctly different wavelengths. These fluorochromes are frequently conjugated to different monoclonal antibodies and may be used to study different antigens on the surface of a single cell.

Some specialized flow cytometers possess the ability to perform *cell sorting*, which allows physical separation of subpopulations of cells. With this feature, cells with specific preselected antigenic characteristics are isolated in individual liquid droplets from the sample column. The cytometer computer identifies cells of interest, and a charge is placed on the droplet, which is then deflected from the sample stream into a collection tube.[3] Collected cells may be further analyzed or used for research purposes. Cell sorting may be technically

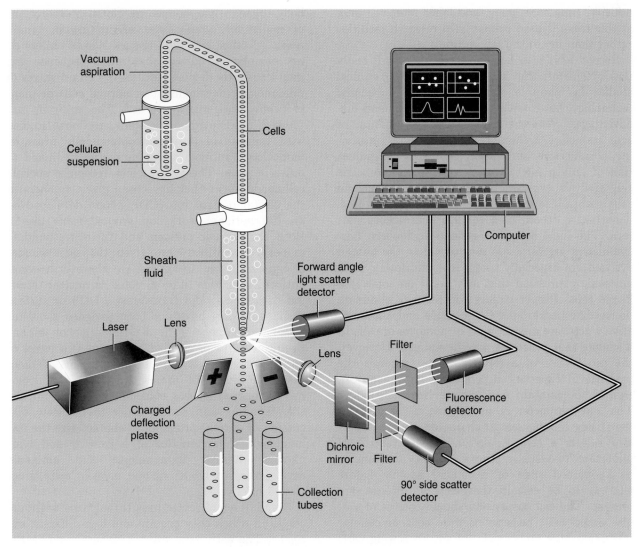

Figure 29–1 Flow cytometry schematic.

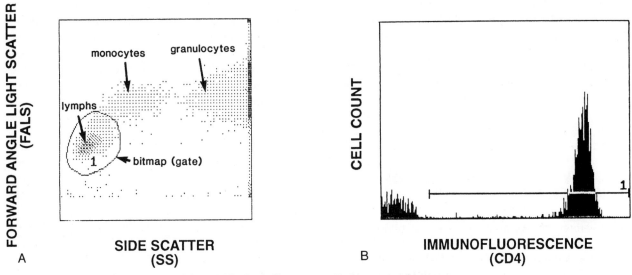

Figure 29–2 *A,* Scattergram; *B,* fluorescence histogram.

difficult, time consuming, and labor intensive and, at this time, is used primarily in research facilities rather than in clinical laboratories.

Recent advances have resulted in user-friendly flow cytometers that are now available for clinical studies in many laboratories. This sophisticated technology, however, has both advantages and disadvantages. Whereas microscopic examination of cells stained with fluorescent dyes is time consuming, is subjective, and usually results in the evaluation of only a few hundred cells, flow cytometric cell analysis typically analyzes several thousand cells within a few minutes and provides a printed, quantitative record of a cellular fluorescence pattern. The light detection systems in modern flow cytometers are far more sensitive than the human eye and are especially useful in quantitating weak antigenic expression that may occur on some leukemic cells. Proper quality control may eliminate nonspecific background fluorescence and allow relatively accurate quantitation of numbers of cells in a sample that possess a specific antigen. However, the proper use of a flow cytometer requires the presence of experienced personnel who have been trained to maintain and operate this instrument. The flow cytometer is, in a sense, a "blind" system; using cellular scatter characteristics, the operator selects a cell population for analysis. It is important to visually scan a Wright- or Romanowsky-stained slide of a cellular sample before analysis to be certain that cells of interest are present. The cell suspension should consist of viable, single cells, because necrotic cells or cellular fragments may nonspecifically adsorb a wide variety of dyes. Cell clumps or debris may obscure analysis and block the narrow sample delivery aperture.[4]

Several manufacturers are currently marketing instruments with different laser light sources and computer analysis systems. Flow cytometers may have the capability to store raw data (listmode data) obtained from cellular analysis on computer discs. Using these hard discs, an operator may "replay" a prior analysis on a computer system and re-gate or otherwise manipulate the information obtained without physically reanalyzing a cellular suspension.[5]

FLOW CYTOMETRIC ANALYSIS OF LEUKEMIAS AND LYMPHOMAS

Leukemias and lymphomas are two major types of malignant hematopoietic proliferations. Leukemias are malignant clonal proliferations of hematopoietic cells originating in the bone marrow that may secondarily involve peripheral blood or other body organs. Lymphomas are clonal proliferations of malignant lymphocytes originating in lymph nodes or other lymphoid tissues. These tumors do not complete a normal maturation sequence and may frequently display features of certain stages of immunologic development of normal cells or inappropriate antigenic patterns.[6] The antigens expressed on hematopoietic cells are now studied with the use of purified, commercially prepared monoclonal antibodies that are directly linked to different dyes. These antibodies recognize specific cellular antigens that have been given numbers in the cluster designation (CD) system developed by an international workshop group (Table 29–1). Both the cellular antigen and the corresponding monoclonal antibody are given the same cluster designation[7] (see Chapter 21). However, several antibodies such as those directed to nuclear terminal deoxynucleotidyl transferase (TdT) or surface immunoglobulin have not been assigned a cluster designation number. The determination of the antigenic features of cells with the use of a panel of antibodies is called immunophenotyping. If more than 20% of cells of interest react with a monoclonal antibody, they are considered positive for the corresponding antigen. In order to facilitate discussion of current attempts to characterize the immunologic characteristics of leukemias and lymphomas, normal immunologic and antigenic development of lymphoid and myeloid cells is reviewed briefly.

B and T lymphocytes pass through maturational stages in which they acquire and lose different antigens. The early *progenitor B cell* is found in the bone marrow and expresses a primitive lymphoid nuclear enzyme called terminal deoxynucleotidyl transferase (TdT) as well as surface HLA-DR. As this cell matures, it sequentially expresses the surface B cell antigens CD19(B4), CD10(CALLA), and CD20(B1), in addition to HLA-DR and nuclear TdT (Fig. 29–3). B cells expressing these additional surface antigens are generally termed *immature B cells*. After the appearance of surface CD20, nuclear TdT expression and the M heavy chain portion of the IgM molecule may be detected in the cytoplasm of this cell, which is now termed a *pre-B cell*. Pre-B cells express cytoplasmic M heavy chain but no surface immunoglobulin. The

Table 29-1. MONOCLONAL ANTIBODY SPECIFICITIES	
T cell markers	CD2, CD3, CD4, CD8, CD5, CD7, CD1
B cell markers	CD19, CD20, CD21, CD22
Myeloid/Monocytic markers	CD13, CD14, CD33

T cell maturation

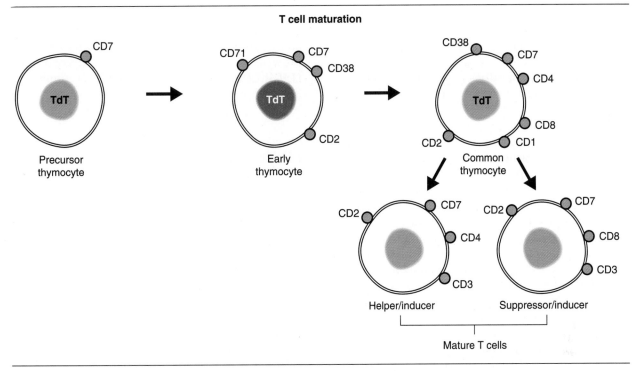

B cell maturation

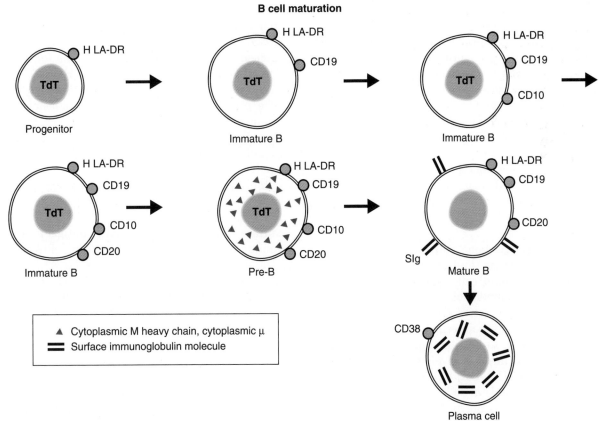

Figure 29–3 T and B cell maturation chart.

final differentiation step results in mature B cells, which express entire immunoglobulin molecules such as IgG, IgM, and IgD on their surface; pan–B surface antigens, including CD19 and CD20, are also present. Cytoplasmic M, nuclear TdT, and CALLA(CD10) are no longer observed. The mature B cells then leave the bone marrow and seed peripheral blood lymph nodes and other lymphoid tissues, in which they may interact with foreign antigens and develop into immunoglobulin-producing plasma cells. Although plasma cells actively secrete and synthesize immunoglobulin molecules, they do not express surface immunoglobulin, CD10, or the pan–B antigens CD19 and CD20. Large quantities of entire immunoglobulin molecules are typically found in the cytoplasm of these cells.[8]

T cell development and maturation occurs in a fleshy, tan, lobulated organ called the thymus (see Fig. 6–12). The earliest T cell is called a *precursor T lymphocyte* or a *precursor thymocyte* and is found in the outer thymic cortex. This early T lymphocyte expresses weak nuclear TdT as well as the T cell surface marker CD7 (Fig. 29–3B). As the T lymphocyte continues to mature, it migrates to the inner thymic cortex, where nuclear TdT expression increases and the surface antigens such as CD38 and CD71 appear. The cell is then termed an *early thymocyte.* The *common thymocyte* expresses several T cell markers, including CD2, CD4, CD8, and CD1; CD1 is considered a specific antigenic marker for the common thymocyte. The T lymphocyte continues its migration into the thymic medulla and loses CD1. Nuclear TdT expression weakens, and the surface antigen CD3 appears. These *mature thymocytes* no longer coexpress both CD4 and CD8 and are divided into two primary groups: CD3+/CD4+ cells (helper cells) and CD3+/CD8+ cells (suppressor cells). When finally released into peripheral blood, mature T cells express pan–T surface markers such as CD2, CD3, and CD7, with either CD4 or CD8 antigens but not both. Approximately two helper cells are released for every suppressor cell in peripheral blood, with a resultant helper:suppressor T cell ratio of 2:1. Mature B and T cells in peripheral blood or lymph nodes should not express nuclear TdT, CD1, or CD10 (CALLA).[6]

Stem cells in the bone marrow give rise to myeloid, megakaryocytic, and erythroid cell series as well as the lymphoid cell line. However, differentiation and development of myeloid, erythroid, and megakaryocytic cell series are not as clearly characterized as the lymphoid cells lines. One precursor cell line gives rise to both granulocytic and monocytic cell series. Blasts of myeloid origin characteristically express HLA-DR, CD33, and CD34. HLA-DR may be found at all stages of monocytic differentiation but is not present on promyelocytes and further mature granulocytic elements. Myeloid antigens such as CD33 and CD13 are acquired during cellular maturation of both neutrophilic and monocytic precursors.[9] However, CD33 expression is generally absent on mature granulocytes. CD33 and CD13 are considered myelomonocytic antigens; however the epitope CD14 is a specific marker for the monocytic cell series. Separate lines of primi-

tive cells give rise to the erythroid and megakaryocytic cell series. The surface antigens CD41, CD42, and CD61 are associated with megakaryocytic cells as well as platelets. The antigen glycophorin A (LICR.LON.R10) has no assigned CD number but is found on erythrocytes and their precursors.[10]

IMMUNOPHENOTYPE OF LEUKEMIAS AND LYMPHOMAS

Acute leukemias are broadly divided into leukemias of lymphoid or myeloid origin (see Chapter 23). Unfortunately, morphologic assessment of leukemias does not consistently differentiate these two major categories of disease. Leukemias may be analyzed with a carefully selected panel of antibodies directed to both myeloid and lymphoid antigens in order to distinguish myeloid from lymphoid leukemias and to distinguish B cell from T cell acute lymphoid leukemias.

Acute leukemias of lymphoid origin (ALLs) have been extensively studied and may be of either B or T cell origin. B cell ALLs are divided into four major immunophenotypic categories. The *early precursor B (null) cell* ALL expresses HLA-DR, nuclear TdT and CD19. Blasts of the *immature B cell* ALL or common ALL express HLA-DR, TdT, and CD10 (CALLA) as well as CD19 and/or CD20. The *pre–B cell* ALL expresses cytoplasmic heavy chain in addition to CD19, CD20, and CD10. *Mature B cell* ALL expresses bright surface immunoglobulin in addition to CD19 and CD20; the blasts are TdT negative and may demonstrate CALLA or cytoplasmic expression. T cell ALL expresses nuclear TdT and varying combinations of pan–T cell antigens such as CD5, CD7, CD2, or CD3 but lacks surface HLA-DR. No specific antigenic pattern immunologically distinguishes French-American-British– (FAB-) classified L1 or L2 ALLs, which may be either B or T cell in origin. However, FAB L3 (Burkitt leukemia/lymphoma) often displays a mature B phenotype with monoclonal surface immunoglobulin.[11]

The majority of acute myeloid leukemias (AML) express HLA-DR, CD33, CD13, and CD15. FAB M1 leukemias are usually CD13 and CD33 positive with HLA-DR; they may also demonstrate a stem cell marker seen on early myeloid precursors (CD34) as well as weak nuclear TdT. The more mature FAB M2 leukemias typically express CD15 in addition to HLA-DR, CD33, and CD13. Nuclear TdT and CD34 are weak or absent.[12] Blasts of either myeloid or lymphoid origin usually express HLA-DR. Both mature and immature monocytic components also demonstrate significant quantities of this surface antigen. HLA-DR is not present on myeloid cells after the myeloblastic stage of cell differentiation; thus it is not surprising that HLA-DR is usually not observed on promyelocytic FAB M3 acute leukemias. FAB M3 leukemia typically demonstrates bright CD33 and CD13 with minimal or no HLA-DR.[13] FAB M4 and M5 may express varying quantities of the monocytic antigen CD14 in addition to HLA-DR, CD33, and CD13.[14]

In the discussion thus far, it has been assumed that both myeloid and lymphoid leukemias are clonal proliferations that express markers only of one specific cell lineage. Recent work with dual- and three-color monoclonal antibodies has demonstrated that up to 30% of acute leukemias may coexpress unexpected surface antigens.[15] These findings have resulted in a confusing array of terms to describe these entities. It is generally agreed that leukemias expressing only one cell lineage of markers are classified as lymphoid or myeloid in origin. However, the simultaneous expression of multiple markers presents a different problem. *Lineage infidelity* generally refers to leukemias with a single aberrant marker. An example of this type of coexpression of markers would be a lymphoid leukemia that expresses a myeloid-associated antigen or vice versa. *Biphenotypic or hybrid* leukemias are a heterogeneous group of tumors that do not fit into a well-defined FAB subgroup. They may be composed of undifferentiated blasts and express at least two aberrant immunophenotypic markers. Biphenotypic leukemias may also appear morphologically to be myeloid leukemias and may coexpress CD10, surface immunoglobulin, or other lymphoid markers, as well as CD33 or CD13, on the same blast population. *Lineage switch* refers to the conversion of a leukemic cell antigenic characteristic from one cell line to another, usually lymphoid to myeloid. Thus blasts from a leukemic relapse need not necessarily re-express a previously identified phenotypic pattern.[16]

Chronic myelogenous leukemia (CML) is composed of a proliferation of mature myeloid elements in the bone marrow. Immunophenotyping is not especially helpful in the treatment of stable-phase disease. However, after approximately 2–3 years, CML may terminate or transform to an acute leukemia. This blast crisis of CML is most frequently myeloid in origin but may also be of lymphoid or mixed cell lineage.[17] Immunophenotyping may be used to identify the origin of these blasts. Chronic lymphocytic leukemias (CLL) consist of malignant proliferations of mature lymphocytes in bone marrow and peripheral blood. These cells usually originate from B cells and coexpress pan–B cell markers CD19 and CD20 and the T cell marker CD5; weak surface immunoglobulin with light chain restriction is also usually observed

(see Chapter 25).[18] The immunologic diagnosis of lymphoma, which may be of B or T cell origin, depends on the ability to demonstrate a clonal cellular proliferation with aberrant antigenic features. Polyclonal or benign lymphocytes display an array of pan–B cell markers such as CD19 and CD20 as well as surface immunoglobulin molecules with both kappa and lambda light chains. Malignant lymphomas of B cell origin, in contrast, frequently express only kappa or lambda light chains, but not both, on the cell surface. This light chain restriction is characteristic of a monoclonal B cell proliferation. Cells that express the B cell antigens CD19 and CD20 without surface immunoglobulin are also considered neoplastic. Mature B cells in peripheral blood and lymph nodes should not express nuclear TdT or surface CALLA (CD10) in significant quantities. The presence of these markers in cell populations undergoing analysis signals the presence of a potentially malignant B cell population. Unusual or unexpected antigenic patterns such as the presence of CD5 on small B lymphocytes would also be compatible with the presence of a population of lymphoma cells.[19]

Demonstration of forthright clonality in T cell disorders is more difficult. Mature T cells in lymph nodes or peripheral blood should demonstrate several pan–T cell antigens (CD2, CD3, CD5, CD7) in combination with CD4 or CD8 antigens. The loss of any of these pan–T cell antigens or coexpression of CD4 and CD8 antigens on the same lymphocyte population is indirect evidence of clonal T cell proliferations. An extremely high or low ratio of CD4 to CD8 cells may be suggestive of a malignant T cell disorder; however, prominent alterations in helper:suppressor ratios should be interpreted with caution, because these results may also occur in reactive processes. The presence of nuclear TdT or surface CD1 on mature lymphocytes in peripheral blood or lymph nodes is presumptive immunologic evidence for a clonal cellular proliferation.[7]

Technical difficulties may be encountered during immunophenotypic analysis of various tissues to rule out the presence of neoplasia. Many lymphomas involve only a portion of a lymph node or may be associated with areas of dense fibrosis. The cells submitted for analysis must therefore be morphologically evaluated in order to be certain that malignant cells are present in the cellular suspension. Some leukemias and lymphomas, especially large-cell lymphomas, are composed of fragile cells that may fragment or lyse during processing. Careful handling of these samples with minimal physical manipulation may be helpful in these cases.[20]

LYMPHOCYTE SUBSET ANALYSIS FOR IMMUNODEFICIENCY STATES

Lymphocyte analysis may be used in the diagnosis of both primary (genetic, hereditary) and secondary (acquired) immunodeficiency states. Many people with hereditary immunodeficiency states have repeated viral and bacterial infections early in life and often manifest decreased numbers of T cells, B cells, or both lymphocyte groups.

Acquired immunodeficiencies may be caused by immunosuppressive therapy, chemotherapy, tumors of various types, or viral infection. Patients who are recipients of heart, kidney, or other solid organ transplants receive drugs that suppress the immune system to prevent organ rejection. The monoclonal antibody OKT3 is administered intravenously to transplantation patients to selectively destroy antigen-receptor CD3 T lymphocytes, which may be involved in graft rejection. Flow cytometry is frequently used to monitor absolute numbers of CD3 T lymphocytes in the peripheral blood of these patients so as to adjust the dosage of OKT3 drug therapy. Lymphocyte subsets are also evaluated in patients who have received chemotherapy for treatment of malignant tumors or preparation for bone marrow transplantation. T and B cells may be observed in these patients to monitor recovery of the immune system after aggressive treatment with immunotoxic drugs.

Acquired immunodeficiency syndrome (AIDS) is caused by infection with the human immunodeficiency retrovirus (HIV) and is associated with selective depletion of CD4 T lymphocytes. This disease is also characterized by immune dysfunction, repeated opportunistic infections, and various forms of neoplasia. HIV-infected patients typically exhibit increased absolute numbers of CD8 suppressor cells and normal or slightly decreased absolute numbers of helper T lymphocytes in peripheral blood. As the disease progresses, CD4 helper cells decrease dramatically, resulting in a very low helper:suppressor T cell ratio. Absolute numbers of peripheral blood CD4 T lymphocytes are thought to most reliably reflect disease progression in AIDS patients and are thus routinely enumerated to determine eligibility for drug protocols and assess efficacy of antiviral therapy. Decreased absolute numbers of peripheral blood CD4 lymphocytes are not exclusively diagnostic of AIDS and are seen in several viral illnesses, including infectious hepatitis, mononucleosis, and cytomegalovirus.[21]

FLOW CYTOMETRIC ANALYSIS OF NUCLEAR DNA

Flow cytometric analysis of cellular DNA content may be performed by staining isolated nuclei with fluorescent dyes. Uptake of a dye, such as propidium iodide, is directly proportional to the nuclear DNA content. The stained cells are then probed with laser light, which excites this nuclear dye and results in emission of fluorescent light. This fluorescence is recorded graphically as peaks that reflect nuclear DNA content. Normal cells that display a characteristic amount of nuclear DNA are termed diploid. Malignant proliferative cells may display abnormal quantities of DNA in comparison with normal cells and are called aneuploid (Fig. 29–4). Ploidy status (diploid or aneuploid) in several hematopoietic disorders has been examined and may have prognostic importance in these diseases.[22]

Malignant lymphomas have been studied by several investigators and may demonstrate either diploid or aneuploid DNA patterns. However, aneuploid DNA stemlines are encountered more frequently in high-grade aggressive lymphomas than in the predominantly diploid low-grade lymphomas.[23] Multiple myelomas with aneuploid DNA stemlines have been associated with shorter survival and resistance to chemotherapeutic regimens.[24] In contrast, researchers in one study who examined a large series of childhood leukemias re-

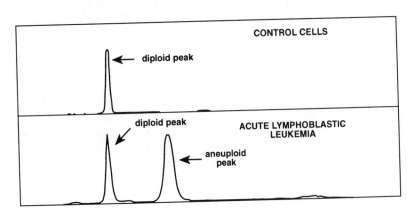

Figure 29–4 DNA ploidy curves.

ported that aneuploid ALL was associated with a good prognosis and a low probability of leukemic relapse after chemotherapy; however, diploid childhood ALL was associated with a poorer prognosis.[25] The clinical significance of DNA ploidy status in childhood AML and adult acute leukemias (both myeloid and lymphoid) is less obvious. One investigator suggested that aneuploid DNA stemlines occurring in AML in young patients with chromosomal translocations may be associated with longer durations of remission and improved survival.[26] The presence of an aneuploid DNA stemline in myelodysplastic syndromes, however, has been associated with a poor prognosis.[27] The prognostic significance of nuclear DNA content varies with the disease state, the patient's age, and chromosomal anomalies.[28] Additional studies are necessary in order to fully understand and confirm many findings that have been reported thus far in the literature.

SUMMARY

A flow cytometer is a sophisticated instrument that may be used to evaluate the antigenic characteristics of individual cells. This emerging technology may provide valuable information that can be used to reproducibly classify hematopoietic disorders such as leukemias and lymphomas and determine appropriate therapeutic protocols.

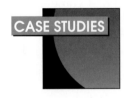
CASE STUDIES

Case 1

A 7-year-old girl was seen by her pediatrician for a persistent upper respiratory tract infection (a cold). Peripheral blood studies demonstrated anemia (hemoglobin, 7.7 g/dL) with thrombocytopenia (59×10^9/L). Review of a peripheral smear revealed nucleated red blood cells and blasts. The bone marrow aspirate contained sheets of small blasts with scant cytoplasm, which demonstrated positivity only for periodic acid Schiff stains. Flow cytometric analysis of bone marrow (Fig. 29–5) demonstrated a population of cells in the scattergram (FALS vs. SS) with the following characteristics:

Antibody	% Positive Cells
TdT	90
CD10(CALLA)	90
HLA-DR	90
CD33(My9)	5
CD13(My7)	5

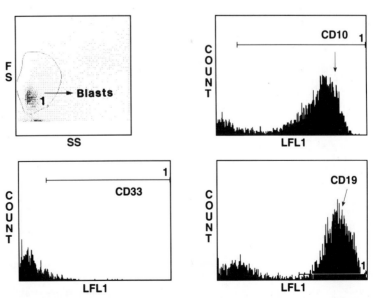

Figure 29–5 Flow cytometric data. Prominent positive peaks present in CD19 and CD10 histograms *(arrow). Abbreviations:* FS, forward-angle light scatter; SS, side scatter; LFL1, log green fluorescence.

CD15(LeuM1)	3
CD14(My4)	2
CD2	4
CD7	6
CD19	90
CD20	5
Kappa	0
Lambda	0

1. What type of acute leukemia does this patient have?

2. What are the characteristic immunophenotypic findings of this disease?

Case 2

A 34-year-old woman reported to her family physician with a fever, weakness, and petechiae. Peripheral blood studies revealed anemia (hemoglobin, 9.6 g/dL), thrombocytopenia (30 × 10⁹/L), and numerous blasts. The bone marrow aspirate and biopsy demonstrated sheets of large blasts with prominent nucleoli and granular cytoplasm with Auer rods. These cells reacted positively to Sudan Black B and myeloperoxidase; all other findings with cytochemical stains were negative.

Immunophenotyping of bone marrow blasts (Fig. 29–6) revealed the following:

Antibody	% Positive Cells
TdT	0
CD10(CALLA)	0
HLA-DR	90
CD33(My9)	95
CD13(My7)	93
CD15(LeuM1)	90
CD14(My4)	2
CD2	3
CD7	5
CD19	6
CD20	2

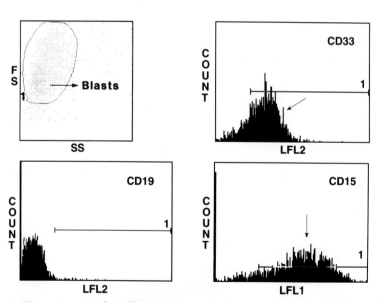

Figure 29–6 Flow cytometric data. Note positive peaks *(arrows)* present in CD33 and CD15 histograms. *Abbreviations:* FS, forward-angle light scatter; SS, side scatter; LFL2, log red fluorescence; LFL1, log green fluorescence.

| Kappa | 2 |
| Lambda | 2 |

1. This case was classified as an AML FAB type M2. How do the flow cytometry findings listed support this diagnosis?

2. Which antibodies in the list differentiate myeloid and lymphoid acute leukemias?

References

1. Shapiro HM: Practical Flow Cytometry, 2nd ed. New York: AR Liss, 1988:21–86.
2. Hansen W, Hoffman R, Healey K: Light scatter as an adjunct to cellular immunofluorescence in flow cytometric systems. J Clin Immunol 1982; 2:32S–41S.
3. Lovett EJ, Schnitzer B, Keren DF, et al: Applications of flow cytometry to diagnostic pathology. Lab Invest 1984; 50:115–140.
4. McCoy JP, Lovett E: Basic principles in clinical flow cytometry. In Keren DF (ed): Flow Cytometry in Clinical Diagnosis. Chicago: ASCP Press, 1989:12–37.
5. Dean PN: Data processing. In Melamed MR, Lindmo T, Mendelsohn ML (eds): Flow Cytometry and Sorting. New York: Wiley-Liss, 1990:415–444.
6. Foon KA, Todd RF: Immunologic classification of leukemia and lymphoma. Blood 1986; 68:1–31.
7. Carey JL: Flow cytometric immunoanalysis of leukemia and lymphoma. J Clin Immunoassay 1989; 12:21–29.
8. Weisenburger DD, Chan WC: Lymphomas of follicles. Am J Clin Pathol 1993; 99:409–420.
9. Carey JL, England BG: Leukocyte antigens and monoclonal reagents: production and characterization. In Keren DF (ed): Flow Cytometry in Clinical Diagnosis. Chicago: ASCP Press, 1989:41–138.
10. Drexler HG: Classification of acute myeloid leukemias—a comparison of FAB and immunophenotyping. Leukemia 1987; 1:697–705.
11. Bennett JM, Catovsky D, Daniel MT, et al: Proposals for the classification of the acute leukaemias (FAB cooperative group). Br J Haematol 1976; 33:451–458.
12. Bain BJ: Leukaemia diagnosis: a guide to the FAB classification. Philadelphia: JB Lippincott, 1990:66–67.
13. Griffin J, Davis R, Nelson D, et al: Use of surface marker analysis to predict outcome of adult acute myeloblastic leukemia. Blood 1986; 68:1232–1241.
14. Neame P, Soamboonsrup P, Browman G, et al: Classifying acute leukemia by immunophenotyping: a combined FAB-immunologic classification of AML. Blood 1986; 68:1355–1362.
15. Del Vecchio L, Schiavoni EM, Ferrara F, et al. Immunodiagnosis of acute leukemia displaying ectopic antigens: proposal for a classification of promiscuous phenotypes. Am J Hematol 1989; 31:173–180.
16. Miller KB: Clinical manifestations of acute nonlymphocytic leukemia. In Hoffman R, Benz EJ, Shattil SJ, et al (eds): Hematology: Basic Principles and Practice. New York: Churchill Livingstone, 1991:725–726.
17. Griffin JD, Todd RF, Ritz J, et al: Differentiation patterns in the blast phase of chronic myeloid leukemia. Blood 1983; 61:85–91.
18. Pangalis GA, Boussiotis VA, Kittas C: Malignant disorders of small lymphocytes. Am J Clin Pathol 1993; 99:402–407.
19. Picker LJ, Weiss LM, Medeiros LJ, et al: Immunophenotypic criteria for the diagnosis of non-Hodgkin's lymphoma. Am J Pathol 1987; 128:181–201.
20. Kotylo PK, Sample B, Redmond NL, Hibner GC: Reference ranges for lymphocyte subsets. Arch Pathol Lab Med 1991; 115:181–184.
21. Giorgio JV: Lymphocyte subset measurements: significance in clinical medicine. In Rose N, Freidman H, Fahey J (eds): Manual of Clinical Laboratory Immunology. Washington, DC: American Society for Clinical Microbiology, 1986:236–246.
22. Kotylo PK: DNA analysis of neoplasia: an introduction for the family physician. Am Fam Physician 1991; 43:1259–1263.
23. Braylan RC: Flow cytometric DNA analysis in the diagnosis and prognosis of lymphoma. Am J Clin Pathol 1993; 99:374–380.
24. Barlogie B, Alexanian R, Dixon D, et al: Prognostic implications of tumor cell DNA and RNA content in multiple myeloma. Blood 1985; 66:338–341.
25. Look AT, Roberson PK, Williams DL, et al: Prognostic importance of blast cell DNA content in childhood acute lymphoblastic leukemia. Blood 1985; 65:1079–1086.
26. Barlogie B, Stass SA, Dixon D, et al: DNA aneuploidy in adult acute leukemia. Cancer Genet Cytogenet 1987; 28:213–228.
27. Peters S, Clark R, Hoy T, Jacobs A: DNA content and cell cycle analysis of bone marrow cells in myelodysplastic syndromes (MDS). Br J Haematol 1986; 62:239–245.
28. Merkel DE, Dressler LG, McGuire WL: Flow cytometry, cellular DNA content, and prognosis in human malignancy. J Clin Oncol 1987; 5:1690–1703.

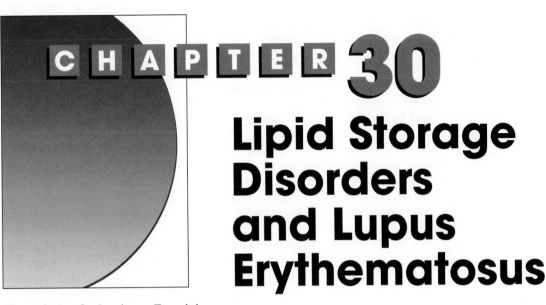

CHAPTER 30

Lipid Storage Disorders and Lupus Erythematosus

Sherri A. Scheirer-Fochler

Outline

Objectives

AFTER COMPLETION OF THIS CHAPTER, THE READER WILL BE ABLE TO

1. Describe the significant clinical features of the major lipidoses.
2. Associate each enzyme deficiency with the specific storage disease that it causes.
3. Describe the appearance of the typical cell in each of the lipid storage diseases.
4. Specify appropriate laboratory tests to confirm the diagnosis of a lipidosis.
5. Discuss current and potential treatments of lipidoses.
6. Recognize the clinical features of systemic lupus erythematosus.
7. Describe the appearance of a typical lupus erythematosus cell on a Wright-stained smear.
8. List both specific and nonspecific laboratory tests used in the diagnosis of lupus erythematosus.

LIPID (LYSOSOMAL) STORAGE DISEASES

Lysosomal storage diseases are rare, autosomally inherited disorders. Although they are uncommon, they are some of the most devastating diseases of childhood. They are caused by various enzyme defects (inborn errors) in lipid metabolism (Fig. 30–1). Lysosomes play a major role in the "intracellular digestive tract," being synthesized in the endoplasmic reticulum and transported to the Golgi apparatus. In the Golgi apparatus, they catalyze the breakdown of a variety of complex macromolecules. Cells of the monocyte/macrophage system phagocytize and digest cell fragments and degenerated and dead cells of all types. For this reason, the lipidoses are sometimes classified as disorders of the monocyte/macrophage system. When there are inherited deficiencies in the production of the enzymes necessary for the catabolism of these ingested cells, various lipids accumulate in the cytoplasm of the phagocytic cells; hence these conditions are termed *lysosomal storage diseases* because of the subcellular accumulation of unmetabolized lipids in the lysosomes. Lipid storage diseases can be of hematologic significance because the bloated macrophages can lead to bone marrow replacement, causing interference with normal cell functions, along with organ involvement, especially massive splenomegaly. Lysosomal storage diseases may closely resemble one another clinically and biochemically. Therefore, to confirm a diagnosis, the accumulated metabolite or the enzyme deficiency must be biochemically identified.

Among certain ethnic groups, most notably the Ashkenazi Jews (whose ancestors came from the Baltic Sea region), the incidence of some lipid storage diseases, particularly Gaucher and Tay-Sachs diseases, is increased, but all ethnic groups are known to be affected.

This group of disorders has a wide range of clinical expression, from essentially asymptomatic to severe and incapacitating with early death. Currently, no completely effective therapy exists; however, newer techniques such as enzyme replacement and gene manipulation have shown success with certain disorders.[1] Gaucher, Niemann-Pick, and Tay-Sachs diseases and sea-blue histiocytosis are the most widely known and well-described of the lipid storage diseases. The clinical features, laboratory diagnosis, prognosis, and treatment of each of these diseases are described in this chapter. Table 30–1 is a summary of storage diseases, enzyme deficiencies, and resultant accumulation products.

Gaucher Disease

The observations of abnormal cells found in a spleen at autopsy were first described in 1882 in the doctoral thesis of Phillippe C. Gaucher. Gaucher disease is the most common of the lipid storage diseases. It is caused by a deficiency of the enzyme β-glucocerebrosidase (EC 3.2.1.45), also known as β-glucosidase, which normally cleaves glucose from glucocerebroside (glucosyl ceramide). The unmetabolized glucocerebroside accumulates primarily in the reticuloendothelial cells of the

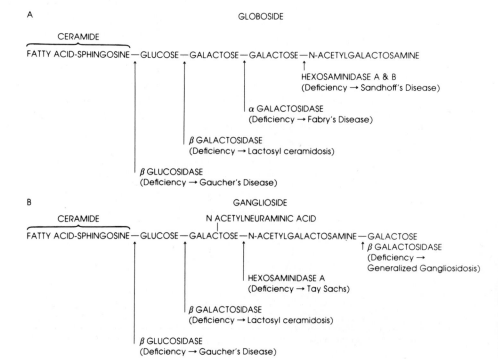

Figure 30–1 Schematic structure of globoside and ganglioside to show site of action of several catabolic enzymes, which when defective result in one of the storage diseases. (From Wintrobe MM [ed]: Clinical Hematology, 8th ed. Malvern, PA: Lea & Febiger, 1981:1341.)

Table 30-1. VARIANTS OF MONOCYTE/MACROPHAGE STORAGE DISEASES*

Name	Enzyme Deficiency	Substance Stored
Hurler syndrome	α-L-iduronidase	Mucopolysaccharide I
Hunter syndrome	Iduronidate sulphatase	Mucopolysaccharide II
Sanfilippo syndrome	Form A: heparin N-sulphatase	Mucopolysaccharide III
	Form B: N-acetyl α-glucosaminidase	
Morquio syndrome	Unknown	Mucopolysaccharide IV
Scheie syndrome	α-L-iduronidase	Mucopolysaccharide V
Maroteaux-Lamy syndrome	Arylsulphatase	Mucopolysaccharide VI
Hand-Schüller-Christian disease		Cholesterol
Gaucher disease	β-glucocerebrosidase	Glucocerebroside
Niemann-Pick disease	Sphingomyelinase	Sphingomyelin
Gangliosidosis	β-galactosidase	G_{m1} ganglioside
Tay-Sachs disease	Hexosaminidase A	G_{m2} ganglioside
Sandhoff disease	Hexosaminidase A	G_{m2} ganglioside
Fabry disease	α-galactosidase	Ceramide trihexoside
Wolman disease	Acid esterase	

* Many dysfunctions result in monocyte/macrophage storage diseases; however, most of them are morphologically quite similar, and cytochemical testing is necessary for determining the specific product stored.
Courtesy of Susan Leclair, University of Massachusetts, Dartmouth, MA.

body, but neurons in the central nervous system may also be involved. Three types of Gaucher disease have been identified; the differences are in severity and age at onset (Table 30-2). All three types are inherited as autosomal recessive disorders.

Type 1 is commonly known as the chronic nonneuronopathic or adult type. This is the most common type of Gaucher disease, accounting for approximately 80% of cases. It is seen most frequently in Ashkenazi Jews. The severity of type 1 is quite heterogenous, which suggests that several genetic mutations are involved. Type 1 is characterized by the absence of cerebral involvement. Affected patients have reduced but detectable levels of glucocerebrosidase. Although it is called the adult type, it may develop any time from early infancy to old age. The diagnosis is not uncommon among older adults who present for medical attention for other reasons and are noted incidentally to have splenomegaly, anemia, or thrombocytopenia. These three symptoms are usually the initial signs of Gaucher disease; however, because they are not

life-threatening, they may go unrecognized for years. On physical examination, patients are often noted to have a jaundiced appearance and pinguecula (yellowish discoloration near the sclerocorneal junction of the eye). Enlargement of the spleen is common, usually accompanied by enlargement of the liver, as a result of the accumulation of Gaucher cells. Episodes of bleeding in the nose or gums are common as a result of thrombocytopenia. A normocytic anemia is usually present. Many patients experience episodic bone pain in the hips, legs, back, and shoulders. These episodes, referred to as *bone crises,* are caused by the accumulation of Gaucher cells in the marrow cavity, which expands and thins the overlying bone. Degenerative changes in the skeleton are the leading cause of disability in patients with type 1 disease. Erlenmeyer flask deformity is often seen.[2] Length of survival of these patients is variable, but most have a reasonably good prognosis, especially if the disease first becomes evident in adulthood.[3]

Type 2, also known as infantile, malignant, or acute neuronopathic Gaucher disease, is much

Table 30-2. GAUCHER DISEASE: CLINICAL SUBTYPES

Clinical Features	Type 1: Nonneuronopathic	Type 2: Acute Neuronopathic	Type 3: Subacute Neuronopathic
Clinical onset	Childhood/adulthood	Infancy	Childhood
Hepatosplenomegaly	+	+	+
Hematologic complications secondary to hypersplenism	+	+	+
Skeletal deterioration	+	−	+
Neurodegenerative course	−	+++	++
Death	Variable	By 2 years	2nd–4th decade
Ethnic predilection	Ashkenazi Jewish	Panethnic	Swedish

From Gaucher disease (1882–1982): Centennial perspectives on the most prevalent Jewish genetic disease. Mt. Sinai J Med 1982; 49:443–453.

more severe because of central nervous system involvement. This form is not very common and is seen in all ethnic groups. Familial intermarriage is frequently found in the history. Manifestation is more uniform than in type 1. In type 2 patients, there is essentially no detectable glucocerebrosidase activity. Early in infancy there is an onset of multiple neurologic signs, including difficulty in swallowing, opisthotonos (extreme arching of the spine), and brain stem involvement. In addition, hepatosplenomegaly is often present, and seizures may occur. As neurologic deterioration proceeds, most patients become apathetic and motionless. Death usually occurs before the age of 2 years, often from anoxia or pulmonary infection.[3]

Type 3 is the juvenile or subacute neuronopathic Gaucher disease. In this third type, the severity of physical symptoms and length of survival range between those of types 1 and 2. Levels of β-glucocerebrosidase are intermediate range between those of types 1 and 2. A history of familial intermarriage is often found. Type 3 is panethnic. Affected patients are usually juveniles, have systemic involvement similar to that of type 1, but have a progressive central nervous system disease with the onset between 6 months and 1 year of age. The neurodegenerative features occur at a later age than in type 2 disease, and the clinical course is more prolonged. Length of survival ranges from late childhood to adolescence. The more severe the neurologic involvement, the shorter the survival.

In all three types of Gaucher disease, the accumulated metabolite, glucocerebroside, is the same; however, the specific patterns of these three types run within families and therefore appear to be distinct types, possibly related to multiple allelism of the affected gene.[4] For example, adults with noncerebral Gaucher disease do not have offspring with the infantile (cerebral) type 2.

LABORATORY DIAGNOSIS

The peripheral blood usually demonstrates a moderate normocytic, normochromic anemia, leukopenia, and thrombocytopenia. The prothrombin and activated partial thromboplastin times may be prolonged because of decreased production of coagulation factors manufactured in the liver. Bleeding tendency is often present as a result of thrombocytopenia, sequestration of platelets by spleen, or coating of platelets with β-glucocerebroside.

A definitive diagnosis can be made by an assay of β-glucocerebrosidase in leukocytes, fibroblasts, or urine. Assay methods have also been employed for the prenatal detection of Gaucher disease and for family counseling. The serum level of acid phosphatase (tartrate resistant) is usually in-

A

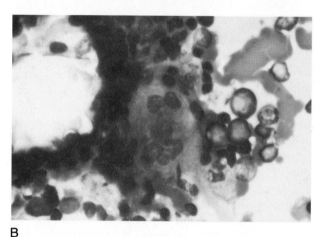

B

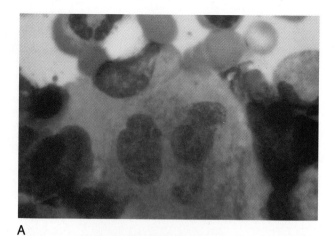

C

Figure 30–2 Three views of a bone marrow aspirate from a child with Gaucher disease. Notice the crumpled cytoplasm with scratch-like lines in it. (Courtesy of Dr. Penchansky, University of Pittsburgh Medical Center.)

creased, and plasma immunoglobulin levels are often high, especially in type 1.[1, 5] These can also be helpful in confirming the disease.

Gaucher cells may be present in the spleen, liver, bone marrow, peripheral blood, and lymph nodes. Bone marrow is often the first tissue in which the diagnostic Gaucher cells are seen (Fig. 30–2). The cells are large: 20–80 μm in diameter. They may be found in clumps or groups of cells. The nuclei are round to oval and relatively small; more than one may be present. The cells have an irregular shape, and the cytoplasm is faintly blue when stained with Wright's stain, with a "crumpled tissue paper" or finely folded appearance. Some authors have described the cytoplasm as "chicken scratch" because of the fine scratch-like lines in it. Electron microscopy has shown that the fibrillar cytoplasm is stuffed with membrane-bound spindles or rod-shaped inclusions of varying length. These inclusions are phagoliposomes, which house lipids in stacks of bilayers.[4]

Gaucher cells react positively to periodic acid Schiff (PAS), acid phosphatase, Giemsa, iron, Sudan black B, and oil red 0 stains.

Molecular techniques have greatly aided in the diagnosis of Gaucher disease. It has been shown through the use of polymerase chain reaction (PCR) that the existence of different subtypes is presumably caused by different gene mutations altering residual acid β-glucosidases. The locus of the gene coding for glucocerebrosidase has been determined to be on chromosome 1q21.[6] The most common mutations occur on exons 5, 9, and 10.[6–8]

Lipid-laden macrophages may be demonstrable in small numbers in bone marrows of patients with diseases other than Gaucher disease. These cells are designated "pseudo–Gaucher cells." The accumulation of glucocerebrosides present in pseudo–Gaucher cells is explained by the fact that in these diseases, there is an increased rate of cellular turnover. Therefore, dead cells are phagocytized at a rate faster than the rate at which the lipids in these cells can be digested. Pseudo–Gaucher cells are seen in diseases with rapid cellular turnover, especially chronic myelogenous leukemia and other disorders such as acute myelocytic leukemia and chronic lymphocytic leukemia (Fig. 30–3). They are also noted in diseases in which there is intermedullary hyperplasia, such as thalassemia major, plasma cell myeloma, and congenital dyserythropoietic anemia. In each of these diseases, however, there is no deficiency of the β-glucocerebrosidase, as there is in Gaucher disease, but simply an overtaxation of a normal system.[9]

PROGNOSIS AND TREATMENT

The length of survival in patients with Gaucher disease is variable and depends on the type. Type 2 is the most severe, and survival beyond the age of two years is rare. Type 3 is intermediate in severity, and patients usually live into adolescence. Patients with type 1 have the longest survival. Their prognosis appears to be better with later age at onset. Many have a relatively normal life span.

Supportive therapy has been the mainstay treatment for the majority of Gaucher patients. Allo-

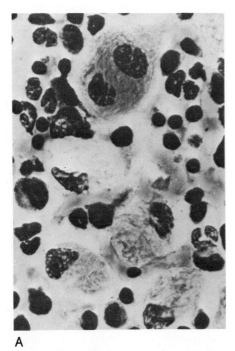
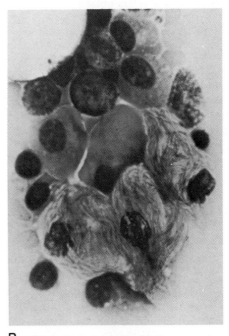

A   B

Figure 30–3 Gaucher cells in the marrow of a patient with Gaucher disease, compared with pseudo-Gaucher cells in CML. *A,* "True" Gaucher cells are huge macrophages, whose fibrillar cytoplasm is stuffed with rod-shaped inclusions, making it appear finely scratched or like crumpled tissue paper. *B,* The pseudo-Gaucher cell is indistinguishable by light microscope from the true Gaucher cell, but the cause of the lipid accumulation is different. (From Jandl JH: Blood: Textbook of Hematology. Boston: Little, Brown, 1987:489.)

geneic bone marrow transplantation has been successful in a few. Trials of enzyme replacement had met with limited success until a commercially prepared enzyme became available. In the original trials, insufficient amounts of enzyme entered the affected cells. In the modified commercial enzyme, mannose residues have been exposed to facilitate targeting of glucocerebroside to tissue macrophages.[10] Macrophages have a surface receptor that recognizes mannose, and so the commercial enzyme with its exposed mannose residues is more readily accepted by the cell.[11] The commercially prepared glucocerebrosidase, Ceredase, is manufactured with purified human placental tissue from France (Genzyme, Cambridge, Massachusetts). Replacement with Ceredase has produced improvement in patients with type 1 disease, but not in patients with types 2 and 3, because of difficulty in delivering the enzyme across the blood-brain barrier.[1]

Niemann-Pick Disease

Niemann-Pick disease is a rare autosomal recessive disorder caused by a deficiency of the enzyme sphingomyelinase. Because of this deficiency, there is a secondary accumulation of the unmetabolized lipid, sphingomyelin, as well as cholesterol. Because sphingomyelin is a constituent of cell membranes and cellular organelles, this deficiency is very serious. The lipid-laden mononuclear phagocytes can be found in the liver, spleen, and bone marrow, and they may also collect in the lungs and nervous system. The incidence of this disease appears increased in the Jewish population. The disease has been divided into five types, A to E, differing on the basis of the particular isoenzyme involved and the clinical manifestations. All are characterized by infiltration of the tissues with the characteristic foamy storage cells. Only types A to C are described, because they account for the majority of the cases.

Type A, also known as infantile or classic Niemann-Pick disease, is the severe form, producing extensive neurologic involvement. It is also the most common form, accounting for up to 85% of all cases.[4] The onset is in early infancy, usually between 3 and 6 months of age. The infants present with mental retardation, difficulty with feeding, hepatosplenomegaly, and sometimes lymphadenopathy in association with a general failure to thrive. Enlargement of the liver and lymph nodes occurs earlier than that seen in Gaucher disease. There is rapid deterioration of motor and intellectual functions, and patients generally become unresponsive by the second year. The skin has a waxy appearance. A cherry-red spot in the macula

of the eye is found in about half of the patients, and other optical and cranial nerve lesions may bring on blindness and deafness. Progressive and severe central nervous system damage usually leads to death within 1–3 years.

Type B is an infantile form that is more chronic and without central nervous system involvement. This type is much less common than type A. The "foam cells" accumulate in the lungs, liver, and spleen, often leading to massive splenomegaly during early childhood. Intellectual development is usually unaffected. Affected patients may live longer than those with type A, but they do not survive beyond early adolescence.

Type C is the chronic neuronopathic form. Clinical symptoms are generally delayed until the ages of 2–4 years. Children show a moderate hepatosplenomegaly but are most affected by neurologic disturbances, including grand mal seizures, muscular incoordination, and impaired mental activity. This relentless neurologic deterioration is usually fatal by the age of 20.

LABORATORY DIAGNOSIS

The diagnosis of Niemann-Pick disease can be made with reasonable certainty on the basis of clinical findings and the appearance of the characteristic foam cells in the bone marrow or spleen (Fig. 30–4). These lipid-choked macrophages or foam cells can also be seen in the liver, lymph nodes, lungs, and brain. Niemann-Pick cells are large, 20–90 μm in diameter, with relatively small, round, inconspicuous nuclei that are often eccentrically located. Niemann-Pick cells are similar to Gaucher cells in size and in nucleus-to-cytoplasm ratio, but the lipid deposits appear as globules or foamy vacuoles. These phagocytic cells have bub-

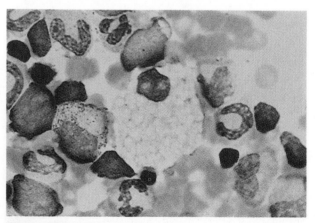

Figure 30–4 Niemann-Pick cell, demonstrating foamy or bubbly cytoplasm. (From Harmening DM [ed]: Clinical Hematology and Fundamentals of Hemostasis, 2nd ed. Philadelphia: FA Davis, 1992:242.)

bly cytoplasm that is greenish-yellow fluorescent in ultraviolet light and is birefringent in polarized light. The cytoplasm is filled with and distended by round, uniformly sized droplets of accumulated lipid, which cause the cell to turn a very pale or light blue with Wright's stain. This cytoplasmic appearance is quite unlike the intertwined fibrillar structures of Gaucher cells. Phase microscopy reveals that the droplets are lipid-filled vacuoles, each consisting of concentrically layered myelin, sometimes creating a striped or zebra-like appearance. Niemann-Pick cells react positively for fat with Sudan black, and oil red 0 stains. They are usually negative or weakly positive for PAS stains and negative for myeloperoxidase. Vacuolated lymphocytes may also be present.

A definitive diagnosis requires proof of sphingomyelinase deficiency in biopsy samples. Enzyme assays may also be successfully performed on frozen sections or with fibroblasts grown in tissue culture. Prenatal diagnosis of type A and possibly type B can be made by analysis of cultured fetal cells via amniocentesis.

In some patients with Niemann-Pick disease, the bone marrow may contain a mixture of Niemann-Pick cells and sea-blue histiocytes. These conditions must be distinguished from the entity of sea-blue histiocytosis, in which histiocytes are distended with blue-staining ceroid when stained with Wright's stain. Other disorders in which bone marrow may contain Niemann-Pick cells are GM_1 gangliosidosis, lactosyl ceramidosis, and Fabry disease.

PROGNOSIS AND TREATMENT

In general, Niemann-Pick disease runs a more rapid course than does Gaucher disease. Patients with type A have a very short life expectancy; death occurs before age 2 years. Those with other types may have a slightly longer survival. Type E, which is very rare and found only in adults, is characterized by a mild chronic course.

No specific therapy for Niemann-Pick disease has been discovered. However, efforts are being made to correct the inborn metabolic defect by enzyme replacement. Research is also being conducted on transplanting human leukocyte antigen–compatible marrow macrophages.[9]

Tay-Sachs Disease

Tay-Sachs disease, also known as amaurotic (having blindness) infantile idiocy and GM_2 gangliosidosis, was first described in 1881 by ophthalmologist Warren Tay and in 1886 by neurologist Bernard Sachs. In the high-risk group, the Ashkenazi Jews, there is a carrier rate of 1 in 30. This autosomal recessive disease is caused by a deficiency of the enzyme hexosaminidase A, while the activity of the other isoenzyme, hexosaminidase B, is increased. Hexosaminidase A catalyzes the degradation of GM_2 ganglioside, and so in Tay-Sachs disease, the unmetabolized ganglioside accumulates in almost all tissues, but its effects are most devastating within the central nervous system and the eye.

Clinical symptoms appear by 6 months of age and include both physical and mental deterioration. Infants have an exaggerated physical response, known as the startle reflex, to noise. Over the span of 1–2 years, a complete vegetative state may develop. An important finding is a cherry-red spot in the macula of each eye, resulting in eventual blindness. There may also be an enlargement (macrocephaly) of the head, seizures, and paralysis. In contrast to the other lipid storage diseases, the spleen, liver, and lymph nodes are not enlarged. The neurons are enlarged by the accumulation of the unmetabolized ganglioside in vacuoles of the cytoplasm.

LABORATORY DIAGNOSIS

The peripheral blood contains vacuolated lymphocytes. The number and size of the vacuoles relate to the duration of disease (Fig. 30–5). These vacuolated lymphocytes, however, are not diagnostic for Tay-Sachs disease, inasmuch as they are also seen in Niemann-Pick disease and in certain leukemias. The major site of pathology is in the central nervous system. Foam cells and vacuolated histiocytes may be found in the bone marrow, which is helpful for characterizing the disease but not diagnostic. Reactions to stains for fat, such as

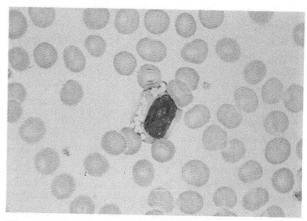

Figure 30–5 A vacuolated lymphocyte from a patient with Tay-Sachs disease. (From Harmening DM [ed]: Clinical Hematology and Fundamentals of Hemostasis, 2nd ed. Philadelphia: FA Davis, 1992:242.)

oil red 0 and Sudan black, are positive. Cytoplasmic inclusions may be seen with the electron microscope, the most prominent being whorled configurations consisting of concentrically arranged membranes surrounding a center of dense material within the lysosomes.[12]

Prenatal detection is important in high-risk groups (Ashkenazi Jews). Decreased hexosaminidase A levels in the fetus can be detected in cultured fibroblasts derived from amniotic fluid.

PROGNOSIS AND TREATMENT

The infantile form is fatal, usually before the age of 4 years. Patients with the juvenile and adult forms have longer survival, which is quite variable. Molecular techniques of RNAase protection assays and PCR have revealed the specific defect to be an amino acid substitution in the alpha subunit of the β-hexosaminidase.[13] This may be of help in genetic counseling for families. Enzyme replacement is being attempted.

Sea-Blue Histiocytosis

Sea-blue histiocytosis, also known as ceroid histiocytosis, is classified as a lipid storage disease because of the accumulation of phosphosphingolipids and glycosphingolipids in the cytoplasm. The storage material in sea-blue histiocytosis is ceroid, which is an oxidation and polymerization product of unsaturated lipids. The lipids accumulate in histiocytes of the spleen, liver, and bone marrow. The exact cause or underlying metabolic defect has not yet been identified, which is why some authors are reluctant to classify this disease as a separate and distinct entity.

This disease or condition is inherited as an autosomal recessive trait and primarily affects adults less than 40 years of age. Patients usually have splenomegaly, hepatomegaly, and thrombocytopenia. Skin conditions may also occur, manifesting as patchy, irregular brownish-gray pigmentation on the face, chest, and shoulders.

LABORATORY DIAGNOSIS

The sea-blue histiocytes can be found in the bone marrow, liver, and spleen. They are large (50–60 μm in diameter) phagocytic macrophages containing prominent granules and fibrillar structures that turn a tropical blue-green after Wright-Giemsa staining. The cytoplasm contains varying amounts of these granules. These colored granules, however, may also be produced by melanin, hemosiderin, and malaria pigment and are not limited solely to sea-blue histiocytosis. The abundant cytoplasm is pinched or curdled and often contains

vacuoles. The nucleus is often eccentric, possessing a single nucleolus. The granules react positively for fat with Sudan black, oil Red 0, and PAS stains.

PROGNOSIS AND TREATMENT

In most patients, the course is benign with few complications. In a few patients, the disease progresses to a fatal outcome, usually resulting from involvement of the bones, lungs, or liver.

AUTOIMMUNE DISEASES

Autoimmune disease occurs when the body produces an immunologic response against itself. Normally the body's immune mechanisms are able to distinguish between a foreign substance and its own substances or tissues. In autoimmune diseases, these mechanisms break down and issue an attack against self, producing antibodies that can cause tissue damage. Tissue injury can be mediated by antibodies or by T cell–mediated reactions. The diseases that result range from those in which a single tissue is targeted (autoimmune hemolytic anemia and anemias caused by increased destruction, discussed in Chapter 17) to those in which several organs are involved (systemic lupus erythematosus [SLE]). SLE is the only autoimmune disease considered here because of the hematologic findings that can occur.

Systemic Lupus Erythematosus

The lupus erythematosus (LE) cell phenomenon was first noted in the bone marrow of patients with SLE by M. Hargraves and associates in 1948. SLE is a multisystem disease of autoimmune origin, characterized by a puzzling array of autoantibodies, particularly anti-nuclear antibodies. The appearance of these limitless numbers of anti-self antibodies indicates that the fundamental defect is a failure of the regulatory mechanisms that maintain self-tolerance. The presence of so many autoantibodies suggests that SLE is caused by polyclonal lymphocyte stimulation rather than antigen-specific stimulation of abnormal clones of autoreactive lymphocytes.[14] The onset may be insidious or may take the form of an acute febrile illness. It is characterized mainly by injury to the skin, joints, kidneys, and serosal membranes. However, virtually every organ in the body may be affected. SLE is predominantly a disease of women (10:1 ratio of women to men), with an incidence of 1 in 700 women between the ages of 20 and 60.

The principal screening test is for anti-nuclear antibodies (ANAs), which are not specific for SLE but are also found in other collagen vascular diseases. More specific tests include anti-DNA antibody to native DNA in abnormal titer and anti-Sm extractable nuclear antigen.[4, 15]

LABORATORY FINDINGS

The principal clinical features include skin rash (butterfly area: across the nose and cheeks), arthritis, and glomerulonephritis. Hematologic features often include an autoimmune hemolytic anemia, leukopenia (often lymphopenia), and thrombocytopenia. The hemolytic anemia and thrombocytopenia are caused by autoantibodies against erythrocytes and platelets. Hemostasis abnormalities in SLE are discussed in Chapter 34.

LE PREPARATION

This is a manual procedure involving the patient's leukocytes and blood or body fluids containing the LE factor. It was a very common procedure years ago but has been replaced by the more sensitive antibody tests. For completeness, the basic principles are included here.

The LE factor is a gammaglobulin that acts as an antibody to nuclear proteins. Blood is subjected to trauma by rotating anti-coagulated blood with glass beads. This action causes extrusion of nuclei from the leukocyte. Three factors must be present in the blood for the LE cell to form: (1) the LE factor, (2) extruded cell nuclei, and (3) phagocytic leukocytes. If the LE factor is present, it causes nuclear lysis, and the phagocytes then engulf this material, causing the LE cell to develop. The LE cell is usually composed of a neutrophil with a large, pale purple, homogenous inclusion (LE body) in the cytoplasm. LE preparations should

be considered positive only if two or more LE cells are seen on a smear. The presence of a single LE cell does not constitute a positive result (Fig. 30–6).

A common source of error with the LE preparation is the presence of "tart cells." A tart cell is formed when phagocytosis of whole nuclei takes place. Tart cells do not indicate a positive result for LE.

The LE cell can occur spontaneously in body fluids other than blood, because all the necessary factors (LE factor, trauma causing extrusion of cell nuclei, and phagocytic leukocytes) are present.

Because the LE procedure is time consuming and the phenomenon cannot always be produced consistently (especially in patients taking steroids), it has essentially been replaced by autoantibody tests.

ANA TEST

The ANA test has replaced the LE preparation as the usual screening test for SLE. It is more sensitive than the LE preparation; however, the results are not specific for SLE. An abnormal ANA result may indicate many other autoimmune disorders such as rheumatoid arthritis, chronic active hepatitis, Sjögren syndrome, and myasthenia gravis; however, virtually every patient with SLE has a positive ANA test result.

ANAs are directed against double- and single-stranded DNA, RNA, histone, and a soluble non-nucleic acid molecule (Smith or Sm antigen). The presence of antibody to native double-stranded DNA is virtually diagnostic for SLE. ANAs are usually detected clinically by immunofluorescence microscopy. Several patterns of nuclear fluores-

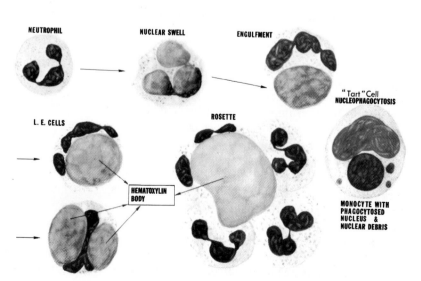

Figure 30–6 Lupus erythematosus phenomenon and nucleophagocytosis. (From Hyun BH, Ashton JK, Dolan K [eds]: Practical Hematology. Philadelphia: WB Saunders, 1975.)

cence are seen, depending on the specific nuclear antigen involved.[4, 15] Patients with SLE have the highest titers of antibody, especially against DNA, which is present in at least 86% of patients. The ANA test is the screening procedure of choice for SLE because of the high sensitivity.

PROGNOSIS AND TREATMENT

This disease has a notoriously variable course, ranging from mild involvement of one or only a few organ systems to a fulminant, life-threatening disease. Therapy is also variable, ranging from aspirin for arthritis symptoms to topical steroids or low-dose anti-malarials when the skin or mucosa are involved to intensive systemic steroids for severe forms. Intensive therapy has been difficult to evaluate because spontaneous remissions do occur. However, systemic corticosteroids are generally recognized as capable of suppressing disease activity and prolonging life. Antigen-antibody components, lymphocyte suppressor function, and other factors that will increase the understanding of autoimmune disorders are under investigation in hopes of developing preventive measures or a cure.

SUMMARY

Lysosomal storage diseases are often classified as disorders of the monocyte/macrophage system because of the "bloated macrophages" that occur in these inborn errors of metabolism. Lysosomal storage disorders may closely resemble one another morphologically, clinically, and biochemically. Differentiation is confirmed by biochemical identification of the metabolite accumulated in the macrophage or by quantitation of enzymes involved in lipid metabolism.

The most widely recognized of these disorders are Gaucher, Niemann-Pick, and Tay-Sachs diseases and sea-blue histiocytosis. In Gaucher disease, because of a lack of the enzyme β-glucocerebrosidase, glucocerebroside is accumulated in the macrophages, causing hepatosplenomegaly, anemia, and thrombocytopenia. The typical Gaucher cell is large with an oval eccentric nuclei. The pale blue cytoplasm has a crumpled tissue paper or chicken scratch appearance. Type 1 entails no cerebral involvement and carries the best prognosis. Type 2 is the most devastating because of central nervous system involvement. Type 3 is intermediate in severity, with some cerebral involvement but not as much as in type 2. Treatment with modified commercially produced glucocerebrosidase has been somewhat successful.

In Niemann-Pick disease, a lack of sphingomyelinase causes the accumulation of sphingomyelin. The Niemann-Pick cell is large with lipid deposits, which cause a foamy or bubbly appearance.

The effects of Tay-Sachs disease are most devastating within the central nervous system and eye. In the bone marrow, foam cells and vacuolated lymphocytes may be found. Hexosaminidase A levels are decreased or absent.

Ceroid is the accumulated metabolite in sea-blue histiocytosis. The disease is much less devastating than the previously discussed disorders; many patients experience a benign course.

SLE is not a hematologic disorder, per se, but one that affects the autoimmune system with some hematologic consequences. For many years, the diagnostic procedure depended on identification of the LE cell buffy coats prepared by traumatizing neutrophils. ANA tests have essentially replaced this procedure, but recognition of the LE cell is important because it may occur spontaneously in body fluids.

REVIEW QUESTIONS

1. Which of the following is/are termed lipid storage diseases?
   a. Tay-Sachs disease
   b. Gaucher disease
   c. Niemann-Pick disease
   d. all of the above

2. Which enzyme is deficient in Gaucher disease?
   a. hexosaminidase A
   b. sphingomyelinase
   c. α-galactosidase
   d. β-glucocerebrosidase

3. What characteristics are typical of Gaucher cells?
   a. macrophages with pale blue, folded cytoplasm
   b. atypical lymphocytes
   c. monocytes with foamy cytoplasm
   d. monocytes with clusters of Auer rods

4. What enzyme is deficient in Niemann-Pick disease?
   a. α-galactosidase
   b. β-glucocerebrosidase
   c. sphingomyelinase
   d. hexosaminidase A

5. Which of the following characteristics are typical of Niemann-Pick Disease?
   a. phagocytic cells with foamy cytoplasm filled with lipid droplets
   b. hypersegmented neutrophils
   c. atypical lymphocytes with foamy cytoplasm
   d. large, granular lymphocytes

6. What enzyme is deficient in Tay-Sachs disease?

a. β-glucocerebrosidase
b. α-galactosidase
c. hexosaminodase A
d. sphingomyelinase

7. An important clinical finding in Tay-Sachs disease is
   a. a cherry-red spot in eye
   b. a rash on the face and neck
   c. bleeding gums
   d. all of the above

8. SLE is characterized by
   a. monoclonal antibodies
   b. autoantibodies
   c. atypical histiocytes
   d. pseudo–Gaucher cells

9. The LE cell characteristically appears as a
   a. large vacuolated histiocyte
   b. neutrophil with a homogenous inclusion in the cytoplasm
   c. monocyte with a pyknotic mass
   d. basophil

10. Clinical and hematologic symptoms of SLE include
    a. a butterfly rash on face
    b. thrombocytopenia
    c. hemolytic anemia
    d. all of the above

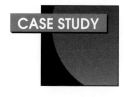
CASE STUDY

A 5-year-old boy was referred to a children's hospital for evaluation of small stature. He had been noted to bruise easily and had experienced nosebleeds at 2- to 3-week intervals since birth. At age 11 months he was noted to have mild splenomegaly, which was not further evaluated at that time. Two older brothers were healthy, and there was no family history of health problems. On physical examination, the child was found to have a noticeably enlarged abdomen. The liver and spleen were markedly enlarged. He had a microcytic, normochromic anemia (Hb 10.2 g/dL) and mild thrombocytopenia, and occasional nucleated red blood cells were noted on the peripheral blood smear. Results of all coagulation factor studies, including a workup for von Willebrand's disease, were normal. The bone marrow was hypercellular, with an M:E ratio of 3:1. Megakaryopoiesis was markedly decreased. Large macrophages with eccentric nuclei and cytoplasm resembling crumpled tissue paper were noted. These cells were periodic acid Schiff stain–positive.

1. What disorder is suggested in this case?

2. What enzyme deficiency is responsible?

3. What is the current treatment for this disease?

References

1. Brady RO, Barton NW: Enzyme replacement therapy for type I Gaucher's disease. *In* Desnick RJ (ed): Treatment of Genetic Diseases. New York: Churchill Livingstone, 199:153–168.
2. Kolodny EH, Ullman MD, Mankin JH, et al: Phenotypic manifestations of Gaucher's disease: clinical features in 48 biochemically verified type I patients and comment on type II patients. *In* Desnick RJ, Gatt S, Grabowski GA (eds): Gaucher's Disease: A Century of Delineation and Research. New York: AJ Liss, 1982: 33–65.
3. Barranger JA, Ginns EI: Glucosylceramide lipidoses: Gaucher's disease. *In* Scriver CR, Beaudet AL, Sly WS, Valle D (eds): Metabolic Basis of Inherited Disease, 6th ed. New York: McGraw-Hill, 1989:1677–1698.
4. Cotran RS, Kumar V, Robbins SL (eds): Robbins Pathologic Basis of Disease, 4th ed. Philadelphia: WB Saunders, 1989:121–162.
5. Robinson DR, Glew RH: Acid phosphatase in Gaucher's disease. Clin Chem 1980; 26:371–382.
6. Tsuji S, Choudary PV, Martin BM, et al: Nucleotide sequence of cDNA containing the complete coding sequence for human lysosomal glucocerebrosidase. J Biol Chem 1986; 261:50–53.
7. Zimran A, Gross E, West C, et al: Prediction of severity of Gaucher's disease by identification of mutations at DNA level. Lancet 1989; 2:349–352.

8. Theophilus B, Latham T, Grabowski GA, Smith FI: Gaucher's disease: molecular heterogeneity and phenotype-genotype correlations. Am J Hum Genet 1989; 45:212–225.
9. Jandl JH: Blood: Textbook of Hematology. Boston: Little, Brown, 1987:424, 488–491.
10. Barton NW, Brady RO, Dambrosia JM, et al: Replacement therapy for inherited enzyme deficiency-macrophage–targeted glucocerebrosidase for Gaucher's disease. N Engl J Med 1991; 324:1464–1470.
11. Doebber TW, Wu MS, Bugianesi RL, et al: Enhanced macrophage uptake of synthetically glycosylated human placental β-glucocerebrosidase. J Biol Chem 1982; 257:2193–2199.
12. Volk BW, Adachi MD, Schneck L: The gangliosidoses. Hum Pathol 1975; 6:555–569.
13. Paw BH, Kaback MM, Neufeld EF: Molecular basis of adult-onset and chronic G_{M2} gangliosidoses in patients of Ashkenazi Jewish origin: Substitution of serine for glycine at position 269 of the α-subunit of β-hexosaminidase. Proc Natl Acad Sci USA 1989; 86:2413.
14. Abbas A: Cellular and Molecular Immunology. Philadelphia: WB Saunders, 1991.
15. Schumacher HR (ed): Primer on the Rheumatic Diseases. Atlanta: Arthritis Foundation, 1988.

PART VI

Hemostasis

CHAPTER 31

Platelet Maturation and Function

Dan Southern and Susan J. Leclair

Objectives

AFTER COMPLETION OF THIS CHAPTER, THE READER WILL BE ABLE TO

1. Describe the origin of platelets and the effect of interleukins and growth factors on the maturation of platelet-producing megakaryocytes.
2. Explain the structural zones of mature platelets and the biologic constituents within each zone.
3. Define the tunica intima, tunica media, and tunica adventitia and explain their association with platelet function.
4. Describe the function of various receptors found on the inner and outer membranes of normal platelets.
5. Describe the physiology of platelets in the resting state and during hemostatic events.
6. Define and discuss activation, adherence, and aggregation of platelets.
7. Explain production of thromboxane A_2 and prostaglandin I_2 and their biologic effect on platelets.

Hemostasis is a balanced process that halts bleeding after blood vessels have been traumatized. Five major components involved in maintaining hemostasis are: vascular integrity, platelet function, fibrin formation (coagulation), control (inhibitory) systems, and lysis (breakdown) of fibrin clots (fibrin lysis). This chapter deals with vascular elements, platelet formation, and the interaction between them. The relationship between platelets and the coagulation schemes are described in more detail in Chapter 32, Normal Hemostasis.

VASCULAR INTEGRITY

The normal vascular wall is composed of three layers: the tunica intima, tunica media, and tunica adventitia. The tunica intima consists of a nonthrombogenic layer of endothelial cells, a basement membrane containing collagen, and an internal elastic membrane. External to the intima is a layer of smooth muscle, collagen, and an external elastic membrane known as the tunica media. Arteries have a thicker tunica media than veins. Less muscle is seen in capillaries and veins than in arterioles (Fig. 31–1). External to the media, collagen and fibroblasts make up the tunica adventitia. This layer is much thicker in veins than arteries.

Normal vessel walls perform three vital functions in hemostasis:

1. They provide a surface resistant to thrombus formation.
2. When disrupted, they provide the initial stimuli for thrombus formation (i.e., platelet activating factor [PAF], tissue factor III, collagen).
3. They provide inhibitors for platelet activity (prostaglandin I_2) and activators for clearance of the thrombus through fibrin lysis (t-PA).

These activities by the vessels make them integral to hemostasis.

Abnormalities of vascular tissue represent a group of hemostatic diseases that includes hypercoagulation and hypocoagulation. A delicate balance exists among the initiators, inhibitors, and clearance properties controlled by the blood vessel wall. Vascular integrity can be compromised through inherited defects, such as hereditary telangectasia, congenital defects such as berry aneurysms, and acquired defects such as those seen in chronic diabetics.

Normal vessels—those with an adequate number of functional platelets—prevent red blood cells from escaping under normal shear forces, thus, bruising, or purpura, is not evident in normal, nontraumatized tissues (Fig. 31–2). Leakage of red blood cells from small pinpoint arterioles and venules is called petechia. A larger loss of blood into soft tissue from veins is ecchymosis. An ecchymosis with significant swelling is termed a hematoma. Bleeding from arteries constitutes a hemorrhage.

Platelet Role in Vascular Integrity

When normal in number and function, platelets maintain vascular integrity by preventing red blood cells from escaping from the blood vessels into the tissue. Too few or dysfunctional platelets result in indiscriminate leakage of red blood cells into subendothelial tissue and failure to repair vessels. Platelets prevent red cell loss through damaged luminal surfaces of blood vessels or with endothelial sloughing.[1] Platelets act as a base upon which circulating coagulation factors combine to form a fibrin clot and also to supply the mitogenic stimulant necessary to initiate cellular division and tissue repair.

PLATELET PRODUCTION AND FUNCTION

Historical Aspects

Platelets were first described by Donne,[2] Gerber,[3] Addison,[4] and Simon.[5] In 1872, Hayem[6] confirmed that platelets were unique cellular elements of the blood. The origin of platelets from megakaryocytes was first described by Julius Bizzozero[7] and was later confirmed by J. Homer Wright.[8] In the 1940s and early 1950s, the ultrastructure of platelets was visualized with electron microscopy. In 1947 Quick and Brinkhous linked platelets to thrombin formation. Since the 1950s, work has continued on the platelet's biochemical and biophysical roles.

Precursor Cell Development

Platelets, also called thrombocytes, are cytoplasmic fragments released from a parent cell known as a megakaryocyte. Megakaryocytes are large cells

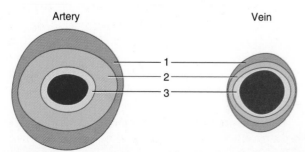

Artery   Vein

Figure 31–1 Cross-sections of an artery (left) and a vein (right) showing the different thicknesses of tunica intima (3), the tunica media (2), and the tunica adventitia (1).

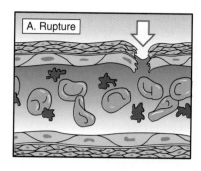

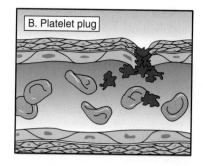

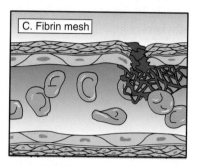

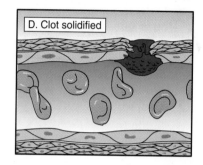

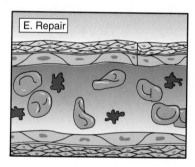

Figure 31–2 General schema for platelet activity. (From Powers LW: Diagnostic Hematology, Clinical and Technical Principles. St. Louis: CV Mosby, 1989:140.)

(80–150 μ in diameter), which are found predominantly in the bone marrow and to a smaller degree in the spleen and lungs. Similar to erythrocytes and leukocytes, megakaryocytes develop from a pluripotential stem cell that has been influenced by colony stimulating factors (CSFs) produced by macrophages, fibroblasts, T lymphocytes, and stimulated endothelial cells. Additional influences, such as interleukin-3 and -6 (IL-3 and IL-6), which appear to be instrumental in differentiation of stem cells into platelet producing megakaryoblasts,[9] and megakaryocyte CSF (Meg-CSF) and granulocyte CSF (G-CSF) synergistically stimulate production of progenitor cells.[10] Meg-CSF is thought to be generated by bone marrow cells in response to megakaryocytic mass. As the number of megakaryocytes decrease, the amount of Meg-CSF increases. Thrombopoietin is generated predominantly by the kidney, and to a lesser amount, by the liver and spleen, in response to a demand for platelets. It stimulates megakaryocyte progenitor cells to mature and release platelets,[11] although its chemical nature is still not completely known.

The spleen is the part of the regulatory system for platelet production wherein approximately 30% of peripheral blood platelets are sequestered. Sudden depletion of platelets, resulting from consumption in clotting or immune and nonimmune destruction, may rapidly empty the splenic pool.[12] In response, thrombopoietin causes maturation of the megakaryoblasts to produce a marrow response equal to the loss of platelets. Because the action of thrombopoietin is similar to that of erythropoietin, any increases in thrombopoietin will speed up the maturation of megakaryocytes.[13] This accelerated maturation results in less platelet production per cell. If the consumption or destruction of platelets continues, the platelet count will fall to a level incapable of maintaining normal vascular and hemostatic integrity and a condition called acute thrombocytopenia.

Platelet production is unique to hematopoietic cells. Erythrocyte and granulocyte precursors usually divide four times during their maturation producing 16 mature cells from each committed stem cell. Megakaryocytes do not experience complete cellular division. A process called endomitosis or endoreduplication, in which normal telophase is missing, creates a cell with a multi-lobed nucleus. Each lobe of the nucleus is diploid (2N), having a full complement of 23 pairs of chromosomes capable of transcription. Megakaryocytes are polyploid, that is, they have more than two complete sets of chromosomes. In the endomitotic divisions of the nucleus, the more ploidy there is, the larger the cytoplasmic volume will be. Megakaryocytes usually achieve 8N to 16N, or 8 to 16 chromosome pairs. Some megakaryocytes will develop 16 lobes (32N), whereas some will only reach two. Megakaryocytes with 64 (128N) have been reported in disease situations but are exceptional. When the turnover rate of platelets is in a steady state, the average megakaryocyte, which is 8N or 16N, produces approximately 1500–2000 platelets.[14]

Megakaryoblast (Figs. 31–3 to 31–7)

The first cell in the maturation sequence is called a megakaryoblast (MK1). Megakaryoblasts are typically 10–15 μ in diameter with a high nu-

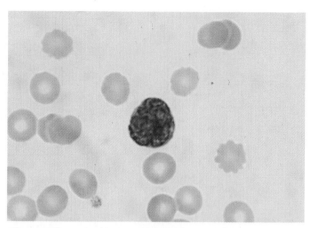

Figure 31–4 Megakaryoblast. Note similarity to other blast cells, which makes identification by morphology alone inadvisable.

clear matter to cytoplasm ratio. They have a single nucleus with two to six nucleoli. The cytoplasm is scanty, blue, and contains no granules. They may resemble lymphocytes or other marrow blast cells and thus cannot be accurately identified by morphology alone. During this stage they may experience nuclear division and gain enough cytoplasm to be up to 50 μ in diameter. Megakaryoblasts occasionally enter the blood and travel to extramarrow sites where they mature further.[15] Occasionally, megakaryoblasts are encountered in normal peripheral blood. In patients with chronic myelocytic leukemia and other myeloproliferative diseases, micro-megakaryocytes with characteristic cytoplasmic "budding" may be seen in the peripheral blood.

Promegakaryocyte

A megakaryoblast matures into a promegakaryocyte (MK2) which enlarges to 80 μ. Three kinds of granules formed in the Golgi apparatus are dense,

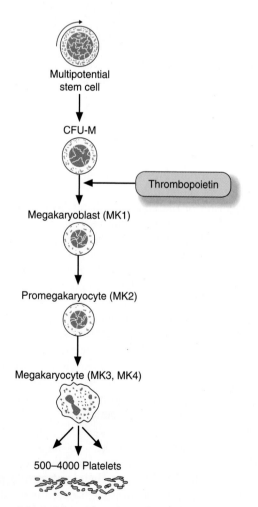

Multipotential
stem cell

CFU-M

Thrombopoietin

Megakaryoblast (MK1)

Promegakaryocyte (MK2)

Megakaryocyte (MK3, MK4)

500–4000 Platelets

Figure 31–3 Maturation of megakaryocytes.

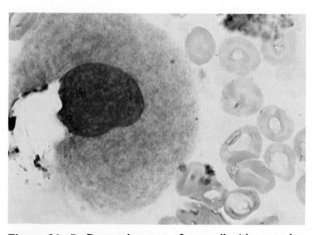

Figure 31–5 Promegakaryocyte. Large cell with no nuclear lobes.

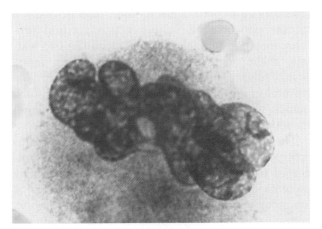

Figure 31–6 Basophilic megakaryocyte. Very blue cytoplasm with evidence of lines of demarcation.

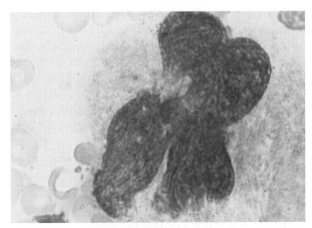

Figure 31–7 Active (platelet-forming) megakaryocyte. Note initial phase of platelet budding.

alpha, and lysosomal. They are dispersed throughout the cytoplasm.[16]

Basophilic Megakaryocyte

Distinct granulation and final divisions of the nucleus occur in the third stage called the basophilic megakaryocyte (MK3). Cytoplasmic lines of demarcation begin to be evident, outlining individual cytoplasmic fragments later to be released as platelets.[17] Each demarcated area consists of a membrane, cytoskeleton, a system of microtubules, canals, and a portion of cytoplasmic granules. Each area also has a store of glycogen that will help

sustain the platelet for 9 to 11 days. The cytoplasmic fragment develops a membrane with several types of glycoprotein (GP) receptors to allow activation, adherence, aggregation, and crosslinking.

Megakaryocyte

In the final stage of maturation, the mature megakaryocyte (MK4) releases cytoplasmic fragments through marrow sinusoid fenestrations in a process called budding or shedding of platelets[18] (Fig. 31–8). When all platelets have been released into the bloodstream, the remaining naked nuclei are phagocytized by marrow histiocytes. Because

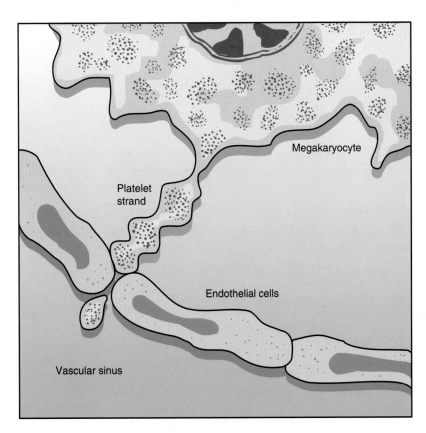

Figure 31–8 Megakaryocyte strand budding platelets. (From Powers LW: Diagnostic Hematology, Clinical and Technical Principles. St. Louis: CV Mosby, 1989: 146.)

thousands of platelets are shed from each mature megakaryocyte, fewer progenitor cells are necessary as compared with other cellular precursors. Because of their size, megakaryocytes can be found quickly on a Wright's stained marrow film, when using either a 4× or 10× objective. Evidence of their presence without much searching usually indicates adequate production. Megakaryocytic hyperplasia indicates a normal response to an increased demand or an autonomous proliferation as found in myeloproliferative diseases.

PLATELET CONSTITUENTS AND STRUCTURE

As platelets enter the peripheral blood circulation, their average diameter is 2.5 microns. Unstimulated platelets are lentiform discs with smooth margins. The platelet structure can be divided into peripheral, sol-gel, organelle, and membrane zones.[19] Figure 31–9 points out these regions and the structures located in each zone.

Peripheral Zone

This includes the platelet membrane, glycocalyx (exterior coat), and cytoskeleton, which is rich in actin and myosin (thrombasthenin) fibrils and in microtubules. The platelet membrane is similar in

structure to most cell membranes, that is, it has a bipolar phospholipid bilayer with structural proteins incorporated below and through the two leaflets. Sialic acid (neuraminic acid) on the membrane surface negatively charges platelets.[20] The traversing integral proteins act as receptors, pumps, enzymes, and cofactors necessary for platelet activity.

The glycocalyx is an exterior coat of side chains protruding beyond the membrane surface and connected to the integral glycoproteins. Many plasma proteins are held there by electrostatic charges or are weakly attached to receptors. The glycocalyx accumulation of plasma proteins is an extension of the inner absorption of the same proteins. The glycocalyx coat may range in width from 10 to 50 nm. Platelet ABO and HLA antigens are expressed in the glycocalyx region as the membrane receptors for thrombin, von Willebrand factor (vWF), epinephrine, ADP, and PAF.[21]

In the resting platelet, fibrils line up under the membrane surface and throughout the cytoplasm in random fashion. During activation, they take on a parallel posture. They are attached to both the platelet cytoskeleton, which is made up of structural proteins of the membrane, and the circumferential microtubules of the cytoskeleton by actin.[22] ATP–assisted contraction of these myosins occurs in the activated platelet and causes the membrane to change its shape from smooth margined discs to spiny projections.

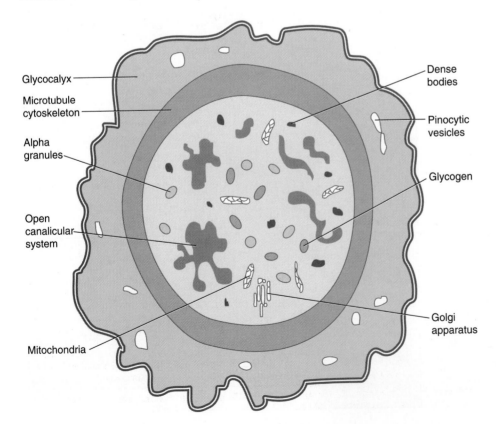

Figure 31–9 A line drawing representing platelet ultrastructure showing significant organelles and zones. Receptor sites may be found on the outer membrane.

Glycocalyx

Microtubule cytoskeleton

Alpha granules

Open canalicular system

Mitochondria

Dense bodies

Pinocytic vesicles

Glycogen

Golgi apparatus

Sol-Gel

The microtubular coil and membrane cytoskeleton represent an extension of the platelet membrane winding inwardly throughout the platelet interior. During activation and constriction of platelets, the open canalicular system (OCS) delivers the granular contents to the surface. The multiple pores of the OCS connect the internal contents with the surface. In the bloodstream, pores allow plasma to enter the microtubule and canal system. Each platelet absorbs plasma coagulation factors. Alpha granules absorb several, especially factor I (fibrinogen) and factor V (labile factor). Recent evidence suggests that megakaryocytes do not synthesize plasma clotting factors; rather, platelets acquire their plasma clotting proteins by endocytosis in the developing megakaryocyte or as they circulate through the blood.[23] Platelets internalize these proteins in proportion to their plasma concentration; thus, fibrinogen, which has the highest concentration (200–400 mg/dL) in the plasma, is the dominant clotting protein in the platelet. Several other blood clotting factors adsorb onto the platelets and are held there by the surface tension of the protruding integral proteins of the platelet membrane. When platelets are activated, most of the clotting factors are readily available.

This zone also includes the dense tubular system (DTS), which is the remnant of the smooth endoplasmic reticulum from the megakaryocyte. The DTS is the primary site for sequestration of internal calcium ions. This calcium is not to be confused with the calcium packaged in the dense bodies released during activation but should be thought of as a source of calcium ions released during activation to drive calcium-dependent mechanisms. Adenylate cyclase, the enzyme responsible for cyclic adenosine monophosphate (cAMP) production, is coupled to surface receptors through G proteins. Cyclic AMP is responsible for phosphorylation of receptor proteins within the DTS, which chelates calcium ions and causes them to accumulate in the dense tubules. Because platelet activation is calcium dependent, the net effect of this activity is to inhibit platelet activity.[24] A high concentration of calcium causes the DTS to appear dense on transmission electron microscopy. A similar effect with calcium-rich dense granules (dense bodies) is seen in the organelle zone.

Organelle Zone

The interior of the platelet contains mitochondria, lysosomes, electron-dense granules, and alpha granules that are released during platelet activity. The mitochondria provide oxidative phosphorylation of ATP energy through its glycolytic and citric acid (Krebs) cycles. In resting platelets, glycogen storage is kept at maximum. After activation and centralization of organelles, breakdown of glycogen (glycogenolysis) is necessary to produce the amount of ATP needed to create a shape change or to produce enough cAMP to reverse the activation and return it to the resting state.

The granules produced by megakaryocytes for each platelet are filled with specific constituents released when platelets participate in various phases of hemostasis (Table 31–1). During activity, dense granules are released after adherence to subendothelial tissue or thrombin. Each normal platelet has up to 10 dense granules. Shape change and intracellular calcium mobilization during platelet activation enable dense granules to release their contents.

A platelet may have over 100 alpha granules whose contents are released next. Calcium mobilization eventually leads to the activation of cyclooxygenase necessary for the production of thromboxane A_2, a powerful vasoconstrictor and platelet agonist necessary to cause the release of granule contents through the open canalicular system. The same pathway exercised in nearby healthy endothelial cells produces inhibitory prostaglandin I_2 that relaxes platelets entering the area and hinders their activation by sequestration of their calcium. Alpha granules also release a platelet derived growth factor (PDGF) that causes proliferation of endothelial, smooth muscle, and fibroblast cells. This mitogen is found in platelets, granulocytes, and endothelial cells. PDGF is chemotactic for smooth muscle cells.

Thrombospondin is a large (450-kD) glycoprotein released from alpha granules that appears to enhance platelet adherence and aggregation by at-

Table 31–1. GRANULAR CONTENTS

Dense granules contain ATP, ADP, ionized calcium (factor IV), magnesium, epinephrine, phosphate and serotonin.

Alpha granules contain platelet derived growth factor (PDGF), heparin neutralizing factor (PF4), plasminogen activator inhibitor (PAI-1), fibronectin, beta-thromboglobulin and thrombospondin protein (TSP), albumin, fibrinogen (factor I), and factor V absorbed from plasma.

Lysosomal granules contain hydrolytic enzymes that may synergistically enhance activation of the intrinsic clotting cascade. Lysosomal granules contain microbiocidal enzymes, neutral proteinases, and peroxidase, along with hexosaminidase, galactosidase, glucuronidase, arabinosidase, glycerophosphatase, and aryl-sulfatase enzymes. Lysosomes also contain cathepsin G and elastase, which are known platelet agonists when their source is from granulocytes.

Abbreviations: ATP, adenosine triphosphate; ADP, adenosine diphosphate.

taching to corresponding platelet receptors. It is released by platelets and endothelial cells. Thrombospondin is classified as an adhesive macromolecule instrumental in facilitating cell-to-cell interactions. Thrombospondin has a unique receptor for its attachment to platelets.[25]

Two other compounds released from alpha granules inhibit heparin released by mast cells and basophils. These are platelet factor 4 (PF4) and beta-thromboglobulin (BTG). Both prevent heparin neutralization of thrombin and other blood clotting enzymes. PF4 has been shown to be released from other disrupted cells such as granulocytes and endothelial cells. PF4 is much more potent than its counterpart BTG. BTG and PF4 are believed to be products of cleavage of a common precursor substance. Another inhibitor released by platelet alpha granules is called plasminogen activator inhibitor 1 (PAI-1), which neutralizes tissue plasminogen activator (TPA) released from traumatized endothelial cells. If not neutralized, TPA would activate the fibrin lysis system before a clot could be formed. Endothelial cells also release a PAI-2 inhibitor that works along the same lines to prevent premature dissolution of the clot.

Acquired Surface Markers

When alpha granules are released, a surface marker appears on the activated platelet that is not detectable on resting platelets. This acquired membrane marker, GMP-140, is found only on activated platelets and is believed to be a part of the alpha granule membrane lodged in the platelet membrane. With flow cytometry, this marker may be used to differentiate resting platelets from activated platelets.

Lysosomal Granule Release

Lysosomal granule release is still not fully understood. Lytic enzymes contained in lysosomes can trigger coagulation as evidenced in persons with myeloproliferative diseases with increased clotting. Recent evidence shows that cathepsin G and elastase released from lysosomes can trigger platelet activation.[26] Like the GMP-140 activation marker, a lysosomal membrane marker, protein 2, has been recognized only on activated platelets.[27]

Finally, lysosomal granules, in response to thromboxane/prostaglandin synthesis, release their enzymes after platelets are activated by a strong agonist such as thrombin or thromboxane A_2.

Receptors

Several glycoprotein receptors have been identified on the platelet membrane and internal sur-

Table 31-2. PLATELET RECEPTORS AND ACTIVITY	
Name	**Function**
Glycoprotein Ia and IIa	Adherence of platelets to charged collagen
Glycoprotein Ib-IX	Adherence to collagen or platelet bound vWF
Glycoprotein IIb-IIIa	Aggregation of platelets in the presence of fibrinogen, fibrin, fibronectin, and vWF
Glycoprotein V	Platelet activation
PAF receptor	Activation, shape change, and secretion
Factor V receptor	Attachment of factor V to platelet phospholipid
ADP receptor	Increases calcium levels by inhibiting adenylate cyclase
Epinephrine receptor	Platelet activation
Thrombospondin receptor	Aggregation of platelets
Thromboxane A_2 and prostacyclin I_2 receptors	Calcium release from DTS and subsequent release of dense, alpha, and lysosomal granules

Abbreviations: vWF, von Willebrand factor; PAF, platelet activating factor; ADP, adenosine diphosphate; DTS, dense tubular system.

faces. Glycoproteins exposed in the resting platelet are receptors for elements not normally present in blood (Table 31–2). Those hidden until activation are capable of reacting with elements found in blood and can cause obvious problems for circulating platelets.[28] The membrane receptors initiate the complex communication system of signal transduction.

Laboratory evaluation of platelet agonists is usually done with only one stimulus at a time. It should be kept in mind, that during vessel trauma in vivo, platelets are simultaneously exposed to multiple stimuli. Understanding each receptor-ligand signal is important, but understanding the synergy of multiple signals is also important. The following section presents the effects of each agonist with the realization that the whole is usually more than the sum of its parts.

Specific Glycoprotein Receptors

Platelets display multiple copies of several specific glycoprotein receptors for ADP, thrombin, vWF, collagen, fibrinogen, fibrin, fibronectin, epinephrine, PAF, thrombospondin, thromboxane A_2, and prostacyclin I_2. The same glycoprotein may contain more than one receptor.

The receptor for vWF is glycoprotein Ib (GPIb). GPIb is a two-chained receptor produced by the megakaryocyte. The alpha chain (143 kD) and the beta chain (22 kD) are held together by a connecting protein (17 kD) named GPIX. Platelets and vWF are both negatively charged by sialic acid residues. In the peripheral blood they repel each other. This repulsive effect keeps platelets from aggregating with plasma vWF in the circulation. Stimulators for glycoprotein Ib receptor is collagen with or without PAF liberated from disturbed endothelial cells in vessel walls.[29] This receptor has also been named the Bernard-Soulier protein because it is missing in Bernard-Soulier syndrome (BSS) (see Chapter 33).

GPV and GPIb-IX act as thrombin and vWF receptor sites. GPIb-IX, with vWF attached, allows platelets to adhere to fibrinogen and fibrin deposited on subendothelial tissues as well as to the extrinsic clot formed outside the wound.[30] During clot lysis, thrombin hydrolyzes GPIb-IX and GPV receptors from platelets releasing their attachment to vWF.[31] GPV is similar in structure to GPIb and, along with GPIb-IX, is also missing in Bernard-Soulier syndrome.[32]

GPIIb-IIIa complex, the receptor for fibrinogen, becomes activated after stimulation by initial activation, adherence, and aggregation. When granules are brought to the surface, the platelet membrane exposes fibrinogen receptors.[33] The GPIIb-IIIa complex also couples fibronectin, with vWF helping platelets adhere and later crosslinking platelets together in a stabilized plug and plasminogen.[34]

The approximately 2500 factor V receptors hold thrombin-modified factor V (V_m) in place on the platelet surface (PF3) so it can act, in conjunction with plasma factor X, as a cofactor for conversion of prothrombin to thrombin in the intrinsic clotting system.[35] Factor V produced by liver cells is absorbed from the plasma into the platelet alpha granules and is secreted when platelets release their alpha granule contents. Factor V released from the platelets clings to the factor V receptors. Thrombin generated from the extrinsic and intrinsic clotting systems modifies platelet-bound factor V to factor V_m.

When epinephrine or norepinephrine (catecholamines) is released during trauma, activation of platelets occurs. This does not cause a shape change but initiates production of thromboxane A_2 synthesis and ADP release. ADP, released from the platelet dense granules, attaches to external ADP receptors on the platelet surface. This allows further aggregation of unbound activated platelets forming a plug of loosely aggregated platelets joined to each other by GIIb-IIIa occupation with fibrinogen.

Thromboxane A_2 and prostaglandin I_2, two other important glycoprotein receptors, both originate from a pathway common to platelets and endothelial cells (Fig. 31–10). The difference in the final product is under control of the enzyme supplied by each particular cell at the termination of the pathway.[36] Platelets contain the enzyme thromboxane synthetase which produces the vasoconstrictive agonist thromboxane A_2 (TXA_2). When TXA_2 couples with its receptor on the platelet, it creates additional calcium mobilization and constriction which releases the second wave–alpha granules. Endothelial cells provide a different terminal enzyme, prostacyclin synthase, which produces the vasodilator prostaglandin I_2 which has inhibitory effects on platelets. PGI_2 sends a second message through activation of adenylate cyclase, which raises the level of cyclic adenosine monophosphate (cAMP) in platelets, thus causing them to return to the resting state. These opposing prostaglandins are produced from the same arachidonic acid precursor derived from their membrane phospholipids when phosphatidylinositol is hydrolyzed by phospholipase C and phospholipase A_2.[37]

PLATELET ACTIVITY

Activation and Adhesion

In the early 1970s, PAF was described as the mediator that caused platelet activation.[38] PAF is produced by endothelial cells, polymorphonuclear neutrophils (PMNs), monocytes, and platelets. It is also liberated during vascular injury.[39] Receptors for PAF can also be found on PMNs and smooth muscle; they are chemotactic for white blood cells. Calcium ions stimulate single stranded actinomyosins (thrombasthenin) to assemble and centralize granules and other organelles of the platelet during the shape change process. Changing shape allows the release of dense granule contents that further activate the platelets. Activated, spiny platelets adhere more readily to each other than to smooth, discoid resting platelets. When platelets reach the point of granule content release, they are irreversibly activated (Fig. 31–11).

Initial adherence between platelets and the subendothelial tissue depends on the GPIb receptor and vWF. A "spreading effect" of the initial platelet monolayer covering exposed subendothelial tissue is caused through GIa-collagen interaction and is independent of vWF, although initial adhesion through vWF and GPIb is a necessary prerequisite. There is some secondary adherence to fibrinogen and fibronectin clinging to the subendothelial surface through the platelet's newly exposed fibrinogen receptors (GPIIb and GPIIIa). After a platelet monolayer is formed on exposed subendothelial tissues, additional blood vWF multimers allow adherence between tissue bound platelets and activated platelets near the wound.[40] Free floating platelets cling to adherent platelets to build a solid platelet plug over the damaged area.

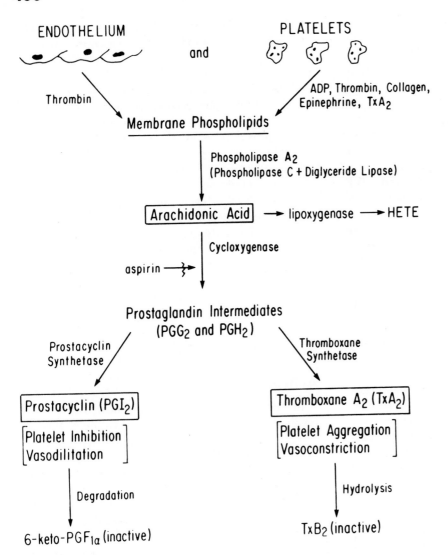

Figure 31–10 Thromboxane A$_2$ and prostaglandin I$_2$ pathways. (From Burns ER: Clinical Management of Bleeding and Thrombosis. Boston: Blackwell Scientific, 1987:5.)

Aggregation

FIRST-WAVE PLATELET INTERACTIONS

Activation and adherence of platelets cause the release of dense granules through the open canalicular system. Among the granular contents released are ADP and ATP.[41] When ADP attaches to its receptor, it has a negative (inhibitory) effect on the second messenger enzyme, adenylate cyclase, which, in resting platelets, increases cAMP levels within the platelet by converting ATP to cAMP to allow phosphorylation of proteins in the dense tubular system (DTS). ADP binding is inhibitory to this process and calcium ions accumulate in the cell cytoplasm.

Serotonin (5 hydroxy-indol acetic acid), a powerful vasoconstrictor, is released from dense granules. This is an ATP dependent reaction with the ATP supplied from the dense granules.[41] Smooth muscle contraction occurs in the tunica media of the injured vessel and in the smooth muscle downstream from the injury site.[42] The resultant vessel contraction slows blood flow (stasis) at the site. In capillaries, venules, and arterioles, the vessel may be completely occluded temporarily by constriction. Blood stasis makes platelets and clotting factors more available while limiting the number of inhibitor proteins flowing into the immediate area.

SECOND-WAVE AGGREGATION OF PLATELETS

Continued aggregation of platelets requires alpha granule release of fibrinogen, fibronectin, and vWF. It also depends upon exposure of fibrinogen and fibronectin receptors on the platelet surface. These two steps rely on intracellular calcium ions. In addition to the calcium raising effects of PAF and ADP, other pathways may be involved in the release of calcium. Before release of alpha granules, aggregation can be reversed. Adherence and release, however, commit the platelet irreversibly.

Several interactive enzymatic pathways occur in activated platelets to accomplish the release of

Circulating
platelet

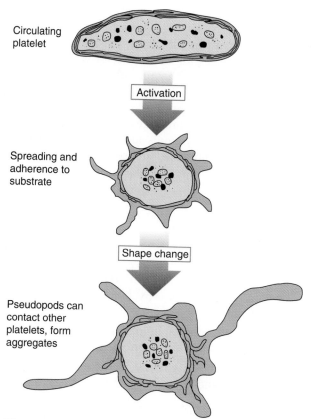

Activation

Spreading and
adherence to
substrate

Shape change

Pseudopods can
contact other
platelets, form
aggregates

Figure 31–11 Summary of platelet shape change. (From Powers LW: Diagnostic Hematology, Clinical and Technical Principles. St. Louis: CV Mosby, 1989:153.)

arachidonic acid from membrane associated phosphatidylinositol or triphosphatidylinositol. The route taken by the platelet is dependent upon the agonist involved. The result in each case is the release of arachidonic acid which is converted to thromboxane A_2 or prostacyclin I_2.[43] These two antithetical products of similar pathways represent a balancing act that allows platelets involved at the clot site to finish their work while inhibiting activation of new platelets coming into the hemostatic zone.

Arachidonic acid enters the pathway for prostacyclin-thromboxane production in either platelets or endothelial cells. Arachidonic acid is converted to endoperoxide by the heme containing enzyme cyclooxygenase.[44] Cyclooxygenase activity is inhibited by aspirin and similar analgesic drugs. Endoperoxides are converted to cell specific end-products by platelets and adjacent healthy endothelial cells. Platelets contain the final enzyme, thromboxane A_2 synthase, to convert the cyclic endoperoxide to a vasoconstrictive, short-lived platelet agonist. Thromboxane A_2 attaches to thromboxane receptors on platelets causing them to further constrict and release their alpha and lysosome granular contents. Thromboxane A_2 spontaneously degrades to an inactive thromboxane B_2 form.

As alpha granules are squeezed from the open canalicular system to the surface to release their contents, they also modulate the GPIIb-IIIa fibrinogen receptor complex at the surface of the platelet. Fibrin monomers and fibrinogen, as well as fibronectin and vWF, help to stabilize the platelet plug. The final result is the formation of a platelet plug that is cohesive enough to prevent further loss of blood. This platelet surface, referred to as platelet factor 3, provides the foundation for an intrinsic clot to form.

Clot Retraction

The final tightly bound platelet plug is constricted when calcium ATP–simulated actin and myosins contract and reduces the plug by expelling trapped fluid. This is analogous, albeit much slower, to clot retraction in vitro. Clot constriction or retraction depends on the presence of fibrinogen receptors occupied by fibrinogen, fibrin, or fibronectin. When contractions occur, aggregated platelets must be tightly attached to each other. Platelets missing these receptors do not retract and the condition is referred to as thrombasthenia.

Effectiveness

Platelet effectiveness in maintaining hemostasis is more dependent on their function than numbers. Persons with normal or elevated platelet counts (thrombocytosis) may exhibit bleeding because their platelets are dysfunctional. Conversely, persons with a low platelet count (thrombocytopenia) may have no bleeding symptoms if their platelets function normally. The reference ranges for platelet count are 150 to 400×10^9/L in SI units or 150,000 to 400,000/mm³ in standard American units. Counts below 50×10^9/L may not always maintain vascular integrity under stress such as surgery but thrombocytopenic patients often do not bleed at counts between $10–50 \times 10^9$/L. Spontaneous bleeding may occur in patients with platelet counts below 10×10^9/L. Very young platelets may possess increased activity that compensates for the lack of numbers. This reinforces the idea that functionality rather than number is the key to maintaining hemostasis.

Platelet Inhibition

Up to the point of alpha granule release, the activation of platelets can be reversed by external signals that stimulate the production of cAMP within the platelet. A major external influence on cAMP production comes from adjacent, healthy endothelial cells. PGI_2 is an inhibitory prostacyclin produced from endoperoxide. Its effect on platelets is to reverse activation and prevent platelets from being activated by raising their level of cAMP to favor calcium sequestration.[45]

When PGI_2 reacts with prostaglandin receptors on platelets, communication with a second messenger enzyme, adenylate cyclase, ensues. This signal transduction is transmitted by a complex activating guanine nucleotide–bound activating protein (G protein).[46] Once activated, this signal causes receptor proteins in the dense tubular system to become phosphorylated and negatively charged. The phosphorylated protein receptors attract cellular calcium and reduce calcium ion levels. PGI_2 is also a powerful vasodilator in opposition to the platelet produced thromboxane A_2. The vasodilation effect causes relaxation of platelets and smooth muscle downstream. This helps reestablish blood flow and provides additional platelets and blood clotting factors at the wound site. An obvious balance between these two mechanisms helps confine platelet activity and clotting to the injured site and helps limit the number of resources used in the process.

Platelet activity can be partially inhibited by drugs that affect cyclooxygenase, like aspirin. This aspirin effect produces an irreversible inhibition of cyclooxygenase in platelets. Aspirin also affects endothelial cell production of PGI_2, but endothelial cells can produce additional cyclooxygenase to neutralize this action. Congenital deficiency of enzymes in the thromboxane/prostacyclin pathways can mimic the aspirin effect and deficiencies are likely restricted to platelets.

SUMMARY

Platelets play major roles in hemostasis by forming a platelet plug at the site of vessel trauma and then serving as the phospholipid foundation for fibrin deposition. The glycoprotein receptors on the platelet surface and sub-surface allow the reception of external messages from vascular and circulatory sources. Signals are transmitted across the platelet membranes to "second messengers" controlled by calcium mobilization or calcium sequestration.

REVIEW QUESTIONS

1. Describe the unique process by which platelets are produced. How is it different from the maturation sequence of red blood cells or white blood cells?
2. List the ingredients in platelet dense granules and describe their function when released.
3. List the ingredients found in the alpha granules in platelets and describe their function.
4. Explain the tunica intima, tunica media, and tunica adventitia of blood vessels. How do these regions differ in arteries, veins, and capillaries?
5. The thromboxane pathway has two major tracks. Describe which path the platelet takes and which path endothelial cells take. How do the activities of their end-products differ?
6. Describe how calcium levels are controlled in the cytoplasm of platelets.

References

1. Bick RL: Disorders of thrombosis and hemostasis; clinical and laboratory practice. Chicago: ASCP Press, 1992: 1–11.
2. Donne AD: L'origine des globules de sang, de leur mode de formation et de leur fin. CK Acad Sco 1842; 14:366.
3. Gerber F: Elements of General and Minute Anatomy of Man and Mammals. London: G. Guliver, 1842.
4. Addison W: On the colorless corpuscles and on the molecules and cytoblasts in the blood. London Med Gaz (NS) 1842; 30:144.
5. Simon JF: Physiologische und pathologische Antropochemie mit Berücksichtigung der eigentlichen Zoochemie. Handbuch der angewandten medizinischen Chemie nach dem neuesten Standpunkte der Wissenschaft und nach zahlreichen eigenen Untersuchungen, Teil II. Berlin: A. Förstner, 1842.
6. Hayem G: Recherches sur l'évolution des hématicies dans le sang de l'homme et des vertébrés. Arch Physiol Norm Pathol 1878; 5:692.
7. Bizzozero J: Über eine neue Formbestand these des Blutes und desen Rolle bei er Thrombose und der Blutgerinnung. Virchows Arch Pathol Anat 1882; 90:261.
8. Wright JH: The origin and nature of the blood platelet. Boston Med Surg J 1906; 154:163.
9. Herodin F, Mestries JC, Janodet D, et al: Recombinant glycosylated human interleukin-6 accelerates peripheral

blood platelet count recovery in radiation induced bone marrow depression in baboons. Blood 1992; 80(3):688–695.
10. Bell A: Hematopoiesis: morphology of human blood cells. In Harmening DM (ed.): Clinical Hematology and Fundamentals of Hemostasis. Philadelphia: FA Davis, 1992:37.
11. McDonald TP, Andrews RB, Clift R, Gottsell M: Characterization of a thrombocytopenic-stimulating factor from kidney cell culture medium. Exp Hematol 1981; 9:288.
12. Hill-Zobel RL, McCandless B, Kang SA, Chillappa G, et al: Organ distribution and fate of human platelets: studies of asplenic and splenomegalic patients. Am J Haematol 1986; 23:231–238.
13. Murphy MJ: Megakaryocyte colony stimulating factor and thrombopoiesis. Hematol Oncol Clin North Am 1989; 3:465.
14. Powers LW: Diagnostic Hematology, Clinical and Technical Principles. St. Louis: CV Mosby, 1989.
15. Thompson AR, Karker LA: Manual of Hemostasis and Thrombosis. Philadelphia: FA Davis, 1981:1–19.
16. Jensen R, Ens GE: Platelet specific proteins. Clin Hemostasis Rev 1991; 5(2):1–4.
17. Hayhoe FGJ, Flemans RJ: Color Atlas of Hematological Cytology. St. Louis: Mosby Year Book, 1992:150–161.
18. Powers LW: Diagnostic Hematology, Clinical and Technical Principles. St. Louis: CV Mosby, 1989:146.
19. Harmening DM: Introduction to hemostasis. In Harmening

DM (ed): Clinical Hematology and Fundamentals of Hemostasis, 2nd ed. Philadelphia: FA Davis, 1992:418.

20. Powers LW: Diagnostic Hematology, Clinical and Technical Principles. St. Louis: CV Mosby, 1989:146.

21. Fristma GA: Platelet production and structure. *In* Corriveau DM, Fristma GA (eds): Hemostasis and Thrombosis in the Clinical Laboratory. Philadelphia: JB Lippincott, 1988:215.

22. White JG, Gerrard JM: Interaction of microtubules and microfilaments in platelet contractile physiology. Methods Achiev Exp Pathol 1979; 9:1–39.

23. Harrison P, Wilbourn B, Debilli N, et al: Uptake of plasma fibrinogen into the alpha granules of human megakaryocytes and platelets. J Clin Invest 1989; 84:1320–1324.

24. Kroll MK, Schafer AI: Biochemical Mechanisms of Platelet Activation. Blood 1989; 74:1181–1195.

25. Asch AS, Barnwell J, Silverstein RL, Nachman RL: Isolation of the thrombospondin membrane receptor. J. Clin Invest 1987; 79:1054–1061.

26. Evangelista V, Rijtar G, deGaetano G, White JG, et al: Platelet activation by FMLP-stimulated polymorphonuclear leukocytes: the activity of cathepsin G is not prevented by antiproteinases. Blood 1991; 77:2379–2388.

27. Silverstein DS, Robinson P, Gerrard JM: Inhibition of intravascular platelet aggregation by endothelium-derived relaxing factor: reversal by red blood cells. Blood 1990; 76:953–958.

28. Southern D: Platelets: maturation, function and laboratory evaluation. Educ Rev 1989; 2:11.

29. Hantgan RR, Hindriks G, Taylor RG, et al: Glycoprotein Ib, von Willebrand's factor and glycoprotein IIb: IIIa are all involved in platelet adhesion to fibrin in flowing whole blood. Blood 1990; 76:345–353.

30. George JN, Pickett EB, Saucerman S, et al: Platelet surface glycoproteins. J Clin Invest 1986; 78:340–348.

31. Adelman B, Rizk A, Hanners ER: Plasminogen interaction with platelets in plasma. Blood 1988; 72:1530–1535.

32. Shimomura T, Fujimura K, Maehama S, et al: Rapid purification and characterization of human platelet glycoprotein V; the amino acid sequence contains leucine-rich repetitive modules as in glycoprotein Ib. Blood 1990; 75:2349–2356.

33. Hiraiwa A, Matsukage A, Shiku H, Takahashi T, et al: Purification and partial amino acid sequence of human platelet membrane glycoproteins IIb and IIIa. Blood 1987; 69(2):560–564.

34. Wiess HJ, Hawiger J, Ruggeri M, Turitto VT, et al: Fibrinogen-independent platelet adhesion and thrombus formation on subendothelium mediated by glycoprotein IIb-IIIa complex at high shear rate. J Clin Invest 1989; 83:288–297.

35. Shimomura T, Fujimura K, Maehama S, et al: Rapid purification and characterization of human platelet glycoprotein V; the amino acid sequence contains leucine-rich repetitive modules as in glycoprotein Ib. Blood 1990; 75:2349–2356.

36. Nowak J, FitzGerald GA: Redirection of prostaglandin endoperoxide metabolism at the platelet vascular interface in man. J Clin Invest 1989; 83:380–385.

37. Jensen R, Ens GE: Platelet activation markers. Clin Hemost Rev 1992; 6(9):1–6.

38. Hardisty R, Pidard D, Cox A, et al: A defect of platelet aggregation with an abnormal distribution of glycoprotein IIb-IIIa complexes with the platelet: the cause of a lifelong bleeding disorder. Blood 1992; 80(3):696–708.

39. O'Flaherty JT, Surles JR, Redman J, Jacobson D, et al: Binding and metabolism of platelet activating factor by human neutrophils. J Clin Invest 1986; 78:381–388.

40. Harrison P, Wilbourn B, Debilli N, et al: Uptake of plasma fibrinogen into the alpha granules of human megakaryocytes and platelets. J Clin Invest 1989; 84:1320–1324.

41. Soslau G, Parker J: Modulation of platelet function by extracellular adenosine triphosphate. Blood 1989; 74(3):984–993.

42. Houston DS, Shepherd JT, Vanhoutte PM: Aggregating human platelets cause direct contraction and endothelium relaxation of isolated canine coronary arteries. J Clin Invest 1986; 78:539–544.

43. Maugeri N, Evangelista V, Piccardoni P, et al: Transcellular metabolism of arachidonic acid: increased platelet thromboxane generation in the presence of activated polymorphonuclear leukocytes. Blood 1992; 80(2):447–451.

44. Schafer AI, Maas AK, Ware JA, Johnson PC, et al: Platelet protein phosphorylation, elevation of cytostolic calcium, and inositol phospholipid breakdown in platelet activation induced by plasmin. J Clin Invest 1986; 78:73–79.

45. Alam I, Smith JB, Silver MJ: Human and rabbit platelets form platelet activating factor in response to calcium ionophore. Thromb Res 1983; 30:71–79.

46. Casey PJ, Gilman AG: G protein involvement in receptor-effector coupling. I Biol Chem 1988; 263:2577.

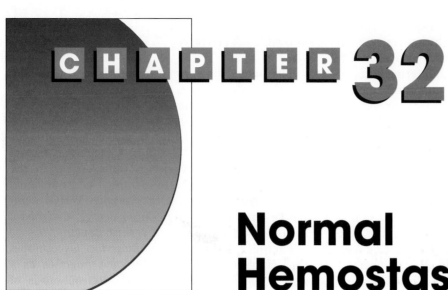

CHAPTER 32

Normal Hemostasis

Dan Southern and Gordon E. Ens

Outline

Objectives

AFTER COMPLETION OF THIS CHAPTER, THE READER WILL BE ABLE TO

1. Describe the nature, origin, and function of each of the tissue and plasma factors necessary for normal coagulation.
2. Explain the role of vitamin K in the production and function of plasma clotting factors in the prothrombin group.
3. Separate the plasma clotting factors into three groups—contact, fibrinogen, and prothrombin—on the basis of their characteristics and function.
4. Establish the role of vascular intima, media, and adventitia in hemostasis.
5. Differentiate the tissue factor pathway from the intrinsic factor pathway.
6. Integrate alternative coagulation pathways into an interactive scheme.
7. Correlate the activity of protein C and protein S with the limitation of thrombus formation.
8. Explain factor XIIIa crosslinking of fibrin and how that relates to D-dimer formation after fibrin lysis.
9. List several possible activators for plasminogen and describe the most likely activator under physiologic conditions.
10. Explain plasmin digestion of fibrin and fibrinogen and distinguish between the degradation products derived from fibrin lysis versus fibrinogen lysis.
11. Characterize plasma and tissue inhibitors associated with hemostasis and identify their origin and function.

Hemostasis is the result of several interactive systems designed to prevent or stop bleeding. Integral parts of the active hemostatic process include platelet activity, intrinsic and extrinsic coagulation (also known as tissue factor pathway), release of vasoconstrictors and vasodilators, and systematic removal of clots by fibrin lysis. Countering each of the active processes is an equally important control or inhibitory process that must be considered in order to appreciate hemostasis in complete terms. Control systems include release of endothelial prostaglandins to inhibit platelet activation and to quiet activated platelets,[1] plasma serine protease inhibitors that neutralize active clotting and lytic factors escaping from the thrombus site, and the protein C and protein S control system[2] that limits clotting by inactivation of pivotal cofactors V and VIII. The balancing act makes normal clotting and repair possible without consuming all of the hemostatic elements in each event. Bleeding disorders occur when the balance is tipped in one direction and cannot rebound. This may be caused by consumption of elements necessary for hemostasis or genetic deficiency in their production.

This chapter presents the individual pieces of the complex hemostasis puzzle and attempts to put them together to reveal a complete picture. Recent discoveries have made the picture clearer but the discovery process continues. (The reader should review Chapter 31, Platelet Maturation and Function, while reading this chapter.) Platelets are intricately involved throughout the normal clotting process. Understanding platelet function is prerequisite to understanding the remainder of the hemostatic process. A thorough knowledge of each

blood and tissue clotting factor is also prerequisite to understanding hemostasis.

COAGULATION FACTORS

The name, the chromosomal origin, and the active form of plasma and tissue clotting factors involved in coagulation are listed in Table 32–1. Table 32–2 summarizes the molecular weight, concentration, and half-life of coagulation proteins and control proteins C and S. Coagulation factors with Roman numeral designations appear in the order in which they were identified and numbered by the World Health Organization (WHO) committee on nomenclature. Those not yet assigned a number are presented by a generic name.

Factor I. Factor I is *fibrinogen*, a glycoprotein that is produced by the liver and migrates as a slow betaglobulin after 8.6 pH electrophoresis of plasma. It has a molecular weight of 340,000 D and acts as the preferred substrate for thrombin in the clotting system. It is also the stabilizing protein that crosslinks platelets by connecting to their glycoprotein IIb and IIIa receptor sites. When converted to fibrin by thrombin, fibrinogen loses four small molecular weight fibrinopeptides that total approximately 10,000 D. Fibrin monomers have distinct electrostatic properties that allow them to polymerize with other fibrin monomers into fibrin polymers.[3]

Fibrinogen is produced by hepatic cells under the control of genes on chromosome 4. The normal plasma reference range is 200 to 400 mg/dL; thus, fibrinogen has the highest concentration of all

Table 32-1. COAGULATION FACTOR SUMMARY

Clotting Factor Designation	Common Name	Chromosome	Active Form	Vitamin K Required
Factor I	Fibrinogen	4	Substrate	No
Factor II	Prothrombin	11	Precursor to thrombin	Yes
	Tissue factor	Unknown	Cofactor surface for factor VII	No
	Calcium	NA	Mineral cofactor	No
Factor V	Labile factor	1	Cofactor	No
Factor VI	No clotting factor assigned			
Factor VII	Stable factor	13	Serine protease	Yes
Factor VIII	Anti-hemophiliac factor	X	Cofactor	No
Factor IX	Christmas factor	X	Serine protease	Yes
Factor X	Stuart-Prower factor	13	Serine protease	Yes
Factor XI	Prothrombin antecedent	4	Serine protease	No
Factor XII	Hageman factor	5	Serine protease	No
Factor XIII	Fibrin stabilizing factor	6	Transglutaminase	No
Fletcher factor	Prekallikrein	Unknown	Serine protease	No
Fitzgerald factor	High-molecular-weight kininogen	Unknown	Cofactor and substrate	No

Table 32–2. MOLECULAR WEIGHT, CONCENTRATION, AND HALF-LIFE OF COAGULATION FACTORS

Clotting Factor	Molecular Weight (D)	Concentration	Half-Life (Hours)
Factor I	340,000	200–400 mg/dL	90
Factor II	69,000	10 mg/dL	60
Tissue factor	45,000	0	Unknown
Calcium	40	8–10 mg/dL	n/a
Factor V	286,000	5–10 μg/mL	12–36
Factor VII	53,000	10–20 μg/mL	5–8
Factor VIII-C	260,000	1–2 mg/dL	8–12
Factor VIII/vWF	1–2 million	7 mg/dL	10
Factor IX	57,100	3–4 μg/mL	48–72
Factor X	59,000	6–8 μg/mL	48–52
Factor XI	160,000	2–7 μg/mL	48–84
Factor XII	84,000	30–40 μg/mL	48–52
Factor XIII	300,000	2.5 mg/dL	72–120
Fletcher factor	100,000	35–50 μg/mL	35
Fitzgerald factor	120,000	70–90 μg/mL	156
Plasminogen	90,000	15–21 mg/dL	24–26
Protein C	62,000	4–6 μg/mL	7–9
Protein S (free)	69,000	20–25 μg/mL	Unknown

blood clotting factors. Early literature postulated that megakaryocytes produced fibrinogen found in platelet alpha granules; whereas results of recent research suggest that platelets absorb plasma fibrinogen into their alpha granules.[4–6]

Fibrinogen is a dimeric molecule consisting of two identical, three-chained proteins attached to each other by disulfide bonds at their N-terminal region. The three polypeptide chains in each half of fibrinogen are named alpha, beta, and gamma. The combined N-terminus of the six chains forms the *E domain,* also referred to as the *disulfide knot region* of the molecule. The separate carboxyl-terminal ends of the alpha, beta, and gamma chains form the two *D domains* of fibrinogen. Thrombin cleavage of low–molecular-weight fibrinopeptides from the N-terminus of the protruding alpha and beta chains results in formation of a fibrin monomer. The cleaved alpha and beta chains in the E domain of fibrin monomers have an affinity for the D domains of other monomers enabling union of the two to form fibrin polymers. Fibrin polymers attach to each other to form an unstable mesh that is soluble in 5-mol urea.

Factor XIIIa catalyzes the formation of peptide-like covalent bonds between the carboxyl terminals of gamma chains from adjacent D domains. Specifically, the crosslink is between the epsilon amino group of lysine and the gamma amide group of glutamine. The reaction frees an NH_2 molecule. Fibronectin is also crosslinked to the mesh by XIIIa, increasing its stability, and alpha$_2$-antiplasmin is attached, limiting clot lysis. Crosslinking of adjacent D domains produces a stable fibrin clot that does not dissolve in 5-mol urea.[7–10] Additional crosslinking of the carboxyl terminal ends of the alpha chains to the crosslinked fibrin provides a three dimensional mesh. Figure 32–1 represents the chemical structure of fibrinogen showing the D and E domains. Polymerization and crosslinking of fibrin into a stable mesh is represented in Figure 32–2.

Fibrinogen is an acute phase reactant and its blood level is increased in many disease states and pregnancy. Smokers have increased levels of fibrinogen, which decreases by as much as 50 mg/dL upon cessation of smoking. Elevated fibrinogen levels are associated with myocardial infarction and stroke.[3]

Low levels of fibrinogen or dysfunctional fibrinogen is associated with bleeding caused by failure to form fibrin clots. Reasons for hypofibrinogenemia are consumption as a result of thrombosis or lack of production by the liver. Dysfunctional fibrinogen mimics hypofibrinogenemia. Dysfibrinogenemia is a qualitative problem where fibrinogen concentration is adequate but non-functional.

Factor II. Factor II, *prothrombin,* is an alpha$_2$ globulin produced in the liver with genetic information coming from chromosome 11. It is produced as a single-chain glycoprotein with a molecular weight of 69,000 D. The prothrombin protein produced by hepatic cells is not functional. A post-synthesis alteration, dependent on vitamin K as a coenzyme, makes prothrombin functional. This alteration and its effect on prothrombin and five other vitamin K–dependent factors are discussed in the section on the role of vitamin K later in this chapter.

Prothrombin is released into the blood stream as *zymogen,* a precursor for the active form, thrombin. Activation of prothrombin to thrombin is a two

Fibrinogen Structure

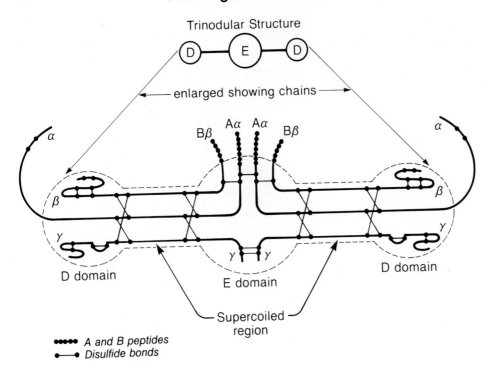

Figure 32–1 Structure of fibrinogen. (From McKenzie SB [ed]: Textbook of Hematology. Philadelphia: Lea & Febiger, 1988:397.)

Formation of Fibrin Polymer

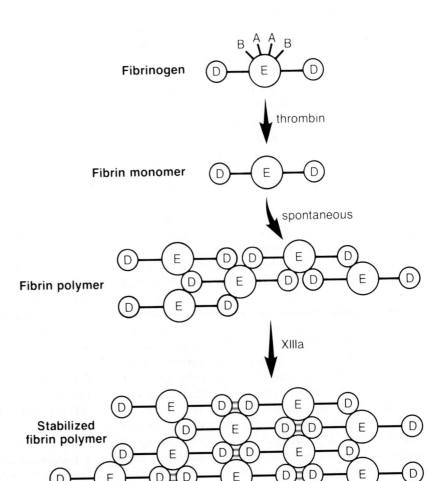

Figure 32–2 Formation of a stabilized fibrin mesh. Fibrin monomers polymerize by affinity of thrombin-cleaved E domain to the D domains. Factor XIIIa crosslinks the gamma chains of adjacent D domains to form a urea-insoluble stable fibrin clot. (Modified with permission from McKenzie SB [ed]: Textbook of Hematology. Philadelphia: Lea & Febiger, 1988:398.)

Prothrombin Conversion to Thrombin

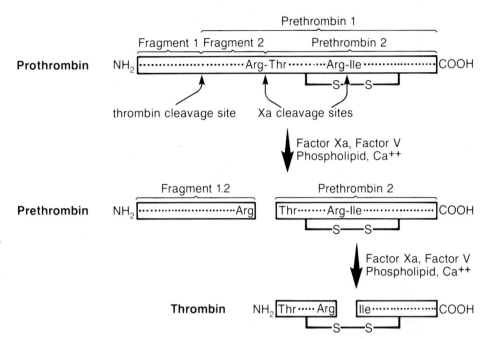

Figure 32–3 Factor VIII/ vWF complex is made up of factor VIIIC coagulant portion bound to multimers of high- and low-molecular-weight von Willebrand factors. (From McKenzie SB [ed]: Textbook of Hematology. Philadelphia: Lea & Febiger, 1988:396.)

step process (Fig. 32–3). Initially, a low-molecular-weight protein, fragment 1.2, is cleaved from the N-terminus to create prethrombin. Prethrombin is further cleaved, exposing the serine active center of the active thrombin molecule. When activated by factor Xa, thrombin becomes an active serine protease capable of catalyzing several important proteolytic reactions related to coagulation and fibrinolysis. It also reacts with thrombin receptors on platelets causing their activation and release. Serine proteases have a serine active center, and hydrolyze arginyl or lysyl peptide bonds on their protein substrates. Thrombin is responsible for conversion of fibrinogen to fibrin and activation of factors V, VIII, XI, and XIII and protein C.[10-12]

Factor III. Originally assigned to *tissue thromboplastin*, factor III is now referred to as tissue factor. A 45,000-D transmembrane lipoprotein, tissue factor is a cofactor found in all tissues but the highest concentrations are found in the brain, liver, lung, and placenta. Both the lipid and protein portions must be present for full effectiveness. Ionized calcium clings to the negatively charged phospholipid surface of tissue factor. Vitamin K-dependent factors bind to the calcium attached to tissue factor. Normally, no tissue factor is found in plasma. It is released from traumatized tissue and carried into the extravascular spaces by escaping blood, where it serves as a cofactor for activation of factor VII in extrinsic coagulation.[10,13,14] Because extrinsic activation of coagulation is dependent

upon tissue factor, it is now termed the *tissue factor pathway*. Platelet phospholipid surfaces, necessary for intrinsic coagulation, are similar in composition and function to tissue factor. Both serve similar roles in clotting by their attraction to calcium ions.

Factor IV. This name was originally given to *calcium*; however, the chemical designation for ionized calcium (Ca^{2+}) is used instead of the Roman numeral IV. Ca^{2+} has a molecular weight of 40 D. Ionized calcium is the mediator of platelet activation and binds vitamin K-dependent factors to phospholipid surfaces (factor III and platelet factor 3 [PF3]). Without calcium ions, vitamin K-dependent factors will not anchor to thrombogenic phospholipids and clotting would be prevented. Chelating agents such as citrate, oxalate, and ethylenediaminetetraacetic acid (EDTA) are used as anticoagulants to remove calcium from blood to prevent clotting. Normal plasma calcium is 8–10 mg/dL with 40% in the ionized form. To ensure that ionized calcium is available, however, platelets release high molar amounts of Ca^{2+} from their dense granules early in the clotting event. Intracellular calcium mobilization leads to platelet aggregation.

Factor V. Factor V is also called *proaccelerin* or *labile factor*. It is a single-chain glycoprotein with a molecular weight of 286,000 D. As its name implies, labile factor diminishes its activity quickly at room temperature. Citrated plasmas should be tested within 30 minutes to avoid deterioration of factor V. It lives up to its generic name, proaccelerin, by acting as a cofactor and accelerating the conversion of prothrombin to thrombin.

Factor V is produced in the liver. It attaches to exposed receptors on activated platelets and tissue factor. In the tissue factor pathway, a small amount of factor V is initially modified by factor Xa until thrombin is generated.[13] Intrinsically, factor V is attached to the PF3 surface in large amounts. Thrombin modification of factor V to factor Vm is the result of limited proteolysis that produces a two-chain version of the molecule, which allows it to serve as a more effective cofactor. Factor Vm holds prothrombin and factor Xa together in an ideal spatial arrangement on the phospholipid surface for factor Xa to activate prothrombin (factor II) to prethrombin and then to thrombin (factor IIa). As part of the common pathway, factor V is necessary for both the tissue factor pathway and the intrinsic pathway conversion of prothrombin to thrombin.[14,15] Ironically, factor Vm is inactivated by thrombin-activated protein C.[2]

Factor VI. Factor VI does not designate any clotting factor. Originally number VI was given to what was thought to be a separate factor. It was subsequently proved that this factor was the same as the modified form (Vm) of factor V and so the number remains vacant.

Factor VII. Factor VII is a single-chain glycoprotein that is vitamin K–dependent. Its generic name is *proconvertin* and its common name is stable factor because it remains stable for several hours in plasma and serum. The gene for factor VII is located on the chromosome 13. Its molecular weight is 53,000. Factor VII is the initiating serine protease enzyme in the tissue factor pathway system. Factor VII changes shape to VIIa by contact with Ca^{2+} anchored to tissue factor. The resulting $VIIa/Ca^{2+}/III$ complex can activate factor X to factor Xa.[16] Interestingly, activated Xa can in turn hydrolyze factor VII enzymatically into the two-chain-activated factor VIIa which has even greater ability to activate factor X than the single chain version created by tissue factor.[15] Factor VIIa can also activate factor IX from the intrinsic pathway.[17-22]

Although heat labile, factor VII activity is stable for 4–5 hours in blood. The zymogen form is stable at refrigerator temperature up to 2 weeks. This liver-produced factor migrates as a fast beta fraction, has a low concentration in plasma, and has the shortest half life (5–8 hours) of the vitamin K–dependent clotting factors. Its short half-life makes it the first factor affected when a vitamin K antagonist such as warfarin is administered.[10] Elevated factor VII levels have been

associated with increased risk for myocardial infarction and stroke.[7] Although no specific inhibitor has been identified for VIIa, tissue factor pathway inhibitor (TFPI) plays an inhibitory role with the VIIa/III complex and inhibits transformation of factor X to factor Xa by this pathway in vivo.[23]

Factor VIII-von Willebrand Factor Complex (VIII:vWF). This factor consists of one factor VIII portion bound to one multimeric von Willebrand factor polymer (vWF). The factor VIII portion is controlled by genes on the X chromosome and has a molecular weight of 260,000 D. Von Willebrand protein is autosomal and controlled by chromosome 12. vWF protein is a multimeric combination of low-, intermediate- and high-molecular weight subunits with varying molecular weights. vWF is produced by megakaryocytes and endothelial cells. Endothelial cells release vWF directly into the plasma or wound site.

Factor VIII is produced in several tissues; however, the major production site is hepatic.[13] Factors VIII and vWF bind together tightly in plasma to form a variable molecular weight complex that weighs over 1 million daltons. The complexing of the two proteins lends stability to the VIII portion, extending its half-life 4- to 6-fold. Megakaryocytes store vWF proteins in their alpha granules but do not have factor VIII attached. DDAVP (1-desamino-8-D-arginine-vasopressin) stimulates the release of vWF from endothelial cells.

Factor VIII/vWF complex is a cold precipitating alpha migrator playing two pivotal roles in hemostasis. Initially, platelets adhere to collagen bound vWF by their glycoprotein Ib (GPIb) receptors after trauma. Subsequently, more vWF in the blood binds to the adherent platelets resulting in platelet aggregates that stop the bleeding. Because factor VIII is bound to vWF multimers, it is present on the surface of platelets involved in the platelet plug. After modification by factor Xa or thrombin, factor VIII becomes an active cofactor (VIIIa) in the coagulation scheme. It serves as a cofactor for factor IXa activation of factor X on the platelet factor 3 surface.[24,25] Factor VIII is similar to factor V in structure.[26]

Factor VIII is heat labile with quickly diminishing activity in plasma at room temperature. Factor VIII is underproduced in hemophilia A, whereas vWF is produced normally. In von Willebrand disease, diminished levels of vWF and dysfunctional factor VIII are seen. Factor VIII is unstable in the circulation when not bound to vWF.

Factor IX. Factor IX, or plasma thromboplastin component (PTC), is commonly called Christmas factor, named for the first family found with this deficiency. Produced in the liver as a single-chain glycoprotein, it is a beta migrator dependent on vitamin K for functionality. Factor IX production is under the control of the X chromosome. Factor IX, bound to calcium ions on phospholipid surfaces, is activated by factors XIa or VIIa producing a two-chain serine protease connected by disulfide bonds. Activated factor IX activates factor X in the common pathway.[12,14,27] Factor IX deficiency is described as hemophilia B or Christmas disease.

Factor X. Factor X is also a vitamin K–dependent glycoprotein produced by the liver under the genetic control of chromosome 13. Consisting of two-chains, one heavy and one light, connected by disulfide bonds, its structure is unique to other single chained glycoprotein vitamin K–dependent factors that become double-chained after activation.[13] Factor X migrates as a fast alpha globulin. Discovered independently in two different families, it is called the Stuart-Prower factor after those families. Factor X can be activated into a serine protease by both factors VIIa and IXa. Factor IXa activation of factor X requires calcium and factor VIII as a cofactor. Factor VIIa activation requires calcium and tissue factor as a cofactor. Factor Xa, along with Ca^{2+}, phospholipid, and modified factor V, forms a complex known as the *prothrombinase* (prothrombin activator) complex.[9,10,13,27]

Factor XI. Factor XI is a dimeric molecule consisting of two identical 80,000 D polypeptide chains linked by disulfide bonds. Its generic name is plasma thromboplastin antecedent and it migrates as a slow beta globulin. Factor XI is a contact factor that clings to negatively charged surfaces such as glass, subendothelial tissue, and activated platelets. It travels in blood complexed in a bimolar arrangement with high molecular weight kininogen (HMWK), another contact factor. Factor XI is activated by factor XIIa or XIIa fragments and becomes an essential serine protease in the intrinsic factor pathway.[28-31] Activation of factor XI by thrombin represents one of the alternate pathways known to exist in vivo. Autoactivation of factor XI on nonphysiologic surfaces, such as glass, has been demonstrated in vitro. It is not yet clear whether a tissue activator for factor XI exists.[30]

Only 15–25% of normal factor XI activity is required to maintain normal hemostasis.[28] Among the four contact factors, factor XI deficiency, also called hemophilia C, is the only one associated with bleeding. Little correlation exists between the percentage activity and the severity of the disease.[13]

Factor XII. Factor XII is called the Hageman factor and was named for the first person known to be deficient in this factor. It is a single-chain glycoprotein produced by the liver and migrates as a beta globulin. Genetic control is on chromosome 5. It is a contact factor that autoactivates upon binding with negatively charged surfaces such as glass, celite, kaolin, dextran sulfate, endotoxins, sulfatides, and subendothelial tissue. Upon contact, factor XII becomes activated into a two-chain molecule wherein a heavy chain is attached to a lighter chain by disulfide bonds. The shape change exposes a serine active center on the light chain. No cofactors are necessary for factor XII autoactivation. Factor XIIa is the initial enzyme in the contact factor system and acts as the catalyst for several important hemostatic events. It is responsible for activation of factor XI to factor XIa, which continues the intrinsic factor system of coagulation. High–molecular-weight kininogen is a necessary cofactor for factor XI activation by XIIa.

Factor XIIa also activates HMWK bound prekallikrein to kallikrein, a serine protease with ability to activate the kinin and fibrinolytic pathways. In addition, factor XIIa and kallikrein activate additional factor XII molecules by enzymatic hydrolysis in a positive feedback loop that amplifies the system. This creates alpha and beta XIIa fragments. Both types of XIIa fragments initiate activation of more prekallikrein while alpha XIIa fragments have more affinity for factor XI activation.[28] Persons with deficiencies in factor XII do not bleed uncontrollably but there is a tendency to develop pulmonary embolism and other thrombotic disorders probably because of lack of activation of the pathway for fibrin lysis. Recent understanding of alternate pathway activation of factor IX by VIIa/tissue factor complex and activation of factor XI by thrombin explains why patients deficient in Hageman factor, prekallikrein, or HMWK do not bleed uncontrollably.[17,28,30,32]

Factor XIII. Factor XIII is a two-chained alpha$_2$-globulin, produced in the liver, that has transglutaminase activity when activated by thrombin.[33, 34] Factor XIII is trapped inside the clot and is activated by thrombin. The enzyme XIIIa forms covalent bonds between adjacent D domains in polymerized fibrin, stabilizing it with formation of crosslinked fibrin. Fibrin crosslinking gives mechanical rigidity to the clot. Because of its function, factor XIII is called the fibrin stabilizing factor. It also crosslinks alpha$_2$–anti-plasmin to the fibrin mesh to protect the clot from premature breakdown.[10 13] Nonstabilized fibrin polymers are soluble in 5-mol urea, whereas crosslinked fibrin is insoluble.

Fletcher Factor. Fletcher factor is also known as prekallikrein (PK). It is a fast gamma globulin with serine protease activity when activated by factor XIIa. Like factor XI, prekallikrein is attached to HMWK, which acts as a cofactor for its activation by factor XIIa. The active enzyme form, kallikrein, activates more factor XII in a positive feedback loop.[28, 30] Kallikrein activates plasminogen to plasmin initiating the fibrin lysis system and it also hydrolyzes low–molecular-weight bradykinins from HMWK to initiate the kinin system. The kinins act as vasodilators and smooth muscle relaxants to reestablish blood flow after serotonin and thromboxane A_2 from platelets have caused vessel constriction. The chromosomal origin of PK is unknown. Its structure is similar to factor XI. PK is produced in the liver and is considered to be a member of the contact group of coagulation proteins.[10, 13, 35]

Fitzgerald Factor. The Fitzgerald factor, also known as HMWK, is a single-chained glycoprotein produced by the liver. Its chromosomal locus is not known. HMWK complexes with factor XI and prekallikrein and is a member of the contact group. It acts as a cofactor to accelerate the activation of factor XI by factor XIIa and acts as a substrate for kallikrein in the production of kinins.[9, 25, 36] Persons with HMWK deficiency are asymptomatic.

Platelet Factor 3. PF3, like tissue factor, is a phospholipid surface that supports coagulation. Platelet activity brings about chemical changes in the platelet membrane phospholipid making it more negatively charged and favorable to Ca^{2+} binding. The calcium-covered phospholipid surface provides binding sites for functional vitamin K–dependent factors that are gamma carboxylated.

THE ROLE OF VITAMIN K IN COAGULATION

Vitamin K plays an important role in the functionality of factors II, VII, IX, and X and of pro-

teins C and S, which are manufactured by the liver. After production, vitamin K participates in an oxidation reaction that adds a second carboxyl group to the gamma carbon of several glutamic acid residues near the N-terminus of these proteins (Fig. 32–4). With two ionized carboxyl groups, the glutamic acids take on a double-negative charge, which allows them to bind more securely to positively charged calcium ions attached to PF3 or tissue factor. Vitamin K antagonists, such as warfarin, prevent this post synthesis addition by interfering with vitamin K activity rendering them non-functional. (See Fig. 32–2 for an illustration of the vitamin K effect on these factors.)

GROUPING OF BLOOD CLOTTING FACTORS

The coagulation factors can be grouped by characteristics and functions. The three groups are the *contact group,* the *prothrombin group,* and the *fibrinogen group.* This classification is helpful for interpretation of mixing studies used to identify factor deficiencies.

The contact group contains the four contact factors: factor XII, factor XI, PK, and HMWK. The contact factors are present in fresh normal plasma and in serum after clotting has occurred. When plasma is adsorbed with barium sulfate or aluminum hydroxide to remove vitamin K–dependent factors the contact factors remain in the supernatant plasma. With the exception of HMWK, which is a cofactor, the contact factors are serine proteases when activated.

The prothrombin group contains the vitamin K dependent factors II, VII, IX, and X and proteins

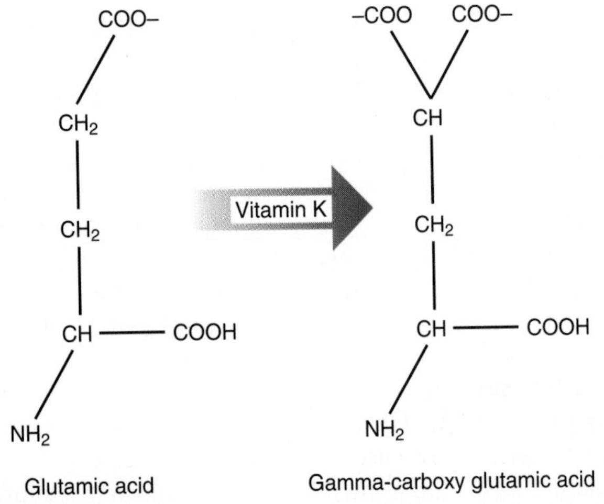

Figure 32–4 Vitamin K plays a major role in the functionality of members of the prothrombin group by facilitating the addition of a second carboxyl group on the gamma carbon of glutamic acid residues near the N-terminus.

Glutamic acid   Gamma-carboxy glutamic acid

Factors	Characteristics of Group
Table 32–3. PLASMA CLOTTING PROTEINS GROUPS	
CONTACT GROUP Factor XII Factor XI Fletcher factor Fitzgerald factor	Found in absorbed plasma; found in serum; contact factors; produced in liver
PROTHROMBIN GROUP Factor II Factor VII Factor IX Factor X Protein C Protein S	Absent in absorbed serum; present in serum except II; produced in the liver; serine proteases except protein S; vitamin K dependent
FIBRINOGEN GROUP Factor I Factor V Factor VIII Factor XIII	Found in absorbed plasma; absent in serum; produced in the liver

C and S. The prothrombin group is dependent upon vitamin K for its functionality. All six prothrombin group factors are precipitated and removed from plasma adsorbed with barium sulfate or aluminum hydroxide. Adsorbed plasma contains the fibrinogen group and the contact group factors. Aged serum contains the prothrombin group proteins with the exception of factor II. Serum, citrated to chelate calcium, is used as a reagent in mixing studies. All prothrombin group proteins are produced in the liver. All are potent serine proteases except protein S, which is a cofactor.

The fibrinogen group is a miscellaneous collection of factors that have several things in common. Factors I, V, VIII, and XIII are placed in this group. They are present in normal and adsorbed plasma whereas they are missing from serum because they are consumed upon clotting. Table 32–3 summarizes the grouping of plasma coagulation proteins.

Plasma serine protease inhibitors (serpins) initially neutralize hemostatic events until their inhibitory capacity is overcome by active clotting factors generated at the local clot site. Overcoming normal inhibitory elements is the first task for normal hemostasis. Inhibitors released by endothelial cells and platelet granules to plasminogen activators (PAI-I) and heparin-antithrombin (PF4-thromboglobulin) play a vital role in allowing initial clot formation.

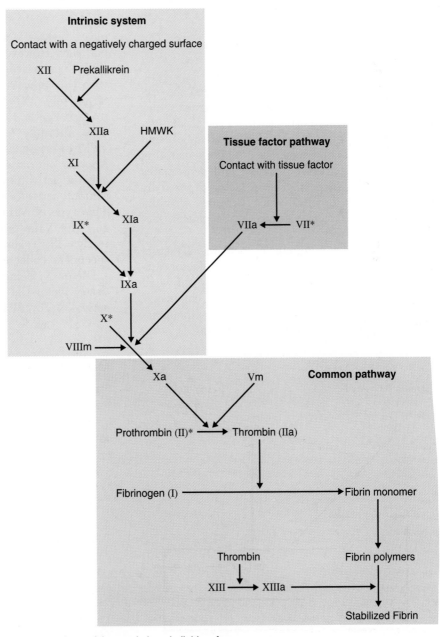

Figure 32–5 Simplistic coagulation scheme.

*requires calcium and phospholipid surface

The original cascade described by McFarland, Davie, and Ratnoff[37, 38] in the early 60s, while no longer a completely accurate summary of hemostasis, remains valid for presenting the basics of hemostasis. Students will benefit from learning a simple cascade first and later adding the more complex interrelated pathways and feedback loops. An inclusive schematic of hemostasis tends to discourage the new learner. Figure 32–5 presents a simplified schema of the coagulation process.

Figures 32–6, 32–7, and 32–8 depict alternate paths leading to fibrin formation. Figure 32–9 better depicts current understanding of the interrelationships and alternate pathways. Control mechanisms, fibrin lysis, and inhibitors have been added to the overall scheme in Figure 32–9.

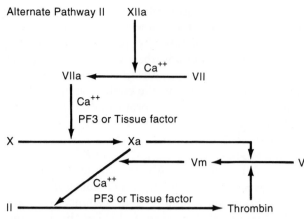

Figure 32–7 Activation of the extrinsic pathway by factor XIIa.

COAGULATION AND PLATELET ACTIVITY

When vessels rupture, blood contacts the exposed subendothelial tissues and extravascular space where clotting begins through the tissue factor pathway. This type of clotting is quick and impedes additional blood loss while generating thrombin that activates platelets and perpetuates the coagulation process. Tissue factor exposed by traumatized endothelial cells becomes calcium coated which attracts vitamin K–dependent factors from the blood.

Even though all vitamin K–dependent factors bind to the calcium ions on the tissue factor surface, only factor VII is conformationally activated by contact with the tissue factor Ca^{2+} complex.[18] Factor VIIa has little protease ability without association with tissue factor. Factor VIIa/TF com-

plex activates factor X to Xa to begin the common pathway. However, tissue factor pathway inhibitor (TFPI), released by traumatized tissue, interferes with this process limiting factor X activation. Alternatively, VIIa/TF complex activates factor IX to IXa. Factor IXa then activates factor X to Xa. This alternate pathway (see Fig. 32–6) to avoid TFPI interference is a normal occurrence in vivo.[23] Another alternate pathway to avoid TFPI interference is activation of factor VII by XIIa through contact activation of factor XII (see Fig. 32–7). This type of VIIa is not interfered with by TFPI and the VIIa product can activate factor X directly. TFPI should not be present in citrated specimens collected by coagulation tests.

Factor X, being vitamin K–dependent, binds to tissue factor-Ca^{2+} complex and allows enzymatic activation by VIIa or IXa. Modified factor VIII

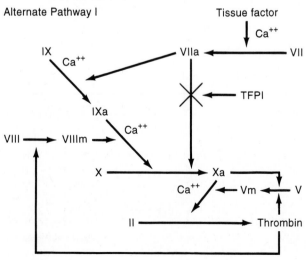

Figure 32–6 Factor VIIa activation of factor IX.

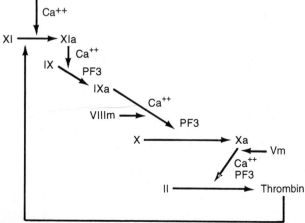

Figure 32–8 Activation of factor XI by platelets and thrombin.

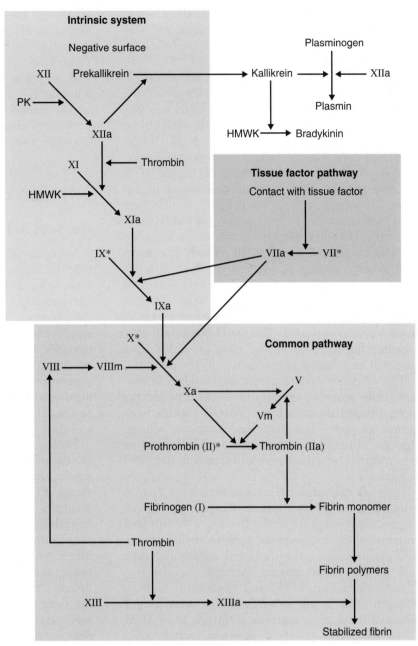

Figure 32–9 Interactive pathways in coagulation.

requires calcium and phospholipid surface

(VIIIm) is a necessary cofactor for the latter reaction. Modified factor V (Vm) is a necessary cofactor in the conversion of prothrombin (II) to thrombin (IIa). Factor V is initially modified by factor Xa until enough thrombin is made.[11, 26] Factor Xa also activates additional factor VII in a positive feedback loop.[39] VIIa created by this positive feedback loop activates factor X in the common pathway and factor IX from the intrinsic pathway.[16, 31] Recent evidence concludes that factor VII plays a much broader role in intrinsic clotting than first believed. Great interest has been shown recently in elevated factor VII levels asso-

ciated with risk of hypercoagulation and cardiac risk.[7, 13, 40]

In the common pathway, Xa activates prothrombin to thrombin with the aid of factor Vm which acts as a cofactor. This is a calcium dependent reaction. Modified factor V is essential for holding all reactants in proper spatial alignment for this reaction. Prothrombin is cleaved in the activation process freeing the active thrombin (factor IIa) from the phospholipid surface. The mobility afforded to thrombin allows it to perform many proteolytic functions (convert fibrinogen to fibrin, activate factor XIII, modify factors V and VIII, activate platelets, and activate protein C). The immediate role for thrombin in the tissue pathway system is to hydrolyze fibrinogen to fibrin monomers and activate factor XIII to XIIIa.

Fibrin monomers are produced when thrombin cleaves low–molecular-weight peptides from the N-terminus of both alpha and beta chains (see Fig. 32–2). This results in a total molecular weight loss of approximately 10, 000 D from the parent fibrinogen molecule. The monomers spontaneously polymerize with each other forming a lattice of E domains attached to D domains of adjacent monomers. The bonds between the E and D domains are weak and unstable. Polymers dissolve easily in 5-mol urea. Stability is given to the fibrin mesh by thrombin-activated factor XIIIa, which enzymatically bonds adjacent D domains together with covalent bonds between the carboxy-terminal ends of their respective gamma chains. This gamma-gamma linkage crosslinks the fibrin and makes it insoluble in 5-mol urea. The D=D bonds will stay together during lysis of the clot, at which time they will be released as D-dimers into the plasma.

The extrinsic system produces thrombus formation while repairing the injured vessel. The thrombin generated initiates many platelet and intrinsic events as well. The extrinsic thrombus will go through fibrin lysis (see section on fibrin lysis in this chapter) and tissue phagocytes will clear the debris.

Platelets activated by platelet activating factors released from injured tissue change their shape, expose their receptors, and adhere to vWF covered collagen along the exposed subendothelial tissue. vWF is present in the disrupted endothelial cells and in the blood moving through the opening. Plasma fibrinogen, vWF, and fibronectin bind to collagen fibers in the subendothelium presenting a cohesive coating for platelets to attach to by their GPIb receptors. Adherent platelets recruit other platelets passing by in an attempt to occlude the opening and stop external flow of blood. Adenosine diphosphate (ADP) released from platelet-dense granules causes platelets to mobilize calcium, which activates phospholipase enzymes generating thromboxane A_2. Thromboxane A_2 causes the platelets to constrict and release their alpha granules containing fibrinogen. The fibrinogen binds to glycoproteins IIb and IIIa (GPIIb and GPIIIa) fibrinogen receptors on platelets causing them to aggregate and crosslink.

Serotonin released from the dense granules causes contraction of the smooth muscle helping to seal the opening and to constrict the vessel downstream. Vessel constriction slows blood flow past the injury site providing the pool of plasma coagulation factors needed for clotting. The altered lipid surface of the stabilized, crosslinked, platelet plug serves as the phospholipid surface for intrinsic clot formation and is known as platelet factor 3 (PF3). Calcium is attracted to the PF3 surface. Factors V and VIII are bound to the platelet by receptors. Vitamin K–dependent factors bind to the calcium on the surface. Contact factors are attracted to the negatively charged PF3 surface and compete with the calcium for binding sites.

INTRINSIC COAGULATION

Contact Activation

Intrinsic pathway clotting is essential for allowing the disrupted tissue to heal while protected from the shear forces of flowing blood. During tissue pathway coagulation and platelet plug formation, contact factor proteins adhere to the exposed negatively charged subendothelium and platelet surfaces. Factor XII auto-activates by undergoing a confirmational shape change exposing its serine protease active center. This begins the classical intrinsic coagulation cascade. Factor XIIa activates factor XI to factor XIa with HMWK acting as a cofactor.

Factor XIIa also activates prekallikrein to the serine protease kallikrein. HMWK acts as a cofactor for this reaction. Kallikrein activates additional factor XII to factor XIIa fragments in a positive feedback loop. It hydrolyzes low molecular weight bradykinin from HMWK. Bradykinin acts as a vasodilator to help re-establish blood flow through blood vessels previously vasoconstricted by serotonin and thromboxane A_2. Kallikrein and XIIa activate *plasminogen proactivator*. Whereas it has not been determined how much of a role this pathway plays in plasminogen activation, it has been demonstrated that in patients with deficiencies in factor XII, HMWK or kallikrein, fibrin clots do not lyse normally. Although there is limited activation of plasminogen by activated contact factors, the major activator of plasminogen is tissue plasminogen activator (tPA) released later by thrombin stimulation of healthy endothelial cells.

Factor XIIa can activate other factor XII molecules by hydrolysis. Persons with factor XII deficiencies clot normally. Alternative pathways explained earlier compensate for a lack of XIIa activation of XI.[31] Factor XIIa also brings about activation of the complement system at the C3 (properdin pathway) level. The complement cascade creates an inflammatory response by bringing white cells into the clotting area by chemotaxis. This response is helpful and regulatory. The white blood cells can release platelet activating factors, can phagocytize neutralized factors, and can stimulate the inhibitory systems to stop clotting.[10, 13] Finally, factor XIIa activates factor VII without the help of tissue factor. The VIIa created is different from the conformationally activated VIIa/TF complex and is more efficient in activating factor X in the common pathway.[28] It can be concluded that XIIa can initiate intrinsic and extrinsic coagulation as well as fibrinolysis and complement activity. It can be further concluded that factor VIIa also plays a vital activation role for both systems. These apparent intersystem relationships make the simple cascade diagrams obsolete, because coagulation is clearly a multi-system event. Terminology must change to describe the more accurate representations of the interdependent pathways.

Intrinsic Factor System

Factor XIa activates factor IX which is vitamin K–dependent. This step requires calcium bound to a phospholipid surface (PF3) in order for factor IX to attach. Factor IXa in turn activates factor X which is also a vitamin K–dependent factor requiring calcium. Modified factor VIII acts as a cofactor to hold the two together in proper spatial arrangement for activation of X to Xa. A limited number of factor VIII molecules are modified initially by Xa. Later, when thrombin is produced, it modifies factor VIII more efficiently. Factor VIII is present on the platelet surface because of its bipolar association with von Willebrand multimers, which are bound to platelet GPIb receptors.

Common Pathway

Factor Xa is the first enzyme in the common pathway. It activates prothrombin with the help of Vm and Ca^{2+} as was described earlier under the tissue factor pathway. Thrombin generated intrinsically forms fibrin monomers that polymerize and are crosslinked by thrombin-activated factor XIIIa.

REGULATION OF HEMOSTASIS BY PROTEINS C AND S

Excess thrombin binds quickly to thrombomodulin on healthy endothelial cells adjacent to the thrombus site. The thrombin-thrombomodulin complex activates plasma protein C, which, along with its cofactor, protein S, inactivates cofactors Vm and VIIIm by degradation. This stops the localized clotting event and signals the beginning of fibrin removal.[41, 42] Figure 32–10 illustrates the activation of the protein C and protein S control

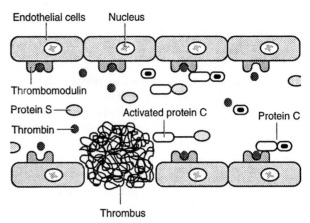

Figure 32–10 Activation of protein C.

system by thrombin and thrombomodulin. This control mechanism for limiting clotting is equally important to creating the clot and achieving a hemostatic balance. Protein C and protein S are vitamin K–dependent proteins produced in the liver. Thrombin, which plays many active roles in coagulation and platelet activities, limits itself through this negative feedback loop. The protein S cofactor is found in the blood in two forms. Approximately 60% is bound to C4, a complement protein. The remaining 40% is free and is the active molecule used to stop clotting. Deficiencies of either protein C or protein S cause hypercoagulable states.

FIBRIN LYSIS

Once a clot has served its useful purpose, it becomes a waste product that must be discarded. The fibrin mesh is too large to be phagocytized. The fibrin mesh is systematically degraded by plasmin, the enzyme form of the zymogen plasminogen. This is called the fibrin lysis system.

Blood plasminogen activators are produced when factor XIIa and kallikrein are produced by contact activation. Plasminogen is a complex molecule produced in the liver. It has five loops in its structure that are heavily populated with carbohydrates attached to the protein backbone. These loops are called kringles because they resemble a Scandinavian pastry of that name. The kringles of plasminogen promote their effectiveness because they bind loosely to the D domains of fibrinogen molecules and tightly to crosslinked fibrin. This allows plasminogen to be attached to fibrin during clot formation.[43, 44]

The major activation of plasminogen to plasmin is mediated by tissue plasminogen activator (tPA)[13] released from nearby healthy endothelial cells. Interestingly, tPA is initially released when the vessel wall is damaged; however, both activated platelets and injured endothelial cells release plasminogen activator inhibitor 1 (PAI-1) to neutralize tPA. tPA is strongly attracted to the site where plasminogen is attached to crosslinked fibrin. Therefore, activation of plasminogen to plasmin by tPA is localized and generally clot specific.[45-48]

tPA hydrolyzes the serine protease enzyme plasmin from plasminogen. Plasmin degrades the fibrin mesh into the most basic units. Figure 32–11 illustrates the digestion process. First, large degradation products that contain three E domains and three crosslinked D domains are carved away from the clot. This fragment is called a YY/DXD fragment. Further degradation cleaves away a DED fragment having one E domain and one crosslinked D domain. This leaves another larger DY/YD fragment consisting of two E domains and two crosslinked D domains. Plasmin hydrolyzes the DY/YD into two additional DED complexes. Plas-

min continues to hydrolyze each DED fragment by splitting it into an E fragment and a D-dimer fragment.[9, 10, 12]

Normal amounts of E- and D-dimer degradation products from fibrin lysis are released into the blood, from which they are removed by liver and spleen macrophages. Activated plasmin enzymes are neutralized by antiplasmins in the blood. Other serine protease inhibitors such as antithrombin and antitrypsin also neutralize plasmin.

Degradation of fibrinogen, which yields D and E fragments, is not a normal process. Fibrinogen lysis without a primary thrombotic event is very rare. Plasmin degrades native fibrinogen into individual D and E domain fragments. These particles are not detectable by plasma D-dimer testing. They can be measured by tests that measure total degradation products such as the serum latex FDP tests or monoclonal tests that measure E fragments. A

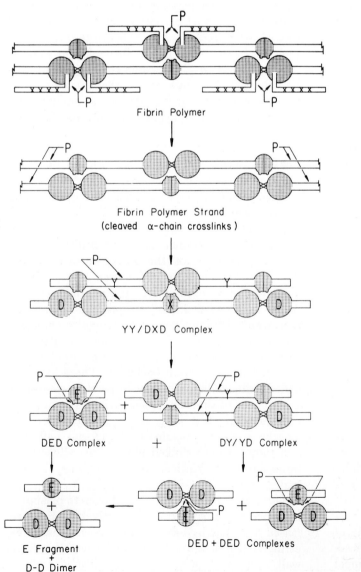

Figure 32–11 Degradation of fibrin by plasmin. (From Thompson AR, Harker LA: Manual of Hemostasis and Thrombosis. Philadelphia: FA Davis, 1983:1–19.)

panel of D-dimer and total FDP tests can differentiate how much of the total is caused by fibrin lysis and how much results from fibrinogen lysis.[49] Both types of degradation products, when elevated, interfere with normal coagulation and many produce a bleeding diathesis. Their anti-coagulant effect is caused by interference of the fragments with the normal polymerization of fibrin and neutralization of some active clotting factors. Plasmin has the ability, when not controlled by inhibitors, to degrade factors VIII and V as well, which adds to the bleeding syndrome.

SERINE PROTEASE INHIBITORS

When thrombin and other activated clotting factors escape the clot site, they are neutralized by inhibitor proteins. Activated clotting factors attach to the inhibitors because the inhibitors have peptide bonds similar to those of their normal substrate. The active enzyme cannot, however, hydrolyze the inhibitor and is irreversibly complexed with it. Active factor-inhibitor complexes are removed by phagocytosis in the spleen, liver, and other organs. Serine protease inhibitors (serpins) include anti-thrombin III (ATIII), heparin cofactor II, C1 inhibitor, alpha$_2$-macroglobulin, alpha$_1$–anti-trypsin, TFPI, PAI, protein C inhibitor, and alpha$_2$–anti-plasmin. Their concentration, molecular weight, and half-life are summarized in Table 32–4. Most serpins have preferred targets but all of them interact with any of the serine proteases (e.g., antithrombin III neutralizes most of the serine proteases as well as thrombin). The normal concentration of inhibitors in plasma is enough to inactivate the normal amount of activated enzymes escaping from routine hemostatic events. When thrombosis increases, however, the consumption of inhibitors increases and the hemostatic balance may become disrupted. Decreased inhibitor function, caused by consumption, lack of production, or production of abnormally functioning proteins, results in a hypercoagulable state.

ATIII is the major inhibitor of activated coagulation proteins. It is a slow inhibitor without its cofactor, heparin. Heparin increases the inhibitory effect of ATIII approximately 1000-fold. Heparin is found in mast cells and tissue basophils. Heparin-like substances are produced by endothelial cells. During trauma leading to clot formation, heparin and heparin-like substances are released in the area of the clot by these cells. ATIII's binding sites are hidden or protected until heparin binds to the opposite side of the molecule, opening up its active binding sites. All vitamin K–dependent serine proteases readily bind to the ATIII heparin complex.[13, 20] After neutralization of a serine protease, heparin dissociates from ATIII and serves as a cofactor for additional ATIII molecules. ATIII enzyme complexes are rapidly cleared from the circulation by hepatic phagocytosis. Heparin therapy may lead to the depletion of ATIII levels after prolonged treatment due to increased utilization. The concentration of ATIII is 18–35 mg/dL, and it has a half-life of 68 hours in plasma.

Heparin cofactor II is synthesized by the liver and has a high specificity for thrombin neutralization. It also has accelerated activity in the presence of heparin. Heparin cofactor II concentration in plasma is considerably lower (6–11 mg/dL). Its half-life in plasma is approximately 60 hours.[50]

C1 inhibitor is a major inhibitor of the complement proteins but also neutralizes the active contact factors XIIa, XIa, and kallikrein. Synthesized in the liver, C1 inhibitor has a half-life of 20 hours and a plasma concentration of 15–35 mg/dL. A similar inhibitor with an affinity for factor XIa has been recognized on the platelet surface.[13]

Alpha$_1$–anti-trypsin is the major inhibitor of activated factor XI and acts as a minor inhibitor for thrombin and plasmin. Alpha$_1$–anti-trypsin is present in the highest concentration of all the serpins in blood. However, deficiency of this inhibitor

Table 32–4. MOLECULAR WEIGHT, CONCENTRATION, AND HALF-LIFE OF INHIBITORS

Name	Molecular Weight (D)	Concentration	Half-Life (Hours)
Protein C inhibitor	57,000	3–7 μg/mL	Unknown
Alpha$_2$-macroglobulin	725,000	150–400 mg/dL	60
Alpha$_1$–anti-trypsin	53,000	100–180 mg/dL	Unknown
Anti-thrombin III	65,000	20–40 mg/dL	68
Heparin cofactor II	65,000	8–10 μg/mL	60
C1 inhibitor	104,000	18–22 mg/dL	20
PAI-1	52,000	14–28 mg/dL	1
Alpha$_2$–anti-plasmin	65,000	5–7 mg/dL	Unknown
Tissue factor pathway inhibitor	39,000	50–140 ng/mL	Unknown

does not cause thrombotic or bleeding problems, which indicates its minor role in hemostasis inhibition.[50] Alpha$_1$–anti-trypsin serves a more useful role in the blood by keeping elastase enzymes from white cells from disrupting the elastic membranes in the subendothelium.[51]

TFPI, formerly known as lipoprotein associated coagulation inhibitor (LACI) or extrinsic pathway inhibitor (EPI), is capable of inactivating VIIa/TF complex and factor Xa. This inhibitor has led to new thinking about extrinsic coagulation with the conclusion that VIIa/TF activation of factor IX plays a critical role in initial clotting. Factor IXa, with factor VIII as its cofactor, carries the initial responsibility for activating factor X until the inhibitory effects of TFPI are overcome. TFPI is associated with high-, low-, and very-low-density lipoprotein fractions in the blood. It is present in such low concentrations in blood that it was difficult to isolate. It appears to be a major regulator of the VIIa/III complex. TPFI is produced in a variety of tissues, including those of the lungs, liver, and bladder, and in endothelial cells. The most important site of production in regulation of coagulation is endothelial cells.[23]

PAI-1 is produced in endothelial cells and megakaryocytes. Platelets carry PAI-1 in their alpha granules. PAI-1 regulates plasminogen activators by preventing their activation of plasminogen. PAI-1 is particularly effective at preventing tPA and urokinase from plasminogen activation, but it has no effect on streptokinase. When vascular injury occurs, PAI-1 is released from injured endothelial cells and activated platelets to provide a localized neutralization of attempts to activate plasminogen to plasmin. This promotes fibrin deposition. After the clot is formed, tPA is released from endothelial cells by activated protein C. No PAI-1 is released and thus plasmin formation occurs.[10,50]

Protein C inhibitor is a small, single-chain protein that can inhibit thrombin, Xa, trypsin, and activated protein C. Its concentration in plasma is similar to protein C concentrations. Protein C inhibitor activity is enhanced by high concentrations of heparin.[50]

Alpha$_2$–anti-plasmin is the major regulator of plasmin. Produced in the liver, alpha$_2$–anti-plasmin readily inactivates free plasmin in the circulation, but has more difficulty with plasmin bound to fibrin because of competitive inhibition. Failure to neutralize free plasmin leads to lysis of native fibrinogen and degradation of factors V and VIII.[50]

Alpha$_2$–macroglobulin can inhibit many serine proteases; however, it does so more slowly than other inhibitors. A large molecule with multiple subunits synthesized in the liver, it is an important backup inhibitor when alpha$_2$–anti-plasmin is not present.[10]

SUMMARY

Normal hemostasis is a complex, interactive group of systems that works in harmony to achieve a hemostatic balance. The systems include platelet function, extrinsic coagulation, intrinsic coagulation, a protein C/protein S control system, fibrin lysis, and the serine protease inhibitors. To understand each part of the total system requires detailed study. Interrelationships, positive and negative feedback loops, autoactivations, and reciprocal activations make up the entire hemostatic mechanism complex.

REVIEW QUESTIONS

1. What is the purpose of coagulation?

2. Which plasma coagulation factor is multimeric in nature? Describe its multimeric make-up.

3. What are the six coagulation factors that depend on vitamin K for gamma carboxylation?

4. What value does gamma carboxylation have for the vitamin K–dependent coagulation proteins?

5. During activation of prothrombin to thrombin, what fragment is cleaved?

6. What role does thrombin play in platelet activity, coagulation, and fibrin lysis?

7. What properties of endothelial cells are responsible for initiation of coagulation, for limitation of the thrombus formation, and for degradation of the fibrin clot?

8. How does factor XIIIa crosslink fibrin polymers?

9. How are D-dimers related to crosslinked fibrin?

10. What are the endogenous mechanisms for activation of plasminogen? Which one is the most likely to happen in normal hemostasis?

11. What is PAI-1? Why is PAI-1 liberated by activated platelets and traumatized tissue?

12. What degradation products are formed from plasmin's digestion of fibrin and fibrinogen?

13. Is degradation of fibrinogen normal? Why or why not?

14. Why are serine protease inhibitors (serpins) present in plasma? What would be the effect if any of them were deficient?

15. Explain protein C activation. What is thrombin's role? What role do endothelial cells and thrombin play in its activation?

16. What is the function of activated protein C? What protein acts as its cofactor? Why are they both vitamin K–dependent?

References

1. Phillips D: Hypercoagulability and thrombosis: the promise of endothelial cells. J Clin Lab Sci 1990; 3:170.
2. Rick ME: Protein C and protein S. Vitamin K–dependent inhibitors of blood coagulation. JAMA 1990; 263:701–703.
3. Jensen R, Ens GE: Clinical significance of fibrinogen. Clin Hemos Rev 1993; 7(Jan):1–4.
4. Harrison P, Wilbourn B, Debilli N, et al: Uptake of plasma fibrinogen into the alpha granules of human megakaryocytes and platelets. J Clin Invest 1989; 84:1320–1324.
5. Louache F, Debili N, Cramer E, et al: Fibrinogen is not synthesized by human megakaryocytes. Blood 1991; 77:311–316.
6. Lange W, Luig A, Dolken G, et al: Fibrinogen γ-chain mRNA is not detected in human megakaryocytes. Blood 1991; 78:20–25.
7. Folsom AR, Wu KK, Davis CE, et al: Population correlates of plasma fibrinogen and factor VII putative cardiovascular risk factors. Atherosclerosis 1991; 91:191–205.
8. Furie B, Furie BC: Molecular and cellular biology of blood coagulation. New Engl J Med 1992; 326:800–806.
9. Powers LW: Diagnostic Hematology: Clinical and Technical Principles. St. Louis: CV Mosby, 1989:161–184.
10. Corriveau DM: Plasma proteins: factors of the hemostatic mechanism. In Corriveau DM, Fritsma GA (eds): Hemostasis and Thrombosis in the Clinical Laboratory. Philadelphia: JB Lippincott, 1988:34–66.
11. Monkovic DD, Tracy PB: Activation of human factor V by factor Xa and thrombin. Biochemistry 1990; 29:1118–1128.
12. Thompson EA, Salem H: Inhibition by human thrombomodulin of factor Xa–mediated cleavage of prothrombin. J Clin Invest 1986; 78(July):13–17.
13. Berg LH: Chemistry of coagulation. In Anderson SC, Cockayne S (eds): Clinical Chemistry—Concepts and Applications. Philadelphia: WB Saunders, 1993:613–632.
14. Jobe MI: Mechanisms of Coagulation and Fibrinolysis. In Lotspeich-Steininger CA, Steine-Martin AE, Koepke JA (eds): Clinical Hematology: Principles, Procedures, Correlations. Philadelphia: JB Lippincott, 1992:579–596.
15. Monkovic DD, Tracy PB: Functional characterization of human platelet-released factor V and its activation by factor Xa and thrombin. J Biol Chem 1990; 265:17132–17140.
16. Ruf W, Miles DJ, Rehemtulla A, Edgington TS: Tissue factor residues 157–167 are required for efficient proteolytic activation of factor X and factor VII. J Biol Chem 1992; 267:22206–22210.
17. Kumar A, Blumenthal DK, Fair DS: Identification of molecular sites on factor VII which mediate its assembly and function in the extrinsic pathway activation complex. J Biol Chem 1991; 266:915–921.
18. Ruf W, Kalnik MW, Lund-Hansen T, Edgington TS: Characterization of factor VII association with tissue factor in solution. J Biol Chem 1991; 266:15719–15725.
19. Wildgoose P, Foster D, Schiodt J, et al.: Identification of a calcium binding site in the protease domain of human blood coagulation factor VII: evidence for its role in factor VII-tissue factor interaction. Biochem 1993; 32:114–119.
20. Mertens K, Briet E, Giles AR: The role of factor VII in haemostasis: infusion studies of factor VIIa in a canine model of factor VIII deficiency. Thromb Haemost 1990; 64:138–144.
21. Rao LVM, Rapaport SI, Hoang AD: Binding of factor VIIa to tissue factor permits rapid antithrombin III/heparin inhibition of factor VIIa. Blood 1993; 81:2600–2607.
22. Morrissey JH, Macik BG, Neuenschwander PF, Comp PC: Quantitation of activated factor VII levels in plasma using a tissue factor mutant selectively deficient in promoting factor VII activation. Blood 1993; 81:734–744.
23. Jensen R, Ens GE: Tissue factor pathway inhibitor. Clin Hemost Rev 1992; 6 (June):1–3.
24. Thompson AR, Harker LA: Manual of Hemostasis and Thrombosis. Philadelphia: FA Davis, 1983:1–19.
25. Bithell TC: Normal hemostasis and coagulation. In Thorup OA (ed): Leavell and Thorup's Fundamentals of Clinical Hematology. Philadelphia: WB Saunders, 1987:137–152.
26. Kane WH, Davie EW: Blood coagulation factors V and VIII: Structural and functional similarities and their relationship to hemorrhagic and thrombotic disorders. Blood 1988; 71:539–555.
27. Bom VJJ, Reinalda-Poot JH, Cupers R, Bertina RM: Extrinsic activation of human blood coagulation factors IX and X. Thromb Haemost 1990; 63(2):224–230.
28. Jensen R, Ens GE: Contact factor mechanisms. Clin Hemost Rev 1994; 8:1–4.
29. Walsh PN: Factor XI: a renaissance. Semin Hematol 1992; 3:189–201.
30. Meijers JCM, McMullen BA, Bouma BN: The contact activation proteins: A structure/function overview. Actions Agents Suppl 1992; 38:219–230.
31. Gailani D, Broze GJ: Factor XI activation in a revised model of blood coagulation. Science 1991; 253:909–1012.
32. Bick RL: Disorders of Thrombosis and Hemostasis: Clinical and Laboratory Practice. Chicago: ASCP Press, 1992:9–22.
33. Catalana PM: Coagulation physiology and hemorrhagic disorders. In Besa EC, Catalano PM, Kant JA, Jefferies LC (eds): Hematology. Malvern, PA: Harwal, 1992:223–227.
34. McKenzie SB: Secondary hemostasis. In McKenzie SB, (ed): Textbook of Hematology. Philadelphia: Lea & Febiger, 1988:381–407.
35. Harmening DM: Introduction to hemostasis. In Harmening DM (ed): Clinical Hematology and Fundamentals of Hemostasis. Philadelphia: FA Davis, 1992:418.
36. Reddigari SR, Kuna P, Miragliotta G, et al: Human high molecular weight kininogen binds to human umbilical vein endothelial cells via its heavy and light chains. Blood 1993; 81(5):1306–1311.
37. Davie WE, Ratnoff OD: Waterfall sequence for intrinsic blood clotting. Science 1964; 145:1310.
38. McFarland RG: An enzyme cascade in blood clotting mechanisms and its function as a biochemical amplifier. Nature 1964; 202:498.
39. Nemerson Y: Mechanisms of coagulation. In Williams W, Beutler E, Erslev A, Lichtman MA (eds): Hematology. New York: McGraw-Hill, 1990:1295–1301.
40. Catalana PM: Coagulation regulation and hypercoagulable states. In Besa EC, Catalano PM, Kant JA, Jefferies LC (eds): Hematology. Malvern, PA: Harwal, 1992:241–243.
41. Stephens CJ: The antiphospholipid syndrome. Clinical correlations, cutaneous features, mechanism of thrombosis and treatment of patients with the lupus and anticardiolipin antibodies. Br J Dermatol 1991; 125:199–210.
42. Marlar RA. The protein C system and its role in hereditary thrombotic disease. Coag Q 1993; 2:1–4.
43. Burns ER: Clinical Management of Bleeding and Thrombosis. Boston: Blackwell, 1987:7–15.
44. Berg DT, Purck PJ, Berg DH, Grinnell BW: Kringle glycosylation in a modified human tissue plasminogen activator improves functional properties. Blood 1993; 81(5):1312–1322.
45. Braaten JV, Handt S, Jerome WG, et al: Regulation of fibrinolysis by platelet-released plasminogen activator inhibitor 1: light scattering and ultrastructural examination of lysis of a model platelet-fibrin thrombus. Blood 1993; 81(5):1290–1299.
46. Christ G, Seiffert B, Hufnagl P, et al: Type 1 plasminogen

activator inhibitor synthesis of endothelial cells is down regulated by smooth muscle cells. Blood 1993; 81(5):1277–1283.

47. Lotspeich-Steininger CA. Introduction to Hemostasis: *In* Lotspeich-Steininger CA, Steine-Martin AE, Koepke JA (eds): Clinical Hematology: Principles, Procedures, Correlations. Philadelphia: JB Lippincott, 1992:564–577.

48. Laposata M, Connoar AM, Hicks DG, Phillips DK: The Clinical Hemostasis Handbook. Chicago: Year Book, 1989: 19–25.

49. Southern DK: Serum FDP and plasma D-dimer testing: What are they measuring? Clin Lab Sci 1992; 5(6):332–333.

50. Jensen R, Ens GE: Serine protease inhibitors. Clin Hemost Rev 1993; 7:1–3.

51. Lindsey BJ: Amino acids and proteins. *In* Bishop ML, Duben-Von Laufen JL, Fody EP (eds): Clinical Chemistry: Principles, Procedures, Correlations. Philadelphia: JB Lippincott, 1992:182–183.

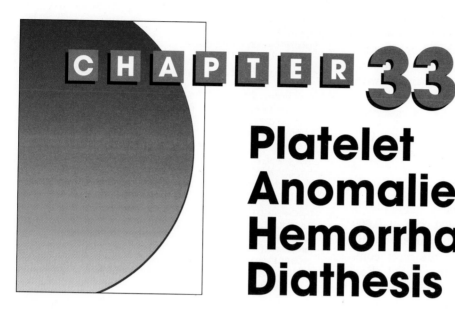

Platelet Anomalies and Hemorrhagic Diathesis

Jeanne M. Clerc

Outline

Objectives

AFTER COMPLETION OF THIS CHAPTER, THE READER WILL BE ABLE TO

1. Define thrombocytopenia, thrombocytosis, and thrombocythemia and state-associated platelet counts.
2. Describe the clinical symptoms of and associated laboratory findings in May-Hegglin anomaly.
3. Name at least four causes of acquired hypoplasia of the bone marrow.
4. Differentiate between acute and chronic idiopathic thrombocytopenia.
5. Describe immunologic and nonimmunologic mechanisms by which drugs may bind to platelet surface membranes.
6. Differentiate between neonatal isoimmune thrombocytopenia and neonatal autoimmune thrombocytopenia.
7. Explain the associated laboratory findings with thrombotic thrombocytopenic purpura (TTP) and hemolytic uremic syndrome (HUS).
8. Describe clinical symptoms of and associated laboratory findings, including platelet aggregation studies, in (a) Bernard-Soulier syndrome, (b) von Willebrand's disease, (c) Glanzmann's thrombasthenia, (d) storage pool diseases and (e) ingestion of aspirin.
9. Describe associated clinical symptoms and causes of the following vascular disorders: (a) hereditary hemorrhagic telangiectasia (HHT), (b) Kasabach-Merritt syndrome, (c) Ehrlers-Danlos syndrome, and (d) acquired vascular disorders.

Clinical manifestations of bleeding disorders can be divided into two broad and rather poorly defined groups: (1) superficial bleeding (such as petechiae, epistaxis, or gingival bleeding), which is usually associated with a platelet defect or vascular disorder, and (2) deep bleeding (such as hematomas or hemarthrosis), which is associated with plasma clotting factor deficiencies.[1] This chapter describes platelet disorders; Chapter 34 describes other coagulation disorders.

THROMBOCYTOPENIA

The reference range for platelets generally is considered to be between 140,000 and 440,000 cells/mm³ ($140-440 \times 10^9$/L). Thrombocytopenia (platelet count < 100,000/mm³) is the most common cause of serious bleeding encountered clinically. Thrombocytopenia may result from any one of four pathophysiologic processes: decreased platelet production, accelerated platelet destruction, abnormal platelet distribution or increased platelet sequestration within the spleen, or loss from the body.[2-5] (Table 33–1).

Small-vessel bleeding attributed to thrombocytopenia results in hemorrhages into the skin of different sizes: 3 mm (petechiae), 1 cm (purpura) or 3 cm (ecchymoses). The clinical importance of thrombocytopenia is related to the bleeding hazard. The clinical bleeding is variable and often not closely correlated with the platelet count. No dysfunction or clinical bleeding, however, is expected with platelet counts higher than 60,000/mm³. Patients with platelet counts as low as 20,000/mm³,

---

Table 33–1. CLASSIFICATION OF PLATELET AND VASCULAR DISORDERS

Quantitative Abnormalities: Changes in Platelet Numbers

THROMBOCYTOPENIA: DECREASE IN CIRCULATING PLATELETS
IMPAIRED OR DECREASED PRODUCTION OF PLATELETS
Congenital: May-Hegglin anomaly
Neonatal
Acquired

INCREASED PLATELET DESTRUCTION
Immune
  Acute and chronic idiopathic thrombocytopenic purpura
  Drug-induced: immunologic
  Neonatal alloimmune (isoimmune neonatal thrombocytopenia
  Neonatal autoimmune thrombocytopenia
  Post-transfusion isoimmune thrombocytopenia
  Secondary autoimmune thrombocytopenia
Nonimmune
  Thrombocytopenia in pregnancy and eclampsia
  Erythroblastosis fetalis
  Thrombotic thrombocytopenic purpura
  Disseminated intravascular coagulation
  Hemolytic-uremic syndrome
  Drugs: nonimmune mechanisms of platelet destruction

DISORDERS RELATED TO DISTRIBUTION OR DILUTION
Splenic sequestration
Hypothermia
Loss of platelets: massive blood transfusions, extracorporeal circulation

THROMBOCYTOSIS: INCREASE IN CIRCULATING PLATELETS
REACTIVE THROMBOCYTOSIS
Associated with blood loss and surgery
Post-splenctomy thrombocytosis
Iron-deficiency anemia
Inflammation and disease
Stress and/or exercise

THROMBOCYTOSIS ASSOCIATED WITH MYELOPROLIFERATIVE DISORDERS
Polycythemia vera, chronic myelocytic leukemia, and myelofibrosis with myeloid metaplasia

THROMBOCYTHEMIA: ESSENTIAL OR PRIMARY THROMBOCYTHEMIA

Qualitative Abnormalities: Changes in Platelet Function (Thrombocytophathy)
DISORDERS OF PLATELET ADHESION
BERNARD-SOULIER (GIANT PLATELET) SYNDROME
VON WILLEBRAND'S DISEASE
ACQUIRED DEFECTS OF PLATELET ADHESION
Myeloproliferative and lymphoproliferative disorders and dysproteinemias
Antiplatelet antibodies
Cardiopulmonary bypass
Chronic liver disease
Drug-induced membrane modification
Hereditary afibrinogenemia

DISORDERS OF PRIMARY AGGREGATION
GLANZMANN'S THROMBASTHENIA (CONGENITAL)
ACQUIRED
Acquired von Willebrand's disease
Uremia

DISORDERS OF PLATELET SECRETION (RELEASE REACTIONS)
STORAGE POOL DISEASES
Dense granule deficiencies
  Hermansky-Pudlak syndrome
  Wiskott-Aldrich syndrome
  Thrombocytopenia with absent radii syndrome
  Chédiak-Higashi syndrome
Alpha granule deficiencies
  Gray platelet syndrome

THOMBOXANE PATHWAY DISORDERS: ASPIRIN-LIKE EFFECTS
Drug inhibition of the prostaglandin pathways
  Cyclooxygenase or thromboxane synthetase deficiency
  Drug inhibition of platelet phosphodiesterase activity
  Hereditary aspirin-like defects

HYPERACTIVE PRETHROMBOTIC PLATELETS
Vascular Disorders
HEREDITARY VASCULAR DISORDERS
Hereditary hemorrhagic telangiectasia (Rendu-Weber-Osler syndrome)
Hemangioma-thrombocytopenia syndrome (Kasabach-Merritt syndrome)
Ehlers-Danlos syndrome and other genetic disorders

ACQUIRED VASCULAR DISORDERS
Allergic purpura (Henoch-Schönlein purpura)
Senile purpura
Paraproteinemia and amyloidosis
Drug-induced vascular purpuras
Vitamin C deficiency (scurvy)

PURPURAS OF UNKNOWN ORIGIN
Purpura simplex (Easy bruisability)
Psychogenic purpura

Sources: Thompson and Harker[6] and Colvin.[9]

and sometimes lower, may have little or no bleeding or purpura, whereas patients with platelet counts below 10,000/mm³ may manifest widespread purpura and bleeding.[5]

Decreased Platelet Production

Abnormalities in platelet production may be divided into two categories: one type is associated with a hypoproliferation or hypoplasia of the bone marrow, and the second type is associated with ineffective thrombopoiesis, the disordered proliferation of the megakaryocytic pool, such as occurs in bone marrow infiltration by malignant cells.

Congenital Hypoplasia

Hypoplasia of the marrow megakaryocytes is seen in a wide variety of clinical situations, including Fanconi syndrome, thrombocytopenia with absent radii (TAR syndrome), and Wiskott-Aldrich and May Hegglin anomalies. The TAR syndrome and Wiskott-Aldrich anomaly produce qualitative as well as quantitative defects and so are described later in this chapter.

The *May-Hegglin anomaly* is an autosomal dominant disorder in which Döhle bodies are present in neutrophils and large platelets (up to 20 μm in length) are seen on the peripheral blood film (Fig. 33–1). Thrombocytopenia is present in about one third of affected patients. In some patients, megakaryocytes are increased in numbers and have abnormal ultrastructure. The thrombocytopenia associated with May-Hegglin anomaly is thought to result from ineffective thrombopoiesis and increased platelet destruction. Most patients are asymptomatic, but bleeding times may be discor-

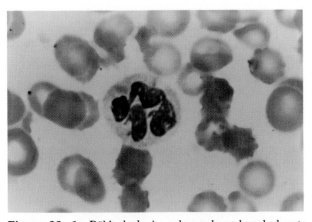

Figure 33–1 Döhle body in polymorphonuclear leukocyte (May-Hegglin anomaly); peripheral blood; May-Hegglin is also associated with the presence of giant platelets as well. (From Amorosi EL: Basic Hematology. Garden Grove, CA: Medcom, 1970.)

dantly prolonged in some patients and associated with clinically significant bleeding.[5, 6]

Several varieties of hereditary thrombocytopenia are well documented. Most of these disorders are caused by deficient platelet production. These disorders may be inherited through either autosomal dominance or X-linkage. The two genetic variants produce similar clinical and laboratory findings. Bleeding usually is mild, platelet function is normal, and the megakaryocytes appear to be normal in number and morphology.[7, 8]

Neonatal Hypoplasia

The thrombocytopenia seen in newborns infected with rubella is severe; platelet counts are as low as 70,000/mm³. Bone marrow examination reveals a marked lack of megakaryocytes.

Chlorothiazide diuretics or tolbutamide ingested by the mother has a direct toxic effect of the thiazide on the fetal marrow megakaryocytes. Recovery usually occurs within weeks after birth. The dyscrasia is slow to develop and slow to regress when the drug is stopped.[2, 5, 8]

Acquired Hypoplasia

Ionizing irradiation and a large number of drugs, including most agents that are used in the treatment of both hematologic and nonhematologic neoplasms, suppress the megakaryocytes, together with other hematopoietic precursor cells, and produce thrombocytopenia. These drugs are generally anti-metabolites or alkylating agents.[2]

Ethanol suppresses megakaryocytopoiesis through an unknown mechanism. Mild thrombocytopenia is a common finding in severely alcoholic patients in whom other causes, such as portal hypertension, splenomegaly, and folic acid deficiency, have been excluded. Thrombocytosis frequently develops when alcohol ingestion is stopped.[8]

Thrombocytopenia presumably caused by megakaryocyte suppression has also been reported to follow the administration of diethylstilbestrol and leukocyte interferon. Other drugs such as certain antibacterial agents (e.g., chloramphenicol, tranquilizers, and anticonvulsants) have also been associated with thrombocytopenia caused by bone marrow depression.[9]

Thrombocytopenia may be an early manifestation of *aplastic anemia* and is a major complication in the management of various forms of this disorder. Both anemia and leukopenia are usually associated with aplastic anemia.

Bone marrow aplasia may be associated with skeletal abnormalities, or it may occur without skeletal abnormalities. The most common example of thrombocytopenia associated with skeletal abnormalities is TAR syndrome, in which the radius is absent, presumably as a result of fetal injury at approximately 8 weeks' gestation. Megakaryocytic hypoplasia has been reported in adults and children without skeletal abnormalities.[6]

Quantitative studies of thrombopoiesis in patients with *pernicious anemia* and *folic acid deficiency* suggest that platelet production, like erythrocyte production, is ineffective. The bone marrow generally contains an increased number of megakaryocytes, but platelet production is deficient. The thrombocytopenia is a result of the impaired DNA synthesis. In megaloblastic anemias, grossly abnormal megakaryocytes with deformed, dumbbell-shaped nuclei are present in large numbers. Stained smears reveal large platelets, which may have a decreased survival time, and may also show abnormal function. Thrombocytopenia is usually mild, and there is evidence of increased platelet destruction. Patients respond to vitamin replacement within 1–2 weeks.[2, 6, 10, 11]

Viruses may cause thrombocytopenia by acting on the megakaryocytes or on circulating platelets, either directly or in the form of viral antigen-antibody complexes. Live measles vaccine can cause degenerative vacuolization of megakaryocytes 6–8 days after vaccination. Viruses readily interact with platelets, in some instances by means of specific platelet receptors. Other viruses associated with thrombocytopenia include cytomegalic inclusion disease, Thai hemorrhagic fever, varicella, rubella, and infectious mononucleosis.[8]

Bacterial infections commonly are associated with thrombocytopenia. This may be a result of toxins of bacterial origin, direct interactions between bacteria and platelets in the circulation, or extensive damage to the endothelium, as in meningococcemia. Many cases of thrombocytopenia in childhood result from infection. Furthermore, purpura may occur in many infectious diseases in the absence of thrombocytopenia, presumably because of vascular damage.[8, 12]

Infiltration of the bone marrow by malignant cells generally results in decreased numbers of megakaryocytes. Abnormal cells crowd out or replace normal bone marrow elements, thereby causing thrombocytopenia. Inhibitors of thrombopoiesis may be produced by these abnormal cells and may also help account for the thrombocytopenia associated with such conditions as myeloma, lymphoma, metastatic cancer, and myelofibrosis.[2, 3, 6]

Increased Platelet Destruction

Thrombocytopenias resulting from platelet destruction can be separated into (1) disorders caused by mechanical damage and consumption (nonimmunologic) and (2) those caused by immunologic responses. An example of consumption is thrombocytopenia associated with sepsis caused by either gram-positive or gram-negative organisms. All serious infections may be accompanied by thrombocytopenia as the result of intravascular coagulation. Regardless of the process, increased production is necessary to compensate for the accelerated loss of platelets.[8, 12, 13]

Immune Mechanisms of Platelet Destruction

ACUTE AND CHRONIC IDIOPATHIC THROMBOCYTOPENIC PURPURAS

The term *idiopathic thrombocytopenic purpura* (ITP) usually refers to cases of thrombocytopenia associated with no apparent etiology or underlying disease states. It is more common than all secondary forms of thrombocytopenia combined. Large but decreased numbers of platelets are typical of ITP[5] (Fig. 33–2).

There is convincing evidence that ITP is caused by platelet destruction as a result of an immunologic process. Antibodies of the ITP type produce thrombocytopenia by attaching to platelets, which, as a result, are removed from the circulation by reticuloendothelial cells, most importantly in the spleen. In addition to removing antibody-sensitized platelets, the spleen may be an important site of antibody synthesis. The shortened life span of the platelet, generally from a matter of hours to 2–3 days, results from a process extrinsic to the platelet. Infusion into a normal recipient of plasma from patients with ITP causes thrombocytopenia. The "ITP factor" is an immunoglobulin G (IgG)

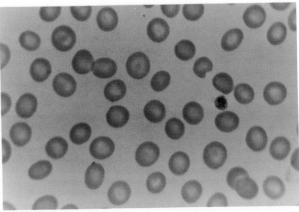

Figure 33–2 Large platelet, idiopathic thrombocytopenic purpura (ITP); peripheral blood. The few platelets which are seen in the peripheral blood film of patients with ITP are usually large and often resemble fragments of megakaryocytes. (From Amorosi EL: Basic Hematology. Garden Grove, CA: Medcom, 1970.)

that can be removed from serum by absorption with normal human platelets and subsequently eluted. However, direct experimental evidence linking immune complexes to platelet destruction in acute ITP is lacking.[5, 8, 14]

Idiopathic thrombocytopenic purpura occurs in acute, chronic, and recurrent forms. The recurrent form is characterized by episodes of thrombocytopenia and periods in which the platelet count is normal.[5]

In the peripheral blood, platelets have a variety of sizes and shapes. In most cases, platelets number fewer than 20,000/mm³. The marrow is characterized by megakaryocytic hyperplasia. Typically, the megakaryocytes are increased in size, and young forms with single nuclei, smooth contour, and diminished cytoplasm are commonly seen. Coagulation test abnormalities include a prolonged bleeding time and deficient clot retraction. Platelet-associated IgG levels are increased in the majority of patients.[5, 8, 14]

Thrombocytopenia is a symptom, and a diagnosis of ITP requires that the numerous secondary causes of thrombocytopenia be ruled out. Treatment consists of steroids, splenectomy, and, in occasional cases, immunosuppressive agents. Platelet transfusions may be of transient benefit in treating severe hemorrhages but should not be given routinely.[5, 14]

Differentiation

There are a number of differences between acute and chronic ITP (Table 33–2). Acute ITP occurs most frequently in children aged 2–9 years and in young adults. Chronic ITP occurs in patients of all ages but is most common in adults aged 20–50 and primarily in women. Of the patients with acute ITP, 60–80% have a history of infection, usually viral (rubella, rubeola, chickenpox, and nonspecific respiratory infections), occurring 2–21 days previ-

ously. Acute ITP may also occur after immunization with live vaccine for measles, chickenpox, mumps, and smallpox. Acute ITP is usually self-limited, and spontaneous remissions occur in 80% of the patients; the duration of the illness may range from days to months. In chronic ITP, there is typically a fluctuating clinical course, with episodes of bleeding that last a few days or weeks; spontaneous remissions are uncommon and usually incomplete.[5, 14]

Symptoms of *acute ITP* are variable, but petechial hemorrhages, purpura, and often bleeding from the gums and gastrointestinal and urinary tracts typically begin suddenly, sometimes over a period of a few hours. Hemorrhagic bullae in the oral mucosa are often prominent in patients with severe thrombocytopenia of acute onset. Usually the severity of bleeding is correlated with the degree of thrombocytopenia.[14]

Presenting symptoms in *chronic ITP* begin with a few scattered petechiae or other minor bleeding manifestations. Occasionally a bruising tendency, menorrhagia, or recurrent epistaxis is present for months or even years before diagnosis. Platelet counts range from 5,000/mm³ to 75,000/mm³ and are generally somewhat higher than those in acute ITP. Bizarre giant platelets and fragmented platelets are commonly seen. Platelet-associated immunoglobulin levels are elevated in more than 90% of the patients.[14]

Chronic ITP occurring in association with human immunodeficiency virus type 1 (HIV-1) infection, with hemophilia, and with pregnancy presents special problems in diagnosis and therapy. Unexplained thrombocytopenia in otherwise healthy members of high-risk populations may be an early manifestation of acquired immunodeficiency syndrome (AIDS).[3, 14]

Treatment also varies for acute and chronic ITP. In *chronic ITP*, initial therapy often consists of

Table 33-2. CLINICAL PICTURE OF ACUTE AND CHRONIC IDIOPATHIC THROMBOCYTOPENIC PURPURA		
Characteristics	**Acute**	**Chronic**
Age at onset	2–6 years	20–50 years
Sex predilection	None	Female over male, 3 : 1
Prior infection	Common	Unusual
Onset of bleeding	Sudden	Gradual
Platelet count	<20,000/mm³	30,000–80,000/mm³
Duration	2–6 weeks	Months to years
Spontaneous remission	90% of patients	Uncommon
Seasonal pattern	Higher incidence in winter and spring	None
Therapy		
Steroids	70% response rate	30% response
Splenectomy	Rare	Under age 45, 90% response; over age 45, 40% response

Sources: Triplett et al.[5] and Quick.[12]

glucocorticoids, which interfere with splenic and hepatic macrophages to increase platelet survival time. However, the resultant immunosuppression and toxicity usually necessitate splenectomy. In *acute ITP*, there is good response to corticosteroids, and rarely is splenectomy required.[5, 11, 13]

DRUG-INDUCED THROMBOCYTOPENIA: IMMUNOLOGIC EFFECTS

Ingestion of quinine, quinidine, and certain other drugs may trigger the formation of antibodies that, in the presence of the drug, react with platelets to cause thrombocytopenia. If the drug is taken by a sensitized pregnant woman shortly before delivery, both she and her offspring may be affected. Quinine, formerly used to facilitate labor, has been implicated as a cause of this type of thrombocytopenia in the newborn.[14]

Other drugs have subsequently been observed to cause acute thrombocytopenia in sensitive persons (Table 33–3). Quinine, quinidine, and stibo-

Table 33–3. COMMON DRUGS CAUSING IMMUNE THROMBOCYTOPENIA
Analgesics
Salicylates
Acetaminophin
Phenylbutazone
Antibiotics
Cephalothin
Penicillin
Streptomycin
Para-aminosalicylic acid (PAS)
Rifampin
Novobiocin
Various sulfa drugs (chlorthalidone, furosemide)
Alkaloids
Quinidine
Quinine
Sedatives, Anti-Convulsants
Methoin
Troxidone
Chlorpromazine
Diphenylhydantoin
Meprobamate
Phenobarbital
Carbamazepine
Oral Hypoglycemics
Chlorpropamide
Tolbutamide
Heavy Metals
Gold
Mercury
Bismuth
Organic arsenicals
Miscellaneous
Chloroquine
Chlorothiazide
Insecticides

Sources: Triplett et al.[5] and Quick.[12]

phen have been studied most extensively with regard to their mechanism of action. The nature of this idiosyncracy is unknown, but it is likely that sensitive persons produce antibodies of unusually high avidity. Small drug molecules (haptens) must first combine with larger (carrier) molecules, usually plasma proteins, to form complete antigens.[8, 14]

Detailed studies of quinidine suggest that the drug first combines with the antibody; the antigen-antibody complex thus formed then attaches to the platelet in an essentially nonspecific manner (the "innocent bystander" hypothesis). However, it now seems clear that the antibodies responsible for drug-induced thrombocytopenia bind to platelets by their Fab regions rather than by attaching nonspecifically as immune complexes. Most drug-induced platelet antibodies are of the IgG class; in rare instances, IgM antibodies have been demonstrated.[8, 14]

Other mechanisms may also be operative in drug-induced thrombocytopenia. In some instances, true autoantibodies that do not require the drug to interact with platelets appear to be produced. This may occur regularly with some drugs such as gold salts and alpha-methyldopa. In other cases, there may be covalent linkage of drug to the platelet membrane with subsequent formation of true hapten-dependent antibodies. Occasional cases of penicillin-induced thrombocytopenia may represent examples of this phenomenon. In some patients, heparin-induced thrombocytopenia may be mediated by heparin–anti-heparin immune complexes.[14] Mechanisms of drug/platelet binding are shown in Figure 33–3.

In drug-induced thrombocytopenia caused by an immunologic mechanism, thrombocytopenia is often very severe initially, platelet levels being less than 10,000/mm³ and sometimes less than 1,000/mm³. The number of megakaryocytes is usually normal or elevated.[14] With common offending drugs such as quinidine, bleeding usually is severe and rapid in onset; hemorrhagic bullae in the mouth may be prominent.[8]

Treatment includes discontinuing ingestion of the offending drug. Drugs are usually cleared from the circulation rapidly, but dissociation of drug-antibody complexes may require longer periods, perhaps 1–2 weeks.[8]

NEONATAL ALLOIMMUNE (ISOIMMUNE) THROMBOCYTOPENIA (NAIT)

The pathophysiology of this disorder is exactly the same as that of erythroblastosis fetalis. The absence of platelet-specific antigens in the mother (usually Pl^A1^, rarely PlGrLy^B1^, and others) that the fetus has inherited from the father results in the

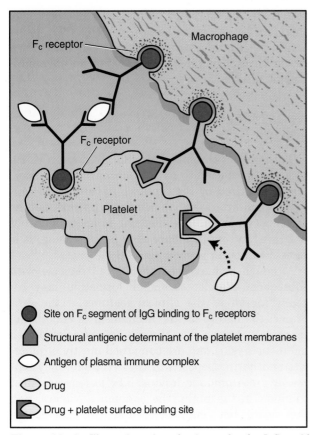

Figure 33–3 Illustration of mechanisms whereby IgG could bind to the platelet surface membrane with resultant removal of the IgG-coated platelet by its binding to the macrophage Fc receptors. (From Rapaport SI: Introduction to Hematology, 2nd ed. Philadelphia: JB Lippincott, 1987:489.)

development of maternal isoantibodies to fetal platelet antigens. If the mother is exposed to the Pl^A1 antigen from the fetal cells, she may make antibodies to the Pl^A1 antigen. The antibodies cross the placenta, attach to the Pl^A1-positive fetal platelets, and produce thrombocytopenia in the fetus. Clinically significant thrombocytopenia develops in an estimated 1 in 5000 newborns and is seen mainly in firstborns.[8, 15]

Affected infants may appear normal at birth but soon manifest scattered petechial and purpuric hemorrhages. In the symptomatic cases, platelet levels are usually less than 30,000/mm³ and may diminish even further in the first few hours after birth.[5, 8]

The diagnosis of congenital isoimmune thrombocytopenia usually is one of presumption. It includes ruling out both history of idiopathic thrombocytopenic purpura in the mother and maternal ingestion of drugs such as the thiazide diuretics. The presence of thrombocytopenia in a neonate with a Pl^A1-negative mother or a history of the disorder in a sibling is strong presumptive evidence in favor of the diagnosis.

Treatment may include administering steroids to the mother, and exchange transfusions have been used with success in some cases. Platelet transfusion may be beneficial even if the platelet count does not rise significantly. Compatible platelets may be prepared by plasmapheresis of the mother. Because the incidence of Pl^A1 antigen–negative platelets is less than 2% in random donor bloods, the mother's platelets are usually the most accessible.[8, 13]

A mortality rate of about 14% among affected infants is reported, but the severity, as in cases of hemolytic disease of the newborn, increases with additional stimulation of the maternal immune response. In many infants with isoimmune thrombocytopenia, serious hemorrhage does not develop, and the infants recover over a 1- to 2-week period as the passively transferred antibody is metabolized.[8, 13]

NEONATAL AUTOIMMUNE THROMBOCYTOPENIA (ITP)

Actually, the prefix *auto* is a misnomer because the autoimmune process occurs in the mother and not in the infant. ITP commonly develops in pregnant women, and if ITP is in remission or partial remission, relapse is common when a woman becomes pregnant. This has been attributed to the facilitation of reticuloendothelial phagocytosis by high estrogen levels. Corticosteroids may be given to the mother without serious danger to the fetus. ITP in the mother tends to remit after delivery.[15]

In order to diagnose autoimmune neonatal thrombocytopenia, ITP must be diagnosed in the mother. In contrast to isoimmune neonatal thrombocytopenia, the mother's nonspecific antibodies of the ITP type cross the placenta and produce thrombocytopenia in the fetus. At birth, many infants of mothers who are thrombocytopenic have thrombocytopenia. For this reason, many obstetricians have recommended that high-risk infants be delivered by cesarean section.[15]

POST-TRANSFUSION ISOIMMUNE THROMBOCYTOPENIA

This disorder develops approximately 1 week after transfusions of platelet-containing blood products and is manifested by the rapid onset of severe thrombocytopenia and moderate to severe hemorrhage. Platelet counts upon initial bleeding are quite low (less than 10,000/mm³). Megakaryocytes are present in the bone marrow in normal or increased numbers. Serologic findings of anti-Pl^A1 antibodies have been reported in each case. This type of thrombocytopenia has been documented in

34 women, more than 90% of whom were multi-gravidas. The natural course of the disease is gradual remission of thrombocytopenia over 1–6 weeks. However, hemorrhage may be life-threatening, and exchange transfusion or plasmapheresis may be used in treatment.[8, 13]

SECONDARY AUTOIMMUNE THROMBOCYTOPENIA

Immune thrombocytopenia develops in about 5–10% of patients with chronic lymphocytic leukemia and in a smaller percentage of patients with other lymphoproliferative disorders. Thrombocytopenia also is noted in 14–26% of patients with systemic lupus erythematosus (SLE). The clinical picture is similar to that of ITP: the bone marrow has a larger than normal number of megakaryocytes, and increased levels of platelet antigen IgG are frequently found.[3, 13]

Nonimmune Mechanisms of Platelet Destruction

Nonimmune platelet destruction may result from exposure of platelets to non-endothelial surfaces, from activation of the coagulation process, or from platelet consumption by endovascular injury with no measurable depletion of coagulation factors.[3]

THROMBOCYTOPENIA IN PREGNANCY AND PREECLAMPSIA

Random platelet counts in pregnant and postpartum women are slightly higher than normal, but about 5% of women in labor or who have delivered within the previous 24 hours are thrombocytopenic (21,000–135,000/mm³). Usually the thrombocytopenia resolves within 1 week of delivery. These findings could be related to low levels of "physiologic" disseminated intravascular coagulation (DIC) that accompanies normal delivery. The acronym HELLP (hemolysis, elevated liver enzymes, and low platelet count) has been used to describe preeclampsia associated with hemolysis, elevated liver enzyme concentrations in serum, and low platelet counts. In most severe cases, DIC can result. HELLP syndrome affects an estimated 4–12% of patients with severe preeclampsia.[14, 16, 17]

ERYTHROBLASTOSIS FETALIS

Thrombocytopenia, usually moderate in degree, occurs frequently in infants with erythroblastosis fetalis. Although the red blood cell destruction characteristic of this disorder is antibody-induced, the antigens against which the antibodies are di-rected are not expressed on platelets. Platelets may therefore be destroyed as the result of their interaction with products of red blood cell breakdown rather than their direct participation in an immunologic reaction.[3]

THROMBOTIC THROMBOCYTOPENIC PURPURA (TTP)

Thrombotic thrombocytopenic purpura (TTP), sometimes referred to as "Moschcowitz syndrome," is characterized by the presence of thrombi in capillaries and arterioles, by hemolytic anemia, and by thrombocytopenia. The disorder is uncommon but not rare, and its incidence may be increasing. It is most common in women aged 30–40 years.[2, 8, 11]

Although primary endothelial cell damage with subsequent platelet thrombus formation may account for all of the clinical features of the syndrome, the nature of the mechanism of endothelial injury is not clear. The thrombi are associated with microaneurysms and are composed mostly of platelets and fibrin. Deposits of these thrombi may represent prethrombotic lesions. The lesions are most common in the brain, the abdominal viscera, and the heart but may be found throughout the body.[6, 8]

The thrombotic lesions give rise to the characteristic manifestations of TTP. Red blood cells and platelets are destroyed mechanically by interactions with the microthrombi in the small vessels (microangiopathic cell destruction). Microspherocytes, shistocytes, and platelet fragments may result. There is evidence of intravascular hemolysis (reduction of haptoglobin, hemoglobinuria, hemosiderinuria) and accelerated red blood cell production (reticulocytosis, nucleated red blood cells, polychromasia, and stippling). The diagnosis of TTP cannot be made unless severely fragmented red blood cells are evident on the peripheral blood smear. The observation of thrombocytopenia (often <20,000 platelets/mm³), reticulocytosis, and fragmented red blood cells makes the blood film the most powerful diagnostic tool for TTP. Reflective of the hemolytic process, lactate dehydrogenase activity levels and unconjugated bilirubin levels are markedly increased. There may be varying manifestations of renal damage, such as proteinuria, hematuria, and a mild elevation of the blood urea nitrogen levels. However, overwhelming renal damage with anuria and fulminant uremia does not occur (which helps distinguish TTP from hemolytic-uremia syndromes).[8, 18]

Before 1990, TTP was fatal in more than 80% of patients. With the advent of exchange plasmapheresis and early diagnosis, 80% of patients who are treated early can be expected to survive TTP.

Plasma exchange may produce dramatic effects within a few hours, and many of the neurologic abnormalities disappear as a result of therapy. The infusion of plasma alone has been beneficial in some patients. Splenectomy and use of anti-platelet drugs and corticosteroids have been effective in a few patients. Platelet transfusions should be avoided.[8, 14]

The exact pathogenic mechanisms responsible for this disorder remain uncertain; however four causes have been suggested: (1) TTP plasma is deficient in a platelet-aggregating factor inhibitor (an immunoglobulin normally found in plasma); (2) large von Willebrand's factor (vWF) multimers promote platelet agglutination; (3) endothelial cell damage through a plasma factor results in platelet adhesion; and (4) as a consequence of endothelial cell damage, there is an abnormality of vascular endothelium caused by a defect in endothelial prostacyclin (PGI_2) metabolism, leading to poor maintenance of blood vessel lining. Other predisposing conditions include deficiency of tissue plasminogen activator, infection, pregnancy, hormones, and hereditary factors.[8, 10, 13, 14]

The majority of patients are between 10 and 60 years old. Two forms of TTP are generally recognized: a chronic type, in which symptoms persist or are recurrent over months or sometimes years, and a much more common acute type, which may be fatal in a few days.[14]

The syndrome includes manifestations of anemia, thrombocytopenia, and neurologic dysfunction (the triad), and fever and renal dysfunction (the pentad) are often present. Anemia and thrombocytopenia commonly are severe at presentation. Headache, confusion, coma, hemiparesis, behavioral changes, aphasia, and seizures are common. Death occurs within a few days to weeks in the majority of untreated persons. TTP and hemolytic-uremic syndrome (HUS) may be variations of the clinical spectrum of a single basic disease. In some cases, TTP is indistinguishable from HUS. However, a definitive diagnosis is needed because treatment varies for the two diseases. The severe intravascular hemolysis of TTP can occasionally trigger DIC.[8, 11, 14]

HEMOLYTIC UREMIA SYNDROME (HUS)

Clinically, HUS resembles TTP except that it predominates in children aged 6 months to 4 years and is self-limiting. It often follows an acute viral infection and it affects males and females in equal numbers. The disease may follow a febrile illness in small children, often associated with vomiting and diarrhea and the demonstrated presence of pathologic gastrointestinal organisms. This infection causing gram-negative endotoxemia can set off an episode of DIC. The childhood form of HUS carries a mortality rate of 33%; the adult form, 61%.

The adult form of HUS is more closely related to TTP than to the "classical," self-limited HUS of infants. More than two thirds of patients with the adult form of HUS are women, and in many the condition develops in association with oral contraceptive use, preeclampsia-eclampsia, or other obstetric complications.

Cardinal signs of HUS are hemolytic anemia, renal failure, and thrombocytopenia. Pathologic changes involving the glomerulus and renal arterioles result in hypertension and renal failure. Thrombocytopenia is mild to moderate. Renal failure is reflected in elevated blood urea nitrogen and creatinine levels. The urine nearly always contains red blood cells, protein, and casts. The hemolytic process is demonstrated by a hemoglobin level of less than 10 g/dL, an elevated reticulocyte count, and the presence of schistocytes in the peripheral blood.[11]

In HUS, platelet consumption occurs primarily in the kidneys. Thrombocytopenia in patients with HUS may be caused by infection-induced immune complex formation, by formation of platelet microaggregates in the kidneys or kidney vasculature, by induced platelet sequestration, or by kidney injury. There is some evidence of genetic predisposition.

Differentiating the adult form of HUS from TTP may be difficult. However, the lack of neurologic symptoms and the prevalence of renal disease suggest HUS. Also in HUS, as opposed to TTP, hypertension is common and renal failure is more common than hepatic involvement.[6, 13]

Patients with HUS are treated with renal dialysis, antihypertensive drugs, and/or transfusions. As uremic symptoms disappear, the platelet count returns to normal. The adult form of HUS responds favorably to heparin therapy. The prognosis for patients with HUS is relatively good.[6, 11, 13]

The most common cause of destructive thrombocytopenia is activation of the coagulation cascade by a variety of agents or conditions, resulting in a consumptive coagulopathy that entraps platelets in intravascular fibrin meshes. This disorder is described in more detail in Chapter 34. In addition to thrombocytopenia, levels of factor V, factor VIII, and fibrinogen are decreased as a result of in vivo thrombin generation. In acute DIC, platelet consumption is rapid, and the resultant thrombocytopenia is severe. In chronic DIC, compensatory thrombocytopoiesis results in a moderately low to normal platelet count.[11, 13]

DRUGS

Heparin-induced thrombocytopenia is being recognized with increasing frequency and is an important cause of hospital-acquired morbidity. Thrombocytopenia seems to occur more often with bovine heparin than with porcine heparin. There appear to be two separate syndromes of heparin-induced thrombocytopenia: (1) most common is a benign, mild thrombocytopenia, the cause of which has been related to the platelet-aggregating property of heparin; (2) less common is a severe thrombocytopenia whose features are characteristic of drug-related immune thrombocytopenia and that is associated with serious thrombotic complications. There is convincing evidence that the more severe form of thrombocytopenia occurring after heparin administration is immunologically mediated.[10, 14]

Ristocetin, an antibiotic no longer in clinical use, is capable of causing thrombocytopenia by direct action on circulating human platelets. Hematin, used for treatment of acute intermittent porphyria, may be followed by transient thrombocytopenia. It appears to be caused by the stimulation of platelet secretion and aggregation. Thrombocytopenia may also follow protamine sulfate and bleomycin therapy.[14]

DISORDERS RELATED TO DISTRIBUTION OR DILUTION

An abnormal distribution of platelets may also cause thrombocytopenia. The normal spleen sequesters approximately one third of the total platelet mass. Mild thrombocytopenia may be present in any of the "big spleen" syndromes. The total body platelet mass often is normal in these disorders, but a large number of platelets are sequestered in the greatly enlarged spleen, with the result that the venous platelet count is low. Such disorders as Gaucher's disease, Hodgkin's disease, sarcoidosis, lymphomas, cirrhosis of the liver, and portal hypertension may result in splenomegaly and lead to thrombocytopenia.[2, 8]

Lowering of the body temperature to less than 25 °C, as with hypothermia for cardiovascular surgery, results in a transient, mild thrombocytopenia secondary to platelet sequestration in the spleen and liver. An associated transient defect in function also occurs with hypothermia. Platelet count and function return to baseline values upon rewarming.[6]

Thrombocytopenia often follows surgery involving extracorporeal circulatory devices, as a consequence of damage and partial activation of platelets in the pump. In a few cases, severe thrombocytopenia, marked impairment of platelet function, and activation of fibrinolysis and intravascular coagulation may develop.[14]

The administration of massive amounts of whole blood containing nonviable platelets may produce a temporary thrombocytopenia by means of a washout phenomenon. This phenomenon is explained by the fact that stored blood contains platelets whose viability is severely impaired by the effects of the requirements for processing and storage temperature. The routine use of some fresh blood or platelet concentrates, together with stored blood, may minimize this problem.[6, 19]

Mild thrombocytopenia may be encountered in many patients with chronic renal failure, severe iron deficiency, postcompression sickness, and chronic hypoxia.

THROMBOCYTOSIS

Thrombocytosis is defined as an abnormally high platelet count (more than 400,000/mm³) in whole blood. In most cases thrombocytosis is secondary to inflammation or trauma and is termed *reactive thrombocytosis,* in which case the platelet count is elevated for a limited period and rarely exceeds 800,000/mm³. A marked and persistent elevation in the platelet count may accompany a myeloproliferative disorder. The platelet count may exceed 1,000,000/mm³ when it is a primary symptom of a myeloproliferative disorder such as polycythemia vera, chronic myelocytic leukemia, or myelofibrosis with myeloid metaplasia. Sometimes the term *thrombocythemia* is used as a synonym for *thrombocytosis.* In this text, *thrombocythemia* is considered to be a separate entity, essential thrombocythemia, in which platelet counts are between 1,000,000/mm³ and 2,000,000/mm³ and that is unassociated with another myeloproliferative disorder.[11, 14]

Reactive (Secondary) Thrombocytosis

Platelet counts between 440,000/mm³ and 800,000/mm³ with no change in platelet function can result from acute blood loss, major surgery (especially splenectomy), childbirth, tissue necrosis, inflammatory disease, exercise, iron deficiency anemia, and administration of epinephrine. Rare patients manifest a platelet count of 1,000,000/mm³ to 2,000,000/mm³. In reactive thrombocytosis, platelet production remains responsive to normal regulatory stimuli (such as thrombopoietin, a humoral factor that is produced in the kidney parenchyma), and morphologically normal platelets are produced at a moderately increased rate. This is in contrast to essential thrombocythemia, which is characterized by unregulated or autonomous platelet production and platelets of variable size.[11, 14, 20]

The bone marrow shows that megakaryocytes are normal. Results of platelet function tests, including aggregation induced by various agents, platelet factor 3 release, and the bleeding time, are usually normal in patients with secondary thrombocytosis but may be abnormal in patients with elevated platelet counts accompanying myeloproliferative disorders.

Reactive thrombocytosis is not associated with thrombosis, hemorrhage, or abnormal thrombopoietin levels. It seldom produces symptoms per se and disappears when the underlying disorder is brought under control.[11, 20]

REACTIVE THROMBOCYTOSIS ASSOCIATED WITH BLOOD LOSS AND SURGERY

Severe or chronic hemorrhage may necessitate multiple transfusions. Because stored blood usually has nonviable platelets, patients may require platelet transfusions; usually, one unit of platelet concentrate is administered for each new unit of cells.

Acute hemorrhage without transfusion therapy is first followed by thrombocytopenia for 2–6 days and then by thrombocytosis that lasts for several days. Major surgery that causes blood loss is followed by a similar pattern of thrombocytopenia and thrombocytosis. The platelet count returns to normal 10–16 days after surgery.[11]

POSTSPLENECTOMY THROMBOCYTOSIS

Removal of the spleen is an exception. The platelet count typically reaches 1,000,000/mm³ regardless of the clinical reason for splenectomy. Intuitively, this is logical because the spleen normally sequesters one third of the circulating platelet mass. Upon its removal, these platelets are free to be in the circulating blood. The platelet count far exceeds levels that could result from equilibration of the physiologic splenic platelet pool. The cause of the accelerated platelet production is unknown. In contrast to blood loss or other surgery, the platelet count reaches a maximum 1–3 weeks after splenectomy and remains elevated for 1–3 months. In some patients who undergo splenectomy for chronic anemia, the count remains elevated for several years.[11, 14]

IRON DEFICIENCY ANEMIA

Mild iron deficiency anemia secondary to chronic blood loss is associated with thrombocytosis in about 50% of cases. The thrombocytosis is likely present only during periods of actual blood loss. It is believed that iron normally is involved in regulating thrombopoiesis by inhibiting thrombopoietin production, thereby inhibiting platelet production. The platelet count may be as high as 2,000,000/mm³. The platelet count returns to normal within 7–10 days after iron therapy is started. In severe iron deficiency anemia, thrombocytopenia is more common than thrombocytosis, particularly in children.[3, 11, 14, 21]

INFLAMMATION AND DISEASE

Like elevated plasma and alpha- and beta-globulin acute-phase reactants, thrombocytosis is an indicator of inflammation. Rheumatoid arthritis, rheumatic fever, osteomyelitis, ulcerative colitis, acute infections, and malignancy are all associated with thrombocytosis. Elevated platelet counts are frequently found in patients with rheumatoid arthritis, in which the presence of thrombocytosis may be correlated with the activation of the inflammatory process. An elevated platelet count may be early evidence of a tumor, as in Hodgkin's disease and various carcinomas. The presence of thrombocytosis appears to be unrelated to the disease. Hemophiliac patients often have platelet counts above normal limits even when there is no active bleeding.[11, 14]

STRESS AND/OR EXERCISE

Strenuous exercise causes relative thrombocytosis, a platelet count increase that is caused by transfer of plasma water to the extravascular compartment, causing hemoconcentration. These increases also occur in red and white blood cell components. All measures return to normal 30 minutes after completion of exercise.[11, 14]

REBOUND THROMBOCYTOSIS

Thrombocytosis follows thrombocytopenia caused by marrow-suppressive therapy, reflecting an increase in thrombocytopoiesis. "Rebound" thrombocytosis usually reaches a peak 10–17 days after withdrawal of the offending drug (e.g., alcohol or methotrexate) or after institution of therapy for thrombocytopenia (e.g., for vitamin B_{12} deficiency).[11, 14]

Thrombocytosis Associated with Myeloproliferative Disorders

Primary or autonomous thrombocytosis is a typical finding in three myeloproliferative disorders: polycythemia vera, chronic myelocytic leukemia, and myelofibrosis with agnogenic myeloid metaplasia. An increased platelet count is often accompanied by an increase in the red and white blood cell lines. In these cases the platelet count seldom reaches the extreme values characteristic of thrombocythemia. A hematocrit higher than 60%, a normal white blood cell count, and enlargement of the spleen in association with thrombocytosis most likely suggests thrombocytosis associated with polycythemia vera, rather than essential thrombocythemia. Chronic myelogenous leukemia usually manifests with anemia, splenomegaly, and leukocytosis far more severe than that seen in primary or essential thrombocythemia. Agnogenic myeloid metaplasia may be associated with an elevated platelet count. However, there is usually marked splenomegaly, teardrop poikilocytosis, and the characteristic reticulin and collagen fibrosis of the marrow (see Chapter 24). Patients with myelodysplastic syndromes usually manifest with anemia and red blood cell macrocytosis that are more pronounced than those seen in patients with primary thrombocythemia.[11, 13, 14, 21]

Thrombocythemia (Essential or Primary)

Thrombocythemia is a clonal disorder pathogenically related to the other chronic myeloproliferative diseases, but it is the least common. It is characterized by proliferation of marrow megakaryocytes and platelet count values between 1,000,000/mm³ and 2,000,000/mm³. There is evidence that it is caused by a clonal proliferation of a single abnormal pluripotential stem cell. Additional evidence that primary thrombocythemia is a disease of a pluripotential stem cell is that a granulocytic leukocytosis is seen in 40–50% of patients. Thrombocythemia is clinically manifested by hemorrhage, platelet dysfunction, and, occasionally, thrombosis. As with most myeloproliferative disorders, it is not congenital or hereditary, is prevalent in middle-aged and older patients, and affects equal numbers of males and females. In contrast to other myeloproliferative disorders, however, other cell lines are not involved.

Bleeding time values are usually normal. Unfortunately, there is no specific clinical sign or laboratory test that establishes the diagnosis. Rather, the diagnosis must be made by ruling out systemic illnesses that produce reactive thrombocytosis and the other myeloproliferative disorders described earlier. However, one unique symptom is the throbbing, aching, and burning sensation in the extremities, particularly in the palms and soles.[11, 13, 14, 21]

Hemorrhagic manifestations are similar to those seen with platelet dysfunction: bleeding from the mucous membranes of the nose and mouth and ecchymoses. Symptoms may be aggravated by aspirin use. In the majority of cases of thrombocythemia, patients experience no clotting disorders. Sometimes there is a paradoxical combination of thromboembolic (clotting) and hemorrhagic episodes associated with this condition, referred to as "double jeopardy."

The bleeding manifestations are related to the many qualitative abnormalities in the platelets, including deficiencies in epinephrine receptors and ultrastructural defects in granules, mitochondria, and microfilaments. Platelets are often agranular or hypogranular and have a clear blue appearance on routine Wright's stain specimens of the peripheral blood. Although their size is heterogeneous, giant, bizarre-shaped platelets are characteristic of myeloproliferative diseases, and it is not uncommon to encounter megakaryocyte fragments or nuclei in the periphery. The platelets may be notably clumped on blood smears, exhibiting marked variation in size and shape. The number and volume of megakaryocytes are increased in the bone marrow, and they are predominantly large, show some cellular atypia, and tend to form clusters. Many of the platelets are functionally defective. Aggregation is absent in response to epinephrine, decreased with adenosine diphosphate (ADP), but normal with collagen. Many of the abnormalities of the platelet aggregation studies can be attributed to abnormalities of platelet surface membrane and receptors (i.e., decreased numbers of alpha-adrenergic receptors and increased numbers of Fc receptors). Platelet adhesion is probably decreased, and thromboplastin activity is subnormal.[11, 13, 14, 21]

The degree of thrombocytosis has not been found reliably predictive of hemorrhagic or thrombotic events; thus the role of lowering platelet counts in this disease is not clearly established. Many clinicians, reasoning that the risks from exposure to mutagenic alkylating chemicals are greater than the risk of thrombosis of hemorrhage, Melphalan, busulfan, or radioactive phosphorus is used if clotting symptoms or splenomegaly is manifested.[14, 21]

QUALITATIVE DISORDERS

A prolonged bleeding time in a patient whose platelet count is normal indicates an acquired or a congenital disorder of platelet function. Congenital disorders have been described as a result of abnormalities of each of the four phases of platelet function: adhesion, aggregation, secretion, and elaboration of procoagulant activity. Rapid progress in this field began in the 1960s mostly as a result of the development of instruments and testing to measure platelet aggregation.[8, 14]

Disorders of Platelet Adhesion

BERNARD-SOULIER (GIANT PLATELET) SYNDROME

Bernard-Soulier syndrome is a moderate bleeding disorder associated with prolonged bleeding time, enlarged platelets, and thrombocytopenia. The primary platelet defects in this syndrome are (1) an inability of platelets to participate in vWF-dependent adhesion to the subendothelium exposed by vascular damage and (2) no response to microfibrils. The result is defective primary hemostasis. There are specific abnormalities and decreased amounts of membrane glycoproteins IbIX, V, and IX. In addition, the platelets do not bind coagulation factor XI normally and bind a decreased amount of thrombin.[6, 8, 13, 14]

Glycoprotein IbIX is the major determinant of the vWF binding site on the platelet and also of the binding site for quinidine-induced platelet antibodies. Results of biochemical studies have suggested that two and possibly three additional glycoproteins may be abnormal in patients with this syndrome. Ristocetin-induced platelet aggregation is deficient presumably because of failure of the platelet membrane to adequately bind vWF. In contrast to von Willebrand's disease (vWD), this abnormality cannot be corrected by the addition of normal plasma or cryoprecipitate, which indicates that the defect resides in the platelets. Aggregation with agonists such as ADP, collagen, thrombin, arachidonic acid, and epinephrine is normal in Bernard-Soulier platelets.[8, 13, 14]

The platelets range from 5 to 8 μm in diameter and usually are obvious in stained blood smears. It has been reported that circulating Bernard-Soulier platelets are of normal size but have increased membrane surface area. In vivo, Bernard-Soulier platelets circulate in a spheric rather than normal discoid shape. The platelet count is usually in the range of 50,000/mm^3–80,000/mm^3. A bleeding time of 20 minutes is a common finding, but clot retraction is normal.[8, 11, 14]

This rare syndrome usually manifests in infancy or childhood with hemorrhage characteristic of defective platelet function: ecchymoses, epistaxis, and gingival bleeding. Hemarthroses and expanding hematomas are unusual features of this disorder.

There is no specific treatment for Bernard-Soulier syndrome. Normal plasma, used to correct the coagulation deficiency of vWD, is ineffective, as is treatment with steroids. Platelet transfusions appeared to be effective in a few cases.[13, 14]

The disorder is inherited as an autosomal recessive trait. Heterozygotes are usually asymptomatic and have a platelet glycoprotein Ib content intermediate between that of normal persons and that of affected patients.[8, 14, 22]

VON WILLEBRAND'S DISEASE

Von Willebrand's disease is the name now given to a wide family of bleeding disorders that result from a quantitative or qualitative abnormality of vWF. In 1926, von Willebrand described a bleeding disorder in 24 of 66 members of a family from the Aland Islands. Both sexes were afflicted, and the bleeding time was prolonged despite normal platelet counts and normal clot retraction.[14, 23]

vWD should be regarded as a syndrome because the disorder is heterogeneous, even with regard to genetics, and several distinct variants and many minor variants have been recognized.[8]

Molecular Biology of von Willebrand's Factor

The vWF is a glycoprotein, synthesized by endothelial cells and megakaryocytes, that circulates in the blood plasma at a concentration of 5–10 μg/mL. The only other cell known to synthesize vWF is the megakaryocyte. The vWF synthesized by megakaryocytes is stored in the alpha granules of platelets. The vWF gene is quite large, spanning approximately 175 kilobases of genomic DNA, and is located on the short arm of chromosome 12.[23]

The messenger RNA transcript of vWF codes for a polypeptide containing a small 22–amino acid signal peptide at the amino-terminal region, followed by a 741–amino acid peptide identical to von Willebrand antigen that is followed in turn by the mature vWF subunit of 2050 amino acids, whose amino acid sequence has been determined.[14, 24]

The precursor molecule M_r forms a high–molecular-weight (260,000-D) multimer in a multi-step process. In the endoplasmic reticulum, glycosylation is initiated by formation of high mannose carbohydrate on the potential n-linked glycosylation sites. Glycosylation is necessary for further processing of the pro-vWF monomers. The pro-vWF monomers then form dimers through interchain disulfide bonds. Dimerization is critical because monomers cannot form multimers and do not progress through the secretory pathway. The vWF dimer is then transferred to the Golgi apparatus. The vWF consists of a series of multimers that range in molecular weight from approximately 800,000 to more than 12,000,000 D.[14, 24]

It has been demonstrated that vWF is stored in endothelial cells in structures called Weibel-Palade bodies. Stimulation by thrombin, calcium iono-phore, or desmopressin acetate (DDAVP), induces the bodies to release the stored vWF.[8, 23]

Factor vWF is a large molecule consisting of two subunits (Table 33–4). Circulating vWF is complexed with factor VIII (coagulant protein), the protein that is decreased in patients with hemophilia A. The coagulant protein is under X-linked control. Although some uncertainly remains as to the precise site or sites of synthesis, there is evidence that it occurs in the liver. The noncovalent association between vWF and factor VIII appears to be stable under physiologic conditions. It has been estimated there may be one molecule of factor VIII for every one or two molecules of vWF.[8, 23]

Pathophysiology

vWD is a disorder of the vWF molecule. Factor vWF is either deficient or aberrant in patients with this disorder. The binding of vWF to specific receptors on the platelet membrane and endothelial surface is impaired. This lack of platelet adherence to the damaged vessel wall is the major defect of vWD and results in a prolonged bleeding time.[8, 17]

Factor VIII also is deficient in patients with most forms of this syndrome, maybe because of a quantitative reduction in vWF and its "carrier protein" function or because of a qualitative aberration of vWF as the result of changes in its multimeric composition. Factor vWF interacts with platelet receptors as a prerequisite to platelet agglutination by the drug ristocetin. Most forms of vWD are associated with deficient vWF and demonstrate deficient ristocetin-induced platelet aggregation (RIPA).[8, 17]

Clinical Symptoms

The van Willebrand syndrome is associated with a mild hemorrhagic diathesis. Mucocutaneous bleeding is the most common symptom in affected patients. Chronic gastrointestinal bleeding is a prominent feature in approximately 10% of patients and may be associated with colonic angiodysplasia or hereditary hemorrhagic telangiectasia. Bruising, epistaxis, and post-traumatic and post-surgical bleeding are common manifestations; for example, mild bleeding may occur after dental extraction or tonsillectomy. Petechiae are rare. Abnormal menstrual bleeding is very common in affected women; in men, the disorder may be virtually asymptomatic, but postsurgical bleeding is a significant hazard. In severely affected patients with the type III variant, the disorder resembles hemophilia A. Dissecting hematomas and severe post-traumatic and postoperative hemorrhage are characteristic. Hemarthrosis may occur after major trauma.[8, 14, 25, 26]

Specific Variants

The exact features and laboratory findings depend on the particular variant. The variants of vWD are described in Table 33–5. The *type I* variant is the most common form of the syndrome. It is inherited as an autosomal dominant trait and is characterized by a moderately prolonged bleeding time and a proportional reduction, to 10–40% of normal, of the major factor VIII/vWF functions: that is, factors VIII and vWF. Although the amount of circulating vWF is decreased, a full range of vWF multimers is present, including those of high molecular weight. The clinical manifestations are primarily those involving systemic hemorrhage; in cases in which factor VIII is decreased to very low levels, however, anatomic hemorrhage may also occur. RIPA may be normal or subnormal. The factor VIII remaining in the plasma is qualitatively normal, as confirmed by agarose electrophoresis or crossed immunoelectrophoresis.[8, 23]

The *type IIa* variant differs from the type I variant in that the plasma levels of VIII and vWF may be either normal or diminished. vWF and

Table 33–4. NOMENCLATURE FOR THE FACTOR VIII–VON WILLEBRAND FACTOR COMPLEX

Current Abbreviation	Previous Abbreviation	Molecule
VIII/vWF	VIII	The combination of factor VIII and von Willebrand factor as they are found in normal plasma
vWF	VIIvWF	Von Willebrand factor, the glycoprotein carrier for factor VIII
vWF:Ag	VIIIR:Ag	An antigenic determinant epitope located on the vWF molecule that is the basis for detection and measurement of plasma vWF by immunoassay
vWFR:Co	VIIIR:RCo	The ristocetin cofactor activity of vWF that is the basis for detection and measurement of plasma vWF by ristocetin-induced platelet aggregometry
VIII	VIII:C	Factor VIII, the protein carried in plasma on vWF that is abnormal or deficient in hemophilia A
VIIIC	VIII:C	Factor VIII coagulant activity as it is measured in a factor-specific clot-based assay
VIIIC:Ag	VIIICAg	Factor VIII coagulant concentration as it is measured by immunoassay

From Montgomery RR, Coller BS: Von Willebrand disease. *In* Colman RW, Hirsh J, Marder VJ, Salzman EW (eds): Hemostasis and Thrombosis: Basic Principles and Clinical Practice, 3rd ed. Philadelphia: JB Lippincott, 1994:135.

Table 33-5. CLASSIFICATION OF VON WILLEBRAND'S DISEASE

Characteristic	Type I	Type IIA	Type IIB	Type IIC	Type III: Autosomal Recessive, Homozygous, or Double Heterozygous
Genetic transmission	Autosomal dominant	Autosomal dominant	Autosomal dominant	Autosomal recessive	
Bleeding time	Prolonged	Prolonged	Prolonged	Prolonged	Prolonged
Factor VIII	Decreased	Decreased or normal	Decreased or normal	Normal	Markedly decreased
Factor vWF	Decreased	Decreased or normal	Decreased or normal	Normal	Absent or minute amounts
Factor vWF	Decreased	Markedly decreased	Decreased or normal	Decreased	Absent
Ristocetin-induced platelet agglutination (PRP)	Decreased or normal	Absent or decreased	Increased	Decreased	Absent
Crossed immunoelectrophoresis	Normal	Abnormal	Abnormal	Abnormal double peak	Variable—usually abnormal
Plasma multimeric structure	Normal	Large and intermediate forms absent	Large multimers absent	Large multimers absent; doublet multimer structure	Variable to absent
Platelet multimeric structure	Normal (quantity of vWF normal)	Large and intermediate forms absent (quantity of vWF normal)	Normal multimers in platelets (quantity normal)	Large multimers absent: doublet multimer structure	Absent
Response to 1-desamino-8-D-arginine vasopressin (DDAVP)	Restore hemostasis to normal	Although vWF increases, multimeric abnormality is not corrected	Transient correction of multimeric abnormality; bleeding time may be corrected		
Possible pathophysiology	Abnormal release from sites of synthesis	Inability to form or stabilize large multimers	Intrinsic abnormality of von Willebrand factor increases tissue binding	Intrinsic abnormality with doublet	Reduced synthesis or rapid breakdown at sites of synthesis

From Triplett DA: Hemostasis: A Case Oriented Approach. New York: Igaku-Shoin, 1985:128.

RIPA are greatly diminished or absent altogether. Crossed immunoelectrophoresis and sodium dodecyl sulfate (SDS) agarose electrophoresis reveal diminished levels of large and intermediate-sized vWF multimers in the plasma and in platelets.[8]

The *type IIb* variant of vWD resembles the type IIa variant, except that crossed immunoelectrophoresis or SDS agarose electrophoresis reveals low levels of high–molecular-weight multimers in the plasma. Platelet vWF multimers are normal in this variant. Levels of vWF are variable and may be normal or abnormal. Tests for RIPA may reveal hyperaggregability of platelets.[14]

The *type III* variant is the most severe form of vWD. Affected patients have very low levels of plasma VIII and vWF. RIPA is deficient. This variant is genetically heterogeneous. It has been described variously as severe, doubly heterozygous type I or as autosomal recessive type III vWD. Use of DNA probes on vWF reveals gross homozygous deletions in patients with recessive vWD.[8, 23]

Platelet-type (or pseudo-) vWD is an autosomal dominant disorder of platelets that produces clinical and laboratory abnormalities closely resembling type IIB vWD. Patients characteristically have mildly to moderately prolonged bleeding times, borderline thrombocytopenia, decreased ristocetin cofactor assay levels, and normal to only mildly decreased levels of vWF antigen and factor VIII. There is an absence of the highest–molecular-weight multimers of vWF. The similarity to type IIB vWD extends to increased RIPA, with a hyperresponsiveness to ristocetin. Studies demonstrating enhanced platelet binding of vWF and the associated finding of thrombocytopenia suggest that this disorder is an intrinsic platelet defect.[8, 23]

Clinical Features

In two large families with vWD, only 65% of persons with both an affected parent and an affected descendent had significant clinical symptoms. Of the unrelated spouses of the patients,

23% were judged to have a positive history of bleeding. In contrast, patients with clinically severe vWD had very strong personal and family histories of excessive bleeding.[14]

Laboratory Diagnosis

Laboratory screening tests reveal a prolonged bleeding time and a variable prolongation of the partial thromboplastin time (APTT), together with a normal platelet count and a normal prothrombin time. The most common laboratory findings are summarized in Table 33–5. In mildly affected patients, the APTT may be normal, and a specific factor VIII assay is required. The plasma level of vWF is usually proportional to the VIII assay level.[8]

A variety of concurrent diseases and drugs may modify the results of the tests. Patients must not take drugs that could affect the bleeding time.

The modified bleeding time test is usually performed when the diagnosis of vWD is considered. In type I vWD, the level of the ristocetin cofactor assay correlates inversely with the bleeding time (i.e., the less cofactor activity, the longer the bleeding time). In general, the concentration of vWF antigen is more closely correlated with the bleeding time than is the platelet ristocetin cofactor activity. In type II vWD, no correlation exists between the bleeding time and the level of platelet ristocetin cofactor activity or platelet vWF antigen.[14]

In most patients with vWD, the APTT is prolonged, and yet the result of this test may be normal in patients with mild clinical disease who have normal or near normal factor VIII levels.[14] In patients with mild vWD, factor VIII levels are variable and may be normal. Of patients with moderate to severe disease, more than 90% have low factor VIII levels. In contrast, patients with a variant of vWD often have normal factor VIII levels, even if severely affected.[14]

vWF antigen is usually measured by electroimmunoassay, immunoradiometric assay, radioimmunoassay, or an enzyme-linked immunospecific assay technique. The Laurell electroimmunoassay technique relies on immunoprecipitation of vWF in gel containing anti-vWF antigen.

The addition of ristocetin to platelet-rich plasma, during platelet aggregation studies causes platelet agglutination. The result of this test is abnormal in 65–70% of patients. It is important that several concentrations of ristocetin be tested, because many patients who have mild vWD may have normal RIPA if levels higher than 1.2 mg/mL are used.[8, 14]

In type IIB vWD and pseudo- or platelet vWD, RIPA is increased. Agglutination of platelet-rich plasma occurs after addition of only 0.2- to 0.8-mg/mL concentrations of ristocetin. These amounts would not induce agglutination of normal platelets.[14]

The *ristocetin cofactor assay* measures the ability of plasma vWF to agglutinate platelets in the presence of ristocetin. Normal platelets, washed free of plasma vWF, are used as fresh platelets or after formaldehyde fixation. The assay is the most sensitive and specific for detection of vWD and has a high degree of reproducibility.

Venom from a snake of the *Bothrops* species causes agglutination of platelets in the presence of vWD, but not in its absence, and has been used to assay ristocetin cofactor.[14]

Crossed antigen-antibody electrophoresis may be employed for the identification of vWF antigen in plasma or cryoprecipitate. With this assay, three major groups of patients with vWD are identified: type I (precipitin is normal), type II (selective decrease of larger multimeric forms of vWF), and type IS/III (no detectable precipitate).[14]

Agarose gel electrophoresis of plasma or platelet lysates separates vWF multimers on the basis of molecular size; the large multimers migrate more slowly than the smaller multimers. The multimers may be visualized by autoradiography. The normal distribution is an orderly progression of size of vWF multimers, from the smallest to the largest.[14]

Aspirin may prolong the bleeding time in some patients with vWF; this phenomenon provides the basis for various *aspirin tolerance tests*. This response to aspirin is not specific and can be demonstrated in patients with platelet dysfunction and those with hemophilia A and B, in whom aspirin may produce serious hemorrhage.[8, 23]

Treatment

In the majority of mildly affected patients, treatment is rarely if ever indicated. In general, the aim of treatment in the case of patients with vWD is to ensure that the levels of hemostatically effective vWF and factor VIII are adequate to prevent significant bleeding.[8, 23]

Human single-donor cryoprecipitate (1 unit/10 kg, once or twice daily) has for many years been the principal treatment for vWD, providing normal multimeric composition and functional activity, together with factor VIII, in a relatively small volume. The therapeutic effect of cryoprecipitate lasts only about 4 hours, presumably because of the removal and catabolism of transfused circulating factor VIII/vWF, as well as the catabolism of the factor VIII/vWF polymers deposited on subendothelium.[14, 23, 27]

Fresh-frozen plasma can be substituted if cryoprecipitate is not available. Commercial factor VIII concentrates, although providing active factor VIII in a minimal volume, do not provide hemostatically adequate vWF because of a loss of the higher–molecular-weight multimers in the manufacturing process.[14, 23]

In severely affected patients with the type III variant, bleeding should be treated with cryoprecipitate in doses much like those used for hemophilia A. For the prevention of postsurgical hemorrhage, cryoprecipitate should be given 24 hours before surgery. The use of epsilon-aminocaproic acid (EACA), a fibrinolytic agent, with cryoprecipitate may be helpful in mildly affected patients.[8]

In the early 1980s the success of DDAVP in raising both the factor VIII and vWF levels in some patients with vWD offered the new possibility of treating mild vWD without the risk of transfusing blood products. DDAVP appears to have the greatest usefulness in cases of mild type I vWD, in which a transient rise in the vWF (and factor VIII) levels occurs. It should not be used to treat patients with the type IIb variant because it may induce thrombocytopenia.[8, 23]

The introduction of a new generation of heat-treated factor VIII/vWF concentrates for clinical use will likely have significant impact on the treatment of vWD. Heat treatment should greatly reduce the risk of viral exposure. In addition, the full range of vWF multimers appears to be present in such concentrates.

Anti–von Willebrand's Factor Antibodies

In approximately 10% of patients with severe vWD (type IS/III), antibodies to vWF develop after transfusion of vWF-containing plasma products. These inhibitors are polyclonal forms of IgG. Patients with such antibodies may have anaphylactoid reactions after plasma or cryoprecipitate therapy. There is a familial tendency for these inhibitors to develop. They prevent optimal response to transfused cryoprecipitate and other blood products.[14]

ACQUIRED DEFECTS OF PLATELET ADHESION

Acquired platelet function defects are seen in patients with autoimmune disorders, including not only SLE, rheumatoid arthritis, and scleroderma but also the immune thrombocytopenias such as ITP.

Fibrinogen degradation products (FDPs) of any etiology, usually DIC or fibrinolysis, often induce platelet dysfunction. The later degradation products (fragments D and E) have a high affinity for the platelet membrane and produce a severe platelet function defect. This defect has been attributed to competition by FDP for fibrinogen-binding sites on platelets.[8, 22]

Patients with severe iron, folate, or cobalamin deficiency may also have platelet function defects. Unlike the rare hereditary platelet function defects, the acquired platelet function defects do not demonstrate typical platelet aggregation abnormalities.[22]

MYELOPROLIFERATIVE AND LYMPHOPROLIFERATIVE DISORDERS AND DYSPROTEINEMIAS

Platelets from patients with chronic myeloproliferative disorders have been reported to have abnormal shapes, decreased procoagulant activity, and decreased aggregation and secretion in response to epinephrine, adenosine diphosphate, and collagen.[28]

These qualitative platelet abnormalities may be attributed to (1) loss of platelet surface membrane alpha-adrenergic receptors; (2) loss of platelet surface membrane receptors for prostaglandin D_2, a minor product of platelet arachidonic acid oxidation; (3) impaired oxidation of arachidonic acid by the lipooxygenase pathway; or (4) an abnormality of dense granules that causes depletion of dense granule ADP.[18]

Platelet dysfunction is observed in approximately one third of patients with IgA myeloma or Waldenström macroglobulinemia, in 15% of patients with IgG multiple myeloma, and occasionally in patients with monoclonal gammopathy of undetermined significance. This dysfunction results from coating of the platelet membranes by paraprotein and does not depend on the type of paraprotein present. In addition to the interaction of the protein with the platelet, a coating of the collagen fibers by the abnormal protein has been reported. Almost all patients with malignant paraprotein disorders demonstrate clinically significant bleeding as well as abnormal platelet function. Other causes of bleeding could include hyperviscosity syndrome, thrombocytopenia, amyloidosis (acquired factor X deficiency), and in rare instances, a circulating heparin-like anti-coagulant or fibrinolysis.[5, 14, 22]

ANTI-PLATELET ANTIBODIES

A normal platelet contains more than 20,000 IgG molecules, of which more than 99% are located within alpha granules. However, immunoglobulin molecules can bind to the platelet membrane in several pathologic conditions, including ITP, SLE, and platelet alloimmunization. Antibody binding (with or without complement binding) accelerates platelet destruction and leads to thrombocytopenia. Besides interfering with the function of the membrane components, some antibodies can activate platelets and induce aggregation and secretion.[14]

CARDIOPULMONARY BYPASS

Cardiopulmonary bypass induces a severe platelet function defect that assumes major importance in surgical bleeding after bypass. This defect most likely results from the effects of platelet activation and fragmentation. Platelet activation may be caused by adherence and aggregation of platelets to fibrinogen (absorbed onto the bypass circuit), mechanical trauma, shear stress, and so forth.[14, 22]

CHRONIC LIVER DISEASE

Chronic liver disease of various etiologies has been reported to cause prolonged bleeding time and reduced procoagulant activity. Mild to moderate thrombocytopenia is seen in approximately one third of patients with chronic liver disease as a result of splenic sequestration secondary to splenomegaly.[10, 14]

Abnormal platelet function tests found in patients with chronic liver disease include reduced platelet adhesion; abnormal platelet aggregation to ADP, epinephrine, and thrombin; and abnormal platelet factor 3 availability. An acquired storage pool deficiency has also been suggested. The thrombocytopenia and platelet abnormalities may result from the direct toxic effects of alcohol on bone marrow megakaryocytes.[10, 14]

The prolonged bleeding time in these patients may respond to infusion of DDAVP. The severe bleeding diathesis associated with end-stage liver disease has many causes, such as decreased coagulation factor production, fibrinolysis, dysfibrinogenemia, thrombocytopenia resulting from hypersplenism, and (occasionally) DIC.[10, 14]

DRUG-INDUCED MEMBRANE MODIFICATION

Many drugs may cause a clinically significant platelet function defect and hemorrhage. The three most common mechanisms by which drugs interfere with platelet function are, in descending order of prevalence, (1) drug interference with the platelet membrane or membrane receptor sites, (2) drug interference with prostaglandin biosynthetic pathways, and (3) drug interference with phosphodiesterase activity. The last two mechanisms are described later in this chapter.[22]

The drugs interfering with platelet membrane function or receptors are amitriptyline hydrochloride (Elavil), imipramine hydrochloride (Tofranil), doxepin hydrochloride (Sinequan), chlorpromazine (Thorazine), cocaine, lidocaine (Xylocaine), iso-proterenol hydrochloride (Isuprel), propranolol, cephalothin sodium (Keflin), ampicillin, diphenhydramine hydrochloride (Benadryl), a combination of promethazine hydrochloride and pseudoephedrine hydrochloride (Phenergan-D), and alcohol. Other drugs inducing platelet dysfunction by this mechanism are phentolamine mesylate (Regitine), phenoxybenzamine hydrochloride (Dibenzyline), reserpine, dihydroergotamine, desipramine hydrochloride (Norpramin), nortriptyline hydrochloride (Aventyl), trifluoperazine hydrochloride (Stelazine), procaine, dibucaine (Nupercainal), nitrofurantoin (Furadantin), nafcillin, moxalactam, ticarcillin, dextran, and hydroxyethyl starch.[22]

Of particular importance to patients undergoing intensive cancer chemotherapy is the effect of antibodies on platelet function. *Carbenicillin,* a drug frequently used in patients with suspected sepsis and limited marrow reserves, is the most extensively studied of the antibiotics reported to cause platelet dysfunction. Most hemostatically normal subjects exposed to carbenicillin have a prolonged bleeding time. The defect appears within 24 hours after the start of therapy and persists for days. *Penicillin G* has also been implicated as a platelet inhibitor but to a lesser degree than carbenicillin, possibly because the dosage is much lower than the typical dosage of carbenicillin. These drugs bind to the platelet surface membrane and interfere with the binding of vWF and other platelet activating agents (e.g., ADP, epinephrine) to platelet surface receptors.[6, 18, 27]

HEREDITARY AFIBRINOGENEMIA

Although this disorder has been documented in more than 100 patients, the nature of the platelet dysfunction remains poorly understood. In many patients, the bleeding time is prolonged and ADP-induced platelet aggregation is deficient. Abnormalities in platelet retention/adhesion studies involving the use of glass beads are also documented. This finding supports the belief that fibrinogen is essential for normal platelet aggregation. These abnormalities are not consistent, and in many cases the bleeding time and platelet function apparently are normal.[8]

Disorders of Primary Aggregation

GLANZMANN'S THROMBASTHENIA

Thrombasthenia was originally described as a bleeding disorder associated with abnormal clot retraction and a normal platelet count. The first and most characteristic laboratory finding is a greatly diminished or total lack of clot retraction. It is associated with prolonged bleeding time, a normal platelet count, and a lack of macroscopic platelet aggregation in response to ADP, collagen, thrombin, and epinephrine.[8, 13, 14, 29]

ADP-induced aggregation is deficient even with very high concentrations of this agonist. However, if the agonist is strong enough (e.g., thrombin or a high concentration of ADP), the platelets undergo a release/secretion reaction, but they do not aggregate. The biochemical lesion responsible for the disorder is a deficiency or abnormality of the platelet membrane glycoprotein IIb/IIIa complex, a membrane receptor for fibrinogen, vWF, and fibronectin. Fibrinogen must bind to the glycoprotein IIb/IIIa complex for normal platelet cohesion. Failure of such binding results in the profound defect in formation of hemostatic plugs and serious bleeding characteristic of thrombasthenia.[8, 13, 14, 18, 29, 30]

Unlike Bernard-Soulier platelets, thrombasthenic platelets adhere normally to subendothelium but fail to show recruitment into hemostatic plug formation. When normal platelets are activated, glycoproteins IIb and IIIa form a heterodimer complex on the platelet membrane, which determines the fibrinogen-binding site. The absence of these glycoproteins impairs the ability of both resting and activated platelets to bind fibrinogen.[6, 8]

Thrombasthenic platelets agglutinate in response to ristocetin, which indicates that they retain the ability to interact with vWF. However, the agglutination is followed by disaggregation rather than the normal secondary wave response. One variant form of thrombasthenia has been identified with poor ristocetin aggregation.[2, 8, 30, 31]

This rare disorder manifests itself in the neonatal period or infancy, occasionally with bleeding after circumcision and frequently with epistaxis and gingival bleeding. Hemorrhagic manifestations include petechiae, purpura, menorrhagia, gastrointestinal bleeding, and hematuria. Extreme variations in the clinical features have been noted, however. Some patients who have a severe inherited abnormality of platelet aggregation may have minimal symptoms, whereas others may have frequent and serious hemorrhagic complications. The severity of the bleeding episodes seems to decrease with age.[28, 32]

The platelet count and platelet morphology are normal in patients with Glanzmann's thrombasthenia, but the bleeding time is markedly prolonged. The platelets have been described as morphologically unusual in that they appear isolated and nonclumped. Platelet factor 3 availability is usually diminished in this disorder.[8, 11, 14]

On the basis of the presence or absence of clot retraction and the presence or absence of platelet alpha granule fibrinogen, thrombasthenia has been classified into types I and II. Type I patients have no clot retraction and no platelet–alpha granule fibrinogen; type II patients have decreased clot retraction and detectable alpha granule fibrinogen.[14]

Glanzmann's thrombasthenia is inherited as an autosomal recessive disorder and is seen in populations with high degrees of consanguinity, particularly the gypsies of France. Heterozygotes are clinically normal, but glycoprotein IIb/IIIa content of the platelets was found to be 50–60% of normal.[5, 14]

Thrombasthenia is one of the few forms of platelet dysfunction in which hemorrhage is severe and disabling. Bleeding of all types, including epistaxis, ecchymoses, subcutaneous hematomas, menorrhagia, and gastrointestinal and urinary tract hemorrhage have been reported. A peculiar clinical observation somewhat similar to that seen in vWD is the fact that the severity of bleeding tends to decrease with age.[5, 8, 14, 31, 32]

Treatment of bleeding in thrombasthenia requires the transfusion of normal platelets. Exchange plasmapheresis or platelet concentrate transfusions (as HLA-compatible as possible) may be necessary in the presence of life-threatening hemorrhage. Unexpected high numbers of transfused circulating normal platelets are required in order to correct the bleeding time. In Glanzmann's thrombasthenia, the defective platelets may interfere with the normal transfused platelets.[5, 8, 14, 31, 32]

Studies on the pathology of glycoprotein IIb/IIIa complexes in acquired disorders of platelet function (acquired thrombasthenia) have progressed. Platelets from patients with familial hypercholesterolemia, retinopathic diabetes, and multiple myeloma are similar to platelets from patients with Glanzmann's thrombasthenia. Few patients have been identified with autoantibodies to the glycoprotein IIb/IIIa complex; the clinical picture is similar to that of Glanzmann's thrombasthenia.[29, 32]

ACQUIRED VON WILLEBRAND'S DISEASE

A number of patients who have an acquired form of vWD have been described. Two important characteristics emphasize the acquired nature of the disorder: a hemorrhagic disorder is observed in patients who had not had a prior bleeding problem even after previous trauma or surgery, and family studies show no evidence of a hereditary bleeding disorder.[14]

Two pathogenic mechanisms have been described. First, a circulating inhibitor directed against vWF has been found in the plasma of these patients. This inhibitor, an IgG antibody prevents ristocetin-induced aggregation of normal platelets but does not bind to washed platelets; therefore, it is not an anti-platelet antibody. In the second mechanism, an inhibitor of vWF activity is not present in the blood, but an antibody that binds to vWF may be present.[14]

In most instances, the development of acquired vWD is related to another disease process. In patients with lymphoproliferative or myeloproliferative disorders, a prolonged bleeding time and bleeding symptoms sometimes develop as a result of an acquired form of vWD. In this syndrome, vWF is inactivated by a plasma inhibitor or absorbed onto malignant tissue. In each of these cases, there is a reduction in the plasma level of the higher–molecular-weight vWF multimers, and in some, the vWF abnormality was corrected by DDAVP and treatment of the underlying disease.[10, 14, 28]

UREMIA

Uremia is commonly accompanied by bleeding caused by platelet dysfunction, and it is proposed that circulating guanidinosuccinic acid or hydroxyphenolic acid interferes with platelet function. Both compounds are dialyzable, and dialysis often corrects or improves platelet function. Other mechanisms of altered platelet function in uremia, including altered prostaglandin metabolism, have also been suggested. Uremic vessels apparently secrete abnormally large amounts of prostacyclin, which could further inhibit platelet function.[8, 22]

The aggregation pattern abnormalities are not uniform, and any combination of defects may be seen. There is evidence of deficient release reaction, such as lack of primary ADP-induced aggregation, and subnormal platelet factor 3 activity.[8, 22]

Bleeding is uncommon in uremic patients who are not concurrently receiving drugs that interfere with platelet function. Platelet concentrates are indicated for life-threatening bleeding in patients with uremia, and other sometimes effective modes of therapy include cryoprecipitate, DDAVP, and estrogen. Maintenance of the hematocrit value above 30% may also help normalize the bleeding times.[8, 22]

Disorders of Platelet Secretion (Release Reactions)

Secondary aggregation disorders are more common than primary aggregation disorders. Of the hereditary platelet function defects, hereditary storage pool disease–type disorders are the most common. The clinical features of secondary aggregation disorders are mucocutaneous hemorrhages and hematuria, epistaxis, and easy and spontaneous bruising. Petechiae are less common than in other qualitative platelet disorders. In patients with storage pool defects, secondary epinephrine and ADP-induced aggregation waves are absent, although the primary waves are present. Collagen-induced aggregation is absent or markedly blunted, and normal RIPA is usually seen. The bleeding time is usually prolonged. Storage pool disorders are associated with mild bleeding disorders.[8, 14, 33]

STORAGE POOL DISEASES: DENSE GRANULE DEFICIENCIES

The platelet dense granules are intracellular storage sites for ADP, adenosine triphosphatase (ATP), calcium, pyrophosphate, and serotonin. The contents of these granules are extruded when platelet secretion is induced, and secreted ADP is thought to be involved in the propagation of the primary platelet response and enlargement of the hemostatic plug. In dense granule deficiencies, the number of dense bodies is decreased, and the amount of ADP secreted when platelets are stimulated is greatly diminished. Consequently, storage pool disease has the overall effect of decreasing platelet ADP to a greater extent than ATP. As a result of this greater decrease of ADP, the ATP:ADP ratio is higher than in normal platelets. This finding is diagnostic for storage pool disease.[5, 8, 14]

Autosomal dominant forms are most common, but other hereditable variations occur. The bleeding times are often very prolonged, aggregation responses to collagen may be markedly abnormal, and the secondary response to ADP and epinephrine is absent. The ATP:ADP ratio is higher than normal, and the uptake of granule-bound nucleotides is greatly diminished.[13]

Acquired forms of dense granule deficiency can be associated with some diseases, such as leukemia and SLE, and with the toxic effects of acute alcoholism. Autoimmune diseases may produce antibodies that promote release of dense granule products, resulting in an ultrastructural appearance that resembles that of the inherited storage pool disorders.

Similar changes in platelet dense granules are seen in patients with various systemic abnormalities. These conditions are associated with prolonged bleeding times and mild to severe bleeding diathesis. This is most likely related to the corresponding thrombocytopenia rather than to the storage pool deficiency.[13]

Hermansky-Pudlak syndrome (tyrosinase-positive oculocutaneous albinism) is an autosomal recessive disorder characterized by ceroid depositions that result in pigmented macrophages. This characteristic indicates a lipid metabolism disorder. A deficient release reaction has been associated with a unique morphologic abnormality of the platelets in four families. This abnormality consists of marked dilatation and tortuosity of the surface-connecting tubular system (the so-called Swiss cheese platelet). The bleeding time is only moderately prolonged, and bleeding problems are usually minor.[8, 11, 13]

Wiskott-Aldrich syndrome is a sex-linked trait characterized by the triad of severe eczema, recurrent infections, and life-threatening thrombocytopenia during the first years of life. It is diagnosed primarily in boys. The triad and a hereditary pattern of sex-linked recessiveness make the diagnosis specific.[5, 11, 12, 13]

The recurrent infections are secondary to both B cell and T cell dysfunction. The serum IgM level is reduced, but serum IgG and IgA levels are normal. A dual mechanism accounts for the thrombocytopenia: ineffective thrombocytopoiesis and increased platelet sequestration and destruction.[5, 11, 13]

Wiskott-Aldrich platelets are structurally abnormal. Small platelets, a feature that appears to be of unique diagnostic importance, are characteristic of this syndrome. The numbers of alpha granules and dense bodies are deficient. Diminished levels of adenine nucleotides are reflected in the lack of dense bodies observed in transmission electron microscopy.[11, 13]

The aggregation curve in Wiskott-Aldrich syndrome is typical of a storage pool deficiency. The platelets of this disorder have defective aggregometry patterns with a lack of a secondary wave of aggregation after administration of the agonists ADP, epinephrine, or collagen. The response to thrombin is normal. Platelet glycolysis and oxidative phosphorylation are also abnormal.[11, 13]

The most effective treatment for the thrombocytopenia is splenectomy. Bone marrow transplantation has been attempted with some success.[11]

TAR syndrome is another, rare autosomal recessive trait characterized by the congenital absence of the radial bones (the most pronounced skeletal abnormality), a number of cardiac and other skeletal abnormalities, and thrombocytopenia (90% of cases). The muscles that are normally inserted into the radius are attached to the carpal bones. The thumbs are always present in this condition. Other hand deformities commonly exist, and the ulna and elbow joint are often abnormal.[13, 34, 35]

TAR syndrome is inherited as an autosomal recessive trait, but the mechanism of thrombocytopenia in this disorder is not clear. The platelets show similar signs of ultrastructural defects in dense granules with corresponding abnormal aggregation responses. Marrow megakaryocytes may be decreased, immature, or normal.[13, 34]

TAR syndrome could be caused by a defect in the pluripotential stem cell or in the committed progenitor cells. However, the course of the disease in most patients suggests that the stem cells are present and that the committed progenitors are capable of producing megakaryocytes.[34]

Life expectancy is normal if the children survive the first year.[35]

Chédiak-Higashi syndrome (CHS) is also a rare autosomal recessive trait characterized by abnormally large lysosomal granules in the leukocytes and megakaryocytes. The disease also features oculocutaneous albinism (inadequate skin and eye pigmentation), susceptibility to bacterial infections, and hemorrhage. The disorder progresses, involving episodes of thrombocytopenia, leukopenia, anemia, macrophage accumulations in tissues, and death at an early age. The bleeding disorder in CHS is caused by defective platelet function. Platelets lack normal dense bodies and have diminished levels of ADP and serotonin. Bleeding varies from mild to moderate as platelet counts decrease.[11, 13]

Alpha Granule Deficiency: Gray Platelet Syndrome

This extremely rare disorder was first described in an 11-year-old boy with thrombocytopenia that was later corrected by splenectomy in 1971, and it has been described in very few patients, most of whom were very young and one who was a 68-year-old male.[36] It is characterized by lifelong mild bleeding tendencies, a prolonged bleeding time, moderate thrombocytopenia, reticulum fibrosis of the marrow, and large platelets whose gray appearance on a Wright-stained blood film is the source of the name of this disorder.[8, 13, 14]

The disorder is hereditary (probably autosomal) and is the result of a marked deficiency of platelet alpha granules and their constituent proteins. The abnormality may be morphologically evident on ordinary blood smears. In electron photomicrographs of platelets and megakaryocytes, the platelets appear virtually agranular and vacuolated and contain an excessively abundant dense tubular system. It is likely that the basic abnormality in this disorder is the inability of megakaryocytes to transfer endogenously synthesized secretory proteins into alpha granules. Dense bodies are normal. Affected platelets do not release normal amounts of acid hydrolases, platelet factor 4 factor VIII R:Ag or beta-thromboglobulin when activated. Platelet membrane glycoprotein Ig (thrombospondin) also is deficient.[8, 14]

DDAVP was found to shorten the bleeding time and has been used as successful prophylaxis in a dental extraction. Severe bleeding episodes may necessitate platelet transfusions. However, a long and relatively uneventful survival can be expected.[8, 14, 36]

Thromboxane Pathway Disorders: Aspirin-Like Effects

Platelet secretion requires activity from several platelet enzymes. A series of phospholipases catalyze the release of arachidonic acid from membrane phospholipids. Arachidonic acid is converted to prostaglandin by cyclooxygenase and to thromboxane A_2 by thromboxane synthase. Thromboxane A_2 binds to adenylate cyclase to regulate production of cyclic adenosine monophosphate.

Several acquired or congenital disorders of platelet secretion are traced to structural and functional modifications of arachidonic acid pathway enzymes. Acquired suppression of cyclooxygenase occurs upon ingestion of such drugs as aspirin and ibuprofen. As a result of the cyclooxygenase enzyme deficiency, less prostaglandin G_2 (PGG_2) and less thromboxane A_2 are produced from arachidonic acid. Thromboxane A_2 is required for stimulating secretion by platelet granules and for maximal cell aggregation in response to epinephrine, ADP, and low concentrations of collagen or thrombin.[11, 13, 27, 28]

Hereditary absence or modification of the same enzymes is usually termed an "aspirin-like syndrome" because the clinical and laboratory manifestations resemble those that follow aspirin ingestion. Aggregometric responses are similar to those in storage pool disorders: primary aggregation followed by disaggregation in response to ADP and epinephrine. In contrast to storage pool disorders, ultrastructure and granular contents are normal.[11]

DRUG INHIBITION OF THE PROSTAGLANDIN PATHWAYS

The most common drugs interfering with platelet prostaglandin synthetic pathways are aspirin and its derivatives. A single 200-mg dose of acetylsalicylic acid (aspirin) irreversibly acetylates 90% of the prostaglandin-producing enzyme cyclooxygenase and completely inhibits its activity. Because platelets are anucleate, they do not synthesize new enzymes, and so the inhibitory effect is permanent for the life span of the platelet (7–10 days). For this reason, aspirin affects the secretory function of platelets for several days after it is discontinued. Aspirin taken by a pregnant woman may lead to a hemorrhagic diathesis in the fetus.[6, 11, 25]

Persons with mild or silent bleeding disorders, such as mild storage pool deficiency, thrombocytopenia, vascular disorder, vWD, or circulating anticoagulant, experience a marked increase in the bleeding time upon aspirin ingestion.[11]

Other drugs with a mechanism of action similar to that of aspirin (i.e., inhibiting the release reaction) include phenylbutazone, ibuprofen (Motrin), naproxen (Naprosyn), sulfinpyrazone, furosemide, and verapamil. With the exception of ibuprofen compounds, these agents do not prolong bleeding times in vivo or cause excessive bleeding.[10, 11, 17, 18]

Less common drugs that share this mechanism of action are hydralazine, quinacrine, fenoprofen calcium (Nalfon), mefenamic acid (Ponstel), tocopheryl acetate, hydrocortisone, methylprednisolone, and cyclosporine (Cyclosporin A). All these inhibit cyclooxygenase, like aspirin, except that the binding of these drugs to the enzyme is reversible. Consequently, their inhibitory effect is more short-lived. Except for their potential to irritate the gastric mucosa, these drugs have not been reported to cause clinically important bleeding.[11, 22, 28]

Prolonged exposure to alcohol, in addition to causing thrombocytopenia, impairs platelet factor 3 release and reduces secondary aggregation. One possible mechanism is the direct impairment of prostaglandin synthesis by ethanol. Thromboxane A_2 release has been reported to be inhibited in alcoholic patients. The reduced platelet count and impaired platelet function may contribute to the increased incidence of gastrointestinal hemorrhage associated with excessive alcohol intake.[3, 11, 22, 28]

Another commonly used drug, dextran, can increase the bleeding time in normal subjects. It has been used as an anti-thrombotic agent, with an efficacy equivalent to that of low-dose subcutaneous heparin. Its mechanism of action is most likely a result of an interaction between dextran and the platelet membrane.[3, 12, 22, 28]

CYCLOOXYGENASE OR THROMBOXANE SYNTHETASE DEFICIENCY

Several patients have been described as having a deficiency of cyclooxygenase or thromboxane synthetase, characterized by the inability to form thromboxane A_2 but retaining the ability to form less potent cyclic endoperoxides. These deficiencies result only in a mild to moderate defect in hemostasis, which suggests that there are other methods of activating the platelet release and aggregation responses, independent of the arachidonate pathway.[6]

Treatment for cyclooxygenase deficiency usually consists of avoiding anti-platelet drugs and use of hormonal therapy to control menorrhagia. Because thrombin causes platelet release through a mechanism other than prostaglandins, the release of normal platelet contents in the presence of thrombin differentiates this condition from a storage pool disease.[3]

The inability to form thromboxane A_2 from endoperoxide intermediates also interferes with aggregation. Aggregation responses to arachidonic acid and PGG_2 are diminished, and the platelets are incapable of responding normally to ADP or epinephrine. The disorder is extremely rare, but it has been shown to be transmitted through autosomal dominance.[13]

DRUG INHIBITION OF PLATELET PHOSPHODIESTERASE ACTIVITY

The drugs interfering with platelet phosphodiesterase activity are caffeine, dipyridamole, aminophylline, theophylline, and papaverine. Vinblastine, vincristine, and colchicine interfere with the platelet contractile protein thrombosthenin.[22]

HEREDITARY ASPIRIN-LIKE DEFECTS

Impairment of the secondary aggregation as a result of abnormalities in the release mechanism has been observed in patients with idiopathic bleeding disorders. The ADP content in the platelets of these patients is normal; however, upon stimulation with collagen and other release-inducing agents, the ADP is not released. Thus, in contrast to patients with storage pool disease, in which there is a deficiency of the content of the dense bodies and an intact release mechanism, patients with an aspirin-like defect have a normal storage pool of ADP but an aberrant release mechanism.[5]

Many individual cases of defects (hereditary) in one of the enzymes of the arachidonic acid metabolic pathway have been described. This aspirin-like defect is inherited through autosomal dominance. It may be a result of hereditary deficiency of cyclooxygenase or thromboxane synthetase (described previously). If bleeding occurs, platelet concentrate infusion is performed. The conditions of some patients have improved with the use of steroids.[22]

Another rare platelet function defect was described in a bleeding patient who demonstrated an inherited impairment of platelet membrane phosphatidylinositol metabolism. The defect was characterized by clinical hemorrhage, delayed platelet aggregation to collagen, lack of an epinephrine-induced second wave of platelet aggregation, and normal arachidonic acid–induced platelet aggregation.[22]

Hyperactive Prethrombotic Platelets

Large bizarre platelets are commonly seen in hypercoagulable patients and in patients undergoing clinical or subclinical thrombotic episodes. Large platelets are young and presumably hemostatically more active. During a thrombotic episode, there is increased fibrin deposition with entrapment of platelets, increased consumption of platelets, a rapid platelet turnover, and decreased platelet survival. In this situation there should be a higher than usual number of young or large platelets. This assumption is valid with a normal functioning bone marrow and spleen. Platelet indices, including platelet hematocrit, platelet distribution, and mean platelet volume, all increase in patients suffering from preclinical or clinical thrombotic events.[22]

VASCULAR DISORDERS

The pathophysiology of disorders of vessels and their supporting tissues remains obscure. Laboratory studies of platelets and blood coagulation usually yield normal results. The diagnosis is often based on medical history and is made by ruling out other sources of bleeding disorders. The usual clinical sign is the tendency to bruise easily or to bleed spontaneously, especially from mucosal surfaces.[14]

Hereditary Vascular Disorders

HEREDITARY HEMORRHAGIC TELANGIECTASIA (RENDU-WEBER-OSLER SYNDROME)

Hereditary hemorrhagic telangiectasia (HHT) is inherited through autosomal dominance. The vascular defect is characterized by thinning vessel walls, and it is developmental as well as structural. At times, the walls of venules or capillaries may be reduced to a single layer of endothelium. The resulting fragile vessels form characteristic telangiectasias in the skin and mucosa. The lesions or telangiectasias are red to purple, are 1–3 mm in diameter, and are most frequently seen on the lips, tongue, conjunctivae, nasal mucosa, face, hands, fingertips, and the palmar and plantar surfaces. The lesions blanch when pressure is applied. The lesions result from decreased content of elastic fibers in the vascular walls, which in turn result in the coiling of capillaries that are dilated with blood.[14]

Patients' complaints are related to recurrent hemorrhage and anemia. Frequent nosebleeds are often the major problem in early childhood. The telangiectasias appear throughout life but are most predominant during the fourth and fifth decades.[14]

The laboratory features relate to the severity of the hemorrhagic tendencies. The bleeding time is usually normal, and the tourniquet test result may be either normal or demonstrate increased capillary fragility. Common features include a hypochromic, microcytic anemia, erythroid hyperplasia, reticulocytosis, and depletion of body iron stores. Abnormal platelet function, factor VIII deficiency, and vWF have also been reported infrequently.[8, 13, 14]

The diagnosis of HHT is based on the characteristic skin or mucous membrane lesions, a history of repeated hemorrhage, and a family history of a similar affliction. Patients with HHT do surprisingly well despite the lack of specific therapy and the seriousness of their hemorrhagic manifestations.[8, 13, 14]

HEMANGIOMA-THROMBOCYTOPENIA SYNDROME (KASABACH-MERRITT SYNDROME)

Kasabach and Merritt orginally described the association of a giant cavernous hemangioma (vascular tumor), thrombocytopenia, and a bleeding diathesis. Other well-recognized features of the Kasabach-Merritt syndrome include acute or chronic DIC and microangiopathic hemolytic anemia. A hereditary basis for this syndrome has not been established, but the condition is present at birth. Several treatment modalities are available for both the tumors and the coagulopathy.[13, 37]

Laboratory features include a low platelet count (10,000–40,000 cells/mm^3). Fibrinogen levels may be very low. External hemangiomas may become engorged with blood and resemble hematomas.[13]

EHLERS-DANLOS SYNDROME AND OTHER GENETIC DISORDERS

The Ehlers-Danlos syndrome is an autosomal dominant disorder. The severity of bleeding problems ranges from easy bruisability to arterial rupture. A defect in fibronectin (an adhesive glycoprotein that crosslinks to collagen) has been described in one family with Ehlers-Danlos syndrome. There also may be an abnormality in platelet factor 3. Common laboratory abnormalities include a positive tourniquet test result and prolonged bleeding time.[13]

Other inherited vascular disorders include pseudoxanthoma elasticum and homocystinuria (both autosomal recessive disorders), as well as the Marfan syndrome and osteogenesis imperfecta (both autosomal dominant). The Marfan syndrome is also characterized by skeletal and ocular defects.[10, 13]

Acquired Vascular Disorders

ALLERGIC PURPURA (HENOCH-SCHÖNLEIN PURPURA)

The term *allergic purpura* or *anaphylactoid purpura* is generally applied to a group of nonthrombocytopenic purpuras characterized by apparently allergic manifestations, including skin rash and edema. Allergic purpura has been associated with allergies to food, drugs, cold, insect bites, and vaccinations. The term *Henoch-Schönlein purpura* is applied when the condition is accompanied by joint pain and abdominal colic.[8, 12, 13, 14]

General evidence implicates autoimmune vascular injury, but the pathophysiology of the disorder remains unclear. Preliminary evidence indicates that the vasculitis is mediated by immune complexes containing IgA antibodies. It has been suggested that allergic purpura may represent autoimmunity to components of vessel walls.[8, 13, 14]

Allergic purpura is primarily a disease of children. It is relatively uncommon among persons under the age of 2 years and over the age of 20. The peak incidence is between the ages of 3 and 7. Twice as many males as females are affected. The onset of the disease is sudden, often following an upper respiratory infection. The organism may damage the endothelial lining of blood vessels, resulting in vasculitis. Attempts have been made to implicate a specific infectious agent, particularly the beta-hemolytic streptococcus.[8, 13, 14]

Malaise, headache, fever, and rash may be the presenting symptoms. The delay in the appearance of the skin rash often poses a difficult problem in differential diagnosis. The skin lesions are urticarial and gradually become pinkish, then red, and finally hemorrhagic. The appearance of the lesions may be very rapid, accompanied by itching. The lesions have been described as "palpable purpura," in contrast to the perfectly flat lesions of thrombocytopenia and most other forms of vascular purpura. These lesions are most commonly found on the feet, elbows, knees, buttocks, and chest. Ultimately a brownish-red eruption is seen. Petechiae may also be present.[8, 13, 14]

As the disease progresses, abdominal pain, polyarthralgias, headaches, and renal disease may develop. Renal lesions are present in as many as 60% of patients during the second to third week of the course of the disorder. Proteinuria and hematuria are commonly present.[8, 13, 14]

The platelet count is normal. Tests of hemostasis, including the bleeding time, tourniquet test, and tests of blood coagulation usually yield normal results in patients with allergic purpura. Anemia is usually not present unless the hemorrhagic manifestations have been severe. The white blood cell count and the erythrocyte sedimentation rate are usually elevated. The disease must be distinguished from other forms of nonthrombocytopenic purpura. A number of infectious diseases that may be associated with purpura must also be considered in the differential diagnosis. Drugs or chemicals may at times be incriminated.[8, 13, 14]

In the pediatric age group, the average duration of the initial attack is about 4 weeks. The initial relapse may be anticipated 6 weeks after the onset of illness, after a period of apparent well-being. Except for patients in whom chronic renal disease develops, the prognosis is usually good. Occasionally, death from renal failure has occurred. Most patients with allergic purpura undergo spontaneous remission after 1–5 weeks, which is often followed by one or more recurrences. There is no effective treatment, but corticosteroids have sometimes been helpful in alleviating symptoms.[8, 13, 14]

PARAPROTEINEMIA AND AMYLOIDOSIS

In many patients with paraprotein disorders and amyloidosis, a diffuse vascular disease with associated hemorrhage and thrombosis develops. In primary amyloidosis, hemorrhage, a result of deposition of amyloid on the endothelium, is the classic hallmark. In secondary amyloidosis, deposits also occur in the perivascular infiltration. The bleeding in patients with amyloidosis is thought to be caused by perivascular infiltration. Platelet function may be abnormal; in rare cases, patients have thrombocytopenia.[10]

SENILE PURPURA

This disorder occurs almost exclusively in older women and as a result of decreased elasticity of the connective tissues surrounding and supporting the superficial blood vessels. The dark blotches are flattened, are about 1–10 mm in diameter, do not blanch with pressure, and resorb slowly. The lesions are limited mostly to the extensor surfaces of forearms and back of the hands. Results of labora-

tory tests are normal, and no other bleeding manifestations are present.[8, 12, 13, 19, 38]

DRUG-INDUCED VASCULAR PURPURAS

Purpura may be associated with normal and functionally adequate platelets in association with various drugs. Sulfonamides and iodides have been implicated most often, but a large number of other drugs, such as aspirin, digoxin, methyldopa and estrogen, have occasionally been implicated. Because the disease is benign and self-limited, many cases are unrecognized and unreported. The lesions vary from a few petechiae to massive, generalized petechial eruptions. Drug-induced vascular purpura is the result of individual idiosyncracy and develops in only an occasional patient who is taking a given drug. The resulting vascular injury is most likely caused by an autoimmune phenomenon.[13, 14]

Tourniquet test results are often positive, but bleeding time, the platelet count, and coagulation tests are normal unless DIC is present.

VITAMIN C DEFICIENCY (SCURVY)

Insufficient dietary intake of vitamin C (ascorbic acid) results in decreased synthesis of collagen and weakening of capillary walls.[13, 14]

Purpuras of Unknown Origin

PURPURA SIMPLEX (EASY BRUISABILITY)

A diagnosis of simple vascular purpura or vascular fragility is made when the cause is undetermined. The ecchymoses are superficial, bleeding is usually mild, and laboratory test results are most often normal.[13]

PSYCHOGENIC PURPURA

Cutaneous bleeding and bruising through intact skin has been observed in patients in whom no vascular or platelet disorders can be diagnosed. Most such patients are women with emotional problems, and the bruising is often accompanied by nausea, vomiting, or fever. Evidence of a psychosomatic origin is equivocal. Laboratory test results are invariably normal.[13]

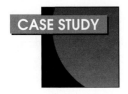
CASE STUDY

A 16-year-old female had experienced easy bruising since early childhood, had frequent nosebleeds, and had heavy menstrual flow. Her brother and father had minor bruising tendencies. Her father's uncle had minor problems with gastrointestinal bleeding, caused by ulcers.

The patient was scheduled for oral surgery to remove wisdom teeth. On the basis of her history, the oral surgeon suggested a full coagulation work-up. The results were as follows:

	Patient Results	*Normal Values*
Bleeding time	12 minutes	2–8 minutes
Prothrombin time	11 seconds	10–12 seconds
APTT	45 seconds	25–35 seconds
Platelet count	200,000/mm³	140,000–400,000/mm³

1. Identify the abnormal results.

2. According to the laboratory results and the patient's history, which of the following should be considered?
   Factor deficiency
   Hereditary disorder
   Acquired disorder
   If hereditary: dominant or recessive

3. What follow-up tests should be performed?

Platelet aggregation studies were performed. Aggregation with epinephrine, ADP, and collagen was normal. Aggregation with ristocetin was decreased.

1. According to the platelet aggregation studies, what is the most likely diagnosis? What variants should be considered? What coagulation factor is involved?

2. What treatment, if any, should be given to the patient before oral surgery?

References

1. Triplett DA: How to evaluate platelet function. Lab Med Pract Phys 1978; July/Aug: 37–43.
2. Brown BA: Hematology: Principles and Procedures, 6th ed. Philadelphia: Lea & Febiger, 1993.
3. Lotspeich-Steininger CA, Stiene-Martin EA, Koepke JA: Clinical Hematology: Principles, Procedures, Correlations. Philadelphia: JB Lippincott, 1992.
4. Miale JB: Laboratory Medicine: Hematology, 6th ed. St. Louis: CV Mosby, 1982.
5. Triplett DA (ed): Platelet Function: Laboratory Evaluation and Clinical Application. Chicago: American Society of Clinical Pathologists, 1978.
6. Thompson AR, Harker LA. Manual of Hemostasis and Thrombosis, 3rd ed. Philadelphia: FA Davis, 1983.
7. Stormorken H, Hellum B, Egeland T, et al: X-linked thrombocytopenia and thrombocytopathia: attenuated Wiskott-Aldrich syndrome. Thromb Haemost 1991; 65:300–305.
8. Thorup OA: Leavell and Thorup's Fundamentals of Clinical Hematology, 5th ed. Philadelphia: WB Saunders, 1987.
9. Colvin BT: Thrombocytopenia. Clin Haematol 1985; 14:661–681.
10. Harmening DM: Clinical Hematology and Fundamentals of Hemostasis, 2nd ed. Philadelphia: FA Davis, 1992.
11. Corriveau DM, Fritsma GA: Hemostasis and Thrombosis in the Clinical Laboratory. Philadelphia: JB Lippincott, 1988.
12. Quick AJ: Hemorrhagic Diseases and Thrombosis, 2nd ed. Philadelphia: Lea & Febiger, 1966.
13. Powers LW: Diagnostic Hematology: Clinical and Technical Principles. St. Louis: CV Mosby, 1989.
14. Williams WJ, Beutler E, Erslev AJ, Lichtman MA (eds): Hematology, 4th ed. New York: McGraw-Hill, 1990.
15. Clerc JM: Neonatal thrombocytopenia. Clin Lab Sci 1989; 2:42–47.
16. Martin JN Jr, Blake PG, Perry KG Jr, et al: The natural history of HELLP syndrome: patterns of disease progression and regression. Am J Obstet Gynecol 1991; 164:1500–1509.
17. Green D: Diagnosis and management of bleeding disorders. Comp Ther 1988; 14:31–36.
18. Rapaport SI: Introduction to Hematology, 2nd ed. Philadelphia: JB Lippincott, 1987.
19. Sirridge MS, Shannon R: Laboratory Evaluation of Hemostasis and Thrombosis, 3rd ed. Philadelphia: Lea & Febiger, 1983.
20. Santhosh-Kumar CR, Yohannon MD, Higgy KE, al-Mashhadani SA: Thrombocytosis in adults: analysis of 777 patients. J Intern Med 1991; 229:493–495.
21. Mitus AJ, Schafer AI: Thrombocytosis and thrombocythemia. Hematol Oncol Clin North Am 1990; 4:157–178.
22. Bick RL, Scates SM: Qualitative platelet defects. Lab Med 1992; 23:95–103.
23. Miller JL: Von Willebrand disease. Hematol Oncol Clin North Am 1990; 4:107–23.
24. Triplett DA: Hemostasis: A Case Oriented Approach. New York: Igaku-Shoin, 1985.
25. Beardsley DS: Hemostasis in the perinatal period: approach to the diagnosis of coagulation disorders. Semin Perinatol 1991; 15(3, Suppl 2):25–34.
26. Colon-Otero G, Cockerill KJ, Bowie EJ: How to diagnose bleeding disorders. Postgrad Med 1991; 90:145–150.
27. Moake JL, Funicella T: Common bleeding problems. Clin Symp 1983; 35:1–32.
28. George JN, Shattil SJ: The clinical importance of acquired abnormalities of platelet function. N Engl J Med 1991; 324:27–39.
29. Meyer M, Kirchmaier CM, Schirmer A, et al: Acquired disorder of platelet function associated with autoantibodies against membrane glycoprotein IIb-IIIa complex—1. Glycoprotein analysis. Thromb Haemost 1991; 65:491–496.
30. Tarantino MD, Corrigan JJ Jr, Glasser L, et al: A variant form of thrombasthenia. Am J Dis Child 1991; 145:1053–1057.
31. Jennings LK, Wang WC, Jackson CW, et al: Hemostasis in Glanzmann's thrombasthenia (GT): GT platelets interfere with the aggregation of normal platelets. Am J Pediatr Hematol Oncol 1991; 13:84–90.
32. Caen JP: Glanzmann's thrombasthenia. Baillieres Clin Haematol 1989; 2:609–623.
33. Pati H, Saraya AK: Platelet storage pool disease. Indian J Med Res 1986; 84:617–620.
34. de Alarcon PA, Graeve JA, Levine RF, et al: Thrombocytopenia and absent radii syndrome: defective megakaryocy-

topoiesis-thrombocytopoiesis. Am J Pediatr Hematol Oncol 1991; 13:77–83.

35. Fromm B, Niethard FU, Marquardt E: Thrombocytopenia and absent radius (TAR) syndrome. Int Orthop 1991; 15:95–99.

36. Berrebi A, Klepfish A, Varon D, et al: Gray platelet syndrome in the elderly. Am J Hematol 1988; 28:270–272.

37. Maceyko RF, Camisa C: Kasabach-Merritt syndrome. Pediatr Dermatol 1991; 8:133–136.

38. Thomas JH, Powell DEB: Blood Disorders in the Elderly. Bristol, UK: J Wright, 1971.

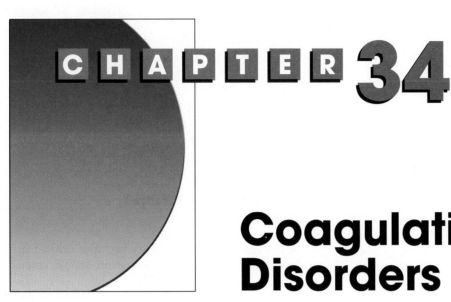

CHAPTER 34

Coagulation Disorders

Jeanne M. Clerc

Outline

Objectives

AFTER COMPLETION OF THIS CHAPTER, THE READER WILL BE ABLE TO

1. Describe the genetics, clinical symptoms, laboratory diagnosis, and blood therapy treatment for hemophilia A and hemophilia B.
2. Describe the genetics, clinical symptoms, laboratory diagnosis, and blood therapy treatment for other factor deficiencies that include factors I, II, V, VII, X, XI, and XII; Fletcher factor; and high–molecular-weight kininogen (HMWK).
3. Describe how acquired factor deficiencies may occur.
4. Describe the clinical symptoms, laboratory diagnosis, and treatment for disseminated intravascular coagulation, liver disease, renal disease, and vitamin K deficiency.
5. Describe how inhibitors or circulating anti-coagulants affect coagulation.
6. Give at least seven examples of inhibitors to coagulation factors.
7. Define fibrinolysis, and describe the clinical symptoms and laboratory diagnosis of primary fibrinolysis.
8. Describe how deficiencies of plasminogen and alpha$_2$–anti-plasmin affect the blood clotting mechanism.
9. Explain the clinical effects that deficiencies of inhibitors to coagulation have on a patient. Describe the laboratory diagnosis of AT III, protein C, and protein S deficiencies.

Deficiency of Factor XIII
  (Fibrin-Stabilizing Factor)
Passovoy Deficiency
Inherited Multiple–
  Coagulation Factor
  Deficiencies
ACQUIRED FACTOR DEFICIENCIES
Disseminated Intravascular
  Coagulation
Chronic Disseminated
  Intravascular Coagulation
Liver Disease
Renal Disease
Vitamin K Deficiency
ACQUIRED CIRCULATING ANTI-
  COAGULANTS
Fibrinogen (Factor I) Inhibitors
Factor II Inhibitors
Factor V Inhibitors
Factor VII Inhibitors
Factor VIII:C Inhibitors
von Willebrand Factor
  Inhibitors
Factor IX Inhibitors
Factor X Inhibitors
Factor XI Inhibitors
Factor XII Inhibitors
Factor XIII Inhibitors
Nonspecific Inhibitors
FIBRINOLYTIC DISORDERS
Primary Fibrinolysis
HYPERCOAGULABILITY
CONGENITAL CLOTTING
  SYNDROMES
Plasminogen Deficiency
Alpha$_2$–Anti-Plasmin
  Deficiency
Defects of Activators
NATURAL INHIBITORS OF
  COAGULATION
Anti-Thrombin III Deficiency
Protein C Deficiency
Protein S Deficiency
Heparin Cofactor II Deficiency
Factor XII and Other Contact
  Factor Deficiencies
DYSFIBRINOGENEMIAS
ACQUIRED CLOTTING STATES

The diverse defects of plasma clotting factors can be divided into two major groups: hereditary and acquired forms. The defects in the clotting factors can be produced by one of the following:

1. Decreased synthesis of the factors.
2. Production of abnormal molecules that interfere with the coagulation cascade.
3. Loss or consumption of the coagulation factors.
4. Inactivation of these factors by inhibitors or antibodies.[1, 2]

Immunologic studies have demonstrated that in some patients with deficiencies of prothrombin (factor II) or of factors VII, VIII, IX, X, XI, or XII, the blood contains a substance that reacts with antibodies to the respective normal factor, which suggests the synthesis of an abnormal factor rather than failure of synthesis of the normal factor. In other patients, there is apparently failure of synthesis of the factor. Molecular abnormalities of fibrinogen (dysfibrinogenemias) as well as afibrinogenemias also occur.[3]

APPROACH TO BLEEDING DISORDERS

A thoughtful, careful history provides critical information. The historical evaluation should establish

1. The type of bleeding present (petechiae, purpura, ecchymosis, single or generalized bleeding sites).
2. The course or pattern of bleeding (spontaneous or postinjury onset, frequency, short-term or lifelong duration, severity).
3. Family history of bleeding and, if positive, whether an X-linked, an autosomal dominant, or an autosomal recessive inheritance pattern.
4. Previous or current therapy (drugs; e.g., aspirin, coumarin, cancer chemotherapy, immunizations, transfusions).
5. Local or systemic associated diseases (such as leukemia, uremia, liver disease, infections, malignancy).[4]

A thorough physical examination should also be conducted.

LABORATORY SCREENING TESTS

Despite the leads derived from the clinical examination, diagnosing the type of hemostatic disorder ultimately depends on laboratory testing. Platelet plug formation reflects the primary hemostatic event and is evaluated through the bleeding time and the platelet count. Abnormalities of coagulation are then screened for by measuring the fibrinogen concentration, thrombin time, prothrombin time (PT), and partial thromboplastin time (PTT). Once screening test results have indicated the type of disorder, additional studies and factor assays are used to establish a specific diagnosis.[4]

HEREDITARY COAGULATION DISORDERS

Hereditary coagulation disorders are the result of a deficiency or functional abnormality of a single factor. They most often result in a lifelong bleeding diathesis that occurs in a consistent genetic pattern. However, some hereditary coagulation disorders may be "silent," whereas others lead to thrombosis.

The most common hereditary disorders of coagulation are hemophilia A, von Willebrand's disease (discussed in Chapter 33), and hemophilia B. These three disorders together constitute more than 90% of the hereditary coagulation disorders, hemophilia A and von Willebrand's disease being the most common. The remaining disorders are thus exceedingly rare.[1, 2]

Hemophilia A (Classic Hemophilia; Factor VIII Deficiency)

This disorder is the most common hereditary coagulation disorder and one of the oldest diseases known to humankind. It occurs in all geographic areas and in ethnic groups with approximately equal frequencies. The genetic abnormality gives rise to deficiency or aberration of the low-molecular-weight subunit of factor VIII, designated VIII:C. Levels of related antigens (factor VIII R:Ag) are normal or elevated.

HISTORY

Hemophilia has influenced history. The disorder affected the royal house of Stuart in Europe and Russia. Queen Victoria of Great Britain, a carrier of the hemophilia gene, was the source of hemophilia in four subsequent generations. She passed the hemophilia gene to two of her five daughters, who transmitted it to the royalty of Spain (both uncles of King Carlos were affected), Germany, and Russia (Alexis, son of Tsar Nicholas II, was affected). Victoria's son Leopold was also a hemophiliac.[2, 5, 6]

Alexis was examined repeatedly by eminent physicians of Russia, but they could not alleviate the problem. His mother, desperate for her son's life, sought the help of Grigori Rasputin, a Siberian peasant priest believed to have many mysterious powers. Rasputin gained influence over the Tsar and Tsarina by his ability to stop bleeding episodes in Alexis. Whether Rasputin really was "magical" or whether he used common sense and possibly hypnosis is still unclear.[7]

The first description of hemophilia in Western medical literature appeared in 1793, and the disease was recognized as a sex-linked disorder by Otto in 1803. Before 1952, X-linked hemophilia was considered a single disease. However, as early as 1947, Pavlovsky observed that when blood from one hemophiliac was transfused into another, the prolonged clotting time in the recipient was normalized. At the time, Pavlovsky did not recognize that two different types of hemophilia accounted for his observation. This was recognized by Aggeler and coworkers in 1952, when they described a patient with a deficiency in plasma thromboplastin component, a blood-clotting factor different from anti-hemophilic factor and later designated factor IX. A deficiency of factor IX was later termed hemophilia B because of the similarities to a factor VIII deficiency (i.e., hemophilia A).[3]

GENETICS

Hemophilia A is inherited as an X-linked recessive trait. The abnormality is fully expressed in men who lack the normal factor VIII allele on their X chromosome. Such men transmit the hemophilia gene to all daughters (generation II). Thus daughters of a hemophilic father are at least obligate carriers. Such carrier females have one defective allele on one X chromosome and one normal allele and have approximately half normal amounts of factor VIII:C because of the phenomenon of random X chromosome inactivation (Lyon hypothesis). These abnormalities seldom lead to bleeding symptoms but do result in the transmission of the genetic defect by carrier females to half their offspring (generation III). Figure 34–1 is a pedigree of a typical family with the hemophilia A gene.[1, 5]

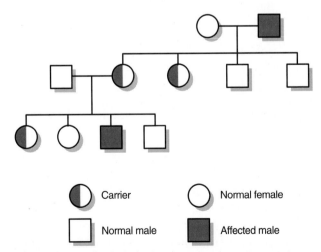

Figure 34–1 Sex-linked inheritance pattern of hemophilia A. All daughters of an affected male are obligatory carriers. Sons of carriers have a 50% chance of being affected with hemophilia A. (From Ruggeri ZM (ed): Clinics in Haematology. Philadelphia: WB Saunders, 1985:360.)

Thus, sex-linked recessive traits appear to skip generations, as generation II females appear not to express the disease. If a daughter of a hemophilic man also inherits a hemophilia gene from her mother (a carrier), she expresses the hemophilia trait, with subsequent bleeding problems. Although this is very rare, it has been documented in hemophilic dog colonies.[1, 5]

Hemophilia is usually seen in white persons, but occasional cases are reported among Chinese and black persons. It is estimated to affect one male per 10,000 people in the whole population. In the familial form, it follows the predicted patterns of inheritance. In the sporadic form, the disease occurs apparently as the result of spontaneous mutation. In approximately 30% of newly diagnosed cases, there is no family history of disease. This suggests either a high mutation rate or several generations of silent carriers.[2, 5, 7]

Fewer than 70% of hemophiliac patients have a family history of the disorder. The rate of detection of female carriers has been greatly improved by the advent of immunoassays. Plasma VIII:C levels in carriers vary widely around a mean level of 50 U/dL (mean of normals: 100 U/dL) and frequently overlap with values obtained in the normal population (range: 50–150 U/dL). The use of factor VIII R:Ag as a means of assisting in the detection of carriers has proved extremely helpful. Because factor VIII R:Ag is controlled by an autosomal chromosome, it would be expected to be normal in carriers and in male patients with hemophilia A. Thus the ratio of level of factor VIII R:Ag to level of factor VIII:C should be approximately 2:1 in the carrier state. Levels of VIII R:Ag are usually higher than 100 U/dL, and so this ratio is more sensitive in the detection of carriers.[1, 8, 9]

For many years hemophilias A and B were considered to be caused by quantitative deficiencies in the respective clotting factor proteins. In 1956, Fantl postulated that some hemophiliacs produce qualitatively abnormal molecules with reduced or no clotting factor activity. Patients have either reduced or no production of normal clotting factor protein, or they produce a molecule so abnormal that the antigenic sites are affected.[7]

About 90% of patients have a deficiency of both factor VIII:C and factor VIII:C:Ag and thus have a true deficiency of cross-reacting material (CRM⁻) or factor VIII:C⁻. The remaining 10% of patients lack factor VIII:C activity but have normal factor VIII:C:Ag; these patients therefore have dysfunctional factor VIII:C and are referred to as CRM⁺ or factor VIII:C⁺ patients. Inactive but immunologically detectable VIII:C:Ag has been found in CRM⁺ patients through the use of homologous human factor VIII inhibitor antibody. However, al-most all these patients were mildly or moderately affected, with measurable levels of factor VIII activity. The absence of factor VIII:C:Ag in most severely hemophilic patients has allowed for the use of a factor VIII:C:Ag immunoassay for prenatal detection of hemophilia A. Patients with deficiencies of factor VIII:C⁻ and factor VIII:C⁺ suffer similar clinical courses.[6, 7]

CLINICAL SYMPTOMS

Hemophilia may be clinically mild or severe. The severity of the disease is closely correlated with the degree of reduction in the amount of procoagulant factor VIII:C in the blood. In the *severe* form of the disease, the factor VIII:C level in plasma is from 0–2 U/dL (1% or less of normal activity of the clotting factor). Hemophilia A is usually characterized by severe and protracted bleeding that follows even minor trauma and by certain spontaneous bleeding manifestations, particularly life-threatening hemorrhage and hemarthrosis (bleeding into the joints). Permanent joint damage is characteristic; any joint may be involved, but repeated hemorrhage into the knees, ankles, and elbows produces the greatest restriction of normal activity. The onset of bleeding may follow very slight joint injury but often appears to be spontaneous. The typical progression is stiffness rapidly followed by pain, swelling, and tenderness. Because the bleeding is into the joint capsule, no discoloration is observed. The blood originates from synovial vessels and rapidly fills the joint space. Recurrent bleeding, often in the same joint, leads to synovial inflammation and thickening.[1, 3, 5, 7, 10]

Bleeding may occur during infancy or may manifest later in life. Severely affected hemophiliacs may experience bleeding without known trauma other than that associated with the usual day-to-day activities. Hemarthroses become frequent at about the time the patient begins to walk. Hemorrhage from the nose, mouth, and lips may be severe.[1, 3, 5, 7, 10]

Another characteristic of hemophilia A is delayed bleeding. After surgical procedures such as tooth extractions, bleeding appears to stop initially, as a result of platelet plug formation. Then bleeding recurs several hours to days later because a fibrin network is not present to seal the injury site. Subcutaneous and intramuscular hematomas are also common manifestations of hemophilia A. Bleeding into the central nervous system is not uncommon in hemophilic patients, is often associated with head trauma, and is usually fatal. Other special bleeding problems include intraabdominal hemorrhage and hemophilic pseudocysts (pockets of liquefied blood in tendons, muscles, and bones). Although most bone lesions in hemophilia are secondary to joint bleeding, a serious complication may arise from pressure necrosis of bone. Hematuria occurs in many cases of severe hemophilia. In some cases, external trauma such as a blow to the groin or back is responsible; in others, a urinary tract stone may be the cause. The urine may be bright red or dark reddish brown.[10]

Injuries to the mouth and pharynx, including local injections for dental anesthesia, can lead to soft tissue hematomas. Additional complications of hemophilia include severe dental and periodontal disease as a result of poor dental care, necessitating extensive extractions at an early age.

The moderate form of the disorder (factor VIII:C levels in plasma of 3–6 U/dL, which is 1–5% of normal factor activity) is associated with serious post-traumatic hemorrhage, but hemarthrosis is less severe, and many patients escape crippling sequelae.[1]

In the mild form of the disorder (factor VIII:C levels in plasma of 7–30 U/dL, which is more than 5% of normal clotting activity), hemarthrosis and other spontaneous bleeding manifestations are uncommon; hemorrhage may be inconspicuous after small injuries and surgical procedures. However, major surgery or injuries can pose a significant hazard.[1]

Within families, the severity of the disease tends to be the same. The disease is clinically more severe and more difficult to treat when a factor VIII inhibitor (antibody) develops.[5]

LABORATORY DIAGNOSIS

The most sensitive screening tool is a complete family history. Patients with hemophilia A usually present with a normal to prolonged PTT, a normal PT, a normal bleeding time, and a normal platelet count. The activated PTT may be normal in mildly affected patients, and specific factor VIII assays are necessary for ruling out the disorder. The bleeding time may be slightly longer in hemophilic patients than in normal persons, but it may nonetheless remain within the normal range. In some patients, the platelet count might be elevated in association with acute bleeding.[1]

The prothrombin consumption test yields abnormal results in severely affected patients. In patients with milder forms of the disorder, this test yields normal results.[1]

Definitive diagnosis is reached by performing a factor VIII assay. The patient's plasma is mixed with plasma from a patient who congenitally lacks factor VIII:C (lyophilized factor VIII–deficient substrate or artificially depleted substrates may also be purchased). The effectiveness of the patient's plasma in shortening the clotting time is compared with that of normal plasma. A standard curve is plotted by mixing dilutions of pooled fresh normal human plasma with the hemophilic plasma substrate and plotting the clotting times against the dilutions on log-log paper. The level of factor VIII:C varies in a normal population from 50–200 U/dL.[11]

TREATMENT

Hereditary coagulation disorders are treated by replacement of the deficient or abnormal factor with a normal factor in amounts sufficient to normalize coagulation. This procedure requires the administration of normal blood or blood products from humans or lower animals. Blood products from lower animals are rarely used and are used only for patients with hemophilia with inhibitors in the United States.[1]

Cryoprecipitate and purified factor VIII are now the mainstays in the replacement therapy of hemophilia A. Plasma, because of its larger volume, is a third choice, although it is still used in the treatment of some other hereditary coagulation disorders.[1]

Cryoprecipitate is prepared by slowly thawing fresh-frozen plasma at 4 °C and collecting the sediment by centrifugation. This sediment represents a 7- to 20-fold concentration of factor VIII. The concentrate contains 50–120 U of factor VIII in a volume of 10–40 mL.[1, 2]

A pool of several units is generally given to a patient. Because blood is screened for human immunodeficiency virus (HIV)–positive donors, it is somewhat safer to use concentrates of human plasma such as anti-hemophilic factor.[1, 2]

Purified factor VIII is marketed by several drug companies. The levels of factor VIII in these concentrates may be up to 400 times higher than those in plasma, and the concentrates have the advantage of uniform potency. A significant risk of transmitting hepatitis and acquired immunodeficiency syndrome (AIDS) exists with the use of these products, although the use of heat treatment appears to inactivate HIV.[1]

Factor VIII:C levels of 10–20% of normal are usually adequate for hemostasis after minor trauma. For major injuries, surgery, or bleeding into dangerous sites (e.g., the central nervous system or respiratory tract), factor VIII:C levels must be maintained at 50–100% of normal for days. The half-life of transfused factor VIII:C is 8–12 hours. Consequently, transfusion must be repeated two or three times a day. In home therapy programs, patients with hemophilia A give themselves transfusions of cryoprecipitate or lyophilized factor VIII concentrates. This usually leads to decreased dependence on hospitals.[12]

Concentrated factor VIII of animal origin is available for clinical use in Great Britain. It may be used for a single treatment only, but it is useful in serious bleeding emergencies.[1]

A synthetic analogue of vasopressin (DDAVP) has been shown to elevate the plasma factor VIII levels in normal subjects, in mildly affected hemophilic patients, and in patients with von Willebrand's disease. The drug appears to act by stimulating the synthesis or release of factor VIII by the hepatic cells. Levels of both factors VIII:C and VIII R:Ag are increased.[1, 12]

Inhibitors of fibrinolysis, such as epsilon-aminocaproic acid and tranexamic acid, have proved useful adjuncts in the treatment of mild hemophilia with minor bleeding manifestations. These agents act to protect labile hemostatic plugs from fibrinolytic degradation.[1, 12]

COMPLICATIONS

Careful preventive dental care is of the utmost importance in hemophiliacs. Serious tooth decay and multiple extractions are more easily prevented than treated. Hepatitis, usually the non-A, non-B type, is relatively common among hemophilic patients because of their extensive exposure to blood products. Many patients have chronically abnormal liver function. A smaller number have chronic hepatitis.[1]

Concentrated factor VIII has been implicated in the transmission of AIDS in a number of cases. The use of purified concentrated factor VIII has declined because of these risks. In the treatment of mild hemophilia, emphasis has switched to the use of DDAVP.

Chronic complications of treatment include inhibitors and liver disease (commonly hepatitis). The development of antibodies or inhibitors to factor VIII:C in hemophilia A occurs in 10–15% of patients with hemophilia A. The first sign may be lack of response to treatment for routine bleeding episodes after an ordinary treatment dose. The inhibitors, usually temperature dependent, are of immunoglobulin G (IgG) class. The potency of the antibody, expressed in inhibitor units, is measured by assay techniques that are based upon determining the dilution of the patient's plasma that neutralizes a set amount of factor VIII under standardized incubation conditions. These inhibitors neutralize factor VIII:C at 37 °C. Inhibitor development is more common among young, severely hemophilic patients who have undergone intense treatment than among mildly hemophilic patients.[1, 2, 4, 5, 6, 11, 13]

The detection of an acquired inhibitor of factor VIII is important because in the presence of the inhibitor, the disease is aggravated and therapy becomes a problem. The anti-VIII:C antibody may incubate in the PTT system for a long time before it is manifested. Thus it is wise to incubate the activated PTT system for 2 hours when the factor VIII:C antibody is sought. The titer of inhibitor falls gradually in the absence of replacement therapy but rises very quickly when cryoprecipitate or other replacement therapy is used. Acquired inhibitors of factor VIII have also been found in hemophilic children without an underlying coagulation abnormality who have not undergone transfusion.[1, 2, 4, 5, 6, 11, 13]

Because hemophilic factor VIII inhibitors are alloantibodies, immunosuppression has not been as useful as in treating the acquired autoantibodies to factor VIII. It is difficult to lower significantly the antibody titer by plasmapheresis. Thus, routine bleeding episodes in patients with such inhibitors are managed as much as possible by immobilization and analgesia. Preventive measures such as exercise programs and dental prophylaxis are therefore even more important for patients with factor VIII inhibitors than for other patients with hemophilia.[4]

In nonhemophilic patients, inhibitors of factor VIII may develop post partum; in association with other diseases, such as rheumatoid arthritis, asthma, colitis, and carcinoma; and in association with drug reactions. Penicillin allergy has acquired a peculiar notoriety in this regard: the inhibitor in cases of penicillin allergy is an IgG globulin that does not appear to be specifically related to penicillin antibody. Although the bleeding tendency caused by inhibitors is often alarming, it does not necessarily afford protection against thrombotic cardiovascular disease.[14]

Immediate complications of blood components include allergic and hemolytic reactions and, for vitamin K–dependent factor concentrates, a thrombotic tendency. Urticaria (hives) is a commonly encountered allergic reaction to infusion with plasma, cryoprecipitate, and sometimes even lyophilized concentrate.[4]

Christmas Disease (Hemophilia B; Factor IX Deficiency)

Hemophilia B is rarer than hemophilia A. The incidence in a normal population is approximately 1/100,000, which is about 15% of the incidence of hemophilia A in the United States. However, in certain areas, such as India, the incidence of hemophilia B equals that of hemophilia A.[2, 5, 11]

Factor IX is a vitamin K–dependent factor. It is synthesized in the liver and is present in serum.

Factor IX is stable in blood or plasma stored at refrigerator temperature (4 °C) as well as in fresh-frozen plasma. Transfused factor IX has a half-life of approximately 24 hours.[2, 12]

GENETICS

Hemophilia B, like hemophilia A, is inherited as a sex-linked recessive trait. The incidence of spontaneous mutation in cases of hemophilia B is less than that in cases of hemophilia A. Excessive bleeding is more common among heterozygous female carriers of the hemophilia B trait than among those of the hemophilia A trait. The obligatory carriers of factor IX deficiency often have factor IX levels of about 35% in plasma. As a consequence, carrier detection through the use of procoagulant assays is easier in persons with factor IX deficiency than in persons with factor VIII deficiency.[5, 11]

Immunologic studies have revealed a variety of abnormal factor IX molecules in patients with this hemorrhagic disorder. Seventy to ninety percent of patients have a true deficiency of factor IX:C and are completely devoid of cross-reacting material (CRM⁻). About 10% of hemophilia B patients have been shown to have the cross-reacting material (CRM⁺). The CRM⁺ dysfunctional variants have been subdivided further into those in which PTs are prolonged when ox brain thromboplastin is used (hemophilia B_m) and those in which PTs are normal with ox brain thromboplastin (hemophilia $B_{Chapel\ Hill}$ and hemophilia $B_{Alabama}$). Hemophilia B_m accounts for about 15% of the cases of hemophilia B. Because most American PT reagents contain rabbit brain tissue factor, the PTs of patients with hemophilia B_m are virtually normal. This apparently "normal" PT may lead to inappropriate management of a patient.[3, 5]

Patients who are CRM⁻ or in whom immunologically detectable protein is reduced in proportion to reduced factor IX activity levels (CRMᴿ) represent cases of genetically deficient production of the protein. In a fifth genetic variant (hemophilia B_{Layden}), factor IX levels tend to increase with age. Screening tests do not distinguish this deficiency from hemophilia A (bleeding time, platelet count, PT, and PTT). It is identified by correction studies and by specific assay.[5]

CLINICAL SYMPTOMS

Although the bleeding abnormality is usually less severe than in factor VIII deficiency, it can be clinically indistinguishable from it. Hemophilia B is identical to the more common hemophilia A in terms of bleeding symptoms, varying degrees of severity, and complications. As in hemophilia A, the severity of factor IX deficiency tends to be the same for affected members of a family.[1, 5]

LABORATORY DIAGNOSIS

The screening tests in hemophilia B reveal essentially the same abnormalities as in hemophilia A. The one exception is the abnormal PT in the B_m variant when bovine brain thromboplastin or Thrombotest is used. One patient has been described as having a prolonged bleeding time. The diagnosis is established by a specific assay for factor IX in which the plasma of a patient with known factor IX deficiency is used as a substrate. An accurate diagnosis is very important because of the widely different clinical regimens for treating factor VIII and factor IX deficiencies.[11]

TREATMENT

The principles of replacement therapy and the general aspects of treatment directed at common complications are the same for hemophilia B as for hemophilia A. Because of the relatively small size of the molecule (60,000 D), there is an initially large extravascular loss of the transfused factor IX. Because of these considerations, a very large initial loading dose of factor IX must be administered in the treatment of major bleeding in patients with hemophilia B. Fresh-frozen plasma is still used in the treatment of minor bleeding in hemophilia B, but the preferred therapeutic material for treatment of major bleeding is one of the commercially available concentrates of vitamin K–dependent factors. In addition to factor IX, these materials contain factors VII and X, prothrombin, and proteins C and S.[1, 12]

COMPLICATIONS

Serious thromboembolic complications have been encountered in patients with liver disease and in premature infants. Hepatitis is a significant risk with factor IX concentrates. Transmission of HIV by concentrates of vitamin K–dependent factors has also been described but is less common than is the case with factor VIII concentrates. Anti–factor IX antibodies develop in about 5–7% of patients with factor IX deficiency. The only therapy for this complication is to neutralize the antibody with prothrombin complex concentrate and then raise the factor IX:C level to achieve hemostasis.[1, 6]

Hereditary Afibrinogenemia

Congenital fibrinogen defects are rare coagulation disorders that reflect absent or defective protein synthesis. They include afibrinogenemia (no measurable fibrinogen), hypofibrinogenemia (plasma levels of fibrinogen less than 100 mg/dL), and dysfibrinogenemia (functionally abnormal fibrinogen). Hypofibrinogenemia is decreased production of fibrinogen, most likely caused by a synthetic defect.[15]

GENETICS

Hereditary afibrinogenemia is a rare autosomal recessive trait in which plasma fibrinogen is totally lacking. Platelet-contained fibrinogen is also deficient. Of the cases reported, over 50% were in the offspring of consanguineous marriages.[1, 3, 15, 16]

CLINICAL SYMPTOMS

Clinical symptoms are mild, considering that the blood is incoagulable in laboratory assays. Hematomas, bruising, and epistaxis are common, but affected women often have normal menstrual periods. Hemarthrosis and other serious spontaneous hemorrhagic manifestations are rare. Patients with afibrinogenemia show manifestations of defective wound healing. Spontaneous rupture of the spleen is fairly common.[1]

LABORATORY DIAGNOSIS

All laboratory tests of coagulation that depend on fibrin clot formation as an end point (i.e., the activated PTT, PT, thrombin time, and whole blood coagulation time) are abnormal. The bleeding time is prolonged in approximately 50% of cases; this finding is attributed to platelet dysfunction. It is imperative to rule out a qualitative defect in addition to a quantitative defect of fibrinogen, because congenital hypofibrinogenemia may be confused with dysfibrinogenemia.[1, 3]

TREATMENT AND COMPLICATIONS

The hemostatic level for fibrinogen is approximately 100 mg/dL (normal range, 200–400 mg/dL). Its biologic half-life ranges from 77 to 106 hours. The disease is treated by administering fibrinogen in the form of cryoprecipitate (4 U/10 kg every other day). Preoperative fibrinogen replacement is important because postsurgical bleeding may be severe. Development of anti-fibrinogen antibodies has been described, and major thrombotic episodes have occurred in a few patients after infusions of fibrinogen concentrates.[1, 3]

Hereditary Hypofibrinogenemia

This appears to be a separate disease because the levels of fibrinogen found in these patients (usually 20–30 mg/dL) are lower than those found in persons heterozygous for the congenital afibrinogenemia trait (usually 150–200 mg/dL). The hereditary transmission is autosomal recessive, but in some families the mode seems to be autosomal dominant. Patients with this disorder have a mild tendency to bleed. The treatment of choice is replacement by infusion of cryoprecipitate.[9, 16]

Hereditary Dysfibrinogenemias

These disorders are characterized by the presence of qualitatively abnormal, functionally defective fibrinogen. More than 100 kinds of dysfibrinogenemias have been identified.

GENETICS

Except in a few families to date, hereditary dysfibrinogenemia is inherited as an autosomal dominant or codominant trait. The majority of persons are heterozygotes.[1, 3]

Diverse functional abnormalities have been documented in the various forms of dysfibrinogenemia and may be classified into three groups: (1) those in which the cleavage of fibrinopeptides by thrombin is defective; (2) disorders in which polymerization of fibrin monomers is retarded; and in rare instances, (3) disorders in which the crosslinking of fibrin polymers by factor XIIIa is deficient.[1]

CLINICAL SYMPTOMS

Most patients with dysfibrinogenemia are asymptomatic and require no treatment. Cryoprecipitates have been effective in patients undergoing major surgery. Commercial fibrinogen preparations have a prohibitively high incidence of transmission of hepatitis and the transmission potential for other viruses. In several varieties, mild bleeding has been reported. In a few others, a thromboembolic diathesis or defective wound healing was apparent. Abnormalities of fibrinopeptide release and crosslinking are most often associated with bleeding, and polymerization defects tend to produce thrombosis.[1, 3]

In many patients with systemic amyloidosis, laboratory coagulation screening results are similar to those in patients with dysfibrinogenemia. Implications are that an inhibitor is responsible for these abnormal results. It has been determined that the prevention (by the inhibitor) of the conversion of fibrinogen to a fibrin clot, rather than dysfibrinogenemia, is the cause of the prolonged thrombin time in patients with primary systemic amyloidosis.[17]

Hereditary Deficiency of Prothrombin (Factor II)

Hereditary prothrombin deficiency is one of the rarest congenital coagulation defects. The defect is caused by decreased synthesis of functionally normal prothrombin (hypoprothrombinemia) or by the synthesis of an abnormal prothrombin molecule (dysprothrombinemia).[1, 3]

GENETICS

Although the amino acid and genetic sequences of normal prothrombin are known, those of the genetic variants of prothrombin are not as fully characterized as those of the variants of factors VIII and IX.[3]

Both hypoprothrombinemia and dysprothrombinemia are inherited as autosomal recessive traits. True hypoprothrombinemia (CRM⁻ variant) apparently is the most common variety. In patients with this disorder, functional assays and immunoassays reveal the same degree of prothrombin deficiency. The second group (the CRM⁺ variants) is characterized by normal levels of prothrombin antigens in association with clear deficiencies in the functional assays. Dysfibrinogenemias have been designated with various proper names: prothrombins Cardeza, Quick, and Houston. Patients with compound heterozygosity (hypoprothrombinemia plus dysprothrombinemia and heterozygosity for two types of dysprothrombinemias) show a high degree of homology with the genes of other vitamin K–dependent factors.[1, 3]

CLINICAL SYMPTOMS

Patients homozygous for a prothrombin defect and those with double heterozygosity may experience mild to moderate bleeding. Patients with some variants, such as prothrombin Cardeza, are asymptomatic. Hemorrhagic episodes in most patients are primarily post-traumatic in origin. Bleeding from mucous membranes is common. Hemarthrosis is very rare. Many heterozygotes are symptomatic or minimally affected.[1, 3]

LABORATORY DIAGNOSIS

Prothrombin deficiency typically results in prolonged PTs and PTTs, but as with other factor deficiencies, the definitive diagnosis must be based on a specific factor II assay along with personal and family histories. The whole blood clotting time may or may not be abnormal, and the Stypven time (coagulation time obtained with Russell viper venom) is abnormal. The clotting time with *Echis carinatus* venom is important because if it is normal, the thrombin region of the prothrombin molecule is normal. Patients with hereditary dysprothrombinemia or hypoprothrombinemia lack the ability to produce normal prothrombin; therefore, vitamin K is of no value. Distinction of hypoprothrombinemia and dysprothrombinemia is based on the results of antigen levels of prothrombin as well as functional assays.[3, 10, 11, 15, 16]

Before a diagnosis of factor II deficiency can be made, an acquired deficiency of prothrombin caused by vitamin K deficiency, liver disease, or warfarin (coumarin) intoxication must be ruled out. This distinction can usually be made from family and personal histories as well as from results of laboratory testing. The presence of an acquired circulating anti-coagulant (anti-prothrombin antibody) must also be ruled out. This inhibitor is associated with systemic lupus erythematosus.[3]

TREATMENT

Treatment of bleeding complications for hypoprothrombinemia or dysprothrombinemia is based on infusion of plasma for minor bleeding episodes (15 mg/kg) for 1 or 2 days or on infusion of prothrombin complex concentrates (Proplex) for major bleeding episodes. Heat-treated prothrombin complex is preferred, because it is treated to inactivate hepatitis and HIV. Circulating prothrombin levels of 10–20% appear to be sufficient for hemostasis in most cases.[3, 15]

Hereditary Deficiency of Factor V

The exact incidence of hereditary factor V deficiency is unknown but is thought not to exceed 1 in 1 million. This hemorrhagic disorder has also been called "parahemophilia," Owren's disease, or labile factor deficiency. Factor V, also referred to as labile factor or proaccelerin, is necessary for the normal conversion of prothrombin to thrombin.[3, 18]

Severe hemorrhagic disease has been observed in association both with reduced synthesis of factor V and with the presence of dysfunctional factor V. Factor V is also found in platelets and is deficient in the platelets of patients with hereditary factor V deficiency. Eighty percent of factor V is in circulation; 20% of body stores are contained in normal platelets. It has been suggested that activated platelet-borne factor V is the binding site for activated plasma factor X (Xa) and factor II (prothrombin).[1, 2, 3, 18]

GENETICS

Factor V deficiency is inherited as an autosomal recessive trait. Symptoms usually occur only in homozygotes. Severely affected patients may have less than 1% functional factor V activity. Both CRM⁻ and CRM⁺ variants of factor V deficiency have been identified. Patients with abnormal factor V antigen have been reported, which suggests that the genetic heterogeneity patients in factor V deficiency is similar to that in patients with other hereditary blood-clotting factor disorders.[1, 3]

CLINICAL SYMPTOMS

Factor V deficiency produces a relatively mild hemorrhagic disorder that varies in severity. Clinical manifestations of factor V deficiency usually consist of post-traumatic bruising, menorrhagia, epistaxis, and bleeding from mucous membranes. Hemarthrosis and dissecting hematomas are uncommon but may occur.[1, 3]

LABORATORY DIAGNOSIS

Both the PT and the PTT are prolonged in patients with factor V deficiency. Both are corrected by the addition of normal plasma adsorbed with barium salts to remove the vitamin K–dependent factors. The Stypven time is abnormal. The whole blood clotting time and prothrombin consumption may or may not be normal. A prolonged bleeding time is also observed in one third of patients, presumably because of decreased platelet factor 5. Diagnosis of factor V deficiency is based on results of the specific assay of factor V functional activity level.[1, 3, 15]

Congenital factor V deficiency must be differentiated from combined deficiency of factors V and VIII. Acquired inhibitors that are specific antibodies against factor V have been reported in postoperative patients and on rare occasions, in patients taking antibiotics.[3]

TREATMENT

The hemostatic level for factor V is approximately 15–25 U/dL, and its biologic half-life ranges from 12 to 36 hours. Fresh or fresh-frozen plasma is the mainstay of therapy in patients with factor V deficiency, because factor V is relatively labile when stored under the usual blood bank conditions. Prophylactic therapy is usually not necessary, except when surgery is anticipated. Factor V is not found in cryoprecipitate, and factor V concentrates are not commercially available.[1, 3]

Hereditary Deficiency of Factor VII

GENETICS

Factor VII deficiency is a rare congenital disease, estimated to occur in 1 of 500,000 persons. It is inherited as an autosomal recessive characteristic. The defective allele is located on chromosome 13. Homozygotes have bleeding symptoms, and heterozygotes are asymptomatic. Factor VII is a stable clotting factor, essential in the extrinsic pathway of coagulation.[3]

The majority of patients with this defect lack factor VII antigens that interact with heterologous antibodies, but both CRM⁺ and CRMᴿ variants have been reported. In patients with CRMᴿ there is some discrepancy between factor VII antigen and factor VII coagulant activity. Further discrepancies have been noted when various investigators have examined patients with a deficiency of factor VII by using thromboplastins of different origins (e.g., human, ox, and rabbit).[1, 9]

CLINICAL SYMPTOMS

The severity of the bleeding is variable and is not correlated with the factor VII level. Most persons with a hereditary deficiency of factor VII have bleeding episodes before they reach adulthood. Homozygotes with factor VII levels below 10% of normal may have only mild symptoms. Patients with less than 1–2% of factor VII activity may experience bleeding as severe as that seen in classic hemophilia or Christmas disease. In these patients, chronic crippling hemarthropathy, repeated hemarthroses, and dangerous hematomas occur. Epistaxis, gingival bleeding, hemorrhage after tooth extractions, and abnormal bruising are common manifestations of factor VII deficiency. Intracranial bleeding, particularly in the neonatal period, is a common and serious manifestation of this disorder. Factor VII deficiency is commonly associated with deficiencies of other vitamin K–dependent coagulation factors, such as factor VII and IX deficiency and factor VII and X deficiency. Despite the bleeding tendency, a few cases of thrombosis (pulmonary emboli and inferior vena caval thrombosis) caused by factor VII deficiency have been reported.[1, 3, 9]

LABORATORY DIAGNOSIS

The PTT is normal and the PT is prolonged in patients with factor VII deficiency. This combination of abnormalities is diagnostic for the disorder. The platelet count and bleeding time are normal. The Stypven time is normal, and the thromboplastin generation test yields normal results. The normal Stypven time is not diagnostic, as it has been demonstrated in a factor X variant (factor X Friuli). Factor VII levels of 0–20 U/dL are found in homozygotes, and heterozygotes have approximately 50% of normal factor VII levels.[1, 3, 16]

TREATMENT

Despite the very short half-life of factor VII (4–5 hours), plasma or prothrombin complex concentrates are effective in the treatment of most forms of hemorrhage in this disorder. Replacement every 12–24 hours is sufficient for hemostasis. Concentrates of the vitamin K–dependent coagulation factors have proved satisfactory and probably are preferable in the management of serious bleeding.[1, 3]

Hereditary Deficiency of Factor X

GENETICS

Factor X deficiency is a rare disorder occurring in fewer than 1/500,000 in the general population. Factor X is a vitamin K–dependent clotting factor synthesized in hepatocytes. Congenital factor X deficiency is inherited as an autosomal recessive trait. The locus of the gene for factor X is on chromosome 13, and the gene has been sequenced. The clinical manifestations may be caused by reduced or absent synthesis of a normal molecule or by an abnormal molecule with decreased functional activity. Four variants have been clearly demonstrated by immunologic and coagulation techniques: two CRM[+] variants (the Prower and Friuli kindreds), a CRM[−] variant (the Stuart kindred), and a CRM[R] variant.

CLINICAL SYMPTOMS

The severity of bleeding complications in hereditary factor X deficiency depends on the degree of depression of factor X clotting activity. Patients with less than 1% factor X activity may have severe bleeding. Patients with 10% factor X activity are only mildly affected. Severely affected patients experience hemorrhage from the umbilical stump and, later, easy bruising, epistaxis, gastrointestinal bleeding, menorrhagia, or bleeding from other mucous membranes. Hematomas are also common. Hemarthroses and post-traumatic hemorrhages are associated with markedly reduced factor X clotting activity. Spontaneous intracranial and intraspinal hemorrhages have also been reported. Mild spontaneous bleeding and postoperative hemorrhage are not uncommon in heterozygotes.[1, 3]

LABORATORY DIAGNOSIS

In patients with factor X deficiency, both the PT and PTT are prolonged, although in one factor X variant, the PTT is reportedly normal. The Stypven time is also abnormal (except in patients with the Friuli variant). The thromboplastin generation test reveals a serum defect in all forms of factor X deficiency. The bleeding time may be prolonged in some severely affected patients, possibly as a result of defective factor Va–factor Xa interactions on the platelet. A specific functional assay for factor X must be performed for specific diagnosis. Assays reveal factor X levels of 6–9% of normal in homozygotes and approximately 50% of normal in heterozygotes.[1, 3, 9]

It is important to rule out acquired coagulation deficiencies whose manifestations might mimic these results (vitamin K deficiency, liver disease, and warfarin intoxication). This can usually be done by history and appropriate laboratory tests.[3]

TREATMENT

Bleeding episodes in factor X deficiency can be managed by infusions of either fresh-frozen plasma or plasma prepared after removal of cryoprecipitate. The biologic half-life of factor X is relatively long (24–60 hours). The hemostatic level for this factor is 10–20 U/dL. Plasma infusions suffice for hemarthroses and minor bleeding episodes. For major bleeding episodes, prothrombin complex concentrates or concentrates of the vitamin K–dependent factors that contain factor X can be used. Concentrates shown to be safe in terms of viral contamination should be used. Infusion of currently available concentrates has been linked to thromboembolic complications and occasional episodes of disseminated intravascular coagulation (DIC).[1, 3]

Hereditary Deficiency of Factor XI

Since 1953, more than 200 cases of factor XI deficiency have been reported. Factor XI deficiency is also referred to as plasma thromboplastin antecedent deficiency, Rosenthal disease, or hemophilia C. Factor XI deficiency is estimated to occur in 1 in 100,000 in the general population. The deficiency occurs primarily in Ashkenazi Jews of eastern European descent. It has been described in several other ethnic groups and in association with Noonan syndrome. A large study in Israel revealed a surprisingly high incidence of the disorder: as many as 5–10% of the population are affected. In Israel, 1 in 1000 Ashkenazi Jews are affected. In the United States, it is confined to geographic areas with large Jewish populations, such as New York and Los Angeles.[1, 3, 6]

Factor XI deficiency may result from a reduced synthesis of the protein, but abnormal factor XI molecules are also thought to exist. CRM[+] variants have been reported.[1,6]

GENETICS

Factor XI deficiency is transmitted as an autosomal recessive trait; therefore, equal numbers of males and females are affected. Homozygotes show factor XI activity levels of less than 1–5% of normal. Half of the heterozygotes have normal factor activity level.[3]

CLINICAL SYMPTOMS

Bleeding in patients with factor XI deficiency is poorly correlated with the plasma level of factor XI. In homozygous patients, epistaxis, hematuria, and menorrhagia are prominent symptoms. In most cases, spontaneous bleeding is lacking and post-traumatic or postoperative bleeding is the only manifestation of the disorder. Hemarthroses and intramuscular hemorrhages are rare. Hemorrhage following tooth extractions, tonsillectomies, and prostatectomies is relatively common. The pattern of delayed bleeding is common in this disorder.[1,3]

LABORATORY DIAGNOSIS

The PTT is prolonged, the PT is normal, and the thromboplastin generation test reveals mild defects of both the serum and plasma reagents. The PTT can be partially corrected with the addition of normal aged serum or plasma absorbed with barium or aluminum salts. The bleeding time usually is normal. The definitive diagnosis is based on results of a specific assay for factor XI.[1,3]

Factor XI deficiency must be distinguished from other hereditary bleeding disorders that produce similar laboratory test results, such as factor XII and factor IX deficiencies. Acquired antibodies to factor XI have been reported in some patients.[3]

TREATMENT

Treatment of factor XI deficiency is rarely required. Postoperative and postextraction bleeding usually responds well to small daily doses of plasma (5–10 mL/kg). Factor XI is relatively labile during storage in the blood bank, and fresh or fresh-frozen plasma is required for treatment of the deficiency. Whole blood loses 80% of its factor XI activity during its first week of storage. Factor XI levels of 20–30% of normal are usually sufficient to maintain hemostasis. The half-life of infused factor XI is thought to be several days. Epsilon-aminocaproic acid may be used as supplemental treatment with plasma. Patients with antibodies to factor XI have been successfully treated with prothrombin complex concentrates.[1,3,13]

Hereditary Deficiency of Factor XII

This disorder is often known as the Hageman factor deficiency after the surname of the first patient identified with this deficiency.[1,3]

Factor XII plays a central role in the surface-activated reactions of the intrinsic pathway and also is involved in numerous host defense processes other than blood coagulation: fibrinolysis, complement activation, regulation of vascular permeability, and chemotaxis.

The disorder is relatively common and is inherited as an autosomal recessive trait. Plasma levels of factor XII in homozygous subjects usually are 0–1 U/dL. Heterozygotes show a bimodal distribution with a mean of 50 U/dL. It is thought that factor XII synthesis is controlled by at least two genes. A high prevalence of partial deficiency of factor XII has been noted in the United States in recent immigrants from southeast Asia. In the majority of subjects, factor XII antigens cannot be demonstrated serologically (CRM⁻ variant); in 2 of 492 families, a CRM⁺ variant of the disorder was demonstrated.[1,3,13]

Complete deficiency of factor XII is not associated with bleeding. The lack of bleeding complications in factor XII–deficient patients remains to be explained. Neither intraoperative nor perioperative excessive bleeding complications have been reported. In fact, both arterial and venous thromboses have been reported in factor XII–deficient patients, although the relationship between factor XII deficiency and thrombosis is not clearly established.[1,3]

LABORATORY DIAGNOSIS AND TREATMENT

Diagnosis of factor XII deficiency is usually made incidentally, as a result of coagulation test screening before surgery. Factor XII–deficient patients exhibit a prolonged PTT, but diagnosis requires a specific factor XII assay. Because there are no bleeding problems, replacement therapy for factor XII deficiency is not required.[3,16]

Prekallikrein (Fletcher Factor) Deficiency

Most of the reported cases of prekallikrein deficiency have been in black families. The deficiency is rare, and the incidence is unknown. Prekallikrein is a major activator of factor XII.[1,3]

GENETICS

The inheritance has been reported to be both autosomal recessive and autosomal dominant. Both

CRM$^+$ and CRM$^-$ variants of prekallikrein deficiency have been identified by immunoassays.[1, 3]

CLINICAL SYMPTOMS

Like patients with a deficiency in Hageman factor, patients with a deficiency in prekallikrein have no bleeding symptoms. Patients with this defect are known to suffer myocardial infarction, which suggests that deficiencies of this protein may lead to lack of protection from thrombosis.[1, 3, 16]

LABORATORY DIAGNOSIS

Prekallikrein-deficient patients present with prolonged PTTs despite normal levels in all known clotting factors. A specific assay is required for detection of prekallikrein deficiency. Acquired deficiencies of prekallikrein have been found in newborns and in patients with severe liver disease and uremia.[1, 3, 8]

High–Molecular-Weight Kininogen Deficiency

High–molecular-weight kininogen (HMWK) functions in coagulation as a cofactor for the action of factor XII on various substrates and in the molecular assembly of the contact system on particulate surfaces. The deficiency was simultaneously recognized in a number of families, so numerous names exist, but *Fitzgerald factor* is the most used synonym for HMWK.[1, 3]

GENETICS

The disorder is inherited as an autosomal recessive trait. Fifty percent of affected subjects also have deficiencies of in low–molecular-weight kininogen (LMWK). This observation suggests that two separate genes code for HMWK: one for a part common to both LMWK and HMWK and one for a portion of the molecule unique for HMWK.[1, 3, 16]

CLINICAL SYMPTOMS

All patients are clinically asymptomatic in terms of bleeding or other known illnesses.

LABORATORY DIAGNOSIS

The results of the primary screening tests are similar to those for factor XII and prekallikrein deficiencies. In specific assays for this factor, fresh-frozen substrate plasma of subjects with deficient HMWK or commercially available lyophilized substrate plasma deficient in HMWK must be used. An immunologic assay for detecting HMWK deficiencies is also available.[1, 3, 6]

Deficiency of Factor XIII (Fibrin-Stabilizing Factor)

GENETICS

The disorder is inherited as an autosomal recessive trait in which heterozygotes are clinically unaffected. Results of studies have suggested that both a qualitative abnormality and a quantitative abnormality of factor XIII are present. Consanguineous marriages have been common among the parents of patients with this disorder. Factor XIII antigens are variable in terms of reactivity to usual heterologous antibodies. Specific immunoassays of the factor XIII molecule have demonstrated complete absence of the A subunit and reduced levels of the S subunit in homozygotes.[1, 3]

CLINICAL SYMPTOMS

The clinical symptoms of factor XIII deficiency differ from most other hereditary coagulation disorders. In most patients, the disorder is manifested in childhood, usually shortly after birth. Bleeding from the umbilical stump or into the central nervous system, slow wound healing, and abnormal scar formation are very common. Spontaneous bleeding is uncommon, but intracranial hemorrhage after trivial head trauma has been reported. Severely affected patients have a lifelong bleeding disorder characterized by ecchymoses, hematomas, and prolonged bleeding after trauma. Hemarthrosis is relatively uncommon. Menorrhagia and spontaneous abortions have been reported by adult female patients.[1, 3]

LABORATORY DIAGNOSIS

Fibrin stabilization is necessary for effective hemostasis. The primary screening tests yield normal results in factor XIII deficiency. A useful screening test is based on the solubility of fibrin clots in 5-M urea from factor XIII–deficient patients. Normal subjects have fibrin clots that are insoluble in 5-M urea. Another satisfactory screening procedure is clot solubility in 1% monochloroacetic acid. More specific assays that are performed with synthetic substrates have been developed. An immunologic assay that makes use of antibodies to the alpha and beta chains is also available. The bleeding time, platelet count, and results of platelet function tests are normal in heterozygotes.[1, 3, 9]

The disorder must be differentiated from other inherited coagulation disorders. The disorder may be sufficiently severe to be confused clinically with classic hemophilia. Acquired deficiencies of factor XIII have been demonstrated in some patients with disorders such as liver disease and tumors have also been noted in patients treated with isoniazid. Deficiencies in factor XIII activity may be caused by inhibitors of factor XIII as well.[1, 3]

TREATMENT

The biologic half-life of factor XIII is 72–96 hours, and its hemostatic level is approximately 1 U/dL. Small doses of plasma (5–10 mL/kg/day) are enough to treat spontaneous hemorrhage and to prevent postoperative bleeding. Replacement therapy in factor XIII deficiency is highly satisfactory because of the small quantities of factor XIII needed for effective hemostasis. Treatment should be administered promptly after head trauma. Prophylactic regimens of cryoprecipitate or plasma at weekly or biweekly intervals may be prescribed for patients preoperatively as well as for pregnant women.[1, 3]

Passovoy Deficiency

Passovoy deficiency is a rare disorder of the intrinsic pathway of coagulation. It appears to be inherited through autosomal dominance. The molecular characteristics are unknown. Patients typically exhibit moderate mucosal membrane bleeding (including epistaxis), easy and spontaneous bruising, and menorrhagia. Severe bleeding may occur with trauma or surgery. The PTT is moderately prolonged, and the PT is normal. Levels of all known clotting factors are normal. Plasma infusions are used for traumatic or surgical hemorrhage.[1, 2, 6]

Inherited Multiple–Coagulation Factor Deficiencies

Two types of multiple-factor deficiencies have been described. The first type is the co-occurrence of more than one disorder and is very rare. The second type is a single heritable disorder associated with deficiencies of two or more factors. The most commonly reported multiple-factor deficiency is combined factor V and factor VIII deficiency, which in most instances is an example of the second type and appears to be caused by a deficiency of an inhibitor of protein C (protein C can inactivate factors V and VIII). Other familial multiple-factor deficiencies have been identified: those of factors VII and IX, factors IX and XI, factors VIII and IX, factors VII and IX, factors VII and VIII, and factors VIII and XI, and factor VII deficiency and von Willebrand's syndrome.[8, 11]

ACQUIRED FACTOR DEFICIENCIES

Acquired coagulation factor defects can occur throughout life. They may be mild and manifest simply as enhanced operative bleeding, in which case they must be distinguished from congenital disorders. They can also manifest as acute generalized bleeding, and are often associated with abnormalities in the results of more than one screening test.[4]

There are four general categories: (1) destructive or consumptive disorders, such as DIC; (2) production defects of synthesis, such as liver disease, renal disease, and vitamin K deficiency; (3) inhibition by circulating anti-coagulants and inhibitors; and (4) massive transfusions.[4]

Disseminated Intravascular Coagulation

DIC is a syndrome characterized by uncontrolled formation and deposition of fibrin thrombi. The generalized activation of the coagulation and fibrinolytic systems causes consumption of coagulation factors and platelets, generation of thrombin, widespread deposition of fibrin in small blood vessels, and formation of large amounts of fibrinogen degradation products. All of these contribute to the bleeding, shock, and vascular occlusion that develop.[15, 19]

DIC and associated fibrinolysis result from excessive activation of the extrinsic or intrinsic coagulation pathway. Extrinsic pathway activation by phospholipoprotein membranes becomes excessive whenever cellular destruction is extensive and surface and organelle membranes intrude into the circulation.[12, 19]

As the rate of fibrin formation exceeds the synthesis rate of coagulation proteins, a net depletion of certain coagulation factors and platelets occurs. This hematologic manifestation of DIC has been referred to as *consumption coagulopathy* and later as *defibrination syndrome*. DIC is not a disease entity but an intermediary mechanism of disease seen in association with well-defined clinical disorders. DIC usually begins with a bleeding diathesis; consumption is a later development of intravascular fibrin formation. In DIC, the fibrin thrombi tend to be microscopic and thus clinically inapparent. Therefore, the early recognition of DIC is largely dependent on laboratory findings.[19, 20]

ETIOLOGY

DIC may be caused by injury involving one or more of the four main components of the hemostatic system: blood vessels, platelets, coagulation, and fibrinolysis. DIC is usually seen in association with well-defined clinical entities; the most common conditions associated with this phenomenon are obstetric emergencies, intravascular hemolysis, septicemia, viremias, disseminated malignancy, leukemia, burns, crush injuries and tissue necrosis, liver disease, prosthetic devices, and cardiac and peripheral vascular disorders.[16, 19, 20]

A consumptive coagulopathy may also be secondary to a localized event, such as the giant hemangioma (Kasabach-Merritt) syndrome in children and large dissecting aneurysms in adults. In these situations, local generation of thrombin results in depletion of coagulation factors and circulating platelets.[9]

Obstetric accidents commonly lead to DIC. Amniotic fluid embolism with associated DIC is the most catastrophic and common of the life-threatening obstetric emergencies. The obstetric complications most commonly associated with DIC include abruptio placentae, placenta previa, retained placenta, amniotic fluid embolism, dead fetus retained in utero, and the hypertensive disorders such as severe preeclampsia and eclampsia. In addition, abortion, septic abortion, or abortion induced by hypertonic sodium chloride may also be associated with acute defibrination.[16, 19]

Intravascular hemolysis of any etiology is a common triggering mechanism for DIC. A frank hemolytic transfusion reaction often triggers DIC, but hemolysis of a milder origin can also cause DIC.[19]

Many viremias, including those caused by HIV, have been associated with DIC, but the most common are varicella, hepatitis, and cytomegalovirus infections.[19]

Malignancy also is often associated with DIC, and most patients with disseminated solid malignancy exhibit at least laboratory evidence of the conditions. In most cases of neoplasia, a malignant rather than benign tumor is present. DIC may develop in patients with acute or chronic leukemias, one of the most common being acute hypergranular promyelocytic leukemia. Sometimes the first clue to DIC in this situation is easy bruising or the appearance of petechiae. Other malignancies commonly associated with DIC are gastrointestinal, pancreatic, prostatic, ovarian, and lung neoplasms; melanomas; myelomas; and myeloproliferative syndromes.[6, 16, 19]

Acidosis and, less commonly, alkalosis may also trigger DIC. It commonly develops in patients with extensive burns and in patients with large crush injuries and tissue necrosis.

On a worldwide basis, DIC caused by venom from snake bites is the predominant cause of death and mortality in the whole range of acquired coagulation disorders. Most snakes whose venom has procoagulant activity belong to the family Viperidae, which includes vipers, rattlesnakes, and

adders. The treatment of choice is anti-venom, not heparin, which is ineffective.[16]

The use of various prosthetic devices also can lead to DIC. An intra-aortic balloon assist is a widely used clinical maneuver to control postmyocardial infarction cardiogenic shock after bypass surgery. Activation of the coagulation system, with an attendant low-grade DIC, can accompany the use of this device. Use of the LeVeen or Denver valve shunting has been found to be associated with generalized DIC.[19]

Many chronic inflammatory disorders, including sarcoidosis, Crohn disease, and ulcerative colitis, may also be associated with compensated DIC. Infections and septicemia are often associated with DIC. The triggering mechanisms are the initiation of coagulation by endotoxin (gram-negative infection) or bacterial mucopolysaccharide (gram-positive infection). Both may activate factor XII to factor XIIa, induce a platelet release reaction, or start a release of granulocyte procoagulant materials.[6, 19]

Purpura fulminans is a form of intravascular coagulation that usually develops several days after an acute infection, most commonly scarlet fever or a viral respiratory disease. The syndrome is most common among infants and children and is manifested by skin infarcts on the lower extremities, genitalia, and buttocks. Gangrene of the digits also is commonly seen. The disorder may be the result of protein C deficiency. Heparin therapy has proved helpful only if given early in the course of the disease.[1]

In many forms of DIC, the factors that initiate the syndrome are multiple and interrelated. For example, in meningococcemia, direct endothelial injury leading to platelet clumping and contact activation, endotoxemia, septic shock, and tissue factor secretion by leukocytes may all act to initiate DIC. In many forms of DIC, the initiating factors are obscure.[1]

PATHOPHYSIOLOGY

After the coagulation system has been activated and both thrombin and plasmin are circulating systemically, the pathophysiology of DIC (Fig. 34–2) is similar in all disorders.[19]

Thrombin causes the cleavage of two pairs of fibrinopeptides (A and B) from fibrinogen. This exposes main sites on the fibrin molecule. Polymerization of this fibrinogen derivative, called fibrin monomer, is prevented by the formation of soluble complexes with the remaining intact molecules of fibrinogen. More than 25% of fibrinogen must be converted to fibrin monomer before polymerization to fibrin takes place. This polymerization results in a fibrin clot in the circulation,

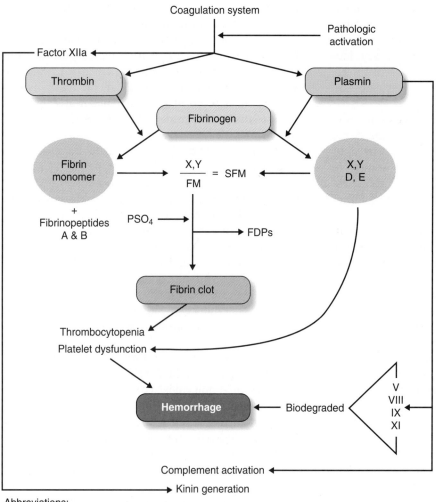

Figure 34–2 The pathophysiology of disseminated intravascular coagulation. *Abbreviations:* PSO_4 = protamine sulfate; FDP = fibrinogen/fibrin degradation products. (From Bick RL, Scates SM: Disseminated intravascular coagulation. Lab Med 1992; 23(3):162.)

Abbreviations:
FM, fibrin monomer
SFM, soluble fibrin monomer

leading to thrombosis, peripheral ischemia, and end-organ damage. As fibrin is deposited, platelets are trapped, and thrombocytopenia results. Plasmin begins to cleave fibrinogen into fibrin (or fibrinogen) degradation products (FDPs) (see Fig. 34–2, upper right). These FDPs may combine with circulating fibrin monomer and become solubilized. The detection of this complex, termed soluble fibrin monomer, is a diagnostic aid. Systemically circulating fibrin (or fibrinogen) degradation products interfere with fibrin monomer polymerization and platelet function, which further impairs hemostasis and contributes to hemorrhage. Plasmin, in addition to biodegrading fibrinogen and fibrin, biodegrades factors V, VIII, IX, and XI and other plasma proteins.[19]

As plasmin degrades crosslinked fibrin, specific fibrin degradation products appear in the circulation; one of these is D-dimer. As plasmin circulates, it often activates C1 and C3, with the subsequent activation of the entire complement sequence, leading to C8 and C9 activation. Activation of the

kinin system is also an important event in DIC. The pathophysiology of DIC explains the paradox of why most patients with the disorder endure hemorrhage plus thrombosis, hypotension, and shock.[19, 20]

CLINICAL SYMPTOMS

In many cases, the clinical picture is dominated by the underlying disease. Specific findings suggestive of include petechiae, purpura, hemorrhagic bullae, acral cyanosis, occasionally gangrene, surgical wound bleeding, traumatic wound bleeding, venipuncture site bleeding, arterial line oozing, subcutaneous hematomas, and deep tissue bleeding.[9, 19]

The average patient with acute DIC typically bleeds from at least three unrelated sites and any combination can be seen. The organ systems include the cardiac, pulmonary, renal, and central nervous system. Venous thromboembolism is also a frequent complication, particularly if antithrombin and protein C are depleted. The major clinical problem in disseminated intravascular coagulation, however, is hemorrhage rather than microthrombosis, because of consumption of coagulation factors.[12, 16, 19]

LABORATORY DIAGNOSIS

Laboratory findings of DIC may be notably variable and difficult to interpret unless the pathophysiology is clearly understood. There is no single laboratory test, or even a small battery of tests, that can reliably detect or rule out the presence of DIC.[7]

Fibrinogen. The fibrinogen concentration in blood is subject to considerable variation because fibrinogen is an acute-phase reactance protein. The normal level is approximately 200–400 mg/dL, depending somewhat on the laboratory method. However, in most of the pathologic states associated with DIC, the fibrinogen concentration is apt to be two or even three times that of normal. Useful information from a single determination is provided only if it is low, as DIC is undoubtedly the most common cause of hypofibrinogenemia.[20]

Platelets. Thrombocytopenia is a common manifestation of DIC, and it has been reported that in 52% of patients with DIC, the level is below 50,000 cells/mm³. The range may be quite variable and as low as 2000 cells/mm³ or greater than 100,000 cells/mm³. The average platelet count in a DIC patient is 60,000 cells/mm³. However, other causes of thrombocytopenia such as bone marrow suppression or ingestion of drugs must be ruled out before DIC may be named as the cause of the low platelet count. In thrombocytopenia, most platelet function test results, including the bleeding time and platelet aggregation, are abnormal in patients with DIC. There is no reason to perform platelet function tests on patients with acute DIC, because results are invariably abnormal. Some diseases (chronic granulocytic leukemia, myeloproliferative syndromes, cancer) are accompanied by high platelet counts; patients with these disorders and DIC may not exhibit thrombocytopenia.[5, 6, 19, 20]

Other Coagulation Factors. The activity of factors II, V, VIII, and X are usually reduced in patients with DIC. Their direct measurement requires the availability of specific, deficient substrate plasma. For the diagnosis of DIC, the performance of these determinations is unnecessary, and their results may be confusing; for example, factors V and VIII may be substantially increased by endotoxin, and so a normal level may be found in the presence of DIC.[20]

Another factor that may be depressed in DIC is plasminogen, which is consumed as the result of ongoing fibrinolysis. It may be measured by a number of assays in which streptokinase is used for the activation of plasminogen to plasmin and casein or fibrin is used as the substrate. Routine measurement of plasminogen for clinical purposes in DIC is difficult and not recommended. Protein C, protein S, and fibronectin levels are also decreased in patients with DIC.[19, 20]

The PT is prolonged in 75% of patients with DIC, and in 25% the PT is normal or shortened. The PT is sensitive to all factors in the extrinsic clotting system (i.e., factors II, V, VII, and X and fibrinogen). Only when the concentration of any one of these factors is below a critical level does prolongation of the PT occur. The PT may also be prolonged by heparin (>0.2 U/mL) or by high concentrations of FDP.[6, 19]

The activated PTT measures clotting in the presence of excess platelet lipids. It is sensitive to all the factors in the intrinsic clotting system. In 25% of cases of DIC, high levels of factor VIII, which may shorten the PTT, are found. However, in 75% of cases of DIC, the PTT is usually prolonged. A normal PTT cannot be used to rule out the diagnosis of DIC.[19, 20]

The thrombin time and reptilase time are prolonged if fibrinogen is grossly depleted (<80 mg/dL). Both tests should be prolonged by the presence of circulating FDPs, by interferences with fibrin monomer polymerization, and by the hypofibrinogenemia commonly present. Heparin or FDP also prolongs the thrombin time.

Intravascular fibrin deposition is followed by secondary fibrinolysis, which results in the elaboration of FDP. However, evidence of increased fibrinolytic enzyme activity is found in the blood of only about 20% of patients with DIC. In some instances, the fibrinolytic activity is actually decreased below normal levels, probably because of the consumption of plasminogen activator. The results of assays of fibrinolytic activity are dependent on the net effect of plasminogen activator release and binding. The euglobulin clot lysis time test separates plasminogen and plasminogen activator from the inhibitors. If plasminogen and fibrinogen levels are adequate, the test measures plasminogen activator. If there is rapid dissolution of the clot (<2 hours) in this test, hyperplasminemia can confidently be diagnosed. Results of the euglobulin clot lysis test may be normal because of depletion of plasminogen.[15, 16, 20]

Peripheral Blood Findings. Schistocytes resulting from fragmentation of red blood cells on fibrin strands are found in about 50% of patients with DIC and may be associated with low-grade hemolysis. Severe hemolysis is rare in patients with DIC. Leukocytosis with an increase in immature forms is common, but leukopenia has been reported in patients with DIC that is secondary to gram-negative septicemia. A mild reticulocytosis may be noted. As noted earlier, thrombocytopenia also occurs. In addition, many large, bizarre platelets representing young platelets are usually seen on the peripheral blood smear of patients with DIC.[6, 19, 20]

FDPs are elevated in 85–100% of patients with DIC. Elevated levels of FDPs are, however, not a diagnostic sign of DIC; they are diagnostic only of plasmin biodegradation of fibrinogen or fibrin. The D-dimer assay is a newer diagnostic test for the presence or absence of DIC. The D-dimer is formed when thrombin initiates the transition of fibrinogen to fibrin; thrombin also activates factor XIII to XIIIa to crosslink the fibrin thus formed. The D-dimer is released to the circulation as a result of plasmin digestion of crosslinked fibrin.[6, 19]

The D-dimer test is specific for crosslinked The D-dimer in plasma, whereas the formation of fibrinolytic degradation products (i.e., X, Y, D, and E fragments), the basis of older FDP tests, may be derived from either fibrinogen or fibrin after plasmin digestion. Monoclonal antibodies against the D-dimer neoantigen DD-3B6/22 have been identified. The presence of D-dimer indicates that thrombin and plasmin were present. This test may replace both the FDP assay and the protamine sulfate (or ethanol gelation) tests in diagnosing DIC. Results of tests for FDPs are positive if the D-dimer test is positive; however, a positive FDP result may not lead to a positive D-dimer test result.[6, 19]

The protamine sulfate and ethanol gelation tests for circulating soluble fibrin monomer are not sensitive tests. Fifteen to twenty percent of patients with DIC may have a negative result on a protamine sulfate test. The anti-thrombin III (AT III) determination is a useful test for aiding in the diagnosis and monitoring of therapy in DIC. In DIC, an irreversible complexing of some circulating activating clotting factors with AT III leads to significant decreases of functional AT III. Immunologic assays for AT III, however, should not be performed on patients with DIC.[6, 19]

Platelet factor IV and beta-thromboglobulin levels are markers of platelet reactivity and release that may aid in the diagnosis or monitoring therapy for DIC. Both assays are readily available for the clinical laboratory, and most patients with DIC have elevated levels of these marker elements. Patients with DIC also have elevated fibrinopeptide A levels; however, the determination of fibrinopeptide A level by itself is not specific for DIC and is laborious for the routine clinical laboratory. A newer modality, also available by radioimmunoassay, is that of B-beta 15-42 and related peptide determinations. Elevation of both fibrinopeptide A and B-beta 15-42 and related peptide levels is a strong indicator of DIC, rather than of primary fibrinolysis.[6, 19]

TREATMENT

The treatment of DIC is confusing and sometimes controversial. There is a scarcity of literature describing the therapy given, morbidity, mortality, and survival of patients with DIC. DIC necessitates an aggressive but reasonable therapeutic approach to first stop and treat the disease process thought to be responsible. Most patients, except those suffering from obstetric emergencies or massive liver failure, usually need some type of anti-coagulant therapy.[19]

Stop the Intravascular Clotting Process. If necessary, the heparin administered intravenously (regular doses, 70–140 U/kg every 4 hours) or subcutaneous low-dose heparin is highly effective against DIC. With continued bleeding, the patient is given subcutaneous calcium heparin at 80–100 U/kg every 4–6 hours as the clinical situation dictates. Anti-coagulant therapy is needed to stop or blunt the underlying condition if significant bleeding or clotting continues for about 4 hours after the initiation of therapy. The hemorrhagic diathesis of DIC is apt to be magnified by heparin treatment, at least temporarily. The risk of serious bleeding has made clinicians understandably reluctant to use heparin for this condition. If heparin is given, it must be given relatively early, and if bleeding is to be minimized, heparin should be given in a dosage no higher than that required to inhibit thrombin elaboration. The dosage of heparin should be adjusted based on measurements of fibrin monomer, fibrinogen levels, and diminishment of FDPs. Effectiveness of treatment is indicated by decreased levels of fibrin monomers, increased fibrinogen levels, and decreased FDPs.[1, 3, 19, 20]

Use Component Therapy as Indicated. If bleeding continues after reasonable treatment of the underlying disease process and after anti-coagulant therapy is started, it is probably the result of coagulation factor depletions. The specific components thought to be deficient and contributing to the hemorrhage should be defined and given. Adequate whole blood may be needed. Fresh-frozen plasma is useful both for providing a plasma expander and for replacing clotting factors, including fibrinogen. Cryoprecipitate is useful for replacing factor VIII and fibrinogen, and platelet concentrates are useful for replacing platelets. Patients with continual DIC should receive only washed packed red blood cells, platelet concentrate, or AT III until the conditions have been controlled.[9, 16, 19]

Consider Inhibition of the Fibrinolytic System. If bleeding continues after the two previously described therapies, this step should be taken. It is necessary in about 3% of patients. Anti-fibrinolytic therapy should never be administered to patients with ongoing DIC because these patients need the fibrinolytic system to keep the microcirculation clear of microthrombi. It should be administered only if the intravascular coagulation process has been stopped and fibrinolysis is continuing. When anti-fibrinolytic therapy is indicated, epsilon-aminocaproic acid is given. A newer, more potent, and possibly safer anti-fibrinolytic agent is tranexamic acid.[19]

Chronic Disseminated Intravascular Coagulation

The differences between acute and chronic DIC are often viewed on a continuum. The onset is usually acute and the course rapid, in most cases being 2 days from onset of DIC to the development of a hemorrhagic diathesis. However, in liver cirrhosis and in many patients with metastatic cancer, the condition may also be low-grade and chronic.[6, 11, 20]

Chronic DIC may also be referred to as compensated DIC. Patients with chronic DIC more commonly have bothersome bleeding and diffuse thromboses, as opposed to acute fulminant life-threatening hemorrhage. In chronic DIC, fibrin deposition and consumption of clotting factors is thought to proceed more slowly: slowly enough to permit hepatic synthesis of clotting factors and even bone marrow production of platelets to keep up. Patients generally present with gingival bleeding, easy and spontaneous bruising, large cutaneous ecchymoses, and mild to moderate mucosal membrane bleeding. However, patients may also present with diffuse or singular thromboses.[6, 11, 20]

Therapy for chronic DIC is very different from that for acute DIC. Therapy for the underlying disease process is most important. In many instances, this will halt the intravascular clotting process and alleviate hemorrhage and thrombosis. Vigorous anti-coagulant therapy may be contraindicated (e.g., in some instances of malignancy, especially intracranial metastases). Combination anti-platelet therapy is often successful in stopping chronic DIC, if attempts to treat the triggering pathophysiology are also used. Replacement therapy and inhibition of the fibrinolytic system are rarely, if ever, indicated.[6]

Liver Disease

Deficiencies of the liver can produce a variety of hemostatic defects: (1) deficiencies in clotting factors and natural protease inhibitors synthesized in hepatic parenchymal cells; (2) production of clotting factor and anti-protease proteins with abnormal structure and/or function; (3) impaired clearance of circulating activated clotting factors; and (4) accumulated plasminogen activators causing or contributing to the development of DIC and/or systemic fibrinolysis, thrombocytopenia, and platelet dysfunction.[7]

Approximately 85% of patients with liver disease have at least one hemostatic abnormality. Fifteen percent have clinically severe bleeding.[7, 11]

PATHOPHYSIOLOGY

The liver normally synthesizes all coagulation factors except factor VIII. Liver failure may thus result in severe multiple coagulation abnormalities. The liver is thought to synthesize the majority of blood coagulation factors, including fibrinogen, factors II, V, VII, IX, and X, and coagulation factors XI, XII, and XIII. The levels of the vitamin K–dependent factors (II, VII, IX, and X) are particularly affected. Factor V is also produced by hepatic cells, but its levels do not usually fall unless liver disease is moderately severe. Similarly, synthesis of plasminogen, as well as that of the inhibitors AT III and alpha$_2$–anti-plasmin, occurs in the liver.[1, 7, 16]

In obstructive liver disease, only vitamin K–dependent coagulation factors are affected, because the absorption of lipid-soluble vitamin K requires bile salts in the gastrointestinal lumen. This defect can be corrected by vitamin K administered parenterally. In contrast, hepatocellular disease impairs synthesis of all coagulation proteins except factor VIII R:WF (ristocetin cofactor).[12]

The liver is also the primary site of synthesis of fibrinogen. The precise site of synthesis of the two components of the factor VIII/von Willebrand factor complex are in the Weibil Pallade bodies. In general terms, levels of VIII:C and VIII:C:Ag are often increased in acute hepatocellular liver disease. In the end stage of chronic liver disease, there often is a low plasma concentration of fibrinogen. In contrast, in uncomplicated cirrhosis, chronic hepatitis, obstructive jaundice, biliary cirrhosis, and hepatoma, a high plasma level of fibrinogen is found.[1, 7, 9]

Patients with liver disease may produce structurally and/or functionally abnormal clotting factor proteins. Acquired dysfibrinogenemia and the presence of abnormal acarboxyprothrombin in the plasma are commonly associated with primary carcinomas of the liver.[1, 7]

A major factor leading to the deficiency of the vitamin K–dependent factors is hepatocellular incompetence, but an additional vitamin K deficiency caused by malabsorption, exocrine pancreatic dysfunction, and poor dietary intake is not uncommon. Deficiencies of AT III, alpha$_2$–antiplasmin, and plasminogen also have been documented in liver disease.[1, 7]

The liver also functions to clear circulating plasminogen activators and activated clotting factors from the plasma. When these activities are impaired in patients with cirrhosis or hepatitis, plasminogen activators and/or activated clotting factors may accumulate and perhaps trigger low-grade DIC and fibrinolysis. Failure of the diseased liver to clear plasminogen activators explains the chronic or acute fibrinogenolysis and fibrinolysis that may arise in patients with severe liver disease. As a result, circulating fibrin degradation products may accumulate in the blood and contribute to hemostatic dysfunction.[1, 7]

Thrombocytopenia is another common cause of bleeding in patients with liver disease. It may result from platelet sequestration in an enlarged spleen, folic acid deficiency in alcoholics, consumption in secondary DIC, or toxic effects of various uncleared metabolites on the bone marrow. Abnormal platelet function with impaired aggregation and platelet factor 3 release in patients with liver disease has been described. Elevated levels of fibrin degradation products can cause platelet dysfunction as well.[7]

Overt DIC has been documented in a few patients, particularly in pregnant women with acute "fatty liver." The severity of the coagulation defect may be diminished by heparin administration, but clinical bleeding is seldom diminished.

CLINICAL SYMPTOMS

Purpura, ecchymoses, recurrent mucosal bleeding, and post-traumatic and postsurgical bleeding are common and familiar manifestations of end-stage liver disease. Bleeding that follows biopsy procedures and tooth extractions is not uncommon. Gastrointestinal hemorrhage from esophageal varices, gastritis, and peptic ulcers can occur. The manifestations of the disease and clinical bleeding cannot often be correlated with laboratory indices.[1, 7]

LABORATORY DIAGNOSIS

With the wide variety of hemostatic abnormalities that occur in patients with liver disease, laboratory testing is important for diagnosis and prognosis. Simple screening tests determine whether a patient with liver disease has a major hemostatic problem. Deficiencies of the vitamin K–dependent factors may develop in patients with mild liver disease, sometimes before there is other evidence of liver disease. The PT has been advocated as a highly sensitive test of liver function. Trace levels of acarboxy-II prothrombin may appear even before the PT is prolonged. Thus acarboxy-II prothrombin can serve as an early marker of liver disease.[7, 16]

There is a strong correlation between the degree of coagulation deficiencies and other tests of hepatic protein synthesis (serum albumin and cholinesterase). Deficiency of fibrinogen indicates severe liver disease or the development of DIC or fibrinolysis.[7]

The thrombin clotting time is sensitive to a number of abnormalities associated with liver disease: hypofibrinogenemia (fibrinogen level usually <50–75 mg/dL), dysfibrinogenemia, and raised levels of FDPs, which interfere with fibrin polymerization. The thrombin clotting time is prolonged in these instances.[16]

A further useful test in hepatic disease is the clotting time with the use of the snake venoms from *Bothrops atrox* (Debfibrase) or *Agkistrodon rhodostoma* (Arvin). These venoms remove fibrinopeptide A, which further exaggerates the fibrin polymerization defect. It is useful to monitor the level of factor V in hepatic disease because this factor is independent of vitamin K, and thus reduced levels reflect pure hepatocellular impairment.[16]

Reduced levels of AT III is characteristic of hepatocellular disease. Tests for plasminogen activator, such as the euglobulin lysis time or fibrin plate test, may show increased fibrinolytic activity. Results of tests for fibrinolysis are abnormal in more than 75% of patients with chronic liver disease and may be abnormal in patients with acute hepatic failure or cholestasis if DIC and secondary fibrinolysis are present.[6, 16]

The thrombocytopenia in patients with liver disease is usually secondary to splenomegaly; the qualitative abnormalities of platelets may be attributed to increased levels of fibrin split products or to the intake of alcohol.[15]

TREATMENT

Treatment of coagulation abnormalities in patients with advanced liver disease is difficult. In general terms, the patients who are not bleeding despite deficiencies of the coagulation factors need no special treatment. The administration of coagulation factors in the form of fresh-frozen plasma or other blood products may produce transitory correction of the laboratory abnormalities, but lasting remission of the disease rarely results. The amount of correction that can be achieved is limited by the volume of plasma that can be infused at one time without risk of circulatory overload. Use of prothrombin-complex concentrates to replace factors II, VII, IX, and X in these patients is not advocated, because these concentrates are known to contain activated clotting factors, which can cause DIC and other thromboembolic disorders because the liver cannot clear these activated factors. These concentrates should be used only in emergencies in which other methods have failed and the patient is still bleeding. Thrombocytopenia caused by impaired platelet production can be temporarily corrected by infusions of platelet concentrates. However, an enlarged spleen or DIC may rapidly consume these transfused platelets.[1, 7, 16]

Heparin administration has produced clinical improvements in a few patients with DIC, but in many others it is ineffective or resulted in accelerated bleeding. A trial of anti-fibrinolytic therapy, such as epsilon-aminocaproic acid and related anti-fibrinolytic agents has been advocated for patients with evidence of excessive systemic fibrinolysis. Anti-fibrinolytic therapy without concurrent heparin therapy is not advocated. Blocking the protective fibrinolysis in DIC can result in massive thrombosis. The use of anti-fibrinolytic agents are most effective when administered prophylactically before minor surgical procedures such as tooth extractions.[1, 7]

The use of AT III concentrates has proved beneficial in a few patients. The administration of vitamin K may be helpful in an occasional patient with a significant superimposed vitamin K deficiency.[1, 7]

Renal Disease

In patients with acute and chronic renal insufficiency, there is a tendency for both thrombosis and bleeding. The bleeding tendency is often characterized by mucosal bleeding: epistaxis, gingival bleeding, hematuria, and gastrointestinal bleeding. Often the bleeding time is prolonged despite a normal platelet count, which suggests a qualitative abnormality of platelet function. Levels of factor VIII, fibrinogen, and inhibitors of plasminogen activation are elevated. Fibrinolytic activity in plasma and elevated factor XIII levels in patients with renal insufficiency have been found.[11]

Altered hemostatic mechanisms play a role in many renal vascular and glomerular diseases. In hemostatic disorders such as DIC, hemolytic-uremic syndrome, and thrombotic thrombocytopenic purpura, there is fibrin deposition in the renal microvasculature.[7]

The presence in the urine of degradation products of fibrinogen or fibrin at a time when degradation products are absent from the blood or present in only very small amounts indicates that localized consumption has occurred in the kidneys, as in rejection of a kidney transplant. Destruction of the donor kidney within minutes to hours after transplantation is associated with extensive deposition of fibrin in the arterioles and glomeruli.[3]

Fibrin degradation products reach concentrations of 2–100 μg/mL in patients with proliferative glomerulonephritis and glomerulonephritis associated with systemic lupus erythematosus and 0.25–2.5 μg/mL in patients with the nephrotic syndrome of membranous glomerulonephritis. The amount of deposited intraglomerular fibrin is correlated with the degree of proteinuria. Patients with autoimmune disorders such as proliferative glomerulonephritis in systemic lupus erythematosus are likely to have fibrin degradation products in the blood as well as the urine, which reflects some degree of disseminated as well as localized consumption.[3]

NEPHROTIC SYNDROMES

A variety of renal diseases can cause a disruption of the normal barriers between blood and urine in the glomeruli, resulting in the loss of low–molecular-weight proteins, including some clotting factors, AT III, and protein C. These proteins have been demonstrated in the urine of nephrotic patients. Plasma deficiencies have been reported for only clotting factors VII, IX, and XIII and for AT III. However, most studies of nephrotic patients show normal plasma levels of these coagulation factors.[7, 11]

Although significant clotting factor deficiencies and bleeding tendencies are uncommon in patients with nephrotic syndromes, thrombotic complications occur in approximately 25% of patients. It is thought that decreased AT III levels predispose the patient to the development of thromboses. However, because AT III is consumed in the formation of thrombin–anti-thrombin complex during clotting, the deficiency may be the result rather than the cause of the thrombosis.[7]

RENAL FAILURE

A variety of hemostatic defects in uremic patients have been described. Thrombocytopenia is present in up to 50% of patients. The most significant coagulation abnormality is impaired platelet function (described in Chapter 33). Marked prolongation of the thrombin time with slight prolongation of the PT and PTT is seen in 25–50% of patients. Fibrinogen levels are usually normal. It is thought that a circulating dialyzable inhibitor of fibrin monomer polymerization is present in these patients. The diagnosis of a uremic inhibitor rests on the demonstration of inhibition of platelet function or fibrin monomer polymerization in a patient with uremia. The correction of these abnormalities after dialysis should be demonstrated whenever possible. The only means of treatment available is the removal of the inhibition by dialysis of plasmapheresis.[7]

Vitamin K Deficiency

A deficiency of vitamin K produces a characteristic abnormality of blood clotting. Vitamin K is present in green vegetables, fish, liver, and tobacco. It is also synthesized by bacteria in the intestine. Bile salts are necessary for its absorption, which occurs primarily in the proximal small intestine. Vitamin K is also synthesized by intestinal bacteria such as *Bacteroides fragilis* and some strains of *Escherichia coli*. These organisms reside primarily in the jejunum and the ileum, beyond the site of maximal vitamin K absorption; therefore, bacterial vitamin K contributes very little after the neonatal period.[7]

Naturally occurring vitamin K_1 is fat-soluble, but synthetic analogues are water-soluble and less efficient than vitamin K_1 in correcting coagulation factor deficiencies. The vitamin K–dependent blood clotting and regulatory proteins are proteins C and S and factors II, VII, IX, and X. When vitamin K deficiency occurs, the inactive precursors of these coagulation factors, which do not bind calcium, continue to be made by the liver and accumulate in the plasma and act as vitamin K antagonists. These were formerly termed PIVKA (protein-induced by vitamin K absence or antagonists). This term has been replaced by the new "acarboxy-" terminology assigned by the International Committee on Thrombosis and Haemostasis. Thus vitamin K deficiency serves as essentially an anti-coagulant. Because it also reduces levels of protein C, a vitamin K deficiency can in addition lead to a dangerous prothrombotic state.[7, 12]

LABORATORY DIAGNOSIS

The diagnosis of vitamin K deficiency has generally been based on the documentation of decreased levels of factor II, VII, IX, and X activity, without deficiencies in other liver-produced factors, and the subsequent correction of these deficiencies after administration of vitamin K. The typical laboratory findings are a prolonged PT and a normal to prolonged PTT. The PTT may be normal in the early stages of vitamin K deficiency. Deficiency of factor VII, which has the shortest half-life, would be the first abnormality to occur and to be detected in the PT. The PT and PTT are corrected by mixing the patient's plasma with normal plasma (this fact excludes the presence of circulating anti-coagulants as a cause), and specific deficiencies in the four vitamin K–dependent clotting factors are corrected by mixing with normal levels of factor V and other liver-produced factors. The thrombin time is normal, because the exogenous thrombin added to the test mixture bypasses the defects produced by vitamin K deficiency.[7, 13, 21]

Several immunoassays for measuring the PIVKA or "acarboxy-" substances have been developed.

ETIOLOGY

Activity levels of vitamin K–dependent factors are depressed during the neonatal period, by treatment with coumarin-type oral anti-coagulants, in severe liver failure, and in conditions that result in impaired dietary intake or absorption of vitamin K (malabsorption syndromes, obstructive jaundice, prolonged antibiotic therapy, and total parenteral nutrition). In these acquired deficiencies, activity of all four factors tends to be diminished simultaneously, although not necessarily to the same extent.[8, 11]

HEMORRHAGIC DISEASE OF THE NEWBORN

In some infants, the synthetic mechanism of the vitamin K–dependent clotting factors in the liver appears to be immature, in association with an inadequate intake of vitamin K during the first few days of life (human milk contains little vitamin K, and the newborn's gut has not yet been colonized by bacteria). Breast-fed babies are more prone to vitamin K deficiency than are babies fed prepared formulas, because breast milk provides less of the vitamin than babies require. Breast milk is also sterile; therefore, seeding of the newborn gut with bacteria is further delayed.[7, 16, 18]

In hemorrhagic disease of the newborn, there is persistent bleeding from sites such as the gastrointestinal tract and umbilical stump, bruising at the sites of birth injury, bleeding after circumcisions, melena, and, occasionally, cerebrovascular hemorrhage. Bleeding is often severe and commonly occurs on the second or third day after birth.[7, 16, 18]

The full-term newborn has physiologically low levels of factors II, VII, IX, and X (in the range of 40–50% of normal adult levels). In hemorrhagic disease of the newborn, the PT and PTT are quite prolonged, and these findings are distinguished from the slight to moderate abnormalities of these tests that are characteristic of normal neonates. Hemorrhagic disease of the newborn is often associated with levels of vitamin K–dependent coagulation factors that are less than 25% of normal. The thrombin time and plasma fibrinogen are normal, as is the platelet count. The amount of citrate anti-coagulant in collection tubes used for venipuncture is appropriate for hematocrits between 25% and 55%. Because many infants have a hematocrit higher than 55%, the proportions may not be adequate, particularly if the tube is not filled completely.[7, 16, 18, 22]

Hemorrhagic disease of the newborn can be corrected by administration of vitamin K. In the event of major hemorrhage, transfusion of fresh-frozen plasma can be given. Since the 1960s, the practice of some obstetric units has been to administer vitamin K_1 (0.5–1.0 mg) to all newborns. Vitamin K_1 should be administered at least to low–birth-weight or premature infants. In addition, infants whose mothers were taking anticonvulsant medications during pregnancy are at high risk for hemorrhagic disease of the newborn.[1, 7, 9, 11, 16]

MALABSORPTION STATES

Pure dietary vitamin K deficiency is rarely a cause of malabsorption. However, malabsorption states may occur in later infancy or at any time in adult life. Symptoms include easy and widespread bruising, hemorrhage from sites of injury or mucous membranes such as the gut and tooth sockets, and gastrointestinal hemorrhage. Patients with poor nutrition, particularly elderly persons who exist on a diet of bread and tea, may not consume enough vitamin K. These persons may exhibit evidence of multivitamin deficiencies, including scurvy, which causes vascular fragility as well as anemia associated with iron and folic acid deficiency. Prolonged therapy with broad-spectrum antibiotics may sterilize the intestine sufficiently to cause hemorrhage.[7, 16]

Intestinal malabsorption can also cause clinically important hemorrhage. This possibility should be considered when an adult exhibits weight loss, muscle wasting, steatorrhea, or diarrhea. The commonest cause of malabsorption syndrome in adults is celiac disease, although other disorders such as tropical sprue, cystic fibrosis, and ulcerative colitis

may cause the same problem. Major resection of the bowel may similarly cause vitamin K deficiency. Severe vitamin K deficiency is seen in patients with obstructive jaundice, in which the lack of bile salts in the small intestine reduces absorption of the fat-soluble vitamin K. Patients with obstructive jaundice should be monitored regularly through the screening coagulation tests to detect vitamin K deficiency.[16]

COUMARINS: ANTI-COAGULANT OVERDOSE

After the severe winter of 1921 in the United States, a previously undescribed hemorrhagic disorder in cattle resulted from the ingestion of spoiled sweet-clover silage. In 1939, Link identified the responsible agent as dicumarol. Warfarin sodium, a dicumarol derivative, is now the most popular vitamin K antagonist used in the United States. Warfarin interferes with the carboxylation of the vitamin K–dependent plasma factors in the liver by interrupting the enzymatic phase of this reaction, with the accumulation of PIVKAs (described earlier).[2, 18]

With the introduction of dicumarol and other anti–vitamin K compounds into anti-coagulant therapy, the monitoring of vitamin K activity depression has been a problem for human medicine. When such drugs are ingested, changes may not be detected in blood coagulation for 1 or 2 days. Because of the differences in the half-lives of vitamin K–dependent factors, their activity levels begin to fall at different times and rates. A decrease in the level of factor VII is noted first, followed by decreases in the levels of factors IX and X and finally of factor II. The most common complication of oral anti-coagulant therapy is hemorrhage, which usually results from overdosage, when the level of vitamin K–dependent factors is too low or when, even in the presence of normal levels, a vascular lesion such as duodenal ulcer may precipitate excess hemorrhage.[8, 10, 16]

Many drugs may increase the biologic effect of oral anti-coagulants and, if the anti-coagulant dosage is not reduced, hemorrhagic complications may occur. Examples of drugs potentiating the effect of coumarin are phenylbutazone, chloramphenicol, quinidine, salicylates, and indomethacin.[16]

To treat anti-coagulant overdosage resulting in mild bleeding, treatment may be withdrawn for 2 or more days and then resumed with a low maintenance dose of the anti-coagulant. If severe bleeding occurs, intravenous vitamin K_1 should be given, followed by oral vitamin K. Anti-coagulants may be discontinued or should be limited.[16]

OTHER DRUG EFFECTS

Several of the new antibiotics, including carbenicillin, moxalactam, cephamandole, cefoxitin, and cefoperazone, have been reported to cause a deficiency in the vitamin K–dependent factors by themselves. Sulfa drugs, neomycin, and other broad-spectrum antibiotics are capable of sterilizing the intestinal tract, which can lead to a vitamin K deficiency.[7, 9]

Decreased sensitivity to oral anti-coagulants can also occur as a result of increased vitamin K in food intake: for instance, when green vegetables are eaten to excess or when chewing tobacco is used. Several drugs can serve as antagonists to coumarin such as barbiturates, phenytoin, meprobamate, phenylbutazone, griseofulvin, and glutethimide that depress the action of the anti-coagulants. A higher anti-coagulant dose may be warranted in these instances.[11, 16]

TREATMENT

Specific therapy for vitamin K deficiency is the administration of vitamin K. The route of administration depends on the severity of the factor deficiencies and clinical symptoms of the patient. When the deficiencies and bleeding are mild, correction over several days is acceptable, and oral vitamin K can be used if there is no impairment of absorption. If the deficiencies and bleeding are severe or if absorption of orally administered vitamin K is impaired, the vitamin can be administered parenterally. With intramuscular administration of vitamin K, correction of the PT may be noted within 24 hours. With intravenous administration, the PT begins to correct within a few hours. In life-threatening hemorrhage, infusions of plasma or prothrombin-complex concentrate may be required.[7]

ACQUIRED CIRCULATING ANTI-COAGULANTS

The presence of excessive circulating inhibitors should always be considered (1) when a known hemorrhagic diathesis suddenly becomes refractory to therapy, (2) when a coagulopathy develops in a previously healthy person, and (3) when results of certain coagulation tests are contradictory results and do not correspond to the pattern known for a typical coagulation-deficiency disease. Some inhibitors result in profound inhibition of in vitro coagulation but are not associated with significant bleeding.[8]

Acquired circulating anti-coagulants (inhibitors, antibodies) may be directed against single or multiple coagulation factors. The presence of acquired circulating anti-coagulants is commonly associated with certain disease entities, ingestion of drugs, and other clinical situations. Other materials such as heparin or FDPs can inhibit the hemostatic mechanism in vivo or in vitro.[2, 6]

Acquired inhibitors occurring in patients with noncongenital deficiencies are classified into three types. The first includes inhibitors that inactivate individual coagulation factors, often in a progressive, usually irreversible, time-dependent manner. Most are immunoglobulins. Subtyping of these factors reveal most of the immunoglobulins to be IgG, and the most common subtype is IgG_4. Kappa chains are more common than lambda light chains.[6]

The second type of circulating inhibitor is characterized by being reversible (or partially reversible) and immediate in action, and it represents a protein-protein interaction (complex formation) with either a specific coagulation factor or a group of factors. These anti-coagulants often do not destroy the coagulation factor, and its biologic activity may be recovered if the complex can be dissociated. These complexes are often seen in patients with malignant or benign paraprotein disorders such as multiple myeloma and with disorders involving high levels of fibrinogen degradation products (anti-thrombin I) in intravascular coagulation, fibrinogenolysis, and liver disease.[1, 6]

The third type includes rare and apparently unique inhibitors of coagulation that have been described in patients with Down syndrome and chronic myelocytic leukemia. Inhibition of coagulation as a result of the endogenous release of heparin-like substances has been documented in patients with multiple myeloma; this finding indicates a possible fourth type of acquired inhibitor.[1, 6]

Fibrinogen (Factor I) Inhibitors

Few cases of acquired inhibitors to fibrinogen have been reported. Of these, some occurred in afibrinogenemic patients who had undergone transfusion. The other cases of noncongenital deficiencies were associated with autoimmune disorders and chronic inflammatory diseases. One case was associated with Down syndrome.[6]

Factor II Inhibitors

Anti-prothrombin (factor II) antibodies are extremely rare in cases of noncongenital factor II deficiency. They have been seen only in patients with systemic lupus erythematosus.

Factor V Inhibitors

The development of a factor V inhibitor is a rare event that can be linked to plasma transfusion in patients with previously normal hemostasis. Antibody to factor V has been acquired in at least 16 patients. In almost 70% of these patients, development of the antibody was preceded by a surgical procedure. Of these surgical patients, 50% reported taking streptomycin as part of their operative course. Development of an anti–factor V antibody has also been linked to the use of streptomycin in several nonsurgical patients. Both IgG and IgM have been incriminated. The inhibitor has been rather short-lived in most patients, lasting for about 2–8 weeks. The therapy is generally limited to fresh-frozen plasma if necessary. If the antibody is persistent, cyclophosphamide and prednisone may be used.[3, 6, 16]

Factor VII Inhibitors

An anti–factor VII antibody has been reported at least once and was associated with a probable carcinoma of the lung. The antibody was IgG.[6]

Factor VIII:C Inhibitors

In hemophilia, the development of these antibodies is a serious complication and may provoke spontaneous bleeding or produce the pattern of severe factor VIII deficiency in a previously mildly affected patient. Two types of factor VIII inhibitors can be distinguished on the basis of their immunologic response to reexposure to the antigen (i.e., factor VIII). In the classic type there is an anamnestic rise in antibody titer after infusion of even trace amounts of factor VIII. Patients with this type of inhibitor are referred to as "high responders." Other patients, however, show little or no rise in titer after factor VIII infusions and are referred to as "low responders." High doses of factor VIII may be effective treatment for acute bleeding episodes in low responders but not in high responders.[7]

In patients without hemophilia, the immunizing event leading to the formation of factor VIII antibodies remains obscure. Factor VIII inhibitors should be suspected in healthy persons who suddenly develop an unexplained hemorrhagic diathesis. In addition, an anti–VIII antibody is the most likely circulating anti-coagulant in the nonlupus patient in whom a circulating anti-coagulant develops. The incidence of the development of factor VIII inhibitors in nonhemophilic patients peaks in the 50- to 80-year age range, in apparently normal persons. Factor VIII inhibitors may develop in persons with apparently no underlying disease, such as in the postpartum patients.[1, 3, 6, 9]

Spontaneous inhibitors of factor VIII:C can arise in a number of different clinical situations, including collagen vascular disease (i.e., systemic lupus erythematosus, rheumatoid arthritis, and ulcerative colitis), certain dermatologic diseases, and after drug reactions (penicillin, sulfa drugs, and gold). Hemorrhagic disorders occurring as a complication of penicillin therapy have been associated with the development of a circulating inhibitor of factor VIII. Affected patients usually have other major manifestations of penicillin allergy. The antibodies do not bind to factor VIII.[1, 3, 6, 9]

Factor VIII inhibitors are occasionally observed in patients with disorders such as multiple myeloma and Waldenström's macroglobulinemia.[1, 3, 6, 9]

CLINICAL MANIFESTATIONS

In nonhemophilic patients, factor VIII antibodies produce a state of acquired hemophilia. Bleeding manifestations include dissecting hematomas; epistaxis; hematuria; in rare instances, hemarthrosis; and post-traumatic and postsurgical hemorrhage. Most nonhemophilic patients in whom an acquired anti–factor VIII antibody develops do not suffer the types of bleeding usually associated with hemophilia A. The clinical course of these inhibitors is variable, but a fatal hemorrhage can occur. The antibodies may disappear within months or years after their appearance.[1, 6, 9, 16]

LABORATORY DIAGNOSIS

The usual laboratory findings are those of hemophilia A: a prolonged PTT and a normal PT. Specific diagnosis depends on the demonstration of time-dependent inactivation of factor VIII in mixtures containing normal factor VIII and the patient's plasma or serum.[1]

With few exceptions, antibodies to factor VIII are IgG and monoclonal in nature. Rare cases of IgM and IgA antibody have been reported. Antibodies to factor VIII react specifically with the coagulant portion of the molecule.[1, 16]

TREATMENT

Treatment of this disorder depends on the titer of the antibody and its avidity for the factor VIII antigen. Replacement therapy is usually ineffective in patients with high titers of antibody because the infused factor VIII is neutralized by the patient's antibody.[1, 3, 6]

In hemophilic patients, amounts of factor VIII sufficient to neutralize all circulating inhibitors should be administered as a bolus in an attempt to attain hemostatic levels for a short time. Continuous infusion with factor VIII concentrates is also a recognized treatment. Better results may be obtained with porcine or bovine factor VIII than with human protein. Exchange plasmapheresis may enhance the response to replacement therapy and lower the antibody titer. Concentrates of vitamin K–dependent factors (Proplex, Autoplex T, Feiba EH Immuno) are alternatives to treatment with high titer factor VIII antibodies. These products contain activated factors, as well as active factor VIII:C. Thrombotic complications, hepatitis, and AIDS are significant risks involved in the use of these therapeutic materials.[1, 3, 6]

The treatment of hemorrhage associated with factor VIII inhibitors in nonhemophilic patients is controversial, but transfusion with washed red blood cells may prevent a rise in inhibitor titer. Immunosuppressive drugs and corticosteroids are useful in nonhemophilic patients in whom an anti–factor VIII antibody develops. Clinical improvement as well as remissions have been documented. Equally good results have been shown in a few patients with cyclophosphamide or azathioprine, either alone or in combination with prednisone.[1, 6]

Spontaneous remissions have been documented in a minority of patients with factor VIII inhibitors, most commonly in postpartum women, in children, and in cases associated with skin diseases and drug reactions.[1]

von Willebrand Factor Inhibitors

Antibodies to factor VIII R:WF may develop in patients with von Willebrand's disease, as described in Chapter 33. Acquired von Willebrand's disease, or development of an acquired anti-coagulant to the von Willebrand portion of the factor VIII macromolecular complex, has been reported. Most have had an autoimmune disorder, lymphoma, myeloproliferative/myelodysplastic syndrome, or a malignant paraprotein disorder. Rare cases have been reported after pesticide exposure and in association with Wilms tumor. In most instances, the bleeding has not been severe. Therapy has consisted of immunosuppression, infusion of cryoprecipitate, or other measures to control the underlying disease process.[6]

Factor IX Inhibitors

The incidence of factor IX inhibitors in patients with hemophilia B is less than half that of factor VIII inhibitors in patients with hemophilia A. In a review of the literature, an incidence of 2.8% was reported. In contrast to the progressive inhibition noted with factor VIII inhibitors, factor IX inhibitors seem to be quite rapid, reaching maximal neutralization within 5 minutes of incubation.[11]

Inhibitors to factor IX arising in previously healthy persons are rare, although several instances have been reported. Anti–factor IX antibodies only rarely occur in patients with rheumatic fever and nonhemophilia B. The most common clinical situations in which they occur are during the postpartum period and in association with systemic lupus erythematosus. Factor IX deficiency has been reported in patients with severe nephrotic syndrome, in at least one patient with congestive heart failure, and in at least one patient with Sheehan syndrome. Like anti–factor VIII antibodies in nonhemophilic patients, the anti–factor IX antibody often abates with immunosuppressive therapy in the form of prednisone, azathioprine, or cyclophosphamide.[1, 11]

Factor X Inhibitors

At least two cases of an anti–factor X antibody have been reported: both occurred in patients with leprosy; one patient had been ingesting dapsone; and neither patient had a clinically significant bleeding diathesis. Of more clinical relevance is the association of selective factor X deficiency associated with systemic amyloidosis. Although an anti–factor X antibody has not been found in the circulation, it is thought that amyloid fibrils may selectively bind with factor X and remove it from the circulation.[6]

Factor XI Inhibitors

Anti–factor XI antibodies in patients with noncongenital factor XI deficiency have been found in at least 11 persons. Ten had an autoimmune disorder, and one had pneumonia thought to be caused by an adenovirus. Laboratory findings have included a prolonged PTT and a decreased factor XI level. The antibody is of the IgG type.[6, 11]

Factor XII Inhibitors

Anti–factor XII antibody has been reported only in patients with systemic lupus erythematosus, Waldenström's macroglobulinemia, and glomerulonephritis. A severe deficiency of factor XII has been found in association with angioimmunoblastic lymphadenopathy, but a circulating anti-coagulant has not been demonstrated.[6]

Factor XIII Inhibitors

Acquired anti–factor XIII antibodies have occurred in at least eight otherwise hemostatically normal persons. Most had been receiving isoniazid, an anti-tuberculosis drug, and in one, an anti-factor XIII antibody developed in the presence of a drug-induced systemic lupus erythematosus–type syndrome. Other drugs such as phenytoin and penicillin have been implicated. These rare antibodies prevent the crosslinking between fibrin monomers and lead to abnormal fragility of fibrin clots. The disorder may cause a persistent and severe hemorrhagic problem that can be fatal in the postoperative period.[3, 6, 15, 16]

Nonspecific Inhibitors

Nonspecific inhibitors like those of the lupus anti-coagulant type are not specific for any single coagulation protein, are usually not associated with bleeding, and are usually not temperature-dependent like those associated with factor VIII:C or factor V. Nonspecific inhibitor antibodies are not directed against specific clotting factor proteins; rather, they interfere with the interaction of clotting factors on a phospholipid surface. Numerous studies have suggested that the nonspecific inhibitors bind to the phospholipid surface in such a way as to inhibit the binding of factor II, and possibly factor Xa, to the surface.[2, 7]

The nonspecific inhibitor tends to inhibit the PTT or PT reactions in one-stage assays. The PTT is almost always affected to a much greater degree than the PT, which often shows little or no prolongation despite marked prolongation of the PTT. That the prolongations are the result of an inhibitor, rather than deficiencies, is demonstrated by the failure of normal plasma to correct the prolongations in mixing tests. The diagnosis of nonspecific inhibitors rests on the demonstration of (1) the inhibitory effect on coagulation screening tests and (2) the presence of normal concentrations of all clotting factors. In documentation of the latter, it is important that the factor assay include several dilutions of the test plasma.[7]

LUPUS INHIBITORS (LUPUS ANTI-COAGULANTS)

The lupus inhibitor is the most common of the acquired inhibitors encountered in the laboratory. Lupus anti-coagulants have been defined as immunoglobulins interfering with phospholipid-dependent tests of coagulation. It acts against the phospholipids that provide the reactive site for the factor X and factor V interaction. The anti-coagu-lant also appears to inhibit prostacyclin production or release.[1, 3, 4, 6, 15]

Unlike the factor specific inhibitors previously described, lupus anti-coagulants do not inhibit activity of specific coagulation factors. Thus, there may be more than one antibody or site of action of these inhibitors. These inhibitors may occur in 5–15% of patients with systemic lupus erythematosus.[1, 3, 4, 6, 15]

Almost one fourth of patients with systemic lupus erythematosus and the lupus anti-coagulant also have a significant prothrombin deficiency. This appears to be a specific feature of the disorder in these patients, but the relationship between the coagulation abnormality and the inhibitor is unclear. More than 40% of patients have significant associated thrombocytopenia. There is no reported increase in surgical hemorrhage in patients with the lupus anti-coagulant alone.[1, 6]

The term *lupus anti-coagulant* is a misnomer, inasmuch as this anti-coagulant is also found in patients who do not have systemic lupus erythematosus. Approximately half of reported cases have been found in patients with disseminated lupus and other collagen vascular disorders. Associated diseases with a lupus anti-coagulant have been reported for various malignancies, gynecologic disorders, various autoimmune states (such as rheumatoid arthritis), cardiovascular problems, and urologic problems. In addition, the lupus inhibitor has been found after viral infections and in some normal, healthy persons. The inhibitor may be associated with AIDS, usually upon the development of inflammation associated with opportunistic infections.[3, 7, 11, 13, 15]

Drug-induced inhibitors of lupus are common. Chlorpromazine and other phenothiazines, quinidine, and procainamide appear to be the drugs most commonly implicated. These inhibitors usually are of the IgM class and often disappear when the drug is withdrawn.[1]

In summary, lupus inhibitors are of the IgG or IgM class, are polyclonal in nature, and usually interfere with the molecular assembly of complex enzymes on phospholipid surfaces. Results of several in vitro studies suggest that the immunoglobulin requires plasma factor in order to be fully inhibitory.[1, 3, 7]

Clinical Manifestations. Lupus inhibitors normally are not associated with significant bleeding or predisposition to hemorrhage. In patients with severe superimposed prothrombin deficiency, thrombocytopenia, or platelet dysfunctions relating to the underlying disease, significant bleeding may be encountered. Lupus inhibitors may, surprisingly, be associated with a tendency for thrombosis and recurrent spontaneous abortions or intrauterine death. Placental insufficiency resulting from thrombosis of placental vessels is the suspected cause for the abortions. Thromboses may involve arteries or veins and may be serious.[1, 6, 13, 23]

Laboratory Diagnosis. All phospholipid-dependent coagulation tests may be prolonged, including the PT (slightly prolonged; usually high-titer inhibitors only), activated PTT (prolonged), and the thrombin time (normal to slightly prolonged). The PTT is considerably more sensitive than is the PT to lupus anti-coagulants. The PTT is not corrected by adding normal plasma. The sensitivity of the activated PTT to the lupus anti-coagulant is highly dependent on the reagents used. Platelet-poor plasma enhances the sensitivity of the phospholipid-dependent tests to the presence of the lupus anti-coagulant. Platelet-rich plasma may diminish the test's sensitivity to lupus anti-coagulants and may mask their presence.[3, 6, 15]

There is no single specific test for the lupus inhibitor. In one technique, which is based on the PT, the thromboplastin is diluted. This thromboplastin inhibition test is based on the lupus anti-coagulant's property of inhibiting highly diluted tissue thromboplastin. The inhibitory effect of the lupus anti-coagulant is potentiated as the thromboplastin is diluted. Diluting the tissue factor reagent of the PT test lengthens the patient's clotting time substantially more than it lengthens the clotting time of normal plasma. This is called a positive dilute thromboplastin inhibition test result. Evidence suggests that there are a number of false-positive results. This test may not detect IgM lupus anti-coagulants, leading to a false-negative result.[1, 5, 6, 13, 23]

It has also been suggested that the Stypven time can be used to detect lupus inhibitors. Again, false-positive results may be obtained. The venom is diluted to give a normal time of 23–27 seconds. The phospholipid is then diluted to a minimal level that will continue to support this range. A prolongation of this system is not corrected with a mixture of the patient's plasma and normal plasma. Both IgG and IgM lupus anti-coagulants are thought to be detected through the Stypven time. Neither the Stypven time nor the tissue thromboplastin inhibition test is recommended for detecting all lupus anti-coagulants. The Stypven time is easy to perform and not affected by inhibitors to factor VIII or IX. It is recommended as a primary screening test for lupus anti-coagulant detection in a hospital clinical laboratory.[1, 5, 6, 13, 23]

The platelet neutralization procedure is another method that is claimed to be highly specific. A third coagulation test commonly used for the detection of lupus anti-coagulants is the kaolin clotting time. A prolonged kaolin clotting time is corrected by addition of phospholipids but not by normal plasma and is considered specific and sensitive.[1, 6, 9, 11, 23]

Among patients with the lupus anti-coagulant, there is also a higher incidence of false-positive results of serologic tests, such as the Venereal Disease Research Laboratories test, as the antibody reacts with cardiolipin, the phospholipid antigen that is used in serologic tests for syphilis. A test for the presence of a specific anti-cardiolipin antibody is available and is highly predictive for the subgroup at risk for a thrombotic tendency.[1, 6, 9, 11, 23]

Treatment. In the great majority of cases, treatment is not required. Steroids may diminish the inhibitory effect in some cases but should not be given to treat the inhibitor. Therapy with corticosteroids and aspirin has helped some women with the lupus anti-coagulant carry their pregnancies to term. The lupus inhibitor should always be clearly identified at the time of presentation. Otherwise, the patient may exhibit a prolonged PTT in an emergency situation and be treated with factor VIII and other blood products, which is potentially dangerous. Plasmapheresis should be reserved for extenuating circumstances but may be helpful for patients with life-threatening, uncontrollable hemorrhages.[1, 4, 7, 16]

Massive Transfusions. Transfusions of large amounts of stored bank blood may produce mild to moderate abnormalities of one-stage screening tests of coagulation but seldom are associated with significant hemorrhage. These abnormalities may be caused by deficiencies of storage-labile factors V and VIII. Use of fresh-frozen plasma may help alleviate the problem.[1, 4, 11]

Citrate toxicity is another consideration in patients who have undergone massive transfusions. This rarely becomes a problem except in newborns or patients with liver disease. Calcium can be given to avoid or reverse this toxicity but is seldom needed clinically.[1, 4, 11]

Thrombocytopenia is much more common than coagulation abnormalities in patients who have undergone massive transfusions and may lead to significant bleeding. Platelets lose their viability in stored blood. Initial therapy should be directed at monitoring and maintaining a count near 100,000 cells/mm[3].[1, 4, 11]

FIBRINOLYTIC DISORDERS

Fibrinolysis results when excess amounts of plasminogen activators convert plasminogen to plasmin within the circulation. Plasminogen activators may be derived from various tissues, secretions, or the vascular endothelium. The contact factors (XIII, Fletcher, and Fitzgerald) are also capable of activating plasminogen. Plasmin digests factors V and VIII and, in addition, breaks down fibrin and fibrinogen to FDP.[15]

When defects of the fibrinolytic system occur, the disrupted balance between procoagulant and anti-coagulant activities in blood may lead to thrombosis (decreased fibrinolytic activity) or a bleeding tendency (increased fibrinolytic activity).

Two major fibrinolytic conditions predisposing patients to *bleeding* are primary fibrinolysis and DIC. Four major conditions predisposing patients to thrombosis have been described: plasminogen deficiency, alpha$_2$–anti-plasmin defect, defects of activators, and plasminogen activator deficiency. Defects of natural inhibitors and dysfibrinogenemias occasionally lead to thrombosis. Acquired clotting states may also lead to thrombosis. Table 34–1 outlines the hypercoagulable disease conditions.[16, 24, 25]

Reduced fibrinolytic activity favors thrombus deposition. The plasma fibrinolytic system can be impaired by inherited deficiencies of plasminogen, by defective release of plasminogen activator from the vascular endothelium, and by high plasma levels of regulatory proteins such as plasma activator inhibitors such as alpha$_2$-macroglobulin, AT III, alpha$_1$–anti-trypsin, and C1 inactivator. In addition, factor XII deficiency may also be responsible for failure of fibrinolysis activation.[9, 24]

Primary Fibrinolysis

The term *primary fibrinolysis* refers to instances in which fibrinogenolysis or inappropriate fibrinolysis apparently arise de novo in the absence of an underlying disease. Primary fibrinolysis is poorly documented and in many cases may represent an inappropriate response to underlying DIC.[1]

Fibrinolysis that follows fibrin deposition is often called *secondary fibrinolysis* because fibrin deposition is the primary event. When an episode of disseminated intravascular clotting results in widespread deposition of fibrin in the microcirculation, secondary fibrinolysis may cause large amounts of FDPs to accumulate in the blood. The most common example of this is DIC.[13]

Increased fibrinolytic activity (primary, not part of the DIC syndrome) is seen in many systemic conditions. These conditions include shock, heat stroke, hypoxia, hypotension, the period after thoracic surgery, acute hemorrhage, cirrhosis of the liver, barbiturate poisoning, methyl alcohol intoxication, and severe anxiety states such as those occurring during examinations. In rare cases, acute leukemia and carcinomas are accompanied by extremely strong fibrinolytic activity without evidence of DIC. Excessive fibrinolytic activity is sometimes seen in normal persons for no apparent reason. Increased fibrinolytic activity can also be a complication of thrombolytic therapy. In general, bleeding is rare in these patients; however, when it does occur, it can be severe and may be fatal.[3, 9, 13, 15]

Pathologic activation of the fibrinolytic system occurs in many patients with liver disease. Decreased inhibitors of the fibrinolytic system, primarily alpha$_2$–anti-plasmin and alpha$_2$–macroglobulin may lead to pathologic activation. The end result of fibrinolysis in patients with liver disease is biodegradation of many coagulation factors (such as factors I, II, and V) by plasmin and creation of FDPs, which have serious deleterious effects on already compromised hemostasis.[6]

In persons without systemic disorders of hemostasis, bleeding can result from localized hyperfibrinolysis. Organs with higher levels of fibrinolytic activity, such as the uterus and the renal pelvis, are presumably most severely affected. Essential menorrhagia, subarachnoid hemorrhages, and gastrointestinal bleeding are all examples of excessive localized fibrinolysis.[3]

Plasminogen activators are sometimes infused intravenously to dissolve thrombi. Unlike tissue plasminogen activator, the agents currently being used—urokinase and streptokinase—are potent activators of circulating plasminogen and of the fibrinolytic process. Large amounts of circulating plasmin are formed and alpha$_2$–anti-plasmin and alpha$_2$-macroglobulin levels fall. Following this, the circulating plasmin can attack the fibrin of the thrombus, but it also can attack circulating fibrinogen and other plasma proteins, such as factors V

Table 34-1. CONGENITAL AND ACQUIRED DEFICIENCIES ASSOCIATED WITH HYPERCOAGULABILITY AND THROMBOSIS

Congenital Deficiencies

FIBRINOLYTIC DISORDERS
Plasminogen deficiency
Alpha$_2$–anti-plasmin deficiency
Defects of activators
Plasminogen activator deficiency

NATURAL INHIBITORS OF COAGULATION
Anti-thrombin III deficiency
Protein C deficiency
Protein S deficiency
Heparin cofactor II deficiency
Hageman factor (factor XII) deficiency

DYSFIBRINOGENEMIAS

Acquired Deficiencies
Tissue and cellular damage
Drug-induced
Disease-induced

and VIII. This creates a potentially hazardous bleeding tendency.[13]

The manifestation of primary fibrino(geno)lysis is *hemorrhage*. Thrombosis does not occur if this is an isolated hemostatic defect.[6]

LABORATORY DIAGNOSIS

The hemorrhagic state is accompanied by a short euglobulin lysis time (unless there is depletion of plasminogen), decreased plasma levels of plasminogen and fibrinogen, and elevated levels of FDPs. Levels of factors V and VIII are generally decreased. The level of factor XIII is also decreased in some patients.[3,15]

In association with elevated levels of FDPs, severe platelet dysfunction, plasmin-induced degradation of clotting factors, and elevation of B-beta 15-42 peptides occurs.[6]

The laboratory patterns are similar to those in DIC, but there are some differences. The PT, PTT, and thrombin time are generally prolonged as a result of the anti-coagulant effect of the FDPs. However, they are seldom as prolonged in hyperfibrinolysis as they are in DIC, for the reduction in levels of factors II and V is not as great as when they are used up in DIC. DIC is usually accompanied by moderate to severe thrombocytopenia. In patients with hyperfibrinolysis syndromes, the platelet count is usually normal, except in cases of high levels of FDPs.[9,15]

Probably the most helpful tests are those that measure the fibrinolytic system. The euglobulin lysis test measures plasminogen activators and plasmin; in primary fibrinolysis, the test reveals rapid lysis, whereas in secondary fibrinolysis in the late stage of DIC, it is only moderately abnormal. Cryofibrinogen and changes in erythrocyte morphology may be found in DIC, but they are not features of the hyperfibrinolytic state.[9]

Treatment for fibrinolysis usually involves administration of an agent, such as epsilon-aminocaproic acid, which inhibits the activation of plasminogen. It must be used only when the increased fibrinolytic activity is primary and not associated with DIC. This drug and related enzyme inhibitors (tranexamic acid, Trasylol) may produce thromboembolic complications in patients with DIC.[1, 9, 15]

HYPERCOAGULABILITY

Fibrinolytic disorders and deficiencies of natural inhibitors may lead to a hypercoagulable state. This is a perturbed but partially contained system that has not yet progressed to fibrin deposition or an unperturbed system in which the threshold re-sistance to thrombogenesis has been decreased. This definition describes the more common situation of a secondary hypercoagulable state (i.e., subclinical activation of coagulation by something else) or the less common primary hypercoagulable state (e.g., an inhibitor deficiency).[26]

Several conditions are associated with an increased tendency for thrombosis to develop (formation of intravascular clots). They are collectively referred to as hypercoagulable or prethrombotic states. This condition may be divided into two categories: (1) primary disorders, in which there is a qualitative or quantitative abnormality of a specific component of the hemostatic system, and (2) secondary disorders, in which the mechanism of the clot formation is not completely known.[15]

Primary disorders are relatively uncommon and include most congenital deficiencies such as deficiencies of AT III and protein C, as well as abnormalities of plasminogen, plasminogen activators, and fibrinogen. The most common of the secondary conditions or states are stasis (inhibition) of blood flow, malignancy, the postoperative state, pregnancy, and the use of oral contraceptives.[15]

The concept of hypercoagulability is generally attributed to Rudolf Virchow. In a lecture in 1845, he postulated that alterations of the blood (later termed *hypercoagulability*), changes in the vessel wall (vascular injury), and impairment of blood flow (stasis) were key conditions leading to thrombosis (Virchow's triad).[26]

Vascular injury leads to the exposure of subendothelial vessel wall components to which platelets adhere, triggering platelet release, platelet aggregation, and development of platelet procoagulant activity. In addition, certain subendothelial structures can directly activate the contact phase of the coagulation system and release small amounts of tissue thromboplastin.[26]

Stasis, or impaired blood flow, may lead to the accumulation of procoagulant substances, such as activated clotting factors, and may facilitate platelet–vessel wall interaction.[26]

Finally, a number of important regulatory factors and mechanisms that prevent excessive platelet aggregation and, in concert with the fibrinolytic system, prevent excessive fibrin deposition have been elucidated.[26]

Platelet numbers may be increased in patients with hypercoagulability, and thrombocytosis is clinically important in the thrombohemorrhagic problems associated with myeloproliferative syndromes. Reactive thrombocytosis does not appear to be pathogenically important. Increased platelet adhesiveness and aggregability may contribute to the thrombotic potential even when platelet numbers are normal. Increased plasma levels of platelet factor 4 and beta-thromboglobulin may be found in patients in whom platelets have been activated in vivo.[8]

Increased levels of almost every known coagulation factor have been described at some time in patients with a tendency for thrombosis to develop; however, there is very little concrete evidence that such increased levels alone lead to an increased rate of fibrin formation. The levels of factors V and VIII and of fibrinogen are increased during the inflammatory processes because they are acute-phase reactant proteins, but this probably represents a response to such processes rather than the cause of thrombosis that may accompany them.[8, 27]

Several methods can be used to detect intravascular fibrin formation through the measurement of products of the fibrinogen-to-fibrin conversion reaction. This is evidence that an episode of intravascular coagulation has occurred, not specific evidence of a hypercoagulable state. Normally, the euglobulin-lysis time in hypercoagulable states is significantly decreased.[8]

No single test can be counted on to detect the prethrombotic state. The following six determinations as a group are recommended: platelet count, hematocrit, PTT, AT III, plasma fibrinolytic activity, and lipoprotein fractionation. A shift of the test values from a patient's baseline may be more informative than one-time testing. It has been shown that a PTT of less than 28 seconds (a reagent produces a normal mean of 37 seconds) in postoperative patients is a strong indication that there is a risk of thrombosis.[9]

CONGENITAL CLOTTING SYNDROMES

Many congenital disorders are characterized by the lack or abnormality of components of the fibrinolytic system. Not only have congenital clotting conditions been identified, but it is now evident that the incidence of congenital clotting problems exceeds that of the bleeding disorders. Most of these conditions have demonstrated the importance of the fibrinolytic system in the pathogenesis of thrombosis.[16, 24, 25]

Plasminogen Deficiency

Plasminogen is normally found in two forms: (1) free in the circulation and (2) incorporated in thrombi bound to fibrin. Under physiologic conditions, when circulating plasminogen is activated, it becomes rapidly inactivated by a circulating inhibitor, alpha$_2$–anti-plasmin, thus preventing fibrino-

genolysis. Plasminogen is an alpha$_2$-protein that plays a central role in the fibrinolytic system. So far no family with a true deficiency of plasminogen has ever been described; however, abnormal plasminogens have been described. Nonetheless, through the availability of reliable and simple plasminogen assays by synthetic substrate methods, this deficiency has been found to be much more common than previously suspected. The disorder is inherited as an autosomal recessive trait. Both the absent form (CRM$^-$) and the dysfunctional form (CRM$^+$) have been described. The dysfunctional form appears to be more common.[6, 7, 9, 16]

The clinical picture appears to be similar to that of a deficiency of AT III and/or of protein C. Patients with congenital deficiencies of plasminogen begin to experience thrombotic events in their late teens. The condition consists of delayed and/or defective activation of plasminogen and seems to be associated with a lifelong tendency for thromboses, including pulmonary embolism.[6, 9]

Inherited plasminogen deficiency is believed to be responsible for about 2–3% of unexplained deep venous thromboses in young patients. The defect is transmitted through autosomal dominance. In heterozygotes, plasminogen activity is about half the normal level (normal range: 75–128%).[25]

Laboratory screening for plasminogen deficiency reveals prolonged euglobulin lysis times after venous occlusion of the arm and/or intravenous infusion of DDAVP. Results of the usual global tests of coagulation, including the platelet count, PT, PTT, thrombin time, and bleeding time, are normal, and the diagnosis depends on specific plasminogen assays for biologic activity performed by synthetic substrate methods. The main laboratory finding is a discrepancy between plasminogen activity, as determined, for example, by means of a chromogenic substrate (S-25511) and plasminogen antigen level. Activation studies with urokinase and/or streptokinase have also been used to characterize the defect. Successful therapy has included heparin, warfarin-type drugs, anti-platelet agents, and urokinase.[3, 6, 16, 25, 28]

Alpha$_2$–Anti-Plasmin Deficiency

Fibrinolysis is a fibrin-oriented process. Activation of plasminogen on the surface of fibrin results in effective fibrinolysis. After lysis of fibrin, plasminogen activator and plasmin are released and bound to their respective plasma inhibitors. The primary physiologic inhibitor of plasmin is alpha$_2$–anti-plasmin. Thus, alpha$_2$–anti-plasmin is a potent inhibitor of the fibrinolytic system. In the absence of alpha$_2$–anti-plasmin, plasmin is free to lyse fibrinogen and other plasmin-sensitive proteins. Physiologic fibrinolysis goes unchecked, and therefore plasmin lysis of a hemostatic plug occurs.[9, 16]

Alpha$_2$–anti-plasmin deficiency is inherited as an autosomal recessive trait and has been described in a few families. Alpha$_2$–anti-plasmin levels are lower than 10% in homozygous patients and around 50% in heterozygous persons.[9]

CLINICAL MANIFESTATIONS

Patients with a hereditary deficiency of alpha$_2$–anti-plasmin have a lifelong history of severe bleeding. In some instances, the pattern of bleeding is suggestive of hemophilia. Umbilical stump bleeding, epistaxis, gingival bleeding, and hemarthrosis have been reported and described frequently. Bleeding can be severe in homozygous patients and typically consists of mucosal membrane bleeding (with hematuria), large subcutaneous hematomas, spontaneous bruising, and severe bleeding with trauma.[6, 9, 16]

Persons who are heterozygous for deficiency of alpha$_2$–anti-plasmin have few bleeding problems. Typically, the results on assays for alpha$_2$–anti-plasmin function and antigenicity are markedly abnormal. Patients rarely demonstrate spontaneous bleeding. Bleeding usually is associated with trauma and often is delayed. Postoperative bleeding is characteristic. Although persons who are heterozygous for the deficiency have few bleeding problems, they are relatively easily detected through the decreased level of alpha$_2$–anti-plasmin.[6, 9]

LABORATORY DIAGNOSIS

Results of laboratory screening tests in patients with a hereditary deficiency of alpha$_2$–anti-plasmin are characteristically normal. However, there is rapid and complete lysis in the whole blood clot lysis test and shortening of the euglobulin clot lysis time. The lack of anti-plasmin activity (chromogenic substrate) and antigen (electroimmunoassay or radial immunodiffusion) are pathognomonic for the abnormality. On occasion, elevated levels of FDPs may be seen.[6, 9, 16]

TREATMENT

Patients with a deficiency of alpha$_2$–anti-plasmin may be treated with fresh-frozen plasma alone or in combination with a plasmin inhibitor, such as epsilon-aminocaproic acid or transexamic acid (cyclokapron).[6, 9]

Defects of Activators

Defective or excessive activation of plasminogen has been recently associated with thrombotic tendency. Defective activator activity has been described in a few families, and several members of these families show a lifelong tendency for thromboses. The main laboratory finding, from the stasis test or DDAVP infusion, was a decrease in activator release from veins. An increased level of activators described in one family, however, seems to be associated with a bleeding tendency.[16]

PLASMINOGEN ACTIVATOR DEFICIENCY

Tissue plasminogen activator is probably the most important plasminogen activator in blood vessels. It has a high affinity for fibrin and converts plasminogen to plasmin, primarily within the fibrin clot. Hereditary deficiency of tissue plasminogen activator release appears to be very rare. The congenital form was first reported in 1978 and is inherited through autosomal dominance. Patients with this deficiency characteristically lack plasminogen activator release in response to venous occlusion or DDAVP therapy. The clinical manifestations are similar to those noted with AT III, protein C, and protein S deficiencies and primarily consist of venous thrombotic disease.[6, 25, 28]

Congenital increases in plasminogen activator inhibitor have also been associated with familial thrombosis but seem to be rare. Plasminogen activator inhibitors serve to regulate fibrinolysis. Two such inhibitors have been purified and are characterized as plasma activator inhibitors I and II. Increased plasma activator inhibitor activity has been measured in a great variety of clinical conditions. Synthetic substrate methods for tissue plasminogen activator and assays for the inhibitor type I are now available to clinical laboratories. Inhibitor type I has been observed in patients with bladder carcinoma, cardiovascular disease, acute or idiopathic thromboembolic disease, hepatic insufficiency, and septicemia and in the postoperative period.[25, 28]

NATURAL INHIBITORS OF COAGULATION

Anti-thrombin III Deficiency

AT III is a single-chain alpha$_2$-globulin that plays an important role in blood coagulation. It is produced in the liver. AT III has mainly an anti–factors IIa and Xa activity and serves to halt the clotting cascade. It also inactivates other serine proteases, including factors IXa, XIa, and XIIa; activated protein C; and kallikrein. It is estimated that about 85% of thrombin potentially generated in plasma and most of the available factor Xa are neutralized by AT III. The primary physiologic target of AT III in preventing thrombus formation is factor Xa rather than thrombin. This action is enhanced considerably by the presence of heparin. In the presence of heparin, inactivation of thrombin and Xa by anti-thrombin III is markedly accelerated and almost instantaneous.[16, 24, 25, 28]

The first family known to have congenital AT III deficiency was seen in 1965 by Egeberg and associates. Since then, several other families have been described. The defect has been described in several parts of the world. AT III deficiency is one of the more common hypercoagulable states. Its incidence in the general population may be as high as 1/2000. The hereditary transmission is autosomal dominant but appears to be heterogeneous. Totally homozygous deficiency in humans is unknown and is most likely incompatible with survival beyond fetal life. The clinical picture is characterized by recurrent episodes of deep venous thrombosis with pulmonary embolization. Arterial thrombosis has only rarely been reported. The most common sites of thrombosis are deep veins of the lower extremities. These events typically appear in the mid to late teens.[16, 24, 25, 28]

The main laboratory finding is a moderate reduction of all AT III activities. The normal range of serum AT III level is 70–125% of reference populations. AT III antigen level is about 50% of normal in heterozygotes. Some patients have deep venous thrombosis and pulmonary emboli between 50% and 70% biologic activity. Crossed immunoelectrophoresis in the presence or absence of heparin shows a qualitatively normal pattern.[1, 6, 11, 16, 18, 28]

Qualitative abnormalities of AT III have been described in at least 15 families. The hereditary pattern is usually autosomal dominant, but variations in hereditary have also been described. Some variants represent a complex and severe AT III molecule defect; others show variably decreased AT III activity with an apparently normal reaction to heparin; still others show only an altered reaction to heparin (decreased or increased affinity). The clinical picture is similar to that of AT III deficiency, although in at least three families no thrombotic tendency has been reported. In two of these cases, the abnormality consisted mainly of a heparin cofactor defect. The main laboratory finding is a discrepancy between variably decreased AT III activity and a normal AT III antigen. The majority of patients with AT III abnormalities also show an abnormal pattern in the crossed immunoelectrophoretic system, usually in the presence of heparin but on occasion only in its absence.[16]

Infants have about half of normal adult AT III levels; however, the adult level is reached at an early age. The mechanisms by which a potential deficiency of AT III may occur are (1) a defect in synthesis that may occur in the congenital form, as well as in several acquired forms such as liver disease; (2) increased consumption of AT III, resulting from pathologic levels of serine proteases, as might be expected to occur in DIC-type syndromes, extensive deep venous thrombosis, massive pulmonary embolization, and diffuse small and large venous and arterial thrombo-occlusive events; (3) loss of AT III from the intracellular compartment, as may occur in certain forms of renal disease; and (4) increased protein catabolism.[6]

Long-term therapy with heparin alone may not prevent recurrent thrombosis. In a number of patients with hereditary AT III deficiency, death from extensive intravascular clotting occurred during heparin administration. In vitro heparin affects adversely the inhibitory capacity of AT III, enhancing its limited proteolysis by thrombin. For all these reasons, intravenous heparin therapy should not be given to patients with AT III deficiency unless normal plasma or AT III concentrates are administered concurrently. Warfarin is the drug of choice for long-term prophylaxis and should be used in dosages sufficient to maintain the PT from one and one-half to two times that of normal. Fresh-frozen plasma that contains AT III can be administered if anti-coagulation is contraindicated. Potent AT III concentrates are available for treating patients with hereditary AT III deficiency.[24, 25, 28]

Protein C Deficiency

Protein C is a vitamin K–dependent factor produced in the liver, and levels therefore decrease during coumarin therapy and/or in vitamin K deficiency. Once activated by thrombin, it acts as a potent inhibitor of activated factors V and VIII:C and, therefore, as an anti-coagulant in the clotting system. Thrombin, which activates protein C to protein Ca, is first bound to endothelial thrombomodulin; then thrombin acquires its ability to activate protein C.[16, 24, 25]

The key regulatory role of activated protein C in blood coagulation is the prevention of thrombin formation through degradation of the heavy chain of factor Va located on the outer surface of platelets, where it serves as the receptor site for factor Xa. By destroying factor Va, activated protein C not only limits further generation of thrombin but also makes factor Xa more accessible to inhibition by AT III. The inhibitory activity of protein C in degrading factors V and VIII:C is markedly enhanced by protein S. It seems also to enhance the fibrinolytic activity of blood. It inactivates a plasma inhibitor of tissue plasminogen activator thus enhancing tissue plasminogen activator release and activity.[16, 24, 25]

Congenital protein C deficiency may account for 6–10% of all patients presenting with venous thrombosis or pulmonary embolus. The normal range is 70–164%. A moderate decrease below 70% is associated with a thrombotic tendency. The hereditary pattern seems to be autosomal dominant, and as in the case of AT III defect, the homozygous state seems incompatible with life: the few patients described have died in infancy.[1, 6, 7, 24, 25]

Most heterozygous persons are at risk for the development of thromboembolic disease. The clinical picture is characterized by recurrent episodes of venous and, less frequently, arterial thrombosis. Three clinical syndromes are commonly attributed to congenital deficiency of protein C: (1) recurrent deep venous thrombosis and pulmonary embolus, happening typically in the late teens; (2) warfarin-induced skin necrosis (purpura fulminans syndrome); and (3) neonatal purpura fulminans. A protein C deficiency seems indistinguishable from that of AT III defect.[7, 16, 24, 28]

Generalized thrombotic manifestations appear in infants homozygous for protein C deficiency shortly after birth. This deficiency is invariably fatal unless protein C is administered by infusion of plasma or concentrates of factor IX that are rich in protein C. Infants with congenital homozygous protein C deficiency are subject to thrombosis of capillaries in association with DIC. This often fatal syndrome is termed *neonatal purpura fulminans*. Relatives of these infants who are heterozygous for the deficiency have usually been asymptomatic; in contrast, most persons heterozygous for protein C deficiency exhibit thrombotic tendencies. Heparin therapy in these infants is ineffective. Anti-coagulation with warfarin is an alternative to the replacement therapy. However, protein C levels drop rapidly when warfarin drugs are used. Only one protein C variant has been described so far.[7, 16, 24, 28]

Recurrent deep venous thrombosis and pulmonary embolus begin in the late teens. Two forms of the disease exist: a CRM⁻ form (absence of the protein) and a CRM⁺ form (a dysfunctional protein). Absence of the protein appears to be more common.[6]

Two immunologic assays are available for measuring two types of protein C. Both assays should be performed to distinguish the CRM⁺ from the CRM⁻ types. Immunologic assays include electroimmunoassay and enzyme-linked immunosorbent assay. It is preferred that both assays be performed, because dysfunctional protein C may otherwise not be detected. Preliminary estimations suggest that congenital protein C deficiency is more common than AT III deficiency and may account for up to 10% of patients presenting with venous thrombosis or pulmonary embolus.[3, 6, 18, 28]

Long-term warfarin therapy has been effective in management. Factor IX concentrates are rich in protein C and have been effective in a number of cases.[18]

Protein S Deficiency

Protein S deficiency was first reported in 1984. With improved laboratory tests for detecting the deficiency, it now appears to be quite common. The function of activated protein C depends to an extent on the presence in plasma of protein S, an additional vitamin K–dependent glycoprotein. Protein S is synthesized by both hepatocytes and megakaryocytes. It serves as a cofactor-enhancing proteolysis of factor Va by activated protein C. Partial deficiency of protein S has been detected in several patients with recurrent thrombosis, and inheritance is thought to be autosomal dominant. Half or more of the heterozygotes have symptomatic thrombotic problems. Homozygotes are severely affected and may exhibit a form of purpura fulminans shortly after birth, similar to that seen with protein C defects. The clinical characteristics appear to be similar to those of congenital AT III and protein C deficiencies. An asymptomatic deficiency state also exists.[6, 7, 24, 25, 28]

The incidence of the deficiency is similar to that for protein C deficiency: about 5–10% of young patients with unexplained venous thrombosis. Protein S exists in plasma in two forms: in 40% of patients, as free protein S, and in 60%, as protein S bound to C4b-binding protein, a component linked to the complement system. The normal range for protein S levels on functional assays is between 63% and 160%. Protein S levels lower than 60% of normal are associated with thrombotic complications. Protein S is active only in the free form, in which it varies quantitatively in individual patients and may decrease considerably in some clinical disorders such as systemic lupus erythematosus. Of the immunologic methods for testing for protein S deficiency, crossed immunoelectrophoresis is most helpful, enabling distinction between the free and bound fractions.[6, 7, 24, 25, 28]

Coumarin-induced skin necrosis is not common

in protein S–deficient patients, probably because protein S has a longer half-life than protein C.[3]

Protein S deficiency exists in two forms: quantitative and qualitative. The majority of persons with protein S deficiency appear to have normal or moderately reduced levels of total protein S antigen, which suggests that the functional protein S deficiency involves the qualitative distribution of protein S between free and bound forms and not an abnormality of the protein S per se.[2, 28]

A classification of the congenital protein S deficiencies based on free protein S, total protein S, and protein S activity levels has been suggested:[29]

Type	Free Protein S	Protein S Activity	Total Protein S
I	Low	Low	Low
IIa	Low	Low	Normal
IIb	Normal	Low	Normal

The mode of inheritance of the type I defect is autosomal dominant.[13]

The treatment of the clotting states related to protein C and protein S deficiencies involves the administration of fresh-frozen plasma or factor IX concentrate. Long-term warfarin or long-term heparin therapy may be appropriate chronic treatment.[25, 28]

Heparin Cofactor II Deficiency

A second heparin-dependent inhibitor of thrombin, distinct from AT III (which is heparin cofactor I), was first identified in 1974. Heparin cofactor II is a glycoprotein that is synthesized by the liver. Like that of AT III, inhibitory activity of heparin cofactor II is markedly accelerated by addition of heparin. In contrast to AT III, heparin cofactor II has a very narrow substrate: only thrombin and chymotrypsin are neutralized efficiently. There appears to be no inhibitory activity against factors Xa, IXa, and XIa. Heparin cofactor II deficiency has thus far proved to be a rare congenital cause of thrombotic disorders. The congenital deficiency was first reported in a patient with left middle cerebral artery thrombosis and a heparin cofactor II level 50% of normal. The clinical manifestations of hereditary heparin cofactor II deficiency can span from arterial or venous thrombosis to asymptomatic states. Many heterozygous patients with the deficiency have been identified and have not yet suffered thrombotic or thromboembolic events. Affected persons may not show symptoms until their fourth decade. Levels of heparin cofactor II have been found to be decreased in most patients with liver disease and in some patients with DIC. Many assays have become available for assessing heparin cofactor II activity in the clinical laboratory. Treatment should be similar to that outlined for AT III deficiency.[6, 25, 28]

Factor XII and Other Contact Factor Deficiencies

Mr. Hageman, who was the index case of factor XII deficiency, died in his early 50s of a massive pulmonary embolus. He was reported to have mild aortic atherosclerosis. Other patients with deficiencies of factor XII have also exhibited thromboembolic phenomena. Persons heterozygous or homozygous for deficiencies of contact factors may be at increased risk for thromboembolic events related to decreased activation of the fibrinolytic system; however, this is yet to be proved. The initial contact activation of factor XII results in the activation of the clotting cascade with generation of thrombin. In addition, plasmin is generated, and the inflammatory response with the generation of kinins, complement, and thromboxane is initiated. Studies of 121 patients with factor XII deficiency showed that 10 (8.2%) experienced thrombotic episodes.[7, 25]

DYSFIBRINOGENEMIAS

Most persons reported to have dysfibrinogens have a bleeding tendency or a thromboembolic disorder or are asymptomatic. A minority, approximately 11%, of the reported patients with dysfibrinogenemias, have clinical features of a recurrent thromboembolic disorder.[1, 25]

Patients with recurrent thrombosis have been reported with any of several functional abnormalities of fibrinogen: defective release of fibrinopeptides A or B or both, defective polymerization of fibrin monomers, and increased resistance to proteolysis by plasmin. The most commonly observed functional defect of the dysfibrinogenemias associated with thrombosis is an abnormality of fibrin monomer polymerization with resistance to fibrinolysis. The fibrinogen associated with thrombosis exhibits decreased binding of plasminogen or a resistance to lysis by plasmin.[1, 25]

The congenital dysfibrinogenemias associated with thrombosis account for about 1% of unexplained venous thromboses occurring in young persons. Both venous and arterial thromboses have been reported in patients with this disease. Patients may have a prolonged PT; in addition, the thrombin time is routinely prolonged. Further assessment with the reptilase test and specific fibrinogen functional assays confirms the diagnosis.

Warfarin may be used to treat thrombosis associated with dysfibrinogenemia.[25]

More than 100 qualitative abnormalities of fibrinogen (dysfibrinogenemia) have been reported. Dysfibrinogenemias are inherited through autosomal dominance; most patients are heterozygous.

ACQUIRED CLOTTING STATES

Acquired hypercoagulable states—those secondary to underlying conditions—are far more common than hereditary forms. Whether a documented hypercoagulable state, such as deficiency of AT III or protein C, is inherited or acquired is important because it affects decisions concerning further clinical investigations and has implications in regard to the validity of the diagnosis itself.[26, 28]

AT III and protein C deficiencies may occur as acquired hypercoagulable states secondary to such conditions as nephrotic syndrome (usually associated with proteinuria), pregnancy, diabetes mellitus, hyperlipidemia, malignancy, and DIC. Oral contraceptives have been reported as decreasing AT III levels, although the research findings are still unclear. Acquired AT III deficiencies are usually caused by consumption of AT III. Chronic liver disease may also lead to an AT III deficiency.[6, 7, 13, 26, 28]

Acquired deficiencies of proteins C and S are commonly seen in patients with DIC, extensive deep venous thrombosis, severe liver disease, and nephrotic syndrome and in patients taking warfarin. In addition, protein C levels may be decreased in the postoperative period, but the role of this decrease in contributing to or causing postoperative deep thrombosis remains unclear. Acquired protein S deficiency also occurs in women using oral contraceptives and in patients with type I diabetes mellitus.[6, 7, 13, 26, 28]

Acquired plasminogen deficiency is seen in patients with severe liver disease and in those with DIC. In addition, decreased plasminogen levels are noted postoperatively after trauma, and in patients with extensive thrombotic or thromboembolic disorders. The deficiency is also found in some infants and adults with respiratory distress syndrome (hyaline membrane disease).[1, 6, 26, 28]

Acquired deficiency of plasminogen activator has been reported in many pathologic conditions, such as unstable angina, acute myocardial infarction, ulcerative colitis, and Crohn's disease. Tissue plasminogen activator activity also decreases with alcohol ingestion and use of estrogen-containing oral contraceptives.[6, 7, 13, 26, 28]

Other thrombosis-inducing clinical conditions include

1. Disorders resulting in *tissue and cellular damage* such as transfusion reactions, surgery, burns, and direct trauma. Tissue necrosis may result in tissue death, which starts a vicious cycle of systemic thrombosis.[25]

2. *Drug-induced hypercoagulability.* Certain chronically administered drugs such as estrogen have been linked to an increased incidence of thrombotic conditions in young women. Drug reactions and interactions can cause intravascular clotting. The risk rises exponentially in relation to the number of medications used. Heparin therapy induces development of an anti-platelet antibody in about 5% of patients. This antibody is now known to be responsible for the thrombotic manifestations after anti-coagulation with heparin. The skin necrosis associated with the initiation of anti-coagulation with warfarin is now believed to be related to the impact of this drug on protein C and protein S. The infusion of prothombin complex can also activate clotting intermediates and is linked to an increased risk of thrombosis.[25]

3. *Disease-induced hypercoagulability.* Blood dyscrasias, particularly those associated with conditions of increased blood viscosity such as polycythemia and leukemia (acute promyelocytic), are well-documented conditions associated with a thrombotic tendency. Measures directed at lowering viscosity such as blood-letting should be used to modify this tendency. In leukemia patients with very high white blood cell counts (greater than $100,000/mm^3$), leukocytes can apparently aggregate or become enclosed in a fibrin mesh, obstructing the microvasculature in vital organs such as the brain. This appears to be more common in patients with myeloid leukemias, particularly myeloblastic, and has been partly attributed to the rigidity of the cell membranes of myeloid precursor cells in comparison with those of other cells.[7, 13, 25]

Hyperviscosity caused by abnormal plasma proteins can lead to thrombosis in small blood vessels. These proteins are usually immunoglobulins that occur in such disorders as Waldenström's macroglobulinemia (IgM), multiple myeloma, and other malignant lymphoproliferative disorders.[7, 13, 25]

Disseminated cancer and some myeloproliferative disorders, such as Budd-Chiari syndrome, are inducers of clotting. Other states of condition-induced hypercoagulability include paroxysmal nocturnal hemoglobinuria, diabetes, hyperlipidemias, systemic lupus erythematosus, and the postpartum period. The presence of lupus anti-coagulants, DIC, atherosclerotic cardiovascular disease, prosthetic heart valves and vascular grafts, congestive heart failure, obesity, and septic states (particularly gram-negative sepsis) are also conditions predisposing to thrombosis.[1, 4, 7, 13, 25]

Another condition associated with hypercoagulability is homocystinemia, an inborn error of me-tabolism caused by a deficiency of the enzyme cystathione synthase, which leads to an accumulation of homocystine in the plasma and tissues. When homocystine is secreted in the urine, the condition is referred to as homocystinuria.[1, 4, 7]

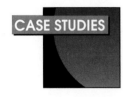

CASE STUDIES

A 20-year-old white woman came in for outpatient laboratory testing after a visit to her physician. She had bruises on her lower legs, arms, and hands. In addition, she noted that if she cut herself, perhaps while cooking or shaving her legs, she seemed to bleed profusely.

Her physician was unaware that she was a chronic alcoholic and had begun drinking at the age of 15. She drank approximately a six pack of beer each evening.

On drawing the patient's blood, the technologist noted a few "track" marks on her arm.

Coagulation Testing Data

PT	22 seconds
Platelet count	100,000/mm³
Activated PTT	50 seconds
Bleeding time	10 minutes

1. Identify the abnormal coagulation test results.

2. Describe the effects that alcohol may have on hemostasis.

3. Identify any follow-up tests that should be ordered related to the abnormal coagulation tests.

4. Describe any follow-up therapy related to correcting coagulation defects.

5. Describe any further laboratory tests that should be ordered.

6. Explain the significance of the tracks on the arm and any special precautions that should be followed.

References

1. Thorup OA: Leavell and Thorup's Fundamentals of Clinical Hematology, 5th ed. Philadelphia: WB Saunders, 1987.
2. Harmening DM: Clinical Hematology and Fundamentals of Hemostasis, 2nd ed. Philadelphia: FA Davis, 1992.
3. Williams WJ, et al. Hematology, 4th ed. New York: McGraw-Hill, 1990.
4. Thompson AR, Harker LA: Manual of Hemostasis and Thrombosis, 3rd ed. Philadelphia: FA Davis, 1983.
5. Miale JB: Laboratory Medicine Hematology, 6th ed. St. Louis: CV Mosby, 1982.
6. Powers LW: Diagnostic Hematology: Clinical and Technical Principles. St. Louis: CV Mosby, 1989.
7. Corriveau DM, Fritsma GA: Hemostasis and Thrombosis in the Clinical Laboratory. Philadelphia: JB Lippincott, 1988.
8. Sirridge MS, Shannon R: Laboratory Evaluation of Hemostasis and Thrombosis, 3rd ed. Philadelphia: Lea & Febiger, 1983.
9. Triplett DA: Hemostasis: A Case Oriented Approach. New York: Igaku-Shoin, 1985.
10. Quick AJ: Hemorrhagic Diseases and Thrombosis, 2nd ed. Philadelphia: Lea & Febiger, 1966.
11. Triplett DA: Laboratory Evaluation of Coagulation. Chicago: American Society of Clinical Pathologists, 1982.
12. Moake JL, Funicella T: Common bleeding problems. Clin Symp 1983; 35:1–32.
13. Rappaport SI: Introduction to Hematology, 2nd ed. Philadelphia: JB Lippincott, 1987.
14. Thomas JG, Powell DEB: Blood Disorders in the Elderly. Bristol, Great Britain: J Write, 1971.
15. Brown BA: Hematology: Principles and Procedures, 5th Ed. Philadelphia: Lea & Febiger, 1988.
16. Ruggeri ZM (ed): Coagulation disorders. Clin Haematol 1985; 14:281–599.
17. Gastineau DA, Gertz MA, Daniels TM, et al: Inhibitor of the thrombin time in systemic amyloidosis: a common coagulation abnormality. Blood 1991; 77:2637–2640.
18. Lotspeich-Steininger CA, Stiene-Martin EA, Koepke JA: Clinical Hematology: Principles, Procedures, Correlations. Philadelphia: JB Lippincott, 1992.
19. Bick RL, Scates SM: Disseminated intravascular coagulation. Lab Med 1992; 23:161–166.
20. Gurewich V: Disseminated Intravascular Coagulation [monograph]. Miami, FL: American Hospital Supply, 1978.
21. Green D: Diagnosis and management of bleeding disorders. Comp Ther 1988; 14:31–36.
22. Beardsley DS: Hemostasis in the perinatal period: approach to the diagnosis of coagulation disorders. Semin Perinatal 1991; 15:25–34.
23. Saxena R, Saraya AK, Kotte VK, et al: Evaluation of four coagulation tests to detect plasma lupus anticoagulants. Am J Clin Pathol 1991; 96:755–758.

24. Marciniak E: Genetic coagulation defects. Adv Exp Med Biol 1987; 214:175–186.
25. Blaisdell FW: Acquired and congenital clotting syndromes. World J Surg 1990; 14:664–669.
26. Joist JH: Hypercoagulability: introduction and perspective. Semin Thromb Hemost 1990; 16:151–157.
27. Ansell JE: Hypercoagulability: a conceptual and diagnostic approach. Am Heart J 1987; 114(4, Part 1):910–913.
28. Bick RL, Kunkel L: Hypercoagulability and thrombosis. Lab Med 1992; 23:233–236.
29. Comp P: Laboratory evaluation of protein S status. Semin Thromb Hemost 1990; 16:178.

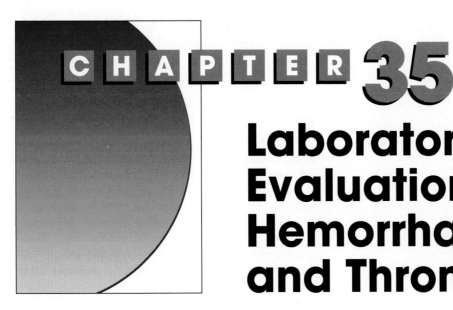

CHAPTER 35

Laboratory Evaluation of Hemorrhage and Thrombosis

George A. Fritsma

Outline

Objectives

AFTER COMPLETION OF THIS CHAPTER, THE READER WILL BE ABLE TO

1. Develop and execute laboratory protocols for hemostasis specimen collection and management.
2. Select appropriate hemostasis laboratory test protocols.
3. Develop and execute laboratory protocols for hemostasis laboratory tests.
4. Observe strict quality assurance principles in performing hemostasis laboratory tests.
5. List circumstances that interfere with clinical interpretation of hemostasis laboratory tests.
6. Communicate the clinical significance of hemostasis laboratory test results.
7. Transmit accurate hemostasis laboratory test reports.

SPECIMEN COLLECTION IN HEMOSTASIS

Most hemostasis laboratory procedures require plasma from a whole blood specimen collected by venipuncture and mixed with a solution of sodium citrate anti-coagulant. Phlebotomists, technologists, and other personnel who collect blood specimens are required to adhere closely to special protocols for the collection, transport, and management of these specimens. The laboratory supervisor is responsible for the current validity of specimen collection and handling protocols and ensures that personnel employ approved techniques.[1]

Patient Management in Hemostasis Specimen Collection

Patients need not fast unless lipemia is anticipated, and no other special patient preparation is required before collection of hemostasis laboratory specimens. Blood collection personnel may manage patients by standard protocol, but if there is a reason to anticipate a bleeding disorder, for example, if the patient has multiple bruises or mentions a tendency to bleed, the phlebotomist should observe the puncture site for several minutes after venipuncture and apply a pressure bandage before dismissing the patient.

Evacuated Hemostasis Specimen Collection Tubes

Most hemostasis specimens are collected in evacuated blue-stoppered sterile blood collection tubes such as Vacutainer (Becton Dickinson, Cockeysville, MD) or Venoject (Terumo, Elkton, MD) brands, containing buffered sodium citrate anti-coagulant.[2] The interior of the tubes and surface of the stoppers are coated with "nonwettable" plastic or silicone. Tubes made from uncoated soda lime or soft glass are unsuitable because they develop a negative surface charge that activates platelets and plasma procoagulants. Certain rules are observed in collection of hemostasis specimens:

■ The blue-stoppered sodium citrate anti-coagulant hemostasis specimen is not the first tube collected because the needle tip accumulates tissue thromboplastin from nonvascular tissue as it passes into the vein, particularly if the venipuncture is traumatic. Thromboplastin activates platelets and plasma procoagulants and shortens coagulation times.
■ If the hemostasis specimen is drawn as part of a series of evacuated tubes from one venipuncture site, it must be the second or third tube in the series, not the last.
■ If the hemostasis specimen is drawn as part of a series of evacuated tubes from one venipuncture site, it must not follow a tube containing heparin, ethylenediaminetetraacetic acid (EDTA), or sodium fluoride, because these may contaminate the specimen and invalidate the results.

■ If the hemostasis specimen is collected alone, it should be preceded by an additive-free "discard" tube into which at least 2 mL of blood is collected from the venipuncture site.

■ At least 90% of the intended whole blood collection volume must be reached. Many sodium citrate tubes are designed to draw 4.5 mL of whole blood to mix with 0.5 mL of sodium citrate contained within. A "short" specimen is any specimen in which less than 90% (4.05 mL in this example) of intended blood volume is drawn. Short specimens must be discarded and a new specimen collected, since the ratio of anticoagulant to plasma in an underfilled tube is increased to a degree that the anticoagulant may prolong test results.

■ Clotted specimens are useless for hemostasis testing. A few seconds after collection the citrate specimen must be inverted gently several times to mix the blood and anti-coagulant and prevent clot formation. Further, the specimen must be visually reexamined just before testing.

■ Agitation causes procoagulant and platelet activation and hemolysis and must be avoided.

■ The results of hemolyzed and lipemic specimens are unreliable using both optical and electromechanical instrumentation. If circumstances dictate that a hemolyzed or lipemic specimen must be used in testing, the technologist appends a note to the report describing the specimen's condition.

■ Excess manipulation of the needle promotes release of tissue thromboplastin, contaminating the specimen and causing procoagulant activation.

■ Slowed or stopped venous circulation, called stasis, results in local concentration of factor VIII/von Willebrand's factor (VWF). Both stasis and tissue fluid contamination may result in false shortening of clot-based coagulation test results, so sparing use of a tourniquet and nontraumatic puncture are essential.[3]

Managers of many specialized hemostasis laboratories insist that specimens from patients from whom blood is difficult to draw and specimens for specialized tests such as platelet aggregometry be collected by syringe, as described in the following section. Many hemostasis laboratories employ technologists and phlebotomists who are specially trained for specimen collection to ensure the integrity of the specimen.

Two-Syringe Hemostasis Specimen Collection

Although it is impractical for high-volume hemostasis screening, the syringe is preferred to the evacuated tube for collecting hemostasis specimens from patients whose veins are small or fragile or who require specialized hemostasis testing such as factor assays or platelet aggregometry. To collect by syringe, the phlebotomist selects sterile syringes with nonthreaded "Luer-slip" hubs and draws a specific volume of anti-coagulant: typically, 10-mL syringes are first charged with 1.0 mL of anti-coagulant. The technologist assembles the prefilled syringes, a scalp vein infusion apparatus, commonly known as a "butterfly" needle set (Fig. 35–1), a tube clamp, standard venipuncture materials, and test tubes. The anti-coagulant may be measured into the test tube rather than the syringe. The phlebotomist then uses the following protocol:

1. Fit the hub end of the needle set loosely to the hub of a 3-mL "discard" syringe.
2. Prepare the patient for venipuncture, then insert the needle. Immobilize the needle set tubing by loosely taping it to the arm about 2 inches below the needle.
3. Remove the tourniquet, then slowly withdraw 2 or 3 mL of blood.
4. Lay the syringe on a clean surface, and clamp the tube near the hub.
5. Remove the 3-mL syringe from the needle set hub and replace it with the hemostasis specimen syringe, taking care to prevent spillage of blood from the needle set.
6. Release the clamp and collect the hemostasis specimen gently. If the syringe is charged with anti-coagulant, mix the anti-coagulant and blood gently with a rotating motion while withdrawing the plunger.
7. Continue to collect blood with additional syringes as needed and complete the venipuncture.

Having seen to the patient's welfare, the phlebotomist transfers the blood specimen to an open, nonwettable tube by slowly pushing the plunger and allowing the specimen to flow gently down the side. The specimen is not forcibly squirted since agitation causes hemolysis and platelet activation. If the anti-coagulant is in the test tube instead of the syringe, the transfer must be accomplished within a few seconds of the time the syringe is filled and the tube must be covered and gently inverted to mix.

Choosing Needles for Hemostasis Specimens

Whether using evacuated collection tubes or syringes, the bore of the needle should be sufficient to prevent activation of platelets and plasma procoagulants. If the overall specimen is less than or equal to 25 mL, a 20-gauge or 21-gauge thin-walled

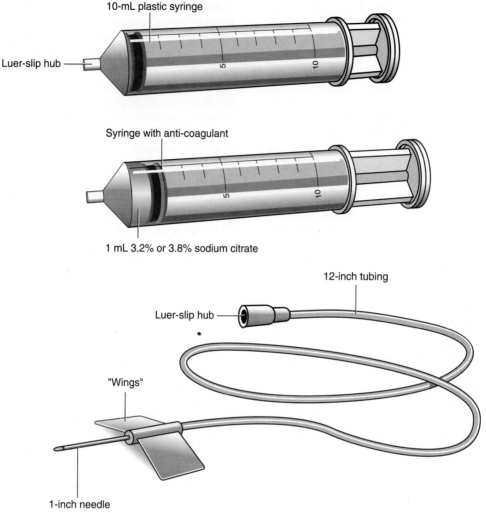

Figure 35–1 Blood collection apparatus for hemostasis specimens.

needle is used. For a larger specimen, a 19-gauge needle is used. A 23-gauge needle is acceptable for pediatric patients or patients whose veins are small.

Indwelling Catheters

Many indwelling catheters are coated with heparin, which contaminates the specimen and invalidates hemostasis results. Before blood is collected for hemostasis testing, the line should be flushed with saline and the first 5 mL of blood collected and discarded.

Capillary Punctures

The Biotrack 512 coagulation monitor (Ciba-Corning Diagnostics, Medfield, MA) and the Thrombolytic Assessment System (Cardiovascular Diagnostics, Durham, NC) provide small-volume capillary techniques for measuring prothrombin

time (PT) and activated partial thromboplastin time (APTT). The techniques compare favorably with standard techniques[4] and provide the capability for point of care and neonatal testing.[5]

Anti-Coagulants for Hemostasis Specimens

BUFFERED SODIUM CITRATE

The only anti-coagulant used for hemostasis testing is 3.2% (0.109 M) or 3.8% (0.129 M) buffered sodium citrate ($Na_3C_6H_5O_7 \cdot 2H_2O$). Sodium citrate binds free calcium ions, while the buffer stabilizes the pH. The anti-coagulant concentration is chosen on the basis of clinical preference. Whether 3.2% or 3.8% sodium citrate is used, the anti-coagulant solution is mixed with blood to produce a 1:10 ratio; 1 part anti-coagulant to 10 parts final solution (9 parts blood). In most cases, 0.5 mL of anti-coagulant is mixed with 4.5 mL of whole blood, the volumes in the most commonly used evacuated collection tubes, but any volumes are valid provided the 1:10 ratio is maintained. The ratio yields a final citrate concentration of 10.9 or 12.9 mmol/L of anti-coagulant in whole blood.

ADJUSTING ANTI-COAGULANT VOLUME FOR HEMATOCRIT

The 1:10 ratio is effective provided the hematocrit is nearly normal. In polycythemia, the decrease in plasma volume relative to whole blood unacceptably raises the anti-coagulant to plasma ratio, causing falsely prolonged clot-based coagulation test results. The technologist provides a tube with a reduced volume of anti-coagulant for collecting blood from a patient whose hematocrit is known to be greater than or equal to 55%. The amount of anti-coagulant needed may be computed for a 5-mL total volume specimen from the graph in Figure 35–2 or by using the following formula, which may be used for any total volume:

$$C = 1.85 \times 10^{-3} (100 - H)\, V$$

where C = volume of sodium citrate in milliliters, V = volume of whole blood–sodium citrate solution in milliliters, and H = hematocrit in percent. There is no evidence to support the need for adding anti-coagulant in anemia.

EDTA AND HEPARIN

Like sodium citrate, disodium (dry) or tripotassium (liquid) EDTA bind free plasma calcium; however, neither type of EDTA is suitable as an anti-coagulant for most hemostasis specimens be-cause factor V is unstable. Furthermore, EDTA inhibits the thrombin-mediated conversion of fibrinogen to fibrin and binds reagent calcium that is added to initiate clot-based tests. EDTA is used for complete blood cell counts, including platelet counts. Heparin, which is used routinely for clinical chemistry specimen collection, is unsuitable as an anti-coagulant for hemostasis tests because it inhibits thrombin and factors XIIa, XIa, Xa, and IXa.

HEMOSTASIS SPECIMEN MANAGEMENT

Hemostasis Specimen Transport and Storage

Specimens collected with sodium citrate for the hemostasis laboratory are kept stoppered to maintain pH and are held in a vertical position with the stopper uppermost. Specimens collected for platelet function tests, such as platelet aggregometry, are maintained at ambient temperature, never chilled. Specimens collected for clot-based plasma tests, such as PT or APTT, may be maintained at ambient temperature or placed in melting ice during transport. Chilling stabilizes the activity of labile procoagulant factors V and VIII but activates factor VII, so its effect in specimens for the PT is equivocal. Specimens collected for special coagulation tests are usually chilled, except in factor VII assays. Specimens maintained at ambient temperatures must be tested within 2 hours of collection, while chilled specimens may be held for up to 4 hours. If the specimen cannot be tested within this interval, it should be centrifuged, the plasma transferred by plastic pipette to a nonwettable

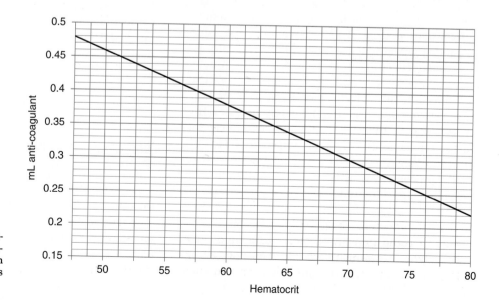

Figure 35–2 Graph for computing the volume of anti-coagulant in a 5-mL specimen when the patient's hematocrit is ≥55%.

tube, stoppered, quick-frozen, and stored at −20 °C for up to 2 weeks or −70 °C for up to 6 months.

Preparation of Hemostasis Specimens for Testing

WHOLE BLOOD

Whole blood platelet aggregometry and lumiaggregometry require at least 4.5 mL of blood collected in 0.5 mL sodium citrate and held at ambient temperature until testing. Chilling diminishes platelet activity. Platelets may be unresponsive in a specimen tested between 0 and 30 minutes after collection, so aggregometry is begun after the specimen has stood for 30 minutes but must be completed before 3 hours has elapsed from the time of specimen collection. The technologist mixes the specimen by gentle inversion, simultaneously checks for clots just before testing, and rejects specimens with clots.

PLATELET-RICH PLASMA

Many aggregometers are designed to test platelet-rich plasma (PRP), or plasma containing platelets at a concentration of $250–300 \times 10^9$/L. Sodium citrate–anti-coagulated whole blood is first visually checked for clots and then centrifuged at 50 g for 30 minutes with the stopper in place to maintain the pH. The supernatant plasma is transferred by plastic pipette to a clean plastic or siliconized tube, and the tube is sealed and stored at ambient temperature until the test is begun. Aggregometry is performed on PRP 30 minutes to 3 hours after the specimen is collected.

PLATELET-POOR PLASMA

Most clot-based plasma coagulation tests require platelet-poor plasma (PPP). Sodium citrate–anti-coagulated whole blood is first checked visually for clots, then centrifuged at 2500 g for 15 minutes with the stopper in place. The supernatant PPP is transferred with a plastic pipette to a clean non-wettable tube and tested immediately or quick-frozen for later testing. The technologist inspects the plasma for hemolysis, lipemia, and icterus. Hemolysis and lipemia may indicate platelet activation or plasma procoagulant activity or may interfere with end-point determination, so the specimen is rejected and a new specimen collected. Icterus may affect photometrically determined end points.

Quick-freezing prevents deterioration of plasma procoagulants. Specimens should be pipetted in small aliquots for quick freezing and placed in vials that are designed to withstand cold. Specimens stored at −20 °C must be tested within 2 weeks of collection, while specimens stored at −70 °C are good for 6 months. The technologist rapidly thaws frozen plasma specimens at 37 °C and tests them immediately.

PLATELET-FREE PLASMA

Tests for the lupus anti-coagulant (anti-phospholipid antibody) require platelet-free plasma (PFP), which is plasma with a platelet count of less than 10×10^9/L.[6] The technologist filters PPP through a 0.22-μm cellulose acetate syringe filter such as the Acrodisc (Gelman Sciences, Ann Arbor, MI) before testing. Double centrifugation is also effective.

PLATELET FUNCTION TESTS

A conscientious hemostasis laboratory protocol requires that the platelet count and a blood film examination be performed before commencing a series of expensive and complex platelet function tests, since thrombocytopenia is the most common cause of platelet-associated hemorrhage.[7] Qualitative platelet abnormalities are suspected only when systemic hemorrhagic symptoms such as easy bruising, petechiae, purpura, or epistaxis are present and the platelet count is at or near the reference interval. Hereditary platelet function disorders are extremely rare; however, acquired disorders, associated with hemorrhage and thrombosis, are common. Acquired defects are often associated with myeloproliferative disorders and myelodysplastic syndromes, myeloma, uremia, autoimmune disorders, anemias, and drug therapy. Platelet morphology is often a clue; for example, Bernard-Soulier syndrome is associated with mild thrombocytopenia and large platelets. On the other hand, large platelets are indicative of rapid platelet turnover, such as in immune thrombocytopenic purpura, and giant or bizarre platelets are seen in myeloproliferative disorders, acute leukemia, and myelodysplastic syndromes.

Bleeding Time Test for Platelet Function

The bleeding time (BT) test is occasionally helpful for diagnosing an unknown bleeding disorder.[8] The adhesion and aggregation components of platelet function are assessed by recording the duration of bleeding from a controlled puncture wound. Results are also prolonged in vascular disease such as scurvy or vasculitis.

Early approaches to BT tests by Duke in 1910[9] and by Ivy[10] in 1941 allowed the critical nonplatelet variables of intracapillary pressure, skin thickness at the puncture site, and size and depth of the wound to cause profound variation. In the current method, the technologist places a blood pressure cuff on the upper arm and inflates it to 40 mm Hg to control intracapillary pressure. A site on the volar surface of the forearm near the antecubital crease is selected and prepared. The skin thickness in this area varies only slightly from one individual to another so the results are comparable provided the area is free of superficial blood vessels, rashes, hair, and scar tissue. A spring-loaded BT lancet that produces a standard wound 5 mm long and 1 mm deep is placed firmly on the site parallel to the long axis of the arm and triggered. Simplate (Organon Teknika, Durham, NC) or Surgicutt (International Technidyne, Edison, NJ) are suitable BT lancets. A stopwatch is started at the same time.[11] The technologist safely discards the lancet and blots the wound with filter paper every 30 seconds, taking care that the paper contacts only the blood and not the wound. Blotting continues until the bleeding stops, then the watch is stopped and the interval is recorded. The technologist must place a pressure bandage over the site to reduce scarring.

The reference range for the standardized lancet BT is 2–9 minutes. The BT is prolonged in thrombocytopenia, hereditary and acquired platelet dysfunction, von Willebrand's disease, afibrinogenemia, severe hypofibrinogenemia, and vascular disorders. A single dose of aspirin will cause a measurable prolongation of the BT in about 50% of normal individuals.[12] Many other drugs may give prolonged results.

Platelet Aggregometry and Lumiaggregometry

Functional platelets adhere to subendothelial collagen, aggregate with each other, and secrete the contents of their alpha granules, lysosomes, and dense bodies. Normal adhesion requires intact platelet membranes and plasma VWF, whereas aggregation requires intact platelet membranes, normal plasma fibrinogen, and normal secretion from platelet organelles. Platelet adhesion, aggregation, and secretion are assessed in vitro through platelet aggregometry.

An aggregometer is an instrument designed to measure platelet aggregation in a suspension of citrated whole blood or PRP. The specimen is collected and managed in compliance with laboratory protocol and maintained at ambient temperature until testing begins. Specimens for aggregometry may first stand 30 minutes after collection while the platelets regain their responsiveness and must be tested within 3 hours to avoid deterioration of labile plasma and platelet procoagulants. After electronically calibrating the instrument in accordance with manufacturer instructions, the operator prepares controls and specimens, pipettes them to instrument-compatible cuvettes, drops in plasticized stir bars, and allows the specimens to warm to 37 °C for 10 minutes in incubation wells before testing. The operator transfers the first cuvette, containing specimen and stir bar, to the instrument's reaction well and starts the stirring device and recording device, often a chart with a pen recorder. The stirring device turns the stir bar at 800–1200 rpm, keeping the platelets in suspension. After a few seconds, an agonist (aggregating agent) is forcibly pipetted into the specimen to start the reaction. Aggregation is complete in 6–10 minutes. The operator then prepares to retest the next specimen cuvette with another agonist.

AGGREGOMETRY WITH PLATELET-RICH PLASMA

PRP aggregometry is performed using an aggregometer that is a specialized photometer. PRP is prepared and adjusted to a count of approximately $300 \times 10^9/L$ by mixing with PPP. The adjusted PRP is placed in a cuvette equipped with a stir bar, warmed to 37 °C, and transferred to the reaction well. Focused white light is directed through the sample cuvette to a photomultiplier. As the PRP is stirred the pen first stabilizes to form the baseline, near 0% transmission. In a normal specimen, after the agonist is added, the platelets' shape changes from discoid to spherical. The intensity of the transmitted light increases slightly in proportion to the degree of shape change. Percent transmittance is continuously monitored and recorded on the strip chart (Fig. 35-3). As platelet aggregates form, more light passes through the PRP and the pen begins to move toward 100% light transmission. Abnormalities are reflected in diminished or absent shape change and aggregation.

WHOLE BLOOD AGGREGOMETRY

In whole blood aggregometry, platelet aggregation is measured by impedance in a saline-diluted whole blood suspension. Parallel electrodes that produce a small current are lowered into the blood suspension. As aggregation occurs, platelets collect on the electrodes, changing the magnitude of the current. The change is directly proportional to the level of platelet aggregation and is amplified and recorded by the instrument. The appearance of a

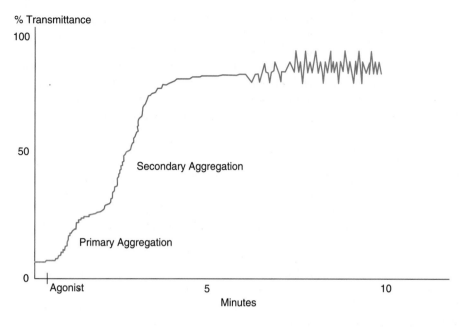

Figure 35-3 Normal aggregometry tracing.

whole blood aggregometry tracing resembles a PRP tracing. Whole blood aggregometry eliminates the need for PRP preparation. The operator pipettes an aliquot of properly mixed whole blood to the cuvette and adds an equal volume of physiologic saline and a stir bar. After 10 minutes, when the specimen has warmed to 37 °C, it is placed in the reaction well, the agonist is added, and the electrodes are suspended within the mixture. A recording device produces an aggregation pattern, such as that shown in Figure 35-3.

LUMIAGGREGOMETRY

The lumiaggregometer may be used to simultaneously measure platelet aggregation and secretion.[13] The procedure for lumiaggregometry differs little from conventional aggregometry and simplifies the diagnosis of platelet dysfunction. The instrument (available from Chrono-log, Havertown, PA) records both aggregation and secretion of dense granule adenosine triphosphate (ATP) that reacts with "firefly luciferin" (Chronolume, Chrono-log, Havertown, PA) to give chemiluminescence. The resulting light emission is detected, amplified, and recorded by the instrument.

Lumiaggregometry may be performed using whole blood or PRP. To perform lumiaggregometry, the operator adds an ATP standard to the first aliquot of specimen, then adds luciferin and tests for full luminescence. A second aliquot is prepared with the luciferin, an agonist is then added, and the specimen is monitored simultaneously for aggregation and secretion. Thrombin is the first agonist used because thrombin induces full secretion independent of the prostaglandin or cyclooxygenase pathway.

Luminescence induced by thrombin addition is measured, recorded, and used for comparison with the luminescence produced by other weaker agonists. Normal secretion induced by other agonists produces luminescence at about 50% of that resulting from thrombin stimulation. Figure 35-4 depicts simultaneous aggregation and secretion responses to epinephrine.

AGONISTS USED IN AGGREGOMETRY

The agonists used most are thrombin, adenosine diphosphate (ADP), epinephrine, collagen, arachidonic acid, and ristocetin. Table 35-1 lists representative concentrations and platelet activation pathways tested by each agonist. Small volumes, 2–5 μL, of concentrated agonist are used so that their dilutional effect in the reaction system is negligible.

Thrombin. Thrombin reacts with several platelet membrane sites to induce full aggregation and secretion of organelle contents independent of the prostaglandin or ADP pathways.[14] In lumiaggregometry, the operator ordinarily begins with thrombin to determine full secretion for a given specimen. Normally, thrombin induces the release of about 2 μmol of ATP. Other less potent agonists such as collagen induce the release of about 50% of the ATP induced by thrombin in a normal specimen. Thrombin-induced secretion may be diminished to less than 1 μmol in severe cyclooxygenase deficiency or storage pool disorders but is relatively unaffected by membrane disorders.

Reagent thrombin is stored at −20 °C and reconstituted with physiologic saline before use. Leftover reconstituted thrombin may be aliquotted and refrozen.

Table 35-1. AGONIST CONCENTRATIONS AND PATHWAYS

Agonist	Typical Final Concentration	Pathway
Thrombin	0.3 unit/mL	Direct secretion
ADP	10 μM	GP IIb-IIIa receptor
ADP	5 μM	ADP secretion
Epinephrine	10 μM	ADP secretion
	2 μM	
Collagen	5–10 μg/mL	Membrane phospholipase
Arachidonic acid	1 mM	Cyclooxygenase
Ristocetin	1.0 mg/mL	Agglutination

ADP, adenosine diphosphate.

Adenosine Diphosphate. ADP binds to a specific platelet membrane receptor to suppress membrane-associated adenyl cyclase activity and induce calcium mobilization to the platelet cytosol. The higher cytosolic free calcium concentration mediates platelet activation and induces secretion of dense-granule stored ADP, which enters the activation reaction and recruits neighboring platelets for aggregation.

ADP has been the most commonly used agonist, particularly in systems that do not measure secretion by luminescence. When specimens from some normal individuals are tested, the ADP concentration may be adjusted to between 1 and 10 μmol to induce "biphasic" aggregation (see Fig. 35-3). At ADP concentrations near 1 μmol, platelets undergo "primary" aggregation, followed by "disaggregation." Primary aggregation means a reversible shape change and formation of microaggregates, reflected in a brief upward deflection of the aggregometry tracing and subsequent return to baseline.

Secondary aggregation identifies full aggregate formation after secretion of platelet contents. At higher concentrations (around 10 μmol), ADP induces simultaneous irreversible shape change, secretion, and formation of aggregates, resulting in a monophasic curve and full deflection of the tracing. In a biphasic tracing, exogenous ADP induces shape change, which is followed by a brief flattening of the curve just before platelet secretion of endogenous ADP begins. Technologists may spend a great deal of effort to get the right ADP concentration for the elusive biphasic curve, since it enables them to use aggregometry to distinguish between membrane-associated and storage pool or release defects; however, this has become less necessary with the advent of lumiaggregometry, which provides a more direct measure of platelet secretion.

When a moderate concentration of ADP is used, aggregation is diminished in membrane disorders, in cyclooxygenase or thromboxane pathway enzyme deficiencies, in nonsteroidal anti-inflammatory agent (NSAIA) (e.g., aspirin) therapy, or in storage pool disorders. ADP at 10 μmol or above induces irreversible aggregation in spite of possible storage pool disorders or release defects.

ADP is stored at −20 °C, reconstituted with physiologic saline, and used immediately. Leftover reconstituted ADP may be subsequently aliquotted and refrozen for later use.

Epinephrine. Epinephrine binds to a specific membrane receptor and causes ADP secretion, inducing the same metabolic pathways as exogenous ADP. The results of epinephrine-induced aggregation match those of ADP except that epinephrine cannot induce aggregation in storage pool disorder or release defects no matter how high its concen-

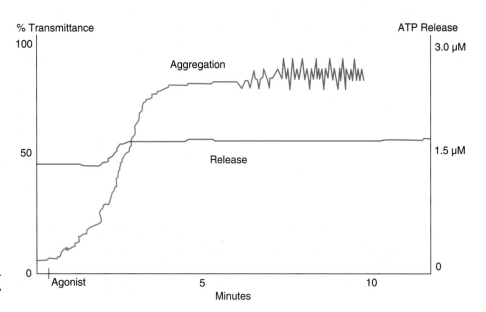

Figure 35-4 Lumiaggregometry tracing. *Abbreviation:* ATP, adenosine triphosphate.

tration. The platelets of about 10% of normal individuals do not respond to epinephrine.

Epinephrine is stored at 2–5 °C, reconstituted with distilled water, and used. Leftover reconstituted epinephrine may be aliquotted and frozen for later use.

Collagen. Collagen induces no primary wave of aggregation. As the agonist is added to the specimen, a brief lag phase follows. Within 30–60 seconds, aggregation begins and a monophasic curve develops, reaching 60–80% light transmission. Collagen-induced aggregation depends on intact membrane receptors, membrane phospholipase pathway integrity, and normal cyclooxygenase and thromboxane pathway function. Loss of collagen-induced aggregation may indicate a membrane abnormality, storage pool disorder, release defect, or the effects of NSAIAs such as aspirin. Most managers purchase lyophilized fibrillar collagen preparations such as Chrono-Par Collagen (Chrono-log, Havertown, PA). Collagen is stored at 2–5 °C and used without further dilution. Collagen may not be frozen.

Arachidonic Acid. Arachidonic acid is used to assess the viability of the thromboxane pathway of platelets. Free acid or sodium arachidonate is added to the specimen to induce a monophasic aggregometry curve with virtually no lag phase. Aggregation is independent of membrane integrity. Deficiencies in thromboxane pathway enzymes or cyclooxygenase result in complete suppression of the curve and no secretion.

Arachidonic acid is readily oxidized and must be stored at −20 °C in the dark. The technologist dilutes arachidonic acid with a solution of bovine albumin for immediate use. Aliquots of arachidonic acid may be thawed and refrozen up to three times.

Ristocetin. Although the platelet test is usually called ristocetin-induced platelet aggregation (RIPA), ristocetin's action on platelets is primarily agglutination since there is no shape change and slight secretion. For ristocetin aggregation to proceed, VWF (ristocetin cofactor) must be in the patient's specimen and the platelets must possess an intact surface membrane, including a functional VWF receptor site glycoprotein Ib (GPIb).

In a normal specimen, ristocetin induces a monophasic aggregation tracing. Specimens from patients with all subtypes of von Willebrand's disease except type IIb have no ristocetin reaction, although all other agonists produce normal tracings. Exogenous VWF in normal plasma restores the ristocetin aggregation reaction, confirming the diagnosis. In patients with Bernard-Soulier syndrome, a congenital change in the membrane includes loss of the GPIbIX receptor and the diminished ristocetin reaction is not corrected by addition of VWF.

Any discussion of von Willebrand's disease must indicate the expected variation in laboratory results both from one patient to another and from time to time in one patient. Ristocetin aggregometry is diagnostic in only about 70% of cases and is nondiagnostic in type IIb von Willebrand's disease. Consequently, the technologist must perform a clot-based factor VIII activity assay and immunometric factor VIII–related antigen assays. Ultimate confirmation and characterization of von Willebrand's disease is based on immunoelectrophoresis for detection of VWF monomers.

Ristocetin Cofactor Assay for von Willebrand's Factor

One refinement of ristocetin aggregometry is the substitution of formalin-fixed or lyophilized normal "reagent" platelets for patients' platelets.[15] When reagent platelets are used the test is called the "ristocetin cofactor," or VWF function, assay. The technologist prepares a patient's PPP, mixes it with reagent platelets, adds ristocetin, and performs aggregometry using the optical, not the electrical impedance, system. The ristocetin cofactor assay yields a proportional relationship between VWF concentration and the aggregometry response of the reagent platelets, so comparison of the aggregation results of patients' PPP to the results of standard dilutions of normal PPP permits for measurement of the VWF level.

Summary of Agonist Responses in Various Platelet Disorders

Thrombin produces maximal ATP release through a direct secretion mechanism. Arachidonic acid tests for cyclooxygenase deficiencies. Collagen, ADP, and epinephrine test for abnormalities in the membrane-associated prostaglandin pathway. Ristocetin checks for abnormalities of plasma VWF. The following conditions may be detected through platelet lumiaggregometry (Table 35–2).

NONSTEROIDAL ANTI-INFLAMMATORY AGENTS AND AGGREGOMETRY

NSAIAs such as aspirin, ibuprofen, indomethacin, and sulfinpyrazone inactivate or inhibit cyclooxygenase; prevent secretion of dense granule serotonin, ADP, and ATP; and suppress secondary aggregation. Secretion and aggregation in response to the agonists ADP, epinephrine, collagen, and arachidonic acid are reduced, but thrombin produces a normal response. Ristocetin induces normal agglutination. Secretion is not measured in the ristocetin reaction.

Table 35-2. LUMIAGGREGOMETRY RESULTS IN NSAIA TREATMENT, RELEASE DEFECT, AND STORAGE POOL DEFECTS

Agonist	NSAIA Treatment or Release Defect	Storage Pool Defect
Thrombin	Normal secretion and aggregation	Diminished secretion and aggregation
Adenosine diphosphate, epinephrine, arachidonic acid, and collagen	Diminished secretion and aggregation	Diminished secretion and aggregation

The physician or technologist must instruct the patient to avoid all drugs for 1 week before blood is collected for aggregometry and particularly to avoid the NSAIAs. If the patient has nevertheless taken an NSAIA, name of the drug, time taken, and dosage are recorded and subsequently noted with the results.

RELEASE DEFECTS: DEFICIENT CYCLOOXYGENASE OR THROMBOXANE PATHWAY ENZYMES AND AGGREGOMETRY

As in NSAIA inhibition, congenital or idiopathic deficiencies of cyclooxygenase or any enzyme in the thromboxane pathway (aspirin-like defects) prevent secretion of dense granule serotonin, ADP, and ATP and suppress secondary aggregation. Thrombin produces normal responses, but secretion and aggregation are diminished in response to the agonists ADP, epinephrine, collagen, and arachidonic acid. Ristocetin induces the expected agglutination.

STORAGE POOL DEFECTS AND AGGREGOMETRY

In a storage pool defect, ATP release in response to thrombin is reduced, as it is to ADP, epinephrine, arachidonic acid, and collagen. Ristocetin induces normal agglutination.

MEMBRANE DEFECTS: THROMBASTHENIA AND AGGREGOMETRY

Thrombasthenia, a membrane defect characterized by loss of the glycoprotein IIb-IIIa receptor site, may be diagnosed by its characteristically diminished secretion and aggregation responses to all agonists except a small response to arachidonic acid and full agglutination to ristocetin.

VON WILLEBRAND'S DISEASE, BERNARD-SOULIER SYNDROME, AND AGGREGOMETRY

In von Willebrand's disease, responses to thrombin, ADP, epinephrine, collagen, and arachidonic acid are normal and the response to ristocetin is often diminished, depending on the severity of disease. Specimens from patients with all subtypes of von Willebrand's disease except type IIb have no ristocetin reaction if the disease is severe but have a normal reaction in mild von Willebrand's disease. Exogenous VWF in normal plasma restores the ristocetin aggregation reaction, confirming the diagnosis. In patients with the rare Bernard-Soulier syndrome, a congenital change in the membrane includes loss of the GPIbIX receptor and the diminished ristocetin reaction is not corrected by addition of VWF.

Ristocetin aggregometry is diagnostic in only about 70% of cases and is nondiagnostic in type IIb VWD. Consequently, the technologist must perform a clot-based factor VIII activity assay and immunometric factor VIII–related antigen assay to confirm the findings suggested by the ristocetin agglutination results. Ultimate confirmation and characterization of von Willebrand's disease is based on immunoelectrophoresis for detection of VWF monomers.

ACQUIRED DISORDERS AND AGGREGOMETRY

Platelets are defective in acquired disorders such as myeloproliferative disorders, leukemia, aplastic anemia, myelodysplastic syndromes, myeloma, uremia, liver disease, and ethanol abuse; however, the lumiaggregometry patterns are variable and nondiagnostic. These disorders must be accounted for in any case where aggregation is abnormal.

Heparin-Associated Thrombocytopenia and Thrombosis Testing

One to five percent of patients receiving bovine heparin for more than 1 week develop a heparin-dependent anti-platelet antibody that is associated with thrombocytopenia and formation of microvascular thrombi.[16] Heparin-associated (or induced) thrombocytopenia and thrombosis is a medical emergency. A drop in platelet count during heparin therapy is an important signal for heparin-associated thrombocytopenia and thrombosis but is mitigated by the fact that about 30% of patients receiving heparin develop an immediate, benign, limited thrombocytopenia.[17] Since 10% of hospitalized patients receive heparin during their stay, the laboratory must provide a procedure to confirm this disorder and differentiate the types. Most use aggregometry or ATP release.

HEPARIN LUMIAGGREGOMETRY TEST FOR HAT

The patient must receive no heparin for at least 4 hours. Blood is collected into a tube with no additives and allowed to clot. The separated serum is heated to 56 °C for 30 minutes to inactivate residual thrombin and prevent a false positive test. The serum is then allowed to cool to room temperature before testing.

A specimen is collected from at least two healthy donors whose platelets are proved to be functional by arachidonic acid–induced aggregometry and unresponsive to therapeutic concentrations of heparin. The platelets of many normal individuals aggregate when heparin is added; these donors must be avoided because a false positive result occurs in the test system. Conversely, donors whose platelets are exceptionally responsive to heparin-dependent anti-platelet antibody should be registered and reused, since responsiveness is variable. Whole donor blood or PRP may be used for the assay.

The technologist prepares the heparin "agonist" by making dilutions in sterile buffered saline from the same lot used for the patient's therapy. The dilutions are prepared so that 5-μL aliquots provide heparin concentrations of 0.1, 0.5, and 100 U/mL of final reaction mixture, respectively.

Approximately equal amounts of patient serum and donor specimen are mixed, then 500 μL is pipetted to a reaction cuvette containing a plasticized stir bar. Heparin dilution or sterile saline (negative control) is added, and the reaction is observed for at least 20 minutes. Aggregation or ATP release may be used as the marker. Saline and each heparin dilution are mixed with specimen aliquots from each donor in separate cuvettes. For any reaction mixture that generates no response after 20 minutes, arachidonic acid is added to recheck for platelet activity.

A response of 10% above control in the 0.1- and 0.5-U/mL dilutions with no response in the 100-U/mL dilution indicates the presence of a heparin-dependent platelet antibody in the patient serum. The 100-U/mL dilution contains enough heparin to neutralize any suspected serum antibody.

Several conditions must be met for the aggregation test to yield valid results. If the saline control is positive, the patient's serum contains therapeutic heparin, a platelet alloantibody, or a platelet autoantibody. If the patient has been off heparin for at least 24 hours, the response is evidence of an alloantibody or autoantibody, which is confirmed immunometrically. The test depends on the presence of free heparin-dependent antibody in the patient's serum. In some cases of patients who have heparin-associated thrombocytopenia and thrombosis and are still receiving heparin, the heparin-dependent antibody becomes fixed to their own platelets during clotting, leaving no detectable antibody in the serum. Although aggregometry is specific for heparin-associated thrombocytopenia and thrombosis, it is about 50% sensitive.[18]

SEROTONIN RELEASE REACTION

The ^{14}C-serotonin platelet release assay is more sensitive than aggregometry and is used in a few laboratories as a screen for heparin-associated thrombocytopenia and thrombosis.[19] PRP from healthy donors is incubated with ^{14}C-serotonin and washed to remove the supernatant radioactive solution. Heat-inactivated patient serum or saline (control) is mixed with one of two heparin concentrations, 0.1 and 100 U/mL (final dilution), and with the ^{14}C-serotonin platelets, and the mixture is allowed to incubate for 60 minutes. EDTA in saline is added to stop the release reaction, and the supernatant is measured for radioactivity in a liquid scintillation counter. The percent release is calculated as follows:

$$\text{Percent Release} = \frac{\text{Release from test sample} - \text{background}}{\text{Total radioactivity} - \text{background}} \times 100$$

IMMUNOMETRIC DETECTION OF HEPARIN-DEPENDENT ANTI-PLATELET ANTIBODY BASED ON PF4 SPECIFICITY

Amiral and coworkers[20] describe a promising new approach to heparin-associated thrombocytopenia and thrombosis screening based on their discovery that platelet factor 4 (PF4) is the target for the heparin-dependent anti-platelet antibody.[20] Test plasma is incubated in microtiter plate wells containing a solid-bound complex of highly purified PF4 and heparin. Heparin-dependent anti-platelet antibodies become bound to the PF4–heparin complex. Bound antibodies are detected using peroxidase-bound goat anti-human IgGAM antibody and the chromophore OPD/H_2O_2. This test appears to be specific, more sensitive than lumiaggregometry or ^{14}C-serotonin platelet release, and able to demonstrate antibodies early in the development of heparin-associated thrombocytopenia and thrombosis.

MEASUREMENT OF PLATELET SECRETIONS

Plasma elevation of the platelet-specific proteins beta-thromboglobulin (β-TG) and platelet factor 4 (PF4) may accompany myocardial infarct.[21] The implication that in vivo platelet activation contributes to the condition or that the measurement of these proteins is of diagnostic or prognostic significance is under investigation.[22] Enzyme immunoassay kits for PF4 and β-TG are produced as thrombotic markers by Diagnostic Stago of Afnières sur Seine, France, and are available in the United States from American Bioproducts Company, Parsippany, New Jersey. Special collection techniques are necessary because PF4 and β-TG test results may be confounded by platelet activation during specimen collection.[23] Evacuated tubes containing the platelet aggregation inhibitors theophylline, adenosine, and dipyridamole are required for specimen collection for these secretions.

CORRECTED PLATELET COUNT INCREMENT DURING THERAPY

Platelet concentrate transfusion effectiveness is assessed using the corrected platelet count increment (CCI) calculation first described by Yankee and associates in 1969.[24] The CCI is especially useful when the patient is suspected of being refractory to platelet therapy and provides more reliable and standardized information than the platelet count. To compute the CCI, platelet counts are performed before and 1 hour after administration of the platelet transfusion, and the following calculation is made:

CCI at 1 hour

$$= \frac{\text{Post-transfusion} - \text{pretransfusion platelet} \\ \text{count} \times \text{body surface area}}{\text{Number of platelets transfused} \\ \text{in multiples of } 10^{11}}$$

where CCI = corrected count increment in platelets/10^{11}/m^2, body surface area (in m^2) is computed from height and weight, and platelets $\times 10^{11}$ = approximate number of platelets/ unit of concentrate.

A CCI of 7500 platelets/10^{11}/m^2 is generally regarded as an adequate post-transfusion response using this formula.[25] The body surface area in square meters is estimated from the nomogram of Sendroy and Cecchini on the basis of the weight and height of the recipient.[26]

CLOT-BASED PLASMA PROCOAGULANT SCREENS

The Lee-White whole blood coagulation time test, described in 1913, was the first laboratory procedure designed to assess coagulation.[27] The Lee-White test is no longer used, but it was the first in vitro clot procedure to employ an important principle: the time interval from initiation of coagulation to visible clot formation reflects the condition of the coagulation mechanism. A prolonged clotting time indicates coagulation inadequacy. The commonly accepted battery of clinical, clot-based coagulation screening tests—PT, APTT, and thrombin clotting time (TCT)—involve the use of the clotting time principle. Many specialized tests, such as specific factor assays, tests of fibrinolysis, inhibitor assays, reptilase time, and tests for acquired coagulation inhibitors, are also based on the relationship between time to clot formation and coagulation function.

Activated Coagulation Time (Point of Care Heparin Monitoring)

The activated coagulation time (ACT) is a 1966 modification of the whole blood clotting time test that is used to monitor heparin therapy. The ACT may be easily performed at the clinic, inpatient bedside, cardiac catheterization laboratory, or surgical suite.[28]

Diatomaceous earth, a particulate activator, is placed in evacuated specimen tubes before blood collection. As soon as an adequate specimen of blood is collected (e.g., 2 mL of whole blood in a tube with 12 mg of activator), a timer is started and the tube is thoroughly mixed to disperse the activator. The tube is then tilted and observed until a clot forms. The median of normal ACT results is 98 seconds. Heparin is administered to yield results of 180–240 seconds in deep vein thrombosis or a median of 400 seconds in cardiopulmonary bypass operations.[29]

The Hemochron Portable Blood Coagulation Timing System (International Technidyne, Edison, NJ) may be used for performing the ACT.[30] After the technologist collects blood in a commercially prepared evacuated tube that contains a measured weight of particulate activator and a plasticized magnet, the tube is placed in the instrument, where it is rotated and continuously monitored. When a clot forms, the magnet is pulled away from a sensing device and the interval to clot formation is recorded automatically. The results of the automated and manual ACT compare favorably with the APTT for heparin monitoring, provided adequate quality control steps are taken. The Hemochron instrument may also be used to measure PT, APTT, TCT, and fibrinogen assays.

Thromboelastography and Sonoclot

Two instruments are designed to measure physical changes in whole blood or plasma during clotting. These are the Thromboelastograph (Haemoscope Corporation, Skokie, IL) and the Sonoclot (Sienco, Morrison, CO).[31] These instruments give point of care information on coagulation and fibrinolysis.[32]

The Sonoclot measures changes in whole blood, PRP, or PPP viscosity over time by a principle termed *dynamic impedance*. A vertically oscillating cylindrical plastic probe attached to a transducer is suspended in the specimen. As plasma viscosity increases, greater voltage is required to maintain the period of oscillation of the probe. Changes in voltage required are recorded on a graph, creating a Sonoclot "signature," as shown in Figure 35–5. The signature provides several measurable parameters: time to onset of clotting, rate of clot formation, time to peak of clot formation, and amplitude of peak clot viscosity. A reference interval has been computed for each of these parameters using whole blood, PRP, and PPP. A variety of reaction situations may be used, including simple recalcification, use of particulate activators, or no reagent. Prolonged onset times, diminished clotting rate and peak amplitude, and delayed time to peak of clot formation are all associated with procoagulant deficiencies. The Sonoclot technique may be used to monitor heparin therapy.

The Thromboelastograph measures changes in clot "stiffness" of whole blood, PRP, and PPP by a principle termed *thromboelastography*. A disposable cylinder is suspended in a specimen held in a stainless steel cup. The distance from the outer wall of the internal cylinder to the inner wall of the cup is 1 mm. The outer cup oscillates 180 degrees about its axis. As the clot forms, forces applied by the oscillating outer cup begin to drive the suspended cylinder in a similar motion. The motion is measured electronically and recorded on a graph. Parameters similar to the Sonoclot parameters are measured, including time to onset, rate of clot formation, and peak amplitude of clot generation. After several minutes the amplitude becomes diminished. The rate at which this occurs is influenced by the fibrinolytic activity. Reagents include calcium chloride and particulate activators. Like the Sonoclot, the Thromboelastograph is sensitive to heparin anti-coagulant therapy and to procoagulant deficiencies. Both the Sonoclot and the Thromboelastograph may provide results that correlate with thrombotic tendency.

Prothrombin Time

PRINCIPLE

Commercially prepared PT thromboplastin reagents are organic extracts of emulsified rabbit brain, lung, or brain and lung suspended in a buffered solution of calcium chloride.[33] When mixed with citrated PPP, the reagent triggers fibrin clot formation by forming a complex with and activating plasma factor VII (Fig. 35–6). Calcium partici-

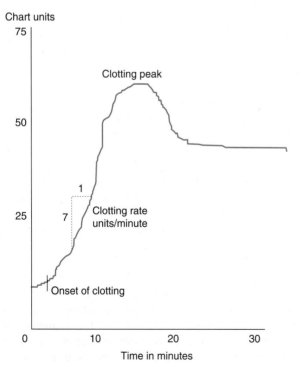

Figure 35–5 Sonoclot signature.

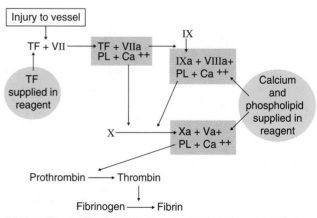

Figure 35–6 Prothrombin time reaction pathway. *Abbreviations:* TF, tissue factor; VIIa, activated factor VII (serine protease); VIIIa, activated factor VIII (cofactor); IXa, activated factor IX (serine protease); PL, platelet surface membrane phospholipid; Xa, activated factor X (serine protease); Va, activated factor V (cofactor).

pates in the formation of the tissue factor–factor VIIa complex, the factor VIIIa–factor IXa complex, and the factor Va–factor Xa complex. The clot is detectable visually or by optical or electromechanical sensors. Although the coagulation scheme implies the PT is prolonged in deficiencies of fibrinogen, prothrombin, and factors V, VII, VIII, IX, and X, the procedure is most sensitive to factor VII deficiencies, moderately sensitive to factor V and X deficiencies, sensitive to severe fibrinogen and prothrombin deficiencies, and insensitive to deficiencies of factors VIII and IX unless the thromboplastin is diluted.[34, 35] The PT is prolonged in multiple factor deficiencies that include deficiencies of factors VII and X and is most often used to monitor the effects of oral anti-coagulant warfarin sodium (Coumadin) therapy.

SPECIMEN REQUIREMENTS FOR PT AND APTT

Specimens for the PT and APTT are collected using the protocol in the section entitled Evacuated Hemostatis Specimen Collection Tubes. Chilling preserves the activity of the labile procoagulants V and VIII but activates factor VII, so its merits are ambiguous for the PT.

PT PROCEDURE

The thromboplastin–calcium chloride reagent is prewarmed to 37 °C. An aliquot of test plasma, usually 0.1 mL, is transferred to the reaction vessel, which is also maintained at 37 °C. The plasma aliquot is incubated at 37 °C for at least 3 and no more than 10 minutes. Aliquots that are incubated more than 10 minutes deteriorate because of degradation of the labile factors V and VIII and also because of evaporation. A premeasured volume of reagent, usually 0.2 mL, is forcibly added to the plasma aliquot, and a timer is started. As soon as the clot forms, the timer stops and the elapsed time is recorded. If the procedure is performed in duplicate, the duplicate values must be within 10% of each other or the test is repeated. Most PT procedures are performed on automated instruments.

QUALITY ASSURANCE FOR BOTH PT AND APTT

The technologist tests normal and prolonged control plasma specimens at the beginning of each shift or with each plasma or batch of patient plasma specimens tested. If a batch exceeds 40 patient specimens, a control specimen is tested with each 40 specimens. Although lyophilized control plasmas are commercially available, the laboratory manager may choose to collect and pool PPP specimens from designated subjects to make controls. In this case the specimens must be collected and managed using the same tubes, anticoagulant, and protocol as is used for patient plasma specimen collection. They are then pooled, tested, and aliquotted. Whether commercial or locally prepared controls are used, the control is tested with patient specimens using the protocol for patient plasma testing.

The normal control result should be within the reference interval, and the abnormal control result should be within the therapeutic range. If the control results fall within the stated limits in the laboratory protocol, the test results are considered valid; but if the results fall outside the control limits, the reagents, control, and equipment are checked, the problem is corrected, and the control is retested. The actions taken are recorded. Control results are recorded and analyzed after regular intervals (e.g., once a week) to determine the long-term validity of results.

REPORTING RESULTS AND THE INTERNATIONAL NORMALIZED RATIO

The technologist reports PT results to the nearest tenth of a second along with the PT reference interval. If the PT is performed in duplicate, the results are averaged and the average is reported. In view of the inherent variations among thromboplastin reagents, most laboratories report the international normalized ratio (INR) for stably anticoagulated patients using the following formula:[36]

$$INR = (PT_{Patient}/PT_{Normal})^{ISI},$$

where $PT_{Patient}$ = PT of patient in seconds, PT_{Normal} = PT of mean of reference interval, and ISI = the international sensitivity index.

Reagent producers generate the ISI for their thromboplastin by performing a linear regression analysis comparing its PT results to those of the international reference thromboplastin (World Health Organization human brain thromboplastin). Automated coagulation timers "request" the reagent ISI from the operator and compute the INR for each test, including specimens from patients who are not stably anti-coagulated. Many physicians base warfarin sodium treatment dosage on the INR result. Others prefer adjusting dosage according to the ratio of PT results to the median of the reference interval. Activity curves or ratios of the PT result to normal control results are no longer used.

REFERENCE INTERVAL

The PT reference interval varies from site to site depending on the patient population, type of thromboplastin, type of instrument, and the pH and purity of the diluent water. One medical center laboratory has established 12–14 seconds as its reference interval. This range is typical, but each center must establish its own range with each new lot of reagent or at least once a year by testing a sample of at least 20 specimens from healthy donors of both sexes spanning the adult age range over several days and computing the 95% confidence interval of the results.

CLINICAL UTILITY

The PT is most often used to monitor the effects of warfarin-based oral anti-coagulant therapy for patients who have deep vein thrombosis, pulmonary embolism, coronary thrombosis, or other thromboembolic diseases. Warfarin is a 4-hydroxycoumarin derivative that inhibits the γ-carboxylation of the vitamin K–dependent procoagulants prothrombin and factors VII, IX, and X, as well as the plasma coagulation inhibitors protein C and protein S. The inactive procoagulants synthesized during warfarin therapy, called proteins induced by vitamin K antagonists (PIVKA), possess fewer γ-carboxyglutamic acid units, are unable to bind calcium ions, do not assemble on phospholipid surfaces with their substrates, and do not participate in coagulation reactions. After warfarin sodium therapy is initiated, the PT begins to lengthen in response to the fall in factor VII activity, the first procoagulant level to fall, then stabilizes at the desired INR value after a few days. The physician adjusts the dosage to achieve an INR of 2–4.5, depending on the severity of the condition. The PT is more sensitive to diminished factor VII deficiency than prothrombin, factor IX, or factor X because factor VII has the smallest plasma concentration and most rapid turnover.

The PT is performed diagnostically in any patient suspected of having a coagulopathy. Acquired multiple deficiencies, such as disseminated intravascular coagulation, liver disease, uremia, and vitamin K deficiency, all affect factor VII activity and therefore are reliably detected through prolonged PT results.

Vitamin K deficiency is seen in malnutrition, during use of broad-spectrum antibiotics that destroy gut flora, and, in malabsorption syndromes. Vitamin K levels are low in the newborn, in whom bacterial colonization of the gut has not begun. Hemorrhage is likely in vitamin K deficiency, and the PT is the best indicator.

The PT is prolonged in congenital single factor deficiencies of factors X, VII, V, prothrombin, and fibrinogen if the fibrinogen level is less than or equal to 1.0 g/L. When the PT is prolonged but the APTT and TCT results are normal, factor VII activity may be deficient. Any suspected single factor deficiency is confirmed through the use of single factor assay techniques. The PT is not affected by diminished levels of factors VIII or IX because the concentration of reagent is high, bypassing the necessity for those factors.

Preoperative PT screening of asymptomatic surgical patients to predict postoperative hemorrhage is not supported by prevalence studies unless the patient is a member of a high-risk population.[37] No clinical data support the use of the PT as a general screening test for low-risk individuals, nor is the PT useful for establishing baseline values in warfarin therapy.[38] The therapeutic target range is based on the INR, not on the baseline PT result or control value.

LIMITATIONS OF THE PT

Specimen variations profoundly affect PT results. The ratio of whole blood to anti-coagulant is critical, so collection tubes must not be underfilled or overfilled by more than 10%. Anti-coagulant volume must be adjusted when the hematocrit is above 55% to avoid false prolongation of the results. Specimens must be thoroughly mixed within seconds after collection to ensure good anti-coagulation, but the mixing must be gentle. Clotted, hemolyzed, icteric, or lipemic specimens are rejected because they give unreliable results. Heparin contamination falsely prolongs the PT results. If the patient is receiving therapeutic heparin, it should be noted with the results. If the technologist or phlebotomist collects a series of evacuated tubes, the citrate tube must not follow any tube with an additive, such as heparin, EDTA, or sodium fluoride, since the additive may carry over to the citrate specimen. Specimen management must follow the protocol given in the section on hemostasis specimen management in this chapter.

Reagents must be reconstituted with the correct diluents and volumes using manufacturer instructions. Reagents must be stored and shipped according to manufacturer's instructions and never used after the expiration date.

Activated Partial Thromboplastin Time

PRINCIPLE

The APTT is performed to monitor the effects of heparin therapy and detect circulating anti-coagulants such as lupus anti-coagulant and anti-factor VIII. The APTT also detects congenital and acquired procoagulant deficiencies, except for factor VII.

The APTT reagent contains a negatively charged particulate activator such as kaolin, ellagic acid, or Celite. The activator provides a surface that mediates a conformational change of plasma factor XII resulting in its activation (Fig. 35–7). Factor XIIa forms a complex with two other plasma components: high-molecular-weight kininogen and prekallikrein. These three plasma proteins, termed *contact activation factors,* initiate in vitro clot formation but are not involved in in vivo coagulation. XIIa, a serine protease, activates factor XI to factor XIa, which in turn, activates factor IX to factor IXa.

Factor IXa binds calcium, phospholipid, and factor VIII to form a complex. In the APTT reaction system, ionic calcium and phospholipid are supplied as reagents, with the phospholipid as partial thromboplastin, an organic extract of rabbit brain tissue. The factor IXa:calcium–factor VIII–phospholipid complex catalyzes factor X to factor Xa. Factor Xa forms another complex with calcium, phospholipid, and factor V, catalyzing the conversion of prothrombin to thrombin.

The factor deficiencies that cause hemorrhage and prolonged APTT results, taken in the order of

reaction, are factors XI, IX, VII, X, and V, prothrombin, and fibrinogen, when it is less than or equal to 1.0 g/L. The APTT reagent is calibrated to be prolonged when the test plasma has less than 0.3 unit/mL of factors VIII, IX, or XI. The APTT is also prolonged in the presence of lupus anti-coagulant, an antibody with affinity for phospholipid, anti–factor VIII antibody, and heparin. Factor VII and factor XIII activity level deficiencies have no effect on the APTT.

SPECIMEN REQUIREMENTS

See Specimen Requirements for PT and APTT.

PROCEDURE

First, 0.1 mL of prewarmed (37 °C) reagent consisting of partial thromboplastin and activator is mixed with 0.1 mL of prewarmed plasma to initiate contact activation.[39] The mixture is allowed to incubate for the manufacturer-specified time, usually 2 or 3 minutes. Next, 0.1 mL of prewarmed 0.025 M calcium chloride is forcibly added to the mixture and a timer is started. When a fibrin clot forms, the timer is stopped and the interval is recorded. Timing may be performed manually or automatically by using an electromechanical or photo-optical device. If the APTT is performed in duplicate, the two results must match within 10%.

QUALITY ASSURANCE

See the section entitled Quality Assurance for PT and APTT. The normal control result should be within the reference interval, and the abnormal control result should be within the therapeutic range, 1.5–2.5 times the median of the reference interval. If the results fall outside the control limits, the reagents, control, and equipment are checked, the problem is corrected, and the control is retested. All actions taken are recorded. Control results are recorded and analyzed after regular intervals (e.g., once a week) to determine the long-term validity of the procedure.

REFERENCE INTERVAL

The APTT reference interval varies from site to site depending on the patient population, type of thromboplastin, type of instrument, and the pH and purity of the diluent water. One medical center laboratory has established 26–38 seconds as its reference interval. This range is typical, but each center must establish its own range with each new lot of reagent or at least once a year by testing a sample of at least 20 specimens from healthy

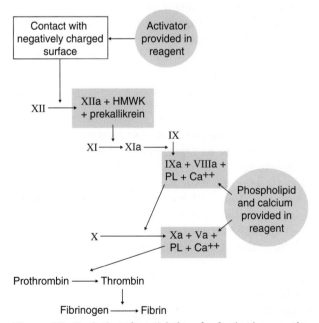

Figure 35–7 Activated partial thromboplastin time reaction pathway. *Abbreviations:* XIIa, activated factor XII (serine protease, not a procoagulant); HMWK, high-molecular-weight kininogen; XIa, activated factor XI (serine protease); TF, tissue factor; VIIa, activated factor VII (serine protease); VIIIa, activated factor VIII (cofactor); IXa, activated factor IX (serine protease); PL, platelet surface membrane phospholipid; Xa, activated factor X (serine protease); Va, activated factor V (cofactor).

donors of both sexes spanning the adult age range over several days and computing the 95% confidence interval of the results.

REPORTING RESULTS AND CLINICAL UTILITY

The technologist reports the results and the reference interval to the physician. If duplicate testing is performed, the average is reported. Because reagent sensitivity varies among producers and from lot to lot, the physician must evaluate results in relationship to the reference interval.[40] No standard partial thromboplastin reagent or INR is established for APTT.

The APTT is most often ordered to measure the effects of heparin therapy. Heparin potentiates the action of anti-thrombin (Fig. 35–8), which covalently neutralizes thrombin and factor Xa.

Thrombin and anti-thrombin bind to heparin and react covalently with each other. The heparin molecule is subsequently released to catalyze another such reaction.[41] Heparin is administered clinically to prevent thromboembolic disorders in those at high risk; in the treatment of venous thrombosis, pulmonary embolism, disseminated intravascular coagulation, and arterial thrombosis; and in patients undergoing surgery involving extracorporeal circulation. Continuous laboratory monitoring is essential because heparin overdose results in hemorrhage. Once heparin administration is begun, the APTT result should reach a

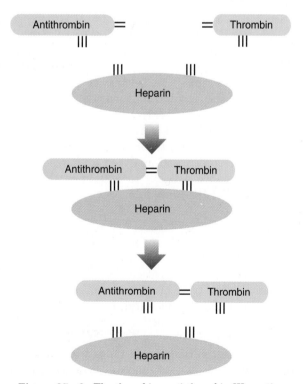

Figure 35–8 The thrombin–anti-thrombin III reaction.

"target range" of 1.5–2.5 times the median of the reference interval. The TCT and ACT are also used to monitor heparin therapy. The APTT is insensitive to the effects of low–molecular-weight heparin therapy.

The APTT is ordered when a hemorrhagic disorder is suspected or when recurrent thrombosis points to a lupus anti-coagulant. The APTT result is prolonged when there is a deficiency of one or more of the coagulation factors: prothrombin and factors V, VIII, IX, X, XI, or XII or when the fibrinogen level is below 1.0 g/L. It is also prolonged in the presence of a specific inhibitor such as anti–factor VIII, a nonspecific inhibitor such as lupus anti-coagulant, and anti-thrombotic substances such as fibrin degradation products (FDP). Disseminated intravascular coagulation gives prolonged results owing to consumption of procoagulants, but the APTT results are not definitive. Vitamin K deficiency results in diminished levels of procoagulant factors II, VII, IX, and X, and thus the APTT is eventually prolonged; however, because factor VII does not affect the APTT and because it is the first coagulation factor to become deficient, the test is not as sensitive to vitamin K deficiency or warfarin sodium therapy as the PT. The APTT is not prolonged in deficiencies of factors VII or XIII or platelet phospholipid.

No clinical data support the use of the APTT as a general screening test for low-risk individuals, nor is the APTT useful for establishing baseline values in heparin therapy for thromboembolic disorders.[42] The therapeutic target range uses the median of the reference range, not the APTT baseline or control result.

LIMITATIONS OF THE APTT

Specimen collection and management follow the same protocol as specimens for the PT test. Reagents must be reconstituted with the correct diluents and volumes using the manufacturer's instructions. Reagents must be stored and shipped using the manufacturer's instructions and never used after the expiration date.

When the APTT is used to monitor heparin therapy, certain interfering factors must be kept in mind. In anti-thrombin deficiency, heparin is ineffective and the APTT remains in the reference range. In individuals with congenital anti-thrombin deficiency, heparin therapy causes anti-thrombin depletion. The therapy is then ineffective and the APTT is normal. In vivo activation of platelets may cause elevated PF4, a heparin-neutralizing protein. The neutralizing function prevents therapeutic heparin from being effective, and the APTT remains unchanged. Hypofibrinogenemia and presence of FDP causes prolongation of APTT that does not reflect heparin levels.[43]

Point of Care PT and APTT

VENOUS WHOLE BLOOD PT AND APTT

The Hemochron Portable Blood Coagulation Timing System (International Technidyne, Edison, NJ) may be used to perform point of care PT and APTT tests through technique similar to the automated ACT.[44] For the PT the distributor provides tubes containing thromboplastin and a plasticized magnet, and for the APTT, tubes containing diatomaceous earth, partial thromboplastin, buffer, calcium chloride, and a plasticized magnet. No anti-coagulant is used in this system. Two milliliters of blood is collected in a syringe and transferred to the reaction tube. The timer is started, and the blood is throughly mixed to disperse the reagents. The tube is then placed in the instrument test well where it is continuously monitored for clotting. The interval to clot formation is recorded automatically. Alternative evacuated tubes designed for direct drawing of a blood specimen are also available.

The reference mean for the Hemochron PT is 55 seconds and that for the APTT is 67 seconds. Although these do not match the ranges for anti-coagulated PPP, they give the advantage of point of care and rapid turnaround of results to the physician. The manufacturer provides whole blood to plasma value conversion charts for both procedures and a whole blood to INR chart for the PT. A control plasma is provided by the company for quality assurance.

CAPILLARY PT AND APTT

PT and APTT may be performed on 50 μL of whole venous or capillary blood, or PPP, using the Thrombolytic Assessment System (TAS) (Cardiovascular, Durham, NC).[45] The TAS uses paramagnetic iron oxide particles combined with PT or APTT test reagents in a flat capillary reaction chamber. A drop of specimen is drawn into the reaction chamber by capillary action. The iron oxide particles are induced to oscillate by a nearby magnet. As clotting occurs, the particle oscillation is restricted. This change is detected by an optical reader, and the timer stops.[46] The timed results are adjusted by internal electronics to match with typical plasma-based APTT or PT reference intervals.[47]

The Endpoint (Edison Institute, Edison, NJ) is an instrument designed for heparin monitoring through the APTT system using approximately 200 μL of whole venous or capillary blood. This system employs a plastic cartridge with a capillary chamber impregnated with kaolin activator and partial thromboplastin. The operator introduces the specimen and starts the timer. The specimen is moved back and forth through the chamber until clotting begins. The movement of the specimen then slows. This is detected optically, and the timer stops. Results are adjusted electronically to match plasma levels.

The 512 Coagulation Monitor (Ciba Corning Diagnostics, Medfield, MA) is another instrument designed for capillary APTT tests. This is a portable laser photometer that also incorporates disposable plastic cartridges with a capillary channel reagent chamber impregnated with activator and phospholipid and is operated similar to the Endpoint. The company provides whole blood controls for quality assurance. The instrument results correlate moderately well with standard APTT results.

THROMBIN CLOTTING TIME

Principle and Reagent

Commercially prepared reagent thrombin at 2 National Institutes of Health (NIH) units/mL cleaves fibrinopeptides A and B from fibrinogen. The resulting fibrinogen reacts to form a fibrin clot, which is detected visually or by electromechanical or optical devices (Fig. 35–9).

Thrombin Reagent

Most laboratory managers prefer commercially manufactured diagnostic lyophilized thrombin reagent, although pharmaceutical topical thrombin may also be used. The reagent is reconstituted ac-

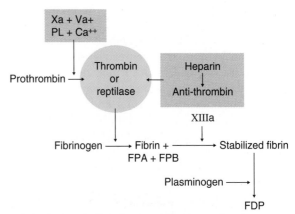

Figure 35–9 Thrombin clotting time and reptilase time pathway.

cording to manufacturer instructions and used immediately or aliquotted and frozen. If thrombin is to be frozen, it should be prepared in a stock solution of 1000 NIH units/mL and frozen at -70 °C until it is ready for use. Once thawed, thrombin is stable for only a few hours and cannot be refrozen for later use.

Procedure

Reagent thrombin is warmed to 37 °C for a minimum of 3 and a maximum of 10 minutes. Thrombin deteriorates during incubation and must be used within 10 minutes of the time incubation is begun. An aliquot, usually 0.1 mL, of normal plasma is allowed to incubate for 3 minutes. The operator forcibly pipettes 0.2 mL thrombin into the plasma aliquot and starts a timer. Thrombin time tests may be performed in duplicate and the results averaged.

Specimen Requirements

TCT specimens are prepared using the same protocol as specimens for the PT or APTT.

Quality Assurance

The technologist tests a normal control and an abnormal control with each batch of TCTs and records the results. The normal control results should fall within the laboratory's reference interval. The abnormal control results should be prolonged to the range that TCT results reach in hypofibrinogenemia. If the results fall outside the laboratory protocol's control limits, the reagents, control, and equipment are checked, the problem is corrected, and the control is retested. The actions taken to correct out-of-control tests are recorded. Control results are analyzed after regular intervals (weekly is typical) to determine the long-term validity of the procedure.

Reporting Results and Clinical Utility

A typical reference range is 25–30 seconds. The TCT is prolonged when the fibrinogen level is less than 1.0 g/L (hypofibrinogenemia) or in the presence of anti-thrombotic materials such as FDP, paraproteins, or heparin. Afibrinogenemia (absence of fibrinogen) or dysfibrinogenemia (fibrinogen that is biochemically abnormal and therefore nonfunctional) also cause a prolonged TCT. Before a prolonged TCT may be considered to be evidence of diminished or abnormal fibrinogen, the presence of anti-thrombotic activity, particularly heparin, must be ruled out.

TCTs may be used instead of APTTs to monitor heparin therapy, although neither is sensitive to the effects of low–molecular-weight heparin fractions. The fibrinogen assay is a simple modification of the TCT in which the concentration of reagent thrombin is greater, at 50 NIH units/mL, and the test specimen is diluted 1:10 to minimize the effects of heparin or anti-thrombotic proteins. The reptilase time procedure is identical to the TCT except that the reagent is insensitive to the effects of heparin.

Point of Care TCT

The Hemochron Portable Blood Coagulation Timing System (International Technidyne, Edison, NJ) may be used to perform a bedside TCT using a technique similar to the automated ACT. The distributor provides evacuated tubes containing lyophilized thrombin, buffer, calcium chloride, and a plasticized magnet. Two milliliters of blood is collected directly in the tube, the timer is started, and the blood is thoroughly mixed to disperse the reagents. The tube is then placed in the instrument test well where it is continuously monitored for clotting. The interval to clot formation is recorded automatically.

The reference mean of the Hemochron TCT is 45 seconds, which, while it does not match the TCT time of PPP, gives the advantage of rapid turnaround of results to the physician. A control plasma is provided by the company for quality assurance.

Reptilase (Atroxin) Time

PRINCIPLE AND REAGENT

Reptilase (Atroxin) is a thrombin-like enzyme, isolated from the venom of *Bothrops atrox*, that catalyzes the conversion of fibrinogen to fibrin in a manner similar to thrombin (see Fig. 35–9), except that reptilase is insensitive to the effects of heparin. The specimen requirements, procedure, and quality assurance protocol for the reptilase time test are the same as for the TCT. Atroxin (Sigma Chemicals, St. Louis, MO) is reconstituted with distilled water and is stable for 1 month when stored at 2–6 °C. Atroxin is a poison that may be fatal if it enters the bloodstream.

CLINICAL UTILITY

A prolonged reptilase time indicates decreased functional fibrinogen. Because the reptilase time test is unaffected by heparin, it is useful in patients receiving heparin therapy. The reptilase test is prolonged in the presence of FDP and paraproteins.

SPECIAL COAGULATION TESTS FOR HEMORRHAGIC DISORDERS

Fibrinogen Assay

PRINCIPLE

The clot-based method of Clauss, a modification of the TCT test, is the recommended procedure for estimating the functional fibrinogen level.[48] Like the TCT test, thrombin reagent is added to plasma and catalyzes the conversion of fibrinogen to fibrin. In the fibrinogen assay, however, the thrombin reagent concentration is 25 times greater at 50 NIH units/mL. Furthermore, the plasma to be tested is diluted 1:10 with Owren's buffer, whereas in the TCT test it is undiluted. The higher reagent concentration and diluted plasma provide an inverse but linear relationship between interval to clot formation and concentration of functional fibrinogen when the concentration is between 1 and 4 g/L. Diluting the plasma also minimizes the anti-thrombotic effects of heparin, FDP, and paraproteins. Heparin levels below 0.6 U/mL and FDP levels below 100 μg/dL do not affect the results of the fibrinogen assay of diluted plasma if the fibrinogen level is greater than or equal to 1.5 g/L.

The interval to clot formation is compared with the results of a reference plasma. A reference curve is prepared in each laboratory and updated regularly using reference plasma or control plasma that has been calibrated to reference plasma.

SPECIMEN REQUIREMENTS

Fibrinogen assay specimens are prepared using the same protocol as specimens for the PT or APTT.

PROCEDURE

Thrombin Reagent. Most laboratory managers prefer commercially manufactured diagnostic lyophilized thrombin reagent, although pharmaceutical topical thrombin may also be used. The reagent is reconstituted according to manufacturer instructions and used immediately or aliquotted and frozen. If thrombin is to be frozen, it should be prepared in a stock solution of 1000 NIH units/mL and frozen at −70 °C until it is ready for use. Once thawed, thrombin is stable for only a few hours and cannot be refrozen for later use.

Reference Curve. A reference curve is prepared with each change of reagent lots, reference plasma, or instrument. The technologist prepares the curve by reconstituting commercially available lyophilized fibrinogen calibration plasma or a reference plasma available from the College of American Pathologists. With Owren's buffer, five dilutions of the calibration plasma are prepared: 1:5, 1:10, 1:15, 1:20, and 1:40. An aliquot, usually 0.2 mL, of each dilution is transferred to each of three reaction tubes or cups, warmed to 37 °C, and tested by adding 0.1 mL of working thrombin reagent at 50 NIH units/mL. Time from addition of thrombin to clot formation is recorded, triplicates are averaged, and the results in seconds are graphed against fibrinogen concentration (Fig. 35–10). Because test plasma samples are diluted 1:10 before testing, the 1:10 calibration plasma dilution is assigned the same fibrinogen concentration as the undiluted reconstituted calibration plasma value.

Test Protocol. The technologist prepares a 1:10 dilution of each patient plasma and control with Owren's buffer. Then 0.2 mL of each of the diluted plasmas is warmed to 37 °C in each of two reaction tubes or cups for 3 minutes. After incubation, 0.1 mL of thrombin reagent is added, a timer is started, and the mixture is observed until a clot forms. The timer is stopped, duplicates are averaged, and the interval in seconds is compared with the graph. Results are reported in grams per liter of fibrinogen.

If the clotting time of the test plasma dilution is short, indicating a fibrinogen level above 4.0 g/L, a 1:20 dilution is prepared and tested. The resulting fibrinogen concentration from the graph must be multiplied by 2 to compensate for the dilution. If the clotting time of the original 1:10 test plasma dilution is prolonged, indicating less than 2.0 g/L of fibrinogen, a 1:5 dilution is prepared. The resulting fibrinogen concentration reading from the graph must be divided by 2 to compensate for the concentrated specimen.

QUALITY ASSURANCE

All duplicate results must agree within a coefficient of variation of less than 7%. The technologist tests a normal control and an abnormal control with each batch of fibrinogen levels and records the results. The normal control results should be within the laboratory's reference interval. The abnormal control results should be in the range of 0.8–1.2 g/L. If either control result falls outside the control limits, the reagents, control, and equipment are checked, the problem is corrected, and the control is retested. The actions taken to correct "out-of-control" tests are recorded. Control results are analyzed after regular intervals (weekly is typical) to determine the long-term validity of the procedure.

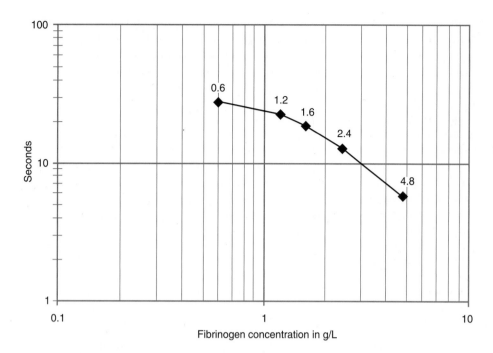

Dilution	Concentration	Seconds
	g/L	
1:5	4.8	6
1:10	2.4	13
1:15	1.6	19
1:20	1.2	23
1:40	0.6	29

Figure 35–10 Fibrinogen reference curve and table.

RESULTS AND CLINICAL UTILITY

One institution's reference interval for fibrinogen concentration is 2.0–4.0 g/L. Hypofibrinogenemia is usually associated with disseminated intravascular coagulation, primary fibrinogenolysis, and severe liver disease. Moderately severe liver disease, pregnancy, and any chronic inflammatory condition may cause an elevated fibrinogen level because fibrinogen is an acute-phase reactant. Congenital afibrinogenemia gives prolonged clotting times and is associated with a mild hemorrhagic disorder. Dysfibrinogenemia may give the same test results as hypofibrinogenemia by this test method because some abnormal fibrinogen species are hydrolyzed more slowly by thrombin than normal fibrinogen. Some forms of dysfibrinogenemia may be associated with thrombosis.[49] Immunometric and turbidimetric (Ellis-Stransky) measures of fibrinogen are normal in dysfibrinogenemia. Although anti-thrombotic effects are minimized by the dilution of plasma specimens, heparin levels above 0.6 U/mL and FDP levels above 100 μg/mL prolong the clotting time and give falsely lowered fibrinogen levels, particularly if a dilution less dilute than 1:10 is used.

LIMITATIONS OF THE FIBRINOGEN ASSAY

Care must be taken that the thrombin reagent is pure and has not degenerated. Exposure to sunlight or oxidation will result in rapid breakdown of thrombin. The working dilution lasts only 1 hour at 2–8 °C and should remain cold until just before testing. Specimens with clots, hemolysis, icterus, or lipemia are unacceptable.

Fibrin or Fibrinogen Degradation Products

PURPOSE AND PRINCIPLE

Bound plasmin is a trypsin-like proteolytic enzyme that cleaves fibrin and yields FDPs, designated X, Y, D, and E. Normally, D and E fragments circulate in concentrations less than or equal to 2 μg/mL. Pathologic degradation of fibrin and fibrinogen, a result of increased fibrin production or unbound plasmin activity, yields FDPs at levels greater than 2 μg/mL. Increased FDP levels are characteristic of acute and chronic disseminated intravascular coagulation, primary fibrinogenolysis, deep vein thrombosis, and pulmonary embolism.[50] Because the D and E fragments from lysis of either fibrinogen or fibrin are structurally identical, the test does not distinguish between disseminated intravascular coagulation and primary fibrinogenolysis. FDPs are also detected in plasma after thrombolytic therapy.[51] FDPs are detected and measured using a latex agglutination immunoassay employing latex particles coated with polyclonal anti-D and anti-E antibodies.

PROCEDURE

Several companies offer kits for rapid semiquantitative latex agglutination immunoassay of serum FDP. Polystyrene latex particles in buffered saline are coated with anti-D and anti-E fragment-specific polyclonal antibodies calibrated to detect FDPs at greater than or equal to 2 μg/mL.

Specimen. The FDP test requires a special specimen collection technique. The technologist collects 2 mL of fresh whole blood and immediately transfers it to a tube containing bovine thrombin and trypsin inhibitor. Most FDP kit distributors provide evacuated tubes containing thrombin and inhibitor. Thrombin promotes rapid and complete clotting while the trypsin inhibitor neutralizes plasmin, preventing in vitro fibrinolysis. These preparations ensure that the serum FDP level does not become elevated by in vitro mechanisms and reflects the in vivo situation.

The anti-thrombotic activity of heparin thwarts the effects of thrombin, so if heparin is expected, reptilase is added to the specimen to trigger clotting. The clotted specimen is centrifuged and supernatant serum is separated from the clot immediately after collection.

Protocol. A 1:5 and 1:20 dilution of test serum is prepared in buffered saline. One drop each of undiluted serum, 1:5 and 1:20 dilutions, respectively, is placed in three labeled circles on a clean glass slide. One drop of well-mixed latex suspension is added to each drop of specimen or dilution and mixed. The slide is rocked for 2 minutes, and the mixture is observed for agglutination. Negative and positive sera, supplied by the manufacturer, are tested with each unknown test serum or batch.

RESULTS

Results of the FDP test are semiquantitative: If only the undiluted serum mixture demonstrates agglutination, the FDP concentration is reported as greater than or equal to 2 but less than 10 μg/mL. This is regarded as a positive result. If the undiluted and 1:5 circles show agglutination, the result is reported as greater than or equal to 10 but less than 80 μg/mL; and if all three wells clump,

the result is greater than or equal to 80 μg/mL. A negative result, absence of agglutination in all three wells, is reported as less than 2 μg/mL. Control results are observed, recorded, and reviewed at regular intervals.

The FDP test result is positive in disseminated intravascular coagulation, deep vein thrombosis, and pulmonary embolism and after thrombolytic therapy. The FDP test result is also positive in primary fibrinogenolysis, a disorder in which plasmin acts on plasma fibrinogen. The D-dimer test, which is specific for fibrinolysis and negative in primary fibrinogenolysis, may be used in tandem with the FDP test to identify fibrinogenolysis when it is suspected.

D-Dimer

PRINCIPLE

As fibrin forms in vivo, it is stabilized by the transpeptidase action of factor XIIIa, which reacts with neighboring chains to form covalent bonds (see Fig. 35–9). As bound plasmin subsequently lyses the stabilized clot, the D-fragment products remain covalently linked to similar D-fragments from neighboring fibrin molecules. These linked D-fragments are released as soluble D-dimers. The D-dimer test incorporates a monoclonal antibody that detects soluble D-dimer molecules. A positive result is specific for the breakdown of stabilized fibrin. Because D-dimer is not released in primary fibrinogenolysis, the D-dimer test is specific for fibrin breakdown, such as occurs in disseminated intravascular coagulation, thrombolytic therapy, and deep vein thrombosis, and is negative in primary fibrinogenolysis.

Several companies offer kits for rapid semiquantitative latex agglutination immunoassay of plasma D-dimers. Polystyrene latex particles in buffered saline are coated with monoclonal anti–D-dimer antibodies that bind D-dimer particles in the test plasma. A positive result is visible agglutination.

Enzyme immunoassay tests are available. These also employ monoclonal anti–D-dimer antibodies in solid phase and provide a colorimetric detection system that is quantitative and designed to be more sensitive than the latex agglutination test.

Specimen. Citrated plasma may be used. The specimen is collected and managed according to the same protocol as for a PT or APTT. EDTA or heparinized plasmas may also be used.

Protocol. The D-dimer latex test is performed as a qualitative or semiquantitative procedure. A drop of test plasma is mixed undiluted with a drop of latex suspension, rocked for 2 minutes, and observed for agglutination. If a semiquantitative test is desired, the test plasma is first serially diluted with glycine-buffered saline and the test is performed on the dilutions. The results are reported as the reciprocal of the last dilution that shows agglutination.

The enzyme immunoassay test for D-dimer employs microtiter plates. The technologist follows the manufacturer's instructions in the performance of this procedure.

Clinical Utility. The D-dimer test result is positive in disseminated intravascular coagulation, deep vein thrombosis, and pulmonary embolism and after thrombolytic therapy but is negative in primary fibrinogenolysis, a disorder in which plasmin acts on plasma fibrinogen but not fibrin. The D-dimer test may be used in tandem with the FDP test to identify primary fibrinogenolysis when it is suspected.

Single Factor Assay with the APTT Test System

PRINCIPLE

If the APTT is prolonged and the PT and TCT are normal, and there is no ready explanation for the prolonged APTT such as heparin therapy, acquired coagulation inhibitor, liver disease, uremia, disseminated intravascular coagulation, or vitamin K deficiency, then the technologist may suspect a congenital single factor deficiency. Three factors that give this reaction pattern and cause hemorrhage are factor VIII (hemophilia A), IX (hemophilia B), and XI, which causes a mild intermittent bleeding disorder primarily found in Ashkenazi Jews.[52] Factor XI deficiency is also called hemophilia C or Rosenthal's syndrome. The next step in diagnosis of a congenital single factor deficiency is performance of a one-stage single factor assay based on the APTT test system.

Although necessary for diagnosis, APTT-based single-factor assays are most often performed on specimens from patients with previously identified single factor deficiencies to monitor supportive therapy during bleeding episodes or invasive procedures. Because hemophilia A is the most common single factor deficiency disorder, our discussion is confined to the factor VIII assay; however, the protocol may be applied to factors IX and XI as well.

The technologist uses the APTT test system to estimate the concentration of functional factor VIII by incorporating factor VIII–depleted plasma in the test system. Factor VIII–deficient plasma may be obtained locally from a hemophilic donor, but most laboratory managers order commercially prepared reagent plasma collected from normal donors and immunodepleted using monoclonal anti-factor VIII antibody.[53]

In the APTT test system, factor VIII–depleted plasma provides normal activity of all procoagulants but VIII. Tested alone, factor VIII–depleted plasma reagent has a prolonged APTT; but when normal plasma is added, the APTT reverts to normal. In contrast, a prolonged result on a patient-factor VIII–depleted plasma mixture implies that the patient plasma is deficient in factor VIII. Furthermore, the clotting time interval of the test plasma factor VIII–depleted plasma mixture may be compared with a previously prepared reference curve that plots time interval against percent factor VIII activity to estimate the level of factor VIII activity in the patient's plasma.

The quantitative factor assay is customarily performed on a 1:10 dilution of test plasma, and the reference curve sets the clotting time for a 1:10 dilution of reference plasma at the assayed factor VIII activity percentage from the package insert.

REFERENCE CURVE FOR FACTOR VIII ASSAY

To prepare a reference curve for the factor VIII assay the technologist obtains a reference plasma such as CAP FVIIIc RM (College of American Pathologists, Northfield, IL) and prepares a series of dilutions with buffered saline.[54] Although laboratory protocols vary, most technologists prepare a series of five dilutions, from 1:5 to 1:500. The results of these dilutions must be linear. Each dilution is mixed with reagent factor VIII–depleted plasma and tested in duplicate according to the APTT system, and the duplicate results are averaged and plotted on log/log or log/linear graph paper (Fig. 35–11). The 1:10 dilution is assigned the factor VIII assay activity value found on the package insert. When patient plasma is tested, the time interval obtained is entered on the vertical coordinate and converted to a percentage.

PROCEDURE FOR FACTOR VIII ASSAY

The technologist prepares 1:10 and 1:20 dilutions of each test plasma and control and then mixes each dilution with equal volumes of factor VIII–depleted plasma and APTT reagent. In most cases, 0.1 mL of APTT reagent is mixed with 0.1 mL each of test plasma dilution and factor-depleted plasma. Both dilutions of each specimen or control are tested in duplicate. After incubation for the manufacturer-specified time at 37 °C, 0.1 mL 0.025 N calcium chloride is added and a timer is started. The interval is recorded in seconds, duplicates are averaged, the mean result is compared

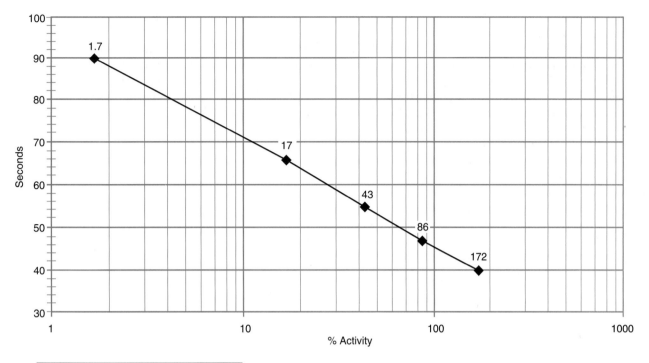

Dilution	Seconds	Percent Activity
1:5	40	172
1:10	47	86
1:20	55	43
1:50	66	17
1:500	90	1.7

Figure 35-11 Factor VIII assay reference curve on linear-log graph form.

with the reference curve, and the percentage of factor VIII activity is reported. Factor activity results of the 1:20 dilutions are multiplied by 2 to compensate for the added dilution factor and should match the results of the 1:10 dilutions within 10%. If the results of the two dilutions do not match, an acquired coagulation inhibitor may be present and the assay cannot provide a reliable estimate of factor VIII activity.

Tests for factors IX and XI are performed according to the same approach, except that the appropriate factor-depleted plasma is substituted for factor VIII–depleted plasma. Tests for the contact factors XII, prekallikrein, or high–molecular-weight kininogen are seldom requested since deficiencies are not associated with bleeding disorders.

EXPECTED RESULTS AND CLINICAL UTILITY OF SINGLE FACTOR ASSAYS

The reference range for factor VIII activity is 50–150%. Symptoms of hemophilia are evident at activity levels of 10% or less. The test is used most often to estimate the plasma level of factor VIII activity during therapy.

QUALITY ASSURANCE

All duplicate results must agree within 10%. The technologist tests a normal control and an abnormal control with each assay and records the results. The normal control results should fall within the reference interval. The abnormal control results should be in the range of 10% factor VIII activity. If either control result falls outside the control limits, the reagents, control, and equipment are checked, the problem is corrected, and the control is retested. The actions taken to correct "out-of-control" tests are recorded. Control results are analyzed after regular intervals (weekly is typical) to determine the long-term validity of the procedure.

LIMITATIONS

Interlaboratory coefficients of variation (CVs) for the factor VIII assay are near 80%, causing undesirable variation in the interpretation of therapeutic monitoring results. To reduce inherent variation, the technologist uses an assayed commercial plasma to prepare the reference curve and selects reference dilutions that comprise only the linear portion of the curve. In addition the technologist must assay two or more dilutions of the patient's plasma to check for the presence of acquired coagulation inhibitors, select a matching reagent-instrument system with a demonstrated control value below 5%, and use factor-depleted substrates that have no trace of the factor.[55] As in the APTT test, good specimen management is essential. Clotted, hemolyzed, icteric, or lipemic specimens are rejected since they give unreliable results. Reagents must be reconstituted with the correct diluents and volumes using manufacturer instructions. Reagents must be stored and shipped according to manufacturer instructions and never used after the expiration date.

Single Factor Assay with the PT Test System

If the APTT and the PT are prolonged and the TCT is normal, and there is no ready explanation for the prolonged test results such as heparin therapy, acquired coagulation inhibitor, liver disease, uremia, disseminated intravascular coagulation, oral anticoagulant therapy, or vitamin K deficiency, the technologist may suspect a congenital single factor deficiency. Three relatively rare factor deficiencies that give this reaction pattern and cause hemorrhage are prothrombin, factor V, or factor X deficiency. If the PT is prolonged and all other test results are normal, factor VII deficiency is suspected. The next step in diagnosis of a congenital single factor deficiency is performance of a one-stage single-factor assay on the basis of the PT test system. The principles and procedure given in the section on single factor assay with the APTT test system may be applied except that tissue thromboplastin reagent replaces the APTT reagent in the test system and the PT protocol is followed. Prothrombin-depleted and factors V, VII, or X-depleted plasmas are available.

Factor XIII Screening Test (Urea Solubility)

Factor XIII, which is activated by thrombin to factor XIIIa, is a transpeptidase that catalyzes the formation of interstrand covalent bonds that stabilize fibrin strands. Patients with congenital deficiency or acquired inhibitor of factor XIII experience a variety of hemorrhagic symptoms, such as poor wound healing, ecchymoses, menorrhagia, and umbilical bleeding. Routine coagulation screening tests do not detect factor XIII deficiency when the remainder of the coagulation system is intact; thus

the decision to perform the factor XIII assay must be clinical. Factor XIII deficiencies may be acquired in metastatic carcinoma, leukemia, hypergammopathy, collagen disease, and liver disease. Congenital factor XIII deficiencies have been described, and anti–factor XIII antibodies have been detected.[56]

PRINCIPLE AND PROCEDURE

The unstable clot that forms in factor XIII deficiency or inhibitor dissolves in a 5 M urea solution, whereas a factor XIIIa–stabilized clot will remain intact for at least 24 hours.

The technologist prepares three tubes. Tube 1 receives 0.3 mL of test PPP and tube 3 receives 0.3 mL of normal PPP. Tube 2 receives 0.2 mL of test PPP and 0.1 mL of normal PPP. The technologist pipettes 0.1 mL 0.025 M calcium chloride to each tube. After clot formation, all three tubes are incubated at 37 °C for 30 minutes. Next, 3 mL of 5 M urea solution is transferred to each tube and the tubes are tapped gently to dislodge the clots from the sides. The tubes are then capped and incubated at ambient temperature for 24 hours but are observed for evidence of clot dissolution at 1, 2, 4, and 24 hours. Decreasing size of clot, fragmentation, and increasing turbidity of the urea solution are evidence for clot dissolution. The clot in the test plasma tube (tube 1) is compared with the normal plasma tube clot (tube 3), and results are reported as "factor XIII present" or "factor XIII absent." If a factor XIII inhibitor is present in the test plasma, dissolution will be seen in both the first and the second tube. A clot in normal PPP remains intact for greater than or equal to 24 hours.

Prothrombin Fragment 1 + 2 Enzyme Immunoassay

Prothrombin fragment 1 + 2 (PF 1 + 2 or PF 1.2) is a soluble fragment released while factor Xa cleaves the prothrombin peptide bond Arg 273–Thr 274. An enzyme immunoassay procedure (available from Organon Teknika, Durham, NC) estimates the plasma level of PF 1 + 2 in comparison to a reference range of 0.32–1.2 nmol/L. Elevated PF 1 + 2 values are seen in deep vein thrombosis and pulmonary embolism, leukemia, severe liver disease, and myocardial infarction, whereas significantly lowered values are seen during heparin and oral anti-coagulant therapy.[57] The PF 1 + 2 is considered to be a marker for coagulation activation and may predict a thrombotic tendency in some patients.[58]

TESTS OF THE FIBRINOLYTIC PATHWAY

Plasminogen

Plasminogen, the precursor of the trypsin-like proteolytic enzyme plasmin, is produced in the liver and circulates as a single-chain glycoprotein. When bound to fibrin, plasminogen is converted to plasmin by the action of tissue plasminogen activator (tPA) or urokinase plasminogen activator (uPA). Bound plasmin degrades fibrin, while free plasmin is rapidly inactivated by a circulating inhibitor, α_2-anti-plasmin.

Congenital plasminogen deficiencies are associated with thrombosis in some families and with hyaline membrane disease in premature infants.[59, 60] Acquired plasminogen deficiencies are seen in disseminated intravascular coagulation and acute promyelocytic leukemia. Thrombolytic therapy is ineffective when plasminogen levels are low. Plasminogen is readily measured in PPP using a chromogenic substrate assay that is available from several manufacturers. The mean plasma level of plasminogen is 125 mg/L.

PRINCIPLE

PPP is mixed with a solution of streptokinase, an exogenous plasminogen activator derived from β-streptococcal cultures (Fig. 35–12). The reagent streptokinase activates the plasma plasminogen by covalently bonding and forming an amidolytic complex. The resulting streptokinase–plasmin mixture reacts with a chromogenic substrate to release a color with an intensity proportional to the original plasminogen concentration. Several substrates are suitable for plasminogen measurement.[61] A control plasma specimen is tested with the patient specimen, and the results are recorded.

Plasminogen Activators

Two plasminogen activators have been described. tPA is synthesized in vascular endothelial cells and released to the circulation where its half-life is approximately 5 minutes and its plasma concentration averages 4 μg/L.[62] uPA is produced in the kidney and vascular endothelial cells and has a half-life of approximately 8 minutes and a concentration of 8 μg/L.[63] Both plasminogen activators are serine proteases that are rapidly taken up by the liver and degraded, and both are inactivated by covalent reactions with plasminogen activator inhibitor-1 (PAI-1). Plasminogen activators form ternary complexes with bound plasminogen at the surface of fibrin, causing localized plasminogen activation to initiate thrombus degradation.

Impaired fibrinolysis, in the form of decreased plasminogen activator release or activity or increased PAI-1, is associated with thromboembolic disease and myocardial infarction.[64]

Plasminogen activator levels are influenced by exercise and diurnal variation and increase as a result of in vitro activation. Patients should be at rest, tourniquet application should be minimal, and immediate acidification of the specimen in acetate buffer is necessary to stabilize the plasminogen activator activity.[65] Blood is collected into citrate tubes according to the protocol given in the section entitled Evacuated Hemostasis Specimen Collection Tubes, acidified within 60 seconds of collection, and centrifuged immediately. Supernatant plasma may be frozen at -70 °C until the assay is performed.

Levels of tPA antigen may be estimated by monoclonal antibody-based enzyme immunoassay. To measure tPA or uPA activity, an indirect chromogenic substrate assay is used. Plasminogen activators are coupled with measured amounts of reagent plasminogen, which is in turn assayed with the plasminogen system. The resulting color intensity is proportional to plasminogen activator activity (Fig. 35–13). The system may incorporate soluble fibrin to increase the plasminogen activator's activity.

Plasminogen Activator Inhibitor-1

PAI-1 is produced by vascular endothelial cells and hepatocytes and circulates in plasma bound to vitronectin at an average concentration of 10 μg/L with diurnal variations.[66] An inactive form of PAI-

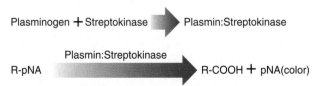

Figure 35–12 Plasminogen assay. *Abbreviation:* R-pNA, chromogenic substrate, where R indicates several choices of amide and pNA is the chromophore para-nitro aniline.

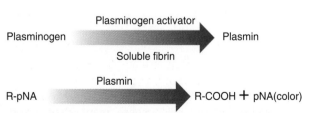

Figure 35–13 Plasminogen activator assay. *Abbreviation:* R-pNA, chromogenic substrate, where R indicates several choices of amide and pNA is the chromophore para-nitro aniline.

1 circulates in high concentrations in platelets.[67] PAI-1 inactivates plasminogen activators by covalent bonding. An elevated level of PAI-1 is associated with thromboembolic disorders and myocardial infarct and may be a cardiovascular risk factor.

Citrated plasma is collected from patients at rest. Immediately after collection, the plasma is prepared to be platelet free to avoid contamination with platelet PAI-1.

Several immunometric and amidolytic methods are available for estimation of PAI-1 antigen concentration and activity in PFP. One sandwich-type enzyme immunoassay for functional PAI-1 converts PAI-1 to a complex with uPA, immobilizes the complex with solid-phase monoclonal anti–PAI-1 and quantitates it with monoclonal anti-uPA as the detecting antibody.[68] Most chromogenic substrate approaches are indirect measures involving the use of tPA or uPA in the plasminogen assay shown in Figure 35–14. The test plasma is mixed with a measured amount of reagent tPA or uPA. Residual activator is then assayed in the plasminogen system as shown in Figure 35–14. The resulting intensity of color is inversely proportional to plasma PAI-1.

Euglobulin Clot Lysis Time

Excessive fibrinolytic activity occurs under a variety of conditions. Inflammation and trauma may be reflected in a radical increase in circulating plasmin that causes hemorrhage. Bone trauma, fractures, and surgical dissection of bone as in cardiac surgery may cause increases in fibrinolysis. A time-honored approach to measurement of fibrinolytic activity is the euglobulin lysis test.

PRINCIPLE AND PROCEDURE

Test plasma is diluted and acidified with cold 1% acetic acid until the solution reaches the pH of 5.35 – 5.40. On refrigeration for approximately 30

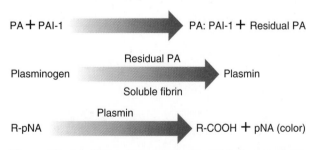

Figure 35–14 PAI-1 chromogenic assay with the use of tPA (tissue plasminogen activator). *Abbreviation:* R-pNA, chromogenic substrate, where R indicates several choices of amide and pNA is the chromophore para-nitro aniline.

minutes a precipitate forms that contains fibrinogen, plasminogen, plasmin, and plasminogen activators. This precipitate is termed the *euglobulin fraction.* Excluded from the precipitate are plasma anti-plasmins, so that fibrinolysis may proceed unchecked. The tubes are centrifuged and the supernate decanted completely. The precipitate is redissolved in borate buffer, and reagent thrombin or calcium chloride is added. A clot should form within a few minutes. A timer is started at the time of thrombin addition, and the clot is observed periodically for dissolution over a period of 90 minutes.

RESULTS

Normal fibrinolysis proceeds slowly in the euglobulin system, so that a firm clot is present after 90 minutes. Disappearance of the clot before 90 minutes has passed indicates increased fibrinolysis.

QUALITY ASSURANCE

Because the euglobulin lysis test is fraught with technical error, both positive and negative plasma controls are included. Fresh or commercial normal plasma is used as the negative control, whereas normal plasma plus streptokinase is used as the positive control. Streptokinase is a humoral activator of plasminogen. Clot dissolution of the test fraction is compared with both the positive and negative controls. Another control, the patient-activated control, is also prepared. This is a specimen of patient euglobulin fraction with streptokinase added. This control ensures against patient specimen plasminogen depletion. When plasminogen levels are diminished, such as in a long-term case of disseminated intravascular coagulation, clot dissolution will not occur. The euglobulin lysis time will appear normal because of the lack of plasminogen. The patient-activated control indicates when this condition exists. Streptokinase-activated plasma from the patient should cause rapid clot dissolution. When plasminogen is depleted, the streptokinase-activated control will give no dissolution and the euglobulin lysis time will appear normal. Thus a normal result in the patient-activated control means the actual test result is untrustworthy.

Hypofibrinogenemia and factor XIII deficiency affect the euglobulin lysis time. In hypofibrinogenemia there is less fibrin to be lysed and a short lysis time may be seen without a genuine increase in fibrinolytic activity. In factor XIII deficiency, the original clot quality is poor and dissolution by normal levels of plasmin is more rapid.

TESTS FOR INHIBITORS

Substitution Screen for Acquired Coagulation Inhibitors

Hemophilia, autoimmune disease, long-term treatment with certain drugs, or collagen disorders are associated with the presence of acquired coagulation inhibitors. Anti–factor VIII, the most common of the specific inhibitors, is detected in 10% of hemophiliacs treated with factor concentrate, cryoprecipitate, or fresh-frozen plasma and may occasionally be present in individuals with immune disorders. The most common nonspecific inhibitor is lupus anti-coagulant, an autoantibody directed against phospholipid-β 2-glycoprotein I complexes, that impairs the in vitro phospholipid-dependent activation of factor X and prothrombin. The APTT is often prolonged in the presence of specific or nonspecific inhibitors. Since the PT results are unpredictable, and the thromboplastin time results are usually normal, the APTT is regarded as a screen for circulating inhibitors (Fig. 35–15).

When the APTT is prolonged on a patient who is not undergoing heparin therapy, the next step is to mix the patient's test plasma with normal PFP by using a ratio prescribed in the laboratory protocol. In most cases, 0.4 mL test plasma is added to 0.1 mL PFP, creating a 4:5 dilution. The mixture is incubated until it reaches 37 °C, then 0.1 mL is tested with the APTT test system. If the result of the test on the mixture is normal, correction has occurred and a factor deficiency may be suspected. Before a factor deficiency is confirmed, however, the incubation of the remaining test plasma–PFP mixture is extended to 120 minutes at 37 °C. Anti–factor VIII reacts more slowly than lupus anti-coagulant, and its effect is enhanced by prolonged 37 °C incubation. If, after the 120-minute incubation, the APTT time interval is again prolonged, anti–factor VIII may be suspected. If correction has occurred in both the 3-minute and 120-minute test specimen–PFP mixture incubation steps, the original prolonged APTT is most likely caused by a factor deficiency. If the prolongation is sustained in either case, an acquired inhibitor is suspected.

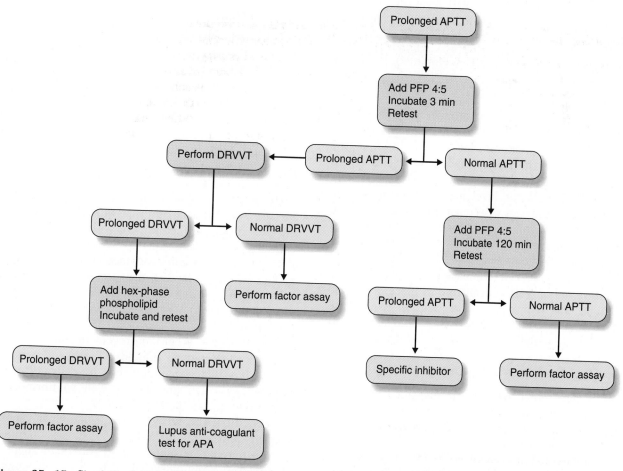

Figure 35–15 Circulating inhibitor detection scheme. *Abbreviations:* APTT, activated partial thromboplastin time; DRVVT, dilute Russell's viper venom time; APA, anti-phospholipid antibody; PFP, platelet-free plasma.

Although others are known, most instances of acquired inhibitor involve either lupus anti-coagulant or anti-factor VIII. The results of the screen must be confirmed with the dilute Russell's viper venom test for lupus anti-coagulant and the Bethesda titer to quantitative anti-factor VIII. Another antibody that is associated with the lupus anti-coagulant, called the anti-phospholipid antibody, may also be suspected and tested for at the same time as the lupus anti-coagulant.

Bethesda Titer for Anti-Factor VIII Inhibitor

Anti-factor VIII antibody is confirmed and quantified by the Bethesda method, in which 0.2 mL of test plasma suspected of containing factor VIII inhibitor is incubated with 0.2 mL normal plasma for 2 hours at 37 °C. A control specimen consisting of 0.2 mL imidazole buffer at pH 7.4 mixed with 0.2 mL of normal plasma is incubated simultaneously. During the incubation period, anti-factor VIII from the test plasma neutralizes a percentage of normal plasma factor VIII activity. The proportion of factor VIII activity neutralized is related to the level of inhibitor activity. After incubation, residual factor VIII level in the pooled normal plasma–test plasma mixture is measured by specific factor assay, as described in the section in this chapter on specific factor assays using the APTT test system.

The level of inhibitor in the specimen is expressed as a percent of the control. If the test specimen–normal plasma mixture retains greater than 75% the residual factor VIII of the control, there is no significant factor VIII inhibitor in the test plasma. If the residual factor VIII level is less than or equal to 25% of control, the test plasma factor VIII inhibitor level is titered using several dilutions of the test specimen in normal plasma. One Bethesda unit of activity is the reciprocal of that titer of antibody that leaves 50% residual factor VIII in the mixture.

The New Oxford modification of this technique employs factor VIII concentrate in place of normal plasma. The reciprocal of the dilution required to leave 50% residual factor VIII in the factor VIII concentrate is defined as a New Oxford unit.

Testing for Lupus Anti-Coagulant

The lupus anti-coagulant is suspected in venous or arterial thromboembolic disease, recurrent unexplained fetal loss, or collagen diseases.[69] It may cause a false positive serologic test for syphilis, and an unexplained prolonged APTT.[70]

If lupus anti-coagulant is suspected because of clinical conditions, the APTT test system de-

scribed in the section entitled Substitution Screen for Circulating Inhibitors may be employed as the initial screening test, but the following points must be kept in mind:[71]

■ Prolongation of any phospholipid-dependent clotting test may indicate the presence of the lupus anti-coagulant provided there is no specific factor deficiency and the patient is not receiving either heparin or oral anti-coagulants. Lupus anti-coagulant tests on patients taking heparin or oral anti-coagulant are unreliable.

■ The APTT is the most frequently used screening test; however, sensitivity to the lupus anti-coagulant varies with the concentration of phospholipid in the reagent. Reagents with low phospholipid content are the more sensitive to lupus anti-coagulant.[72]

■ The lupus anti-coagulant is neutralized by the presence of platelets or platelet membranes in the patient's plasma. Tests should be performed on PFP for greatest sensitivity. If the specimen is to be frozen before testing, it must be free of platelets before freezing.

■ Mixing studies must be sensitive to low levels of lupus anti-coagulant activity. Normal plasma must be free of platelets, and four parts test plasma must be mixed with one part fresh or pooled normal plasma, since a 1:1 ratio neutralizes weak lupus anti-coagulant causing a false negative result.

The dilute Russell's Viper venom (DRVVT) tissue thromboplastin inhibition (TTI), and kaolin clotting time (KCT) tests are employed as screening tests for lupus anti-coagulant.

DILUTE RUSSELL'S VIPER VENOM TEST

Principle. Russell's viper venom, the reagent for the Stypven time test, activates factor X without the need for factors VII, VIII, IX, or XI or contact factors and thus is prolonged only when fibrinogen, prothrombin, or factors V or X are deficient. If these factors are present and provide normal levels of activity, the dilute Russell's viper venom test (DRVVT) is sensitive to lupus anti-coagulant.

The DRVVT is an improvement on the TTI test, which employed diluted PT reagent because the TTI results were influenced by deficiencies of factors VII, VIII, and IX as well as fibrinogen, prothrombin, and factors V and X.

Procedure for DRVVT. Russell's viper venom reagent and cephalin reagent may be obtained from a number of sources (e.g., American Bioproducts, Parsippany, NJ). The Russell's viper venom reagent is diluted 1:2000 with *tris*-buffered saline and may be refrigerated for up to 1 week before use. Cephalin reagent without an activator, such as the reagent used in the (nonactivated) PTT test is prepared and diluted 1:20 with Owren's buffer just before use.

In this test, 0.1 mL of test PFP is mixed with 0.1 mL dilute Russell's viper venom and 0.1 mL dilute cephalin reagent and incubated for a prescribed period of time (e.g., 30 seconds to 2 minutes). A normal control plasma is assayed at the same time as test PFP samples. At the end of the incubation, 0.1 mL of 0.025 M calcium chloride is forcibly added and the time interval to clot formation is measured. The test is performed in duplicate, and the duplicate results are averaged.

DRVVT Results. The control plasma result should be less than or equal to 30 seconds. Normal test plasma results give a ratio of less than or equal to 1.1 times control value. If the test PFP result is greater than 1.1 times control, lupus anti-coagulant may be present. To confirm the presence of lupus anti-coagulant, the test is repeated on PFP that has been incubated with a reagent containing a high concentration of phospholipid such as the platelet neutralization reagent or the hexphase phospholipid suspension.

Confirmation of Lupus Anti-Coagulant with DRVVT and Phospholipid Reagent. Platelet neutralization procedure reagents, prepared by freezing and thawing washed PRP, may be obtained commercially and used as a source of phospholipid. Hex-phase phospholipid is also available. A plasma suspected of containing lupus anti-coagulant is incubated for a few minutes with the phospholipid reagent, then the DRVVT is repeated. If the result is shortened by at least 10%, the presence of lupus anti-coagulant is confirmed.

KAOLIN CLOTTING TIME

Principle of the Kaolin Clotting Time (KCT). Kaolin initiates clotting through the contact factors XII, high–molecular weight kininogen, and prekallikrein. If all coagulation factors are present and provide normal levels of activity, the KCT is sensitive to lupus anti-coagulant. No phospholipid is present in the KCT reagent.

Procedure for KCT. Kaolin may be obtained from a number of sources (e.g., American Bioproducts, Parsippany, NJ) and diluted to 20 mg/dL with Owren's buffer. The test is performed on test PFP, normal PFP, and a 4:1 mixture of test PFP and normal PFP.

In this test, 0.1 mL of test PFP or 4:1 test PFP:normal PFP mixture is mixed with 0.1 mL kaolin reagent and incubated for a prescribed period of time (e.g., 30 seconds to 2 minutes). A

normal control plasma is assayed at the same time as test plasma. At the end of the incubation, 0.1 mL of 0.025 M calcium chloride is forcibly added and the time interval to clot formation is measured. The test is performed in duplicate, and the duplicate results are averaged.

KCT Results. The control plasma result should be greater than 60 seconds. Normal test plasma results will give a ratio of less than or equal to 1.1 times control value. If the test PFP result is greater than 1.1 times control, and the mixture of test PFP with normal PFP is less than or equal to 1.1 times control, then lupus anti-coagulant is suspected. As in the DRVVT, phospholipid neutralization is employed to confirm the presence of lupus anti-coagulant.

Anti-Phospholipid Antibody

Anti-phospholipid antibody is often present with lupus anti-coagulant, and both may be found in venous or arterial thromboembolic disease, recurrent unexplained fetal loss, or collagen diseases.[73] The test for anti-phospholipid antibody is often ordered with the test for lupus anti-coagulant and has the advantage of being performed on serum requiring no special preparations; it is quantitative, may be standardized, and has no interference from heparin or oral anti-coagulants. Enzyme immunoassay or radioimmunoassay techniques are available, and both are more sensitive in detecting antibodies than the lupus anti-coagulant test.

Bovine heart cardiolipin (Sigma Diagnostics, St. Louis, MO) is used as the solid-phase antigen. Serum is incubated with the antigen, then antibodies binding the cardiolipin are detected by using enzyme-labeled goat anti-IgG and anti-IgM. The results may be expressed quantitatively, in GPL units, in which 1 unit is equivalent to 1 μg/mL of an affinity-purified standard IgG anti-phospholipid specimen, or MPL units, in which 1 unit is equivalent to 1 μg/mL of an affinity-purified standard IgM anti-phospholipid specimen. Both IgG and IgM antibodies are tested for, to increase sensitivity, although there seems to be no clinical relationship of one or the other to disease process. The cutoffs for negative and positive sera are 5 GPL and 5 MPL, respectively.

Anti-Thrombin Assay

CHROMOGENIC ANTI-THROMBIN ASSAY

Anti-thrombin (formerly called anti-thrombin III and ATIII) is a plasma glycoprotein serine protease inhibitor that suppresses the activity of thrombin and factor Xa through covalent bonding.[74] The inhibitory action of anti-thrombin is potentiated by the effects of heparin binding.[75] The normal plasma concentration of anti-thrombin is 2.5 μm/L, and deficient anti-thrombin function is associated with recurrent venous thromboembolic disease. Acquired anti-thrombin deficiencies may be associated with oral contraceptive use, liver disease, disseminated intravascular coagulation, and nephrotic syndrome.[76] Congenital anti-thrombin deficiencies have been described.[77] Heparin therapy is ineffective when anti-thrombin activity is diminished.

Anti-thrombin activity is measured using a chromogenic substrate technique.[78] An aliquot of a plasma specimen, collected in citrate, transported, and centrifuged at 4 °C, is mixed with a solution of heparin. The resulting anti-thrombin–heparin complex is mixed with either thrombin or factor Xa and allowed to react. The residual substrate, either thrombin or factor Xa, is next allowed to react with a chromogenic substrate (S2238 for thrombin or S2765 for factor Xa). The intensity of the resulting color reaction is inversely proportional to the plasma anti-thrombin activity (Fig. 35–16).

Other assay systems for anti-thrombin include immunometric systems employing enzyme immunoassays, radioimmunoassays,[79] and Laurell rocket electroimmunoassays.[80] There is also a clot-based anti-thrombin assay.

Protein C Assay

Protein C is a vitamin K–dependent proenzyme that, when converted to an enzymatically active serine protease, becomes an anti-coagulant that cleaves factors Va and VIIIa.[81] In vivo, thrombin combines with thrombomodulin on the endothelial cell surface to convert circulating protein C to protein Ca. For protein Ca to bind to factor Va or factor VIIIa, a cofactor, protein S, must be present.[82] Protein C and protein S assemble with their target procoagulants Va and VIIIa on a phos-

pholipid surface such as a platelet or endothelial cell membrane (Fig. 35–17).[83]

The reference range for protein C is 70–130%, with 100% being equal to 4 μg/mL.[84] Patients with heterozygous congenital deficiencies have protein C levels of 30–65%, and many experience deep venous thrombosis or pulmonary embolus. Unless treated, homozygous deficiency is not compatible with life.[85] Acquired protein C deficiency is associated with liver disease, vitamin K deficiency, and disseminated intravascular coagulation and may occur in patients receiving oral anti-coagulants. Protein C levels are also lowered in patients with thrombotic disease, after surgery, in patients taking contraceptives, and during pregnancy. Deficiency is expected during the first month of life. Dysfunctional forms of protein C have been described.[86]

PROTEIN C IMMUNOASSAY

Immunoassay measures protein C antigen, which includes nonactivated or dysfunctional protein C, and therefore does not reflect protein C activity but is more sensitive than activity measurement techniques. Immunoassay is performed by Laurell rocket electroimmunassay or enzyme immunoassay using citrated plasma specimens.

Laurell Rocket Electroimmunoassay for Protein C. In the Laurell rocket electroimmunoassay for protein C, an agarose gel contains polyclonal anti–protein C antibody. Plasma is placed in a well and an electric current is applied, causing migration of the plasma proteins, including protein C, toward the cathode. The anti-serum reacts with the protein C to form a precipitate, and the distance from the well to the tip of protein C migration is proportional to protein C concentration.[87] Standards and controls are measured with each batch of specimens.

Enzyme Immunoassay for Protein C. Monoclonal antibodies to protein C may be linked to a solid-phase material such as a microtiter plate.[88]

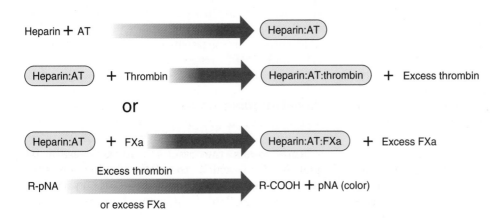

Figure 35–16 Chromogenic substrate assay for anti-thrombin III. *Abbreviations:* FXa, activated Factor X; R-pNA, chromogenic substrate, where R indicates several choices of amide and pNA is the chromophore para-nitro aniline.

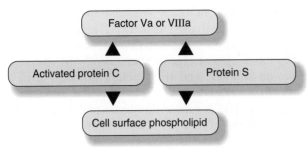

Figure 35–17 Activated protein C complex.

The test plasma is incubated with the antigen and washed away, and an enzyme-labeled anti–protein C antibody is added, forming a complex that gives a color that is proportional to protein C concentration. Standards and controls are measured with each batch of specimens. This is the most sensitive protein C assay, detecting as little as 1% of normal activity.[89]

CHROMOGENIC SUBSTRATE ASSAY FOR PROTEIN C

Functional studies for protein C require an activation step. A specific activator venom, derived from the southern copperhead snake *(Agkistrodon contortrix contortrix)*, is available commercially and is now employed in most chromogenic techniques in place of a less specific thrombin–thrombomodulin complex. Plasma is incubated with the activator so that protein C is converted, then substrate specific for activated protein C is added (S2366). The intensity of the colored product is proportional to protein C activity as it relates to factor Va or VIIIa inactivation (see Fig. 35–17). The results of the chromogenic substrate assay are low when the ability of protein C to bind and inactivate factor Va or VIIIa is diminished, but are not sensitive to dysfunctions involving the parts of the protein C molecule that react with the phospholipid membrane or protein S, instances that may contribute to thrombosis.

CLOT-BASED ASSAY FOR PROTEIN C

The clot-based assay, although more cumbersome than chromogenic substrate, detects all possible defects of the protein C molecule. After activation with *Agkistrodon* snake venom, activated protein C is mixed with a protein C–deficient plasma to ensure the presence of all other procoagulants and anti-coagulants at full strength. An APTT is then performed on the mixture, and the results are compared with the median of the normal range. The amount of activated protein C in the plasma is directly proportional to the clotting

time interval. Neither the chromogenic substrate assay nor the clot-based assay is useful when the patient is on oral anti-coagulant therapy.[90] Reagents for this assay are available from American Bioproducts, Parsippany, New Jersey.

Protein S Assay

Like protein C, protein S is a vitamin K-dependent plasma protein, but unlike protein C, protein S is a cofactor that has no enzymatic properties.[91] Protein S circulates in plasma either free or bound to C4b binding protein, a large complement-binding protein.[92] For protein Ca to bind to factor Va or VIIIa, free protein S must be present. Protein Ca and protein S assemble with their target procoagulant Va or VIIIa on a phospholipid surface such as a platelet or endothelial cell membrane (see Fig. 35–17).

The reference range for total protein S is 65–140% of normal plasma mean protein S levels, is higher in men than in women, and increases with age. Patients with heterozygous congenital deficiencies have protein S levels of near 50%, and many experience thromboembolic disorders; however, the relationship of symptoms to protein S levels is confounded by the ratio of bound and free protein S.[93] Acquired protein S deficiency occurs in liver disease, vitamin K deficiency, and disseminated intravascular coagulation, in patients receiving oral anti-coagulants, and during pregnancy and contraceptive therapy and is expected during the first month of life.[94] In newborns the concentration of C4b binding protein is low so the level of free protein S is normal.[95] C4b binding protein is an acute phase reactant. In inflammatory disorders, including episodes of deep vein thrombosis, C4b binding protein levels increase, diminishing the level of free protein S and making the interpretation of protein S assays difficult.

PROTEIN S IMMUNOASSAY

Immunoassay measures the presence of protein S antigen, including free and bound protein S. Immunoassay may be performed using Laurell rocket electroimmunoassay or enzyme immunoassay using citrated plasma specimens. Immunoassay is more sensitive than activity measurement techniques. The Laurell rocket assay technique for protein S is performed like the assay for protein C; however, free and bound protein S have different electrophoretic properties, and the level of C4b binding protein lowers the results.[96] Rocket assays on plasma from which the C4b binding protein–protein S complex are precipitated by polyethylene glycol are available.[97] Enzyme immunoassay for protein S is conducted as for protein C and should not be affected by the level of C4b binding protein. Commercial kits are available.

FUNCTION ASSAY FOR PROTEIN S

A clot-based assay for functional protein S is marketed by American Bioproducts (Parsippany, NJ). The test is performed using citrated plasma maintained at 4 °C until the plasma is separated from the cells. Plasma may be frozen at −70 °C until testing is performed, and is diluted 1:10 with Owren's buffer just before testing.

The clot-based assay employs lyophilized protein S–deficient plasma, activated protein C reagent, and activated factor V reagent, all three of which are reconstituted just before use. The plasma dilution is first mixed with protein S–deficient plasma to ensure that all other coagulation proteins are present. The activated protein C reagent is then added, followed by the activated factor V reagent. After a 2-minute incubation, 0.025 M calcium chloride is added and the reaction is timed until a clot forms. Time to clotting is proportional to protein S activity. A reference curve involving at least four dilutions of normal plasma is performed with each batch of plasmas tested. The range of linearity is 20–120%, so if the results are less than 20% the test is performed again on a 1:5 dilution and the results divided by 2. If the results are above 120%, the test is performed on a 1:20 dilution and results multiplied by 2. All dilutions should be tested within 30 minutes after preparation. High levels of heparin, greater than or equal to 1 IU/mL plasma, cause overestimation of protein S.

References

1. National Committee for Clinical Laboratory Standards: Collection, Transport, and Processing of Blood Specimens for Coagulation Testing and Performance of Coagulation Assays, 2nd ed. Approved Guideline. NCCLS document H21-A2. Villanova, PA: NCCLS, 1991.
2. National Committee for Clinical Laboratory Standards: Procedures for the Collection of Diagnostic Blood Specimens by Venipuncture, 3rd ed. Approved Standard. NCCLS document H3-A3. Villanova, PA: NCCLS, 1991.
3. Palkuti HS: Specimen collection and quality control. In Corriveau DM, Fritsma GA (eds): Hemostasis and Thrombosis in the Clinical Laboratory. Philadelphia: JB Lippincott, 1988:67–91.
4. Rose VL, Dermott SC, Murray BF, et al: Decentralized testing for prothrombin time and activated partial thromboplastin time using a dry chemistry portable analyzer. Arch Pathol Lab Med 1993; 117:611–617.
5. McGlasson DL, Paul J, Shaffer KM: Whole blood coagulation testing in neonates. Clin Lab Sci 1993; 6:76–77.
6. Machin SJ, et al: Guidelines on testing for the lupus anticoagulant: Lupus anticoagulant working party on behalf of the BCSH haemostasis and thrombosis task force. J Clin Pathol 1991; 44:885–889.
7. Bick RL: Platelet function defects: A clinical review. Semin Thromb Hemostas 1992; 18:167–185.
8. Lind SE: The bleeding time does not predict surgical bleeding. Blood 1991; 77:2547.
9. Duke WW: The pathogenesis of purpura haemorrhagica with especial reference to the part played by the blood platelets. Arch Intern Med 1912; 10:445.
10. Ivy AC, Nelson D, Bucher G: The standardization of certain factors in the cutaneous "venostasis" bleeding time technique. J Lab Clin Med 1941; 26:1812.
11. Kumar R, Ansell JE, Canoso RT, Deykin D: Clinical trial of a new bleeding device. Am J Clin Pathol 1978; 70:642.
12. Mielke CH, et al: The standardized normal Ivy bleeding time and its prolongation by aspirin. Blood 1969; 34:204.
13. Ingerman-Wojenski CM, Silver MJ: A quick method of screening platelet dysfunctions using whole blood lumiaggregometry. Thromb Haemostas 1984; 51:154–156.
14. Bick RL: Platelet function defects: A clinical review. Semin Thromb Hemostas 1992; 18:167–185.
15. Allain JP, Cooper HA, Wagner RH, et al: Platelet fixed with paraformaldehyde: A new reagent for assay of von Willebrand factor and platelet aggregating factor. J Lab Clin Med 1975; 85:318–328.
16. Brace LD: Testing for heparin-induced thrombocytopenia by platelet aggregometry. Clin Lab Sci 1992; 5:80–81.
17. Isenhaart CE, Brandt JT: Platelet aggregation studies for the diagnosis of heparin-induced thrombocytopenia. Am J Clin Pathol 1993; 99:324–330.
18. Messmore HL, Sucha N, Godwin J: Heparin-induced thrombocytopenia and platelet activation in cardiovascular surgery. In Pifarre R (ed): Anticoagulation, Hemostasis, and Blood Preservation in Cardiovascular Surgery. Philadelphia: Hanley and Belfus, 1993.
19. Sheridan D, Carter C, Kelton JG: A diagnostic test for heparin-induced thrombocytopenia. Blood 1986; 67:27–30.
20. Amiral J, Bridey F, Dreyfus M, et al: Platelet factor 4 complexed to heparin is the target for antibodies generated in heparin-induced thrombocytopenia. Thromb Haemostas 1992; 68:95–96.
21. Sadayasu T, Nakashima Y, Yashiro A, et al: Heparin-releasable platelet factor 4 in patients with coronary artery disease. Clin Cardiol 1991; 14:725–729.
22. Rapold HJ, Grimaudo V, Declerck PJ, et al: Plasma levels of plasminogen activator inhibitor type 1, beta-thromboglobulin, and fibrinopeptide A before, during, and after treatment of acute myocardial infarction with alteplase. Blood 1991; 78:1490–1995.
23. Papp AC, Hatzakis H, Bracey A, Wu KK: ARIC hemostasis study: I. Development of a blood collection and processing system suitable for multicenter hemostatic studies. Thromb Haemostas 1989; 61:15–19.
24. Yankee RA, Grumet FC, Rogentine GN: The selection of compatible platelet donors for refractory patients by lymphocyte HL-A typing. N Engl J Med 1969; 22:1208–1212.
25. Friedberg RC, Donnelly SF, Boyd JC, et al: Clinical and blood bank factors in the management of platelet refractoriness and alloimmunization. Blood 1993; 81:3428–3434.
26. Sendroy J, Cecchini LP: Determination of human body surface area from height and weight. J Appl Physiol 1954; 7:1–12.
27. Lee RI, White PD: A clinical study of the coagulation time of blood. Am J Med Sci 1913; 243:279–285.
28. Hattersley P: Activated coagulation time of whole blood. JAMA 1966; 136:436.
29. Najman DM, Walenga JM, Fareed J, Pifarre R: Effects of aprotinin on anticoagulant monitoring: Implications in cardiovascular surgery. Ann Thorac Surg 1993; 55:662–666.
30. Grill HP, Spero JE, Granato JE: Comparison of activated partial thromboplastin time to activated clotting time for adequacy of heparin anticoagulation just before percutaneous transluminal coronary angioplasty. Am J Cardiol 1993; 71:1219–1220.
31. von Kaulla KN, Schultz RL: Comparative studies for evalu-

ating fibrinolysis: Studies with two combined techniques. Am J Clin Pathol 1985; 29:104–109.

32. Sugiura K, Ono IF, Watanabe K, Ando Y: Detection of hypercoagulability by the measurement of dynamic loss modulus of clotting blood. Thromb Res 1982; 27:161–166.

33. National Committee for Clinical Laboratory Standards: One-Stage Prothrombin Time Test (PT): Tentative Guideline. NCCLS document H28-T. Villanova, PA: NCCLS, 1992.

34. Talstad I: Which coagulation factors interfere with the one-stage prothrombin time? Haemostasis 1993; 23:19–25.

35. Biggs R, MacFarlane RG: Reaction of haemophilic plasma to thromboplastin. J Clin Pathol 1951; 4:445–459.

36. Poller L: Laboratory control of anticoagulant therapy. Semin Thromb Hemostas 1986; 12:13–19.

37. Eisenberg JM, Clarke JR, Sussman SA: Prothrombin and partial thromboplastin times as preoperative screening tests. Arch Surg 1982; 117:48–51.

38. McKinly L, Wrenn K: Are baseline prothrombin time/partial thromboplastin time values necessary before instituting anticoagulation? Ann Emerg Med 1993; 22:697–702.

39. National Committee for Clinical Laboratory Standards: Activated Partial Thromboplastin Time Test (APTT): Tentative Guideline. NCCLS document H29-T. Villanova, PA: NCCLS, 1992.

40. Brandt JT, Arkin CF, Bovill EG, et al: Evaluation of APTT reagent sensitivity to factor IX and factor IX assay performance. Arch Pathol Lab Med 1990; 114:135–141.

41. Tollefsen DM: Laboratory diagnosis of antithrombin and heparin cofactor II deficiency. Semin Thromb Hemostas 1990; 16:162–168.

42. McKinly L, Wrenn K: Are baseline prothrombin time/partial thromboplastin time values necessary before instituting anticoagulation? Ann Emerg Med 1993; 22:697–702.

43. Estry DW, Wright L: Laboratory assessment of anticoagulant therapy. Clin Lab Sci 1988; 1:161–164.

44. Vacek JL, Hibiya K, Rosamund TL, et al: Validation of a bedside method of activated partial thromboplastin time measurement with clinical range guidelines. Am J Cardiol 1991; 68:557–559.

45. Oberhardt BJ, Dermott SC, Taylor M, et al: Dry reagent technology for rapid, convenient measurements of blood coagulation and fibrinolysis. Clin Chem 1991; 37:520–526.

46. Rose VL, Dermott SC, Murry BF, et al: Decentralized testing for prothrombin time and activated partial thromboplastin time using a dry chemistry portable analyzer. Arch Pathol Lab Med 1993; 117:611–617.

47. Ansell J, et al: Measurement of the activated partial thromboplastin time from a capillary (fingerstick) sample of whole blood: A new method for monitoring heparin therapy. Am J Clin Pathol 1991; 95:222–227.

48. National Committee for Clinical Laboratory Standards: Procedure for the Determination of Fibrinogen in Plasma: Tentative Guideline. NCCLS document H30-T. Villanova, PA: NCCLS, 1991.

49. Comp PC: Overview of the hypercoagulable states. Semin Thromb Hemostas 1990; 16:158–161.

50. Southern DK: Serum FDP and plasma D-dimer testing: What are they measuring? Clin Lab Sci 1992; 5:332–333.

51. Lawler CM, Bovill EG, Stump DC, et al: Fibrin fragment D-dimer and fibrinogen B beta peptides in plasma as markers of clot lysis during thrombolytic therapy in acute myocardial infarction. Blood 1990; 76:1341–1348.

52. Seligsohn U: High gene frequency of factor XI (PTA) deficiency in Ashkenazi Jews. Blood 1978; 51:1223–1228.

53. Rothschild C, Amiral J, Adam M, Mayer D: Preparation of factor VIII depleted plasma with antibodies and its use for the assay of factor VIII. Haemostasis 1990; 20:321–328.

54. Arkin CF, Bovill EG, Brandt JT, et al: Factors affecting the performance of factor VIII coagulant activity assays: Results of proficiency surveys of the College of American Pathologists. Arch Pathol Lab Med 1992; 116:908–915.

55. Hirst CF, Hewitt J, Poller L: Trace levels of factor VIII in substrate plasma. Br J Haematol 1992; 81:305–306.

56. Krumdieck R, Shaw DR, Huang ST, et al: Hemorrhagic disorder due to an isoniazid-associated acquired factor XIII inhibitor in a patient with Waldenström's macroglobulinemia. Am J Med 1991; 90:639–645.

57. Bruhn HD, Conard J, Mannucci M, et al: Multicentric evaluation of a new assay for prothrombin fragment F 1+2 determination. Thromb Haemostas 1992; 68:413–417.

58. Estivals M, Pelzer H, Sie P, et al: Prothrombin fragment 1 + 2, thrombin-antithrombin III complexes and D-dimers in acute deep vein thrombosis: Effects of heparin treatment. Br J Haematol 1991; 78:421–424.

59. Lottenberg R, Dolly FR, Kitchens CS: Recurring thromboembolic disease and pulmonary hypertension associated with severe hypoplasminogenemia. Am J Hematol 1985; 19:181.

60. Ambrus CM, Weintraub DH, Dunphy D, et al: Studies on hyaline membrane disease: I. The fibrinolytic system in pathogenesis and therapy. Pediatrics 1963; 32:10.

61. Walenga JM: Molecular and automated assessments of coagulation. In Corriveau DM, Fritsma GA (eds): Hemostasis and Thrombosis in the Clinical Laboratory. Philadelphia: JB Lippincott, 1988.

62. Wiman B, Hamsten A: The fibrinolytic enzyme system and its role in the etiology of thromboembolic disease. Semin Thromb Hemostas 1990; 16:207–216.

63. Patrassi GM, Sartori MT, Casonato A, et al: Urokinase-type plasminogen activator release after DDAVP in von Willebrand disease: Different behaviour of plasminogen activators according to the synthesis of von Willebrand factor. Thromb Res 1992; 66:517–526.

64. Dawson S, Henney A: The status of PAI-1 as a risk factor for arterial and thrombotic disease: A review. Atherosclerosis 1992; 95:105–117.

65. Chandler WL, Schmer G, Stratton JR: Optimum conditions for the stabilization and measurement of tissue plasminogen activator activity in human plasma. J Lab Clin Med 1989; 113:362–371.

66. Juhan-Vague I, Alessi MC, Raccah D, et al: Daytime fluctuation of plasminogen activator inhibitor 1 (PAI-1) in populations with high PAI-1 levels. Thromb Haemostas 1992; 67:76–82.

67. Macy EM, Meilahn EN, Declerck PJ, Tracy RP: Sample preparation for plasma measurement of plasminogen activator inhibitor-1 antigen in large population studies. Arch Pathol Lab Med 1993; 117:67–70.

68. Philips M, Juul A, Selmer J, et al: A specific immunologic assay for functional plasminogen activator inhibitor 1 in plasma: Standardized measurements of the inhibitor and related parameters in patients with venous thromboembolic disease. Thromb Haemostas 1992; 68:486–494.

69. Hughes GRV: An immune mechanism in thrombosis. Q J Med 1988; 258P:753–754.

70. Mannucci PM, Canciani MT, Mari D, Meuycci P: The varied sensitivity of partial thromboplastin and prothrombin reagents in the demonstration of lupus-like anticoagulants. Scand J Haematol 1979; 22:423–432.

71. Machin SJ, Giddings JC, Greaves M, et al: Guidelines on testing for the lupus anticoagulant: Lupus anticoagulant working party on behalf of the BCSH haemostasis and thrombosis task force. J Clin Pathol 1991; 44:885–889.

72. Kaczor DA, Bickforn NN, Triplett DA: Evaluation of different mixing study reagents and dilution effect in lupus anticoagulant testing. Am J Clin Pathol 1991; 95:408–411.

73. Triplett DA: Laboratory diagnosis of lupus anticoagulants. Semin Thromb Hemostas 1990; 16:182–192.

74. Seeger WH: Antithrombin III: Theory and clinical applications. Am J Clin Pathol 1978; 68:367.

75. Rosenberg RD: Actions and interactions of antithrombin and heparin. N Engl J Med 1975; 292:146.

76. Kauffman RH, et al: Acquired antithrombin III deficiency and thrombosis in nephrotic syndrome. Am J Med 1978; 65:607–613.

77. Marciniak E, Farley CH, DeSimone PA: Familial thrombosis due to antithrombin III deficiency. Blood 1974; 43:219.

78. Odegard OR: Evaluation of an amidolytic heparin cofactor assay method. Thromb Res 1975; 7:351–360.

79. Chan V, Chan TK, Wong V, et al: The determination of

antithrombin III by radioimmunoassay and its clinical application. Br J Haematol 1979; 41:563.

80. Laurell CB: Electroimmunoassay. Scand J Clin Lab Invest 1972; 29(suppl 124):21.

81. Clouse LH, Comp PC: The regulation of hemostasis: The protein C system. N Engl J Med 1986; 314:1298–1304.

82. Walker FJ: Protein S and the regulation of activated protein C. Semin Thromb Hemostas 1984; 10:131–138.

83. Marlar RA, Kleiss AJ, Griffin JH: Mechanism of action of human activated protein C, a thrombin-dependent anticoagulant enzyme. Blood 1982; 59:1067–1072.

84. Marlar RA: Protein C in thromboembolic disease. Semin Thromb Hemostas 1985; 11:387–393.

85. Bertina R, Broekmans A, van der Linden I, et al: Protein C deficiency in a Dutch family with thrombotic disease. Thromb Haemostas 1982; 48:1–5.

86. Marlar RA, Adcock DM: Clinical evaluation of protein C: A comparative review of antigenic and functional assays. Hum Pathol 1989; 20:1040–1047.

87. Laurell CB: Electroimmunoassay. Scand J Clin Lab Invest 1977; 29:21–32.

88. Boyer C, Rothschild C, Wolf M, et al: A new method for the estimation of protein C by ELISA. Thromb Res 1984; 36:579–589.

89. Vigano D'Angelo S, Esmon CT, Comp PC, et al: Measurement of protein C and protein S in plasma samples. *In* Albertini A, Lenfant C, Paoletti R (eds): Biotechnology in Clinical Medicine. New York: Raven Press, 1987:163–173.

90. Vigano D'Angelo S, Comp PC, Esmon CT, et al: Relationship between protein C and anticoagulant activity during oral anticoagulation and in selected disease states. J Clin Invest 1986; 77:416–425.

91. de Fouw NJ, Haverkate F, Bertina RM, et al: The cofactor role of protein S in the acceleration of whole blood clot lysis by activated protein C in vitro. Blood 1986; 67:1189–1192.

92. Dahlback B: Interaction between vitamin K–dependent protein S and the complement protein, C4b-binding protein: A link between coagulation and the complement system. Semin Thromb Hemostas 1984; 10:139–148.

93. Broekmans AW, Bertina RM, Reinalda-Poot J, et al: Hereditary protein S deficiency and venous thromboembolism: A study in three Dutch families. Thromb Haemostas 1985; 53:273–277.

94. Comp PC: Laboratory evaluation of protein S status. Semin Thromb Hemostas 1990; 16:177–181.

95. Schwarz HP, Muntean W, Watzke H, et al: Low total protein S antigen but high protein S activity due to decreased C4b-binding protein in neonates. Blood 1988; 71:562–565.

96. Malm J, Laurell M, Dahlback B: Changes in the plasma levels of vitamin K–dependent proteins C and S and of C4b-binding protein during pregnancy and oral contraception. Br J Haematol 1988; 68:437–443.

97. Dahlback B: Purification of human vitamin K–dependent protein S and its limited proteolysis by thrombin. Biochem J 1983; 209:837–846.

PART VII

Specific Age Groups

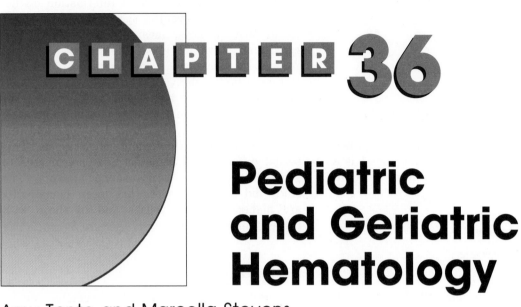

CHAPTER 36

Pediatric and Geriatric Hematology

Amy Tonte and Marcella Stevens

Outline

Objectives

AFTER COMPLETION OF THIS CHAPTER, THE READER WILL BE ABLE TO:

1. List normal reference ranges in the newborn and child.
2. Compare the peripheral blood smear of the newborn and child with the adolescent and adult.
3. List common diseases of childhood.
4. Provide a definition of the geriatric hematology patient, including reference values and variation from the average adult population.
5. Describe the hematologic disorders most often encountered in the geriatric population and the diagnostic test(s) of choice for each disorder.
6. Explain the problems encountered due to age-associated changes in the geriatric patient that influence testing and diagnosis of disorders in this population.

Reference ranges for hematologic values are fairly stable from approximately 14–60 years of age. Two populations that necessitate special discussion are infants and children (pediatric) and senior citizens (geriatric).

PEDIATRIC HEMATOLOGY

Determining reference ranges for the pediatric population is especially difficult, because children mature at different rates, and as they develop, reference ranges change constantly.[1] Table 36–1 is a compilation of reference ranges from standard sources.

Erythrocyte Parameters

RED BLOOD CELL COUNT AND HEMOGLOBIN

Two parameters that are relatively high at birth are the red blood cell count ($5.0-6.0 \times 10^{12}$/L) and the hemoglobin (14–19 g/dL). After the first week, hemoglobin and red blood cells of peripheral blood decline. The changes are targeted for the establishment of hematopoietic equilibrium. This decrease in hemoglobin is an adjustment to increased oxygen saturation of the blood, which occurs when the placenta is replaced by the lungs as an oxygen source. Red blood cell formation is at a minimum until the hemoglobin level reaches 11 or 12 g/dL. During the first few months, as the red blood cell count and hemoglobin decrease in equal degrees, physiologic anemia of the newborn occurs. At 6 weeks to 2 months, hemoglobin reaches its lowest levels and remains fairly constant throughout infancy. During the first 2 years, the normal hemoglobin value is approximately 10–12 g/dL. After this, it gradually rises until it reaches its maximum of 16 g/dL for males and 14 g/dL for females by 14 years of age.[2] The red blood cell count average is $4.44 \pm 0.4 \times 10^{12}$/L by the end of the first year and $4.80 \pm 0.5 \times 10^{12}$/L by age 10.[1] Adult red blood cell counts are usually obtained by age 14.[2]

HEMATOCRIT

At birth the average hematocrit is 0.55 L/L (55%). This declines to around 0.30 L/L by the second month and gradually increases to 0.36 L/L by one year of age. Normal adult values of about 0.45 L/L for males and 0.42 L/L for females are reached in adolescence. On occasion, normal children will have a marked increase in red blood cells, hematocrit levels, and hemoglobin levels during adolescence. Such changes are transient and return to normal in the post-adolescent period.[2] From 1966 to 1970, a large survey was performed in the United States which provided information on hematocrit levels in youths aged 12 to 17. It was found that in boys, mean hematocrits increase consistently with age, about one percent each year. At age 12, they have a low average of 0.41 L/L that goes to a high average of 0.46 L/L by age 17. This increase of the hematocrit with age in males does not occur in females. Girls have mean hematocrits ranging from 0.40 L/L to 0.41 L/L, and this remains constant throughout adolescence. This sexual difference in hematocrits is not related to geography, race, or socioeconomic factors. The study did show, however, that mean hematocrits are higher in white youths and in those with higher family incomes.[2]

RED BLOOD CELL INDICES

A useful means of designating anemias can be provided by the calculation of red blood cell indices based on ratios of the red blood cell count, packed red blood cell volume, and hemoglobin concentration.[2] Red blood cells are unusually large at birth; the average mean corpuscular volume (MCV) is 119 ± 9.4 fL.[3] The lower limit of normal (80 fL) for children and adults is reached at ages 4 to 5. The mean corpuscular hemoglobin concentration (MCHC) remains fairly constant throughout infancy and childhood. The normal adult average MCHC of approximately 33 g/dL is reached at about 6 months of age.[2]

RETICULOCYTES

At 12 weeks of gestation, there are about 90% reticulocytes in the blood of the human fetus. This percentage drops to 5–10% by 24 weeks gestation. At birth, reticulocytes range from 4–6%. This reflects active red blood cell formation in fetal life and explains why polychromasia is seen on the Wright stained smears of peripheral blood of newborns. This reticulocytosis which occurs at birth remains for about 3 days. There is a definite drop from days 4 to 7 to a low level of 0.5%.[2] The reticulocyte count remains low during the first 2 months of life because of low red blood cell production. By age 2 months, the number of reticulocytes again increases slightly. There is a large capacity for red blood cell production around the fourth month that maintains hemoglobin levels and compensates for shorter life span of the fetal red blood cell and the rapid growth of the infant.[4] From ages 3 months to 2 years, there is a slight decline until adult levels are attained.[2]

Table 36-1. REFERENCE RANGES FOR HEMATOLOGY

Test	0-1 Day	2-4 Days	5-7 Days	8-14 Days	15-30 Days	1-2 Months	3-5 Months	6-11 Months	1-3 Years	4-7 Years	8-13 Years	Adult Female	Adult Male
Hb (g/dL)	16.5-21.5	16.4-20.8	15.2-20.4	15.0-19.6	12.2-18.0	10.6-16.4	10.4-16.0	10.4-15.6	9.6-15.6	10.2-15.2	12.0-15.0	12.0-15.0	14.0-18.0
Hct (L/L)	0.48-0.68	0.48-0.68	0.50-0.64	0.46-0.62	0.38-0.53	0.32-0.50	0.35-0.51	0.35-0.51	0.34-0.48	0.34-0.48	0.35-0.48	0.35-0.49	0.40-0.54
WBC (×10⁹/L)	9.0-37.0	8.0-24.0	5.0-21.0	5.0-21.0	5.0-21.0	6.0-18.0	6.0-18.0	6.0-18.0	5.5-17.5	5.0-17.0	4.5-13.5	4.5-11.5	4.5-11.5
RBC (×10¹²/L)	4.10-6.10	4.36-5.96	4.20-5.80	4.00-5.60	3.20-5.00	3.40-5.00	3.65-5.05	3.60-5.20	3.40-5.20	4.00-5.20	4.00-5.20	4.00-5.40	4.60-6.00
MCV (fL)	95-125	98-118	100-120	95-115	93-113	83-107	83-107	78-102	76-92	78-94	80-94	80-94	80-94
MCH (pg)	30-42	30-42	30-42	30-42	28-40	27-37	25-35	23-31	23-31	23-31	26-32	26-32	26-32
MCHC (%)	30-34	30-34	30-34	30-34	30-34	31-37	32-36	32-36	32-36	32-36	32-36	32-36	32-36
RDW (%)	11.5-14.5	11.5-14.5	11.5-14.5	11.5-14.5	11.5-14.5	11.5-14.5	11.5-14.5	11.5-14.5	11.5-14.5	11.5-14.5	11.5-14.5	11.5-14.5	11.5-14.5
Bands (%)	4-14	3-11	3-9	1-9	0-5	0-5	0-5	0-5	0-5	0-5	0-5	0-5	0-5
Polys (%)	37-67	30-60	27-51	22-46	20-40	20-40	18-38	20-40	22-46	30-60	35-65	50-70	50-70
Lymphs (%)	18-38	16-46	24-54	30-62	41-61	42-72	45-75	48-78	37-73	29-65	23-53	18-42	18-42
Monos (%)	1-12	3-14	4-17	4-17	2-15	3-14	2-11	2-11	2-11	2-11	2-11	2-11	2-11
Eos (%)	1-4	1-5	2-6	1-5	1-5	1-4	1-4	1-4	1-4	1-4	1-4	1-3	1-3
Baso (%)	0-2	0-2	0-2	0-2	0-2	0-2	0-2	0-2	0-2	0-2	0-2	0-2	0-2
ANC (×10⁹/L)	3.7-30.0	2.6-17.0	1.5-12.6	1.2-11.6	1.0-9.5	1.2-8.1	1.1-7.7	1.2-8.1	1.2-8.9	1.5-11.0	1.6-9.5	2.3-8.6	2.3-8.6
NRBC (per 100 WBC)	2-24	5-9	0-1	0	0	0	0	0	0	0	0	0	0
Retic (%)	1.8-5.8	1.3-4.7	0.2-1.4	0-1.0	0.2-1.0	0.8-2.8	0.5-1.5	0.5-1.5	0.5-1.5	0.5-1.5	0.5-1.5	0.5-1.5	0.5-1.5
Platelets (×10⁹/L)	150-450	150-450	150-450	150-450	150-450	150-450	150-450	150-450	150-450	150-450	150-450	150-450	150-450

Abbreviations: Hb = hemoglobin; Hct = hematocrit; WBC = white blood cells; RBC = red blood cells; MCV = mean corpuscular volume; MCH = mean corpuscular hemoglobin; MCHC = mean corpuscular hemoglobin concentration; RDW = red blood cell distribution width; Polys = polymorphonuclear cells; Lymphs = lymphocytes; Monos = monocytes; Eos = eosinophils; Baso = basophils; ANC = absolute neutrophil count; NRBC = nucleated red blood cells; retic = reticulocytes.
From Riley Hospital for Children, Indianapolis, IN; compiled from standard sources.

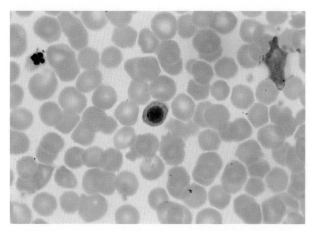

Figure 36-1 Peripheral blood smear of a newborn, demonstrating two nucleated red blood cells and a lymphocyte.

NORMOBLASTS

Frequently, normoblasts are observed in the normal infant on the first day of life. In most instances, they are gone, however, by the third to fifth day. At birth the average number ranges from 3–10 nucleated red blood cells (NRBCs) per 100 white blood cells (WBCs). With acute infection associated with anemia, NRBCs can be seen in older infants. Figure 36–1 illustrates a typical peripheral blood film of a newborn, containing a lymphocyte and two NRBCs. The presence of normoblasts in the blood of older patients, along with pancytopenia, indicates bone marrow stress and often the invasion of the marrow by tumor or replacement by leukemia.[2]

Leukocyte Parameters

WHITE BLOOD CELL COUNT

The total leukocyte count is high at birth, ranging from 9.0 to 30.0 × 10⁹/L. During the first

week, the WBC count drops to 5.0–21.0 × 10⁹/L. At one year, the normal value ranges from 6.0 to 18.0 × 10⁹/L.[5]

DIFFERENTIAL VALUES

Neutrophils. The percentage of neutrophilic leukocytes averages around 60% at birth. This average drops to about 40% by day 10 and then to 30% between the fourth and sixth months. It remains at that level until age 4, when the percentage rises to around 40%. In the sixth year, adult values of 55–60% are reached.[2]

Lymphocytes. Lymphocytes constitute about 30% at birth and rise to 60% in the fourth to sixth month. In the fourth year, the average percentage drops to 50% and drops further to 30% by the eighth year.[2] It is not uncommon for lymphocytes in infants and children to appear "reactive." This morphology, however, is normal at this age and many laboratories do not report reactive lymphocytes on children less than 2 years of age (Fig. 36–2).

Monocytes. At birth the average monocyte count is 6%. An average of about 5% is maintained throughout infancy and childhood except in the second and third week when it rises to around 9%.[2]

Eosinophils and Basophils. The percentage of eosinophils (2–3%) and basophils (0.5%) are consistent throughout infancy and childhood.[2]

Platelets

At birth, the normal range for platelets is 150–350 × 10⁹/L. Adult values of 250–350 × 10⁹/L are reached at about age 6 months. The lower number of platelets at birth has been attributed to the trauma caused by the birth process. Platelets of a newborn infant show greater variation in size and

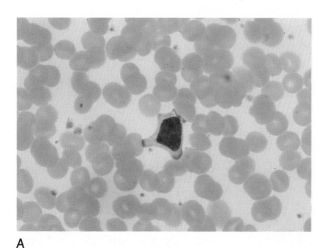

A

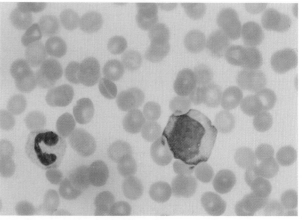

B

Figure 36-2 Reactive lymphocytes (*A* and *B*). These blood cells are common in children less than 2 years of age.

shape than those of adults as well. Large platelets are often considered to represent young platelets.[2] Obtaining an accurate platelet count on a child is difficult if a venipuncture is not possible, and blood must be collected by capillary puncture. This method often takes more time, and the flow of blood is often not as good; therefore it is not unusual for clumped platelets to be found.

COMMON DISEASES OF CHILDHOOD

Common hematologic disorders of childhood include anemia due to ABO-Rh incompatibility or iron deficiency, bacterial and viral infections, and acute lymphocytic leukemia.

GERIATRIC HEMATOLOGY

Definition of the Geriatric Patient

The age at which a patient is termed geriatric varies from 50 to 65 years old, but the most common reference point is over 60.[6-8] Currently a greater percentage of patients fall within this range than ever before. Between the years 2020 and 2030, 75% of health care providers' time will be spent with geriatric patients.[9, 10] Clinical laboratory scientists must become aware of the changes in hematologic parameters that result from advancing age. There is still controversy concerning reference ranges for the elderly. Some studies have shown that healthy individuals over 60 demonstrate reference values equivalent to those of younger adults; however, other studies suggest lower reference ranges for this group.[11-16] Bone marrow changes take place with aging. There is a decrease in the lymphocyte count and an increase in chromosomal abnormalities, which may be related to the increased incidence of myelodysplastic syndrome.[17] Additional sources state that the elderly have higher bone marrow iron and serum ferritin concentrations resulting from impaired utilization.[17-20]

Hematopathologies most commonly seen in the elderly result from or are influenced by decreased bone marrow reserve, poor nutrition, increased neuropsychiatric changes, increased incidence of anemia, myeloproliferation, malignancy, abnormal coagulation, and alterations of immune function.[7, 13, 14, 15, 21] A better understanding of the hematologic diseases associated with the elderly will aid in early and correct diagnosis to determine whether the hematologic manifestation is primary or secondary, and if treatment is necessary and appropriate (Table 36-2).[22]

Table 36-2. GERIATRIC HEMATOPATHOLOGIES
Anemias
Vitamin B_{12} deficiency (pernicious anemia)
Folic acid deficiency
Iron deficiency
Sideroblastic anemia
Anemia of chronic disease
HEMOLYTIC
Malignancies
MYELOPROLIFERATIVE DISEASE
Polycythemia vera (PV)
Agnogenic myeloid metaplasia
MYELODYSPLASIA (MDS)
LEUKEMIAS
Acute myeloblastic (AML)
Acute lymphoblastic (ALL)
Chronic lymphocytic (CLL)
MULTIPLE MYELOMA (MM)
Coagulopathies
Coumarin ingestion
Antibody-like inhibitors
Acquired coagulopathies (disseminated intravascular coagulation (DIC))

Geriatric Phlebotomy

Phlebotomists, faced with fragile rolling veins and autoimmune disorders that impair platelet and coagulation function, resort to syringe and butterfly techniques in the old more often than in the younger population.[23] A method of stabilizing the rolling vein is to place a hair pic on the skin with the vein between the central prongs parallel to the vein. This holds the vein in place without flattening or stretching the fragile skin (Fig. 36-3).[11]

Another concern is the inability of the geriatric patient to maintain pressure on the venipuncture site. This can result in an increased incidence of hematomas, so the patient's arm should not be bent. The geriatric patient should be clearly instructed to actively put pressure on the venipuncture site. If this is not possible, the aid of the phlebotomist, healthcare worker, or an accompanying relative may be necessary.

Geriatric Hematopathology

ANEMIAS

Anemia is common in the elderly.[14] Diagnosing and defining the anemia may be difficult because baseline values for elderly patients may be different from that of the younger population.[12] Factors involved are a physiologic decrease in bone marrow function, a decline in physical activity, and an increase in cardiovascular and chronic inflammatory disorders. These not only alter red blood cell production but also plasma volume, thus leading to

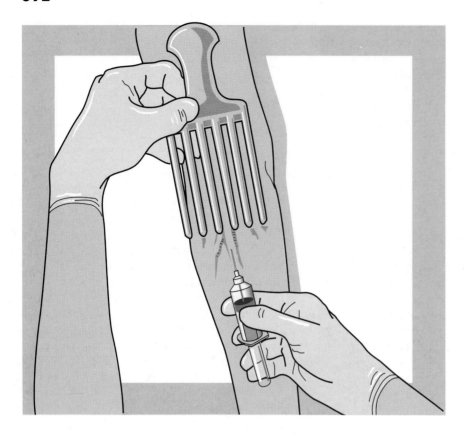

Figure 36-3 A hair pic may be used to stabilize rolling veins in elderly patients. (From Bischof RD: [Letter in "Practical Pointers"]. Consultant 32[4]: 42, 1992.)

lower hemoglobin concentrations and hematocrit values. A classification of anemias seen in the geriatric patient is listed in Table 36–3 along with the appropriate red blood cell morphology indicators.

Hypoproliferation of red blood cells is the most common form of anemia in the geriatric patient. Bone marrow reserves decrease and hormonal response to hematologic stress diminishes in the elderly patient, influencing the development of anemia.[17, 20] The anemia is often secondary to *chronic disease* or *iron deficiency*.[14] Chronic diseases resulting in a secondary anemia include chronic inflammatory diseases such as rheumatoid arthritis, renal failure, infections, liver disease, and malignancy. *Anemia of chronic disease* is similar morphologically to iron deficiency anemia, but differs in a decreased transferrin level and normal red cell distribution width (RDW).[16] Some tests to aid diagnosis are those measuring reticulocyte counts, erythrocyte indices, transferrin levels, serum ferritin, and free erythrocyte protoporphyrin assays (FEP)[6] (see Chapters 16 and 19). Older people tend to have a higher *baseline* ferritin; therefore, it is possible that depletion can occur while ferritin is still within the normal range.[18] As an acute phase protein, serum ferritin rises with chronic inflammation and so a normal ferritin reading does not exclude an iron-depleted state. As a person becomes iron-deficient without anemia, serum iron falls and the transferrin levels rise. In older individuals, however, serum transferrin and serum iron decrease as a result of the decreased body activity and requirements, which may make the results of these tests unreliable.[13]

Iron requirements seem to decrease with age, particularly in women.[24] The elderly have higher levels of liver iron,[18] bone marrow iron,[19] and serum ferritin.[18, 20] A low serum ferritin level always indicates iron deficiency, as does the absence of iron in the bone marrow. The ferritin

MCV	RDW	Disorder
Normal	Normal	Chronic disease
		Hemorrhage
		Leukemia
Normal	High	Early iron deficiency
		Mixed deficiency
		Sideroblastic anemia
Low	Normal	Chronic disease
Low	High	Iron deficiency
High	Normal	Myelodysplastic syndrome
High	High	Vitamin B$_{12}$ deficiency
		Folic acid deficiency
		Immune hemolytic deficiency

Table 36-3. CLASSIFICATION OF GERIATRIC ANEMIA WITH MCV AND RDW INDICES

Abbreviations: MCV, mean corpuscular volume; RDW, red blood cell distribution width.

values may be within the normal range even in an iron-deficient person with a concomitant anemia of chronic disease, however, so results in an older patient may be confusing.

When iron deficiency occurs in the elderly, it usually results from bleeding rather than nutritional lack or malabsorption. Although it is important to prevent iron deficiency, indiscriminate use of iron could conceivably lead to iron overload.[24] Once iron deficiency is diagnosed, it is important to replace body iron while the source of bleeding is being sought and treated.[25]

Primary acquired *sideroblastic anemia* is seen most frequently in patients over 50 years of age.[17] This anemia presents with a dimorphic blood picture with both normochromic and hypochromic red blood cells. Peripheral blood cells may be microcytic or megaloblastic. The presence of ringed sideroblasts in the bone marrow is necessary for diagnosis[17, 26] (see Chapter 16).

The primary hematologic finding in *megaloblastic disorders* is a macrocytic anemia with an MCV above 95 fL. This is accompanied by hypersegmented polymorphonuclear leukocytes and decreased reticulocyte and platelet levels.

Megaloblastic anemia caused by *vitamin B_{12} deficiency* occurs most often in persons over 60 years old and is rarely associated with poor diet.[26, 27] The most common cause of vitamin B_{12} deficiency is the production of autoantibodies which interfere with vitamin B_{12} absorption. This leads to pernicious anemia, which develops slowly and insidiously and can result in a late diagnosis because of neuropsychiatric abnormalities in the absence of the anemia. Treatment with parenteral vitamin B_{12} may correct the anemia but not reverse the neurologic aspects of the disease; thus early detection and treatment are important.[26, 27]

A second megaloblastic anemia prevalent among the elderly population results from *folate deficiency*. When older chronically ill patients suffer from hematologic or neuropsychiatric disorders, folate deficiency caused by poor diet may be present.[28] Although certain studies support this, others conclude that folic acid has no effect on the progression of neurologic symptoms typical of a vitamin B_{12} deficiency.[28, 29] In order to determine if neuropsychosis is a result of folate deficiency, cerebrospinal fluid levels of indole can be measured if previous diagnostic tests remain inconclusive. Indole levels will be normal in patients with primary disorders and lower in patients with neuropsychiatric disorders caused by folate or vitamin B_{12} deficiencies.

The peripheral blood analysis of folate deficiency may be quite similar to that of vitamin B_{12} deficiency; however, folate levels will decrease. The most meaningful diagnostic test measures erythrocyte folate levels. The folate content of red blood cells reflects liver stores whereas the serum folate level is dependent on recent dietary changes and so lacks a fixed criterion.[27, 28]

A previously undiagnosed *hemolytic anemia* in the older patient is most likely to be one of the acquired type, of which immune hemolytic anemias are the most common. Their presence can usually be suspected on clinical grounds and, in the vast majority, readily confirmed by simple laboratory tests. The reticulocyte count and direct anti-human globulin test (DAT) or direct Coombs test results are usually decisive, but false negative results do occur. Chronic lymphocytic leukemia, malignant lymphoma, collagen vascular disease, and drugs administered for other illnesses may result in immune hemolytic anemia. In drug-induced immune hemolytic anemia, it may be necessary to rule out nonimmune mechanisms, such as glucose-6-phosphate dehydrogenase (G6PD) deficiency or the presence of unstable hemoglobins.[16, 30]

Malignancies. Hematologic malignancies are also common in the geriatric patient. The median age for acute leukemia ranges from 55 to 65 years and 90% of diagnosed cases of chronic lymphocytic leukemia are in patients over 50 years old.[31, 32] The presence of an abnormal serum protein as seen in multiple myeloma increasingly occurs in individuals over the age of 80.[33]

Of all geriatric hematologic diseases, *myeloproliferative disorders* are most consistently associated with this age group and occupy an important position among the geriatric hematopathologies.[34] Myeloproliferative disease is a monoclonal proliferation of the hematopoietic pluripotent precursor cell. The specific cell phenotype varies and results in a broad group of diseases which may involve the erythroid (polycythemia), megakaryocytic (thrombocythemia), myeloid (myeloid metaplasia), and granulocytic (basophilia, polymorphonuclear neutrophil dysfunction) phenotypes. Establishing the involvement of all three cell lineages is most helpful in diagnosing myeloproliferative disease. Peripheral blood should be examined to determine abnormalities associated with each phenotype. All patients should have a bone marrow aspiration and a biopsy and direct analysis of the chromosomes of the hematopoietic cells. Red blood cell mass and plasma volume should be measured to evaluate the polycythemic and anemic phenotypes of myeloproliferative disease.[34] Myeloproliferative disorders are further discussed in Chapter 24.

Elderly patients often develop acute or chronic leukemia and myelodysplasia. On the basis of morphology, histochemical staining, and immunologic markers, the leukemias are categorized according to the French-American-British (FAB) classification of acute leukemias and myelodysplasia. Recent advances in chromosome banding techniques and protein two-dimensional gel techniques allow more accurate classification of malignancies resulting in more appropriate treatment.[35] Treatment protocols for acute lymphocytic leukemia (ALL) which have been successful in patients aged 15–59 have had poorer outcomes in the geriatric patient with similar disease.[7]

The *myelodysplastic syndromes* (MDS) are a heterogenous group of disorders in which the hematopoietic precursors may be abundant but morphologically abnormal. Hematopoiesis is ineffective and normal numbers of mature peripheral blood cells are not produced.[31]

Acute myeloid leukemia (AML) is predominantly a disease of the elderly. Approximately 13% initially present with previous hematologic disorders such as myelodysplastic syndrome, hypoplastic bone marrow, polycythemia, or myelofibrosis. Geriatric AML differs from AML in the younger population in blast cell phenotype and morphology (decreased number of Auer rods) as well as other factors related to geriatric disease mentioned previously.[27] The geriatric patient is more likely to succumb to treatment toxicity or become resistant to therapy. Predictive factors for favorable prognosis include blast counts $<50 \times 10^9$/L, serum albumin readings >33 g/L, and an absence of hepatosplenomegaly.[21] Although ALL in the elderly is less common, many of the same problems of poor tolerance to the necessary intensive therapies exist.[7, 8]

In *chronic lymphocytic leukemia* (CLL), the initial presentation is often in an individual over 50 years old with fatigue, malaise, or an infection or unrelated disease. Over 25% of patients are asymptomatic; usually CLL is discovered upon routine physical examination or blood count. The diagnosis of CLL requires the demonstration of sustained lymphocytosis and bone marrow lymphocyte infiltration in the absence of other causes. The absolute lymphocyte count is generally above 15×10^9/L. These cells appear mature and are usually indistinguishable from normal lymphocytes, although they may be slightly smaller. Many patients are hypogammaglobulinemic or agammaglobulinemic because of the primary involvement of the B cell.[36]

Monoclonal gammopathies such as *multiple myeloma* (MM) are one of the most strikingly age-related phenomena among the immunologic and other neoplastic disorders in man. Diagnosing the bone manifestations in the older patient may be difficult. The pain associated with bone lesions is frequently the initial presenting symptom and this may be attributed to "arthritis of old age." Hypercalcemia is a frequent complication of myeloma, in part related to the increased absorption of bone, as well as from subsequent impairment of renal calcium excretion, which may become a vicious cycle in such patients. The primary characteristic of MM is a circulating serum M (myeloma) protein or the excretion of free monoclonal light chains (Bence-Jones protein), which is seen in 99% of all patients. IgG protein is seen in 50% of patients, and IgA in 25%, whereas 20% produce only light chains, which are found in the urine. A smaller percentage demonstrate IgD, IgE, and IgM proteins. These elevated proteins result in an increased sedimentation rate, which may be attributed to the increase in autoimmune proteins often seen in old age and therefore not investigated.[31]

Coagulopathies. Conflicting studies make the normal coagulation status in the elderly uncertain. It has been stated that there is no difference in coagulation factors in individuals from 50–80 years of age compared with younger people. Other investigators, however, have reported mild elevation of factors XIII, XII, XI, X, and V and anti-thrombin III, with a decline after the eighth decade of life.[37]

A frequent bleeding disorder seen in the elderly is associated with ingestion of coumarin-like drugs. Most elderly patients also take a variety of other drugs that may influence the action of the coumarin.

Bleeding also occurs secondary to the altered immune system of the elderly and involves increased production of antibody-like proteins which act as inhibitors of coagulation factors or procoagulants. Disorders in which this occurs are systemic lupus erythematosus, multiple myeloma, and macroglobulinemia.

Many bleeding disorders of the elderly are acquired. These include vitamin K–deficiency states, hepatocellular disease, massive blood replacement, heparinization, circulating anti-coagulants, fibrinolysis, and disseminated intravascular coagulation (DIC). One study of DIC patients with other underlying diseases demonstrated that 40% were over age 60, and of those, 90% died of DIC.[37] This is a striking example of the need to recognize and diagnose hematologic disorders of the elderly early to avoid a fatal outcome.

SUMMARY

Reference ranges for hematologic values remain stable from approximately 14 to 60 years of age. Two groups who deserve special discussion are infants and children (pediatric) and senior citizens (geriatric).

At birth the erythrocyte count and hemoglobin and hematocrit levels are relatively high, but decline to their lowest level at 6 weeks to 2 months.

After this they gradually rise until adult levels are reached at approximately 14 years of age. The MCV of a newborn is unusually high at an average 119 fL, reaches a low of average 80 fL at approximately 4–5 years, and then levels out at adult ranges.

The leukocyte count is high at birth (9–30 × 10^9/L) and quickly drops to 5–21 × 10^9/L during the first week. Young children normally have higher WBCs than adults and, as with all parameters, reference ranges should be established within each institution. At birth the percentage of lymphocytes is in the adult range, but after 4–6 months, it has risen to 60%. Adult ranges are usually reached by age 8. It is so common to find reactive lymphocytes in infants and children, especially those under 2 years of age, that many laboratories do not report them as reactive in that age group.

The newborn may have 3–10 NRBC/100 WBC.

The NRBCs usually disappear by the third to fifth day. Normoblasts that develop after that time usually indicate a pathologic condition. As a result of this active red blood cell formation, the newborn's peripheral blood smear exhibits polychromasia.

There are no current reference values available for the geriatric population and very little documentation of phlebotomy techniques specific to this group. Although the anemias, malignancies, and coagulopathies are the same diseases found in younger people, the concurrence of other diseases as well as the physiologic changes in aging alter the test values, treatment, and prognosis.

The increased awareness of preventive medicine, as well as new medical technologies, have resulted in an increased life span. This increase in the percentage of patients over 60 years of age will be paralleled by an increase in hematopathologies reflecting a unique relationship with the aging process.

References

1. Johnson TR: How growing up can alter lab values. Diagn Med 1982; 5(Special Issue):12–18.
2. Miller DR: Normal blood values from birth to adolescence. *In* Miller DR, Baehner RL, Miller LP (eds): Blood Diseases of Infancy and Childhood, 6th ed. St. Louis: CV Mosby, 1990:26–51.
3. Oski FA: The erythrocyte and its disorders. *In* Nathan DG, Oski FA (eds): Hematology of Infancy and Childhood, 4th ed. Philadelphia: WB Saunders, 1993:18–43.
4. Brown MS: Physiologic anemia of infancy: normal red cell values and physiology of neonatal erythropoiesis. *In* Stockman JA, Pochedly C (eds): Developmental and Neonatal Hematology. New York: Raven Press, 1988:249–274.
5. Willoughby ML: Paediatric Haematology. New York: Churchill Livingstone, 1977: xiv.
6. Guyatt GH, Patterson C, Ali M, et al: Diagnosis of iron deficiency anemia in the elderly. Am J Med 1990; 88:205–209.
7. Delannoy A, Ferrant A, Bosly A, et al: Acute lymphoblastic leukemia in the elderly. Eur J Haematol 1990; 45:90–93.
8. Whitely R, Hannah P, Holmes F: Survival in acute leukemia in elderly patients, no improvement in the 1980's. J Am Geriatr Soc 1990; 38:527–530.
9. Selker LG: Introduction. J Allied Health. 1987; 16:283–284.
10. Brotman AC: Chart Book on Aging in America. Washington: White House Conference on Aging, 1981.
11. Bischof RO: Stabilizing a rolling vein. Consultant 1992; 32(4):42.
12. Cavalieri TA, Chopra A, Bryman PN: When outside the norm is normal: interpreting lab data in the aged. Geriatrics 1992; 47(5):66–70.
13. Freedman ML, Marcus DL: Anemia and the elderly: Is it physiology or pathology? Am J Med Sci 1980; 280:81–85.
14. Besa EC: Approach to mild anemia in the elderly. Clin Geriatr Med 1988; 4(1):43–55.
15. Daly MP, Sobal J: Anemia in the elderly, a survey of physicians' approaches to diagnosis and workup. J Fam Pract 1989; 28(5):524–528.
16. Stander PE: Anemia in the elderly. Symptoms, causes and therapies. Postgrad Med 1989; 85(2):85–90, 92, 96.
17. Baldwin JG Jr: True anemia: incidence and significance in the elderly. Geriatric 1989; 44(8):33–36.
18. Casale G, Bonor AC Migliavacca A, et al: Serum ferritin and aging. Age Ageing 1981; 10:119–122.
19. Benzie, R McD: The influence of age upon the iron content of bone marrow. Lancet 1963; 1:1074–1075.
20. Lipschitz DA, Cook JD, Finch CA: A clinical evaluation of serum ferritin as an index of iron stores. N Engl J Med 1974; 290:1213–1216.
21. Tucker J, Thomas AE, Gregory WM, Ganesan TS, et al: Acute myeloid leukemia in elderly adults. Hemat Oncol 1990; 8:13–21.
22. Stevens ML, Stevens RL: Geriatric hematology: blood disorders in the elderly. Clin Lab Sci 1988; 1:347–349.
23. Stevens ML: Unpublished data.
24. Marcus DL, Freedman, ML: Clinical disorders of iron metabolism in the elderly. Clin Geriatr Med 1985; 1:729–745.
25. Freedman ML: Common hematological problems: diagnosis and treatment. Geriatrics 1983; 38:119–131.
26. Daly MP: Anemia in the elderly. Am Fam Pract 1989; 39(3):129–136.
27. Crantz JG: Vitamin B_{12} deficiency in the elderly. Clin Geriatr Med 1985; 1:701–714.
28. Grinblat J: Folate status in the aged. Clin Geriatr Med 1985; 1:711–728.
29. Robbins SL, Cotran RS, Kumar V: Pathologic Basis of Disease. Philadelphia: W.B. Saunders, 1984.
30. Javid J: Immune hemolytic anemia in the aged. Clin Geriatr Med 1985; 1:747–772.
31. Antin JH, Rosenthal DS: Acute leukemias, myelodysplasia, and lymphomas. Clin Geriatr Med 1985; 1:795–826.
32. Stahl RL, Silber R: Chronic lymphocytic leukemia. Clin Geriatr Med 1985; 1:857–867.
33. Cohen HJ: Multiple myeloma in the elderly. Clin Geriatr Med. 1985; 1:827–855.
34. Gilbert HS: Myeloproliferative disorders. Clin Geriatr Med 1985; 1:773–793.
35. Hanash SM: New polypeptide markers in leukemia: identification by 2D-gel-electrophoresis. Lab Mgmt 1987; 25(5):33–38.
36. Takkunen H, Sappanen R: Iron deficiency in the elderly population in Finland. Scand J Soc Med (Suppl) 1979; 14:151–162.
37. Stemerman MB: Coagulation in the elderly. Clin Geriatr Med 1985; 1:869–885.

PART VIII

Instrumentation

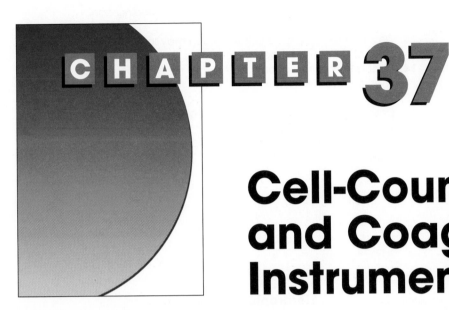

CHAPTER 37

Cell-Counting and Coagulation Instrumentation

Martha K. Miers,* Maralie G. Exton,*
and Christine Daniele

Outline

Objectives

AFTER COMPLETION OF THIS CHAPTER, THE READER WILL BE ABLE TO

1. Explain the different principles of automated cell counting.
2. Explain how the general principles are used on the different instruments discussed.
3. Identify the hemogram parameters directly measured on the four analyzers presented.
4. Explain the derivation of calculated or indirectly measured hemogram parameters for the four analyzers presented.
5. Explain the derivation of the white blood cell differential count on the different instruments discussed.
6. Interpret patient data, including white and red blood cell histograms and cytograms, for the major hematology instruments.
7. Explain the general principles of automated reticulocyte counting.
8. Identify sources of error in automated cell counting and determine appropriate corrective action.
9. Describe the mechanical method of clot detection and the different types of instruments that use this method.
10. Describe the optical density method of clot detection.

* The authors wish to thank the Hematology Laboratories of Baptist Hospital, Memphis, as well as St. Thomas Hospital; Specialized Assays; Diaclin Laboratories; and Vanderbilt University Medical Center, all of Nashville, Tennessee, for assistance in using the different analyzers to test the specimens presented in this chapter.

11. Explain the difference between the turbidimetric and nephelometric optical density methods.
12. Explain guard time and how its misunderstanding can lead to erroneous results.
13. Describe specimen conditions which may interfere with optical density methods.
14. Discuss sampling options used to cut reagent costs and specimen requirements.
15. Explain the principle of chromogenic testing.
16. Describe the principle of platelet aggregation in whole blood and platelet rich plasma.
17. Describe options for performing whole blood point-of-care testing.

Automation provides both greater accuracy and greater precision than manual methods. Over the past 20 years, instrumentation has virtually replaced manual cell counting, with the possible exception of phase platelet counting as a confirmatory procedure.[1] Hematology analyzers have been developed and are marketed by multiple instrument manufacturers. These analyzers typically provide data on the eight standard hematology parameters (complete blood count, or CBC) plus a three- or five-part differential leukocyte count in less than 1 minute on 100 μL of whole blood. Automation thus allows for more efficient workload management and more timely diagnosis and treatment of disease.

GENERAL PRINCIPLES OF HEMATOLOGY INSTRUMENTATION

Despite the number of hematology analyzers available from different manufacturers and with varying levels of sophistication and complexity, two basic principles of operation are primarily used: electronic impedance (resistance) and light scatter. Electronic impedance, or low-voltage direct current (DC) resistance, was developed by Wallace Coulter in the 1950s[2] and is the most common method used. Radio frequency, or high-voltage electromagnetic current resistance, is sometimes used in conjunction with DC electronic impedance. Technicon Instruments introduced darkfield optical scanning in the 1960s, and Ortho Diagnostics Systems followed with a laser-based optical instrument in the 1970s.[3] Optical scatter, which uses both laser and nonlaser light, is frequently used on today's hematology instrumentation.

Electronic Impedance

The impedance principle of cell counting is based on the detection and measurement of changes in electrical resistance produced by cells as they traverse a small aperture. Cells suspended in an electrically conductive diluent, such as saline, are pulled through an aperture (orifice) in a glass tube. In the counting chamber, or transducer assembly, low-frequency electrical current is applied between an external electrode (suspended in the cell dilution) and an internal electrode (housed inside the aperture tube). Electrical resistance between the two electrodes, or impedance in the

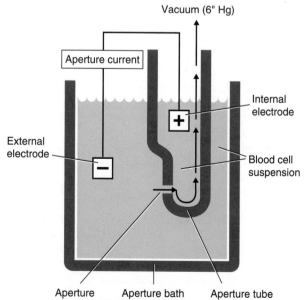

Figure 37–1 Coulter principle of cell counting. (From Coulter Electronics: Coulter STKR Product Reference Manual (PN 4235547 E). Hialeah, FL: 1988.)

current, occurs as the cells pass through the sensing aperture, causing voltage pulses that are measurable (Fig. 37–1).[4, 5] Oscilloscope screens on some instruments display the pulses generated by the cells as they interrupt the current. The number of pulses generated is proportional to the number of cells counted. The size of the voltage pulse is directly proportional to the size (volume) of the cell, thus allowing discrimination and counting of specifically sized cells through the use of threshold circuits. Pulses are collected and sorted (channelized) by pulse height analyzers according to their amplitude. The data are plotted on a frequency distribution graph, with relative number on the y-axis and size (the channel number is equivalent to specific size) on the x-axis. The histogram produced depicts the volume distribution of the cells counted. Figure 37–2 illustrates the construction of a frequency distribution graph. Size thresholds

separate the cell populations on the histogram, with the count being the cells enumerated between the lower and upper set thresholds for each population. Size distribution histograms may be used for the evaluation of one cell population or subgroups within a population.[5] The use of proprietary lytic reagents, as used on the Coulter S-Plus IV and STKR or the Sysmex E-5000, to control shrinkage and lysis of specific cell types allows for separation and quantitation of white blood cells (*WBCs*) into three populations (lymphocytes, mononuclear cells, and granulocytes for the "three-part differential") on one size distribution histogram.[6-8]

Several factors may affect size or volume measurements in impedance or volume displacement instruments. Aperture size is critical, with the red blood cell/platelet (RBC/PLT) aperture smaller than the WBC aperture to increase platelet-counting sensitivity. Protein build-up on the aperture decreases the size of the orifice, thereby decreasing the flow of cells and increasing the electrical resistance as the cells are pulled through. This phenomenon results in lower cell counts and falsely elevated cell volumes. Older impedance instruments required frequent cleaning of the apertures, but newer instruments have incorporated "burn circuits" or other internal cleaning systems to prevent or slow down protein build-up.[6, 7] Carry-over of cells from one sample to the next is also minimized by these internal cleaning systems. Coincident passage of more than one cell at a time through the orifice causes artificially large pulses, resulting in falsely increased cell volumes and falsely decreased cell counts. This count reduction, or coincident passage loss, is statistically predictable (and, therefore, mathematically correctable) because of its direct relationship to the cell concentration and the size or effective volume of the aperture.[7, 8] Coincidence correction is typically completed by the analyzer computer before the final printout of cell counts is obtained from the instrument. Other factors affecting pulse height include orientation of the cell in the center of the aperture and deformability of the red blood cell, which may be altered by decreased hemoglobin content.[9, 10] Recirculation of cells back into the sensing zone creates erroneous pulses and falsely elevates cell counts. A backwash or sweep-flow mechanism has been added to prevent recirculation of cells back into the sensing zone, and anomalously shaped pulses are edited out electronically.[6, 7]

The use of hydrodynamic focusing avoids many of the potential problems inherent in a rigid-aperture system. The sample stream is surrounded by a sheath fluid as it passes through the central axis of

Oscilloscope

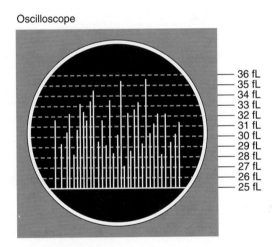

Histogram

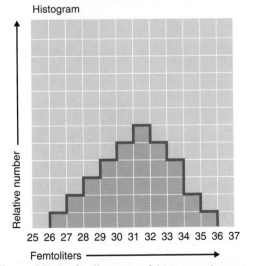

Figure 37–2 Oscilloscope and histogram demonstrating the construction of a frequency distribution graph. (From Coulter Electronics: Significant Advances in Hematology: Hematology Education Series (PN 4206115 A). Hialeah, FL: 1983.)

the aperture. Laminar flow allows the central sample stream to narrow sufficiently to separate and align the cells into single file for passage through the sensing zone.[11] The outer shealth fluid minimizes protein build-up and plugs, eliminates recirculation of cells back into the sensing zone with generation of spurious pulses, and reduces pulse height irregularity since off-center cell passage is prevented and better resolution of the blood cells is obtained. Coincident passage loss is also reduced because blood cells line up in the direction of the flow.[12] A more complete discussion of laminar flow and hydrodynamic focusing can be found in Chapter 29.

Radio Frequency

Low-voltage DC impedance may be used in conjunction with radio frequency (RF) or high-voltage electromagnetic current flowing between both electrodes at the same time. Whereas the total volume of the cell is proportional to the change in DC, the cell nuclear volume is proportional to pulse size or change in the radio frequency signal. Conductivity, as measured by this high-frequency electromagnetic probe, is attenuated by the nuclear-to-cytoplasmic ratio, the nuclear density, and the cytoplasmic granulation. Both DC and RF voltage changes may be detected simultaneously and separated by two different pulse-processing circuits.[12] Figure 37–3 illustrates the simultaneous use of DC and RF current.

Two different cell properties, such as impedance and conductivity, can be plotted against each other for the formation of two-dimensional cytograms or scatterplots. Such plots display the cell populations as clusters, with the number of dots in each cluster representing the concentration of that cell type. Computer cluster analysis can then determine absolute counts for specific cell populations. The use of multiple methods on a given instrument for the determination of at least two cell properties allows the separation of white cells into a five-part differential (neutrophils, lymphocytes, monocytes, eosinophils, and basophils). DC and RF resistance are the two methods used on the Sysmex NE-8000 to determine the WBC differential.[12]

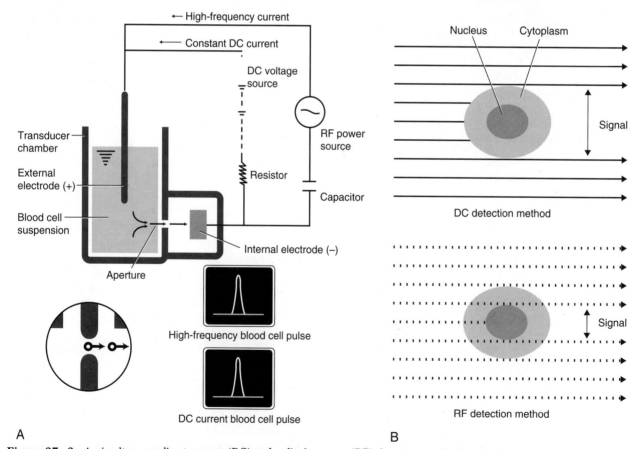

Figure 37–3 *A*, simultaneous direct current (DC) and radio frequency (RF) detection on the Sysmex NE-8000. *B*, measurement of cell size and volume with DC voltage change versus measurement of cell nuclear volume with change in the RF signal. (From Toa Medical Electronics Company: Sysmex NE-8000 Operator's Manual (CN 461-2326-5). Kobe, Japan: 1990.)

Optical Scatter

Optical scatter may be used as the primary method or in combination with other methods. In optical scatter systems (flow cytometers), a hydrodynamically focused sample stream is directed through a quartz flow cell past a focused light source. The light source is generally a tungsten halogen lamp or a helium neon laser (*light amplification by stimulated emission of radiation*). Laser light, termed *monochromatic light* because it is emitted as a single wavelength, differs from brightfield light in its intensity, its coherence (i.e., it travels in phase), and its low divergence, or spread. These characteristics allow for the detection of interference in the laser beam and enable enumeration and differentiation of cell types.[11, 13] Optical scatter may be used to study RBCs, WBCs, and platelets.

As the cells pass through the sensing zone and interrupt the beam, light is scattered in all directions. Light scatter results from the interaction between the processes of absorption, diffraction (bending around corners or surface of a cell), refraction (bending because of a change in speed), and reflection (backward rays caused by obstruction).[14] The detection and conversion of scattered rays into electrical signals is accomplished by photodetectors (photodiodes and photomultiplier tubes) positioned at specific angles. Lens fitted with blocker bars to prevent nonscattered light from entering the detector are used to collect the scattered light. A series of filters and mirrors separates the varying wavelengths and presents them to the photodetectors. Photodiodes convert light photons to electronic signals that are proportional in magnitude to the amount of light collected. Photomultiplier tubes (PMTs) are used to collect the weaker signals produced at 90° and to multiply the photoelectrons into stronger, useful signals. Analog-to-digital converters change the electronic pulses to digital signals for computer analysis.[11, 13]

Forward-angle light scatter (0°) correlates with cell volume or size, primarily because of diffraction of light. Orthogonal light scatter (90°), or side scatter, results from refraction and reflection of light from larger structures inside the cell and correlates with the degree of internal complexity of the cell.[15] Forward low-angle scatter (2°–3°) also correlates with cell volume, and forward high-angle scatter (5°–15°) correlates with refractive index or internal complexity of the cell.[16] Differential scatter is the combination of this low- and high-angle forward light scatter, which is primarily used on Technicon H systems for the evaluation of red cells and the quantitation of basophils. The angles of light scatter measured by the different flow cytometers are manufacturer specific.

Scatter properties at different angles may be plotted against each other for the generation of two-dimensional cytograms or scatterplots. Multiple-angle analysis is the primary technology for the evaluation of white cells on the Abbott Cell-Dyn (CD) 3000 and 3500.[17, 18] Optical scatter may be plotted against absorption, as on the Technicon H systems,[19, 20] or, likewise, scatter may be plotted against volume, as on the Coulter STKS.[21] Computer cluster analysis of the cytograms may yield both quantitative and qualitative information.

PRINCIPAL CELL-COUNTING INSTRUMENTS

Overview

Hematology analyzers are produced by many manufacturers, including Abbott Laboratories, Coulter Corporation, Instrumentation Laboratory, Miles, Roche Diagnostic Systems, Serono-Baker Diagnostics, and TOA Medical Electronics Company. The following discussion is limited to the instrumentation produced by four of these suppliers. Emphasis is not placed on sample size or handling, speed, level of automation, or comparison of instruments or manufacturers. Instead, a detailed description of the methods used by these manufacturers is given to demonstrate the usage of, and to further clarify, the principles presented earlier as well as to better enable the technologist to interpret patient data, including instrument-generated histograms and cytograms, in the hematology laboratory. Table 37–1 summarizes the methods used for hemogram determination on four major hematology instruments. Table 37–2 summarizes the methods used for WBC differential determination on the same four analyzers.

Hematology instruments have some common basic components or systems, including hydraulics, pneumatics, and electrical systems. The hydraulics system includes the aspirating unit, dispensers, diluters, mixing chambers, aperture baths and/or flow cells, and the hemoglobinometer. The pneumatics includes the vacuums and pressures required for operating the valves and moving the sample through the hydraulic system. The electrical system controls the operational sequences of the total system and includes the electronic analyzers and the computing circuitry used to process the data generated. Some instruments have oscilloscope screens that display the electric pulses in real time as the cells are counted. A data display

Table 37-1. METHODS FOR HEMOGRAM DETERMINATION ON FOUR MAJOR HEMATOLOGY INSTRUMENTS

Parameter	COULTER STKS	SYSMEX NE-8000	ABBOTT CELL-DYN 3000	MILES/TECHNICON H SYSTEMS
WBC	Impedance	RF, DC detection: electrical resistance or impedance	Optical scatter	Hydrodynamic focusing, optical scatter and absorption
RBC	Impedance	Hydrodynamic focusing, DC detection	Impedance	Hydrodynamic focusing, laser low-angle (2°–3°) and high-angle (5°–15°) scatter
HGB	Modified cyanmethemoglobin (525 nm)	Cyanmethemoglobin (540 ± 5 nm)	Cyanmethemoglobin (540 nm)	Modified cyanmethemoglobin (546 nm)
HCT	(RBC × MCV) ÷ 10	Cumulative pulse height detection	(RBC × MCV) ÷ 10	(RBC × MCV) ÷ 10
MCV	Mean of RBC size distribution histogram	(HCT ÷ RBC) × 10	Mean of RBC size distribution histogram	Mean of RBC volume histogram
MCH	(HGB ÷ RBC) × 10	(HGB ÷ RBC) × 10	(HGB ÷ RBC) × 10	(HGB ÷ RBC) × 10
MCHC	(HGB ÷ HCT) × 100	(HGB ÷ HCT) × 100	(HGB ÷ HCT) × 100	(HGB ÷ HCT) × 100
PLT	Impedance (2–20 fL): least square fit of size distribution histogram (0–70 fL)	Hydrodynamic focusing, DC detection (≈2–30 fL)	Impedance (≈2–30 fL)	Hydrodynamic focusing, high-angle (5°–15°) scatter
RDW	CV (%) of RBC histogram: (SD ÷ MCV) × 100	RDW – SD (fL) or RDW – CV (%) available	Relative value, equivalent to CV	CV (%) of RBC histogram: (SD ÷ MCV) × 100

Abbreviations: CV, coefficient of variation; DC, direct current; HCT, hematocrit; HGB, hemoglobin; MCH, mean cell hemoglobin; MCHC, mean cell hemoglobin concentration; MCV, red blood cell mean cell volume; PLT, platelet; RBC, red blood cell; RDW, red blood cell distribution width; RF, radio frequency; SD, standard deviation; WBC, white blood cell.

unit receives information from the analyzer and prints results, histograms, and/or cytograms.

Sample handling varies from instrument to instrument based on the degree of automation, ranging from discrete analyzers to walkaway systems with "front-end load" capability. The newest Sysmex HS system robotically links the NE-8000, the R-3000 (Sysmex's automated reticulocyte analyzer), and an automatic slide maker and stainer for complete automation. Computer functions also vary, with the larger instruments having extensive microprocessor capability. Computer programs may include quality control (with automatic review of quality control data, calculations, graphs, moving averages, and storage of quality control files); patient data storage and retrieval (with delta checks, panic or critical value flagging, and automatic review of results, for which acceptance or rejection is based on user-defined criteria); automatic start-up and shutdown (with internal diagnostic self-checks and some maintenance); and even animal software.

Table 37-2. METHODS FOR WHITE BLOOD CELL DIFFERENTIAL DETERMINATION ON FOUR MAJOR HEMATOLOGY INSTRUMENTS

Parameter	COULTER STKS	SYSMEX NE-8000	ABBOTT CELL-DYN 3000	MILES/TECHNICON H SYSTEMS
Neutrophils	Volume, conductivity, scatter (VCS)	RF, DC detection	Multiangle (0°, 90°,10°, 90° depolarized) polarized scatter separation (MAPSS)	Peroxidase staining, optical scatter and absorption
Lymphocytes	VCS	RF, DC detection	MAPSS	Peroxidase staining, optical scatter and absorption
Monocytes	VCS	RF, DC detection	MAPSS	Peroxidase staining, optical scatter and absorption
Eosinophils	VCS	Differential lysis/shrinkage, DC detection	MAPSS	Peroxidase staining, optical scatter and absorption
Basophils	VCS	Differential lysis/shrinkage, DC detection	MAPSS	Differential lysis, laser low-angle (2°–3°) and high-angle (5°–15°) scatter

Abbreviations: DC, direct current; RF, radio frequency.

Coulter Instrumentation

The Coulter Corporation manufactures an extensive line of hematology analyzers, from the single-aperture Z series to the automated, walk-away MAXM and STKS. Coulter instruments typically have two measurement channels in the hydraulics system for determining the hemogram data. The RBC and WBC counts and the hemoglobin (HGB) determination are considered to be measured directly. The aspirated whole blood sample is divided into two aliquots and mixed with an isotonic diluent. The first dilution is delivered to the RBC aperture bath, and the second is delivered to the WBC aperture bath. In the RBC chamber, both the RBCs and the platelets (PLTs) are counted and discriminated by electrical impedance as the cells are pulled through each of three sensing apertures (50-μm diameter, 60-μm length). Particles between 2 and 20 fL are counted as platelets, and those greater than 36 fL are counted as RBCs. A reagent to lyse RBCs and release hemoglobin is added to the WBC dilution before the WBCs are counted by impedance in each of three sensing apertures (100-μm diameter, 75-μm length) in the WBC bath. After the counting cycles are completed, the WBC dilution is passed to the hemoglobinometer for hemoglobin determination (light transmittance read at a wavelength of 525 nm). The electrical pulses obtained in the counting cycles are sent to the analyzer for editing, coincidence correction, and digital conversion. Two of the three counts obtained in both the RBC and the WBC baths must match within specified limits for the counts to be accepted by the instrument.[5, 21] This multiple counting procedure prevents data errors resulting from aperture obstructions or statistical outliers and allows for excellent reproducibility on the Coulter instruments.

The digital information obtained from each aperture is channelized by pulse height analyzers; 256 channels are used for WBC and RBC analysis, and 64 channels are used for platelet analysis. Size-distribution histograms of WBC, RBC, and platelet populations are generated. The RBC mean cell volume (MCV) is the average volume of the RBCs taken from the size distribution data. The hematocrit (HCT), mean cell hemoglobin (MCH), and mean cell hemoglobin concentration (MCHC) are calculated from measured and derived values. The RBC distribution width (RDW) is directly calculated from the histogram as the coefficient of variation (CV) of the RBC volume distribution, with a reference range of 11.5–14.5%.[5] The RDW is an index of anisocytosis but may be falsely skewed because the RDW reflects the ratio of standard deviation and MCV. That is, an RBC distribution histogram with normal divergence but with a decreased MCV may imply a high RDW, falsely indicating increased anisocytosis. The MCV and RDW are used by the instrument to flag possible anisocytosis, microcytosis, and macrocytosis.[21]

Platelets are counted within the range of 2–20 fL, and a size distribution histogram is constructed. If the platelet size distribution meets specified criteria, a statistical least-squares fit is applied to the raw data, fitting the data to a log-normal curve. The curve is extrapolated from 0–70 fL, and the final count is derived from this extended curve. This fitting procedure eliminates interfering particles in the noise region, such as debris, and in the larger region, such as small red cells. The mean platelet volume (MPV), analogous to the red cell MCV, is also derived from the platelet histogram. Reference values for the MPV are about 7.8–11.0 fL, and the MPV increases slightly as the sample sits in ethylenediaminetetraacetic acid (EDTA).[5] Normally, platelet size varies inversely with platelet count, as visualized on the larger Coulter systems on a platelet nomogram devised by Bessman and coworkers (Fig. 37–4).[22]

Many Coulter instruments, such as the S-Plus IV or the STKR, provide three-part leukocyte subpopulation analysis, which differentiates the white cells into lymphocytes, mononuclear cells, and granulocytes. In the WBC channel, a special lysing reagent causes differential shrinkage of the leukocytes, allowing the different cells to be counted and sized based on their impedance. A WBC histogram is constructed from the channelized data. Particles between approximately 35 and 90 fL are considered lymphocytes; those between 90 and 160 fL, "mononuclears" (monocytes, blasts, immature granulocytes, and atypical lymphocytes); and those between 160 and 450 fL, granulocytes, thus allowing the calculation of both relative and abso-

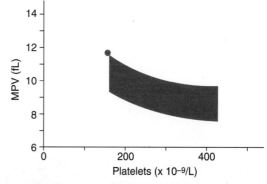

Figure 37–4 Platelet nomogram showing the inverse relationship of platelet size and number. (From Coulter Electronics: Significant Advances in Hematology: Hematology Education Series (PN 4206115 A). Hialeah, FL: 1983.)

lute numbers for these three populations.[6] Proprietary computerized algorithms further allow flagging for increased eosinophils and/or basophils as well as interpretation of the histogram differential to include flagging for abnormal cells such as atypical lymphocytes and blasts.[7] When cell populations overlap or a distinct separation of the populations does not exist, a region alarm (R flag) may be triggered, indicating the area of interference on the size distribution histogram. For example, an R1 flag represents excess signals at the lower-threshold region of the WBC histogram and a questionable WBC count. This interference is visualized as a "high take-off" of the curve and may indicate the presence of nucleated RBCs, clumped platelets, unlysed RBCs, or electronic noise.[6, 7] Figure 37–5 shows composite printouts from the Coulter STKR that include the "interpretive differential."

More recent Coulter instruments, the STKS and the MAXM, generate hemogram data (including the WBC count) exactly as before but use the Coulter VCS technology in a separate channel to evaluate white cells for the determination of a five-part differential. The VCS technology includes *volumetric* sizing of cells by impedance, conductiv-ity measurements of cells, and laser light *scatter*, all performed simultaneously for each cell. After the RBCs are lysed and the WBCs are treated with a stabilizing reagent to maintain them in a near-native state, a hydrodynamically focused sample stream is directed through the flow cell past the sensing zone. Low-frequency DC measures size while a high-frequency electromagnetic probe measures conductivity, an indicator of cellular internal content. Each cell is scanned with monochromatic laser light, which reveals information about cell surface, such as structure, shape, and reflectivity. Approximately 8000 cells are analyzed in each sample. The combination of technologies provides a three-dimensional plot or cytograph of the WBC populations, which are separated by computer cluster analysis. Two-dimensional scatterplots of the three measurements represent different views of the cytograph. Discriminate function 1 (DF 1) scatterplot of volume (y-axis) versus light scatter (x-axis) shows clear separation of lymphocytes, monocytes, neutrophils, and eosinophils. Figure 37–6 represents a standard patient printout from the Coulter STKS showing a DF 1 scatterplot. Basophils, hidden behind the lymphocytes in this

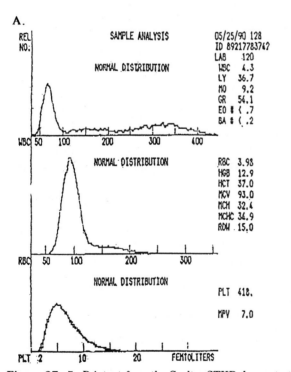 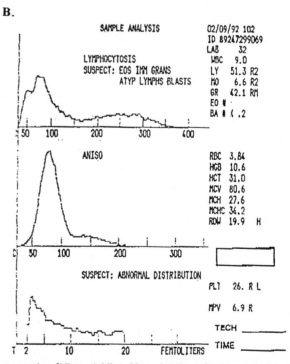

Figure 37–5 Printout from the Coulter STKR demonstrating the "interpretive differential." *A,* Note the three distinct white blood cell (WBC) populations, normal gaussian or bell-shaped distribution of red blood cells (RBCs) and the left-shifted or log-normal distribution of platelets (PLTs). *B,* Note the left shift in the WBC histogram and the possible interference at the lower threshold region. *R2 flag* indicates interference and loss of valley resulting from overlap or insufficient separation between the lymphocyte and mononuclear populations at the 90-fL region. *RM flag* indicates interference at more than one region. Eosinophil data have been suppressed. Also note the abnormal platelet size distribution and the low platelet count. Manual 200-cell differential counts: *A,* 42.5% neutrophils (37% segmented neutrophils, 5.5% bands), 41.5% lymphocytes, 4.5% monocytes, 1% basophils, 0.5% metamyelocytes, 9.5% myelocytes, and 0.5% atypical lymphocytes; *B,* 51% neutrophils (23% segmented neutrophils, 28% bands), 12% lymphocytes, 9.5% monocytes, 1% metamyelocytes, 1.5% myelocytes, 25% atypical lymphocytes, and 17 NRBCs/100 WBCs.

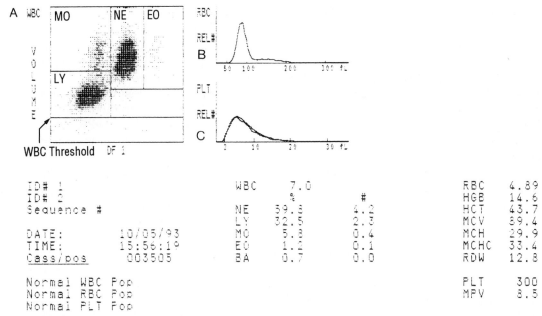

ID# 1		WBC	7.0			RBC	4.89
ID# 2			%	#		HGB	14.6
Sequence #		NE	59.8	4.2		HCT	43.7
		LY	32.5	2.3		MCV	89.4
DATE:	10/05/93	MO	5.8	0.4		MCH	29.9
TIME:	15:56:19	EO	1.2	0.1		MCHC	33.4
Cass/pos	003505	BA	0.7	0.0		RDW	12.8
Normal WBC Pop						PLT	300
Normal RBC Pop						MPV	8.5
Normal PLT Pop							

Figure 37–6 Composite scatterplots-histograms from the Coulter STKS on the same normal specimen demonstrated in Figures 37–7, 37–9, and 37–12. The white blood cell (WBC) two-dimensional scatterplot in *panel A* shows volume as determined by impedence on the y-axis versus light scatter on the x-axis (discriminate function 1 [DF 1]). Computer-generated floating discriminators separate lymphocyte (LY), monocyte (MO), neutrophil (NE), and eosinophil (EO) regions. Data below the WBC threshold represent non–white cell debris. Large or clumped platelets, nucleated red blood cells (NRBCs), white cell fragments, or unlysed RBCs in abnormal samples should fall below this threshold. DF 2 and DF 3 scatterplots, not shown, are both derived from volume (y-axis) versus conductivity (x-axis). Basophils (BA) are best visualized on the DF 3 display from which the neutrophil population has been removed. All two-dimensional scatterplots, single-parameter histograms, or the three-dimensional (3-D) cytograph may be reviewed at operator request. The relative value (%) of each of the five white cell populations derived from this three-dimensional analysis is multiplied by the WBC count derived in a separate impedance channel for determination of the absolute count (#). *B* and *C*, Relative number (y-axis) versus size distribution (x-axis) histograms for red blood cells (RBCs) and platelets (PLTs), respectively. Note the normal Gaussian or bell-shaped distribution of the RBCs in *panel B* and the left-shifted or log-normal distribution of PLTs in *panel C*. The small population of larger RBCs on the right of the RBC curve represents coincident passage of doublets and/or triplets through the impedance aperture, creating larger pulses. This portion of the RBC curve is excluded from the calculation of the red cell distribution width (RDW). Manual 200-cell differential count: 58.5% neutrophils (53.5% segmented neutrophils, 5% bands), 35% lymphocytes, 4.5% monocytes, 0.5% eosinophils, 0.5% basophils, and 1% atypical lymphocytes.

scatterplot, are separated by conductivity because of their cytoplasmic granulation. The basophil population can be visualized on the DF 3 display, which is visible when the neutrophil population is removed from the DF 2 scatterplot. The DF 2 scatterplot, which has volume on the y-axis and conductivity on the x-axis, shows lymphocytes, monocytes, and neutrophils as the prominant populations. The DF 2 and DF 3 scatterplots are available at operator request. Single-parameter histograms of volume, conductivity, and light scatter are also available.[21, 23]

Two types of WBC flags (alarms or indicators of abnormality) are generated on all hematology instruments that provide a WBC differential count: (1) user defined, primarily set for distributional abnormalities, such as eosinophilia or lymphocytopenia (based on absolute eosinophil or lymphocyte counts, respectively); and (2) instrument specific and primarily set for morphologic abnormalities. For distributional flags, the user establishes reference ranges and programs the instrument to flag each parameter as high or low. Morphologic flags,

or suspect flags indicating the possible presence of abnormal cells, are triggered when cell populations fall outside expected regions or when specific statistical limitations are exceeded. Instrument-set flags on the STKS include immature granulocytes/bands, blasts, variant lymphocytes, nucleated RBCs (NRBCs), and platelet clumps. Inadequate separation of the cell populations may disallow reporting of differential results by the instrument and may elicit a subsequent "review slide" message.[21]

Sysmex Instrumentation

Sysmex instruments, manufactured by TOA Medical Electronics Company, include a full line of hematology analyzers from the smallest, the K-1000, to the larger walkaway systems, such as the E-5000, which provides a three-part differential, and the NE-8000, which performs a complete blood cell count and five-part differential. The WBC, RBC, hemoglobin, hematocrit, and platelet counts are considered to be measured directly.

Three hydraulic subsystems are used to determine the hemogram: the WBC channel, the RBC/PLT channel, and a separate hemoglobin channel. In the WBC and RBC transducer chambers, the diluted WBC and RBC samples are aspirated through the different apertures and are counted by using the electronic resistance (impedance) detection method for counting and sizing cells. Two unique features enhance the impedance technology: (1) in the RBC/PLT channel, a sheathed stream with hydrodynamic focusing is used to direct the cells in single file through the aperture, thereby reducing coincident passage and pulse height irregularities, and (2) in both the WBC and RBC/PLT channels, "floating thresholds" are used to discriminate each cell population.[8, 12]

As the cells pass through the apertures, the signals are transmitted in sequence to the analog circuit and then to the particle size distribution analysis circuits for conversion to cumulative cell size distribution data. Particle size distribution curves are constructed, and the optimal position of the autodiscrimination level (i.e., the threshold) is then set by the microprocessor for each cell population. For example, the lower platelet threshold may be set between 2 and 6 fL, and the upper threshold anywhere from 12 to 30 fL, based on the particle size distribution. Likewise, the RBC lower and upper thresholds may be set between 25 and 75 fL and 200 and 250 fL, respectively. This floating threshold circuitry allows for discrimination of cell populations on a sample-by-sample basis. The cell counts include the pulses between the lower and upper autodiscriminator levels, with dilution ratio, volume counted, and coincidence error accounted for in the final computer-generated counts. In the RBC channel, the floating discriminator is particularly useful in separating platelets from small RBCs. The hematocrit is also determined from the RBC/PLT channel, based on the principle that pulse height of the red cells is proportional to cell volume. The hematocrit is then the cumulative pulse height and is considered a true relative percentage volume of erythrocytes. In the hemoglobin flow cell, the concentration of cyanmethemoglobin is measured as absorbance at 540 nm for the hemoglobin concentration.[8, 12]

The following indices are calculated in the microprocessor using the directly measured or derived parameters: MCV, MCH, MCHC, RDW standard deviation (RDW-SD), RDW-CV, MPV, platelet distribution width (PDW), and platelet–large cell ratio (P-LCR). The RDW-SD is the red blood cell arithmetic distribution width measured at 20% of the height of the RBC curve, reported in femtoliters with a reference interval of 37–54 fL. RDW-CV is the red blood cell distribution width reported as a coefficient of variation. PDW is the platelet arithmetic distribution width, also measured at 20% of relative height level, reported in femtoliters. The P-LCR represents the proportion of large platelets (those > 12 fL) to the total platelet count and may be an indicator of possible platelet clumping, giant platelets, or cell fragments.[8, 12] Neither the PDW nor P-LCR is reportable in the United States, and their usefulness is yet to be determined.

The Sysmex NE-8000 uses differential shrinkage and lysis along with impedance and radio frequency to obtain a five-part differential analysis. WBCs are analyzed simultaneously by low-frequency DC and high-frequency current (radio frequency) in the transducer chamber. A plot (scattergram) of RF-detection signals (y-axis) versus DC detection signals (x-axis) yields separation of the white cells into lymphocytes, monocytes, and granulocytes. Floating discriminators determine the optimal separation between these populations. Eosinophils and basophils are counted by impedance in separate channels in which the RBCs are lysed and WBCs other than eosinophils or basophils are selectively shrunk by temperature and chemically controlled reactions. Eosinophils and basophils are subtracted from the granulocyte count derived from the scattergram analysis for the determination of the neutrophil count. User-defined distributional flags may be set, and instrument-specific suspect flags, similar to those described on the Coulter STKS, are triggered for the possible presence of morphologic abnormalities.[12] Figure 37–7 is a patient report obtained from the NE-8000 on the same sample represented in Figure 37–6, which shows the analysis performed by the Coulter STKS.

Cell-Dyn Instrumentation

Instruments offered by Abbott Laboratories include smaller analyzers, like the Cell-Dyn (CD) 1600 and larger walkaway systems, the CD 3000 and 3500. The CD 3000 has three independent

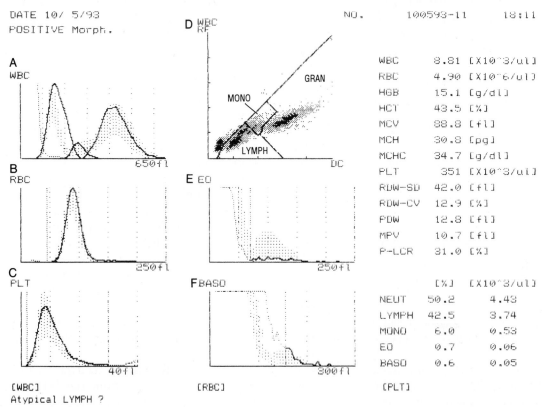

Figure 37–7 Composite histograms/scattergram from the Sysmex NE-8000 on same normal specimen demonstrated in Figures 37–6, 37–9, and 37–12. *A, B,* and *C* are relative number (y-axis) versus size distribution (x-axis) histograms for white blood cells (WBCs), red blood cells (RBCs) and platelets (PLTs), respectively. The three peaks in *panel A* represent, from left to right, lymphocyte, mixed, and neutrophil populations. Note the bell-shaped RBC curve in *panel B* with little interference on the right side from coincident passage, minimized by hydrodynamic focusing in the RBC/PLT channel. The red blood cell distribution widths (RDW-SD and RDW-CV) are determined at the 20% relative height level, thus excluding any possible interference. *Panel C* shows the normal left-shifted or log-normal distribution of platelets. The platelet distribution width (PDW) and the mean platelet volume (MPV) are analogous to the RDW-SD and the mean cell volume (MCV), respectively. P-LCR, or platelet–large cell ratio, represents the percentage of total platelets greater than 12 fL. In the WBC scattergram (*panel D*), the y-axis shows radio frequency (RF) detection signals plotted against the direct current (DC) detection signals on the x-axis. Floating discriminators determine optimal separation of lymphocytes (LYMPH), monocytes (MONO), and granulocytes (GRAN). The WBC count includes all cells below the main discriminator line. Eosinophils (EO) and basophils (BASO) are determined in separate differential lysis reactions. *E* and *F*, EO and BASO distribution curves, respectively, with RBC ghosts and WBC fragments other than EOs (or BASOs) to the left of a computer-determined autodiscrimination line. EO and BASO counts are determined by enumerating cells between the autodiscriminator level and an upper fixed discriminator position. The absolute neutrophil count (NEUT) (×10³/μL) is computed by subtracting EO and BASO counts from the GRAN result derived from the scattergram analysis. Relative differential results (%) are computed by dividing absolute numbers by total WBC count. Manual 200-cell differential count: 58.5% neutrophils (58.5% segmented neutrophils, 5% bands), 35% lymphocytes, 4.5% monocytes, 0.5% eosinophils, 0.5% basophils, and 1% atypical lymphocytes. Note the atypical lymph suspect flag triggered by the instrument.

measurement channels for determining the hemogram and the differential: (1) the optical channel for WBC count and differential data, (2) the impedance channel for RBC and platelet data, and (3) the hemoglobin channel for hemoglobin determination.[17] (The CD 3500 has an additional impedance channel for determining a WBC impedance count; this channel is used as an internal check against the primary WBC optical count.)[18] The WBC, RBC, hemoglobin, and platelet counts are considered to be measured directly. A 60- $\times$ 70-μm aperture is used in the RBC/PLT transducer assembly for counting and sizing of the RBCs and platelets by the aperture impedance method. Pulses are collected and sorted in 256 channels according to their amplitude: particles between 1 and 35 fL are included in the initial platelet data, and those greater than 35 fL are counted as red cells. Floating thresholds are then used to determine the best separation of the platelet population and to eliminate interference, such as noise or debris or small red cells, from the count. Coincident passage loss is corrected for in the final RBC and platelet counts. Red cell pulse editing is applied before MCV derivation to compensate for aberrant pulses produced by nonaxial passage of RBCs through the aperture. The MCV is the average volume of the red cells derived from the RBC size distribution data. Hemoglobin is directly measured using a modified hemiglobincyanide method that measures absorbance at 540 nm. Hematocrit, MCV, and MCHC are calculated from the directly measured or derived parameters. The RDW, equivalent to the coefficient of variation, is a relative value, derived from the RBC histogram by using the 20th and 80th percentiles. Other indices available include MPV, plateletcrit or PCT (which is analogous to the hematocrit), and platelet distribution width.[17] The platelet distribution width and the plateletcrit are not reportable parameters.

The WBC count and differential are derived from the optical channel through multiangle polarized scatter separation (MAPSS). A hydrodynamically focused sample stream is directed through a quartz flow cell past a focused light source, a vertically polarized helium neon laser. Scattered light is measured at multiple angles: 0° forward light scattering is used for determination of cell size; 90° orthogonal light scattering, for determination of cellular lobularity; 10° narrow angle scatter, which correlates with cellular complexity; and 90° depolarized (90°D) light scattering for evaluation of cellular granularity. Orthogonal light scatter is split, with one portion directed to the 90° photo-

multiplier tube and the other portion directed through a polarizer to the 90°D photomultiplier tube. Only light that has changed polarization (depolarized) can be detected by the 90°D photomultiplier tube. Various combinations of these four measurements are used to differentiate and quantitate the five major WBC subpopulations: neutrophils, lymphocytes, monocytes, eosinophils, and basophils.[17, 24]

The light scatter signals are converted into electrical signals, sorted into 256 channels on the basis of amplitude for each angle of light measured, and graphically presented as scatterplots, with two angles plotted against each other in various combinations. Lobularity or orthogonal scatter (90°) plotted on the y-axis against complexity (10°) on the x-axis yields separation of the mononuclear subpopulation, including basophils, and the polymorphonuclear subpopulation. Basophils cluster with the mononuclear subpopulation in this analysis because the basophil granules dissolve in the sheath reagent and the degranulated basophil is a less complex cell. When size (0°) for the mononuclear subpopulation is plotted on the y-axis against complexity (10°) on the x-axis, the mononuclear subpopulation can be separated into lymphocytes, monocytes, and basophils. Nucleated RBCs, unlysed RBCs, giant platelets, and platelet clumps fall below the lymphocyte cluster on this scatterplot and are excluded from the WBC count and differential. (Information from the WBC impedance channel on the CD 3500 is additionally used to discriminate these particles.)[18] When granularity (90°D) for the polymorphonuclear subpopulation is plotted on the y-axis against lobularity or orthogonal scatter (90°) for the same population, the polymorphonuclear subpopulation is separated into neutrophils and eosinophils. Because of the unique nature of eosinophil granules, eosinophils scatter more 90°D light, allowing clear separation of eosinophils and neutrophils. Dynamic thresholds are used for best separation of the different populations in the various scatterplots. Each cell type is identified with a distinct color so that after all classifications are made and size (0°) is plotted against complexity (10°), each cell population can be easily visualized on the data terminal screen by the operator. Other scatterplots (90°/0°, 90°D/0°, 90°D/10°) are available and may be displayed at operator request. As on the previously described instruments, user-defined distributional flags may be set, and instrument-specific suspect flags may alert the operator to the presence of abnormal cells.[17, 24] Figure 37–9 represents a patient printout from the CD-3000.

Technicon Instrumentation

The Technicon H·1, H·2, and H·3 systems, manufactured by Miles are modifications of older Technicon analyzers, namely the Hemalog 8, D-90, and H-6000, which are no longer manufactured. The H systems extend the technology of the previous instruments while greatly simplifying the hydraulics and operation of the analyzers.[25] The H systems all provide a complete hemogram and WBC differential; the H·2 and H·3 have automated sample handling capability, and the H·3 additionally provides an automated reticulocyte count.[19, 20]

Four independent measurement methods or channels are used in the determination of the hemogram and differential: (1) RBC/PLT channel, (2) hemoglobin channel, (3) peroxidase (PEROX) channel for WBC and differential data, and (4) basophil-lobularity (BASO) channel for WBC and differential data. The WBC, RBC, hemoglobin and platelet counts are measured directly. Hemoglobin is measured using a modified cyanmethemoglobin method that measures absorbance in a colorimeter flow cuvette at approximately 546 nm. The RBC/PLT method uses flow cytometric light-scattering measurements that are determined as the cells pass through a sheath-stream flow cell past a helium neon laser. RBCs and platelets are isovolumetrically sphered before they enter the flow cell. Laser light scattered at two different angular intervals, low angle (2°–3°), correlating with cell size, and high angle (5°–15°), correlating with internal complexity (i.e., hemoglobin concentration), are measured simultaneously (Fig. 37–10). This unique "differential scatter" technique, in combination with isovolumetric sphering, eliminates the adverse effect of variation in cellular hemoglobin

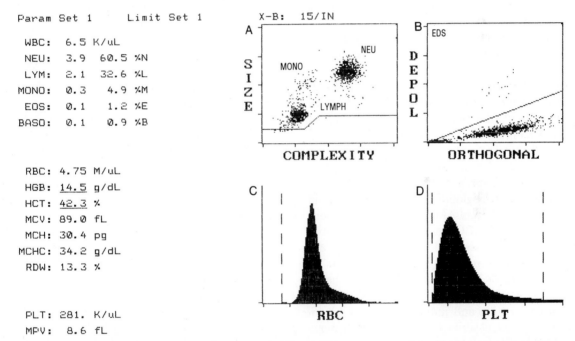

Figure 37–9 Composite scatterplots-histograms from the Cell-Dyn 3000 on same normal sample demonstrated in Figures 37–6, 37–7, and 37–12. A, White blood cell (WBC) data derived by multiangle polarized scatter separation (MAPSS). Zero-degree forward light scatter correlating with size (y-axis) is plotted against 10° narrow-angle light scatter correlating with complexity (x-axis). Neutrophil (NEU), monocyte (MONO), lymphocyte (LYM), eosinophil (EOS), and basophil (BASO) population clusters are indicated. Not shown: 90° versus 10° scatterplot separating mononuclear from polymorphonuclear cell populations, and 0° versus 10° scatterplot of the mononuclear population separating it into lymphocytes, monocytes, and basophils. (Basophils cluster with mononuclears because the cytoplasmic granules dissolve in the sheath fluid.) B, Separation of the polymorphonuclear population using 90° depolarized (90° D or Depol) light scatter (y-axis) correlating with granularity, plotted against 90° orthogonal light scatter (x-axis) correlating with lobularity or internal complexity. Eosinophils with their unique granulation scatter more 90° D light. A dynamic threshold is used to determine the best separation between the EOS and NEU populations. After the cells are classified into five subpopulations as shown on the 0°/10° scatterplot, the number of pulses above the dynamic range in the 0° channel is enumerated for determination of the WBC count. Computer algorithms determine the WBC count and relative number (%) of each subpopulation. The absolute number (K/μL) is calculated by multiplying the percentage of each subpopulation by the WBC count. C and D, Red blood cell (RBC) and platelet (PLT) data determined in the impedance channel. The small population of larger RBCs on the right of the RBC curve represents coincident passage of doublets and/or triplets through the aperture, creating larger pulses. The red cell distribution width (RDW) is derived from the 20th and 80th percentiles of the RBC histogram, thus excluding these artificially large pulses from the calculation. Manual 200-cell differential count: 58.5% neutrophils (58.5% segmented neutrophils, 5% bands), 35% lymphocytes, 4.5% monocytes, 0.5% eosinophils, 0.5% basophils, and 1% atypical lymphocytes.

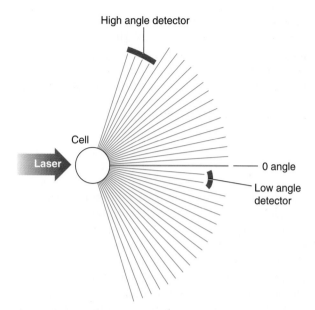

Figure 37–10 Differential scatter detection as used on the Technicon H systems, showing forward high-angle (5°–15°) and forward low-angle (2°–3°) scatter detection for RBC and WBC analysis. (From Technicon H Systems Training Guide Tarrytown, NY, 1993.)

concentration on the determination of RBC volume (as seen when differences in cellular deformability affect the pulse height generated on impedance instruments.)[9, 26] The Mie theory of light scatter of dielectric spheres[14] is used to plot the scatter-intensity signals from the two angles against each other for a cell-by-cell RBC volume (y-axis) versus a hemoglobin concentration (x-axis) cytogram, or RBC map (Fig. 37–11).[16] Independent histograms of RBC volume and hemoglobin concentration are also plotted. Platelets are counted and sized from the high-angle signals at high-gain setting (×10), and a platelet size distribution histogram is generated.[19, 20]

Several parameters and indices are derived from the measurements described in the previous paragraph. The MCV and the MPV are the mean of the RBC volume histogram and the platelet histogram, respectively. Hematocrit, MCH, and MCHC are mathematically computed using the RBC, hemoglobin, and MCV values. RDW is calculated as the coefficient of variation of the red cell volume histogram, and hemoglobin distribution width (HDW), an analogous index, is calculated as the standard deviation of the RBC hemoglobin concentration histogram. The reference interval for HDW is 2.2–3.2 g/dL. The corpuscular hemoglobin concentration mean, or CHCM, which is analogous to the MCHC, is derived from the cell-by-cell direct measurement of hemoglobin concentration. Interferences in the hemoglobin colorimet-

ric method, such as lipemia or icterus, affect the calculated MCHC but do not alter the measured CHCM. The CHCM is not printed on the patient report but is used by the instrument as an internal check against the MCHC and is available to the operator for back-calculation of the hemoglobin, if interferences are present. Unique RBC flags derived from this direct measure of hemoglobin concentration include variation (VAR) in cellular hemoglobin concentration; hypochromia (HYPO); and hyperchromia (HYPER).[19, 20]

The H·1, H·2, and H·3 analyzers determine the WBC count and a six-part WBC differential (neutrophils, lymphocytes, monocytes, eosinophils, basophils, and large unstained cells, or LUCs) by cytochemistry and optical flow cytometry, using the peroxidase and basophil-lobularity channels.

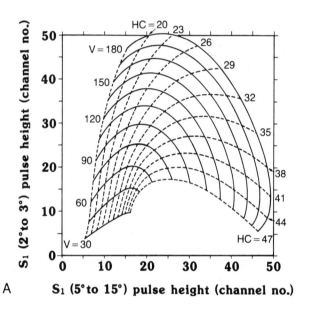

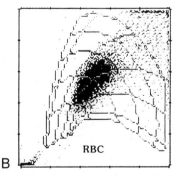

Figure 37–11 Cytograms, or red blood cell (RBC) maps, demonstrating the Mie theory of light scatter of dielectric spheres. *A*, Transformation between two scatter angles (2°–3° and 5°–15°) illustrated as a nonlinear plot, with red cell volume (V) on the y-axis and hemoglobin concentration (HC) on the x-axis. *B*, RBC map of patient sample. (*A* and *B* from Golin J, Panyko L, Tabachnick E [eds]: Proceedings of Technicon H·1™ Hematology Symposium, October 11, 1985. Tarrytown, NY: Technicon Instruments Corporation, 1986:5.)

PEROXIDASE (PEROX) CHANNEL

In the peroxidase PEROX channel the RBCs are lysed, and the WBCs are stained for their peroxidase activity. The following reaction is catalyzed by cellular peroxidase, converting the substrate to a dark precipitate in the peroxidase-containing cells (neutrophils, monocytes, and eosinophils):

$$H_2O_2 + 4\text{-chloro-1-naphthol} \xrightarrow[\text{peroxidase}]{\text{cellular}} \text{dark precipitate}$$

A portion of the cell suspension is fed to a sheath-stream flow cell, where a tungsten halogen dark-field optics system is used to measure absorbance (which is proportional to the amount of peroxidase content in each cell) and forward scatter (which is proportional to the size of each cell). Absorbance is plotted on the x-axis of the cytogram and scatter is plotted on the y-axis. A total WBC count (WBC-PEROX, or WBCP) is obtained from the optical signals in this channel, and computerized cluster analysis allows for classification of the different cell populations.[19, 20, 25]

Neutrophils and eosinophils contain the most peroxidase and cluster to the right of the cytogram. Monocytes stain weakly and therefore cluster in the mid-region of the cytogram. Lymphocytes, basophils, and large unstained cells (LUCs) (variant or atypical lymphocytes and blasts) contain no peroxidase and appear on the left of the cytogram, with the LUCs appearing above the lymphocyte area. Basophils cluster with the small lymphocytes and require further analysis for classification.[19, 20, 25]

BASOPHIL-LOBULARITY CHANNEL

In the basophil-lobularity channel the cells are treated with a reagent containing a nonionic surfactant in an acidic solution. The basophils are particularly resistant to lysis in this temperature-controlled reaction, whereas the RBCs and platelets lyse and the other leukocytes (nonbasophils) are stripped of their cytoplasm. Laser optics, using the same two-angle (2°–3° and 5°–15°), forward-scattering system of the RBC/PLT channel, allows quantitation of basophils by their large low-angle scatter (y-axis). The remaining nuclei are classified as mononuclear (MN) or polymorphonuclear (PMN) based on their nuclear complexity and high-angle scatter (x-axis).[19, 20, 25]

Basophils fall above a fixed horizontal threshold on the cytogram. The stripped nuclei fall below this threshold, with polymorphonuclear nuclei to the right and mononuclear nuclei to the left of a computer-set threshold along the x-axis. The ratio of signals from the two nuclear classes forms a cellular lobularity index (LI) and provides an indication of WBC maturity or suspected left shift. Additionally, this channel provides a second total WBC count (WBC-BASO, or WBCB). Internal check of the WBCP against the WBCB allows for alert of possible interferences in the WBCP and may result in the WBCB being reported by the instrument. Relative differential results (%) are computed by dividing absolute numbers of the different cell classifications by the total WBC count.[19, 20, 25]

Information from the peroxidase and basophil-lobularity channels is used to generate differential morphology flags indicating the possible presence of atypical (ATYP) lymphocytes, blasts, left shift (L shift), immature granulocytes (IG), nucleated RBCs or large platelets (N), and abnormal clustering, or "no-fit" (NF), conditions.[19, 20] Figure 37–12 represents a patient printout from the Technicon H·2.

AUTOMATED RETICULOCYTE COUNTING

Reticulocyte counting is the last of the manual cell counting procedures to be automated. The imprecision and inaccuracy in manual reticulocyte counting are due to multiple factors, including stain variability, slide distribution error, statistical sampling error, and inter-observer error.[27] All of these potential errors, with the possible exception of stain variability, are correctable with automated reticulocyte counting. Increasing the number of red cells counted results in increased precision,[28] as was evidenced with the 1993 College of American Pathologists pilot reticulocyte proficiency survey (Set RT-A, Sample RT-01) on which the coefficient of variation for the reported manual results was 35.0%, compared with 8.3% for the flow cytometry method.[29] Automated reticulocyte methods may count as many as 30,000 RBCs, as compared with 1000 cells counted by the routine manual procedure.[30]

The following automated reticulocyte analyzers are available: flow cytometry systems, such as the Becton Dickinson FACS or Coulter EPICS; Sysmex R-3000, made by TOA Medical Electronics Company; Coulter MAXM and STKS, made by the Coulter Corporation; and the Technicon H·3 RTC and RTX systems, made by Miles. All of these analyzers evaluate reticulocytes based on optical scatter or fluorescence after treating the red cells with either fluorescent dyes or nucleic acid stains to stain the RNA in the reticulocytes.[20, 30, 31] Because neither the FACS nor the EPICS is gen-

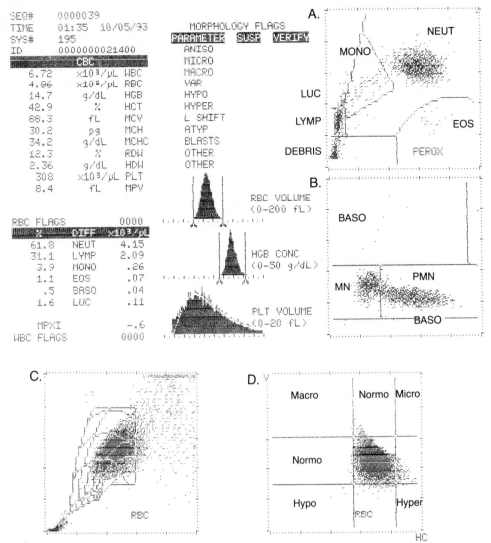

Figure 37–12 Composite cytograms-histograms from the Technicon H-2 on same normal specimen demonstrated in Figure 37–6, 37–7, and 37–9. *A,* White blood cell (WBC) cytogram derived from the peroxidase (PEROX) channel in which the WBCs have been stained for their peroxidase activity. Darkfield optical scatter correlating with size is plotted on the y-axis against light absorbance proportional to staining intensity on the x-axis. Computer cluster analysis separates the WBCs into neutrophils (NEUT), eosinophils (EOS), monocytes (MONO), lymphocytes (LYMPH), and large unstained cells (LUC). Basophils cluster with small lymphocytes in the PEROX channel. *B,* WBC cytogram derived from the laser-based basophil-lobularity (BASO) channel in which the cells have been treated with a differential lysis reagent. Low-angle (2°–3°) scatter correlating with size is plotted on the y-axis against high-angle (5°–15°) scatter correlating with nuclear complexity on the x-axis; the comparison shows nonlysed basophils with their large, low-angle scatter falling above a fixed horizontal threshold on the cytogram. Stripped nuclei (nonbasophils) fall below this threshold and cluster into polymorphonuclear (PMN) and mononuclear (MN) populations based on their nuclear complexity and high-angle scatter. Blasts, when present, fall to the far left below channel 8. Basophils are subtracted from the LYMPH count for the final absolute counts (×10³/μL). Relative differential results (%) are computed by dividing absolute counts by the total WBC count. The red blood cell (RBC) map based on Mie's theory of light scatter is seen in *panel C,* with *panel D* representing a linear plot of volume (V) on the y-axis versus hemoglobin concentration (HC) on the x-axis. The direct measure of hemoglobin concentration allows classification of RBCs as macrocytic, hypochromic (1); macrocytic, normochromic (2); macrocytic, hyperchromic (3); normocytic, hypochromic (4); normocytic, normochromic (5); normocytic, hyperchromic (6); microcytic, hypochromic (7); microcytic, normochromic (8); or microcytic, hyperchromic (9). *Panels C* and *D* were not printed on the patient report form above but were available on different report screens. Single-parameter histograms for RBC volume, hemoglobin concentration (HGB CONC), and platelet (PLT) volume are generated. The RBC histogram has markers at the 60-fL and 120-fL channels for visualization of microcytosis or macrocytosis, respectively. Likewise, the HGB CONC curve has markers at the 28-g/dL and 41-g/dL channels for visualization of hypochromia and hyperchromia. Hemoglobin distribution width (HDW), analogous to the red cell distribution width (RDW), is derived from the HGB CONC histogram. Manual 200-cell differential count: 58.5% neutrophils (53.5% segmented neutrophils, 5% bands), 35% lymphocytes, 4.5% monocytes, 0.5% eosinophils, 0.5% basophils and 1% atypical lymphocytes.

erally available in the routine hematology laboratory, the remaining discussion is limited to the other three systems listed.

The Sysmex R-3000 is a stand-alone reticulocyte analyzer that uses an auramine O fluorescent dye and measures forward scatter and side fluorescence as the cells pass through a sheath-stream flow cell past an argon laser. The signals are plotted on a scattergram with forward-scatter intensity (correlating with size) plotted against fluorescence intensity (which is proportional to RNA content). Automatic discrimination separates the populations into mature RBCs and reticulocytes. The reticulocytes fall into a low-fluorescence ratio region, a middle-fluorescence ratio region or a high-fluorescence ratio region, with the less mature reticulocytes showing higher fluorescence. Platelets fall below a lower discriminator line.[31]

Coulter and Technicon have incorporated reticulocyte methods into primary cell counting instrumentation, namely the MAXM or STKS and H-3 RTC or RTX systems, respectively. Off-line staining preparations are required for both methods, but the same laser optics used for counting cells are used for enumerating reticulocytes. The operator must simply change computer functions on the instrument before aspirating the reticulocyte preparation. The Coulter method uses a new methylene blue stain and the VCS technology described earlier. Two scatterplots are generated: (1) Volume is plotted against scatter on the DF 5 scatterplot, and (2) volume is plotted against conductivity, correlating with opacity of the RBC, on the DF 6 scatterplot. Stained reticulocytes show greater optical scatter and greater opacity than mature RBCs. Relative and absolute reticulocyte counts are reported, along with mean reticulocyte volume and maturation index.[30]

The Technicon H·3 enumerates reticulocytes in the same laser optics flow cell used in the RBC/PLT and BASO channels described earlier. The reticulocyte reagent isovolumetrically spheres the RBCs and stains the reticulocytes with oxazine 750, a nucleic acid-binding dye. Three detectors measure low-angle scatter ($2°-3°$), high-angle scatter ($5°-15°$), and absorbance simultaneously as the cells pass through the flow cell. Three cytograms are generated: (1) high-angle scatter versus absorption, (2) low-angle scatter versus high-angle scatter (Mie cytogram or RBC map), and (3) volume versus hemoglobin concentration. The absorption cytogram allows separation and quantitation of reticulocytes, with additional subdivision into low-, medium-, and high-absorbing cells based on amount of staining. Volume and hemoglobin concentration for each cell are derived from the RBC map by use of Mie scattering theory.[32] Unique reticulocyte indices (MCV of reticulocytes, or MCVr, CHCMr, RDWr, HDWr, hemoglobin content of reticulocytes, or CHr, and hemoglobin content distribution width of reticulocytes, or CHDWr) are provided. Hemoglobin content of each cell is calculated as the product of the cell volume and the cell hemoglobin concentration. A single-parameter histogram of hemoglobin content is constructed and a corresponding distribution width calculated.[20] These reticulocyte indices are not available on the routine patient printout but are available to the operator. Figure 37–13 is a reticulocyte printout from the H-3 that shows the cytograms and reticulocyte indices.

Automated counting of reticulocytes has allowed for increased precision and accuracy and has greatly expanded the analysis of immature RBCs, providing new parameters and indices that may be useful in the diagnosis and treatment of anemias. The clinical utility of the new data is still being defined. The reticulocyte indices, as derived on the Technicon H-3, appear valuable in the monitoring of erythropoietin therapy response, and CHr, in particular, may be useful in the early detection of iron-deficient erythropoiesis.[33] The release of new, young macroreticulocytes, as indicated by hyperfluorescent reticulocytes (HFR) on the Sysmex system or the MCVr on the Technicon H·3, is considered an early predictor of bone marrow transplantation engraftment.[34] Widespread use of the new parameters may be limited by instrumentation availability.

LIMITATIONS AND INTERFERENCES

Establishing automation in the hematology laboratory requires critical evaluation of the instrument's methods, limitations, and performance goals for the individual laboratory. The National Committee for Clinical Laboratory Standards (NCCLS) has proposed a standard for performance goals for the internal quality control of multichannel hematology analyzers.[35] This standard provides guidelines for instrument calibration and assessment of performance criteria, including accuracy, precision, linearity, sensitivity, and specificity. The clinical sensitivity and specificity of the methods should be such that the instrument appropriately identifies patients who have disease and those who do not have disease, respectively.[36] Quality control systems should reflect the laboratory's established performance goals and provide a high level of assurance that the instrument is working within its specified limits.

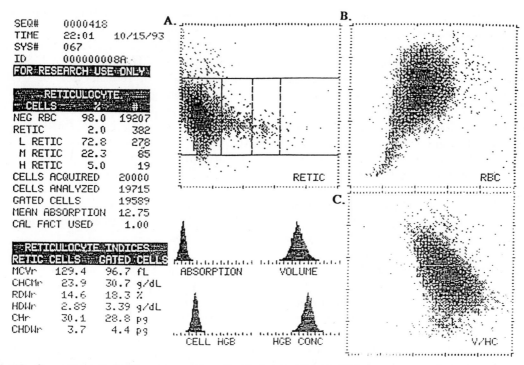

SEQ# 0000418
TIME 22:01 10/15/93
SYS# 067
ID 000000008A
FOR RESEARCH USE ONLY

RETICULOCYTE
CELLS	%	#
NEG RBC	98.0	19207
RETIC	2.0	382
L RETIC	72.8	278
M RETIC	22.3	85
H RETIC	5.0	19
CELLS ACQUIRED		20000
CELLS ANALYZED		19715
GATED CELLS		19589
MEAN ABSORPTION		12.75
CAL FACT USED		1.00

RETICULOCYTE INDICES
	RETIC CELLS	GATED CELLS	
MCVr	129.4	96.7	fL
CHCMr	23.9	30.7	g/dL
RDWr	14.6	18.3	%
HDWr	2.89	3.39	g/dL
CHr	30.1	28.8	pg
CHDWr	3.7	4.4	pg

Figure 37-13 Composite reticulocyte cytograms from the Technicon H·3. *A,* High-angle (5°-15°) scatter on the y-axis versus absorption on the x-axis, allowing separation of low-, medium-, and high-absorbing cells based on amount of staining. *B,* Low-angle (2°-3°) scatter on the y-axis versus high-angle (5°-15°) scatter on the x-axis (red blood cell [RBC] map). *C,* volume (y-axis) versus hemoglobin concentration (x-axis). Because the RBCs are evaluated by the instrument on a cell-by-cell basis, the unique reticulocyte indices can be derived.

Calibration

Calibration is critical in defining the accuracy (as contrasted to precision) of the data produced. Calibration, or the process of electronically correcting an instrument for analytical bias (numerical difference from the "true" value), may be accomplished by the appropriate use of reference methods, reference materials, and/or commercially prepared calibrators.[35] Because few instruments are precalibrated by the manufacturer, calibration must be performed at initial installation and verified at least every 6 months under Clinical Laboratory Improvement Act 1988 (CLIA'88) requirements.[37] Periodic recalibration may be required after major instrument repair requiring optical alignment or part replacement is performed.

Whole blood calibration using fresh whole blood specimens requires the use of reference methods, materials, and procedures to determine true values.[2, 38, 39] The International Committee for Standards in Hematology (ICSH) has established guidelines for selecting a reference blood cell counter for this purpose,[2] but the cyanomethemoglobin method remains the only standard available in hematology for calibration and quality control.[40] Whole blood calibration, which historically has been considered the preferred method for calibra-

tion of multichannel hematology analyzers, has virtually been replaced by the use of commercial calibrators assayed against reference methods. Calibration bias is possible with the use of these calibrators because of inherent differences in stabilized and preserved cell suspensions.[41] Therefore, calibrations must be properly carried out and verified by comparison to reference methods or review of quality control data after calibration and by external comparison studies, such as proficiency testing.[2]

Instrument Limitations

The continual improvement of automated technologies has resulted in greater sensitivity and specificity of instrument flagging and detection of possible interferences in the data. However, the parallel improvement in instrument walk-away capabilities has increased the importance of the technologist's awareness and understanding of instrument limitations and of his or her ability to recognize factors that may interfere and cause erroneous laboratory results. Limitations and interferences may be related to methodology or to inherent problems in the blood sample.

Each instrument has limitations related to methodology that are clearly defined in instrument operation manuals and in the literature. A common method limitation is an instrument's inability to reliably distinguish cells from other particles or cell fragments of the same size. For example, cell fragments may be counted as platelets in samples from chemotherapy-treated patients who have increased white cell fragility.[1, 2] Likewise, schistocytes or small RBCs may interfere in the platelet count. Larger platelet clumps may be counted as WBCs, resulting in a falsely decreased platelet count and a potentially increased WBC count. Micromegakaryocytes may be counted as nucleated RBCs or WBCs. RBCs containing variant hemoglobins, such as S or C, are often resistant to lysis. These unlysed cells are falsely counted as nucleated RBCs or WBCs and interfere with the hemoglobin reaction.[42] This phenomenon has become more apparent with the gentler diluent and lysing reagents of the new analyzers with automated WBC differential technology. Nonlysis may also be seen on the Sysmex instruments[12] in neonates (increased levels of hemoglobin F), in patients with severe liver disease, in those who undergo chemotherapy treatment, and on the Technicon H instruments[20] in those with markedly elevated serum urea nitrogen levels. The Technicon H systems are able to provide a correct WBCB count from the basophil-lobularity channel because of its stronger lysing reagent. An extended lyse cycle may be used on the CD 3500 if interference from lysis-resistant RBCs occurs.[18] TOA's next-generation instrument, the Sysmex SE-9000, will have an additional WBC channel that should eliminate interference in the WBC count from nonlysis on that instrument.[43]

Suppression of automated data, particularly WBC differential data, may occur when internal instrument checks fail or cast doubt on the validity of the data. Some manufacturers release results with specific error codes or flags for further review. The rejection rate of the different instruments varies, with the Coulter STKS and the Sysmex NE-8000 showing the highest suppression of data (10.4% and 18.0%, respectively) and the Technicon H-2 and CD 3000, the lowest (1.2% and 0%, respectively) in one study.[44] The suppression of automated differential data ensures the performance of a manual differential count, whereas the release of data with appropriate flagging mandates the need for careful data and possibly blood film review. This suggests a difference in philosophy among the manufacturers and obviously affects the workflow in different ways.[44] More importantly, each laboratory must establish its own criteria for directed blood film review based on established performance goals, instrument flagging, and inherent instrument limitations. Table 37–3 outlines

one reported review criteria algorithm for a Technicon H system.[45]

Sample Limitations

Limitations resulting from inherent sample problems include factors such as cold agglutinins, icterus, and lipemia. Cold agglutinins present with a classic pattern of increased MCV (frequently > 130 fL), markedly decreased RBC count, and increased MCHC (frequently > 40 g/dL). Careful examination of the histograms-cytograms from the instruments may yield clues to this abnormality.[46] Icterus and lipemia directly affect hemoglobin measurements and related indices.[42] Table 37–4 summarizes conditions that cause interference on most hematology analyzers and offers suggestions for obtaining correct patient results.

Sample age and improper sample handling can have a profound effect on the reliability of hematology test results. These factors have even greater significance as hospitals move toward more off-site testing by large reference laboratories. Specific problems with older samples include increased WBC fragility, swelling and possible lysis of RBCs, and deterioration of platelets.[12] In addition, viable RBCs continue to mature with age, causing a decrease in the reticulocyte count. Stability studies should be performed before the use of an instrument, and specific guidelines should be established for specimen handling and rejection.

CLINICAL UTILITY OF AUTOMATED HEMATOLOGY INSTRUMENTATION

Automated cell-counting analyzers have directly affected the availability, accuracy, and clinical usefulness of the CBC and WBC differential count. Some parameters available on hematology instrumentation, but not available manually, have provided further insight into various clinical conditions. The RDW, a quantitative estimate of erythrocyte anisocytosis, has been used with the MCV in anemia classification. Various discriminants (mathematical formulas or discriminant functions) using these two values have been proposed for the differentiation of iron deficiency from thalassemia minor, based on the typical pattern of iron deficiency having a low MCV and a high RDW, and beta thalassemia minor having a low MCV and a normal RDW.[48-52] RDW has been shown to be unreliable as a sole discriminator of microcytic anemias.[53] The direct measure of RBC hemoglobin concentration on the Technicon H systems has proved a valuable tool in the early detection of iron deficiency anemia and in the dis-

Table 37-3. TECHNICON H-1 WHITE BLOOD CELL DIFFERENTIAL REVIEW CRITERIA

Flagging	Lab Action
Abnormal cytograms (with or without other flags)	Review smear* if any abnormal clustering, excess noise, or valley failures occur on perox or baso channel.
LUC %	Accept <4% with no WBC flags; with flags, follow criteria listed below. If LUCs >4%, review smear; if atypical lymphocytes, append LUCs with ''atypical lymphs'' comment; if large lymphocytes or agranular monocytes, add back to lymph or mono % and absolute counts, respectively; if abnormal cells, do manual differential count, >4% LUCs should be reported only when commented as atypical lymphs.
LS	If + in combination with normal absolute neutrophil count and normal cytogram verify H-1 results. Review + + or + in combination with absolute neutrophil <1.5 × 10⁹/L or >10.5 × 10⁹/L or abnormal cytogram, or other WBC flags. If smear review confirms that left shift is due to bands only or <2% metamyelocytes, add ''slight left shift'' comment to the differential report. Greater than 2% metamyelocytes or any less mature cells such as myelocytes or promyelocytes must be enumerated and reported separately.
Atyps	If LUCs ≤4% and normal cytogram, verify H-1 results. If LUCs >4%, review smear. If atypical lymphocytes seen, append LUCs with ''atypical lymphs'' comment. If blasts or abnormal cells present, perform manual differential count.
Blasts	Review smear. If blasts or abnormal cells present, perform manual differential count. Otherwise, verify H-1 results.
Other N	Scan for NRBCs or large or clumped platelets. Correct WBCB (WBC basophil lobularity channel) if NRBCs >5/100 WBCs and report manual differential count. Report WBCB instead of the WBCP (WBC peroxidase channel) if giant platelets are present and do not report the H-1 absolutes if the WBC substitution did not occur.
IG	Review smear. Perform manual differential count, if necessary.
NFB/NFP	Review smear. Perform manual differential count, if necessary.
NFH	Dilute, rerun, correct results.
NFL	If WBC count <1.0 × 10⁹/L, comment as ''insufficient cells for differential.'' If WBC count >1.0 × 10⁹/L, review smear. Perform manual differential count, if necessary.
WBC	If WBC count >80 × 10⁹/L, dilute for H-1 differential count.
Asterisked differential	Review smear. Perform manual differential count, if necessary.

(From Miers MK, Exton MG, Hurlbut TA, et al: White blood cell differentials as performed by the Technicon H-1: Evaluation and implementation in a tertiary care hospital. Lab Med 1991; 22:99–106.)

+, Instrument flag.

* Atyps, atypical lymphocytes; B, basophil lobularity channel; H, high; IG, immature granulocytes; L, low; LS, left shift; LUCs, large unstained cells; NF, no fit; NRBCs, nucleated red blood cells; P, peroxidase channel; WBC, white blood cell.

† Manual smear review will be defined as follows: WBC review—scan approximately 50 WBCs on 50× oil. A 100-cell manual differential count should be performed only when necessary. If a manual differential count is necessary, absolute counts should *not* be calculated and reported.

crimination of iron deficiency from thalassemia minor.[54, 55] Directly measured hemoglobin concentration has also been used in the detection of iron-deficient erythropoiesis in iron-replete subjects treated with recombinant erythropoietin.[56] The MPV may be useful in detecting whether or not bone marrow megakaryopoiesis is normal. A low MPV may indicate marrow hypoproduction, whereas a high MPV may be suggestive of a myeloproliferative disorder.[57] However, methodology, anti-coagulation, and storage time all influence the MPV, making the parameter less useful.[58]

Automation of the WBC differential has had significant impact on laboratory workflow because of the labor-intensive nature of the manual differential count. The three-part differential available on earlier instruments generally proved suitable as a screening leukocyte differential to identify those samples that required further evaluation or a manual differential count.[59-61] However, partial differential counts do not substitute for a complete differential in abnormal populations.[62-64] The five-part automated differentials now available on the

larger instruments have been evaluated extensively and appear to have acceptable clinical sensitivity and specificity for the detection of distributional and morphologic abnormalities.[65-72] Abnormal cells, such as blasts and nucleated RBCs in low concentration, may not be detected by the instruments but likewise may be missed by the routine 100-cell manual-visual differential count.[73, 74]

Instrument evaluations based on the NCCLS H20-T or H20-A standard[75] with the use of either an 800- or a 400-cell manual leukocyte differential count, respectively, as the reference method have shown acceptable correlation coefficients for all WBC types, with the possible exception of monocytes.[44, 76-78] Further studies using monoclonal antibodies as the reference method for counting monocytes suggest that automated analyzers yield a more accurate assessment of monocytosis than do manual methods.[79, 80]

Histograms and cytograms along with instrument flagging provide valuable information in the diagnosis and treatment of RBC and WBC disorders. Multiple reports indicate the efficacy

Table 37-4. CONDITIONS THAT CAUSE INTERFERENCE ON MOST HEMATOLOGY ANALYZERS

Condition	Parameter(s) Affected	Cause	Instrument Indicators	Corrective Action
Cold agglutinins	RBC ↓, MCV ↑, MCHC ↑, grainy appearance	Agglutination of RBCs	Dual RBC population on RBC map or right shift on RBC histogram	Warm sample to 37 °C and rerun
Lipemia icterus chylomicrons	HGB ↑, MCH ↑	↑ Turbidity affects spectrophotometric reading	HGB × 3 ≠ HCT ± 3, abnormal histogram/cytogram*	Plasma replacement†
Hemolysis	RBC ↓, HCT ↓,	RBCs lysed and not counted	HGB × 3 ≠ HCT ± 3, may show lipemia pattern on histogram/cytogram*	Request new sample
Lysis-resistant RBCs with abnormal hemoglobins	WBC ↑, HGB ↑	RBCs with HGB S, C, or F may fail to lyse and be counted as WBCs	Interference at noise/WBC interface on histogram/cytogram	Manual dilutions, allowing incubation time for lysis
Microcytosis or schistocytes	RBC ↓	Size of RBCs or RBC fragments < lower RBC threshold	Left shift on RBC histogram, MCV flagged if below limits	Smear review
NRBCs, megakaryocyte fragments, or micro-megakaryoblasts	WBC ↑	NRBCs or micro-megakaryoblasts counted as WBCs	NRBC/N‡ flag resulting from interference at noise lymphocyte interface on histogram/cytogram	Count NRBCs or micro-megakaryoblasts per 100 WBCs and correct§
Platelet clumps	PLT ↓, spurious WBC ↑	Large clumps counted as WBCs	Platelet clumps/N flag interference at noise/lymphocyte interface on histogram/cytogram	Redraw specimen in sodium citrate
WBC > 50,000/μL	HGB ↑, RBC ↑, HCT incorrect, abnormal indices	↑ turbidity on HGB, WBCs counted with RBC count	HGB × 3 ≠ HCT ± 3 If WBC > 100,000/μL, count may be above linearity and may not be reported	Spun microhematocrit, manual HGB (spin/read supernatant)†, correct RBC count, recalculate indices; if above linearity dilute for correct WBC
Leukemia, especially with chemotherapy	Spurious WBC ↓ spurious PLT ↑	Fragile WBCs, fragments counted as platelets	Inconsistent PLT count with previous results	Smear review, phase PLT count
Old specimen	MCV ↑, MPV ↑, PLT ↓, automated differential may be incorrect	RBCs swell as sample ages, platelets swell and degenerate, WBCs effected by prolonged exposure to EDTA	Abnormal clustering on WBC histogram/cytogram	Establish stability and sample rejection criteria

CHCM, corpuscular hemoglobin concentration mean; EDTA, ethylene diaminetetra-acetic acid; HCT, hematocrit; HGB, hemoglobin; MCH, mean cell hemoglobin; MCHC, mean cell hemoglobin concentration; MCV, mean cell volume; MPV, mean platelet volume; NRBC, nucleated red blood cell; RBC, red blood cell; PLT, platelet; WBC, white blood cell.

 * Lipemia shows signature pattern on Technicon H cytogram.

 † HGB can be back-calculated from directly measured CHCM on Technicon H Systems.

 ‡ N flag is specific for Technicon H systems; indicates interference at noise-lymphocyte valley; possible NRBCs, platelet clumps, lipids, excess noise.

 § Correct WBCB on Technicon H systems. Small NRBCs thresholded out of WBC count on Sysmex NE-8000 and Cell-Dyn 3000/3500; correction for NRBCs may not be necessary. Semiautomated Sysmex instruments have adjustable lower thresholds to allow inclusion of all nucleated cells in the white cell count.[47]

 For other analyzers, alternate WBC counts may be necessary before correction.

of the histograms-cytograms in the characterization of various abnormal conditions, including RBC disorders, such as cold agglutination, and WBC diseases, like leukemias and myelodysplastic disorders.[46, 81-83] The major instrument manufacturers have published case study books that include histograms-cytograms to aid the technologist in the interpretation of the instrument data.[23, 84, 85]

Selection of a hematology analyzer for an individual laboratory requires careful evaluation of the laboratory's needs and scrutiny of several probing instrument questions and issues, including instru-

(Text continued on page 626)

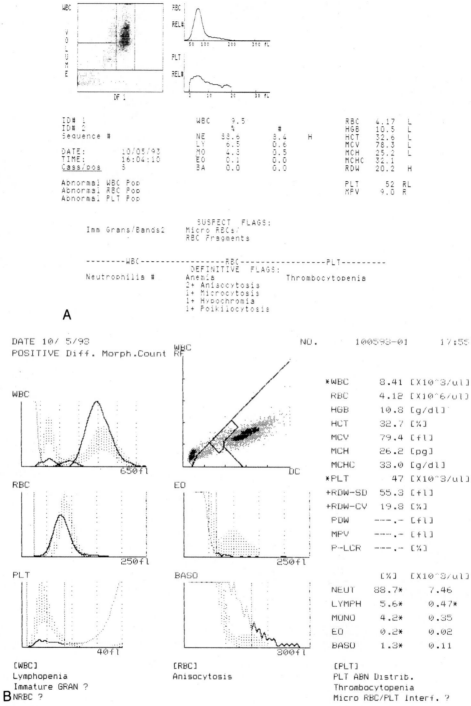

Figure 37–14 Histograms-cytograms from the four major instruments assessing the same patient sample. *A,* Coulter STKS; *B,* Sysmex NE-8000.

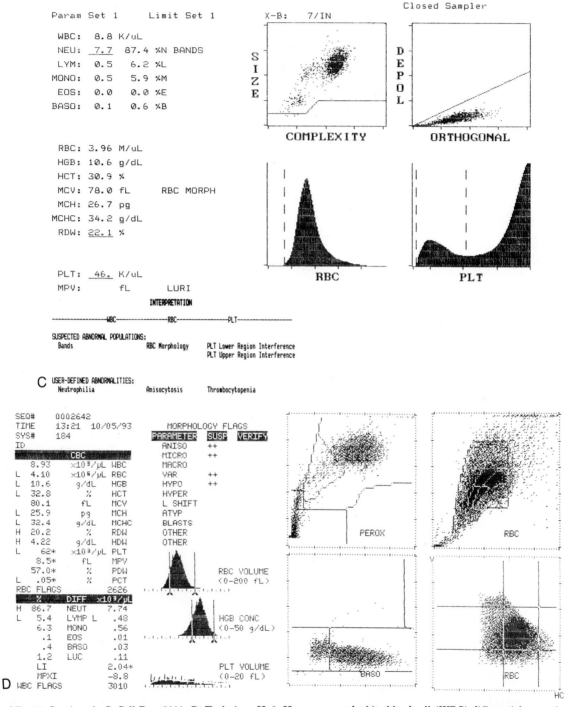

Figure 37–14 *Continued C*, Cell-Dyn 3000; *D*, Technicon H·3. Hemogram and white blood cell (WBC) differential numerical data are the same on all instruments. Note the difference in the flags generated, with only one instrument giving a nucleated red blood cell (NRBC) flag. All instruments called significant abnormal RBC morphology, indicating the need for a smear review. Manual 200-cell differential count: 87% neutrophils (85.5% segmented neutrophils, 1.5% bands), 7.5% lymphocytes, 3.5% monocytes, 2.0% myelocytes, and 3.5% NRBCs. RBC morphology: anisocytosis, poikilocytosis, polychromasia, and schistocytes.

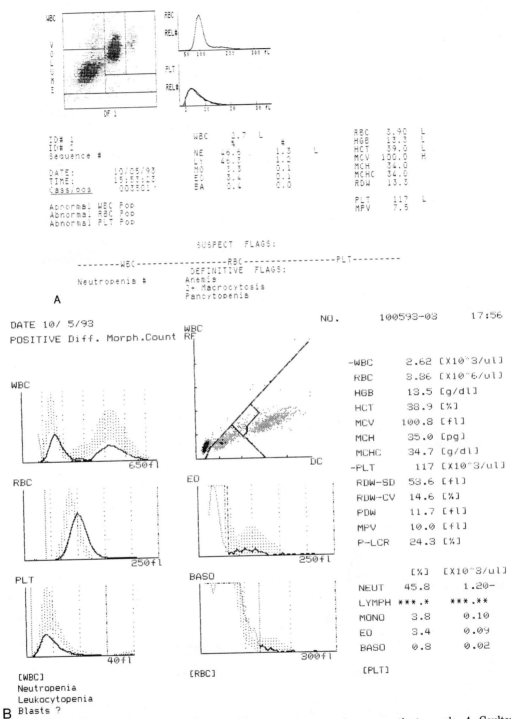

Figure 37-15 Histograms-cytograms from the four major instruments assessing the same patient sample. *A*, Coulter STKS; *B*, Sysmex NE-8000.

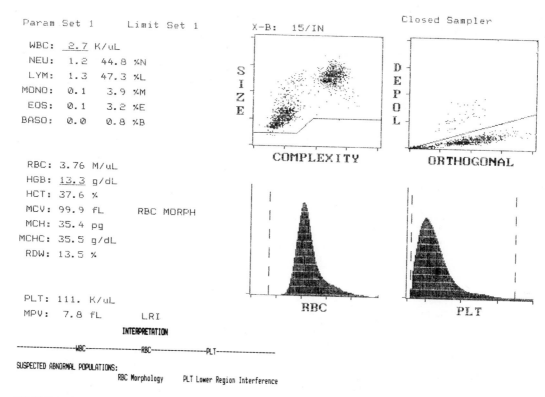

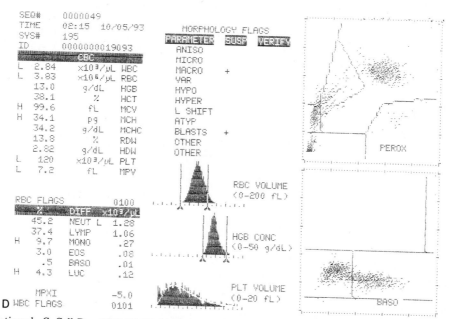

Figure 37–15 *Continued C*, Cell-Dyn 3000; *D*, Technicon H·3. Hemogram and white blood cell (WBC) differential numerical data show little variance on the different instruments. Flagging is somewhat different, with only two of the instruments giving a BLAST flag. Manual 200-cell differential count: 57.5% neutrophils (47% segmented neutrophils, 10.5% bands), 28% lymphocytes, 3% monocytes, 2% eosinophils, 0.5% basophils, 0.5% promyelocytes, and 8.5% blasts. Red blood cell (RBC) morphology: slight anisocytosis and macrocytosis.

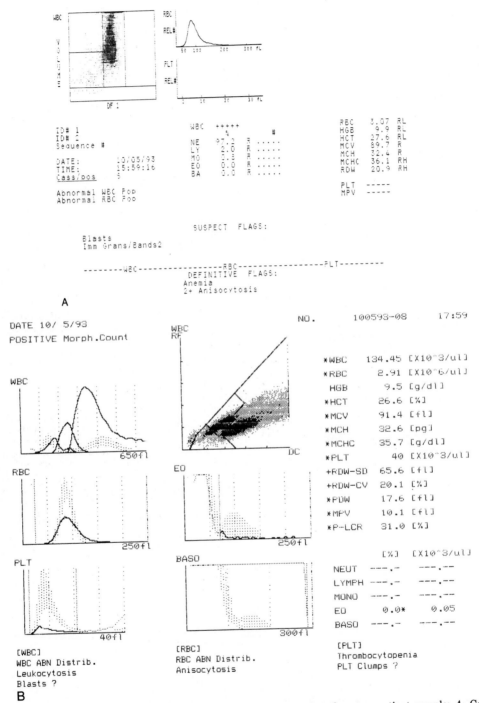

Figure 37–16 Histograms-cytograms from the four major instruments assessing the same patient sample: *A,* Coulter STKS; *B,* Sysmex NE-8000.

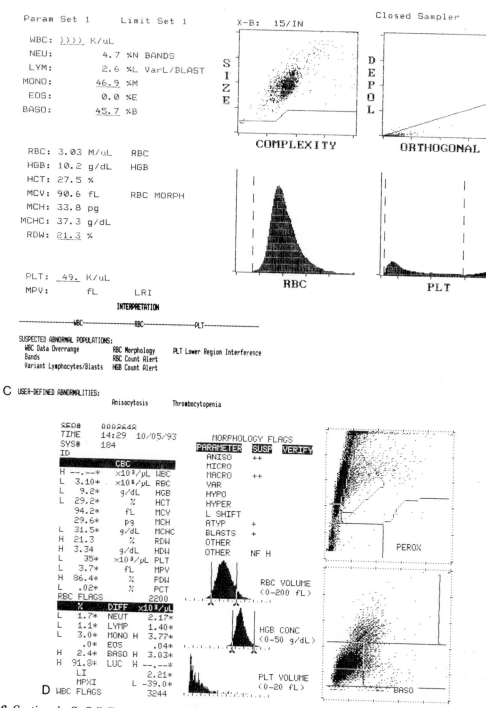

Figure 37–16 *Continued* *C,* Cell·Dyn 3000; *D,* Technicon H·3. Hemogram data show little variance. White blood cell (WBC) differential data are markedly different on two analyzers, and two of the instruments suppress the differential results. All of the cytograms show abnormal WBC distribution. Manual 200-cell differential count: 1% segmented neutrophils, 2% lymphocytes, 0.5% monocytes, 1% promyelocytes, and 95.5% blasts. Red blood cell (RBC) morphology: slight anisocytosis and macrocytosis, few schistocytes.

626

ment specifications and system requirements, methods, training requirements, maintenance, reagent usage, data management, staff response, and short- and long-term expenditures.[86] The instrument selected should be appropriate for the workload and patient population and should positively affect the laboratory's workflow. Ultimately, the instrument decision may be swayed by individual preferences.[44]

CASES

Figures 37–14 through 37–16 represent composite cases of patient samples run on (or performed on) by the Coulter STKS, the Sysmex NE-8000, the CD 3000, and the Technicon H-2. The cases are presented to compare how the different analyzers handle abnormal data and to show representative examples of RBC and WBC flagging.

GENERAL PRINCIPLES OF COAGULATION INSTRUMENTS

The coagulation laboratory evaluates patients for hemorrhagic and thrombotic status. A full explanation of testing in hemostasis is given in Chapter 35.

Mechanical Clot Detection Methods

Coagulation instruments detect clot formation either mechanically or photo-optically. One mechanical method uses *electrical impedance,* which is the principle employed in the fibrometer (BBL Microbiology Systems, Division of Becton Dickinson, Cockeysville, MD) and the Dataclot 2 (Helena Laboratories, Beaumont, TX).[87] These semi-automatic instruments have two probes that are suspended in a reaction cup. One probe is stationary while the other moves to detect the clot. Clot formation breaks the current and stops the timer. These instruments are basic and do not need much maintenance. Probes must be cleaned between analyses of each specimen to prevent specimen carryover. Curves determined by use of these instruments must be constructed manually and the results read from the curves.

Another method of mechanical clot detection uses increased plasma viscosity on an iron ball in an electromagnetic field (ST4, American Bioproducts Corporation, Parsippany, NJ).[88] When placed in an electromagnetic field, the iron ball swings in a pendulum motion. As the plasma becomes more viscous, the ball stops, thus signaling clot formation. The ST4 has the capacity to store curves for

several tests and to convert the curves to patients' results.

Photo-Optical Methods

Instruments using the *photo-optical* principle detect clot formation by measuring the change in the plasma optical density. Light from a controlled beam passes through a collimator, which illuminates the plasma. The light beam is detected by a photodetector that monitors the intensity of the light beam. As a clot forms, the light intensity decreases, triggering the end point.[89] The clot can be detected by use of turbidity or nephelometry, depending on the angle of the light beam to the photodetector. In *turbidimetric* systems, the light is parallel to the photodetector. In the *nephelometric* method, the light beam is at a 90° angle to the photodetector and scattered light is measured.[90]

Sources of Error

The addition of reagents may affect the initial optical density. Most instruments have a guard time during which the specimen and the reagents equilibrate.[89] This is important to remember when dealing with hypercoagulable human and animal samples. If the sample is already clotted when the initial optical density is read, there will be no change so the instrument will indicate incorrectly that there was no clot formation.

In some extreme circumstances, photo-optical instruments may give falsely elevated results. This could occur with viscous plasmas, such as are found in hyperlipidemia, hyperbilirubinemia, or hyperalimentation fluid. This viscosity hampers the ability of the photo-optical system to detect any change in optical density. However, many of the newer photo-optical instruments have been improved to eliminate the interference from turbidity. Plasma with a low fibrinogen content forms a clear clot that can also hamper detection. Both turbid and clear plasmas will provide accurate results with instruments using mechanical clot detection.

OPTIONS ON PRIMARY INSTRUMENTS

Most automated instruments use the photo-optical principle. The diversity of these instruments should make it easy for a laboratory to find one to suit its unique situation. With computer capabilities increasing and the number of personnel decreasing, efficient sample handling has become an important consideration.

Automated Pipettors and Dilutors

Automated plasma pipettors are standard on many instruments. The pipettor can sample directly from the Vacutainer tube or sample cup, for example, the ACL system (Instrumentation Laboratory, Lexington, MA),[90] MLA 1000 (Medical Laboratory Automation, Inc., Pleasantville, NY),[91] MDA (Organon Teknika, Durham, NC),[92] and Koagulab 40A (Ortho Diagnostic Systems, Inc., Raritan, NJ).[93] Dilutions for fibrinogens and factor assays are also performed by the instrument. Instruments that do not have built-in pipettors or dilution capabilities have additional units to perform these tasks (such as some manufactured by Helena Laboratories,[94] Organon Teknika,[95] and Ortho[93]).

When instruments with automatic pipettors or separate pipetting units are evaluated, specimen carryover should be considered. Carryover can be evaluated by testing a series of normal specimens following one that had an elevated activated partial thromboplastin time caused by heparin, or by running a factor-deficient specimen after a normal one. If there is more than a 10% change in the results, carryover should be suspected. Additional consideration should be given to the operable condition of the instrument when the autopipette is disabled.

Bar Codes

Bar code reading capabilities make workflow most efficient, but incorrect patient identification numbers on instruments without positive identification capabilities encourage clerical errors.

Sample Requirements

Laboratories that deal with a large pediatric population must consider the minimal amount of sample necessary for tests. Some instruments are set to pipette smaller volumes. Other instruments offer the option of using half volumes, which reduces the sample and the amount of reagents required.

Another option is single testing. The guidelines of the NCCLS state that the decision to use single or duplicate testing depends on the end-point method. Single testing can be considered only with fully automated instruments. Sufficient data must be gathered to document the precision of the instrument to do single testing. Furthermore, controls, both normal and abnormal, must be run more often.[96]

Quality Control and Data Management

Quality control has been streamlined with the addition of disk drives and personal computers to the instruments. Controls are automatically added to files. By use of internal running clocks, the control results can be identified for each shift. Westgard rules (see Chapter 5) can be activated on some instruments to detect trends and problems. Quality control results can be printed out at the end of the month with the calculated mean, standard deviation, and coefficient of variation.

Data management has reduced the amount of time required to perform specialized tests. The instruments construct curves for each test and convert patients' times into results, which saves time and reduces errors during manual calculations.

CHROMOGENIC SUBSTRATES

The standard clot-based tests are being complemented with synthetic chromogenic substrate assays. The synthetic substrate is linked to the chromophore *p*-nitroaniline. During the reaction, *p*-nitroaniline is cleaved from the substrate, which produces a yellow color that can be read at 405 nm on a spectrophotometer. The MLA 900C and 1000, the ACL 1000, 2000, and 3000, and the MDA instruments have added chromogenic optics. In the MLA and ACL series, the reagents must be changed to run the chromogenic assays. Thus, routine prothrombin times, activated partial thromboplastin times, and fibrinogens can be analyzed. If there is only one instrument in the laboratory and changing reagents would cause a workflow problem, manual methods for chromogenic assays should be considered. The CSA 1200 Chromogenic Analyzer (Helena)[97] is a spectrophotometer that can read small volumes at 405 nm. If platelet aggregation studies must be performed, the PACKS-4 (Helena)[98] and the PAP-4 (Bio-Data, Hatboro, PA)[99] aggregometers are equipped to perform kinetic and end-point chromogenic assays.

AGGREGOMETRY

Platelet function studies are used as an indicator of thrombosis and hemorrhage. Platelet aggregation measures the ability of platelets to adhere to one another. Whole blood or platelet-rich plasma can be used for testing. With platelet-rich plasma, a change in turbidity, caused by the addition of aggregating agents, is measured by a spectrophotometer. With whole blood, an impedance method is used to measure the change in blood viscosity on addition of aggregating agents.[100] PACKS-4, PAP-4, and ChronoLog (Chrono-Log Corporation, Havertown, PA)[101] have multiple-channel instruments. PACKS-4 and PAP-4 have programs to perform ristocetin cofactor testing for the von Willebrand molecule. The Chronolog instrument can use either whole blood or platelet-rich plasma. The whole blood option decreases the time needed for test completion. The Chronolog series also includes an instrument that can measure ATP release with luminescence during platelet aggregation.[102]

WHOLE BLOOD TESTING

The concern for rapid turn around time, especially by surgeons, has initiated the reconsideration of whole blood bedside testing. Cardiovascular surgeons and cardiologists performing angiography and angioplasty have used the activated clotting time (ACT) to monitor heparin administration. In this test, unanticoagulated whole blood is added to an activator such as kaolin, Celite, or diatomaceous earth. The test can be done manually or inserted into an instrument for mixing and detection of clot formation.[103] The Hemachron (International Technidyne Corp., Edison, NJ) detects clot formation with a magnetic detector. The tubes have an aligned magnet within them. After whole blood is added, the tube is inserted into the instrument, which slowly rotates the tube. As the clot forms, the magnet is displaced and cannot be detected. This signals clot formation.

This concept has been adapted to a bedside testing unit for whole blood prothrombin time, activated partial thromboplastin time, and thrombin time. The Factor VI instrument (International Technidyne Corporation, Edison, NJ)[104] can use anticoagulated whole blood or blood drawn directly into special Vacutainer tubes that contain the reagents necessary to perform these assays.

The Biotrack 512 (Ciba-Corning, Medfield, MD)[105] takes whole blood testing even further. Prothrombin time or activated partial thromboplastin time can be tested with one drop of blood applied to a cartridge in a hand-held instrument. This instrument uses capillary motion to move the blood through the cartridge, where blood mixes with the appropriate reagents. A laser detects cessation of flow. The monitor converts this time to the test result.

Whole blood testing provides results within minutes and is particularly useful in surgery and critical care units. It also offers the advantage that the cellular elements present in whole blood provide a more accurate in vivo picture.[103] However, whole blood testing requires strict adherence to proper technique.

SUMMARY

Two basic principles of operation are used for cell-counting instrumentation: electronic impedance (resistance) and optical light scatter. Impedance is based on the detection and measurement of changes in the electrical resistance created as cells pass through an aperture. Low-voltage impedance is used to measure cell size and number, whereas high voltage impedance is used to measure nuclear size and internal complexity of the cell. Impedance may also be used in combination with optical light scatter. Light scatter is the result of interactions between light absorption, diffraction, and reflection. Photodetectors convert the scattered rays into electrical signals. Forward angle scatter correlates with cell volume, and orthogonal (or side) light scatter correlates with the degree of internal cell complexity. The combined use of these principles allows for a more accurate evaluation of blood cell size and identification.

Analyzers on the market today offer a wide range of possibilities. Some systems provide an eight-parameter hemogram, whereas others have walk-away systems with hemogram, a complete five-part differential, and automated reticulocyte count. The final selection of a hematology analyzer should reflect a careful evaluation of the laboratory's workflow, expectations, personnel, and resources.

Coagulation instruments operate on the basis of two primary principles: photo-optical and electromagnetic. The majority of laboratories use photo-optical instruments for routine testing.

References

1. Nelson DA, Morris MW: Basic examination of blood. In Henry JB (ed): Clinical Diagnosis and Management, 18th ed. Philadelphia: WB Saunders, 1991:553–603.
2. Koepke JA: Quantitative blood cell counting. In Koepke JA (ed): Practical Laboratory Hematology. New York: Churchill Livingstone, 1991: 43–60.
3. Watson JS, Dotson MA: Multiparameter hematology instruments. In Lotspeich-Steininger CA, Stiene-Martin EA, Koepke JA (eds): Clinical Hematology: Principles, Procedures, Correlations. Philadelphia: JB Lippincott, 1992:496–514.
4. Coulter WH: High speed automatic blood cell counter and cell size analyzer. Proc Natl Electron Conf 1956; 12:1034.
5. Coulter Electronics: Significant Advances in Hematology: Hematology Education Series, PN 4206115A. Hialeah, FL: Coulter Electronics, 1983.
6. Coulter Electronics: Coulter Counter Model S-Plus IV With Three-Population Differential: Product Reference

Manual (PN 423560B). Hialeah, FL: Coulter Electronics, 1983.

7. Coulter Electronics: Coulter® STKR Product Reference Manual (PN 4235547E). Hialeah, FL: Coulter Electronics, 1988.

8. TOA Medical Electronics Company: Sysmex™ Model E-5000 Operator's Manual (CN 461-2104-2). Kobe, Japan: Toa Medical Electronics Company, 1985.

9. Mohandas N, Clark MR, Kissinger S, et al: Inaccuracies associated with the automated measurement of mean cell hemoglobin concentration in dehydrated cells. Blood 1980; 56:125–128.

10. Arnfred T, Kristensen SD, Munck V: Coulter counter model S and model S-plus measurements of mean erythrocyte volume (MCV) are influenced by the mean erythrocyte haemoglobin concentration (MCHC). Scand J Clin Lab Invest 1981, 41:717–721.

11. Johnson KL: Basics of flow cytometry. Clin Lab Sci 1992; 5(1):22–24.

12. Toa Medical Electronics Company: Sysmex™ NE-8000 Operator's Manual (CN 461-2326-5). Kobe, Japan: Toa Medical Electronics Company, 1990.

13. Shapiro HM: How a flow cytometer works. In Shapiro HM (ed): Practical Flow Cytometry, 2nd ed. New York: AR Liss, 1988:21–86.

14. Jovin TM, Morris SJ, Striker G, et al: Automatic sizing and separation of particles by ratios of light scattering intensities. J Histochem Cytochem 1976; 24:269–283.

15. McCoy JP, Lovett EJ: Basic principles in clinical flow cytometry. In Keren DF (ed): Flow Cytometry In Clinical Diagnosis. Chicago, ASCP Press, 1989:12–40.

16. Tycko DH, Metz MH, Epstein EA, et al: Flow-cytometric scattering measurement of red blood cell volume and hemoglobin concentration. Appl Opt 1985; 24:1355–1364.

17. Abbott Laboratories: Cell-Dyn® 3000 System Operator's Manual (LN 92420-01). Abbott Park, IL: Abbott Laboratories, 1993.

18. Abbott Laboratories: Cell-Dyn® 3500 System Operator's Manual (LN 9140285A). Abbott Park, IL: Abbott Laboratories, 1994.

19. Technicon Instruments Corporation: Technicon H-2™ System Operation (PN UA9-0759B00). Tarrytown, NY: Technicon Instruments Corporation, 1990.

20. Miles: Technicon H-3 RTX™/RTC™ System: System Reference Guide (PN TK9-2823-10). Tarrytown, NY: Miles, 1993.

21. Coulter Corporation: Coulter® STKS Operator's Guide (PN 4235928H). Hialeah, FL: Coulter Corporation, 1992.

22. Bessman D, Williams LJ, Gilmer PR: Mean platelet volume: The inverse relation of platelet size and count in normal subjects and an artifact of other particles. Am J Clin Pathol 1981; 76:289–299.

23. Coulter Electronics: Coulter VCS Technology Casebook (PN 4206281-2A). Hialeah, FL: Coulter Electronics, 1989.

24. Abbott Diagnostics: Cell-Dyn® Rainbow™ Classification Program (PN 97-9427/R3-20). Abbott Park, IL: Abbott Diagnostics, 1992.

25. Groner W: New developments in flow cytochemistry technology. In Simson E (ed): Proceedings of the Technicon H-1™ Hematology Symposium, October 11, 1985. Tarrytown, NY: Technicon Instruments Corporation, 1986:1–8.

26. Mohandas N, Kim YR, Tycko DH, et al: Accurate and independent measurement of volume and hemoglobin concentration of individual red cells by laser light scattering. Blood 1986; 68:506–513.

27. Koepke J: Current limitations in reticulocyte counting: Implications for clinical laboratories. In Porstmann B (ed): The Emerging Importance of Accurate Reticulocyte Counting. New York: Caduceus Medical Publishers, 1993:18–22.

28. National Committee for Clinical Laboratory Standards: Reticulocyte counting by flow cytometry: Proposed guideline (NCCLS document H44-P). Villanova, PA: National Committee for Clinical Laboratory Standards, 1993.

29. College of American Pathologists: CAP Surveys: Reticulocyte (Pilot) Survey Set RT-A, 1993. Northfield, IL: College of American Pathologists, 1993.

30. Coulter Corporation: Introducing a new reticulocyte methodology using Coulter® VCS technology on Coulter STKS and MAXM hematology systems (Product brochure TC93003201). Miami, FL: Coulter Corporation, 1993.

31. TOA Medical Electronics Company: Sysmex™ R-3000 Automated Reticulocyte Analyzer (Product brochure lit. no. SP-9620). Los Alamitos, CA: TOA Medical Electronics (USA), 1991.

32. Colella G: Technical advancements of the H-3 hematology analyzer. In Balzac F, Chapman S, Verderese C (eds): Conference Proceedings: H-3 New Perspectives for Hematology. New York: Caduceus Medical Publishers, 1993:28–29.

33. Goldberg M: Recombinant erythropoietin therapy and the detection of iron-deficient erythropoiesis in iron-replete individuals. In Balzac F, Chapman S, Verderese C (eds): Conference Proceedings: H-3 New Perspectives for Hematology. New York: Caduceus Medical Publishers, 1993:16–18.

34. d'Onofrio G: Simultaneous H-3 RBC and reticulocyte measurement: Is it clinically useful? In Balzac F, Chapman S, Verderese C (eds): Conference Proceedings: H-3 New Perspectives for Hematology. New York: Caduceus Medical Publishers, 1993:23–27.

35. National Committee for Clinical Laboratory Standards: Performance goals for the internal quality control of multichannel hematology analyzers: Proposed standard (NCCLS publication H26-P). Villanova, PA: National Committee for Clinical Laboratory Standards, 1989.

36. National Committee for Clinical Laboratory Standards: Assessment of clinical sensitivity and specificity of laboratory tests: Proposed guideline (NCCLS document GP10-P). Villanova, PA: National Committee for Clinical Laboratory Standards, 1987.

37. Rules and regulations. Federal Register February 28, 1992; 57(40): 7165.

38. Gilmer PR, Williams LJ, Koepke JA, et al: Calibration methods for automated hematology instruments. Am J Clin Pathol 1977; 68:185–190.

39. Koepke JA: The calibration of automated instruments for accuracy in hemoglobinometry. Am J Clin Pathol 1977; 68:180–184.

40. International Committee for Standardization in Haematology: Recommendations for reference method for haemoglobinometry in human blood (ICSH Standard EP 6/2:1977) and specifications for international haemiglobincyanide reference preparation (ICSH Standard EP6/3:1977). J Clin Pathol 1978; 31:139–143.

41. Savage RA: Calibration bias and imprecision for automated hematology analyzers: An evaluation of significance of short-term bias resulting from calibration of an analyzer with S Cal™. Am J Clin Pathol 1985; 84:186–190.

42. Cornbleet J: Spurious results from automated hematology cell counters. Lab Med 1983; 14:509–514.

43. Tsuda I, Tatsumi N: Evaluation of detection of immature WBC by the new Sysmex SE-9000 automated hematology analyzer. Poster presentation at the International Society for Laboratory Hematology, Seventh International Symposium on Technology Innovations in Laboratory Hematology. Lake Tahoe, NV: April 7–10, 1994.

44. Bentley SA, Johnson A, Bishop CA: A parallel evaluation of four automated hematology analyzers. Am J Clin Pathol 1993; 100:626–632.

45. Miers MK, Exton MG, Hurlbut TA, et al: White blood cell differentials as performed by the Technicon H-1: Evaluation and implementation in a tertiary care hospital. Lab Med 1991; 22:99–106.

46. Strobel SL, Panke TW, Bills GL: Cold erythrocyte agglutination and infectious mononucleosis. Lab Med 1993; 24:219–221.

47. Culp NB, Fritsma G: New approaches to nucleated RBC correction of WBC counts. Clin Lab Sci 1990; 3(4):239.

48. Bessman JD, Feinstein DI: Quantitative anisocytosis as a

discriminant between iron deficiency and thalassemia minor. Blood 1979; 53:288–293.

49. Bessman JD, Gilmer PR, Gardner FH: Improved classification of anemias by MCV and RDW. Am J Clin Pathol 1983; 80:322–326.

50. Fossat C, David M, Harle JR, et al: New parameters in erythrocyte counting: Value of histograms. Arch Pathol Lab Med 1987; 111:1150–1154.

51. Green R, King R: A new red cell discriminant incorporating volume dispersion for differentiating iron deficiency anemia from thalassemia minor. Blood Cells 1989; 15:481–495.

52. Fernandes B, Houwen B: A new algorithm for classification of microcytic anaemias. Presented at the International Society for Laboratory Hematology, Seventh International Symposium on Technology Innovations in Laboratory Hematology. Lake Tahoe, NV: April 7–10, 1994.

53. Duca D, Green R: Red cell distribution width is a poor discriminator for distinguishing iron deficiency anemia from thalassemia minor or the anemia of chronic disease (abstract). Poster Presentation at the 1993 Fall Meeting of the American Society of Clinical Pathologists (ASCP) and the College of American Pathologists (CAP). Orlando, FL: October 16–22, 1993.

54. Green R, King R, Greenbaum A, et al: Early detection of iron deficiency by direct measurement of red cell hemoglobin concentration: Sequential studies in phlebotomized normal volunteers. Blood 1990; 76(Suppl 1):122A.

55. Mohandas N, Greenbaum A, Green R: Variability in cell hemoglobin content of individual red cells can be used to discriminate iron deficiency from thalassemia minor. Blood 1990; 76(Suppl 1):155B.

56. Brugnara C, Chamber LA, Malynn E, et al: Red blood cell regeneration induced by subcutaneous recombinant erythropoietin: Iron-deficient erythropoiesis in iron-replete subjects. Blood 1993; 81:956–964.

57. Coulter Electronics: Proceedings of the Coulter Automated Differential International Symposium, September 26, 1986. Hialeah, FL: Coulter Electronics, 1987.

58. Reardon DM, Hutchinson D, Preston FE, et al: The routine measurement of platelet volume: A comparison of aperture-impedance and flow cytometric systems. Clin Lab Haematol 1985; 7:251–257.

59. Allen JK, Batjer ID: Evaluation of an automated method for leukocyte differential counts based on electronic volume analysis. Arch Pathol Lab Med 1985; 109:534–539.

60. Pierre RV, Payne BA, Lee WK, et al: Comparison of four leukocyte differential methods with the National Committee for Clinical Laboratory Standards (NCCLS) reference method. Am J Clin Pathol 1987; 87:201–209.

61. Payne BA, Pierre RV, Lee WK: Evaluation of the TOA E-5000® automated hematology analyzer. Am J Clin Pathol 1987; 88:51–57.

62. Ross DW, Watson JS, Davis PH, et al: Evaluation of the Coulter three-part differential screen. Am J Clin Pathol 1985; 84:481–484.

63. Cornbleet J, Kessinger S: Evaluation of Coulter S-Plus three-part differential in population with a high prevalence of abnormalities. Am J Clin Pathol 1985; 84:620–626.

64. Miers MK, Fogo AB, Federspiel CF, et al: Evaluation of the Coulter S-Plus IV differential as a screening tool in a tertiary care hospital. Am J Clin Pathol 1987; 87:745–751.

65. Ross DW, Bentley SA: Evaluation of an automated hematology system (Technicon H-1). Arch Pathol Lab Med 1986; 110:803–808.

66. Bollinger PB, Drewinko B, Brailas CD, et al: The Technicon H-1: An automated hematology analyzer for today and tomorrow. Am J Clin Pathol 1987; 87:71–78.

67. Watson JS, Davis RA: Evaluation of the Technicon H-1 hematology system. Lab Med 1987; 18:316–322.

68. Warner BA, Reardon DM: A field evaluation of the Coulter STKS®. Am J Clin Pathol 1991; 95:207–217.

69. Hallawell R, O'Malley C, Hussein S, et al: An evaluation of the Sysmex NE-8000® hematology analyzer. Am J Clin Pathol 1991; 96:594–601.

70. Cornbleet PJ, Myrick D, Judkins S, et al: Evaluation of the Cell-Dyn 3000 differential. Am J Clin Pathol 1992; 98:603–614.

71. Cornbleet PJ, Myrick D, Levy R: Evaluation of the Coulter STKS five-part differential. Am J Clin Pathol 1993; 99:72–81.

72. Brigden ML, Page NE, Graydon C: Evaluation of the Sysmex NE-8000 automated hematology analyzer in a high-volume outpatient laboratory. Am J Clin Pathol 1993; 100:618–625.

73. Rumke CL: The statistically expected variability in differential leukocyte counting. In Koepke JA (ed): Differential Leukocyte Counting. Skokie, IL: College of American Pathologists, 1978:39–45.

74. Koepke JA, Dotson MA, Shifman MA: A critical evaluation of the manual/visual differential leukocyte counting method. Blood Cells 1985; 11:173–181.

75. National Committee for Clinical Laboratory Standards: Reference leukocyte differential count (proportional) and evaluation of instrumental methods: Approved standard (NCCLS document H20-A). Villanova, PA: National Committee for Clinical Laboratory Standards, 1992.

76. Warner BA, Reardon DM, Marshall DP: Automated haematology analysers: A four-way comparison. Med Lab Sci 1990; 47:285-296.

77. Swaim WR: Laboratory and clinical evaluation of white blood cell differential counts: Comparison of the Coulter VCS, Technicon H-1, and 800-cell manual method. Am J Clin Pathol 1991; 95:381–388.

78. Buttarello M, Gadotti M, Lorenz C, et al: Evaluation of four automated hematoogy analyzers: A comparative study of differential counts (imprecision and inaccuracy). Am J Clin Pathol 1992; 97:345–352.

79. Goossens W, Hove LV, Verwilghen RL: Monocyte counting: Discrepancies in results obtained with different automated instruments. J Clin Pathol 1991; 44:224–227.

80. Seaberg R, Cuomo J: Assessment of monocyte counts derived from automated instrumentation. Lab Med 1993; 24:222–224.

81. Watson JS, Ross DW: Characterization of myelodysplastic syndromes by flow cytochemistry with the Technicon H-1. J Med Technol 1987; 4(1):18–20.

82. Krause JR, Costello RT, Krause J, et al: Use of the Technicon H-1 in the characterization of leukemias. Arch Pathol Lab Med 1988; 112:889–894.

83. Penchansky L, Krause JR: Flow cytochemical study of acute leukemia of childhood with the Technicon H-1. Lab Med 1991; 22(3):184–189.

84. Walters JG, Garrity PF: Case Studies in the New Morphology. McGaw Park, IL: American Scientific Products, 1987.

85. Simson E, Ross DW, Kocher WD: Atlas of Automated Cytochemical Hematology. Tarrytown, NY: Technicon Instruments Corporation, 1988.

86. Camden TL: How to select the ideal hematology analyzer. Medical Laboratory Observer 1993; 25(2):29–33.

87. Coagulation analyzers; automated, semi-automated. Product Comparison System, Product codes 15-098, 17-176, 1991.

88. Ledford MR, Kaczor DA. Evaluation of the ST4 clot detection instrument. Lab Med 1992; 23:172–175.

89. MLA 700 Instrument Manual. Pleasantville, NY: Medical Laboratory Automation. p 4-3.

90. ACL 3000 instrument manual. Hialeah, FL: Coulter Electronics, undated.

91. MLA 1000 instrument manual. Pleasantville, NY: Medical Laboratory Automation.

92. MDA product information. Durham, NC: Organon Teknika Corporation.

93. Ortho auto dilutor unit video. Raritan, NJ: Ortho Diagnostic Systems.

94. Cascade auto sample processor product information. Beaumont, TX: Helena Laboratories.

95. Gayzuetta FG, Billett HH: Evaluation of an automated sampler for routine coagulation testing. Lab Med 1992; 23:667–669.

96. National Committee for Clinical Laboratory Standards: Collection, transport and preparation of blood specimens for coagulation testing and performance of coagulation assays. Approved guideline (NCCLS document H21-A). Villanova, PA: National Committee for Clinical Laboratory Standards, 1986.

97. CSA 1200 Chromogenic analyzer instrument manual. Beaumont, TX: Helena Laboratories, undated.

98. PACKS-4 Aggregometer instrument product information. Beaumont, TX: Helena Laboratories, undated.

99. PAP-4 Aggregometer instrument product information. Hatboro, PA: Bio-Data Corporation, undated.

100. Ens GE. Laboratory observation. Clin Hemost Rev, 1992; 6:9.

101. Chrono-Log Aggregometer product information. Havertown, PA: Chrono-Log Corporation, undated.

102. Ingerman-Wojenski CM, Silver MJ: A quick method for screening platelet dysfunction using the whole blood lumi-aggregometer. Thromb Haemost 1984; 51:154–156.

103. Jensen R, Ens GE: Whole blood coagulation monitoring. Clin Hemost Rev 1992; 6:2.

104. Factor VI instrument manual. Edison, NJ: International Technidyne Corporation, undated.

105. Biotrack 512 instrument manual. Medfield, MA: Ciba-Corning, undated.

PART IX

Body Fluids

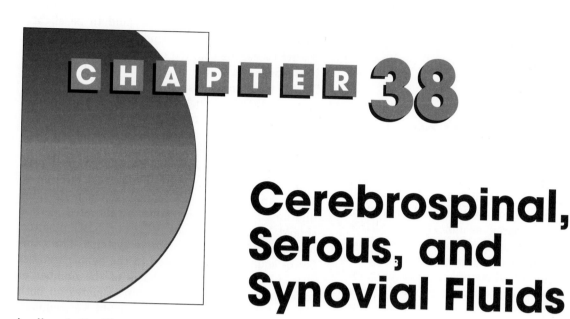

CHAPTER 38

Cerebrospinal, Serous, and Synovial Fluids

Leilani Collins

Outline

Objectives

AFTER COMPLETION OF THIS CHAPTER, THE READER WILL BE ABLE TO

1. Perform cell counts on body fluids, including choice of diluting fluid for appropriate cells, selection of counting area, counting of nucleated cells and red blood cells, and calculation and corrections (if necessary) of counts.

2. Discuss the gross appearance of body fluids, its significance, and its practical use in determining cell count dilutions.

3. Discuss the advantages and disadvantages of cytocentrifuge preparations.

4. Differentiate between traumatic spinal tap and cerebral hemorrhage on the basis of cell counts and appearance of uncentrifuged and centrifuged specimens.

5. Identify normal cells found in cerebrospinal, serous, and synovial fluids.

6. Describe the characteristics of benign versus malignant cells in body fluids.

7. Identify crystals in synovial fluids, using polarization.

The examination of body fluids, including blood cell count and differential, can provide valuable diagnostic information. The fluids to be discussed in this chapter include cerebrospinal fluid (CSF), serous or body cavity fluids (pleural, pericardial, and peritoneal fluids), and synovial (joint) fluids.

PERFORMING CELL COUNTS ON BODY FLUIDS

Examination of all fluids should include color, turbidity, cell counts, and differential. Blood cell counts should be performed and cytocentrifuge slides should be prepared as quickly as possible after collection of the specimen since white blood cells (WBCs) begin to deteriorate within 30 minutes after collection.[1] Cell counts on fluids are usually performed on a hemacytometer (see Chapter 12); however, some automated instruments are now capable of performing blood cell counts on fluids. Care should be taken to observe operating limits of these instruments as well as volume limits of the fluid received.

Cell counts are performed with undiluted fluid if the fluid is clear. If the fluid is hazy or bloody, appropriate dilutions should be made to provide accurate counts of both WBCs and red blood cells (RBCs). The diluting fluid for RBCs is isotonic saline. Diluting fluids for WBCs include Turk's solution, which contains glacial acetic acid to lyse RBCs and methylene blue to stain the nuclei of the WBCs. Dilutions should be based on the turbidity of the fluid or on the number of cells seen on the hemacytometer. A WBC count of approximately 200/mm³ or an RBC count of approximately 400/mm³ will cause a fluid to be slightly hazy. If the fluid is blood tinged to slightly bloody, the RBCs can be counted using undiluted fluid, but it is advisable to use a small (1:2) dilution with Turk's solution to lyse the RBCs and provide an accurate WBC or nucleated cell count. If the fluid is bloody, it will be necessary to use a 1:200 dilution for RBCs (standard dilution in RBC Unopettes [Becton Dickinson, Rutherford, NJ]) and either a 1:2 dilution with Turk's solution or a 1:20 (standard dilution in WBC Unopettes) dilution to obtain an accurate WBC count. When performing dilutions for blood cell counts, a calibrated method should be used, such as WBC or RBC pipettes, MLA pipettes, or the Unopette systems. The number of squares to be counted in the hemacytometer should be decided on the basis of the number of cells present. In general, all nine squares on both sides of the hemacytometer should be counted. However, if the number of cells is high, fewer squares may be counted. Each square equals 1 mm². The formula for calculating the number of cells is

$$\frac{\text{cells counted}}{\text{area counted (mm}^2)} \times \text{depth factor} \times \text{dilution factor}$$

Guidelines for counting are summarized in Table 38–1.

Table 38-1. GUIDELINES FOR COUNTING FLUIDS

| Test | Gross Appearance | | | | |
	CLEAR	HAZY	BLOOD-TINGED	CLOUDY	BLOODY
WBCs	0–200/mm³	200+/mm³	Unknown	High	Unknown
Dilution for counting cells	None	1:2 Turk's	1:2 Turk's	1:20 WBC Unopette	1:2 Turk's or WBC Unopette
No. of squares to count on hemacytometer	9	9	9	9 or 4	9 or 4
RBCs	0–400/mm³	Unknown	400+/mm³	Unknown	6000+/mm³
Dilution for counting cells	None	None	None	None	1:200 RBC Unopette
No. of squares to count on hemacytometer	9 large	9 large	9 or 4 large	4 large or 5 small	5 small
Cytospin dilution (0.25 mL (5 drops) of fluid)*	Straight	Dilute with saline to 100–200/mm³ nucleated cell count	Straight or by nucleated cell count	Dilute with saline to 100–200/mm³ nucleated cell count	Dilute by nucleated cell count; if RBC >1 million/mm³, make a pushed smear and differentiate cells that are pushed out on the end

Abbreviations: WBC, white blood cell; RBC, red blood cell.
* Expected cell yield (WBC count for no. cells recovered on slide): 0/mm³ for 0–70, 1–2/mm³ for 12–100, 3+/mm³ for 100+.

PREPARATION OF CYTOCENTRIFUGE SLIDES

The cytocentrifuge enhances the ability to identify the kinds of cells present in a fluid. This centrifuge spins at a low rate of speed, which minimizes distortion of the cellular elements and provides a "button" of cells that are concentrated into a small area. The cytocentrifuge assembly consists of a cytofunnel, filter paper to absorb excess fluid, and a glass slide. These three elements are clipped together in a clip assembly; a few drops of well-mixed specimen are dispensed into the cytofunnel, and the entire assembly is centrifuged slowly. The cells are deposited onto the slide while excess fluid is absorbed into the filter paper, producing a monolayer of cells in a small button.

Although there is some cell loss into the filter paper, this is not selective and, therefore, an accurate representation of the types of cells present in a fluid is provided. There may also be some distortion of cells due to the centrifugation process or to crowding of cells when high cell counts are present. To minimize distortion due to overcrowding of cells, appropriate dilutions should be made with normal saline before centrifugation. The basis for this dilution should be the WBC count or the nucleated cell count. A nucleated cell count of 200/mm³ or less will provide a good preparation for the differential. If the RBC count is very elevated, a larger dilution may be necessary; however, an RBC count of up to 5000/mm³ will not cause significant nucleated cell distortion. For example, if a fluid has a nucleated cell count of 2000/mm³ and an RBC count of 10,000/mm³, a 1:10 dilution should be made, producing a nucleated cell count of 200/mm³ and an RBC count of 1000/mm³ for the cytocentrifuge slide. If the RBC count of a fluid is greater than 1 million/mm³, it is best to make a "push" slide to perform the differential. In this case, unlike performing differentials on peripheral blood smears, the differential should be performed on the end of the smear where the cells are pushed out since that is where the larger, and possibly more significant, cells will be deposited.

If a consistent amount of fluid is used when preparing cytocentrifuge slides, a consistent yield of cells can be expected. This can be used as a confirmation for the WBC or nucleated cell count. For example, if 5 drops of fluid (undiluted or diluted) is always used to prepare cytocentrifuge slides, a 100-cell differential should be obtainable if the WBC or nucleated cell count is equal to or greater than 3/mm³. In all cases, the entire cell button should be scanned before performing the differential to be sure that significant clumps of cells are not overlooked. The area of the cell button that is used for performing the differential is not important, but if the number of nucleated cells present is small, a "systematic meander" starting at one side of the button and working toward the other is best. In case the number of cells recovered is small, the area around the cell button should be marked on the back of the slide with a wax pencil or premarked slides should be used to prepare cytocentrifuge slides.

CEREBROSPINAL FLUID

CSF is the only fluid that exists in quantities sufficient to sample in healthy individuals. CSF is present in volumes of 90–150 mL in adults and 10–60 mL in newborns.[2] This fluid bathes the brain and spinal column and serves as a cushion to protect the brain, as a circulating nutrient medium, as an excretory channel for nervous tissue metabolism, and as lubrication for the central nervous system.

Gross Examination

Normally, CSF is a thin, crystal clear, colorless liquid. A cloudy or hazy appearance may indicate the presence of WBCs (>200/mm³), RBCs (>400/mm³), microorganisms, or an increased protein level.[2] A bloody fluid may be caused by a traumatic tap in which blood is acquired as the puncture is performed or by a pathologic hemorrhage within the central nervous system. If more than one tube is received, the tubes can be observed for clearing from tube to tube. If the first tube contains blood but the remaining tubes are clear or progressively clearer, the blood is the result of a traumatic puncture. If all tubes are uniformly bloody, the probable cause is a subarachnoid hemorrhage. When a bloody sample is received, an aliquot should be centrifuged and the color of the supernatant observed. A clear, colorless supernatant indicates a traumatic tap, while a yellowish or pinkish yellow tinge indicates a subarachnoid hemorrhage. This yellowish tinge in CSF is called xanthochromia and is caused by the breakdown of RBCs (Fig. 38–1; Table 38–2).

Cell Counts

Normal cell counts in CSF are 0–5 WBC/mm³ and 0 RBC/mm³. If a high RBC count is obtained, one may determine if the source of RBCs is peripheral blood contamination by utilizing the peripheral blood ratio of 1 WBC per 500–900 RBCs. A high WBC count may be found in patients with infective processes such as meningitis. In general,

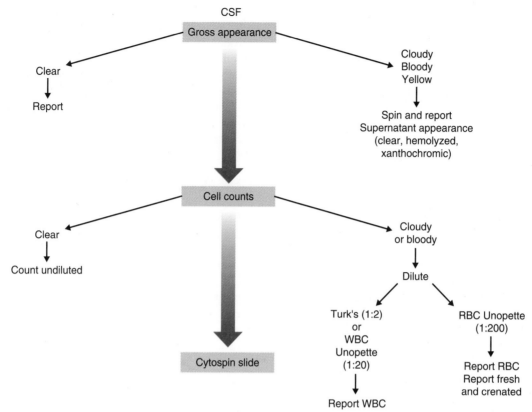

Figure 38–1 Flow chart for examination of cerebrospinal fluid (CSF).

WBC counts are much higher (in the thousands) in patients with bacterial meningitis than in those with viral meningitis (in the hundreds).[3] However, the predominant cell type present on the cytocentrifuge slide—neutrophils or lymphocytes—is a better indicator of the type of meningitis. Elevated WBCs or nucleated cell counts may also be obtained in patients with inflammatory processes and malignancies.

Differential

The normal cells seen in CSF are lymphocytes and monocytes (Fig. 38–2). In adults, the predominant cells are lymphocytes; in newborns, the pre-

dominant cells are monocytes.[2] Neutrophils are not normal in CSF by may be seen in small numbers owing to concentration techniques. When the WBC count is elevated and large numbers of neutrophils are seen, a thorough and careful search should be made for bacteria since organisms may be present in very small numbers early in bacterial meningitis (Fig. 38–3). In viral meningitis, the predominant cells seen are lymphocytes, including reactive or viral lymphocytes and plasmacytoid lymphocytes (Fig. 38–4). Eosinophils and baso-

Table 38–2. CHARACTERISTICS OF CEREBROSPINAL FLUID	
Traumatic Tap	**Pathologic Hemorrhage**
Clear supernatant	Xanthochromic or hemolyzed supernatant
Clearing from tube to tube	Same appearance in all tubes
Fresh RBCs	Crenated RBCs
Bone marrow contamination	Erythrophages
Cartilage cells	Siderophages (may have bilirubin crystals)

Abbreviation: RBC, red blood cell.

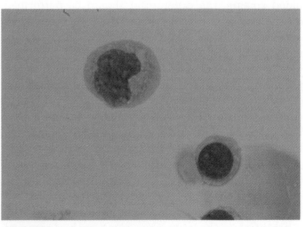

Figure 38–2 CSF (1000×): monocyte *(left)* and lymphocyte *(right)* seen in normal CSF.

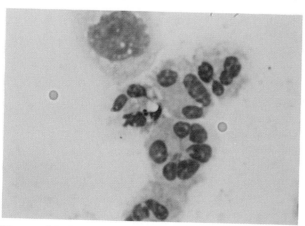

Figure 38–3 CSF (1000✕): neutrophil with bacteria (Wright's stain) from a patient with bacterial meningitis.

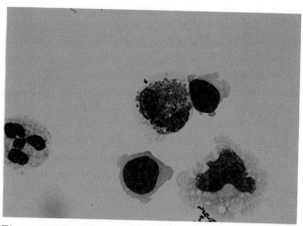

Figure 38–5 CSF (1000✕): eosinophil, lymphocytes, monocyte, and neutrophil from a patient with a shunt.

phils may be seen as a reaction to foreign materials such as shunts or as a result of an allergic reaction (Fig. 38–5).[2] When nucleated RBCs are seen, bone marrow contamination due to accidental puncture of the vertebral body during spinal tap should be suspected. In case of bone marrow contamination, other immature neutrophils and megakaryocytes may also be seen.

Ependymal and choroid plexus cells may be seen. These are the lining cells of the central nervous system. They are large cells with abundant cytoplasm that stains lavender with Wright's stain. They most often appear in clumps; and although they are not diagnostically significant, it is important not to confuse them with malignant cells (Figs. 38–6 and 38–7).

Cartilage cells may be seen if the vertebral body is accidentally punctured. These cells usually occur singly, are medium to large, and have cytoplasm that stains wine red with a deep wine-red nucleus with Wright's stain (Fig. 38–8).

Siderophages are macrophages (i.e., monocytes or histiocytes) that have ingested RBCs and, as a result of the breakdown of the RBCs, contain hemosiderin. Hemosiderin appears as large, rough-shaped, dark blue or black granules in the cytoplasm of the macrophage. These cells may also contain bilirubin or hematoidin crystals, which are golden yellow and are a result of further breakdown of the ingested RBCs. The presence of siderophages indicates a pathologic hemorrhage. Siderophages appear approximately 48 hours after hemorrhage and may persist for 2–8 weeks after the hemorrhage has occurred (Fig. 38–9).

A high percentage of patients with acute lymphoblastic leukemia or acute myelocytic leukemia have central nervous system involvement.[2] Therefore, it is always important to look carefully for leukemic cells (i.e., blast forms) in the CSF of patients with leukemia. Patients with lymphoma, myeloma, and chronic myelocytic leukemia in blast crisis may also have blast cells in the CSF. These blast cells have the characteristics of blast forms in the peripheral blood, including a high nuclear:cytoplasmic ratio, a fine "stippled" nuclear chromatin pattern, and prominent nucleoli. They are usually large cells that stain basophilic with

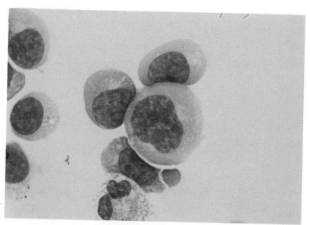

Figure 38–4 CSF (1000✕): transformed (viral) lymphocytes from a patient with viral meningitis.

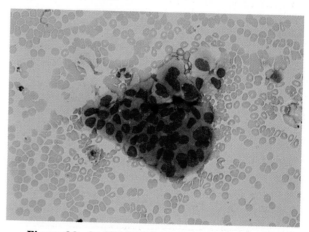

Figure 38–6 CSF (200✕): clump of ependymal cells.

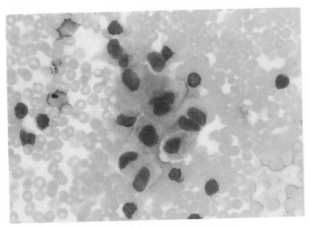

Figure 38–7 CSF (400×): clump of ependymal cells.

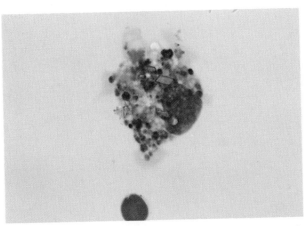

Figure 38–9 CSF (400×): siderophage with bilirubin crystals (hematoidin).

Wright's stain and have a fairly uniform appearance (Fig. 38–10).

Malignant cells due to metastases to the central nervous system may be found. The most common primary tumors that metastasize to the central nervous system are breast, lung, and gastrointestinal tract tumors and melanoma.[2] These malignant cells are usually large with a high nuclear:cytoplasmic ratio and are often basophilic or hyperchromic. They often occur in clumps but may occur singly. Within clumps of malignant cells there is dissimilarity between cells, and in multinucleated cells there may be variation in nuclear size. Clumps of malignant cells may appear three-dimensional, requiring up and down focusing to see the cells on different planes, and there are usually no "windows" between the cells. The nucleus of these cells is usually large, often with abnormal distribution of chromatin, and it may have an indistinct or jagged border or there may be "blebbing" at the border. Increased mitosis may be demonstrated by the presence of several mitotic figures in the cell button. Malignant cells fre-

quently have a bizarre appearance (Fig. 38–11; Table 38–3).[4]

SEROUS FLUID

Serous fluids, including pleural, pericardial, and peritoneal fluids, normally exist in very small quantities and serve as lubricant between the membranes of an organ and the sac in which it is housed. It would be very difficult to remove these fluids from a healthy person; therefore, the presence of these fluids in detectable amounts indicates a disease state.

Transudates vs. Exudates

The accumulation of a large amount of fluid in a cavity is called an effusion. Effusions are further subdivided into transudates and exudates to distinguish whether disease is present either within or outside the body cavity. In general, transudates develop as part of systemic disease processes such as

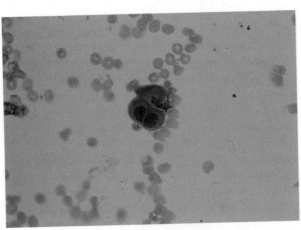

Figure 38–8 CSF (400×): cartilage cells.

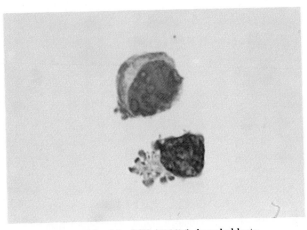

Figure 38–10 CSF (1000×): lymphoblasts.

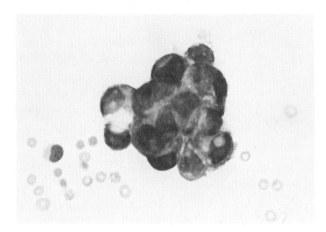

Figure 38–11 CSF (400X): clump of breast tumor cells.

chronic heart failure while exudates indicate disorders associated with bacterial or viral infections, malignancy, pulmonary embolism, or systemic lupus erythematosus. There are several parameters that can be measured to determine if an effusion is a transudate or an exudate (Table 38–4).

Gross Examination

Normally, serous fluid should appear straw colored and clear. A cloudy or hazy fluid may indicate an infectious process; a bloody fluid may be the result of trauma or malignancy, and a milky fluid may indicate effused chyle in the thoracic cavity.

Differential

The cells found in normal serous fluid are lymphocytes, monohistiocytes (macrophages), and mesothelial cells. Neutrophils are commonly seen in the fluid sent to the laboratory for analysis but would not be present in normal fluid. When neutrophils are seen, they have more segments and longer filaments than in peripheral blood (Fig. 38–12).

Table 38-3. CHARACTERISTICS OF BENIGN AND MALIGNANT CELLS

Benign	Malignant
Occasional large cells	Many cells may be very large
Light to dark-staining	May be very basophilic
Rare mitotic figures	May have several mitotic figures
Round to oval nucleus; nuclei are uniform size with varying amounts of cytoplasm	May have irregular or even bizarre nuclear shape
Smooth nuclear edge	Edges of nucleus may be indistinct and irregular
Nucleus intact	Nucleus may be disintegrated at edges
Nucleoli are small, if present	Nucleoli may be large and prominent
In multinuclear cells (mesothelial), all nuclei have similar appearance (size and shape)	Multinuclear cells have varying sizes and shapes of nuclei
Moderate to small N/C ratio	May have high N/C ratio
Clumps of cells have similar appearance among cells, are on the same plane of focus, and may have "windows" between cells	Clumps of cells contain cells of varying sizes and shapes, are "three-dimensional" (have to focus up and down to see all cells), and have dark staining borders

Abbreviation: N/C, Nuclear/cytoplasmic.

Mesothelial cells are the lining cells of body cavities and are shed into these cavities constantly. These are large (12–30 μm) cells and have a "fried egg" appearance with basophilic cytoplasm, oval nucleus with smooth nuclear borders, stippled nuclear chromatin pattern, and 1–3 nucleoli.[2] Mesothelial cells may vary in size, may be multinucleated (including giant cells with as many as 20–25 nuclei), and may have frayed cytoplasmic borders and/or cytoplasmic vacuoles. They may occur singly, in small or large clumps, or even in

Table 38-4. SEROUS FLUID

Characteristic	Transudates	Exudates
Specific gravity	Less than 1.016	Greater than 1.016
Protein	Less than 3.0 g/dL	Greater than 3.0 g/dL
Lactate dehydrogenase	Less than 200 IU	Greater than 200 IU
WBCs	Less than 1000/mm³ (predominant cell type mononuclear)	Greater than 1000/mm³
Protein fluid/serum ratio	Less than 0.5	Greater than 0.5
Lactate dehydrogenase fluid/serum ratio	Less than 0.6	Greater than 0.6
Color	Clear/straw	Cloudy/yellow, amber, or grossly bloody
Volume		Extremely large

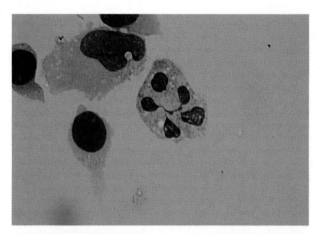

Figure 38–12 Hypersegmented neutrophil with prominent filaments: normal appearance of neutrophils in body fluids.

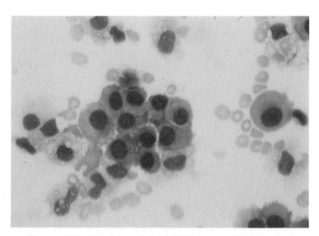

Figure 38–14 Pleural fluid (400X): mesothelial cells.

sheets. When they occur in clumps, there are usually "windows" between the cells. The nuclear:cytoplasmic ratio is 1:2–1:3, and this is generally consistent despite the variability in cell size.[2] They tend to have a similar appearance to each other on a slide. Mesothelial cells are seen in the majority of effusions and are increased in sterile inflammations and decreased in tuberculous pleurisy and bacterial infections (Figs. 38–13 through 38–15).[2]

Macrophages appear as monocytes or histiocytes in serous fluids and may contain RBCs (erythrophages) or siderotic granules (siderophages) or may appear as "signet ring" cells when lipid has been ingested and the resulting large vacuole pushes the nucleus to the periphery of the cell (Figs. 38–16 and 38–17).

Eosinophils and basophils are not normally seen but may be present in large numbers as a result of allergic reaction or sensitivity to foreign material.

When large numbers of neutrophils are seen, a thorough search should be made for bacteria and, if possible, a Gram stain should be performed on a second cytocentrifuge slide to aid in rapid identification if bacteria are found. Table 38–5 lists Gram-stained organisms most commonly seen in body fluids.

Lupus erythematosus (LE) cells may be seen in serous fluids of patients with systemic lupus erythematosus since all the factors necessary for the formation of these cells—presence of the LE factor, incubation, and trauma to the cells—exist in vivo. These cells indicate systemic lupus erythematosus and should be reported (Fig. 38–18).

Malignant cells are seen in serous fluids from primary or metastatic tumors. They have the characteristics of malignant cells found in CSF (Figs. 38–19 through 38–24).

A flow chart for examination of serous fluids is found in Figure 38–25.

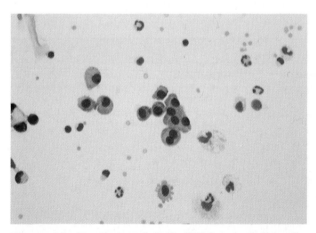

Figure 38–13 Peritoneal fluid (200X): mesothelial cells. Note "fried egg" appearance.

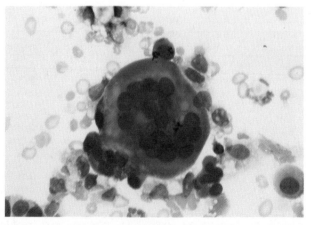

Figure 38–15 Pleural fluid (400X): mesothelial cell with 21 nuclei.

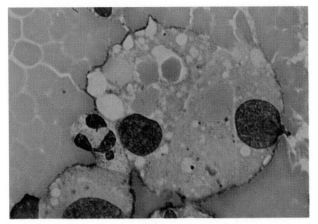

Figure 38–16 Peritoneal fluid (1000×): erythrophage.

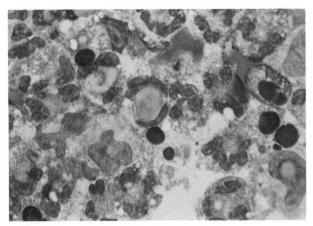

Figure 38–18 Pleural fluid (1000×): lupus erythematosus cell.

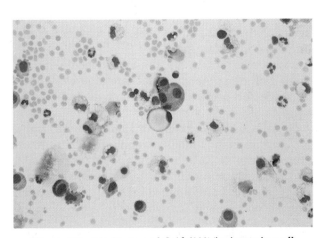

Figure 38–17 Peritoneal fluid (200×): signet ring cell.

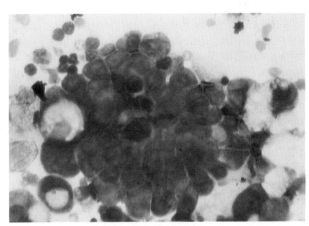

Figure 38–19 Pleural fluid (200×): Clump of tumor cells.

Table 38–5. GRAM-STAINED ORGANISMS MOST COMMONLY SEEN IN BODY FLUIDS

Fluid	Organism
Cerebrospinal	Gram-negative diplococci
	Gram-positive cocci
	Gram-negative coccobacilli
	Yeast—will stain gram positive
	Cryptococcus—look for capsule
Serous	Gram-positive cocci
(peritoneal,	Gram-negative bacilli
pleural, or	Gram-positive bacilli
pericardial)	Yeast
Synovial	Gram-positive cocci
(joint)	Gram-negative bacilli
	Gram-negative diplococci
	Gram-negative coccobacilli

Note: If the Gram-stained organisms you are seeing on a fluid are not listed above for that fluid, do *not* report Gram stain results—save the slide for review.

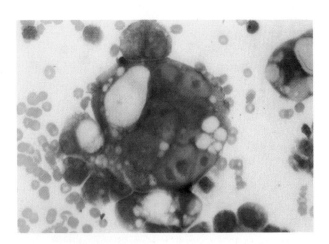

Figure 38–20 Pleural fluid (200×): tumor cells.

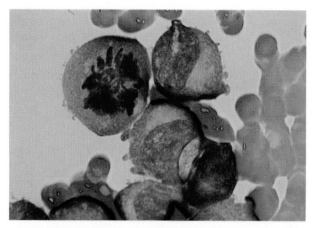

Figure 38–21 Pleural fluid (1000X): tumor cells and mitotic figure.

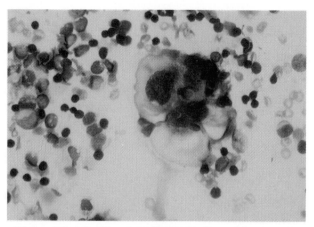

Figure 38–23 Pleural fluid (200X): adenocarcinoma cells.

SYNOVIAL FLUID

Gross Examination

Synovial fluid is normally present in very small amounts in the synovial cavity surrounding joints. When fluid is present in amounts large enough to aspirate, there is a disease process in the joint. Normally this fluid is straw colored and clear. Synovial fluid contains hyaluronic acid, which makes it very viscous. A small amount of hyaluronidase powder should be added to all joint fluids before cell counts are performed or cytocentrifuge slides are prepared to liquefy these fluids. If a crystal analysis is to be performed, an aliquot of fluid should be removed for this purpose before the hyaluronidase is added.

Differential

Cells that are normal in synovial fluid are lymphocytes, monocytes/histiocytes, and synovial cells. Synovial cells line the synovial cavity and are shed into the cavity. They resemble mesothelial cells but are usually present in smaller numbers (Fig. 38–26).

LE cells may be present in synovial fluid just as in serous fluid. Malignant cells are rarely seen in synovial fluid but, when present, resemble tumor cells seen in serous fluids or CSF.

Many neutrophils are present in acute inflammation of joints. As always, a careful search should be made for bacteria when many neutrophils are seen.

Crystals may be present in synovial fluid, and it is very important to look carefully for them. These crystals may be intracellular and/or extracellular and will not stain with Wright's stain. All synovial fluids should be examined carefully for crystals using a polarizing microscope with a red compensator.

The most common crystals seen in synovial fluids are cholesterol, calcium pyrophosphate, and monosodium urate.

Cholesterol crystals are large, flat extracellular crystals with a notched corner.[5] They are seen in

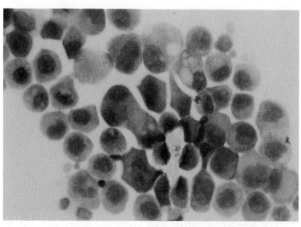

Figure 38–22 Pleural fluid (200X): tumor cells.

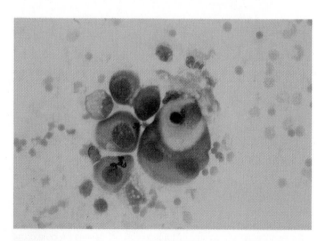

Figure 38–24 Peritoneal fluid (200X): tumor cells (note cannibalism).

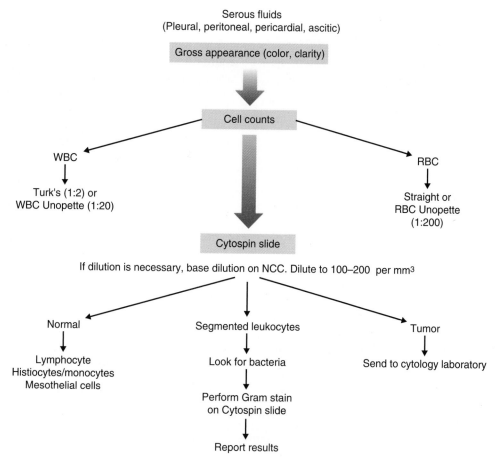

Serous fluids
(Pleural, peritoneal, pericardial, ascitic)

Gross appearance (color, clarity)

Cell counts

WBC

Turk's (1:2) or
WBC Unopette (1:20)

RBC

Straight or
RBC Unopette
(1:200)

Cytospin slide

If dilution is necessary, base dilution on NCC. Dilute to 100–200 per mm³

Normal

Lymphocyte
Histiocytes/monocytes
Mesothelial cells

Segmented leukocytes

Look for bacteria

Perform Gram stain
on Cytospin slide

Report results

Tumor

Send to cytology laboratory

Abbreviation: NCC, nucleated cell count

Figure 38–25 Flow chart for examination of serous fluid.

patients with chronic effusions, particularly those with rheumatoid arthritis.

Calcium pyrophosphate crystals are seen in pseudogout. These crystals are intracellular and are small rhomboid, plate-like, or rod-like.[5] These crystals are weakly birefringent when polarized (i.e., they do not appear very bright when polarized). When the red compensator is used, calcium pyrophosphate crystals appear blue when the longitudinal axis of the crystal is parallel to the slow component of the compensator (y-axis) (Fig. 38–27).[5]

Monosodium urate crystals are seen in gout. They are large, needle-like crystals that may be intracellular or extracellular. These crystals are strongly birefringent when polarized. When the red

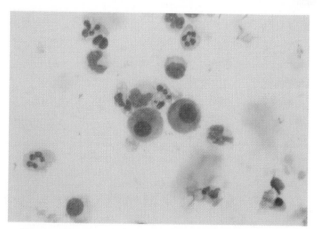

Figure 38–26 Synovial fluid (400×): synovial cells (note similarity to mesothelial cells).

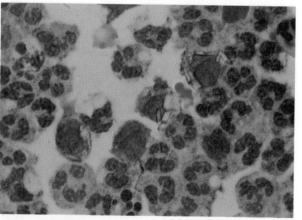

Figure 38–27 Synovial fluid (1000×): intracellular calcium pyrophosphate crystals.

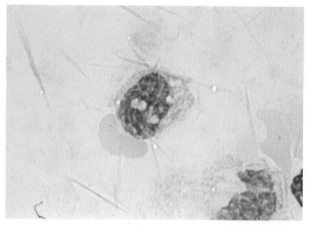
Figure 38–28 Synovial fluid (1000X): intracellular and extracellular monosodium urate crystals.

compensator is used, monosodium urate crystals appear yellow when the longitudinal axis of the crystal is parallel to the *y*-axis (Fig. 38–28).[5]

A flow chart for synovial fluid is found in Figure 38–29.

SUMMARY

The examination of body fluids, including cell counts and examination of cells on cytocentrifuge preparations, can provide valuable diagnostic information. Cerebrospinal fluid is present at all times in a quantity sufficient to allow withdrawal and examination. Therefore, both normal and abnormal conditions can be detected. However, all other fluids (serous and synovial) normally exist in very small quantities. The fact that a quantity of these fluids is obtained, implies an abnormal condition. This chapter has described methods for cell counting, cytocentrifuge preparation, and identification of normal and abnormal cells in cerebrospinal fluid, serous fluids, and synovial fluid.

REVIEW QUESTIONS

1. Calculations:
   A spinal fluid is diluted 1:2 with Turk's solution to perform the nucleated cell count. Undi-

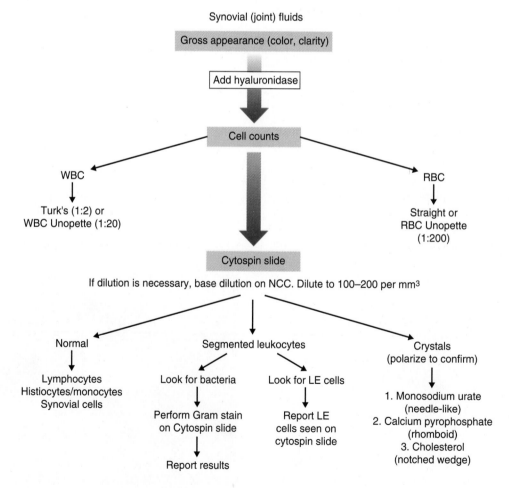

Abbreviations: NCC, nucleated cell count
LE, lupus erythematosus

Figure 38–29 Flow chart for examination of synovial (joint) fluid.

luted fluid is used to perform the RBC count. A total of 6 nucleated cells were counted on both sides of the hemacytometer, counting all nine squares on both sides.

A total of 524 RBCs were counted on both sides of the hemacytometer, counting four large squares on both sides.

What is the nucleated cell count?

What is the RBC count?

What would the appearance of the fluid be?

2. What are the normal cells seen in CSF, serous and synovial fluids?

3. A 33-year-old semi-conscious female presented in the Emergency Room. The previous day she had complained of a headache and had left work early, taken some aspirin and a nap, and felt better later in the evening. The next morning, her husband stated that "she couldn't talk" and brought her to the Emergency Room. A spinal tap was performed. The fluid that arrived in the laboratory was cloudy. The WBC was 10.6×10^9/L. The majority of the cells seen on the Cytospin slide were neutrophils.

   a. What dilution should be made to obtain a satisfactory Cytospin slide?

   b. What do you look for on the Cytospin slide?

   c. What is the most likely diagnosis for this patient?

4. A 56-year-old male presented in his doctor's office complaining of pain and swelling in his left great toe. Fluid was aspirated from the toe that was straw-colored and cloudy. The WBC count was 2543/mm³. The differential consisted mainly of neutrophils and monohistiocytes. Both intracellular and extracellular crystals were seen on the Cytospin slide. The crystals were needle-shaped, and, when polarized, appeared yellow on the Y-axis. What is the diagnosis?

5. A 49-year-old male presented in the Emergency Room with a severe headache and a stiff neck. A spinal puncture was performed and the fluid obtained was cloudy. The WBC count was 854/mm³. On the Cytospin slide, the majority of the cells seen were lymphocytes with several large, transformed lymphocytes and several plasmacytes. What is the diagnosis?

6. A 34-year-old female with a history of breast cancer developed a pleural effusion. The fluid obtained on thoracentesis was bloody and had a nucleated cell count of 284/mm³. On the Cytospin slide there were several neutrophils and a few mono/histiocytes. There were also several clusters of large, dark-staining cells. These cells appeared "three-dimensional" and contained some mitotic figures. What is the most likely identification of the cells in clusters?

7. A 19-year-old male developed difficulty in breathing and a feeling of heaviness in his chest following an upper respiratory infection. On x-ray, his heart was found to be enlarged. Pericardial fluid was obtained which had a nucleated cell count of 445/mm³. The predominant cells seen on the differential performed on a Cytospin slide were mono/histiocytes. Was this fluid a transudate or an exudate? What criteria did you use in making your decision?

8. Spinal fluid was obtained on a 26-year-old female who was undergoing a myelogram. Upon receipt in the laboratory, the fluid was noted to be slightly bloody. When a portion of the fluid was centrifuged, the supernatant was clear. The cell counts were: RBC-5200/mm³ and WBC-24/mm³. On the Cytospin slide, several nucleated red blood cells were seen. The differential was 52% lymphocytes; 20% neutrophil segmented cells; 22% monocytes; 4% myelocytes; 2% blasts. What is the most likely explanation for the presence of the nucleated RBCs and immature granulocytes?

References

1. Glasser L: Cells in cerebrospinal fluid. Diagn Med 1981; 4(2):33–50.
2. Kjeldsberg C, Knight J: Body Fluids. Chicago: American Society of Clinical Pathologists Press, 1986.
3. Krueger R: Meningitis: A case study. Lab Med 1987; 18:677–681.
4. Cornbleet J: Microscopy of CSF and body fluids. Workshop material presented before the national meeting of the American Society of Clinical Pathologists, 1991.
5. Strasinger S: Urinalysis and Body Fluids, 3rd ed. Philadelphia: FA Davis, 1994.

PART X

Management

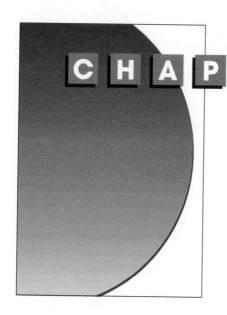

CHAPTER 39

Management and Supervision in the Hematology Laboratory

John R. Snyder

Objectives

AFTER COMPLETION OF THIS CHAPTER, THE READER WILL BE ABLE TO

1. Discuss strategies for a successful transition to management.
2. Describe the four functions of management from a systems approach.
3. Develop policies and procedures for the clinical laboratory.
4. Apply principles of organization and delegation.
5. Analyze the test requisition–report cycle and laboratory space layout for effectiveness and efficiency.
6. Participate in the employee selection process and conduct performance appraisals.
7. Determine staffing needs and schedule personnel according to text complexity.
8. Describe the budgeting process, including cost accounting, break-even analysis, and use of financial ratios.
9. Apply cost-containment principles to the maintenance of supplies inventory.

The vast majority of this textbook is devoted to the theory and application of clinical laboratory procedures performed in hematology laboratories. This body of knowledge, coupled with similar works in other laboratory disciplines, forms the scientific basis for academic preparation and credentialing of clinical laboratory personnel. This combined knowledge and technical skill is essential for quality laboratory testing. Many clinical laboratory scientists, however, are given responsibilities for managing and supervising laboratory services early in their careers. Although appropriate degrees and professional certification are fairly reliable indicators of technical competence, these alone do not connote the knowledge and skills to manage.

The purpose of this chapter is to provide an overview of management and supervision activities. These activities complement the hematology body of knowledge, converting technical proficiency into the efficient and effective delivery of laboratory services for quality patient care. The chapter begins with a case study describing a competent and experienced practitioner about to make the transition to management. How does one prepare for this change? Suggested strategies for becoming an effective laboratory manager or supervisor follow. A foundation for understanding managerial responsibilities is laid in the global view of laboratory services as a system. Practical strategies for planning, organizing, and controlling test analysis are covered by describing policy and procedure development, delegation, and layout flow charting, just to name a few. The chapter then focuses on developing the human resources in the laboratory and ends with financial management and inventory control.

THE TRANSITION TO MANAGEMENT

The following case study is fairly typical of a clinical laboratory practitioner about to make the transition to being a manager:

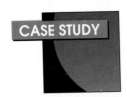
CASE STUDY

Cheryl A. graduated from a medical technology program 9 years ago. She stayed on to work for about a year at the institution where she did her clinical practicum. After marrying, she and her husband moved and she accepted an evening position in a 500-bed hospital. This position required that she do a variety of analyses, including chemistry and hematology, and a few immunology and microbiology, tests. She preferred the hematology procedures and by mutual agreement with her co-worker usually divided the workload that way. After 14 months on the evening shift, Cheryl took a full-time day position in the hematology laboratory. She enjoyed doing the special hematology procedures performed only on the day shift and also became the "resident expert" on the automated cell counter. Subsequently, she was chosen for special training when a Coulter STKS Hematology System was purchased. Over time, she had the opportunity to help write some of the new and revised procedures for the laboratory. She was also chosen to help implement a change in which some of the bone marrow tests would be done by select technical staff. She stayed on in the laboratory during several years when turnover seemed an ongoing problem, helping to orient two laboratory assistants and several technicians and technologists. Before long, she was one of three staff technologists with the greatest seniority. Cheryl had not thought much about managing or supervising; the technical work seemed a more satisfying challenge. Yet when her hematology supervisor retired, she was suggested as the logical replacement. Because she had seniority, got along well with the other technical staff, and was recognized for her hematology expertise, she was offered the job. She accepted, thinking how difficult could it be? After all, she'd watched her supervisor competently handle things for years. Cheryl knew the hematology laboratory operations well—now it was up to her to become a manager.

The key to Cheryl's success as a manager or supervisor does not rest on the reasons that she was chosen for the job. True, her longevity in the institution gave her the advantage of knowing how things were done there. Also true, she had shown that she could work well with the existing staff— but as a colleague and not as their supervisor. Her hematology expertise would be an asset for her, but she must now prepare someone else to take her place as the "resident expert" in the performance of testing. Cheryl was about to give up that which her whole career and satisfaction had centered around—doing testing. She was faced with a *new role:* managing the resources (people, time, space, equipment, and budget) to ensure that efficient and effective hematology analyses were provided for quality patient care. To be successful, Cheryl must make the transition from doing testing to managing the testing process.

Selection of Managers

The selection of Cheryl A. to be a supervisor as described in the case study is fairly typical. LaCroix and Seidel[1] refer to this selection process as the trickle-up school of laboratory management. Typically an individual who has worked in a particular laboratory for many years is selected as a manager primarily on the basis of longevity, sort of a reward for having spent time on the bench and becoming a technical expert. These individuals may accept the position out of obligation or be motivated to accept the position as a means of promotion or release from weekend work. By contrast, there is also a growing trend for selecting laboratory managers who have expertise in management but lack credentials as a laboratory practitioner. The disadvantage to this latter approach is in the general manager's lack of understanding about the interworkings of the laboratory that comes from having a clinical background.

Noteworthy also in the case study is that Cheryl A. is embarking on a new set of relationships with technical staff who used to be her peers. In a survey of what laboratory personnel like in supervisors, Ramsey[2] found that the most important characteristic of a supervisor was organization and consistency. In addition, employees valued supervisors who were fair and impartial, willing to come out of the management role and assist with bench testing when staffing and workload demanded it, sought out the opinions of employees on laboratory matters, supported employees when dealing with physicians or hospital administrators, and were willing to admit errors. Some of these characteristics can be exhibited by a practitioner before being selected as a manager; others require time and experience in the managerial position to cultivate.

Management Tasks

The duties of a laboratory manager are many, including planning for how the work in the hematology laboratory will be done, developing a work force to perform the analysis, supervising the activities of the laboratory, controlling and evaluating the process for efficiency and effectiveness, and managing the financial aspects of the department. In a study conducted by Karni and Seanger,[3] managers and supervisors ranked a variety of skills required for the clinical laboratory science practitioner at entry level management (Table 39–1). The top ranking task by both managers and supervisors was the ability to communicate effectively with coworkers, superiors, subordinates, patients, and the public. Other high-ranking management tasks included understanding and responding to the mission of the institution, managing laboratory data, developing a quality assurance program, and ensuring that laboratory methods were appropriate for the services offered. Entry-level management skills such as developing a plan and objectives for the hematology laboratory, writing procedures and policies, and developing position descriptions were also ranked in the top 10 tasks in which a practitioner making the transition to management should have competency.

Management Skills

A manager must exhibit a variety of skills somewhat unique to this new role. These skills are not task specific but rather overlap for many of the responsibilities of a laboratory manager.

Umiker[4] has identified six skills that are required for an effective manager or supervisor.

Table 39-1. ENTRY-LEVEL MANAGEMENT SKILLS FOR CLINICAL LABORATORY SCIENCE PRACTITIONERS

Management Skill	Managers' Rankings (n = 25)	Supervisors' Rankings (n = 20)
Communicate effectively (orally and in writing) with coworkers, superiors, subordinates, patients, and the public	1	1
Understand and respond appropriately to the mission of the institution in which one works	2	2
Manage data through input, storage, and retrieval	3	3
Establish and use a quality assurance program to include statistics, proficiency samples, and check samples.	4	4
Perform method evaluation of laboratory procedures	5	6
Write a personal résumé and evaluate one's individual strengths in terms of employment	6.5	5
Participate in and provide professional activities (e.g., membership in professional organizations and attendance at continuing-education programs)	6.5	9
Develop a plan and objectives for laboratory unit/section	8.5	8
Write procedures and policies appropriate for the laboratory and the institution	8.5	7
Write a job description including education and experience specifications, tasks of the job, and levels of accountability	10	
Use appropriately various federal or state laws, regulations, and guidelines (e.g., labor laws, OSHA, and EEO)		10

From Karni KR, Seanger DG: Management skills needed by entry-level practitioners. Clin Lab Sci 1988; 1:296–300.
Abbreviations: OSHA, Occupational Safety and Health Administration; EEO, Equal Employment Opportunity (Commission).

First, the manager must be able to motivate employees, adopting an appropriate leadership style that sets an example, minimizes dissatisfiers, and creates a desire to achieve results. Communication is an essential skill to keep everyone informed. The manager must also be able to make the best use of time, organizing one's own work, establishing priorities, and delegating effectively. The manager must be able to make decisions, seeking advice when necessary, establishing policies and procedures, and applying problem-solving techniques as necessary. Coordination and integration are necessary, whether it be for linking the laboratory activities with services provided by other health care departments, bridging between shifts of personnel in the laboratory, or matching people and laboratory instrumentation. And finally, the manager is required to be involved in training and education for new employees, for existing employees when new procedures and new instruments are added, and possibly in the educational preparation of students and others.

Resources

Making a successful transition to laboratory management can be facilitated by acquiring and studying a variety of resources that are not typically of interest to someone involved in the technical aspects of laboratory testing. Two specific resources are beneficial: a copy of the Management and Administrative Services Section of the current Joint Commission on Accreditation of Health Care

Organization's *Standards*[5] and the Clinical Laboratory Improvement Amendments (CLIA) of 1988 *Final Rule*.[6] From the latter, the personnel standards by laboratory test complexity is an important section. This is reproduced in Table 39-2. Also, the responsibilities of a technical supervisor under CLIA reinforce the management tasks and skills described earlier in this section. These responsibilities are shown in Table 39-3.

A SYSTEMS APPROACH TO UNDERSTANDING MANAGEMENT

With this background of how managers are selected, the required tasks and skills, and the resources beneficial for making an effective transition from bench technologist to manager, focus can now be shifted to understanding laboratory management from a systems viewpoint.

Management Defined

Management has been variously defined as getting things done through other people and coordinating actions that lead to the accomplishment of objectives.[7] Perhaps a more comprehensive, albeit flowery, definition is the guiding of human, physical, and financial resources into dynamic organization units that lead to the accomplishment of goals and objectives to the satisfaction of the client and with a sense of accomplishment by those rendering the service. A helpful way to visualize this defini-

Table 39-2. PERSONNEL STANDARDS BY LABORATORY TEST COMPLEXITY UNDER CLIA '88

Laboratories Performing only Waived Tests
No personnel requirements

Moderate Complexity Laboratories

DIRECTOR

M.D./D.O.: If not board certified in anatomic or clinical pathology: 1 year directing or supervising nonwaived testing, or by August 2, 1993, have 20 hours of continuing education (for laboratory directors, consistent with 493.1407); or residency training equivalent to the 20 hours specified above, or

Ph.D.: Department of Health and Human Services–recognized boards; or 1 year of training or experience or both plus 1 year's experience as a supervisor, or

Master's degree with 1 year of training or experience or both plus 2 years as a supervisor; or previously qualified under 493.1415 (March 14, 1990) before February 28, 1992; or, before February 28, 1992, qualified under state law to direct a laboratory in the state

TECHNICAL CONSULTANT

M.D./D.O.: If not board certified in anatomic or clinical pathology, having 1 year of training or experience in the designated specialty or subspecialty of service, or

Ph.D. or master's degree with 1 year of training or experience or both in the designated specialty or subspecialty of service, or

Bachelor's degree with 2 years of training or experience or both in the designated specialty or subspecialty of service

CLINICAL CONSULTANT

Qualified as a director (M.D./D.O. or board-certified Ph.D.) or M.D./D.O.

TESTING PERSONNEL

M.D./D.O., Ph.D., master's degree, bachelor's degree, associate's degree, or high school diploma or equivalent

Must have successfully completed a military laboratory procedures course of at least 50 weeks and held an enlisted occupational specialty of medical laboratory specialist or high school diploma (or equivalent) with documented training in eight specified areas

High-Complexity Laboratories

DIRECTOR

M.D./D.O.: If not board certified in anatomic or clinical pathology: 1 year of laboratory training during residency or 2 years of experience directing or supervising high-complexity testing; by September 1, 1994, be certified by national boards or be serving as laboratory director and previously qualified or could have qualified (that is, was eligible to qualify) as director under 42 CFR 493.1415 (published March 14, 1990) on or before February 28, 1992; or on or before February 28, 1992, be qualified under state law as a laboratory director for the state

TECHNICAL SUPERVISOR

The director may function as technical supervisor, or the laboratory may perform anatomic and clinical laboratory procedures if the director qualifies as an M.D./D.O.

The laboratory may perform tests in the specialities/subspecialities in which the technical supervisor is specifically qualified as follows:

M.D./D.O., Ph.D., master's degree, or bachelor's degree with 1 to 4 years of training and/or experience and at least 6 months of experience in many subspecialities.

CLINICAL CONSULTANT

M.D./D.O. (board certified) or Ph.D. qualified as a director and having HHS-approved national boards, or M.D./D.O.

GENERAL SUPERVISOR

Qualified as a laboratory director or technical supervisor for high-complexity testing, or

M.D./D.O., Ph.D., or Master's degree, or

Bachelor's degree with 1 year of training, experience, or both in high-complexity testing, or

Associate's degree with 2 years of training, experience, or both in high-complexity testing, or

Previously qualified under 42 CFR 493.1427 (March 14, 1990)

TESTING PERSONNEL

M.D./D.O., Ph.D., master's degree, bachelor's degree, or associate's degree or have previously qualified or could have qualified (that is, was eligible to qualify) as a technologist under 42 CFR 493.1433 (March 14, 1990)

High school diploma: Until September 1, 1997, have a high school diploma and documented training prior to performing testing on any patient's specimens that includes eight specific items (See 493.1489(b)(4)(ii))

From Clinical Laboratory Improvement Amendments of 1988: Final rule: 42 CFR subpart M: Personnel for moderate and high complexity testing, 493.1401–1495. U.S. Department of Health and Human Services, HCFA/PHS. Fed Register 1992; 57:7172–7183.

tion is to consider the clinical laboratory from a systems view in relationship to health care delivery.

A Systems View

Becan-McBride[8] has described the clinical laboratory in relationship to health care delivery from a systems perspective having three distinct components: *input*—that which arrives at the laboratory to initiate work in the form of requisitions and samples; *process*—specimen analysis within the clinical laboratory; and *output*—reports and consultation as the service effecting health care. This systems view is illustrated in Figure 39–1.

The traditional systems view of the clinical laboratory was a flow process in which each component led directly to the next, such as input to

Table 39-3. RESPONSIBILITIES OF A TECHNICAL SUPERVISOR

The technical supervisor is responsible for the technical and scientific oversight of the laboratory. The technical supervisor is not required to be on site at all times testing is performed; however, he or she must be available to the laboratory on an as needed basis to provide supervision.

A. The technical supervisor must be accessible to the laboratory to provide on-site, telephone, or electronic consultation; and

B. The technical supervisor is responsible for —
1. Selection of the test methodology that is appropriate for the clinical use of the test results;
2. Verification of the test procedures performed and establishment of the laboratory's test performance characteristics, including the precision and accuracy of each test and test system;
3. Enrollment and participation in an HHS-approved proficiency testing program commensurate with the services offered;
4. Establishing a quality control program appropriate for the testing performed and establishing the parameter for acceptable levels of analytic performance and ensuring that these levels are maintained throughout the entire testing process from the initial receipt of the specimen, through sample analysis and reporting of test results;
5. Resolving technical problems and ensuring that remedial actions are taken whenever test systems deviate from the laboratory's established performance specifications;
6. Ensuring that patient test results are not reported until all corrective actions have been taken and the test system is functioning properly;
7. Identifying training needs and assuring that each individual performing tests receives regular in-service training and education appropriate for the type and complexity of the laboratory services performed;
8. Evaluating the competency of all testing personnel and assuring that the staff maintain their competency to perform test procedures and report test results promptly, accurately, and proficiently. The procedures for evaluation of the competency of the staff must include, but are not limited to —
   a. Direct observations of routine patient test performance, including patient preparation, if applicable, specimen handling, processing, and testing;
   b. Monitoring the recording and reporting of test results;
   c. Review of intermediate test results or worksheets, quality control records, proficiency testing results, and preventive maintenance records;
   d. Direct observation of performance of instrument maintenance and function checks;
   e. Assessment of test performance through testing previously analyzed specimens, internal blind testing samples, or external proficiency testing samples; and
   f. Assessment of problem-solving skills; and
9. Evaluating and documenting the performance of individuals responsible for high complexity testing at least semiannually during the first year the individual tests patient specimens. Thereafter, evaluations must be performed at least annually unless test methodology or instrumentation changes, in which case, prior to reporting patient test results, the individual's performance must be reevaluated to include the use of the new test methodology or instrumentation.

From Clinical Laboratory Improvement Amendments of 1988: Final rule: 42 CFR subpart M: Personnel for moderate and high complexity testing, 493.1401–493.1495. U.S. Department of Health and Human Services, HCFA/PHS. Fed Register 1992; 57:7172–7183.

process or process to output. There were several shortcomings to this arrangement, as identified by Barr[9] and Mass,[10] that detracted from both efficiency and effectiveness of laboratory testing on health care. In the traditional flow process, communication and interaction was almost nonexistent before the receipt of the test order or after the release of the results. This allowed the laboratory to function somewhat in isolation of those using the service. The two-way arrows shown in Figure 39-1 at the input component suggest that the laboratory has a responsibility in influencing the appropriateness of the test ordered as well as, at the output component, the test interpretation. To be most effective and efficient in providing laboratory services, the clinical laboratory has an obligation to consider the appropriateness of the test ordered for the clinical condition as well as the time of specimen collection. During specimen analysis in the process component, the laboratory must be concerned not only with the accuracy and precision of analyte measurement but also with clinical rele-

vance and turnaround time. At the output component, the interaction focuses on the impact of the laboratory results on patient care considering whether the laboratory information was properly interpreted and integrated into a care plan.

Managerial Functions

Figure 39-1 also elaborates on the process component by showing the managerial functions of planning, organizing, directing, and controlling. These functions are appropriately illustrated as a continuous cycle since each is related. These functions are carried out by the laboratory manager, who is entrusted with three types of resources: *human resources*—the technical and support staff in the laboratory; *physical resources*—space and equipment to do the laboratory testing; and *financial resources*—a budget to support the activities of specimen analysis. The planning function includes identifying goals and objectives; establishing policies and procedures; estimating space, personnel,

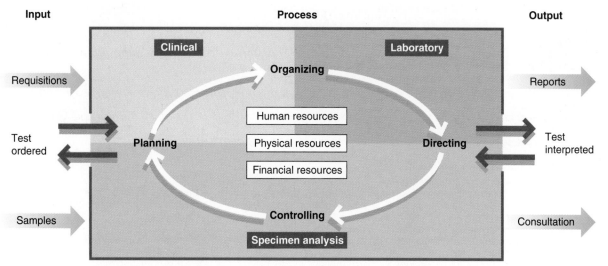

Figure 39–1 A systems view of laboratory management.

and equipment needs; and preparing budgets. The organizing function calls for the grouping of related work activities, establishing lines of communication and authority, staffing and scheduling, and arranging the equipment and work flow in the space provided. The directing function includes supervising daily work, creating a challenging work environment, delegating responsibility, communicating, and training. The controlling function includes establishing standards, measuring performance against goals, developing feedback mechanisms, and correcting deviations.

Managerial functions are by design described in global terms. These are occasionally elaborated in more detail in the form of a position description for a manager or supervisor. Table 39–4 contains a job description for a supervisor of hematology. Under the supervisor's duties, a number of tasks related to planning, controlling, and decision-making are elaborated. In light of previously described personnel standards and technical supervisor responsibilities, it is appropriate to point out the section of the job description that specifies qualifications for the position (section I) and the level of authority to act either independently or with consultation (section II).

PLANNING: ESTABLISHING POLICIES AND PROCEDURES

As described earlier, the planning function of management includes defining and selecting a course of action. There are various types of plans. After a general introduction to these plans, this section focuses on the development of policies and procedures for the hematology laboratory.

Types of Plans

Plans can be classified by scope. The broadest category of a plan is put forth in the institution's mission statement, philosophy, and goals. This provides the purpose for the institution or department, hence its reason for existence. To accomplish the institution's mission and the department's goals, a series of objectives are prepared as a second type of plan. Objectives are tangible, concrete plans stated in terms of results to be achieved. To be functional, the laboratory's objectives need to specify dimensions of quality, time, accuracy, and/or priority. To accomplish the laboratory's objectives, a series of policies are written that spell out that which is required, prohibited, or suggested courses of action. Even more specifically, procedures provide a guide to action within a section. Procedures detail the sequence of steps to be followed in accomplishing a specific task or policy. And finally, the focus of plans classified by scope narrows to include rules and methods. These are designed to guide thinking, to channel behavior, and to predetermine issues.

Developing Policies

Often a manager finds it beneficial to develop policies that specify the purposes, principles, and appropriate actions to guide the laboratory department. Policies are directives and may be both explicit and implied.

Individual policies will vary by importance and level of determination, specifying action or consequences appropriate to the topic. For example, when patient care is threatened by an employee who is performing analysis while chemically dependent, immediate discharge may be the sanction.

Table 39-4. JOB DESCRIPTION: SUPERVISOR OF HEMATOLOGY

Qualification
Must be certified Medical Technologist (M.S. preferred, B.S. required) with at least 6 years' laboratory experience, including a minimum of 3 years in Hematology.

Authority
Act and report to no one as long as consistent with the policies of the Hematology Laboratory, the Department, and the Hospital. (Level I)

Act as long as consistent with the Laboratory, the Department, and the Hospital, but inform the Manager of Hematology. (Level II)

Act only after consultation with specific approval from the Manager of Hematology. (Level III)

Duties
PLANNING
Space needs and space utilization within the area of supervision (Authority III)*

Annual requirements, for budgetary purposes, of capital equipment, supplies, wages, and salaries. (Authority II)*

Programs for instruction and evaluation of new personnel and students and cross-training of personnel in all sections of Hematology. (Authority II)

Organize work-flow pattern for Hematology. (Authority III)

Develop and maintain an organization plan showing the number, types, and duties of personnel in all sections of Hematology. (Authority I)†

Evaluate and finalize position descriptions for personnel within the incumbent's direct authority. (Authority III)*

Maintain adequate personnel files on each individual under the incumbent's direct authority to include attendance records, evaluation records, and documentation relevant to employee performance. (Authority I)

Organize and update programs on quality control of laboratory tests, preventive maintenance of instruments, and safety in the laboratory. (Authority III)

Evaluate and implement new procedures and instruments and update existing methodologies. (Authority III)

Review, update, and write laboratory technical procedures and instrument preventive maintenance procedures. (Authority III)

Maintain good communications within all divisions of Clinical Pathology, and meet personnel needs within the areas of the incumbent's authority. (Authority I)

Review present functions of areas of the incumbent's direct authority, and revise and optimize functions to better meet the goals and objectives of the Department.

CONTROLLING
Monitor the time records of personnel within the incumbent's area of authority. Institute corrections when necessary. (Authority I)†

Monitor the rotation of personnel to all sections of Hematology.

Monitor straight overtime needed to fill staffing needs. (Authority I)†

Monitor for accuracy and acceptable turnaround time of all testing done in all sections of Hematology. (Authority I)

Monitor preventative maintenance schedules on all laboratory equipment. (Authority I)

Schedule and conduct regular meetings of personnel within the incumbent's area of direct authority for purposes of information and general communication. (Authority II)

Monitor the timely handling of all proficiency-testing surveys within all sections of Hematology. (Authority I)

DECISION-MAKING
Conduct performance evaluation for personnel within the incumbent's area of direct authority. (Authority III)*

Hiring of personnel within incumbent's area of direct authority. (Authority III)*

Additions to the table of organization or personnel roster in the incumbent's area of direct authority. (Authority III)*

Initiate requests and conduct follow-ups on orders for equipment and medical supplies for the incumbent's area of direct authority:
- Capital equipment (Authority III)*
- Supplies up to $500 per order (Authority I)*
- Supplies above $500 per order (Authority III)*
- Renewals of orders for reagents and expendables (Authority II)*
- Maintenance contracts (Authority III)*

Recommend personnel for the participation of continuing education programs and workshops on a local level that involve no special funds and absence of no longer than 1 day. (Authority II)*

Recommend personnel for the participation of continuing education programs and workshops involving special funds and absence of more than 1 day. (Authority III)*

OTHER DUTIES
Perform clinical tests at work station(s) where help is required, i.e., scheduled rotation, heavy workload, instrument breakdown, or personnel shortage.

Working Relationship
Report to Manager of Hematology

Also to Director of Clinical Pathology

Has reporting to him/her:
  All Assistant Supervisors of Hematology.
  All technologists, technicians, and technical assistants in Hematology

---

* Act only after consultation with specific approval from the Hematology Laboratory Manager.
† Inform the Director of Clinical Pathology.

Individual policies will also vary by specificity. For example, the hours of work may be specifically defined whereas the department's support of continuing education may be less detailed. The timing or frequency stated in the policy may vary, as in the case of a mandatory dress code during regular working hours but a relaxation of the policy if an individual is called in during off hours to handle a specific problem.

Sometimes policies originate from formal decisions made by the institution. Other times, government regulation (e.g., Occupational Safety and Health Administration requirements) or a union contract will be the basis for establishing a policy. Regardless, policies must be reasonable and enforceable, properly communicated so that they can be understood, and flexible in light of possible unusual circumstances.

Developing Procedures

To ensure accuracy and precision of laboratory testing, procedure manuals are usually written with a high degree of detail outlining the steps to be followed. The National Committee for Clinical Laboratory Standards[11] has developed a set of requirements for technical procedure manuals. These guidelines suggest that procedures for the clinical laboratory be divided into four sections: (1) general information; (2) specimen requirements; (3) quality control; and (4) the detailed components of the procedure.

The general aspects of the procedure manual requirements note that the procedure should have a section for documenting review and annual approval. Changes should be dated and approved and accurately reflect only those procedures done in the hematology section. The manual must be written and available at the bench for testing personnel.

The specimen requirement section of the procedure should detail any patient preparation that is required, particularly if it is out of the ordinary phlebotomy. Specimen collection, handling, and storage specifications should all be included. In addition, the criteria for an unacceptable specimen need to be defined.

Under quality control, the procedure should detail the preparation of controls, the lot number and date of preparation, and mean value and lower and upper limits. In addition, remedial action to be taken with unacceptable results needs to be defined.

In detailing the steps of the procedure, the methodology, calibration and linearity, and derivation of results must be written. The preparation and storage of reagents and standards should be included. If there is an alternate procedure for automated tests, this should be noted in this section. Reference ranges for results as well as criteria for handling abnormal or critical values should be noted. The procedure should also include any flow sheets, keys, or tables that will facilitate performance of the procedure as well as specific notes and references for the procedure.

ORGANIZATION AND DELEGATION

The organizing function of management brings together the three categories of resources (human, physical, and financial) to accomplish the goals and objectives of the hematology laboratory. This section specifically focuses on the principle of organization as applied to organizational structure with emphasis on delegation.

Organizational Structure

An organizational structure is a chart that details lines of communication, authority and delegation, and focused activities. Figure 39–2 illustrates a traditional hematology department organizational structure. The chart shows a laboratory manager responsible for the hematology area assisted by three supervisors and an administrative assistant. Each of the supervisors is responsible for a defined area or function. This is the principle of specialization or departmentation. Under the principle of specialization, work is confined to a single function or focus. The specialization within this hematology department includes phlebotomy, general hematology, and hemostasis.

The vertical and horizontal lines in an organizational chart detail the difference between line and staff decision-making responsibility. For example, the supervisor of hemostasis is in a decision-making role related to those technical personnel reporting to him or her, while the administrative assistant is in a staff position serving as an "assistant to" or consultant or advisor in decisions that affect hemostasis under the overall direction of the laboratory manager.

Hematology departments can be organized as either "tall" or "flat" structures. Figure 39–2 illustrates a "tall" structure in that there are several layers of "management," including the supervisors, assistant supervisors, and senior technologists. In defining these activities, the concept of lead technical staff member reduces the number of employees for which any immediate supervisor is responsible. In a "flat" structure, the number of employees or span of control is increased.

The organizational structure details unity of

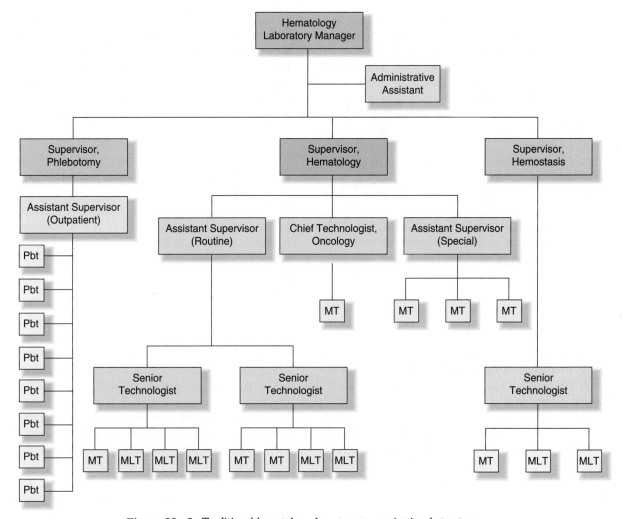

Figure 39–2 Traditional hematology department organizational structure.

command (subordinates being responsible to only one supervisor) as well as chain of command (supervisors having direct responsibility only for their subordinates).

The organizational structure also implies delegation of authority, that is, that activities are performed at the lowest possible level in the organization. Authority and responsibility flow in a direct line vertically from the highest to the lowest individual shown on the chart. This is known as the scalar principle. An important corollary to the delegation of authority is the concept of parity, which states that responsibility cannot be greater than the authority granted.

Organizational Structure in the Future

Organizational hierarchies are always in somewhat of a state of flux. These bureaucratic structures have in some cases led to duplication of resources and unnecessary specialization and isolation. Current trends toward patient-focused testing

and point of care testing suggest that matrix organizational structures involving the clinical laboratory and a patient unit of the institution may be more effective. With matrix organizations, the principles of unity of command and chain of command are modified in that both the manager and employee have dual responsibility and reporting lines, respectively. In an effort to make organizations more "lean" and empower employees, middle management positions such as the assistant supervisor level within the Figure 39–2 illustration are being eliminated. This movement tends to flatten organizational structures, increasing the span of control for those who would typically have been on the top rungs of an organizational structure. To improve communications both within a department and across an organization as well as reduce delays in decision-making, Mills and Friesen[12] suggest that cluster organizations may be a better structure to meet client needs. In addition, the rapidly changing technology of the clinical laboratory and increased automation specifically in areas of hematology and chemistry may herald organizational structures with less specialization or departments along traditional lines. Markin[13] proposes that a major core laboratory defined by highly automated analyses such as the general hematology and chemistry areas might in the future become a more logical single department.

Delegation

To be effective as a manager or supervisor, one must learn to delegate. As described under organizational structure, delegation enables decisions and performance of activities to occur at the lowest level in the organization. Yet, delegation is fraught with a variety of barriers both to the delegator and delegate. Managers and supervisors describe a host of reasons not to delegate, including "it takes longer to teach someone to do it than to do it myself," "someone else cannot do it as well," and "no one is willing to do it," to name a few. Responses of employees about why delegation is ineffective range from not having sufficient information or authority to accomplish the delegated task to not being sure what is expected.

An excellent way to get the full import of delegation is to treat it like a legal contract. The parties, the supervisor, and the employee in this instance, to the delegation (the contract), must reach a meeting of the minds as to the content and meaning of a "contract's" provisions. There must be agreement on (1) the scope of the job (responsibilities); (2) the specific results the employee is to achieve (accountability); (3) the time schedule; (4) the authority needed to carry out the delegation; (5) the means used to measure performance (control and feedback); and (6) that the supervisor and employee each accepts his or her part of the "contract" and will live up to it.

ANALYSIS OF SERVICE OPERATIONS

The hematology laboratory manager as illustrated in the systems view described earlier (see Fig. 39–1) has responsibility for analyzing the effectiveness and efficiency of testing in relationship to both the input and output components as well as the process component. In this section, the test requisition–report cycle is addressed followed by layout flow charting within the laboratory.

The Test Requisition–Report Cycle

A sometimes overlooked opportunity for improving the efficiency and effectiveness of the clinical laboratory is the careful analysis of demands for testing on the laboratory and the impact that test results have on patient care. This adds the dimension of quality management.[14] Krieg[15] describes the test requisition–report cycle as the integration of two decision systems: (1) the attending physician making clinical decisions and (2) the laboratory decision system by the technologist performing the specimen analysis. In initiating the clinical decision component, the physician selects laboratory procedures that will improve the diagnostic and/or therapeutic aspects of patient care. Given specific "orders" for laboratory procedures, the technologist makes decisions in performing the analyses and reporting the laboratory data. This laboratory information then reaches the attending physician, again contributing to the clinical decision-making process.

The opportunity for the laboratory manager to improve service operations is at both the input and output phases of the system. First, the manager can evaluate the selection of laboratory procedures by critically analyzing the impact of requisition formatting. Second, the manager can evaluate the use of data generated by the laboratory.

In some small hospitals and ambulatory clinics, a single printed form serves as both the requisition and the report. The attending physician merely checks the procedure requested and ultimately receives back the results written directly on the same form. More often, requisitions and reports are handled electronically through a hospital information system interfaced with the clinical laboratory's information system. With the use of a computer terminal in the patient care area, laboratory tests are ordered from a menu screen. When this electronic requisition is sent to the laboratory, phlebotomy lists and patient sample labels can be printed as well as worksheets for different analyte clusters. After the tests are completed, data can be verified on a computer terminal in the laboratory if an analyzer is connected on line with the laboratory information system. Manual entry of results is also possible at this terminal, of course. The report back to the patient area can be presented in print or electronic media or both.

At the input phase, the hematology manager can evaluate the selection of laboratory procedures. Is it possible that the requisition form is designed in such a way that a complete blood cell count is ordered when only a white blood cell count or hemoglobin or hematocrit is really desired? A careful analysis of both utilization and intended use of the data can prove beneficial in reducing unnecessary testing. It is also helpful to look at utilization patterns, such as standing orders. Studnicki and colleagues[16] found that by implementing a procedure for monitoring excessive laboratory tests and developing standing order guidelines, test volumes decreased by 55% and test outlyers (tests that violated compliance with guidelines) decreased by 95%.

At the output phase, questions about the contribution of laboratory information to quality patient care should be considered. The laboratory report, presented by either print, electronic, or voice media, is an essential component of the total testing process. Spackman and Beck[17] suggest that computer-generated graphic reports drawing on advances in medical informatics and clinical pathology can be improved through modifications in laboratory information systems. Kent[18] reports that comprehensive assessment of the clinical value of laboratory tests should include demonstration of technical capacity (able to detect a condition with reproducible results), diagnostic accuracy (sensitivity, specificity, and receiver operating characteristic statistics), and therapeutic efficacy.

Laboratory Space Layout Flow Charting

The placement of work stations and instrumentation in the hematology laboratory can be analyzed for efficiency of service operations. This is not a highly sophisticated strategy but is often overlooked since placement is frequently a function of what instrumentation was acquired when and technical staff personal preferences for location of work areas.

At the onset it may be helpful to gain a perspective of space allocation in relation to test volume and type, instrumentation, and other functions, such as teaching, which may also be required in the area. McCutchen[19] recommends that 1200 work units per square foot be allocated for hematology laboratories with large teaching responsibilities and 1700 work units per square foot for hematology laboratories in institutions with small teaching efforts.

Figure 39-3 illustrates a hematology laboratory layout flow chart as an example of efficiency assessment. The layout includes locations of equipment and work stations. The flow of work and reports is indicated by dotted lines. Although the placement of routine and automated hematology procedures appears appropriate, the placement of the centrifuge for coagulation testing could be more appropriately located closer to the hemostasis analyzer.

DEVELOPING HUMAN RESOURCES

From a budgeting perspective, the human resource entrusted to the laboratory manager or supervisor's care represents 50-70% of the total financial resource. This percentage of the budget, however, does not adequately reflect the true value of the human resource. Rather, this reflects wages and fringe benefits to perform laboratory testing, but the expertise inherent in the individuals represents an additional financial investment. To understand this, if a laboratory manager needed to replace a portion or all of the current technical staff, the financial outlay would exceed considerably the budgeted dollar amount for wages and fringe benefits.

The Human Resource Cycle

Figure 39-4 illustrates the human resource cycle in the clinical laboratory. It identifies two categories of individuals at the preemployment stage: applicants and candidates. After the selection process is complete, the employee is oriented to the new testing environment and assumes responsibilities for analyte testing. His or her performance is monitored over time and becomes the basis for documentation at a preestablished appraisal period. During the appraisal, a discussion about the employee's performance naturally leads to two categories of action. The employee may receive an adjustment in salary (reward system) perhaps based on merit, and a development plan to guide enhancement activities during the upcoming year may be established. This development plan then becomes the basis for monitoring performance responsibilities during the subsequent year, and the cycle is repeated.

Recruitment, Hiring, and Orientation

The employee selection process can be divided into four components: (1) advertising and recruitment, (2) receipt of applications, (3) reference checks and an interview with qualified candidates, and (4) selecting the best candidate. The steps of advertising and recruitment and receipt of applications are typically handled by the institution's human resources department. The laboratory manager or supervisor may have a role in designing the advertisement based on a position description and that which is required on the job. It is important in the advertisement to include only those expectations that are bona fide occupational qualifications. Assuming the recruitment is successful, a variety of applicants submit paperwork to be considered for the position. A subsequent screening process by the human resources department will net the top candidates for further consideration by the laboratory manager or supervisor. Throughout the screening process as well as during the preemployment interview, the goal is to identify the best

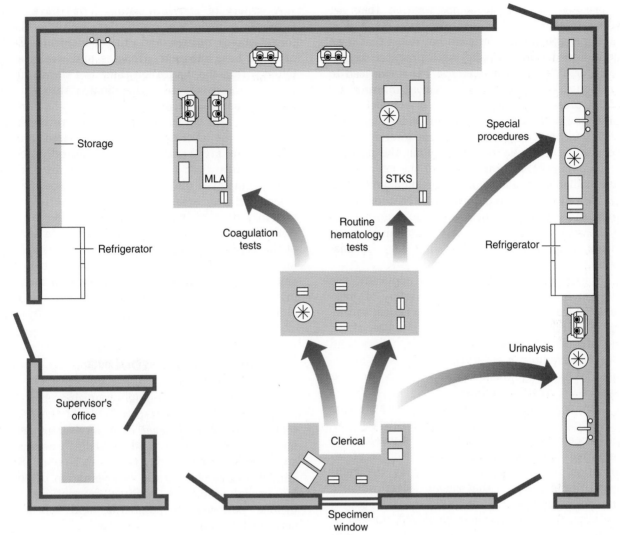

Figure 39–3 Hematology laboratory layout flow chart. (Note: microscopes are disproportionately large for clarity in this illustration.)

match between the candidate and the vacant position.[20]

As part of the preparation for a preemployment interview, references should be checked. The information that is available is often limited with an intent to protect the applicant. The purpose of the reference check is to validate the applicant's employment record as well as educational background and certification. With regard to a candidate's previous employment record, institutions are ap-

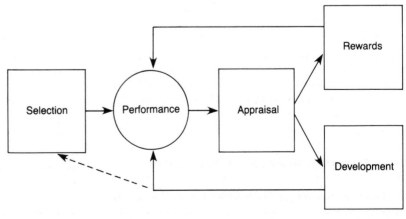

Figure 39–4 Human resource cycle in the clinical laboratory. (From Levy S, Loomba NP: Health Care Administration: A Managerial Perspective, 2nd ed. Philadelphia: JB Lippincott, 1984:464.)

The Human Resource Cycle

propriately cautious about information they are willing to share. Parks[21] identifies risks involved in issuing employment references but notes that if an institution develops a policy with practical suggestions for a "controlled reference," this can lead to a responsible exchange of employment information.

The preemployment interview is conducted for candidates who have already been deemed qualified by a screening of applicants. This interview provides an opportunity to fully explain the position to the applicant, making a copy of the job description available. In addition, the preemployment interview offers a first-hand exchange of information about the candidate. There are clearly limitations to the selection interview since impressions made during such a short period of time may be misleading.

To gain information about the applicant, the manager or supervisor can plan a variety of questions.[22] Ideally these should be open ended, soliciting insight into the candidate's knowledge, skills, and attitudes by asking what, when, where, and why. For example, a supervisor might ask a candidate, "What do you consider to be your strongest asset? . . . greatest liability?"

There are a number of laws that govern the type of information that may be posed during the preemployment interview. The Uniform Guidelines in Employee Selection[23] is an excellent source of information to guide questions posed by the manager. In brief, subjects that violate federal uniform guidelines include nationality, marital status, spouse's occupation or where employed, number of children or babysitting arrangement, religious affiliation, personal finances, handicaps not related to job performance, arrest record, and organizational affiliations not related to work.[20]

Once the best candidate is selected, a pre-service orientation is necessary. This would introduce the new employee to particular policies and procedures of the institution, methods used in the laboratory, types of equipment and their operation, and other aspects to ensure that the new employee begins to become productive as soon as possible.

Performance Appraisals

The purposes of employee performance appraisals are to ensure competent performance, substantiate modifications of the reward system, and provide guidance to the employee for development and advancement.[24] The appraisal process includes both measurement and judgment. The measurement is accomplished by comparison with a standard, typically the position description. The manager or supervisor conducting the appraisal then exercises judgment based on that measurement.

A variety of standard rating forms have been developed, including rating scales, checklists, forced choice ratings, and critical incidents. Each of these have inherent strengths and weaknesses. Often within the institution there is a standardized rating form developed and validated through the human resources department. Perhaps the clinical laboratory as a whole has developed a rating form specific to the laboratory. If a standardized form is used, there are limitations that naturally occur. These standardized forms do not allow for distinction of employee differences related to specific job responsibilities, areas of technical expertise, professional development, or personal career aspirations. Consequently, it is helpful to have a section of the appraisal form that allows for the establishment of mutually beneficial objectives to help the employee to become a more valuable staff member in the institution as well as to prompt the employee to "grow" personally and professionally.

STAFFING AND SCHEDULING

The functions of planning, organizing, and controlling overlap is the responsibility of the hematology laboratory manager or supervisor to determine staffing needs and schedule personnel appropriate for the testing that is to be done. Specific strategies include the determination of staffing needs, developing position descriptions that include performance standards, and scheduling personnel to adequately cover the test menu and volume on a daily basis.

Determining Staffing Needs

In today's cost-containment environment, it is important to justify staffing needs on the basis of work to be accomplished. Often this is done using workload historical data as measured by the College of American Pathologists (CAP) workload recording units. From a broad perspective, if the volume of work as measured by workload recording units is known, the number of full-time equivalent (FTE) staff can be calculated. To do this, the following formula is implied:

$$FTE = \frac{Workload}{7800 \ units}$$

This calculation assumes a 75% productivity level (or 45 productive minutes each hour), and the rationale for this calculation is as follows:

40 hours/week × 60 minutes

= 2400 minutes/week

2400 minutes/week × 52 weeks/year

$$= 124,800 \text{ minutes/year}$$

124,800 minutes/year ÷ 12 months/year

$$= 10,400 \text{ minutes/month}$$

10,400 minutes/month × 0.75 = 7800 units/FTE

Other approaches have been used to determine staffing needs by forecasting volume based on either the average number of tests per census or using a formula that considers the average severity of patient illness. Barletta[25] reported on the use of projectional analysis to determine staffing needs, using the following formula:

$$\frac{\text{Average test}}{\text{Census}} \times \text{Projected census}$$

$$= \text{Projected test volume}$$

Projected test volume
× Average CAP workload units (in minutes)
= Projected required employee time (in minutes)

$$\frac{\text{Projected required employee time (in minutes)}}{\text{8-hour day} \times 60 \text{ minutes} \times \text{productivity goal}}$$

$$= \text{Projected required FTEs/day}$$
(maximum required staffing)

The hospital census is not always a reliable indicator of test volume, however. Harper[26] found that a more pertinent formula to project staffing needs is derived when the average severity of patient illness is considered. With this approach, a staffing estimate can be determined using patient acuity (determined by the number of nursing hours per 24 hours required) to adjust a work index as a way of forecasting the number of laboratory procedures that would be performed.

Developing Position Descriptions and Performance Standards

To be sure that adequate coverage for all hematology procedures is available to match the scope of testing done in the laboratory, position descriptions become an essential tool. The sample position description for the hematology supervisor (see Table 39–4) serves as a useful template for a model technical staff position description. A position description should include the qualifications required in terms of education and experience. The authority granted in the position for both the test performance and the reporting of results needs to be specified. When consultation with either a senior technologist, laboratory supervisor, or pathologist is necessary, this should be spelled out. The duties section of the position description lists the

range of tasks expected of the employee. These should be comprehensive, covering responsibilities from specimen preparation and test performance through reporting of results. Identifying working relationships will help to clarify lines of communication and delegated authority.

Performance standards need to be similarly specified. Performance standards are qualitative or quantitative measures of expected results (productivity) or behaviors that delineate a level of performance. These are useful in the delineation of position responsibilities, provide a basis for performance evaluation and feedback, and serve to supplement coaching and counseling. The characteristics and criteria of performance standards include (1) they are linked to a specific duty of the employee; (2) they contain expected results in observable behavior terms; (3) they state conditions for and constraints of task accomplishment; and (4) they include measurable criteria that indicate satisfactory performance.

Scheduling Personnel

Under CLIA '88, hematology tests have been categorized by complexity. These are shown in Table 39–5. For each of the three major categories (waived tests, moderate complexity tests, and high complexity tests) specific personnel standards have been defined for managerial and testing personnel as contained in Table 39–2. Assuming that the staff available to schedule include a mixture of technicians and technologists, a job skills inventory (i.e., what tests each individual can do) can be prepared. This then becomes the basis for scheduling technical staff in the hematology laboratory.

When scheduling technical staff, the manager or supervisor needs to consider both the volume and complexity of procedures to be done.[27] It is sometimes helpful to schedule staff in staggered shifts, with several individuals beginning ahead of others, to match the volume of work to be done at any given time with the number of personnel available. In recent years, a variety of innovative scheduling techniques have proven successful. These include, for example, 10-hour days/4-day work weeks, shift sharing, use of part-time employees, and 7 days on/7 days off scheduling.

FINANCIAL PLANNING AND CONTROL

Historically, under a retrospective reimbursement system, clinical laboratories were viewed as profit centers since the more testing a laboratory performed, the more revenue was generated. With

Table 39-5. HEMATOLOGY TESTS CATEGORIZED BY COMPLEXITY UNDER THE CLINICAL LABORATORY AMENDMENTS OF 1988

Waived Tests
1. Dipstick or tablet reagent urinalysis for the following: bilirubin, glucose, hemoglobin, ketone, leukocytes, nitrate, pH, protein, urobilinogen, specific gravity
2. Ovulation tests: visual color tests for human luteinizing hormone
3. Urine pregnancy tests - visual color comparison test
4. Erythrocyte sedimentation rate (nonautomated)
5. Hemoglobin copper sulfate (nonautomated)
6. Fecal occult blood
7. Spun microhematocrit

Moderate Complexity Tests
1. Automated hematology procedures without differentials that do not require operator intervention during the analytic process
2. Automated hematology procedures with differentials that do not require operator intervention during the analytic process and that do not require an analyst to interpret a histogram or scattergram
3. Manual white blood cell differential counts when the analyst is not required to identify atypical cells
4. Automated procedures that do not require operator intervention during the analytic process
5. Manual hematology procedures with limited steps and with limited sample or reagent preparation
6. Manual coagulation procedures with limited steps and with limited sample or reagent preparation

High Complexity Tests
1. Manual reticulocyte counts
2. Hemoglobin electrophoresis
3. Bone marrow evaluation
4. Manual coagulation procedures with multiple steps in sample or reagent preparation or the analytic process
5. Manual cell counts
6. Automated or semi-automated procedures that do require operator intervention during the analytic process
7. Manual white blood cell differential counts when the analyst is required to identify atypical cells
8. Manual hematology procedures with multiple steps in sample or reagent preparation or the analytic process
9. Flow cytometry
10. Manual platelet counts

From Clinical Laboratory Improvement Amendments of 1988: Final rule: 42 CFR subpart A: General provisions, 493.1–493.25. U.S. Department of Health and Human Services, HCFA/PHS. Fed Register 1992; 57:7172–7183.

today's emphasis on prospective payment based on diagnosis-related groups, managed care, and negotiated financial contracts between health care provider organizations, the hematology laboratory is considered a cost center. Consequently, the manager and supervisor need to have a clear understanding of strategies appropriate for financial planning and control.

An Economic Overview

To be a good steward of the financial resources under a manager's control, one must understand both the revenue and costs associated with providing laboratory services. Revenue by definition is the income derived in exchange for laboratory information from specimen analysis. Revenue is obviously related to the volume of testing performed. Managers must understand that the revenue generated is defined as the total dollars received (not billed).

The costs associated with performing laboratory analyses can be divided into two major categories: (1) direct costs and (2) indirect costs. Direct costs are those that are directly attributable to the production of laboratory test data. For example, direct costs may include technical staff salaries, reagents and supplies, and instrument costs. Indirect costs

are those costs associated with maintaining a facility for doing laboratory testing. Examples of indirect costs include salaries of administrative officers in the institution, janitorial services, and food services.

Both direct and indirect costs can be further subdivided into fixed or variable costs. Fixed costs are those that are incurred regardless of whether the laboratory performs any analyses. For example, the institution's human resource department is an indirect fixed cost that must be paid for regardless of whether the laboratory is busy. A hematology analyzer is a direct fixed cost that must be paid for regardless of whether the analyzer is being used. Variable costs are those that increase proportionally to the volume of testing performed. So, if the laboratory is not performing any hematology testing, variable costs are zero; as volume increases, the costs increase proportionally. An example of an indirect variable cost is electricity for the instrumentation. An example of a direct variable cost is reagents used in testing.

Cost Accounting

Cost accounting enables the manager or supervisor to track and control costs of laboratory operations. By calculating cost per test analysis, financial information is available to facilitate pricing and contract negotiations for fee setting, differential costing for alternative capital equipment and methods, and analysis for continuous improvement in technology methods.

To calculate costs per test, the manager or supervisor must include the direct and other labor per procedure, direct and other materials per procedure, equipment expense per procedure, and overhead expense. Direct labor is the cost of technical employees' time required to complete a test. Other labor costs include the cost of support and supervisory (administrative) personnel within the cost center. Direct materials costs are those identifiable materials, reagents, and supply items consumed in the delivery of the procedure. Other materials costs are those not directly traceable to a procedure (e.g., general purpose chemicals, office supplies). Equipment costs usually include depreciation for the cost of the major equipment used in the performance of the procedure. Overhead costs are those costs of non–revenue-producing cost centers apportioned to revenue-producing cost centers (e.g., housekeeping, employee health, operation of the facility).

Break-Even Analysis

Occasionally a manager or supervisor will wish to know how many tests of a given procedure need to be performed at a fixed revenue amount to determine whether the laboratory is making a profit or losing money on a procedure, or if a procedure ought to be sent to a reference laboratory. This calculation is a break-even analysis and considers both direct and indirect and fixed and variable costs in doing the procedure as well as revenue. To calculate a break-even point, the following formula is used:

$$\text{Break even} = \frac{\text{Total fixed cost} + \text{net income contribution}}{\text{Revenue per unit} - \text{variable cost per unit}}$$

In this formula, the net income contribution is a defined profit margin typically included to ensure that the laboratory has sufficient capital to advance with new technologies.

Budgeting

Both the planning and control functions come into play with the budgeting process. Inherent in this process is a forecasting to predict revenue and expenses in the hematology laboratory. Table 39–6 shows an example of a hematology department budget.

The three major columns of this example of a monthly budget include categories labeled budgeted, actual, and variance. The budgeted column

Table 39-6. EXAMPLE OF MONTHLY HEMATOLOGY DEPARTMENT BUDGET

	Budget	Actual	Variance (%)
Volume			
Patient admissions	756	723	−4.4
Patient days	1,134	1,105	−2.6
Procedure/patient day	3.3	2.75	−1.7
Procedure/patient admission	5	4.2	−1.6
Procedures	3,780	3,037	−19.6
Revenue	$37,780	$33,407	−11.6
Expenses			
Salaries			
Technical labor	$9,445	$8,760	−7.2
Nontechnical labor	4,600	4,100	−10.9
Professional fees	2,644	2,338	−11.6
Supplies	3,780	3,100	−18.0
Equipment			
Depreciation	1,134	1,134	0
Service contracts	950	950	0
Repairs	480	600	+25.0
Other	1,467	1,125	−23.3
Direct costs	24,500	22,107	−9.7
Indirect costs	10,000	9,024	−9.7
Total costs	$34,500	$31,131	−9.7
Net Income	$3,280	$2,276	−30.6
Financial Ratios			
Total cost/procedure	$9.13	$10.25	+12.3
Labor/procedure	3.72	4.23	+13.7
Supply cost/procedure	1.00	1.02	+ 2.0
Revenue/procedure	10.00	11.00	+10.0
Margin/procedure	$0.87	$0.75	−13.8

shows estimated revenue and expenses resulting from forecasting. In this example, forecasts were based on patient admissions to the institution at five procedures per admission, average revenue of $10 per procedure, and 1.5 days per patient admission. The actual column shows the actual revenues realized and expenses incurred. The variance column shows a percentage of overage or shortfall between budgeted and actual. A review of the table shows that the actual work performed was less than that budgeted. Even though revenue per procedure increased slightly, this still resulted in a net reduced revenue because of the fewer numbers of patients admitted and tests performed.

The last section of the budget example includes a variety of financial ratios.[28] These financial ratios bring together key pieces of financial information from earlier in the budget as a quick method for monitoring the budget on an ongoing basis. Because the actual and to some extent the budgeted volume, revenue, and costs will vary on a monthly basis, it is wise not to attempt to make corrections in a budget in which variance is consistently negative or positive until several months have elapsed.

PURCHASING AND INVENTORY CONTROL

The purpose of purchasing and inventory control is to maintain sufficient supplies so that patient care is not compromised. The inability to perform hematology analysis because inventory has been depleted could delay treatment or surgery, resulting in an increased length of stay.

If this were a perfect world, a back door of the hematology laboratory would lead directly to a vendor's warehouse so that no inventory was required in the laboratory, no pre-payment was necessary, and supplies were readily available at all times. This is the basis for the current trend to order supplies with a "just in time" delivery. But we live in an imperfect world. Problems encountered in purchasing and inventory maintenance include the fact that supplies become outdated before being used up, delays occur in receiving supplies and processing orders, and occasionally vendors report out-of-stock or back-ordered items.

Inventory Management

As background, it is helpful to look at the process of supplies depletion and replenishment.[29] Figure 39–5 graphically illustrates this process for a single supply. In this example, demand is defined as the number of units of supply used per month (40 per month). In this illustration it takes 30 days between the time an order is placed and the supply arrives in the laboratory. This is referred to as the lead time. This particular laboratory has established that every 10 days the amount of stock in inventory will be reviewed. To ensure that the laboratory will not run out of the supply, a safety stock of 20 units is planned to be on hand at all times. This illustration also shows that a reorder

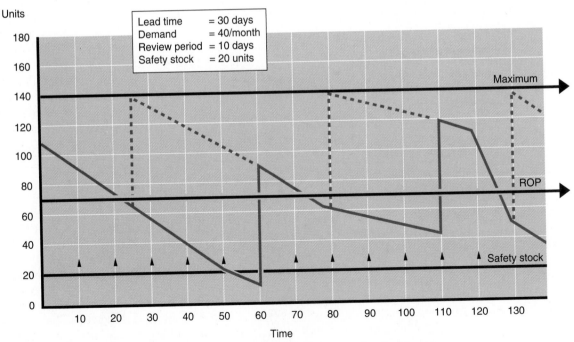

Figure 39–5 A view of supplies depletion and replenishment.

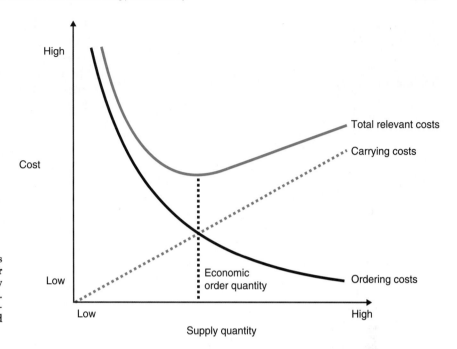

Figure 39–6 Ordering costs versus holding costs. (From Noel SA, Snyder JR: Forecast comparisons in inventory management. Lab Med 1990; 21:91–96. Copyright © 1990 by the American Society of Clinical Pathologists. Reprinted with permission.)

point has been established when the supplies in inventory reach 70. The volume ordered depends on the amount in inventory at a given time to bring the stock up to a total of 140. Hence, the volume ordered is consistent each time but the demand in the illustration varies somewhat over the 130 days shown.

Opposing Costs: Ordering and Holding

A hematology manager or supervisor might wonder why not to order a large quantity at a reduced rate so the laboratory supply will not run out, or perhaps why not to place an order every week so that the laboratory is always anticipating a smaller shipment. The reason for not doing this is illustrated in Figure 39–6, which shows the opposing cost pressures associated with ordering versus holding.[30]

Costs associated with placing a purchase order include direct and indirect expenses such as stationery, postage, and telephone costs involved in order preparation, accounting, and paying the invoice. There are also paper costs related to review, purchasing, expediting, receiving, inspection, and warehousing of supplies. Although a precise measurement of these costs is generally not possible, a reasonable approximation can be made for purposes of comparison. The cost of an average purchase order can range from $25 to $50 in a health care institution, although some institutions report much higher ranges.

Carrying costs are those costs associated with holding supplies in inventory from the time an item is purchased until it is used. These costs include taxes and insurance related to inventory; rental or depreciation of space and fixtures devoted to inventory; security and janitorial costs to maintain this storage space; shrinkage and obsolescence of supplies due to non-movement, excess, and outdating; and the interest costs of money tied up in inventories. Carrying costs are stated as a percentage of the actual unit cost, usually 20–30%.

From Figure 39–6 it is evident that ordering costs per unit decrease as the size of the order in number of units increases. It is also evident that carrying costs per unit increase as the size of the order increases. To minimize ordering costs, the manager must place fewer orders; to minimize carrying costs, the manager must keep inventory as long as possible. This ideal mix between minimal ordering costs and holding costs is termed the *economic order quantity.*

Inventory Analysis

One of the strategies that a manager or supervisor can employ is a careful look at the volume of inventory on hand within the storeroom. An assessment of the day's inventory on hand, which includes a tabulation of the total carrying costs associated with maintaining that inventory, can often lead to improved finances. The analysis of inventory on hand will show how often the inventory is turned over.

Strengthening Inventory Management

In light of the opposing costs for ordering and holding inventory as well as characteristics associated with supplies depletion and replenishment, several strategies can be used to strengthen inventory management. First, the usual rule for rotating stock in terms of first unit in/first unit used is prudent. For problematic supplies and delivery, the manager will want to plan by knowing the usual demand, calculating the lead time for delivery, and establishing a safety stock. Standing orders should be used whenever possible for high volume supplies. With standing orders, however, it is important to review storeroom stock periodically and to set up a maximum number of units as the limit when ordering. Some managers and supervisors have used visiting vendors effectively to go through their supplies inventory, checking receipt of orders and conducting follow-up if a particular order has not arrived on time. Finally, it is occasionally beneficial to review the inventory on hand and turnover of supplies within the storeroom.

SUMMARY

This chapter began with a case study describing a competent hematology practitioner faced with making the transition to management. To help this individual make this transition and be effective, a systems approach to understanding management was described. The managerial functions of planning, organizing, directing, and controlling were elaborated in the form of strategies to establish policies and procedures, develop an organizational chart and strengthen delegation, and analyze the service operations of the laboratory. Strategies specific to the human resources in the laboratory included recruitment, employee selection, and performance appraisals. Ways to determine staffing needs and schedule personnel were suggested. The strategies of cost accounting, break-even analysis, and budgeting prepare the manager or supervisor for financial planning and control responsibilities. Finally, the related financial aspects of purchasing and inventory control were described. Clearly, the key to effective management is recognizing that the manager's role, tasks, and skills required are different than those required of a technical staff member.

REVIEW QUESTIONS

1. When making the transition from practitioner to manager, a medical technologist/clinical laboratory scientist must avoid the trap of
   a. hiring staff with more expertise than the manager
   b. continuing to concentrate on performing testing, rather than managing
   c. looking at the contribution of laboratory testing in the total context of quality health care delivery
   d. balancing the expectations of both the institution and the employees

2. The organizational principle that states that activities should be performed at the lowest feasible level in the organization is the principle of
   a. span of control
   b. unity of command
   c. delegation of authority
   d. chain of command

3. The four functions of management include all of the following, *except*
   a. directing
   b. scheduling
   c. planning
   d. controlling

4. Which of the following types of plans is most detailed for guiding activities in the laboratory?
   a. mission/philosophy/goals
   b. policies
   c. objectives
   d. rules/methods

5. The concept of "formal organization" refers to
   a. the deliberately planned relationships among members of an organization
   b. the ceremonial aspects of the superior-subordinate relationship
   c. the unplanned, spontaneous relationships among members of an organization
   d. the policy-making level of the organization

6. The means by which a laboratory documents its costs for performing a particular procedure and then establishes its charges based on the direct and indirect costs is known as
   a. cost per test
   b. budget setting

c. break-even point

d. priority rating

7. Which of the following is a direct cost in a laboratory budget?
   a. building depreciation
   b. heating and air conditioning
   c. technical staff salary
   d. institution's personnel (human resources) department

8. The term *variance* on a budget sheet refers to
   a. excess manpower
   b. category of expense or revenue
   c. forecasted amount of revenue or expense
   d. overage or shortfall between budgeted and actual

9. Which of the following inventory terms refers to the amount of time between placing an order and the time the order will arrive for use in the laboratory?
   a. demand
   b. safety stock
   c. lead time
   d. review time

10. Failure to delegate can be attributed to one or more of the following:
    a. fear of competition from employees
    b. lack of experience among subordinates
    c. enjoyment of doing the work
    d. lack of time

11. When designing a reporting system, which one or more of the following should be considered?
    a. conciseness
    b. understandability
    c. identification of patient, patient location, and physician
    d. administrative and record-keeping value

References

1. LaCroix KA, Seidel LF: Management in action: What a university can do when the route to effective laboratory management is reconsidered. Clin Lab Sci 1991; 4:196–197.
2. Ramsey MK: What laboratory personnel like in supervisors. Clin Lab Sci 1989; 2:214–215.
3. Karni KR, Seanger DG: Management skills needed by entry-level practitioners. Clin Lab Sci 1988; 1:296–300.
4. Umiker WO: The Effective Laboratory Supervisor. Oradell, NJ: Medical Economics Books, 1982:24–25.
5. 1992 JCAHO Standards. MA 1.4.4, Management and Administrative Services. Chicago: Joint Commission on Accreditation of Healthcare Organizations, 1992.
6. Clinical Laboratory Improvement Amendments of 1988: Final rule: 42 CFR Subpart M: Personnel for moderate and high complexity testing, 493.1401–493.1495. U.S. Department of Health and Human Services, HCFA/PHS. Fed Register 1992; 57:7002–7228.
7. Snyder JR, Senhauser DA: The nature of management in the clinical laboratory. *In* Snyder JR, Senhauser DA (eds): Administration and Supervision in Laboratory Medicine, 2nd ed. Philadelphia: JB Lippincott, 1989:3–19.
8. Becan-McBride K: Textbook of Clinical Laboratory Supervision. New York: Appleton-Century-Crofts, 1982:1–28.
9. Barr JT: Clinical laboratory utilization: The role of the clinical laboratory scientist. *In* Davis BG, Bishop ML, Mass D (eds): Clinical Laboratory Science: Strategies for Practice. Philadelphia: JB Lippincott, 1989:31–46.
10. Mass D: Medical technologists of the future: New practice, new service, new function. Lab Med 1993; 24:403–406.
11. National Committee for Clinical Laboratory Standards. Clinical Laboratory Procedure Manuals; Approved Guidelines. NCCLS publication GP2-A. Villanova, PA: NCCLS, 1984.
12. Mills DQ, Friesen GB: Clusters: A new style of organization. Clin Lab Man Rev 1992; 6:499–513.
13. Markin RS: Clinical laboratory automation: A paradigm shift. Clin Lab Man Rev 1993; 7:243–247.
14. Statland BE: Quality management: Watchword for the '90s. MLO. 1989; 21:33–40.
15. Krieg AF: Lab Communication. Oradell, NJ: Medical Economics Company, 1978.
16. Studnicki J, Bradham DD, Marshburn J, et al: Measuring the impact of standing orders on laboratory utilization. Lab Med 1992; 23:24–28.
17. Spackman KA, Beck JR: Approaches to improving laboratory test reporting. Lab Med 1991; 22:725–727.
18. Kent DL: Decision analysis and assessment of the clinical impact of diagnostic tests. Lab Med 1991; 22:718–724.
19. McCutchen G: Space allocation guidelines for the clinical laboratory. J Med Tech 1985; 2:772–777.
20. Long IW: Employee selection and orientation as a determinant of performance assessment. Clin Lab Sci 1992; 5:212–214.
21. Parks DG: Employment references: Defamation law in the clinical laboratory. Clin Lab Man Rev 1993; 7:103–110.
22. Umiker WO: Selection interviews of health care workers. Healthcare Supr 1988; 6(2):62–64.
23. Uniform Guidelines in Employee Selection (1978). Equal Employment Opportunity Commission. Fed Register 1978; 43:28290–38315.
24. Laudicina RJ: Successful implementation and use of performance assessment. Clin Lab Sci 1992; 5:215–217.
25. Barletta JM: Using projectional analysis to reach your staffing goals. MLO 1984; 16(3):81–90.
26. Harper SS: The key to predicting laboratory workload. MLO 1984; 16(11):65–67.
27. Passey RB: How to meet the new personnel requirements (while continuing to operate your laboratory). MLO 1992; 24(9):47–51.
28. Sharp JW: Financial ratios for laboratory management decision-making. *In* Snyder JR, Senhauser DA (eds): Administration and Supervision in Laboratory Medicine, 2nd ed. Philadelphia: JB Lippincott, 1989:475–486.
29. Luchhetti RV, Snyder JR: Inventory management and cost containment. *In* Snyder JR, Senhauser DA (eds): Administration and Supervision in Laboratory Medicine, 2nd ed. Philadelphia: JB Lippincott, 1989:487–509.
30. Noel SA, Snyder JR: Forecast comparisons in inventory management. Lab Med 1990; 21:91–96.

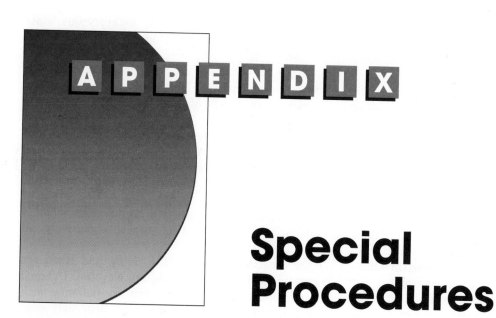

APPENDIX

Special Procedures

Doris McGhee and
Bernadette F. Rodak

FREQUENTLY USED TESTS FOR IDENTIFYING HEMOGLOBIN ABNORMALITIES

The most commonly used tests for the diagnosis of the hemoglobinopathies are complete blood cell count with red blood cell evaluation; sickle cell solubility testing; hemoglobin electrophoresis using cellulose acetate (pH 8.4–8.6); and hemoglobin electrophoresis using citrate agar (pH 6.0–6.2).

The *fetal hemoglobin (HbF) alkali denaturation test* is helpful in identifying conditions in which HbF is elevated, such as sickle cell anemia and hemoglobin S (HbS)–thalassemia conditions.

Hemoglobin A_2 quantitation helps rule out thalassemia and double heterozygous HbS–thalassemia. Hemoglobin A_2 is normal in HbSS– and HbAS–thalassemia but is increased in HbS–thalassemia and other thalassemia syndromes.

The *Heinz body stain, isopropanol stability test, and heat precipitation test* may be used for the identification of unstable hemoglobins.

Globin chain electrophoresis is a highly specific test and used when routine electrophoresis is not adequate.

Tests for common membrane disorders that may cause hemolysis include osmotic fragility, sucrose hemolysis, and acidified serum tests.

The *osmotic fragility* is increased in red blood cells that have a decreased surface-to-volume ratio, primarily spherocytes.

The *sucrose hemolysis,* or sugar water, test is a screening test for paroxysmal nocturnal hemoglobinuria. Positive results should be confirmed by the *acidified serum test.*

THE MOST COMMON HEMOGLOBIN ABNORMALITIES*

At birth, the most prevalent hemoglobin in the erythrocyte of the normal infant is fetal hemoglobin. Some hemoglobin A (HbA), the major adult hemoglobin, and a small amount of hemoglobin A_2 (HbA$_2$) are present. Levels of HbF decline after birth, and adult levels of HbA and HbF are reached by the first year of life. The major hemoglobin present after the age of 1 year is HbA; up to 3.4% is HbA$_2$, and less than 2% is HbF.

Sickle cell anemia is a homozygous state manifesting almost exclusively with HbS. A very small amount of HbF may be present.

Sickle cell trait is a heterozygous state manifesting with HbA and HbS and a normal amount of HbA$_2$ on electrophoresis on cellulose acetate. Re-

---

* See Chapter 18 for a complete discussion.

sults on citrate agar show hemoglobins in the A and S migratory positions.

Sickle cell–C disease is a heterozygous state demonstrating HbS and hemoglobin C (HbC) in combination.

Sickle cell–thalassemia, type HbS/beta$^+$, is a condition in which HbA, HbS, HbF, and HbA$_2$ are all present, but levels of HbA$_2$ and HbF levels are elevated.

Sickle cell–thalassemia, type HbS/beta^0, is a condition in which HbA is absent and levels of HbS, HbF, and HbA$_2$ are elevated.

In *thalassemia–C disease*, HbA, HbF, and HbC are present.

Hemoglobin C disease is a homozygous state in which the hemoglobin is almost exclusively all HbC.

In *thalassemia major*, HbF, HbA, and HbA$_2$ are present, and HbF and HbA$_2$ are elevated. Unequal bands of hemoglobin are seen in patients with thalassemia, transfusion, and iron deficiency anemia and with unstable hemoglobins.

METHODS

Hemoglobinopathies

HEMOGLOBIN SOLUBILITY TEST[1-3]

The solubility test is a screening test for determining the presence of sickling hemoglobin. The test is rather inexpensive, has a high degree of accuracy, and yields rapid results. A number of prepackaged test kits are available.

Principle

Sickle hemoglobin in the deoxygenated state is less soluble than in the oxygenated state and forms a precipitate when placed in a high-molarity phosphate buffer solution. The precipitate results when the deoxygenated hemoglobin molecules form tactoids (liquid crystals) that refract and deflect light rays, thus producing a turbid solution.

Specimen

Whole blood is collected in ethylenediaminetetraacetic acid (EDTA) and held at 4 °C until testing is performed. Specimens may be refrigerated for up to 3 weeks.

Reagents

K_2HPO_4 (dibasic potassium
phosphate, anhydrous)   216 g

KH$_2$PO$_4$ (monobasic potassium
phosphate, crystals)   169 g
Saponin   1 g
Sodium hydrosulphite (dithionite)   10 g

Place approximately 500–800 mL of distilled water into a 1-L volumetric flask. Add the dibasic potassium phosphate and mix until dissolved. Add the monobasic potassium phosphate and saponin, one at a time, dissolving after each addition. Dilute to 1000 mL with distilled water. Solution is stable for approximately 3–4 weeks at 4 °C.

Equipment

12 × 75 mm tubes
Special rack with black lines (or card with thin black lines) for observation of turbidity

Equipment and reagent can be obtained prepackaged. Manufacturer's instructions should be followed exactly.

Quality Control

1. Positive and negative control blood samples must be tested with each group of solubility tests performed.
2. The positive control should have a hemoglobin content of 10–14 g/dL and 30–45% of HbS.

Procedure

1. Pipette 2 mL of reagent into a labeled 12 × 75 mm test tube.
2. Allow reagent to warm to room temperature (approximately 22–25 °C).
3. Add 20 µL (0.02 mL) of blood. Mix and let stand for 5 minutes.
4. Using a special rack (or a card with black lines), observe turbidity against black lines.

Interpretation

A positive test result for sickling hemoglobin is indicated by a very turbid solution. The black lines on the rack cannot be seen through the solution. HbC-Harlem, HbS-Travis, and HbC-Ziquinchor, as well as HbS, produce positive solubility test results. Thus the test is not totally specific for HbS but should be reported as positive or negative for sickling hemoglobin.

A negative test result for sickling hemoglobin occurs when the black lines can be seen through the blood reagent solution, even if the solution appears slightly cloudy. Most hemoglobins, including A, F, C, D, G, and A$_2$, produce negative results.

Sources of Error and Comments

1. Polycythemia, the addition of too much blood in relation to reagent, dysglobulinemia, recent transfusion of blood containing a sickling hemoglobin, hyperlipidemia, and leukemia with an extremely high white blood cell or platelet count can produce false positive results.
2. Inactive or outdated reagents, recent transfusions of normal blood to a person with a sickling hemoglobin, tests on newborns and infants less than 6 months of age, and anemia in which the hemoglobin concentration is less than 7 g/dL may produce a false negative result.
3. Cold and improperly mixed reagents may produce inaccurate results.
4. Poor grades of saponin and failure to use anhydrous salts and dithionite in the reagent lead to inaccurate results.
5. The mixture of blood and reagents is light red to pink. Light orange indicates deteriorated reagent, usually caused by oxidation of the sodium hydrosulfite in the reagent.
6. This is only a screening procedure; thus cellulose acetate electrophoresis must be completed on each positive sample.

CELLULOSE ACETATE ELECTROPHORESIS[4-7]

This is a screening test that detects the presence of some abnormal hemoglobin variants. The test is very useful in the diagnosis of S and C hemoglobinopathies, as well as several other hemoglobinopathies.

Principle

Electrophoresis is the movement of charged particles in an electrical field. At an alkaline pH, hemoglobin is a negatively charged protein. Therefore, the hemoglobin migrates toward the anode in an electrical field. During electrophoresis, various hemoglobins separate because of differences in charges caused by structural variations of the hemoglobin molecule. This separation allows detection of many of the different hemoglobins. Electrophoresis with cellulose acetate as a support medium is often used for the initial screening because the equipment can be easily obtained and the method is rapid and relatively easy.

Electrophoresis equipment may be obtained from one of the suppliers.

Specimen Requirements

A whole blood specimen is collected in EDTA or heparin. When refrigerated at 4 °C, specimens are stable for up to 10 days. When the volume of blood drawn from the patient is of major concern, several heparinized capillary tubes are sufficient. However, this type of specimen should be analyzed within 2–3 days.

Reagents

Buffer

1. Stock buffer (Tris, EDTA, Boric Acid [pH 8.2–8.6])
2. Working buffer

Buffer may be purchased prepackaged. Store at 15–30 °C. Expiration date is printed on the box.

Dilute 20 mL of stock buffer with 980 mL of de-ionized water. The solution is stable for 2 months at 15–30 °C.

Ponceau S Stain

Store at room temperature. Expiration date is on the label. (This reagent may be used many times. Refill as needed. Cover to prevent evaporation.)

Solution for Destaining

To 475 mL of de-ionized water, add 25 mL of glacial acetic acid.

Note: Always add acid to water, not water to acid. This solution is stable for 1 month in a tightly sealed container.

Clearing Solution (Clear Aid, Helena)

To 70 mL of absolute methanol, add 30 mL of glacial acetic acid. (This is done under a hood.) Then add 4 mL of Clear Aid. This solution is stable for 1 month in a tightly sealed container.

Hemolysate Reagent (Helena)

Store at room temperature. Expiration date is printed on the label.

Quality Control

A control sample containing at least two different known hemoglobins (HbAS is preferred, but HbAC could be used) must be applied to each strip with the unknown samples. Slight current fluctuations, different buffer lots, or different application variables cause the same sample to vary slightly in migration rate with each run. The patterns of unknown samples must be compared with those of known samples.

Procedure

1. Dissolve one package of buffer in 980 mL of de-ionized water.
2. Properly code the required number of cellulose acetate plates by marking on the glossy hard side with a permanent marker in the bottom right corner when the plate is positioned, so that the longest side is from left to right rather than up and down.
3. Soak the required number of plates in buffer for 5 minutes. The plates may be wetted by slowly and uniformly lowering each plate into the buffer. Take care in placing the strip in the buffer in order to prevent air from being trapped as bubbles in the strip. (This causes uneven migration of hemoglobins, making patterns difficult to interpret.) The same soaking buffer may be used for soaking as many as 12 plates or for approximately 1 week if stored tightly closed. If used for a prolonged period, residual solvents from the plates may build up in the buffer and cause poor separation of the proteins, or evaporation may cause higher buffer concentration.
4. Pour 100 mL of buffer into each of the outer sections of the electrophoresis chamber.
5. Wet the two disposable wicks in the buffer, and drape one over each support bridge, ensuring that the wicks make contact with the buffer and that there are no air bubbles under the wicks.
6. Cover the chamber to prevent buffer evaporation. Discard buffer after use.
7. Prepare a hemolysate of the control and patient samples according to the following procedure (alternatively, the procedure in the citrate agar gel electrophoresis procedure may be used):
   a. Mix sample tube by inversion.
   b. Pipette 0.2–0.5 mL into a 12 × 75 tube; fill with 0.9% NaCl; cover and mix by inversion.
   c. Centrifuge 5 minutes, remove wash solution, and repeat wash.
   d. After second wash, remove wash solution and pipette a small volume of packed cells into a clean 12 × 75 tube. Add a volume of hemolyzing reagent to make a 1:5 dilution (e.g., 0.05 mL of washed cells plus 0.20 mL of hemolyzing solution).
   e. Mix well using a vortex; let sit 5 minutes and wash again.
8. Using a 20-μL pipette and a rubber bulb, fill the sample well plate with the control sample in position 1 and hemolysates of patient samples in the remaining wells. (For Helena systems, use 5 μL of sample.)
9. To prevent evaporation, cover the sample well plate with a glass slide if the samples are not used within 2 minutes.
10. Prime the applicator by depressing the tips

into the sample wells five or six times. Fill applicator tips to the indented margin, but do not overfill. Apply this loading to a piece of blotter paper. If it is necessary to wipe tips, do so carefully so as not to damage them. (Priming the applicator makes the second loading much more uniform.) Do not load the applicator again at this point, but proceed quickly to the next step.

11. Remove the wetted cellulose plate from the buffer and blot once firmly between two blotters. Place the plate in the aligning base, the cellulose acetate side up, aligning the edge of the plate with the black scribe line marked "cathode application." The identification mark should be aligned with sample number 1 on the underside of the top left corner. Before placing the plate in the aligning base, place a drop of water or buffer on the center of the aligning base. This prevents the plate from shifting during the sample application.

12. Apply the sample to the plate by depressing the applicator tips into the sample well three or four times and promptly transferring the applicator to the aligning base. Press the button and hold it down for 5 seconds.

13. Quickly place the plate in the electrophoresis chamber, cellulose acetate side down with application point closest to cathode (−) pole. Place a weight (e.g., a glass slide or a coin) on the plate to ensure contact with the wicks.

14. Subject the plate to electrophoresis for 25 minutes at 350 V.

15. Remove the plate from the electrophoresis chamber. Submerge in Ponceau S stain for 5 minutes.

16. Destain in three successive washes of 5% acetic acid. Allow the plate to stay in each wash 2 minutes. One wash may be reused from run to run, but at least two must be prepared fresh for each run.

17. Dehydrate the plate in two successive washes of absolute methanol. Destaining and dehydrating work better if the staining dish is agitated or rotated.

18. Place the plate in clearing solution for 5–10 minutes. Prepare this solution fresh daily.

19. Remove the plate from the clearing solution and drain off excess solution. (Care must be taken in this step, because the cellulose acetate is very soft and can be easily damaged until it is dried.)

20. Place the plate, cellulose acetate side up, on a blotter pad and allow to air dry, or place in the laboratory drying oven at 56 °C for 10 minutes or until dry. Drying can be facilitated by leaning the plate against something so that the clearing solution can drain off while it is drying.

21. Label the plates appropriately and store in plastic envelopes that come with the kit.

22. For a qualitative evaluation, the hemoglobin plate may be inspected visually for the presence of abnormal hemoglobin bands. The control sample provides a marker for band identification.

23. If a quantitative measurement of hemoglobin bands is desired, quantitation by a densitometer method should be performed.

24. The dried plates are stable for an indefinite period of time and may be stored in plastic envelopes. Prolonged exposure to light may cause fading.

Interpretation

The migration patterns of hemoglobins on cellulose acetate and the results of hemoglobin solubility tests are compared. Both the solubility and the cellulose acetate pattern should be reported.

Migration patterns on cellulose acetate for the most common hemoglobins are seen in Figure 18–29.

Further testing is frequently necessary in order to correctly interpret the hemoglobin patterns.

Sources of Error and Comments

1. Buffer of improper pH; cloudy or contaminated buffer.
2. Hemolysates that are old, discolored, or contaminated.
3. Improper presoaking (trapped air bubbles) or blotting of cellulose acetate strips.
4. Improper sample application (too much or too little).
5. Delay in applying sample to blotted strip.
6. Improper placement of samples on medium or of medium in chamber.
7. Poor contact with wicks.
8. Faulty power supply (350 V should yield 3 mA per electrophoresis strip).

Hemoglobin solubility is done on all electrophoresis samples and correlated with migration patterns. Some abnormal hemoglobins have similar electrophoretic mobilities and must be differentiated by other methods.

CITRATE AGAR GEL ELECTROPHORESIS[4, 8–10]

The citrate agar gel electrophoresis performed at acid pH allows for further differentiation between hemoglobins that migrate at the same rate on cellulose acetate electrophoresis. Electrophoresis in citrate agar at a pH of 6.0–6.2 allows HbS to be distinguished from HbD and HbG and allows HbC to be distinguished from HbE and HbO. There are four major zones on citrate agar: F, A, S, and C. HbF is the fastest moving hemoglobin (cathode to anode) and is easily separated from HbA. All hemoglobin variants except S and C move in the same general zone as HbA. HbS and HbC move into distinct and independent areas.

Citrate agar gel electrophoresis is a useful procedure for detecting small amounts of HbA in the presence of large volumes of HbF and vice versa, and in detecting small amounts of adult HbA and HbS in umbilical cord blood at birth.

Principle

As in standard electrophoretic techniques, the agar gel method is based on the principle that a charged ion or protein will migrate in an electrical field. However, with the standard techniques such as cellulose acetate electrophoresis, HbS, HbD, and HbG all have identical migration rates, as do HbC, HbC-Harlem, HbE, and HbO-Arab.

Specimen Requirements

The specimen should be whole blood collected with the use of any of the following anti-coagulants: EDTA, sodium citrate, or heparin. If refrigerated at 4 °C, the specimen is stable for up to 10 days. Heparinized capillary tubes may be used when the volume of blood from the patient is a concern; however, this is *not* the specimen of choice, and it should be analyzed immediately.

Reagents

Buffer

1. Stock buffer (pH 6.0–6.3, 0.5 mol/L); 147 g of sodium citrate; 4.3 g of citric acid; 1 L of de-ionized water
2. Working citrate buffer

Pour 100 mL of citrate buffer into a 1000-mL volumetric flask and add de-ionized water up to the scribed line. Adjust the pH to 6.0–6.3 by adding drops of citric acid. Refrigerate at 2–8 °C. The buffered solution remains stable for 1 month. Discontinue use if microbial growth is visible.

Stain

5.0%	acetic acid	10.0 mL
0.2%	O-dianisidine in methanol	5.0 mL
1.0%	sodium nitroferricyanide	1.0 mL
3.0%	hydrogen peroxide	1.0 mL

Hemolysate Reagent (Helena)

A commercial hemolysate can be obtained through Helena Laboratories. The expiration date is provided by the manufacturer. Regardless of this expiration date, however, use of the product should be discontinued immediately if microbial growth or any form of contamination becomes apparent.

Quality Control

A control sample containing at least two different known hemoglobins (HbAS, HbAC, etc.) must be applied to each strip with the unknown samples. Slight current fluctuations, different buffer lots, or different application variables cause the same sample to vary slightly in migration rate with each run. The patterns of unknown samples must be compared with those of known samples.

Procedure

1. Remove the citrate agar plate from its plastic and remove the tape and coverslide. Allow the plate to come to room temperature.
2. Fill each side of the electrophoresis chamber with 100 mL of citrate buffer (pH of buffer should be checked before use).
3. Soak 2 precut sponges in buffer and place one in each of the outer compartments so that the top surface protrudes approximately 2 mm above the inner chamber ridges. Replace the chamber cover.
4. Prepare a hemolysate of patients and controls according to the following procedures (alternatively, the procedure for cellulose acetate electrophoresis can be used):
   a. Centrifuge whole blood for 10 minutes at a relative centrifugal force of about 2000 × g (gravity).
   b. Remove plasma, and wash cells three times with 0.85% NaCl.
   c. After three washings, completely remove all saline.
   d. Lyse cells by adding five volumes of distilled water.
   e. Add one volume of chloroform or toluene, shake vigorously, and centrifuge at 3000 × g for 15 minutes. (Caution: These solvents are toxic and should be handled under a hood).
   f. Remove the clear hemolysate at the top of the tube, and filter through a layer of Whatman No. 1 filter paper.
5. Using a disposable micropipette, streak a small drop of each hemolysate in the corresponding sample well.

6. Place the agar plate into the aligning base so that application may be made at one end of the plate.
7. Remove the spring from the applicator. Load the applicator by gently depressing the tips into the sample wells several times. The first several loadings should be wiped off in order to make the application clearer and more uniform. Once the applicator is loaded, it should be used immediately.
8. Transfer the loaded applicator to the aligning base. Gently allow the tips to rest against the agar plate for 60 seconds.
9. Place the plate gel side down in the chamber so that the gel layer makes contact with the top surface of the sponges and with the application nearest the anode (+).
10. Tightly close the chamber, attach the electrodes, and plug into the power supply. Set the voltage at 50 for 45 minutes.
11. After electrophoresis, unplug the power supply and remove the gel plate from the chamber. Place the plate in a staining tray and cover the entire surface of the plate with the staining solution for 5–10 minutes.
12. Rinse the plate for 10 minutes with 5.0% acetic acid. Remove the plate from the staining dish.
13. Allow the plate to dry by air or in an oven at 100 °C for 2 hours. Replace the cover, reseal with tape, and label appropriately.

Interpretation

Normal adult hemoglobin migrates as a single A band. The mobilities of various mutant hemoglobins on citrate agar and cellulose acetate are shown in Figure 18–7.

Sources of Error and Comments

1. Buffers of improper pH; cloudy or contaminated buffers.
2. Hemolysates that are old, discolored, or contaminated.
3. Improper sample application; imperfections in the agar plate.
4. Improper placement of plate in the chamber.

FETAL HEMOGLOBIN DETERMINATION[7, 11–14]

Levels of HbF (alkali-resistant hemoglobin) are increased in several conditions: various hemoglobinopathies, unstable hemoglobins, infancy, pregnancy, thalassemia, hereditary persistence of HbF, and doubly heterozygous conditions such as HbSD, HbSC, HbS–thalassemia, and HbC–thalassemia.

Principle

The amount of HbF is expressed as a percentage of the total hemoglobin concentration. Most human hemoglobins denature readily at an alkaline pH and can be precipitated when an ammonium sulfate solution is added to make a 40% solution. However, HbF is not so denatured. This technique permits a rapid and relatively simple quantitative measurement of the amount of HbF present in human blood.

Specimen Requirements

The specimen may be anti-coagulated with any anti-coagulant (usually EDTA or heparin). Specimens are stable at 4 °C for 1 week if the anti-coagulant is EDTA or heparin and for 3–4 weeks if collected with acid citrate dextrose (ACD) solution. This procedure requires a minimum of 1.0 mL of whole blood. Avoid freezing the specimen, because a completely hemolyzed specimen cannot be used.

Reagents

Betke's Solution

Potassium cyanide	200.0 mg
Potassium ferricyanide	200.0 mg

Dilute to 1000 mL with de-ionized water. The solution is stable indefinitely when stored in a brown bottle at room temperature.

Caution: Betke's solution has approximately four times the cyanide concentration of Drabkin's solution. It should be handled with appropriate care.

Saturated Ammonium Sulfate

Ammonium sulfate [$(NH_4)_2SO_4$]	375.0 g
De-ionized water	500.0 mL

Add the ammonium sulfate to de-ionized water; warm, and agitate to bring into solution. Crystals reappear upon cooling, which indicates saturation. The solution is stable indefinitely at room temperature.

1.2 N Sodium Hydroxide

To 24.0 g of NaOH, add distilled water until the total volume is 500 mL. The solution is stable indefinitely at room temperature.

Quality Control

A second sample that has a normal hematocrit and a normal white blood cell count is processed along with the patient's sample. If the control sample is not within the normal range for HbF, another control sample is selected, and the test is repeated.

Procedure

1. Hemolysate is prepared according to the following procedure:
   a. Place approximately 1 mL of whole blood in a centrifuge tube, and add cold isotonic saline to a volume of approximately 10 mL.
   b. Centrifuge at 4 °C, 2500 rpm, for 15 minutes and discard the supernatant, including the buffy coat.
   c. Transfer 0.2 mL of packed cells to 4 mL of Betke's solution. Let stand 15 minutes.
2. Transfer 2.8 mL of the hemolysate to a test tube.
3. Add 0.2 mL of 1.2 N NaOH and mix. Begin timing when the sodium hydroxide solution is added.
4. Exactly 2 minutes after the addition of sodium hydroxide, add 2.0 mL of saturated ammonium sulfate and mix. Incubate 5 minutes to allow protein to coagulate.
5. Filter through a small-sized filter paper (Whatman No. 42 is recommended). If the filtrate is not absolutely clear, refilter through the same paper (HbF fraction, or FF).
6. Read absorbance of the filtrate at 540 nm in a spectrophotometer, using a cuvette with a 1-cm light path. If the absorbance exceeds 1.0, dilute to 1:2 or 1:3 with distilled water and reread.
7. Transfer 0.4 mL of the original hemolysate (not the one treated with sodium hydroxide) to another tube, and add 6.75 mL of distilled water. Agitate to mix, and read the optical density of this in the same manner as in step 6. This provides a 10% dilution of the total hemoglobin fraction (TF).

Calculations

% alkali resistant hemoglobin

$$= \frac{\text{absorbance of FF} \times 100}{\text{absorbance of diluted TF} \times 10}$$

Example: Absorbance reading of FF = 0.009; absorbance reading of diluted TF = 0.356. Therefore,

$$\frac{0.009 \times 100}{0.356 \times 10} = 0.25\%$$

Interpretation

In adults, the normal range for the HbF concentration is 0.2–1.0%. The HbF concentration is usually between 5% and 15% of the total hemoglobin in the high HbF or delta/beta type of thalassemia minor. In beta–thalassemia major, the HbF concentration may be 30–90% or even more of the total hemoglobin. Slight increases in HbF concentration are also found in a variety of unrelated hematologic disorders, such as aplastic anemia, hereditary spherocytosis, and myeloproliferative disorders. In homozygous sickle cell disease, HbF concentration is often slightly increased. Higher concentrations of HbF occur in patients with HbS/beta^0–thalassemia and in patients who are doubly heterozygous for the HbS gene and a gene for hereditary persistence of HbF (HPFH). These disorders may be differentiated by family studies or by acid elution (Kleihauer-Betke) test for HbF, which reveals uniform intra-erythrocytic distribution of HbF in HPFH and nonuniform distribution in HbS/beta–thalassemia. The electrophoretic finding of a moderate increase in HbF and small quantities of HbA in a patient who has mostly HbS is strong evidence of HbS/beta–thalassemia (if the patient has not had a transfusion).

Sources of Error and Comments

1. For anemic patients, it may be necessary to use 0.1 ml of packed red cells in step 1c. Results are satisfactory with this half volume. No other adjustments in volume are required.
2. There are several published variations of the alkali denaturation test of hemoglobin. The following are two important advantages of this (Betke) procedure:
   a. It is a sufficiently sensitive method for measuring concentrations of fetal hemoglobin in the range of 1–10% of the total hemoglobin.
   b. It does not give erroneously high values when carboxyhemoglobin is present, as do other alkali denaturation tests (because the carbon monoxide is released in this procedure).
3. It must be recognized that this procedure and other rapid tests for fetal hemoglobin give erroneously low results when HbF comprises 30% or more of the total hemoglobin in a specimen. For example, these techniques underestimate by about 50% the actual HbF concentration of umbilical cord blood.
4. In addition to HbF, the rare Hb Rainier appears to be alkali-resistant and Hb Bethesda also appears to be somewhat alkali-resistant.

HEMOGLOBIN A$_2$ QUANTITATION BY MICROCOLUMN[15, 16]

A very rapid and accurate method for determining the percentage of HbA$_2$ in hemolysate is Sickle-Thal by Helena Laboratories.

Principle

The Helena Sickle-Thal Quik Column Method quantitates HbA$_2$ by an anion exchange chromatography method. The anion exchange resin is a product of cellulose covalently coupled to small, positively charged molecules. In the anion exchange chromatography of HbA$_2$, buffer and pH levels are controlled to cause different hemoglobins to display varying net negative charges. These negatively charged hemoglobins are attracted to the positively charged resin and consequently bind. After binding, the hemoglobins are removed discerningly from the resin by changing the pH or ionic strength of the elution buffer (developer). HbA$_2$ (also HbC and HbE, if present) is eluted, and this fraction is equated to the total hemoglobin by measuring the absorbance of each, by using a spectrophotometer and then calculating the percentage of HbA$_2$.

Specimen Requirements

Whole blood is collected in EDTA. The specimen may be refrigerated at 4 °C for 3–5 days before preparation of hemolysate.

Reagents

Sickle-Thal Quik Column (Helena)

The reagent should be stored at 2–6 °C. Bacterial contamination is indicated by a yellow or yellow-green color.

HbA$_2$ Developer
Hemolysate Reagent C
(Sickle-Thal Column Kit)

These clear, colorless solutions should be stored at 2–6 °C.

HbA$_2$ Quik Column Control Samples
(Normal and Abnormal)

Store at −20 °C. Reconstitute with 1 mL of type I de-ionized water. After reconstitution, control samples are stable for 14 days at 2–6 °C.

Quality Control

Two control samples, one normal and the other abnormal, are set up with each batch. The control results should fall within the manufacturer's expected range of results. If the control results do not fall within that range, no patient results are reported. All controls are reconstituted, used, and stored according to the manufacturer's directions. No further dilution is necessary before application to the Sickle-Thal Column.

Procedure

1. For each patient or control quantitation to be performed, the following are required:
   a. One Sickle-Thal Quik Column.
   b. One small collection tube, labeled A$_2$.
   c. One large collection tube, labeled TF (total fraction).
   d. One small test tube for hemolysate.
2. Bring the appropriate number of columns and reagents to room temperature before performing the test.
3. Pour 50 μL of whole blood into a small test tube. Add 200 μL of hemolysate reagent C to the test tube and shake. Let stand 5 minutes. (Note: The reconstituted controls do not need to be diluted with hemolysate reagent C.)
4. Prepare the Sickle-Thal Quik Columns, by inverting each column twice to remove any resin from the top cap closure.
5. Remove the top cap closure and, using a Pasteur pipette with a small rubber bulb, resuspend the contents of the column.
6. Immediately after resuspension of each column, hold the column over a sink or absorbent paper and remove the bottom cap closure, allowing the buffer to elute. If the column is allowed to stand with the bottom cap closure in place, resuspension must be repeated.
7. As the resin repacks, a slurry interface slowly moves up the tube. As soon as the slurry settles, aspirate the remaining supernatant (making sure not to disturb the resin) and discard, flushing the sink with running water. (It is very important to remove all the buffer from the column. Excess buffer going into the collection tube will cause erroneous HbA$_2$ results.)
8. Carefully apply 100 μL of the hemolysate (patient sample preparation) to the Sickle-Thal Quik Column. During application, do not allow bubbles to form in the sample or to run down the side of the column. Use of excessive force during application will disturb the resin and may cause erroneous results.
9. Immediately after sample application to the column, add 100 μL of the sample preparation to the large collection tube labeled total fraction (TF). Fill the tube to the scribed line with de-ionized water so that the total volume is 15 mL.
10. Allow the sample to be completely absorbed into the resin. The hemolysate will have a glossy appearance until the sample is completely absorbed by the resin. Upon complete absorption, the top of the resin will have a dull matte-like appearance.

11. Upon completion of absorption of the hemolysate into the resin, place the column in the Quik Column rack aligned over the small collection tube.

12. Slowly apply 3.0 mL of HbA$_2$ developer to the column. Excessive force will cause a disturbance of the resin, producing erroneous results. The developer above the resin should be clear. If the developer contains hemoglobin, the column should be discarded and the test repeated with a fresh column.

13. Allow all the developer to pass through the column into the small collection tube (approximately 30 minutes). This eluate contains the HbA$_2$.

14. The eluate in the small collection tube should reach the scribed line (3-mL volume); if it does not, add de-ionized water to adjust the level to the scribed line. The volume should never be above the scribed line; otherwise, erroneous values will result.

15. Invert all tubes several times to ensure thorough mixing.

16. Set the spectrophotometer at 415 nm. Properly zero the instrument, using water as a blank.

17. Read and record the absorbance of each eluate (HbA$_2$ fraction) and each total fraction. Absorbance values for both fractions are stable for 24 hours at 2–5 °C.

Calculations

$$\% \text{ HbA}_2 = \frac{100 \text{ (absorbance HbA}_2 \text{ fraction)}}{5 \text{ (absorbance total fraction)}}$$

Interpretation

Normal values are in the range of 1.7%–3.4%. Values between 3.5% and 8% are indicative of beta-thalassemia trait. However, HbA$_2$ levels may be normal if iron deficiency coexists. HbE and HbC, if present, will elute with HbA$_2$, indicating HbA$_2$ concentrations higher than 8%. When values are above 8%, there is a strong probability that HbC or HbE is present. This should be confirmed by other tests (such as cellulose acetate and agar gel electrophoresis).

Hemoglobin Defects

HEINZ BODY PREPARATION[4, 17, 18]

Heinz body preparations are helpful in the diagnosis of anemias caused by oxidative stress resulting from enzyme deficiencies, by abnormal synthesis of reducing agents (such as glutathione), or by an unstable hemoglobin. The hexose monophosphate shunt, in addition to glucose metabolism, provides reducing agents to protect the red blood cell from oxidative stress.

Principle

When red blood cells deficient in reducing capacity are subjected to an oxidizing agent such as acetylphenylhydrazine, the hemoglobin molecule and other cellular components are oxidized and precipitated as denatured hemoglobin known as Heinz bodies. These bodies are then stained with crystal violet, a vital stain, which allows them to be seen with brightfield microscopy. They can also be viewed on a wet preparation in phase microscopy.

Specimen Requirements

Blood collected in heparin, EDTA, or acid citrate dextrose is satisfactory, but the blood specimen must be no more than 4 hours old. Crenation of cells causes difficulty in interpretation. The fresher the specimen, the easier and more reliable the result.

Reagents

Phosphate Buffer, 0.067 M, pH 7.6

Potassium phosphate, monobasic (KH$_2$PO$_4$)	0.1186 g
Sodium Phosphate, Dibasic (Na$_2$HPO$_4$–12 H$_2$O)	0.2083 g

Dissolve in 100 mL of de-ionized water.

Buffer-Glucose-Acetyl Phenylhydrazine (APH) Solution

Glucose (dextrose, anhydrous granular)	20 mg
Acetylphenylhydrazine (APH)	10 mg
Phosphate buffer	10 mL

Mix well. Prepare fresh before each use.

Crystal Violet Solution

Crystal violet	2 g
0.85% NaCl	100 mL

Add the crystal violet to the NaCl and stir for approximately 20 minutes. Filter through Whatman No. 42 filter paper. Mixture is stable indefinitely.

Quality Control

A normal blood sample is tested simultaneously with the patient specimen. If red blood cells of the normal control contain Heinz bodies before incubation with acetylphenylhydrazine or five or more Heinz bodies after incubation, another control must be selected, fresh reagents prepared, and the procedure repeated.

Procedure

1. In a 12×75 mm tube, add 20 μL of whole blood and 50 μL of crystal violet solution. Incubate at room temperature for 10 minutes.
2. Prepare and examine films and moist preparations without further staining.
3. If Heinz bodies are attached to the red blood cell membrane, refer to the "Interpretation" section. If Heinz bodies are not present, proceed with step 4.
4. In a 13×100 mm tube, add 2 mL of the buffer-glucose-APH solution and 0.1 mL of whole blood.
5. Immediately mix the suspension, aerate with gentle bubbling of air through the solution, and place in a 37 °C water bath.
6. After 2 hours, mix and aerate the suspension. After 4 hours, repeat aeration.
7. After the last aeration, mix 0.02 mL of the suspension with 0.05 mL of crystal violet in a 12×75 mm tube and incubate at room temperature for 10 minutes.
8. Prepare and examine films and moist preparations without further staining.
9. Count 100 red blood cells, recording the number containing five or more Heinz bodies per cell and the number containing fewer than five Heinz bodies per cell.

Interpretation

Normal: Before incubation with acetylphenylhydrazine, no Heinz bodies should be detected. After incubation with acetylphenylhydrazine, 68% or more red blood cells contain one to four Heinz bodies per cell, and 0%–32% contain five or more Heinz bodies per cell. (These values permit no false negative results.) In a susceptible individual, greater than 32% of the red blood cells will contain 5 or more Heinz bodies.

Heinz bodies stain deep purple and vary from 1 to 4 μm in diameter. They tend to be attached to the red blood cell membrane. Heinz bodies are usually caused by excess alpha chains in beta thalassemia, excess beta chains in HbH disease, unstable hemoglobin resulting from structural defects, and precipitation of normal hemoglobin after an exposure to an oxidant, as in glucose-6-phosphate dehydrogenase (G-6-PD) deficiency.

RED BLOOD CELL DENATURATION TEST[4, 17, 19]

Some abnormal hemoglobins are unstable and precipitate within the red blood cells when these cells are heated.

Principle

A phosphate buffer is added to red blood cells that were hemolyzed with water and incubated at 50 °C for 3 hours. Unstable hemoglobins that are heat-sensitive denature, and a flocculent precipitate results within 1 hour of incubation. Normal blood shows little, if any, precipitation.

Reagents

Phosphate Buffer

0.1 mol/L of NaH_2PO_4 (13.8 g of $NaH_2PO_4 \cdot 2H_2O$ in 1 L of distilled water)
0.1 mol/L of Na_2HPO_4, anhydrous (14.2 g in 1 L of distilled water)

Add 19.2 mL of 0.1 mol/L of NaH_2PO_4 to 80.8 mL of 0.1 mol/L of Na_2HPO_4. Mix and let stand for 10 minutes. Adjust pH to 7.4.

Quality Control

Test a normal control sample along with the specimen.

Procedure

1. In separate test tubes, wash 1 mL of the patient sample and 1 mL of control blood with 0.85% saline four times. Discard supernatant after each wash.
2. Lyse the cells by adding 5 mL of distilled water to each tube.
3. Add 5 mL of phosphate buffer to each tube; mix and centrifuge for 10 minutes at 3000 rpm.
4. Remove upper 2 mL of clear supernatant and incubate for 1 hour at 50 °C.
5. Record the appearance of the test and control solutions.
6. Incubate for 2 hours, and again record the appearance of both solutions.

Interpretation

Normal Control—little or no precipitation.
Patient—flocculent precipitation after 1 hour; greatly increased flocculation after 2 hours.

Results will be negative if only a small amount of abnormal hemoglobin is present or if hemoglobin is insensitive to heat. The results can be quantitated through calculation of the percentage of unstable hemoglobin present, based on the difference in absorbance of the unheated sample and the heated sample divided by absorbance of the unheated sample.

UNSTABLE HEMOGLOBIN SCREEN[7, 20, 21, 22]

This test, also called the isopropanol stability test, is used to diagnose the presence of unstable hemoglobins, thus aiding in their identification.

Principle

By making the solvent in a hemoglobin solution more nonpolar, the internal bonding forces of the hemoglobin molecule are weakened and its stability decreases. Thus in a 17% isopropanol solution at 37 °C, normal hemoglobin is of borderline stability and will begin to precipitate after approximately 40 minutes. The presence of a significant molecular instability will produce much more rapid precipitation, usually evident within 5 minutes, and flocculation within 20 minutes.

Specimen Requirements

Any anti-coagulated specimen is acceptable; however, an EDTA specimen is preferable. Blood specimens containing most unstable hemoglobins may be stored at 4 °C for several days before hemolyzing.

Reagents

Isopropanol-Tris Buffer

Tris (hydroxymethyl) aminomethane	12.11 g
Distilled water	700 mL
100% isopropyl alcohol	170 mL

Mix well and adjust pH to 7.4 with concentrated hydrochloric acid. Bring volume to 1 L with distilled water. Keep in a tightly stoppered bottle at room temperature.

Quality Control

A normal blood sample must be run simultaneously with the patient specimen. If the normal blood demonstrates precipitation within 20 minutes, repeat the procedure, using another control blood sample.

Procedure

1. Prepare fresh hemolysate:
   a. Pour approximately 2–3 mL of EDTA blood into a conical centrifuge tube.
   b. Remove the plasma from the cells by centrifuging at 3000 rpm for 18 minutes. Aspirate and discard supernatant off the cells.
   c. Wash the red blood cells by adding up to 10 mL (mark 10 mL line on centrifuge tube) of isotonic saline. Mix well and centrifuge at 3000 rpm for 10 minutes.
   d. Remove and discard the saline layer and repeat the step twice more. After the third washing, remove as much supernatant as possible.
   e. Add an equal volume of de-ionized water to the cells, and mix well.
   f. Add a 0.5 volume of organic solvent (toluene, chloroform, or carbon tetrachloride), and mix by vortex. Let the solution stand for 20 minutes. Centrifuge for 10 minutes at 3000 rpm.
   g. Transfer the hemoglobin solution to a clean tube, and label immediately.
2. Equilibrate two small stoppered tubes containing 2 mL of the isopropanol buffer at 37 °C in a water bath.
3. Add 0.2 mL of fresh control hemolysate to one tube and 0.2 mL of fresh test hemolysate to the other tube. Restopper the tubes, mix by inversion, and replace in the 37 °C water bath.
4. The tubes are observed at 0, 5, 20, and 40 minutes for the presence and type of precipitation.

Interpretation

Normal hemoglobin will not precipitate until about 30–40 minutes. Unstable hemoglobin will show signs of precipitation by 5 minutes and flocculation by 20 minutes.

Sources of Error and Comments

1. Using a 17% isopropanol solution and temperature control at 37 °C is critical.
2. The pH is not critical, but it should not fall below 7.2.
3. Hemolysates should be freshly made, although cells may be several days old without affecting the test.
4. The presence of large amounts of methemoglobin may produce false positive results, because methemoglobin is considerably less stable than oxyhemoglobin.
5. Increased HbF (5% or greater) may produce false positive results.

Membrane Defects

ERYTHROCYTE OSMOTIC FRAGILITY[23, 24]

The erythrocyte osmotic fragility is useful in detecting hereditary spherocytosis, especially in mildly affected patients.

Principle

Whole blood is added to saline diluents that have concentrations equivalent to 0.00%–0.85% NaCl. When red blood cells are placed into a hypotonic solution, water is taken into the cells, causing them to swell, to become spherical, and eventually to lyse, releasing hemoglobin. The critical volume for cells from patients with spherocytosis is reached much closer to the isotonic concentration (0.85%) than is that for normal cells.

The percentage of hemolysis of the patient sample is determined after a 20-minute incubation at room temperature and is plotted against that of a normal control sample. For normal samples, an almost symmetric sigmoid-shaped curve results. This procedure may also be performed on whole blood that has been incubated at 37 °C under sterile conditions in order to detect mild spherocytosis.

Specimen Requirements

Whole blood that has been defibrinated or collected in heparin

A normal control sample collected in the same manner

Reagents

Stock Saline

One percent NaCl solution: Add 1 g of NaCl crystals, analytic grade, to 100 mL of distilled water in a volumetric flask. Shake to dissolve.

Working NaCl Concentrations

Tube No.	1% NaCl (mL)	Distilled H₂O (mL)	NaCl %, Final Concentration
1	8.5	1.5	0.85
2	6.5	3.5	0.65
3	6.0	4.0	0.60
4	5.5	4.5	0.55
5	5.0	5.0	0.50
6	4.5	5.5	0.45
7	4.0	6.0	0.40
8	3.5	6.5	0.35
9	3.0	7.0	0.30
0	0.0	10.0	0.00

Quality Control

1. Control blood should be treated in same manner as the patient sample.
2. No visible hemolysis should be seen in the 0.85% tube.
3. Values for the control blood must fall within the expected normal curve.

Procedure

1. Label 10 tubes for patient and control samples as follows: 0, 0.30, 0.35, 0.40, 0.45, 0.50, 0.55, 0.60, 0.65, and 0.85. Each tube represents the corresponding concentration of NaCl; the tube labeled 0 contains only distilled water.
2. Using a 20-μL positive displacement pipette, add 20 μL each of patient and control blood to corresponding tubes.
3. Cover with parafilm and invert several times to mix.
4. Incubate at room temperature for 30 minutes.
5. At the end of 30 minutes, centrifuge all tubes at 2000 rpm for 5 minutes. Be careful not to disturb the cell button when removing tubes from the centrifuge.
6. Read and record the absorbance, or optical density (OD) of the supernatant of each tube at 540 nm in a spectrophotometer against a distilled water blank.
7. Plot % hemolysis for patient (tube X) against % hemolysis of control (tube 0).

Calculations

$$\% \text{ lysis} = \frac{\text{OD of tube X} - \text{OD of tube 1}}{\text{OD of tube 0} - \text{OD of tube 1}} \times 100$$

Interpretation

An increased osmotic fragility is seen in spherocytosis. A decreased osmotic fragility is seen in thalassemia (see Fig. 17–4).

SUCROSE HEMOLYSIS TEST[25, 26]

The sucrose hemolysis test is a screening procedure for the presence of paroxysmal nocturnal hemoglobinuria (PNH). Positive test results should be confirmed with the acidified serum test.

Principle

The sucrose hemolysis test depends on the activation of complement at low ionic strengths. When normal red blood cells are suspended in an isotonic sucrose solution, osmotic lysis does not occur, whereas cells from patients with PNH hemolyze. In the normal red blood cell, the sucrose does not penetrate the cell membrane; PNH cells, however, are sensitive to complement, which may cause lysis by one of two mechanisms: either the PNH cells develop membrane defects through which sucrose can pass and cause hemolysis, or complement itself may cause large enough defects to allow the loss of red blood cell contents.

Specimen Requirements

Patient—Whole blood defibrinated or collected in citrate or EDTA

Control—Whole blood defibrinated or collected in citrate, plus 20 mL non–anti-coagulated blood (to provide serum). Must be of same ABO group as the patients blood and contain no unusual antibodies. Serum must be fresh or have been stored at −4 °C for no longer than 1 week.

Reagents

Sucrose (Stock)

Sucrose	486 g
Sodium barbital	5.1 g
Distilled water	1000 mL

Dissolve the reagents in 500 mL of distilled water. Adjust pH to 7.3–7.4 with hydrochloride, and add water to achieve a volume of 1 L. Stable for 1 year at 4 °C.

Sucrose (Working Solution)

0.90% NaCl
0.01 M NH$_4$OH

Dilute 2 parts working solution with 8 parts stock (2 mL plus 8 mL or 20 mL plus 80 mL.

Quality Control

The control sample must be of the same ABO type as the patient sample and not show more than 5% lysis. Failure of the control sample to demonstrate the expected value requires trouble-shooting and repetition of the test.

Procedure

1. Preparation of cells: Centrifuge whole blood from both patient and control. Remove the plasma and buffy coat. Wash cells three times in 0.9% NaCl. After last washing, resuspend in 0.9% NaCl to make an approximately 50% suspension.
2. Prepare serum: After complete clotting of specimen, centrifuge and separate serum from the control sample. Repeat centrifugation to ensure that serum that is free of red blood cells.
3. Label eight tubes (1–4 for patient and 1–4 for control samples) and prepare the test mixture as follows:

Tube 1—0.90 mL of sucrose, 0.05 mL of cells, 0.05 mL of serum
Tube 2—0.95 mL of sucrose, 0.05 mL of cells
Tube 3—0.95 mL of sucrose, 0.05 mL of serum
Tube 4—0.05 mL of cells, 0.95 mL of 0.01 M NH$_4$OH

4. Incubate at room temperature for 60 minutes.
5. Add 4 mL of 0.9% NaCl to each tube.
6. Centrifuge for 5 minutes at 2000 rpm.
7. Read and record the optical density (OD) of the supernatant of each tube at 540 nm against a distilled water blank in a controlled spectrophotometer.
8. Calculate the percentage of lysis.

Calculations

$$\% \text{ lysis} = \frac{\text{OD of tube 1} - (\text{OD of tube 2} + \text{OD of tube 3})}{\text{OD of tube 4} - \text{OD of tube 2}} \times 100$$

Interpretation

The normal range of hemolysis is less than 5%. If more than 5% lysis occurs, the diagnosis of PNH is strongly suggested and should be confirmed by Ham's acidified serum test.

Sources of Error and Comments

1. Equivocal results may occur in other hematologic diseases, especially megaloblastic anemias, autoimmune hemolytic anemia, and myeloproliferative syndromes.
2. False negative results may occur if the proportion of PNH cells is low as a result of destruction in the circulation.

ACIDIFIED SERUM TEST[25, 27]

The acidified serum test should be used to confirm a diagnosis of paroxysmal nocturnal hemoglobinuria.

Principle

Erythrocytes from patients with PNH are hemolyzed by fresh serum acidified to a pH of 6.5–7.0 at 37 °C.

Specimen Requirements

Patient—Whole blood defibrinated, or collected in citrate or EDTA

Control—Whole blood defibrinated or collected in citrate, plus 20 mL non–anti-coagulated blood (serum). Must be of the same ABO group as the patient sample and contain no unusual antibodies.

Reagents

0.90% NaCl
0.15 N HCl
0.01 M NH$_4$OH

Quality Control

Control sample must be a normal EDTA or citrate blood of the same ABO type as the patient, and tube 1 of the control sample should not exhibit more than 1% hemoloysis.

Procedure

1. Preparation of cells: Centrifuge whole blood samples of both patient and control. Remove the plasma and buffy coat. Wash cells three times in 0.9% NaCl. After the last washing, prepare an approximate 50% suspension of cells in 0.9% NaCl.
2. Prepare the serum: After clotting is complete, centrifuge and separate the serum from the ABO-compatible control. Repeat centrifugation to ensure that the serum is free of red blood cells.
3. Divide serum of the control into three aliquots and treat as follows:
   a. Unacidified serum: Store approximately 1.3 mL at room temperature until time of testing (not more than 2 hours).
   b. Acidified serum: Using a properly calibrated pH meter to determine the endpoint, add 0.15 N HCl drop by drop to remaining serum until the pH is between 6.4 and 6.6. Store at room temperature until time of testing.
   c. Heated-acidified serum: Place approximately 1.3 mL of acidified serum (step 3b) at 56 °C for 30 minutes.
4. Label twelve 12 × 75 mm glass tubes 1–6 for both patient and control samples and prepare test mixture as follows:

Tube 1—0.5 mL of acidified serum, 0.05 mL of cells (patient or control)
Tube 2—0.5 mL of unacidified serum, 0.05 mL of cells (patient or control)
Tube 3—0.5 mL of heat-acidified serum, 0.05 mL of cells (patient or control)
Tube 4—0.5 mL of acidified serum, 0.05 mL of 0.9% NaCl
Tube 5—0.05 mL of cells (patient or control), 0.5 mL of 0.9% NaCl
Tube 6—0.05 mL of cells (patient or control), 0.5 mL of 0.01% M NH$_4$OH

5. Incubate the tubes for 60 minutes at 37 °C.
6. Add 4 mL of 0.9% NaCl to each tube.
7. Centrifuge 5 minutes at 2000 rpm.
8. Read and record the OD of the supernatant of each tube at 540 nm in a controlled spectrophotometer, using distilled water as a blank.
9. Calculate the percentage of lysis for tubes 1, 2, and 3 for both patient and control samples

Calculations

The percentage of lysis in tubes 1, 2, and 3 is calculated as follows:

$$\% \text{ lysis} = \frac{ODi - (OD5 + OD4)}{OD6 - OD5} \times 100,$$

where ODi represents the absorbance reading of tube 1, 2, or 3 and OD4, OD5, and OD6 are the absorbance readings for tubes 4, 5, and 6.

Interpretation

Normal acidified serum lysis is less than 1%.

If significant lysis (>1%) occurs in tube 1 and no lysis occurs in tube 2 or tube 3, the diagnosis of PNH is probable. The percentage of lysis is commensurate with, but usually less than, the percentage of complement sensitive cells. The test result may also be positive in aplastic anemia, leukemia, and some myeloproliferative disorders.

Sources of Error and Coments

1. It is essential to use fresh serum to prevent false negative results.
2. Heat inactivation of the serum must be complete to prevent incorrect or questionable results.
3. False positive results can be caused by noncompatible serum: If serum contains iso-antibodies capable of reacting with the test cells, the test result may appear positive when the cells are normal. Using serum from an AB donor or

carefully typing the cells to be tested can prevent this problem.

4. False negative results can be caused by impotent serum: Serum from some individuals may not readily lyse PNH cells. It is advisable to run known PNH cells (if available) in parallel the first time a new donor is used to be certain that the serum is able to lyse PNH cells. Great care must be taken in storing the serum at proper temperature if fresh serum is not used.

5. Over-acidification: If the pH of the serum is rendered too low, lysis may occur. With over-acidification, lysis usually occurs in the tube containing heated serum.

6. Congenital dyserythropoietic anemia (CDA): The cells of certain patients with CDA, sometimes designated by the acronym HEMPAS (*h*ereditary *e*rythrocytic *m*ultinuclearity with

positive *a*cidifed *s*erum test), will be lysed by the serum of many normal donors. If CDA is suspected, absorb the serum at 0 °C with washed packed red blood cells from the patient. If the absorption markedly reduces the amount of lysis, CDA should be suspected. No reduction in lysis of PNH cells is seen if serum is absorbed similarly by PNH or normal cells.

7. Small complement-sensitive population: If the population of complement-sensitive cells is so small as to make detection of lysis difficult, the amount of lysis may be increased by using the lighter red blood cells (reticulocytes), because the proportion of complement-sensitive cells is higher in this population. In order to obtain the lighter portion, centrifuge cells in a hematocrit tube and repeat the test, using only the cells at the top of the centrifuged tube.

References

1. National Committee for Clinical Laboratory Standards (NCCLS): Standardized Method for Confirmation of Sickling Hemoglobins in Whole Blood (TSH-10). Villanova, PA: NCCLS, 1980.

2. Greenberg MS, Harvey HA, Morgan C: A simple and inexpensive screening test for sickle hemoglobin. N Engl J Med 1972; 286:1143.

3. Kim HC, Schwartz E: Laboratory techniques—Sickle hemoglobin procedure. *In* Williams WJ, Beutler E, Erslev AJ, Lichtman MA (eds): Hematology, 4th ed. New York: McGraw-Hill, 1990:1722–1723.

4. Pearce CJ, Dow P: Anemia of abnormal globin development—Hemoglobinopathies. *In* Lotspeich-Steininger CA, Stiene-Martin EA, Koepke JA (eds): Clinical Hematology: Principles, Procedures, Correlation. Philadelphia: JB Lippincott, 1990:185–211.

5. Helena Laboratories: Hemoglobin Electrophoresis Procedure Using Cellulose Acetate Plate in Alkali Buffer. Beaumont, TX: Helena Laboratories, 1985.

6. National Committee for Clinical Laboratory Standards (NCCLS): Abnormal Hemoglobin Detection by Cellulose Acetate Electrophoresis (Publication H8-A), vol 6(9). Villanova, PA: NCCLS, 1979.

7. Fairbanks, V: Hemoglobinopathies and Thalassemias: Laboratory Methods and Case Studies. New York: BC Decker, 1980.

8. National Committee for Clinical Laboratory Standards (NCCLS): Citrate Agar Electrophoresis for Confirming the Identification of Variant Hemoglobins (Publication H23-T), Vol. 8(6). Villanova, PA: NCCLS, 1988.

9. Helena Laboratories: Titan IV Citrate Hemoglobin Electrophoresis (Product literature). Beaumont, TX: Helena Laboratories, 1983.

10. Schneider RG, Hightower BJ, Barwick RC: Laboratory identification of the hemoglobinopathies. Lab Manage 1981; 19(8): 29–42.

11. Betke K, Marti HR, Schlicht I: Estimation of small percentages of foetal haemoglobin [Letter to the Editor]. Nature 1959; 184:1877–1878.

12. Fairbanks VF: Hemoglobinopathies and thalassemias. *Laboratory Methods and Case Studies.* New York: BC Decker, 1980:96–98.

13. Pembrey ME, McWade P, Weatherall DJ: Reliable routine estimation of small amounts of foetal haemoglobin by alkali denaturation. J Clin Pathol 1972; 25:738–740.

14. Singer K, Shernoff A, Singer L: Studies of abnormal hemoglobins: I. Their demonstration in sickle cell anemia and other hematologic disorders by means of alkali denaturation. Blood 1951; 6:413–428.

15. Helena Laboratories: Sickle-Thal Quik Column Method. Beaumont, TX: Helena Laboratories, 1988.

16. Kim HC, Adachi K, Schwartz E: Separation of hemoglobins—Quantitation of HbA$_2$. *In* Williams WJ, Beutler E, Erslev AJ, Lichtman MA (eds): Hematology, 4th ed. New York: McGraw-Hill, 1990:1717–1719.

17. Beutler E, Dern RJ, Alving AS: The hemolytic effect of primaquine: VI. An in vitro test for sensitivity of erythrocytes to primaquine. J Lab Clin Med 1955; 45:40.

18. Henry JB: Clinical Diagnosis and Management by Laboratory Methods, 6th ed. Philadelphia: WB Saunders, 1979.

19. Huchns ER: Disease due to abnormalities of hemoglobin structures. Am Rev Med 1970; 21:157.

20. Kim HC, Schwartz E: Unstable hemoglobins—Isopropanol stability test. *In* Williams WJ, Beutler E, Erslev AJ, Lichtman MA (eds): Hematology, 4th ed. New York: McGraw-Hill, 1990:1708–1709.

21. Carrell RW, Kay R: A simple method for the detection of unstable hemoglobins. Br J Hematol 1972; 23:615.

22. National Committee for Clinical Laboratory Standards (NCCLS): Standardized Method for Confirmation of Sickling Hemoglobins in Whole Blood (Publication H13-T). Villanova, PA: NCCLS, 1986.

23. Beutler E: Osmotic fragility. *In* Williams WJ, Beutler E, Erslev AJ, Lichtman MA (eds): Hematology, 4th ed. New York: McGraw-Hill, 1990:1726–1728.

24. Hyun BH, Ashton JK, Dolan K: Practical Hematology. Philadelphia: WB Saunders, 1975:240–243.

25. Beutler E. Sucrose hemolysis and acidified serum tests. In: Williams WJ, Beutler E, Erslev AJ, Lichtman MA (eds): Hematology 4th ed. New York: McGraw-Hill, 1990:1729–1730.

26. Hartmann RC, Jenkins DE Jr, Arnold AB: Diagnostic specificity of sucrose hemolysis test for paroxysmal nocturnal hemoglobinuria. Blood 1970; 35:462–475.

27. Leclair SJ: Acquired nonimmune anemia of increased destruction. *In* Lotspeich-Steininger CA, Stiene-Martin EA, Koepke JA (eds): Hematology: Principles, Procedures, Correlations. Philadelphia: JB Lippincott, 1992:257–266.

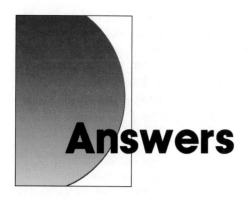

Answers

CHAPTER 2

Review Questions

1. b
2. c
3. a
4. d
5. b

Case Studies

1. First the phlebotomist should have the mother verify the patient's identity. Then try to calm and reassure the child. He or she should not tell the child that it will not hurt, but explain that it will hurt a little. The child may be coaxed with a "reward," such as a special adhesive bandage or "brave patient" sticker. A nurse may be asked to assist in positioning and holding the child. Sometimes it is easier to control a child if the parents leave the room. If no one is available to hold the patient, assistance should be sought from the laboratory; collection from an uncooperative patient should not be attempted without assistance.

2. The phlebotomist should ask the patient if he or she could just look at his or her arms for possible sites. Asking the patient where other phlebotomists have had the most success in drawing blood may help. If the phlebotomist is unable to find a good site, the patient should be told that someone else will come to draw blood. A venipuncture should never be attempted "blindly." If a potential site is found but fails to yield blood after two attempts, another phlebotomist should be sent for.

CHAPTER 3

1. The Bloodborne Pathogen Standard requires that
   ■ Hands must be washed under the following circumstances: (a) hands are visibly contaminated with blood or body fluids; (b) after the completion of work and before leaving the laboratory; (c) after gloves are removed and between glove changes; (d) before eating, drinking, smoking, applying cosmetics or lip balm, changing contact lens, and using the lavatory; and (e) before all other activities that entail hand contact with mucous membranes, eyes, or breaks in skin.
   ■ Eating, drinking, smoking, and applying cosmetics or lip balm must be prohibited in the laboratory work area.
   ■ Hands, pens, and other fomites must be kept away from the worker's mouth and all mucous membranes.
   ■ Food and drink must not be kept in the same refrigerator as laboratory specimens or reagents or where potentially infectious materials are stored or tested.
   ■ Mouth pipetting is prohibited.
   ■ Needles and other sharp objects contaminated with blood and other potentially infectious materials should not be manipulated in any way.
   ■ Contaminated sharps must be placed in a puncture-resistant container that is appropriately marked.
   ■ Personal protective clothing should be provided to the worker.
   ■ Procedures that involve manipulation of specimens should be performed in a manner that would prevent splashing, spraying, or the production of droplets.
   ■ Phlebotomy trays should be appropriately labeled to indicate potentially infectious materials.
   ■ When specimens are transported in a pneu-

matic tube system, the specimens should be placed in a special leakproof bag labeled with the biohazard symbol.

■ Contaminated equipment requiring service must be decontaminated before service begins.

2. Universal precautions require that potentially infectious materials be treated as if they were infectious. Universal precautions apply to the following potentially infectious materials: blood, semen, vaginal secretions, cerebrospinal fluid, synovial fluid, pleural fluid, any body fluid with visible blood, any unidentified body fluid, and saliva from dental procedures.

3. The proper procedure for handwashing:
■ Wet hands and wrists thoroughly under running water.
■ Apply germicidal soap and rub hands vigorously for 10–15 seconds.
■ Rinse hands thoroughly under running water.
■ Dry hands with paper towel. Use the paper towel to turn off the faucet.

4. Sharps must be placed in a puncture-resistant, leakproof container that is appropriately labeled with the biohazard symbol.

CHAPTER 4

1. b
2. c
3. a
4. b
5. c
6. d
7. a

CHAPTER 5

1. a
2. b
3. c
4. a
5. c
6. 7.4 g/dL
7. 0.17

CHAPTER 6

1. Mesenchyme is primitive tissue with hematopoietic potential. In cases of red blood cell loss or invasion of the bone, mesenchyme can become involved in hematopoiesis.

2. Primitive erythroblasts serve the developing embryo and fetus. They are large and short-lived, and their progeny are not anucleated. Definitive erythroblasts give rise to anucleated red blood cells, which have an extended life of 120 days.

3. The thymus of an 83-year-old man would be atrophied, hardly visible.

4. Yellow marrow is composed mostly of fat, which can be converted to energy.

5. Hematopoiesis takes place in the flat bones, the sternum, the pelvis, the vertebrae, the ribs, the skull, and the proximal ends of the long bones.

6. Agents that can destroy red marrow are certain rays (x-rays, gamma rays) and many chemicals.

7. The cords of Billroth is a specialized area in the spleen through which red blood cells must pass to get to the sinusoids. The area slows down the red blood cells, which results in increased number of red blood cells, which almost deplete the glucose. The cells are phagocytosed by macrophages that reside in the area.

8. A splenectomy is advised in cases of severe red blood cell destruction, specific cases of autoimmune hemolytic anemias, and cases of hereditary spherocytosis.

9. The mitotic index is used to measure the percentage of marrow cells engaged in mitosis.

10. Till and McCullock discovered new growth units and stimulating factors.

11. c

12. In medicine, the new information regarding colony stimulating factors is being used therapeutically in cases of bone cancer and leukemias. It is also used analytically to link specific conditions to the absence of certain factors.

CHAPTER 7

1. b
2. c
3. a
4. b
5. d
6. a
7. d
8. d

CHAPTER 8

1. The "feedback mechanism" is a schematic used to illustrate the balance among production, use, and destruction of the red blood cell. Conditions that can alter balance include hemolysis and hypersplenism.

2. If hemolysis is excessive, the bone marrow responds with increased production (i.e., assumes a hyperplastic state). In cases of hypersplenism, with destruction of normal cells, the bone marrow responds with increased production of cells.

3. Erythropoietin can stimulate normoblasts to undergo mitosis; it can shorten mitotic/maturation divisions; and it can assist reticulocytes to egress through the walls of the sinusoids.

4. A. c
   B. e
   C. d
   D. b
   E. a

5. Integrity of the RBC membrane is derived from spectrin, which forms tetramers bound by interactions with band 4.1 and actin-tropomyosin to provide the scaffolding for the lipid bilayer. This network is attached to the lipid bilayer by ankyrin, which binds to the spectrin β chain, linking it to protein 3.

6. Characteristics of the RBC that contribute to senescence include biochemical shutdowns; the non-oxidative pathway with no production of ADP; methemoglobin reductase, which allows accumulation of methemoglobin; and accumulation of increased cholesterol or other phospholipids on the membrane.

7. Extravascular hemolysis is the route of normal, controlled day-by-day hemolysis of senescent red blood cells. Macrophages in the spleen remove the senescent cells from the circulation and disassemble the components that direct the storage of recycling elements and the disposal of non-usable parts. Intravascular hemolysis involves a system of transport proteins that bind to the component parts of the RBC when hemolysis takes place within the lumen of the blood vessel. These proteins are stored until needed for recycling.

8. ■ *PNH (paroxysmal nocturnal hemoglobinuria):* condition in which membrane proteins are both structurally and functionally abnormal.
   ■ *Hereditary pyropoikilocytosis and hereditary elliptocytosis:* defective spectrin self-association.
   ■ *Hereditary spherocytosis:* condition in which the amount of newly assembled spectrin in the membrane of a reticulocyte is quantitatively reduced, thus affecting the synthesis of ankyrin.

CHAPTER 9

1. d
2. a
3. a
4. a
5. a
6. d
7. c
8. d
9. b
10. a
11. a

CHAPTER 11

1. d
2. b
3. d
4. c
5. c
6. d
7. a
8. a
9. c

Case Study

1. The initial CBC was probably a result of the leukoerythroblastic (or stress neutrophilia) picture that sometimes is seen in patients with malignancies.

2. Auto-infection becomes a concern when the absolute neutrophil count drops below 1×10^9/L, which occurred in this patient 4 days after the initiation of therapy. $(2.1 \times 10^9$/L $* 35\% = 0.74 \times 10^9$/L) and is almost a certainty when the count is below 0.5×10^9/L. That number was reached the next day with an absolute value of 0.32×10^9/L.

3. G-CSF stimulates granulocyte commitment and maturation, and so shortens the time during which the patient has an excessively low neutrophil count. By shortening the nadir caused by the oncologic therapy, the time during which the patient is at risk for infection is shortened.

CHAPTER 12

1. $\frac{100 \times 10 \times 20}{4} = 5.0 \times 10^9/L$

2. $\frac{20.0 \times 10^9/L \times 100}{25 + 100} = 16.0 \times 10^9/L$

3. Potassium cyanide, potassium ferrocyanide.

4. ■ Lipemia: make a blank, using patient plasma.
   ■ WBC greater than $30.0 \times 10^9/L$: subject dilution to centrifugation, and read transmittance of supernatant.
   ■ Hemoglobins that are resistant to hemolysis, such as hemoglobins S and C: make an equal-parts dilution with distilled water, read outcome on spectrophotometer, and multiply hemoglobin value by 2.
   ■ Precipitation of abnormal globulins: no longer a problem if commercial reagent is used.

5. $8 \times 3 = 24$. Hematocrit should be between 0.21 and 0.27 L/L.

6. ■ MCV = $\frac{30 \times 10}{5.0} = 60$ fL
   ■ MCHC = $\frac{9 \times 100}{30} = 30$ g/dL

7. Indices indicate that the erythrocytes are microcytic and hypochromic. Potential diagnoses include iron deficiency anemia, thalassemia, and some anemias associated with defective iron use.

8. The reticulocyte count gives an estimate of erythropoiesis.

9. $6 \times \frac{30}{45} = 4$; RPI $= \frac{4}{2} = 2$

10. The ESR gives an indication of inflammation and is used to differentiate diseases, such as rheumatoid arthritis and osteoarthritis, and to monitor therapy in some diseases.

CHAPTER 13

1. d
2. c
3. a
4. c
5. b
6. c

CHAPTER 14

1. c
2. d
3. a
4. d
5. b

6. Tumor cells are often found in clusters near the edge of the slide or coverslip; they tend to form syncytia; nuclei are often hyperchromatic; and vacuoles may be seen in the cytoplasm.

7. Bone marrow aspirates provide specimens for cytologic examination of cells; therefore, they are useful when immature or abnormal cells are observed in the peripheral blood; in the presence of a -cytosis or -penia; or when the proportions of hematopoietic cells are abnormal. Biopsy specimens allow a better determination of cellularity. They are the preferred specimens in the evaluation of the presence or extent of diseases such as Hodgkin's disease, non-Hodgkin's lymphoma, multiple myeloma, and vessel or stromal abnormalities.

8. A systematic approach (i.e., examination of the peripheral smear, the bone marrow aspirate, and bone marrow biopsy) forces the correlation of all facets of the bone marrow, instead of focusing on one abnormality and missing associated findings. Supplemental clinical and laboratory data should be considered when a differential diagnosis and recommendations for further studies are suggested.

CHAPTER 15

1. No, anemia is not a disease or a diagnosis. Anemia is a manifestation of an underlying disease.

2. Anemia is a decrease in erythrocytes, hemoglobin, and hematocrit to levels below the previously established normal values for healthy persons of the same age, gender, and race as a particular patient and under similar environmental conditions.

3. The two essential clinical features that are performed by the physician in an approach to the diagnosis of anemia are a complete history and physical examination.

4. The essential hematology tests needed in the workup of a patient with anemia are a complete blood count on a hematology cell analyzer to determine the RBC count, hemoglobin, hematocrit, RBC indices, WBC count, and platelet count; an RBC histogram and a calculated value for RDW (available on some electronic counters); and reticulocyte count, thorough peripheral blood smear examination, and, if necessary, a bone marrow examination. Other tests may be ordered on the basis of information obtained from results of the aforementioned tests (serum iron, TIBC, folate, vitamin B_{12}, hemoglobin electrophoresis, and so forth).

5. The three morphologic classification of anemia are normocytic, normochromic; microcytic, hypochromic; and macrocytic, normochromic.

6. ■ Normocytic anemia: MCV = 80–100 fL
   ■ Microcytic anemia: MCV < 80 fL
   ■ Macrocytic anemia: MCV > 100 fL

7. ■ Increased destruction of RBCs by hemolysis, or loss of blood by bleeding
   ■ Decreased production of RBCs

8. One anemia that is caused by a disorder of hemoglobin synthesis is thalassemia.

9. The laboratory procedure that is the most important in the workup of a patient with anemia is the careful and complete examination of the well-stained peripheral blood smear.

CHAPTER 16

Case 1

1. Red blood cell count, hemoglobin, hematocrit, MCV, MCH, MCHC, RDW, serum iron level, percentage of saturation, ferritin, NRBC, and reticulocytes.

2. Gastrointestinal blood loss.

3. Nonsteroidal anti-inflammatory drugs have been shown to cause erosion, gastrointestinal discomfort, and bleeding.

4. The offending medication should be removed, and the patient should receive oral iron supplementation.

Case 2

1. WBC, RBC, hemoglobin, hematocrit, MCV, MCH, platelet count, differential, LDH, AST level, and vitamin B_{12} level.

2. Hypersegmented neutrophils.

3. Megaloblastic RBC precursors and erythroid hyperplasia.

4. Perform tests for antibody to intrinsic factor and/or parietal cells and the Schilling test.

5. Vitamin B_{12}, given parenterally in the Schilling test, would be measured by vitamin B_{12} assays and would cause the bone marrow to appear normal within 6–12 hours.

Review Questions

1. a
2. c
3. b

4. d
5. a
6. a

CHAPTER 17

Case 1

1. Conditions such as thrombotic thrombocytopenic purpura (TTP), disseminated intravascular coagulation (DIC), incompetent artificial heart valve, hemolytic uremic syndrome (HUS), and March hemoglobinuria produce mechanical red blood cell injury with fragmentation and intravascular hemolysis.

2. The combination of thrombocytopenia with severely fragmented RBCs and increased reticulocytes makes the blood film the most powerful diagnostic tool. The diagnosis is untenable if fragmented cells are absent. Biopsies to demonstrate characteristic microvascular lesions are supportive but not necessary in order to make an initial diagnosis and begin treatment.

3. In the absence of an underlying explanation for the illness, the diagnosis can be made with the presence of routine and immediate data that yield a pentad of clinical and laboratory features: the apparent hemolytic anemia; the thrombocytopenia (denoting that the platelet survival is severely curtailed as the result of intravascular consumption); the fluctuating neurologic dysfunction (which can result from platelet thrombotic occlusions of small vessels of the CNS); the renal dysfunction (present because of microthrombi in the renal vasculature); and the fever (which may be the result of lesions in the hypothalamus). A normal prothrombin time and a normal partial thromboplastin time tend to rule out DIC.

4. Improvement can be measured by the clearing of neurologic signs, a rising platelet count and hematocrit, a decrease in reticulocyte level, and lower LDH and total bilirubin, which reflect the diminished hemolysis. Most patients recover totally and permanently with the current use of plasma infusion and plasmapheresis. Fifteen percent of patients suffer relapses, which may occur up to 12 years after the initial episode. Patients should undergo follow-up examinations after recovery, with careful attention to the platelet count and blood film.

   ■ Diagnosis: thrombotic thrombocytopenic purpura.

Case 2

1. This type of hemolytic anemia is caused by extracorpuscular defects with the damage to the RBCs, resulting in an immunologic event on the surface of the cells and not involving any known abnormality intrinsic to the cells.

2. A positive, direct Coombs test result denotes an antibody, complement, or both on the RBC surface and is confirmation of an immune hemolytic anemia. The direct Coombs test result is usually negative in patients with hemolytic anemias induced from snake and spider bites and other poisons.

3. Four mechanisms that lead to a drug-immune hemolytic anemia are an immune complex mechanism, a drug adsorption (hapten) mechanism, a nonimmune protein adsorption mechanism, and an idiopathic mechanism.

4. The essential feature is that the drug is nonspecifically bound to or absorbed by the patient's RBCs and remains firmly attached to the cells. If an anti-drug antibody develops, it will react with the RBC-bound drug protein. The strong DAT result is caused by IgG sensitization and a high titer of IgG antibody present in the serum. The indirect Coombs is positive for drug-treated but not normal RBCs. RBC eluate reacts only with drug-treated RBCs. The drugs most commonly involved in this response include the penicillins, some cephalosporins, and some streptomycins.

5. In the presence of a hemolytic state, treatment focuses on the discontinuation of the drug.

   ■ Diagnosis: drug-induced hemolytic anemia.

Case 3

1. On the basis of morphology in the peripheral smear, the high MCHC, and the predominance of microspherocytes, hereditary spherocytosis would be suspected. In this condition, there is an intrinsic defect in the membrane of the RBC. As the cells repeatedly go through the spleen, they suffer loss of membrane and plasticity. Excess Na leaks into the cells, causing the formation of microspherocytes.

2. Laboratory tests that establish the presence of hemolysis and suggest increased erythrocyte destruction and increased production would be desirable:

   ■ A *reticulocyte count* indicates the rate of erythrocyte production and compensation of the bone marrow. The slight polychromatophilia that is reported indicates qualitatively that there is blood regeneration and increased bone

marrow activity. The larger-than-normal polychromatophilic erythrocyte also explains the increased RDW. An increased reticulocyte count would be expected in this case.

   ■ Measurement of *haptoglobin* is also useful in assessing intravascular destruction and is decreased or absent in acute hemolysis.

   ■ An increased *serum bilirubin* level (indirect fraction), a breakdown of hemoglobin products, and an increase in urine and fecal urobilinogen would be expected with increased destruction of erythrocytes.

   ■ An increased *lactate dehydrogenase* (LDH) level indicates intravascular or extravascular RBC lysis.

   ■ A *Coombs test* would detect antibodies and thus an autoimmune hemolytic anemia. Antibodies can attach to erythrocytes, destroy the membrane, and form spherocytes. In hereditary spherocytosis, no antibodies are present; a negative Coombs test result would be expected.

   ■ An *osmotic fragility* test would detect an intrinsic defect in the membrane of the RBC that causes the formation of microspherocytes. Spherocytes are fragile because they are smaller and filled with hemoglobin. They are not able to take in much water and lyse more readily than normal cells, and thus they produce increased osmotic fragility.

   ■ An *erythrocyte autohemolysis* test is useful in confirming a diagnosis of hereditary spherocytosis. In hereditary spherocytosis, autohemolysis is almost always increased and corrected by the addition of glucose. Other conditions are not corrected by glucose.

3. This condition is congenital and may be diagnosed at any age. The inheritance mode is autosomal dominance, and the condition occurs most often in persons of European ancestry.

4. A splenectomy (removal of the spleen) allows the cells to circulate longer and relieves the anemia, although the inherited abnormal appearance of the erythrocyte persists.

   ■ Diagnosis: hereditary spherocytosis.

Case 4

1. The CBC showed a mild leukopenia (WBC count, 4300) with relative neutrophilia, moderate normochromic, normocytic anemia with marked elevated RDW, and a normal platelet count. The smear showed marked erythrocytic anisocytosis and poikilocytosis. Scattered spherocytes were also noted.

2. This condition is characterized by an inherited structural membrane defect that causes the

RBCs to take the form of an elliptocyte or an ovalocyte. The transmittance is through autosomal dominance. The results vary from those corresponding to a mild anemia to those corresponding to hereditary spherocytosis. At least 25% of the RBCs in the blood smear are elliptocytes. The osmotic fragility and autohemolysis test results are usually normal, but they are abnormal in conditions with a hemolytic variant. This patient is noted to have elevated LDH and bilirubin levels, which are indicators of hemolysis.

3. The prime morphologic feature of this disorder is the presence of the predominant elliptocytes, which are seen in a variety of conditions, including chronic hereditary elliptocytosis, iron deficiency, thalassemia, megaloblastic anemia, myelophthisic anemia, myelofibrosis, pyruvate kinase deficiency, hemoglobin C disease, and sickle cell trait. With the magnitude of the elliptocytosis and poikilocytosis present, the findings in this case are consistent with hereditary elliptocytosis.

4. Clinical correlation is required. The patient and family members should be investigated for a family history of anemia. Anemia is usually corrected by splenectomy.

■ Diagnosis: hereditary elliptocytosis with a hemolytic component.

CHAPTER 18

Case 1

1. Confirmatory tests that should be performed are a hemoglobin solubility test and citrate agar electrophoresis at a pH between 6.0 and 6.2. On the citrate agar test, hemoglobin C is separated from hemoglobins A, O, and E as a result of mode of migration: hemoglobin C migrates more toward the anode, whereas hemoglobins A, O, and E migrate toward the cathode. Likewise, hemoglobin S migrates anodally, whereas hemoglobins D and G migrate cathodally.

2. Characteristically, red blood cells that contain crystallized aggregates of hemoglobin that protrude through the cell membrane are seen.

3. On the basis of the electrophoretic pattern, the diagnosis of presence of hemoglobin SC can be made.

4. According to Mendelian law, the genotype can be depicted by the following chart:

	A	S
A	AA	AS
C	AC	SC

Of the offspring, 25% would be of each genotype: AA, AS, AC, and SC.

Case 2

1. The family history revealed a Mediterranean ethnic background; both alpha and beta thalassemia were common in the Mediterranean. It is a common mistake to treat a thalassemic individual for iron deficiency anemia because both iron deficiency and thalassemia are microcytic, hypochromic anemias, especially in areas in which thalassemia is not common in the general population. His mother's gallbladder "attacks" were probably caused by pigment stones, which resulted from the mild hemolytic anemia of heterozygous thalassemia. She underwent a cholecystectomy in 1977, which did reveal pigment stones. The student also had his gallbladder removed in 1983 because of pigment stones. Because Cooley's anemia, which is beta thalassemia major, had been diagnosed in his first cousin's children, it was quite likely that the student had beta thalassemia trait.

2. The elevated level of hemoglobin A_2, which is a marker for beta thalassemia minor, helped establish the diagnosis. Iron studies, which would have revealed normal or increased serum levels of iron in a non–iron-deficient patient with beta thalassemia minor and decreased serum levels of iron in iron-deficiency anemia, would also have differentiated the two conditions. The family history and the elevated Hb A_2 level in this situation made iron studies an unnecessary expense.

3. A microcytic, hypochromic anemia could be alpha or beta thalassemia, HbE, iron-deficiency anemia (IDA), or, more rare, sideroblastic anemia, lead poisoning, or anemia of chronic disease. Iron deficiency is the most common of these, and thalassemia patients often receive misdiagnoses of IDA. This patient's mother had periodically been given iron therapy. In this area of the United States, thalassemia is rather rare because of the small number in the ethnic groups in which this disorder is present, and so the mistake has been fairly common among these patients.

4. His spouse should have a complete blood count, and microcytosis and anemia should be sought. If they are present, further testing should be conducted. If his spouse is found to carry the thalassemia gene, the couple should be advised that according to Mendelian law, the genotypes of their offspring would be normal for 25%, thalassemia trait for 50%, and thalassemia major for 25%.

CHAPTER 19

1. The erythrocytes are typical echinocytes seen in renal disease.

2. The anemia in this case is caused by several mechanisms, including an inflammatory process, anemia of renal disease, and blood loss from lack of platelets.

CHAPTER 20

Study Questions

1. b
2. a
3. c
4. d
5. c
6. c
7. d

Case Study

1. The elevated hemoglobin and hematocrit were caused by the decrease in plasma volume that resulted from the blister formation that occurs in second-degree burns. The WBC count and differential were reflective of a stress reaction, perhaps to the movement of cells within granulocyte pools.

2. Two responses were at work: (1) Her hemoglobin and hematocrit had been modified by the probable use of intravenous fluids such as saline. This fluid absorption countered the decreases in the plasma volume and may have returned the child's hemoglobin and hematocrit back to pre-accident levels or slightly below. (2) The fever and positive wound cultures indicate that an infection was present. The demand for granulocytes to aggressively defend against the bacteria produced a strain on the productive capacity of the bone marrow that was manifested in the increased numbers of prematurely re-

leased granulocytes. This assumption of prematurity can be supported by the presence of the Döhle bodies and the toxic granulation, both of which result from stress at the promyelocyte, myelocyte, and metamyelocyte stages of development.

3. Because the mild anemia was still present, either the intravenous fluids were still being used or the hemoglobin and hematocrit reflected her "normal" state. The declining WBC count, coupled with the presence of more mature granulocytes without the toxic granulation or Döhle bodies, indicates that the WBCs together with the antimicrobial agent have prevented the spread of the infection and are in the process of removing it as a significant event in this child's recuperation.

CHAPTER 21

Case 1

Acute lymphoblastic leukemia

Case 2

1. 12
2. Chronic myelogenous leukemia
3. Leukemoid reaction

Case 3

Acute myelomonocytic leukemia (M4).

Case 4

1. Hairy cell leukemia.
2. Isoenzyme 5

Case 5

Characteristics of FAB M6:
■ More than 30% non-erythroid blasts in the bone marrow
■ More than 50% erythroid precursors in the bone marrow
■ Megaloblastic and binucleated erythroid precursors
■ Hemoglobin positive; glycophorin C positive

Case 6

Most likely diagnosis is Hodgkin's lymphoma (nodular sclerosing). Factors that contributed to diagnosis: CD30+; CD15+; CD20−; Reed-Sternberg cells present on hematoxylin and eosin-stained specimen.

Case 7

Plasma cell or multiple myeloma (kappa) is the most likely diagnosis. Diagnostic features in this case included increased immature and atypical plasma cells within the bone marrow; positive kappa cells in most plasma cells; also, increased serum level of calcium, which caused lethargy and cardiac arrhythmia due to increased viscosity, was found in the patient.

CHAPTER 22

1. Reasons for performing chromosome analysis include investigation of mental retardation, infertility, ambiguous genitalia, short stature, fetal loss, risk of genetic or chromosomal disease, and diagnosis and prognosis of certain types of malignancies.

2. "Beads on a string" represent chromatin wrapped around histone proteins. This is one stage of DNA packaging.

3. Chromosome 1; long arm; region 2; band 1.

4. Tissues used for chromosome analysis must be either spontaneously dividing cells, like bone marrow cells, or cells that can be stimulated to divide, such as peripheral blood lymphocytes.

5. Potassium chloride swells the cells; Colcemid arrests the cells in metaphase by disrupting the mitotic spindle.

6. Aneuploidy is the loss or gain of chromosomes, such as 47,XY,+21. Polyploidy is the gain of any multiple of the basic haploid number other than diploid, such as 3n or 4n.

7. A translocation is the exchange of chromatin material between chromosomes. The translocation characteristic of CML is t(9;22)(q34;q11.2)

8. The syndrome association with the loss of chromatin from the short arm of chromosome 5 is cri du chat. Clinical features include mental retardation, a small head, and a high-pitched cry in infancy that sounds like a cat's cry.

CHAPTER 23

Case 1

1. This is a case of chronic lymphocytic leukemia, determined from the patient's age, lymphade-

nopathy, and splenomegaly. He is mildly anemic and not thrombocytopenic, as would be expected in ALL. Thrombocytosis would be expected in CML.

2. Most cases of CLL have a B cell immunophenotype.

3. The median length of survival is 6 years.

4. The blast count would be low, except in the rare (<1%) cases of blast transformation. Bone marrow transplantation is generally not used as a therapeutic modality in this age group.

Case 2

1. This is a case of acute lymphoblastic leukemia. The chronic leukemias or myeloproliferative disorders usually occur in adults and are rarely associated with thrombocytopenia at presentation. The blasts pictured are small "L1" type lymphoblasts.

2. This child has clinically good prognostic features: age, female sex, and low white blood count. A poor prognostic finding is the headache, which may represent CSF involvement.

3. The most common phenotype of childhood ALL is CD10-positive, TdT-positive immature B lineage ALL, which is also the best phenotype prognostically. T cell ALL, which usually develops in older male children in association with mediastinal involvement, is a less favorable phenotype, as is surface immunoglobulin-bearing ALL (mature B cell ALL). Cytoplasmic immunoglobulin is present in pre−B cell ALL, which carries a prognosis intermediate between those of immature B cell ALL and B cell ALL.

Case 3

1. This is a case of acute myelogenous leukemia. The patient has a disease of short duration and symptoms of anemia and thrombocytopenia, and there are Auer rods in the blasts in the peripheral smear. Other clinical indications that this is of myeloid instead of lymphoid origin is the lack of lymphadenopathy or organomegaly.

2. Gingival infiltration usually signals a monocytic component (acute myelomonocytic leukemia [FAB-M4] or acute monocytic leukemia [FAB-M5]).

3. Bruising is caused by thrombocytopenia.

4. Bone marrow findings are those that would be seen in any acute myeloid leukemia. The M:E ratio would be greater than 1. Blasts constitute more than 30% of all nucleated cells. In the case of monocytic leukemias, a significant monocytic component must be proved.

Case 4

1. This is an illustrative case of acute myelogenous leukemia of the FAB-M3 subtype (acute promyelocytic leukemia.) Note the reniform contours of the blasts and the heavy granulation in the cytoplasm. These cells characteristically lose HLA-DR on their surfaces and do not express CD34, although they are not invariably associated with the FAB-M3.

2. A common chromosome phenotype is t(15;17) translocation.

3. Although acute promyelocytic leukemia is fairly characteristic, other entities to consider in the differential diagnosis are acute myelogenous leukemia with maturation (FAB-M2) or acute myelomonocytic leukemia (FAB-M4).

CHAPTER 25

Case 1

1. The presence of unilateral cervical or supraclavicular lymphadenopathy in a young patient with unexplained fever, weight loss, and night sweats is suggestive of Hodgkin's disease. Peripheral blood eosinophilia and normocytic, normochromic anemia may also be present in this disorder.

2. The biopsy material demonstrates cellular nodules separated by thick bands of fibrous tissue (large arrow, Fig. 25–8A). Reed-Sternberg cells and associated variants are present in the nodular areas of the biopsy (small arrow, Fig. 25–8B). The clinical and morphologic findings in this case are those of nodular sclerosis Hodgkin's disease.

Case 2

1. The lymph node biopsy specimen from this patient demonstrated characteristics of non-Hodgkin's follicular lymphoma. Note the vaguely nodular pattern at low power and replacement of the lymph node with a cellular proliferation. Unlike the follicles in reactive lymphadenopathy (see Fig. 25–1), the follicles in malignant lymphoma are of uniform size and shape and lack a mantle or rim of small, mature lymphocytes (see Fig. 25–9). The cells within the follicles are a mixture of both small and large neoplastic cells. According to the Working Formulation classification system, the diagnosis is malignant follicular lymphoma with mixed small cleaved and large cell type.

2. Flow cytometric analysis of this case could be useful in distinguishing florid reactive lymphadenopathy from nodular malignant lymphoma. Nodular or follicular lymphomas are usually of B cell origin and typically demonstrate several pan–B surface antigens (CD19, CD20, or CD22) as well as bright CD10 (CALLA) and monoclonal surface immunoglobulin. Reactive hyperplasia may also display pan–B antigens, but bright CD10 or monoclonal surface immunoglobulin are absent.

CHAPTER 26

1. d
2. c
3. b
4. d
5. c
6. a

CHAPTER 27

1. The malignant phenotype, uncontrolled cell division, must be inherited by the progeny cells, or they would cease to be malignant. DNA is the heritable code from parent to progeny, so there must be a mutation in this DNA that allows for the uncontrolled cell growth.

2. An oncogene stimulates uncontrolled cell growth, whereas a tumor suppressor gene represses it.

3. Benzene, radiation, alkylating agents.

4. Persons with Down syndrome (trisomy 21), Klinefelter syndrome (XXY), neurofibromatosis, Bloom syndrome, Fanconi anemia, or ataxia-telangiectasia and monozygotic twins have an increased risk of developing acute leukemia.

5. Epstein-Barr virus, HTLV-1.

6. Biphenotypic leukemia, which shares characteristics of both ALL and AML. VP-16 can cause 11q23 abnormalities.

7. *myc* can cause ALL L3 and Burkitt's lymphoma. It is involved in t(8;14), t(8;22), and t(2;8). *myc* is on chromosome 8 and is translocated to one of the immunoglobulin genes.

8. CML and ALL. In ALL the t(9;22) produces a shorter fusion tyrosine kinase, which is a more active growth signal.

9. Growth factors (e.g., basic fibroblast growth factor), signal transducers (e.g., *ras*), and transcription factors (e.g., *myc*).

10. Follicular lymphomas over-express *bcl*-2, which prevents lymphocytes programmed to die (called apoptosis) from doing so.

11. *ras* is the most commonly mutated oncogene in MDS and AML.

CHAPTER 29

Case 1

1. This is an example of acute lymphoblastic leukemia (ALL) of childhood. Note the location of these relatively small, agranular blasts in the area of low FALS and low SS in the scattergram (see Fig. 29–5). The blasts also demonstrated TdT and surface CD10 (CALLA) positivity, which is frequently observed in cells of lymphoid lineage. The HLA-DR test result was also positive; this marker is not lineage specific and is typically present on blasts of either lymphoid or myeloid origin. The B cell surface antigen CD19 was also strongly positive. T cell antigens (CD2, CD7) and myeloid antigens (CD33, CD13, CD14) were not expressed.

2. The findings of HLA-DR/TdT/CD10/CD19 positive blasts are typical immunologic features of an immature B, non–T cell acute leukemia of lymphoid origin or acute lymphoblastic leukemia. The surface light chains (kappa and lambda) were negative in this case and are observed only in mature B cell leukemias.

Case 2

1. The presence of Sudan black B and myeloperoxidase-positive granular blasts with Auer rods is entirely consistent with acute myeloid leukemia (AML). As in the previous case, HLA-DR is present on blasts and does not distinguish ALL from AML.

2. The myeloid markers CD33 and CD13 are strongly positive and suggest a myeloid lineage; the lymphoid markers CD19, CD20, kappa, lambda, CD2, and CD7 are negative. CD15 is a surface marker that is associated with myelomonocytic cells but may also be associated with lymphoid cells. Although CD15 does not distinguish ALL from AML, it may be coexpressed with CD33 or CD13 in FAB M2 leukemia.

CHAPTER 30

Review Questions

1. d
2. d
3. a
4. c
5. a
6. c
7. a
8. b
9. b
10. d

Case Study

1. Gaucher disease
2. *β*-glucocerebrosidase
3. Commercially prepared glucocerebrosidase administered intravenously has been successful in treating type 1 Gaucher disease. Because of the difficulty in delivering enzymes across the blood-brain barrier, treatment has not been successful in types 2 and 3 Gaucher disease.

CHAPTER 31

1. Megakaryocytes are cells produced in the bone marrow by the hematopoietic process originating from the same pluripotential stem cell as red blood cells, granulocytes, and monocytes. However, unlike the other cells, they do not produce daughter cells by cellular division. Rather, the parent megakaryocyte undergoes several unique nuclear duplications without cell division. Each time the nucleus divides, twice the chromosomal power is gained to produce platelets. The number of platelets produced by a megakaryocyte is directly related to the number of nuclei.

2. Platelet dense granules contain serotonin, calcium, ADP, and ATP. When released, serotonin acts as a vasoconstrictor, causing smooth muscle to constrict. This is an ATP-dependent activity. Calcium ions released help raise the level of intracellular calcium necessary to initiate the thromboxane A_2 pathway and provide calcium to coat the lipid surfaces of the platelet plug. ADP attaches to platelet ADP receptors, sending a second message to inhibit adenylate cyclase activity, which lowers cAMP levels within the platelet, allowing mobilization of intracellular calcium. Dense granule release prepares the platelet for thromboxane A_2 production, alpha granule release, and aggregation.

3. Alpha granules contain several platelet-produced proteins and some absorbed proteins. Platelet-specific proteins are platelet-derived growth factor, a mitogen that stimulates tissue repair, and

thrombospondin, a large protein that helps platelets aggregate, and heparin neutralizing factors PF4 and BTG. Platelet vWF may help in the aggregation process. Absorbed platelet proteins are fibrinogen and fibronectin, which participate in platelet aggregation and crosslinking. Absorbed plasma factor V attaches to exposure factor V receptors on the platelet surface and participates in the common pathway of coagulation.

4. The tunica intima consists of endothelial cells, a basement membrane containing collagen, and an internal elastic membrane. The tunica media consists of smooth muscle, collagen, and an external elastic membrane. The tunica adventitia is made up of collagen and fibroblasts. The tunica adventitia is thicker in veins than arteries, whereas the tunica media is thicker in arteries than in veins. Arterioles have more muscle (tunica media) than do veins and capillaries.

5. The thromboxane pathway is similar in active platelets and responding endothelial cells through production of cyclic endoperoxide from arachidonic acid. However, the result of each pathway is controlled by a specific enzyme produced by each cell type. Platelets produce thromboxane synthetase, which causes the pathway to terminate in thromboxane A_2, whereas endothelial cells produce prostacyclin synthetase that produces prostaglandin I_2. The end products of both pathways are antithetical in their activities. Thromboxane A_2 is vasoconstrictive and encourages platelet activity by attaching to its platelet receptor. Prostaglandin I_2 is a vasodilator and quiets platelets by enhancing adenylate cyclase activity in resting platelets.

6. Calcium levels are raised and lowered within the platelet by two opposing mechanisms. Normal or PGI_2-enhanced adenylate cyclase activity in platelets produces cAMP from ATP and causes calcium ions to be bound to protein in the dense tubular system. ADP, released from dense granules of activated platelets, attaches to ADP receptors and inhibits adenylate cyclase activity, causing lowered cAMP and increased release of calcium ions from the dense tubular system. Other mechanisms allowing calcium influx into the cell contribute to the sudden rise in calcium levels within the activated platelet.

CHAPTER 32

1. The purpose of coagulation is to prevent or stop bleeding.

2. Factor VIII–von Willebrand factor complex is made up of a factor VIII:C portion linked to a vWF portion that is made up of various molecular-weight parts. Each part is under separate genetic control. The two parts bind to each other before being released into the plasma. The molecular weight of VIII:vWF varies, depending on the molecular weight of the vWF multimers included.

3. The six vitamin K–dependent plasma proteins are vitamin factors II, VII, IX, and X; protein C; and protein S. The first four are involved in producing a fibrin clot; the latter two are involved with halting thrombus formation.

4. Gamma carboxylation of glutamic acid residues near the N-terminus of the vitamin K–dependent factors is essential for the functionality of the factors and allows them to bind to calcium-coated surfaces at the wound site.

5. Activation of thrombin is a two-step process. Fragment 1.2 is cleaved from prothrombin by factor Xa, producing prethrombin. Prethrombin is further altered by factor Xa to produce the active thrombin form.

6. Thrombin binds to thrombin receptors on platelets, causing immediate mobilization of intracellular calcium, which activates the thromboxane A_2 pathway and leads to release of alpha granules. Platelets aggregate irreversibly in response to thrombin activation, providing a PF3 surface for fibrin formation to occur. Thrombin converts fibrinogen to fibrin in coagulation and activates factor XIII. Thrombin also activates factor XI, which further promotes thrombin on healthy epithelial cells, causing activation of protein C, which halts coagulation by inactivating factors V and VIII. The thrombin-thrombomodulin complex also stimulates the release of tissue plasminogen activator (tPA) from healthy endothelial cells, which activates plasminogen to the fibrin-lysing plasmin enzyme.

7. Traumatized endothelial cells liberate PAF, tPA, PAI-1, tissue factor, and vWF. PAF activates platelets; tissue factor initiates thrombin production and fibrin formation; PAI-1 neutralizes tPA so that the thrombus will not be degraded too quickly; and vWF binds collagen and active platelets together to plug the hole and prevent bleeding. Healthy endothelial cells provide thrombomodulin surface proteins for thrombin to attach. The thrombin-thrombomodulin complex activates protein C to limit fibrin formation and causes release of tPA for fibrin degradation.

8. Thrombin-activated factor XIII forms a stable covalent bond between adjacent D regions in the fibrin polymer.

9. When plasmin digestion of fibrin occurs, the covalent bond between adjacent D domains remains in place, causing the release into the blood of two D regions attached to each other. These are called D-dimers.

10. Endogenous activators for plasminogen include factor XIIa, kallikrein, and tPA. Contact factors XIIa and kallikrein are not believed to play a major role in vivo to activation of plasminogen. In vitro, they are responsible for clot lysis. After thrombi formation, thrombin-thrombomodulin complexes stimulate release of tPA from healthy endothelial cells, which provides the major activator of plasminogen.

11. PAI-1 is plasminogen activator inhibitor. It is released during trauma from tissue and active platelets to neutralize tPA that is released as a result of the injury. Without PAI-1, tPA would activate fibrin lysis and prevent fibrin formation at the wound site.

12. Plasmin digestion of crosslinked fibrin yields the waste products E fragment and D-dimers to the blood for removal by phagocytosis. Plasmin digestion of fibrinogen yields D and E fragments because there is no crosslinking of D domains in fibrinogen.

13. Under normal hemostatic conditions, native fibrinogen is not degraded because plasmin is localized to the thrombus site. When digestion is complete and active plasmin escapes, t-serine protease inhibitors are available to neutralize its activity before it can degrade plasma fibrinogen.

14. Serpins are present in plasma to bind active serine protease enzymes escaping the clot site into the blood stream. A deficiency of Serpins would allow excessive enzymatic activity and thrombi formation downstream.

15. When a thrombus is formed, thrombin escapes the wound site and becomes complexed with thrombomodulin on the surface of nearby endothelial cells. The thrombin-thrombomodulin complex activates protein C by enzymatic action.

16. Activated protein C enzymatically inactivates factor Vm and factor VIIIm, halting formation of the thrombus. Protein S is an essential cofactor. Both proteins are vitamin K–dependent, which helps them bind to Ca^{2+} at the clot site.

CHAPTER 33

1. The bleeding time and APTT are prolonged.

2. Hereditary disorder, most likely autosomal dominant, according to family history. The prolonged APPT suggests a possible factor deficiency.

3. Platelet aggregation and platelet adhesion studies should be conducted to more clearly define the platelet abnormality. Substitution studies and a specific factor assay could be undertaken to determine the cause of the prolonged APTT.

4. The most likely diagnosis is von Willebrand's disease. The most likely variants would be types IA, IIA, and IIB. The coagulation factor involved is factor VIII.

5. Cryoprecipitate or fresh or frozen plasma could be given prophylactically before surgery or after surgery if bleeding occurs.

CHAPTER 34

1. Prothrombin time, APTT, platelet count, and bleeding time.

2. Chronic alcohol consumption can affect production of coagulation factors made by the liver. Of the 15 factors identified in the coagulation cascade, 13 are produced in the liver. The liver is the primary producer of the vitamin K–dependent factors: II, VII, IX, and X. Alcohol can also cause a prolonged bleeding time as a result of vasculature abnormalities and/or decreased platelets.

3. Follow-up coagulation tests that should be ordered include substitution studies, to see whether normal plasma corrects the patient's values and to rule out circulating inhibitors. If normal plasma corrects the patient's PT and APTT, specific factor assays should be performed and deficiencies identified. Most likely, multiple deficiencies will be identified.

4. If the coagulation defects are severe, transfusion of fresh-frozen plasma may be needed. If the patient is very anemic, it may be necessary to administer packed RBCs. The patient should be assisted in obtaining help for the alcohol problem. This case study reinforces the importance of the complete history and physical examination.

5. Complete blood count (CBC), including RBC indices to determine whether macrocytes (common in alcoholism) or other RBC abnormalities are present. Because nutrition in alcoholics is

often poor, measurement of vitamin B_{12}, folic acid, and ferritin levels may be helpful. A biochemical profile to detect liver involvement would also be useful. In this patient, drug studies and alcohol levels may provide additional information.

6. The tracks on this patient's arms indicate drug abuse. The technologist should follow universal precautions, as with drawing blood from all patients. Drug users are likely to transmit infectious diseases, such as hepatitis and AIDS.

CHAPTER 38

1. The nucleated count is 7/mm³. The RBC count is 655/mm³. The fluid would appear hazy or slightly bloody.

2. Normal cells seen in CSF are lymphocytes and monocytes. Normal cells seen in serous fluid are lymphocytes, monocytes/histiocytes, and mesothelial cells. Normal cells seen in synovial fluids are lymphocytes, monocytes/histiocytes, and synovial cells.

3. A. 1:53 dilution with saline.
   B. Bacteria.
   C. Bacterial meningitis.

4. Gout

5. Viral meningitis

6. Metastatic breast cancer

7. Transudate, according to the low cell count and the presence of monocytes/histiocytes as opposed to neutrophils.

8. Traumatic tap with bone marrow contamination.

CHAPTER 39

1. b
2. c
3. b
4. d
5. a
6. a
7. c
8. d
9. c
10. a, b, c, d
11. a, b, c, d

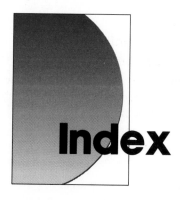

Index

Note: Page numbers in *italics* refer to illustrations; page numbers followed by t refer to tables.

Aberrations, of lenses, 31
Abetalipoproteinemia, 213
Abnormal localization of immature precursors, in myelodysplastic syndromes, 394
ABO erythroblastosis, 242
Acanthocytes, *176*, 213
in anemia of chronic renal failure, 289
Acanthocytosis, 213–214
Accuracy, definition of, 40, *41*
Acetylcholinesterase, deficiency of, in paroxysmal nocturnal hemoglobinuria, 224
Achromatic objective lens, 31
Acid elution slide test, 281–282
Acid phosphatase stain, 311–312, *312*
Acidified serum lysis test, 226, 227t, 686–688
Acquired immunodeficiency syndrome (AIDS), anemia in, 128–129
lymphocyte subset analysis in, 432
malignant lymphoma in, 384–385
Actin, of erythrocyte membrane, *84*, 85t, 86
Activated partial thromboplastin time (APTT), 564–567, 572
capillary, 567
clinical utility of, 566
limitations of, 566–567
point of care, 567
principle of, 564–565, *565*
procedure for, 565
quality assurance for, 565
reference interval for, 565–566
results reporting for, 566, *566*
Active transport, 83
Additives, in specimen collection, 8–9, 10t
Adenocarcinoma cells, on pleural fluid differential, *644*
Adenosine deaminase, deficiency of, 105
Adenosine diphosphate (ADP), in platelet aggregometry, 557, 557t
Adenosine triphosphate (ATP), generation of, 104, 104t
Adrenal cortex, disorders of, anemia in, 128
AEC reaction, 317
Aerobic glycolysis, 104–105, 104t
Afibrinogenemia, 500, 517–518
Agammaglobulinemia, sex-linked, 304
Agar gel electrophoresis, 677–679
Agglutinins, cold, instrumentation interference from, 619t

Aggregometry, platelet, 555–558, *556*
adenosine diphosphate in, 557, 557t
agonists in, 556–558, 557t
arachidonic acid, 557t, 558
collagen in, 557t, 558
epinephrine in, 557–558, 557t
instrumentation for, 627–628
ristocetin in, 557t, 558
specimen collection for, 555
thrombin in, 556, 557t
with platelet-rich plasma, 555, *556*
with whole blood, 555–556
Agnogenic myeloid metaplasia, 368–370, *369*, 369t
extramedullary hematopoiesis in, 368
immune response in, 369
incidence of, 369
morphologic changes in, 368–369, *369*, 369t
myelofibrosis in, 368
prognosis for, 369
treatment of, 369–370
AIDS. See *Acquired immunodeficiency syndrome (AIDS)*.
Albinism, oculocutaneous, tyrosinase-positive, 502–503
Alcohol, in sideroblastic anemia, 193
Alcoholism, anemia of, 130
Alder-Reilly anomaly, 299
Aldolase, deficiency of, 220t
Aldomet, hemolytic reaction with, 240
Alkali denaturation test, for hemoglobin F, 281, 679–680
Alkaline phosphatase–anti-alkaline phosphatase method, 316, *316*
Alkaloids, plant, 413, 414t
Alkylating agents, 413, 414t
ALL. See *Leukemia, lymphoblastic, acute (ALL)*.
Allergic purpura, 506–507
Allergy, with venipuncture, 14
Alpha granule deficiency, 503–504
Alpha thalassemia. See *Thalassemia, alpha*.
Alpha$_2$–anti-plasmin, 479t, 480
deficiency of, 541–542
Alpha$_1$–anti-trypsin, 479–480, 479t
Alpha-interferon, in leukocyte neoplasia, 415
Alpha$_2$–macroglobulin, 479t, 480
Alpha-methyldopa, thrombocytopenia with, 488, 488t
Alpha-naphthyl acetate esterase reaction, 309–310, *309*, *310*

Alpha-naphthyl butyrate esterase reaction, 309–310, *310*
Amaurotic infantile idiocy, 443–444, *443*
Amniocentesis, 331
Amyloidosis, 507
systemic, vs. dysfibrinogenemia, 518
ANA (anti-nuclear antibody) test, 445–446
Anaerobic glycolysis, 102–104, 102t, *103*, 104t
Analyzer. See *Instrumentation*.
Anaphylactoid purpura, 506–507
ANC, 589t
Ancylostoma duodenale, in iron deficiency anemia, 184
Androgens, in erythropoiesis, 128
Anemia. See also at *Hemoglobin; Thalassemia*.
adaptations to, 179
aplastic, 194–197
bone marrow findings in, 197, *197*
classification of, 194–195, 195t
clinical findings in, 196–197
differential diagnosis of, 194, 195t
familial, 196
hereditary, 196
idiopathic, 194–195, 195t
incidence of, 194
laboratory findings in, 196–197
pathophysiology of, 196
prognosis for, 197
secondary, 195, 195t
thrombocytopenia in, 485
treatment of, 197
blood loss, 126, 288
bone marrow examination in, 176–177
classification of, 177–179, *178*
by red blood cell distribution width, 179
morphologic, 177–179, *178*
pathophysiologic, 179, 179t
clinical findings in, 174–175
definition of, 174
diagnosis of, 175–177
blood smear examination in, 175, *176*, 176t
complete blood count in, 175
reticulocyte count in, 175
dyserythropoietic, congenital, 197–198
endocrine disorders and, 127–128
Fanconi's, 196
Heinz body, congenital, 265–266
hemolytic, alloimmune, 240–241
autoimmune, 237–240

ISBN 0-7216-4727-8

90071

9 780721 647272